MW00990902

The American Cancer Society's Oncology in Practice
Clinical Management

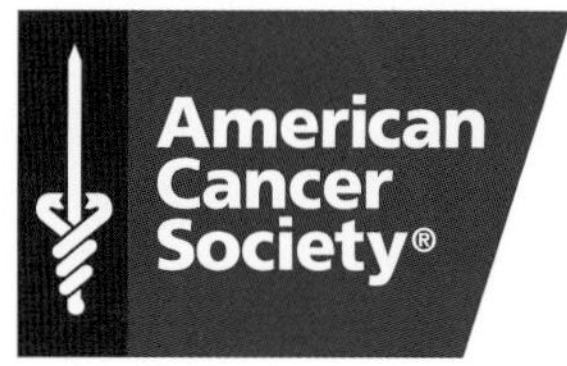

The American Cancer Society is a global grassroots force of nearly 2 million volunteers dedicated to saving lives, celebrating lives, and leading the fight for a world without cancer. From breakthrough research, to free lodging near treatment, a live helpline, free rides to treatment, and convening powerful activists to create awareness and impact, the Society is the only organization attacking cancer from every angle. For more information go to www.cancer.org.

The American Cancer Society's

Oncology in Practice

Clinical Management

Edited by The American Cancer Society

Atlanta, Georgia, USA

WILEY Blackwell

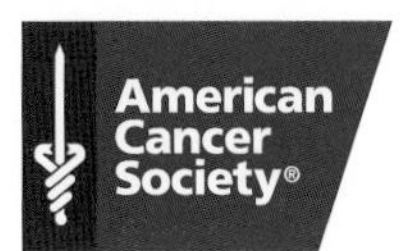

Registered Office(s)
John Wiley & Sons, Inc., 111 River Street, Hoboken, NJ 07030, USA
John Wiley & Sons Ltd, The Atrium, Southern Gate, Chichester, West Sussex, PO19 8SQ, UK

Editorial Office
9600 Garsington Road, Oxford, OX4 2DQ, UK

For details of our global editorial offices, customer services, and more information about Wiley products visit us at www.wiley.com.

Wiley also publishes its books in a variety of electronic formats and by print-on-demand. Some content that appears in standard print versions of this book may not be available in other formats.

Library of Congress Cataloging-in-Publication Data

Names: American Cancer Society, editor.
Title: The American Cancer Society's Oncology in Practice : clinical management / edited by American Cancer Society.
Other titles: American Cancer Society textbook of clinical oncology (2018) | Textbook of clinical oncology
Description: Hoboken, NJ : Wiley, 2018. | Includes bibliographical references and index. |
Identifiers: LCCN 2017027177 (print) | LCCN 2017028088 (ebook) | ISBN 9781118592076 (pdf) | ISBN 9781118591963 (epub) |
ISBN 9781118517642 (cloth)
Subjects: | MESH: Neoplasms
Classification: LCC RC263 (ebook) | LCC RC263 (print) | NLM QZ 200 | DDC 616.99/4–dc23
LC record available at https://lccn.loc.gov/2017027177

Cover design by Wiley
Cover image: © Tendo/Shutterstock

Set in 9.5/11.5 pt Warnock by SPi Global, Pondicherry, India
Printed and bound in Singapore by Markono Print Media Pte Ltd

10 9 8 7 6 5 4 3 2 1

Contents

Editorial Board

Reviewers

Robert Benjamin, MD
Antonia Bennett, PdD
Andy Berchuck, MD
Destin Black, MD
Hearn Jay Cho, MD
Grace K. Dy, MD
Paul Finger, MD
Matthew Galsky, MD
Kris E. Gaston, MD
Mark A. Henderson, MD
Joan Kramer, MD
Robin A. Lacour, MD, MPH
Edward R. Laws, Jr., MD, FACS
Alexander Olawaiye, MD
Christy Russell, MD
Sonali Smith, MD
Mary Kay Washington, MD
Lynn Westphal, MD
Karen Winkfield, MD, MGH

American Cancer Society Content Staff

Chuck Westbrook
Eleni Berger
Esmeralda Galan Buchanan
Jin Hee Kim

List of Contributors

Costantine Albany, MD
Assistant Professor
Indiana University School of Medicine
Simon Cancer Center
Indianapolis, Indiana, USA

Khaldoun Almhanna, MD, MPH
Medical Oncologist
Department of Gastrointestinal Oncology
Moffitt Cancer Center
Tampa, Florida, USA

Richard Ambinder, MD, PhD
Professor of Oncology
Departments of Medicine and Oncology
Johns Hopkins University School of Medicine
Baltimore, Maryland, USA

Kenneth C. Anderson, MD
Professor of Medicine
Department of Medical Oncology
Dana Farber Cancer Institute
Boston, Massachusetts, USA

Celina Ang, MD
Assistant Professor
Division of Hematology and Medical Oncology
The Tisch Cancer Institute
Mount Sinai Medical Center
New York, New York, USA

Christina Appin, MD
Assistant Professor
Department of Pathology
Northwestern University
Feinberg School of Medicine
Chicago, Illinois, USA

Stanley W. Ashley, MD
Chief Medical Officer and Senior Vice President for Medical Affairs
Brigham and Women's Hospital
Frank Sawyer Professor of Surgery
Harvard Medical School
Boston, Massachusetts, USA

Pratiti Bandopadhayay, MD
Professor
Department of Pediatric Oncology
Dana-Farber/Boston Children's Cancer and Blood Disorders Center
Boston, Massachusetts, USA

Leon Bernal-Mizrachi, MD
Assistant Professor
Department of Hematology and Medical Oncology
Winship Cancer Institute
Emory University
Atlanta, Georgia, USA

Matthew Biagioli, MD
Radiation Oncologist
Department of Radiation Oncology
Moffitt Cancer Center
Tampa, Florida, USA

Giada Bianchi, MD
Instructor in Medicine
Department of Medical Oncology
Dana Farber Cancer Institute
Boston, Massachusetts, USA

Erkut Borazanci, MD
Professor
Department of Surgery
Feist-Weiller Cancer Center
Louisiana State University Health Sciences Center
Shreveport, Louisiana, USA

Alexandros Bouras, MD
Associate Scientist
Department of Neurosurgery
Icahn School of Medicine at Mount Sinai
New York, New York, USA

David Bowes, MD, FRCPC
Associate Professor
Department of Radiation Oncology
Nova Scotia Cancer Center
Dalhousie University
Halifax, Nova Scotia, Canada

Daniel Brickman, MD
Assistant Professor
Department of Otolaryngology – Head and Neck Surgery
Levine Cancer Institute
Carolinas HealthCare System
Charlotte, North Carolina, USA

Maria E. Cabanillas, MD
Associate Professor
Department of Endocrine Neoplasia and Hormonal Disorders
The University of Texas MD Anderson Cancer Center
Houston, Texas, USA

Richard Carvajal, MD
Associate Professor
Columbia University Medical Center
Herbert Irving Comprehensive Cancer Center
New York, New York, USA

Emily Chan, MD, PhD
Associate Professor
Department Medical Oncology
Vanderbilt University
Nashville, Tennessee, USA

Devron H. Char, MD
Director
The Tumori Foundation;
Department of Ophthalmology
University of California San Francisco
San Francisco, California, USA

Mehee Choi, MD
Assistant Professor
Department of Radiation Oncology
Loyola University Chicago School of Medicine
Chicago, Illinois, USA

Quyen D. Chu, MD, MBA, FACS
Professor
Department of Surgery and Division of Surgical Oncology
Feist-Weiller Cancer Center
Louisiana State University Health Sciences Center
Shreveport, Louisiana, USA

Michael D. Chuong, MD
Radiation Oncologist
Department of Radiation Oncology
University of Maryland
Baltimore, Maryland, USA

Tia B. Cole, MScPH
Research Associate
The Tumori Foundation
San Francisco, California, USA

Domenico Coppola, MD
Pathologist
Gastrointestinal Division
Moffitt Cancer Center
Tampa, Florida, USA

Aimee Crago, MD, PhD
Attending Physician
Department of Medicine
Memorial Sloan Kettering Cancer Center and
Weill Cornell Medical College
New York, New York, USA

Juanita Crook, MD, FRCPC
Professor
Department of Radiation Oncology
University of British Columbia
British Colombia Cancer Agency
Cancer Center for the Southern Interior
Kelowna, British Columbia, Canada

Ramona Dadu, MD
Assistant Professor
Department of Endocrine Neoplasia and
Hormonal Disorders
The University of Texas MD Anderson Cancer Center
Houston, Texas, USA

Stephanie B. Dixon, MD
Pediatric Hematology-Oncology Fellow
Department of Pediatric Oncology
St. Jude Children's Research Hospital
Memphis, Tennessee, USA

Robert Dreicer, MD, MS, MACP, FASCO
Section Head, Division of Hematology/Oncology
Professor, Department of Medicine
University of Virginia School of Medicine
Charlottesville, Virginia, USA

Kathleen M. Egan, ScD
Instructor
H. Lee Moffitt Cancer Center
Tampa, Florida, USA

Lawrence H. Einhorn, MD
Professor
Indiana University School of Medicine
Simon Cancer Center
Indianapolis, Indiana, USA

Mark H. Einstein, MD, MS
Gynecologic Oncologist
Rutgers New Jersey Medical School
Newark, New Jersey, USA

Cathy Eng, MD
Professor
Department of Gastrointestinal Medical Oncology
The University of Texas MD Anderson Cancer Center
Houston, Texas, USA

Nicola Fabbri, MD
Professor
Department of Surgery
Memorial Sloan Kettering Cancer Center and
Weill Cornell Medical College
New York, New York, USA

Christopher R. Flowers, MD, MS
Professor
Department of Hematology and Oncology
Winship Cancer Institute
Emory University
Atlanta, Georgia, USA

Lisa M. Force, MD
Instructor in Pediatrics
Department of Pediatric Oncology
St. Jude Children's Research Hospital
Memphis, Tennessee, USA

Clifton D. Fuller, MD, PhD
Associate Professor
Division of Radiation Oncology
The University of Texas MD Anderson Cancer Center
Houston, Texas, USA

Ted Gansler, MD, MPH, MBA
Strategic Director
Intramural Research
American Cancer Society
Atlanta, Georgia, USA

Jorge A. Garcia, MD
Assistant Professor of Medicine
Department of Hematology and Medical Oncology
Cleveland Clinic Lerner College of Medicine
Cleveland, Ohio, USA

Matthew Gary, MD
Emory Healthcare Network Physician
Emory Clinic
Atlanta, Georgia, USA

Christina Gauthreaux, MD
Internal Medicine Resident
Washington University School of Medicine/
Barnes Jewish Hospital
St Louis, Missouri, USA

Alan C. Geller, MPH, RN
Senior Lecturer
Department of Social and Behavioral Sciences
Harvard TH Chan School of Public Health
Director, Melanoma Epidemiology
Massachusetts General Hospital
Boston, Massachusetts, USA

Ben George, MD
Associate Professor of Medicine
Medical College of Wisconsin
Milwaukee, Wisconsin, USA

David E. Gerber, MD
Associate Professor of Internal Medicine
(Hematology-Oncology) and Clinical Sciences
Department of Clinical Science
Harold C. Simmons Comprehensive Cancer Center
The University of Texas Southwestern Medical Center
Dallas, Texas, USA

Nilanjan Ghosh, MD, PhD
Director, Lymphoma Division
Department of Hematologic Oncology and
Blood Disorders
Levine Cancer Institute
Carolinas HealthCare System
Charlotte, North Carolina, USA

Ivana Gojo, MD
Associate Professor of Oncology
Division of Hematologic Malignancies,
Department of Oncology
Sidney Kimmel Comprehensive Cancer Center
Johns Hopkins University
Baltimore, Maryland, USA

Mrinal Gounder, MD
Attending Physician and Assistant Professor
Department of Medicine
Memorial Sloan Kettering Cancer Center and
Weill Cornell Medical College
New York, New York, USA

F. Anthony Greco, MD
Director
Sarah Cannon Cancer Center
Nashville, Tennessee, USA

Neil D. Gross, MD, FACS
Associate Professor
Department of Head and Neck Surgery
The University of Texas MD Anderson Cancer Center
Houston, Texas, USA

Michael R. Grunwald, MD
Associate Director, Leukemia Division
Department of Hematologic Oncology and
Blood Disorders
Levine Cancer Institute
Carolinas HealthCare System
Charlotte, North Carolina, USA

Constantinos Hadjipanayis, MD, PhD
Professor
Department of Neurosurgery
Icahn School of Medicine at Mount Sinai
New York, New York, USA

John D. Hainsworth, MD
Senior Investigator
Sarah Cannon Research Institute
Nashville, Tennessee, USA

Alireza Hamidian Jahromi, MD, MRCS
Professor
Department of Surgery
Louisiana State University Health Sciences Center
Shreveport, Louisiana, USA

Ehab Hanna, MD
Professor
Department of Head and Neck Surgery
The University of Texas MD Anderson Cancer Center
Houston, Texas, USA

Nasser Hanna, MD
Professor
Indiana University School of Medicine
Simon Cancer Center
Indianapolis, Indiana, USA

Rian M. Hasson Charles, MD
Fellow in Cardiothoracic Surgery
Mayo Clinic
Rochester, Minnesota, USA

Susan Hedlund, MS
Professor
Social Work and Survivorship
Knight Cancer Institute
Oregon Health and Science University
Portland, Oregon, USA

H. William Higgins II, MD
Assistant Professor of Dermatology
Department of Dermatology
Brown University School of Medicine
Providence, Rhode Island, USA

Sarah E. Hoffe, MD
Section Head
Gastrointestinal Radiation Oncology
Moffitt Cancer Center
Tampa, Florida, USA

Randall F. Holcombe, MD
Professor
Division of Hematology and
Medical Oncology
The Tisch Cancer Institute
Mount Sinai Medical Center
New York, New York, USA

Emma B. Holliday, MD
Assistant Professor
Division of Radiation Oncology
The University of Texas MD Anderson Cancer Center
Houston, Texas, USA

Adriana G. Ioachimescu, MD, PhD, FACE
Associate Professor of Medicine and Neurosurgery
Co-Director, The Emory Pituitary Center
Emory University School of Medicine
Atlanta, Georgia, USA

Candice A. Johnstone, MD
Associate Professor
Medical College of Wisconsin
Milwaukee, Wisconsin, USA

Fadlo R. Khuri, MD
Professor of Hematology and Medical Oncology
Adjunct Professor of Medicine, Pharmacology and Otolaryngology
Winship Cancer Institute
Emory University School of Medicine
Atlanta, Georgia, USA

Roger H. Kim, MD, FACS
Associate Professor of Surgery
Program Director, General Surgery Residency
Division of General Surgery/Department of Surgery
Southern Illinois University School of Medicine
Springfield, Illinois, USA

Joseph Klink, MD
Urologist
Deaconess Clinic Gateway Health Center
Newburgh, Indiana, USA

Merieme Klobocista, MD
Gynecologic Oncologist
John Theurer Cancer Center
Hackensack University Medical Center
Hackensack, New Jersey, USA

Justin M. Ko, MD, MBA
Associate Professor of Dermatology
Department of Dermatology
Stanford University Medical Center
Stanford, California, USA

Jean L. Koff, MD
Instructor
Department of Hematology and Medical Oncology
Winship Cancer Institute
Emory University
Atlanta, Georgia, USA

Badrinath R. Konety, MD, MBA
Professor and Department Chair
Department of Urology
University of Minnesota
Minneapolis, Minnesota, USA

Lauren Kosinski, MD, MS
Managing Partner
The Seed House
Chestertown, Maryland, USA

Anna Kuan-Celarier, MD
Resident House Officer
Department of Obstetrics and Gynecology
Louisiana State University Health Sciences Center
New Orleans, Louisiana, USA

Michael E. Kupferman, MD
Professor
Department of Head and Neck Surgery
The University of Texas MD Anderson Cancer Center
Houston, Texas, USA

Benjamin D. Li, MD, FACS
Director
MetroHealth Cancer Center
Cleveland, Ohio, USA

Bobby C. Liaw, MD
Assistant Professor
Hematology and Medical Oncology
Icahn School of Medicine at Mount Sinai
Mount Sinai Downtown Chelsea Center
New York, New York, USA

John R. Lurain, MD
Marcia Stenn Professor of Gynecologic Oncology
Northwestern University Feinberg School of Medicine
Robert H. Lurie Comprehensive Cancer Center
Chicago, Illinois, USA

Mohammad Mahmoud, MD
Professor
Department of Urology
University of Chicago
Chicago, Illinois, USA

Peter Manley, MD
Assistant Professor of Pediatrics
Department of Pediatric Oncology
Dana-Farber/Boston Children's Cancer and
Blood Disorders Center
Boston, Massachusetts, USA

Avinash V. Mantravadi, MD
Assistant Professor
Department of Otolaryngology – Head and Neck Surgery
Indiana University School of Medicine
Indianapolis, Indiana, USA

Karen J. Marcus, MD
Associate Professor and Division Chief
Pediatric Radiation Oncology
Dana-Farber/Boston Children's Cancer and
Blood Disorders Center
Boston, Massachusetts, USA

Jonathan Mathias, MD
Professor
Department of Internal Medicine
Cleveland Clinic
Cleveland, Ohio, USA

Kenneth L. Meredith, MD
Professor
Department of Gastrointestinal and Surgical Oncology
Sarasota Memorial Hospital
Sarasota, Florida, USA

Kriti Mittal, MD
Hematologist
Division of Hematology/Oncology
University of Massachusetts Medical School
Worcester, Massachusetts, USA

Michael G. Moore, MD
Associate Professor of Otolaryngology and Head and Neck
Surgery and Director of Head and Neck Surgery
The University of California at Davis Medical Center
Sacramento, California, USA

Michael Moore
Department of Neurosurgery
Emory University School of Medicine
Atlanta, Georgia, USA

Burt Nabors, MD
Co-Leader
Neuro-Oncology Program
University of Alabama at Birmingham
Birmingham, Alabama, USA

Loretta J. Nastoupil, MD
Assistant Professor
Department of Lymphoma/Myeloma
The University of Texas MD Anderson Cancer Center
Houston, Texas, USA

William K. Oh, MD
Professor
The Tisch Cancer Institute
Icahn School of Medicine at Mount Sinai
New York, New York, USA

Jeffrey J. Olson, MD
Professor
Department of Neurosurgery
Emory University School of Medicine
Atlanta, Georgia, USA

Ruth O'Regan, MD
Professor
Department of Medicine
University of Wisconsin School of Medicine and
Public Health
Madison, Wisconsin, USA

D. Ryan Ormond, MD
Assistant Professor
Department of Neurosurgery
University of Colorado School of Medicine
Aurora, Colorado, USA

Moshe C. Ornstein, MD, MA
Hematology/Oncology Fellow
Department of Hematology and Medical Oncology
Taussig Cancer Institute
Cleveland, Ohio, USA

Nelson M. Oyesiku, MD, PhD
Professor of Neurosurgery and Medicine (Endocrinology)
Emory University Co-director
Emory Pituitary Center
Emory University
Atlanta, Georgia, USA

Alok Pant, MD
Professor
John I Brewer Trophoblastic Disease Center
Northwestern University
Feinberg School of Medicine
Chicago, Illinois, USA

Elisavet Paplomata, MD
Assistant Professor
Department of Hematology and Medical Oncology
Winship Cancer Institute of Emory University
Atlanta, Georgia, USA

Jamie M. Pawlowski, MD
Radiation Oncology Resident, PGY-3
Department of Radiation Oncology
UT Health San Antonio Cancer Center
The University of Texas Health Science Center at San Antonio
San Antonio, Texas, USA

Michael L. Pearl, MD, FACOG, FACS
Professor and Director
Division of Gynecologic Oncology
Stony Brook Medicine
Stony Brook, New York, USA

Lorraine C. Pelosof, MD, PhD
Medical Officer
Harold C. Simmons
Comprehensive Cancer Center
The University of Texas
Southwestern Medical Center
Dallas, Texas, USA

Alexander Perl, MD, MS
Associate Professor of Medicine
Department of Medicine
Perelman Center for Advanced Medicine
University of Pennsylvania
Philadelphia, Pennsylvania, USA

Mario Javier Pineda, MD, PhD
Professor
Division of Gynecologic Oncology
Department of Obstetrics and Gynecology
Robert H. Lurie Comprehensive Cancer Center
Northwestern University Feinberg School of Medicine
Chicago, Illinois, USA

Roshan Prabhu, MD
Radiation Oncologist
Southeast Radiation Oncology Group
Charlotte, North Carolina, USA

Christopher Przybycin, MD
Associate Staff Pathologist
Robert J Tomsich Pathology and Laboratory Medicine Institute
Cleveland, Ohio, USA

Suresh S. Ramalingam, MD
Professor of Hematology and Medical Oncology
Roberto C. Goizueta Chair for Cancer Research
Deputy Director, Winship Cancer Institute
Emory University School of Medicine
Atlanta, Georgia, USA

Srikant Rangaraju, MD
Vascular Neurologist
Emory Clinic
Atlanta, Georgia, USA

Chandrajit P. Raut, MD, MSc
Professor
Department of Surgery
Brigham and Women's Hospital
Center for Sarcoma and Bone Oncology
Dana-Farber Cancer Institute
Associate Professor of Surgery
Harvard Medical School
Boston, Massachusetts, USA

Vinod Ravi, MD
Associate Professor of Medicine
Department of Sarcoma Medical Oncology
The University of Texas MD Anderson Cancer Center
Houston, Texas, USA

Sonia Reichert, MD
Oncologist
Division of Hematology and Medical Oncology
The Tisch Cancer Institute;
Mount Sinai Medical Center
New York, New York, USA

Jordan Reynolds, MD
Associate Staff Pathologist
Robert J Tomsich Pathology and Laboratory Medicine Institute
Cleveland, Ohio, USA

Brian Rini, MD
Oncologist
Taussig Cancer Institute
Cleveland, Ohio, USA

Michael C. Risk, MD, PhD
Assistant Professor
Department of Urology
University of Minnesota
Minneapolis VA Medical Center
Minneapolis, Minnesota, USA

Kyle Robinson, MD
Assistant Professor of Clinical Medicine
Hematology and Medical Oncology
Hospital of the University of Pennsylvania
Philadelphia, Pennsylvania, USA

Carlos Rodriguez-Galindo, MD
Director, International Outreach Program
Department of Pediatric Oncology
St. Jude Children's Research Hospital
Memphis, Tennessee, USA

David I. Rosenthal, MD
Professor
The University of Texas MD Anderson Cancer Center
Division of Radiation Oncology
Houston, Texas, USA

Darshan Roy, MD
Assistant Professor of Pathology
Department of Pathology
Rowan School of Medicine
Stratford, New Jersey, USA

Carolyn D. Runowicz, MD
Executive Associate Dean for Academic Affairs
Professor, Department of Obstetrics and Gynecology
Florida International University
Herbert Wertheim College of Medicine
Miami, Florida, USA

Guillermo Sangster, MD
Professor
Department of Radiology
Feist-Weiller Cancer Center
Louisiana State University Health Sciences Center
Shreveport, Louisiana, USA

Satish Shanbhag, MBBS, MPH
Assistant Professor of Medicine and Oncology
Departments of Medicine and Oncology
Johns Hopkins University School of Medicine
Baltimore, Maryland, USA

Ravi Shridhar, MD PhD
Associate Professor
Department of Radiation Oncology
Moffitt Cancer Center
Tampa, Florida, USA

Nataly Silva, MS
Associate Professor
Department of Gastrointestinal Medical Oncology
The University of Texas MD Anderson Cancer Center
Houston, Texas, USA

Lewis B. Silverman, MD
Associate Professor of Pediatrics
Department of Pediatric Oncology
Dana-Farber/Boston Children's Cancer and
Blood Disorders Center
Boston, Massachusetts, USA

Blaine D. Smith, MD
Clinical Resident
Department of Surgery Division of Head and
Neck Surgery and Communication Sciences
Duke University Medical Center
Durham, North Carolina, USA

Ayman Soubra, MD
Resident
Department of Urology
University of Minnesota
Minneapolis, Minnesota, USA

Erin E. Stevens, MD
Gynecologic Oncologist
Billings Clinic Cancer Center
Billings, Montana, USA

Jonathan Strosberg, MD
Associate Professor
Department of Gastrointestinal Oncology
H. Lee Moffitt Cancer Center and Research Institute
Tampa, Florida, USA

Susan M. Swetter, MD
Professor of Dermatology
Director, Pigmented Lesion and Melanoma Program
Physician Leader, Cancer Care Program in
Cutaneous Oncology
Stanford University Medical Center and
Cancer Institute
VA Palo Alto Health Care System
Stanford, California, USA

Charles R. Thomas, Jr, MD
Professor and Chair
Department of Radiation Medicine
Knight Cancer Institute
Oregon Health and Science University
Portland, Oregon, USA

Brandon H. Tieu, MD, FACS
Associate Professor of Surgery
Division of Cardiothoracic Surgery
Knight Cancer Institute
Oregon Health and Science University
Portland, Oregon, USA

Liana Tsikitis, MD
Associate Professor
Division of Gastrointestinal and General Surgery
School of Medicine
Knight Cancer Institute
Oregon Health and Science University
Portland, Oregon, USA

Kiran K. Turaga, MD, MPH
Associate Professor
Department of Surgery
University of Chicago
Chicago, Illinois, USA

Joyce Varughese, MD
Assistant Professor
Division of Gynecologic Oncology
Stony Brook Medicine
Stony Brook, New York, USA

Alfredo Voloschin, MD
Associate Professor
Department of Hematology and Medical Oncology
Winship Cancer Institute
Emory University School of Medicine
Atlanta, Georgia, USA

Paula Province Warren, MD
Assistant Professor
Neuro-Oncology Program
University of Alabama at Birmingham
Birmingham, Alabama, USA

Martin A. Weinstock, MD, PhD
Professor of Dermatology
Dermatoepidemiology Unit
VA Medical Center
Providence, Rhode Island, USA

Steven P. Weitzman, MD
Assistant Professor
Department of Endocrine Neoplasia and
Hormonal Disorders
The University of Texas MD Anderson Cancer Center
Houston, Texas, USA

Jocelyn L. Wozney, MD
Hematologist
Lancaster General Health
Lancaster, Pennsylvania, USA

Yoshiya Yamada, MD
Professor
Department of Radiation Oncology
Memorial Sloan Kettering Cancer Center and
Weill Cornell Medical College
New York, New York, USA

Mark Zafereo, MD
Associate Professor
Department of Head and Neck Surgery
The University of Texas MD Anderson Cancer Center
Houston, Texas, USA

Joshua F. Zeidner, MD
Assistant Professor of Medicine
Division of Hematology/Oncology
Lineberger Comprehensive Cancer Center
University of North Carolina
Chapel Hill, North Carolina, USA

Introduction

The American Cancer Society (ACS) published its first textbook in 1963 with the objective of introducing students and practicing clinicians to the rapidly emerging field of oncology. Since then, eleven editions of this book have been published under a variety of titles. Due to the growing body of cancer information available, we have divided the content into two books to cover the information we considered most essential.

This book, *The American Cancer Society's Oncology in Practice – Clinical Management,* applies the principles of multidisciplinary care to specific forms of cancer. Each chapter begins with sections that summarize the population burden of that disease, risk factors, screening, and diagnosis. The chapters focus on treatment for persons with each type of malignancy, and then conclude with a summary of follow-up and survivorship considerations.

This textbook and its companion (*The American Cancer Society's Principles of Oncology – Prevention to Survivorship*) are comprised of the contributions of myriad authors, editorial board members, and reviewers. The most essential contributors are, of course, the distinguished chapter authors who took time from their busy clinical and/or research schedules to organize and summarize their knowledge on a particular aspect of cancer control. Relative to these other components of their work, contributing a chapter to this book yields much less recognition (and, absolutely no remuneration). These dedicated, hard-working, geniuses have been a pleasure to work with and we appreciate their patience through the inevitable revisions and delays inherent in the publication of a book of this magnitude.

This work also would not have been possible without the advice, time, and expertise of our editorial board of prominent experts. They selected chapter authors, reviewed and edited chapter manuscripts, and helped keep the work moving. There were some chapter topics for which our editorial board recommended review by additional experts. These peer reviewers are listed in the frontmatter and I sincerely appreciate their valuable contribution to this book.

Once the authors and editors are finished, the work of the publisher still continues. A good publisher is a delight to work with. The converse is even more true, and I appreciate the expertise and dedication of our colleagues at Wiley-Blackwell.

Finally, this work could not have been initiated and completed without the work of many American Cancer Society staff and volunteers. I especially want to thank Ms. Jin Kim who as managing editor of this project skillfully coordinated and organized the work of everyone else. And of course, this book and everything else done by the American Cancer Society depends on the support of our volunteers and donors, and is inspired by our constituents.

Ted Gansler, MD, MBA, MPH

Section 1

Thoracic Cancers

1

Lung Cancer

Suresh S. Ramalingam and Fadlo R. Khuri

Emory University School of Medicine, Atlanta, Georgia, USA

Incidence and Mortality

Lung cancer is the most commonly diagnosed cancer worldwide with an estimated 1.8 million new cases each year. This accounts for approximately 13% of all cancers in the world. With an estimated 1.6 million deaths each year, lung cancer is also the leading cause of cancer-related mortality globally [1, 2]. Among men, lung cancer is the most common malignancy, whereas in women, lung cancer incidence is exceeded only by breast and colorectal cancers. The estimated incidence rates of lung cancer in more developed countries are 18.6 per 100,000 women per year and 47.4 per 100,000 in men per year. The corresponding rates for less developed countries are 11.1 and 27.8 for women and men, respectively. The mortality related to lung cancer in men has declined in the past two decades in the Western countries, but is increasing rapidly in the developing world. However, in women the incidence and mortality related to lung cancer continues on an upward trend in most regions of the world. In the United States (US), an estimated 222,500 cases of lung cancer will be diagnosed in the year 2017 and approximately 155,870 deaths will result from lung cancer [3]. In Europe, an estimated 417,000 cases of lung cancer are diagnosed annually with approximately 367,000 deaths each year [4]. China has experienced a 465% increase in the deaths related to lung cancer over the past 30 years [5]. With approximately 500,000 new cases annually, lung cancer is the most common cancer in China in both men and women. Based on the increasing incidence of cigarette smoking in the developing world, it is estimated that most lung cancers cases will occur outside the US and Europe by the year 2030.

Risk Factors

Cigarette smoking is the most common risk factor for lung cancer. Nearly 85% of patients with lung cancer have a history of smoking tobacco products. Among them, approximately 50% are former smokers, defined as being free from smoking for at least 12 months before the diagnosis of lung cancer. The risk of developing lung cancer is proportional to the number of cigarettes smoked per day and the cumulative duration of smoking time. Patients with a smoking history of more than 20–30 pack years are considered to be at high risk for developing lung cancer. Though the prevalence of cigarette smoking is declining in the US, it is increasing at an alarming rate in developing and third world countries. Consequently, the number of cases of lung cancer diagnosed annually is likely to rise over the next few decades. Smoking cessation is associated with a gradual reduction in risk of lung cancer, though it does not reach that of a never-smoker. Since fewer than 20% of heavy smokers develop lung cancer, genetic susceptibility to lung cancer also appears to play a risk. Women appear to be at a higher risk of developing lung cancer compared to men. In recent years, there are an increasing number of never-smokers diagnosed with lung cancer. The tumors in these individuals are more likely to harbor certain genetic alterations such as mutations in the epidermal growth factor receptor (*EGFR*) gene, and rearrangement in the anaplastic lymphoma kinase (*ALK*) gene [6]. Second-hand exposure to smoke is another risk factor that contributes to nearly 1% of all cases of lung cancer.

Occupational exposure to asbestos is a known risk factor for lung cancer [7, 8]. It is estimated that in patients without a smoking history, there is a fourfold higher risk of lung cancer with asbestos exposure. Cigarette smoking has an additive effect on increasing the risk of lung cancer associated with asbestos exposure [9]. Although the use of asbestos is banned in nearly 50 countries in the world, it is on the rise in China, India, Russia, and many other countries. The Environmental Protection Agency (EPA) and the World Health Organization consider all forms of asbestos as carcinogenic. There is a latency of a few decades between asbestos exposure and the development of lung cancer. The risk of developing lung cancer from asbestos is related to the duration of exposure, quantity, and the type of asbestos fiber.

The American Cancer Society's Oncology in Practice: Clinical Management, First Edition. Edited by The American Cancer Society.

Radon exposure has also been implicated in the development of lung cancer [10]. Radon results from the radioactive decay of uranium. Household exposure to radon in certain geographical regions is high and contributes to nearly 20,000 new cases of lung cancer each year, according to an EPA estimate [11]. The EPA recommends that household radon levels should be <4 picocuries/L of air to minimize the risk of developing lung cancer. Simple remedial methods are available to reduce radon exposures above this threshold. Exposure to ionizing radiation in the form of therapeutic radiation, or frequent diagnostic radiographic tests is also associated with a higher risk of developing lung cancer. Industrial exposure to metals such as arsenic, nickel, chromium, and general air pollution have all been linked to a higher risk of lung cancer. There are no known familial genetic syndromes associated with lung cancer.

Pathology

Historically, lung cancer was broadly subdivided into nonsmall cell lung cancer (NSCLC) and small cell lung cancer (SCLC), based on the distinct behavior and response to chemotherapy between these two subsets of patients. NSCLC constitutes adenocarcinoma, squamous cell carcinoma and large cell carcinoma subtypes. In the past few years, distinct differences between the various subhistologies of NSCLC have been recognized and an increasing emphasis is placed on the identification of subtypes from diagnostic specimens.

Adenocarcinoma is the most common histological subtype of lung cancer. It has gradually increased in incidence, surpassing squamous cell cancer in the past two decades. In the US, adenocarcinoma represents nearly 50% of all cases of lung cancer. Adenocarcinoma has a higher predilection for distant metastasis compared to squamous cell histology. Never-smokers that develop lung cancer most frequently have the adenocarcinoma subtype. Since 2011, a new classification system for lung adenocarcinoma has been in use [12]. Under this system, adenocarcinoma is divided into preinvasive, minimally invasive, and invasive types (Table 1.1). Atypical adenomatous hyperplasia refers to a localized proliferative lesion consisting of atypical type II pneumocytes or Clara cells and measuring <5 mm. Adenocarcinoma *in situ* (AIS) refers to lesions measuring <3 cm in size that do not have any invasive characteristics. This was previously referred to as bronchioloalveolar carcinoma. Lesions ≤3 cm with a predominant lepidic pattern (referring to growth along alveolar structures) and invasion of <5 mm in greatest dimension are referred to as minimally invasive adenocarcinoma (MIA). AIS and MIA have a >95% 5-year survival rate when treated with surgical resection. Invasive adenocarcinoma represents nearly 90% of cases of adenocarcinoma. Based on the predominant growth pattern, it is categorized as lepidic, acinar, papillary, micropapillary, or solid predominant with mucin production. In addition to morphological features, immunohistochemistry studies are helpful in establishing the histological subtype of NSCLC. Adenocarcinoma specimens tend to be positive for cytokeratin 7, napsin A and thyroid transcription factor-1 (TTF-1) and are negative for cytokeratin 20 [13]. TTF-1 is considered a strong marker of adenocarcinoma based on positivity in nearly 75–85% of cases [14].

Table 1.1 IASLC/ATS/ERS classification of lung adenocarcinoma in resection specimens.

Preinvasive lesions
Atypical adenomatous hyperplasia
Adenocarcinoma *in situ* (≤3 cm formerly BAC)
Nonmucinous
Mucinous
Mixed mucinous/nonmucinous
Minimally invasive adenocarcinoma (≤3 cm lepidic predominant tumor with ≤5 mm invasion)
Nonmucinous
Mucinous
Mixed mucinous/nonmucinous
Invasive adenocarcinoma
Lepidic predominant (formerly nonmucinous BAC pattern, with >5 mm invasion)
Acinar predominant
Papillary predominant
Micropapillary predominant
Solid predominant with mucin production
Variants of invasive adenocarcinoma
Invasive mucinous adenocarcinoma (formerly mucinous BAC)
Colloid
Fetal (low and high grade)
Enteric

Source: Travis *et al.* [12]. Reproduced with permission of Elsevier.
ATS, American Thoracic Society; BAC, bronchioloalveolar carcinoma; ERS, European Respiratory Society; IASLC, International Association for the Study of Lung Cancer [28].

Squamous cell lung cancer is decreasing in incidence in the US, most likely due to the changing smoking habits of the population. Squamous cell tumors are often centrally located and are almost always seen in patients with smoking history. Squamous dysplasia and squamous cell carcinoma *in situ* are preinvasive lesions that can develop into invasive cancers. The majority of squamous cell tumors stain positive for p63 and p40 markers; these markers can be tested in diagnostic specimens of lung cancers lacking apparent squamous differentiation on routinely stained slides. A panel of markers including TTF-1, p63 and p40 is increasingly evaluated in diagnostic specimens of patients with lung cancer to identify the histological subtype [14].

Large cell carcinoma represents 3–4% of NSCLC and is characterized by a high mitotic rate, necrosis, and morphological features of NSCLC [15, 16]. The tumors stain positively for neuroendocrine markers such as chromogranin A and synaptophysin. Accurate diagnosis of this histological subtype requires an abundance of specimen tissue. Large cell carcinoma is associated with an aggressive clinical course and poor survival rates even with early-stage disease. Large cell carcinoma is strongly associated with smoking history.

SCLC is diagnosed in approximately 13% of lung cancer cases in the US. The incidence of SCLC has gradually declined over the past three decades in the US. SCLC is strongly associated with smoking and is rare in never-smokers. Pathological diagnosis is established by light microscopy that demonstrates characteristic features such as a high degree of mitosis and necrosis. Diagnostic workup of SCLC includes immunostaining for TTF-1, chromogranin, synaptophysin, and CD-56. Approximately 15% of SCLC specimens have mixed morphology with components of NSCLC [15, 17].

Molecular Pathology

In recent years, a number of molecular abnormalities have been identified in lung cancer (Figure 1.1) [18]. Many of these represent targets for therapy and therefore obtaining adequate tumor tissue to conduct molecular studies is an essential component of the diagnostic workup for lung cancer. The heterogeneity of lung cancer in terms of presenting features and clinical course has been recognized for a long time. Now, a greater understanding of the molecular features that account for the heterogeneity is leading to individualized treatment approaches. In lung adenocarcinoma, nearly two-thirds of patients harbor an oncogenic mutation that can potentially be targeted with specific agents. The most common among these are mutations involving *K-RAS, EGFR, B-RAF, HER-2, PIK3CA* and gene rearrangements involving the *ALK, RET* and *ROS1*. *K-RAS* mutations are present in approximately 25% of lung adenocarcinoma patients and are often associated with cigarette smoking. The most common sites of mutation in *K-RAS* include codon 12, 13 and 61 that results in an amino acid substitution [19]. This results in impaired GTPase activity, which confers constitutive activation of *RAS* signaling. The prognostic value of *K-RAS* mutation in patients with lung cancer is controversial, despite early reports that it portends a poor overall outcome and reduced sensitivity to chemotherapy.

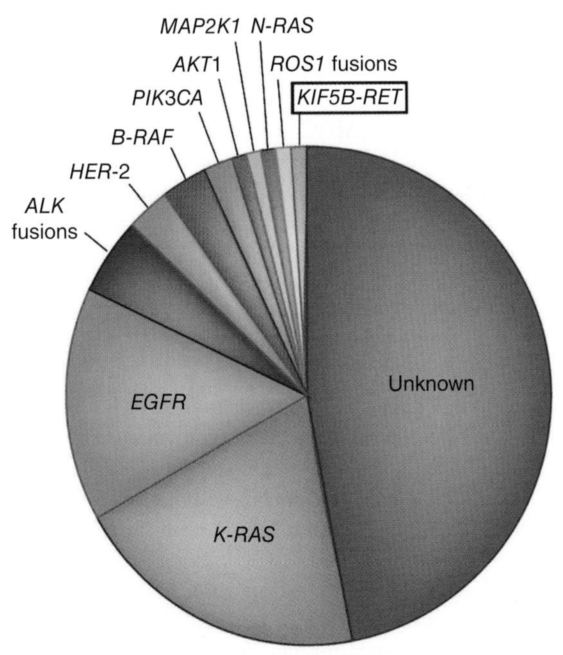

Figure 1.1 Molecular drivers in lung adenocarcinoma. *Source:* Pao and Hutchinson [18].

Mutations in *EGFR* are observed in nearly 15% of White lung cancer patients and 40% of Asians. Deletion mutation in exon 19 and a point mutation in exon 21 are the most common *EGFR* mutations. These mutations are located in the tyrosine kinase-binding domain of the receptor and result in constitutive activation of the pathway, leading to proliferation, evasion of apoptosis and angiogenesis. Patients with *EGFR* activating mutations derive robust clinical benefits with EGFR tyrosine kinase inhibitors (TKI) [20, 21]. Nearly 60% of patients with an *EGFR* mutation will develop a secondary mutation in exon 20 (T790M) upon continued exposure to an EGFR TKI [22]. This mutation is the most common mechanism of resistance to EGFR TKI therapy, but can also be found *de novo* in certain patients with lung adenocarcinoma along with an exon 19 or 21 mutation prior to exposure to EGFR TKI therapy. In approximately 5% of patients with lung adenocarcinoma, gene rearrangement involving *ALK* is observed. This fusion gene results in activation of downstream signals that can be inhibited by specific ALK kinase inhibitors. Crizotinib, an ALK inhibitor, induces objective tumor response in nearly two-thirds of patients [23]. It is noteworthy that *EGFR* and *K-RAS* mutations and *ALK* gene rearrangement are mutually exclusive. *ALK* gene rearrangement is detected by the fluorescent *in situ* hybridization (FISH) test using the Vysis break-apart assay. Immunohistochemistry can be used as a screening step before conducting the FISH test. Other fusion abnormalities involving the *RET* and *ROS1* genes are each present in 1% of lung adenocarcinoma specimens [24]. In addition to these molecular events, *p53* mutation and **LKB1** loss are commonly observed in lung adenocarcinoma patients [24].

Squamous cell carcinoma has an entirely different spectrum of molecular abnormalities. Recent studies from the Cancer Genome Atlas (TCGA) project indicate common mutations including *TP53, PTEN* loss, *PIK3CA, KEAP1, DDR2,* and *RB1* [25]. Amplification of the fibroblast growth factor receptor (*FGFR*) gene is also noted in 10–20% of squamous cell lung cancers. Many of these abnormalities provide potential opportunities for targeted therapies. In SCLC, the common genetic changes include *RB1* and *TP53* mutations, which are observed in nearly 90% and 50% of patients respectively. The availability of highly sophisticated methods to sequence the genome allows for the ability to detect hitherto unidentified molecular abnormalities and thus uncover new therapeutic targets for lung cancer. With present technology, it is increasingly possible to conduct 'multiplex' testing for a number of molecular markers with limited tissue specimens. Guidelines issued by the IASLC recommend routine testing for *EGFR* mutation and *ALK* translocation for all newly diagnosed patients with lung adenocarcinoma. In squamous cell histology, routine molecular testing is not yet recommended.

Diagnosis

Presenting symptoms of lung cancer include cough, dyspnea, pain, hemoptysis, and weight loss. Since most patients with lung cancer have other tobacco-related cardiopulmonary diseases, these overlapping symptoms often result in a delay in diagnosis of the underlying malignancy. Symptoms could also result from local invasion or metastasis of the tumor such as headache, bone pain, bronchial obstruction, etc. Paraneoplastic syndromes associated with lung cancer include syndrome of inappropriate anti-diuretic hormone (SIADH), hypercalcemia, pulmonary hypertrophic osteoarthropathy, Eaton-Lambert myasthenic syndrome (ELMS), and Cushing syndrome. Some of the paraneoplastic syndromes are associated with specific histologies; hypercalcemia is common in squamous cell carcinoma, whereas SIADH, ELMS, and Cushing syndrome are common in SCLC. Diagnosis of lung cancer at an early stage is often made as an incidental finding during evaluation for other conditions. With the advent of computed tomography (CT) screening, it is anticipated that a greater subset of patients with lung cancer will be detected before the onset of symptoms.

In patients with clinical or radiographic findings suspicious of lung cancer, CT scans of the chest and abdomen are indicated to determine the location of the primary tumor, involvement of mediastinal lymph nodes, and spread to other anatomic sites. The most common sites of metastasis with lung cancer include mediastinal lymph nodes, contralateral lung, liver, adrenal gland, bones, and the brain. Imaging of the brain is recommended to evaluate for metastasis in patients with suggestive symptoms and signs, or those with lung adenocarcinoma >3 cm and evidence of mediastinal nodal involvement. Magnetic resonance imaging (MRI) or CT scan with contrast are acceptable modalities to evaluate for brain metastasis. Radionuclide study of the bones is indicated in patients with symptoms of bone pain or an unexplained elevation in serum alkaline phosphatase level. Positron emission tomography (PET) utilizing ^{18}fluorodeoxyglucose (FDG) is included as part of staging for lung cancer in patients with localized lung cancer or for evaluation of solitary pulmonary nodules. The use of an FDG-PET scan to assess response to anticancer therapy and in surveillance following curative therapy is not recommended. An MRI scan of the chest may be useful in determining invasion of surrounding structures such as the brachial plexus in patients with tumors involving the superior sulcus of the lung.

A biopsy is necessary to establish diagnosis, and in recent years, to conduct molecular studies (for NSCLC) that can guide therapy. The most accessible site with the least invasive method is the preferred approach to obtaining diagnostic tissue. A fine-needle aspiration procedure is often adequate for establishing the diagnosis of lung cancer, and can be accomplished by a transthoracic approach or by bronchoscopy. However, the yield from a fine-needle aspiration is often inadequate to conduct molecular studies. Therefore, in recent years, a core-needle biopsy to obtain sufficient tissue is recommended for patients with suspected lung cancer. For patients presenting with pleural or pericardial effusions, transthoracic aspiration of the fluid is sufficient to establish the diagnosis and to complete staging workup. Cell blocks prepared by centrifuging the fluid, and processing the pellet as a histological specimen, can be used to conduct molecular studies, though the success rate depends on the number of viable cancer cells in the specimen. The diagnostic yield of pleural fluid in patients with a malignant effusion is approximately 50–70% [26]. In instances where repeated aspiration of pleural fluid is nondiagnostic, a video-assisted thoracoscopy procedure might be necessary to establish the diagnosis. For patients with localized lung tumors that are suspicious for cancer, it is reasonable to proceed with surgical resection without a diagnostic biopsy if all other potential etiologies are excluded.

In recent years, with the utilization of molecularly targeted therapies, understanding the mechanism of resistance has emerged as an important determinant of subsequent therapies. Therefore, obtaining additional tumor biopsies at various time-points during the course of treatment is recommended.

Early Detection

Decades of research on screening high-risk individuals for earlier detection of lung cancer have finally met with success. The National Lung Cancer Screening Trial randomized subjects to screening with low dose CT scans or chest radiographs that were performed at baseline and after 1 and 2 years from enrollment [27]. Positive scans were observed in nearly 25% and 7% of the subjects screened with CT and chest radiograph, respectively. Among patients with a positive CT scan, 96.4% were deemed false positive after appropriate additional evaluation. Adverse events were uncommon with approximately 1.5% of patients with an abnormal scan developing complications related to further diagnostic workup. Screening with annual low dose CT scans in high-risk individuals was associated with a 20% reduction in lung cancer mortality. All-cause mortality was also reduced by 6.7%. Nearly 80% of patients diagnosed with lung cancer with low dose CT had stage I, II, or IIIA disease that is amenable to curative therapy. These results have now led to the adoption of low dose CT for early detection of lung cancer by major relevant health organizations including the American Cancer Society (see *The American Cancer Society's Principles of Oncology: Prevention to Survivorship*, Chapter 11).

Staging

Stage is the most important determinant of prognosis in patients with lung cancer. The 7th Edition of the American Joint Committee on Cancer (AJCC) and the Union for International Cancer Control (UICC) system introduced in 2010 is in use until the end of 2017 [28]. The 8th Edition of the AJCC staging system has a number of changes to the 7th Edition and will be implemented on January 1, 2018 [29] (Table 1.2). The descriptors are based on analysis of nearly 95,000 cases from 16 countries around the world. Notable changes included introduction of new 'T' and 'M' descriptors to the TNM system. Individual 'T' descriptors were defined based on tumor size of: <1 cm (T1a), 1–2 cm (T1b), 2–3 cm (T1c), 3–4 cm (T2a), 4–5 cm (T2b), 5–7 cm (T3) and >7 cm (T4). Nodal staging has also been revised and new descriptors include: single station N1 (N1a), multiple station N1 (N1b), single station N2 without N1 (N2a1), single station N2 with N1 (N2a2), multiple station N2 (N2b), and N3. Patients with metastatic disease will be categorized based on the number and location of metastasis into: malignant pleural or pericardial effusion, separate tumor nodule in a contralateral lobe (M1a), single extrathoracic metastasis in a single organ (M1b) and multiple extrathoracic metastasis (M1c) (Figure 1.2) [30]. This staging system applies to both NSCLC and SCLC.

Table 1.2 American Joint Committee on Cancer (AJCC) TNM staging system for lung cancer.

Definition of primary tumor (T)

T category	T criteria
TX	Primary tumor cannot be assessed, or tumor proven by the presence of malignant cells in sputum or bronchial washings but not visualized by imaging or bronchoscopy
T0	No evidence of primary tumor
Tis	Carcinoma *in situ* Squamous cell carcinoma *in situ* (SCIS) Adenocarcinoma *in situ* (AIS): adenocarcinoma with pure lepidic pattern, ≤3 cm in greatest dimension
T1	Tumor ≤3 cm in greatest dimension, surrounded by lung or visceral pleura, without bronchoscopic evidence of invasion more proximal than the lobar bronchus (i.e., not in the main bronchus)
T1mi	Minimally invasive adenocarcinoma: adenocarcinoma (≤3 cm in greatest dimension) with a predominantly lepidic pattern and ≤5 mm invasion in greatest dimension
T1a	Tumor ≤1 cm in greatest dimension. A superficial, spreading tumor of any size whose invasive component is limited to the bronchial wall and may extend proximal to the main bronchus also is classified as T1a, but these tumors are uncommon
T1b	Tumor >1 cm but ≤2 cm in greatest dimension
T1c	Tumor >2 cm but ≤3 cm in greatest dimension
T2	Tumor >3 cm but ≤5 cm or having any of the following features: • Involves the main bronchus regardless of distance to the carina, but without involvement of the carina • Invades visceral pleura (PL1 or PL2) • Associated with atelectasis or obstructive pneumonitis that extends to the hilar region, involving part or all of the lung T2 tumors with these features are classified as T2a if ≤4 cm or if the size cannot be determined and T2b if >4 cm but ≤5 cm
T2a	Tumor >3 cm but ≤4 cm in greatest dimension
T2b	Tumor >4 cm but ≤5 cm in greatest dimension
T3	Tumor >5 cm but ≤7 cm in greatest dimension or directly invading any of the following: parietal pleura (PL3), chest wall (including superior sulcus tumors), phrenic nerve, parietal pericardium; or separate tumor nodule(s) in the same lobe as the primary
T4	Tumor >7 cm or tumor of any size invading one or more of the following: diaphragm, mediastinum, heart, great vessels, trachea, recurrent laryngeal nerve, esophagus, vertebral body, or carina; separate tumor nodule(s) in an ipsilateral lobe different from that of the primary

Definition of regional lymph node (N)

N category	N criteria
NX	Regional lymph nodes cannot be assessed
N0	No regional lymph node metastasis
N1	Metastasis in ipsilateral peribronchial and/or ipsilateral hilar lymph nodes and intrapulmonary nodes, including involvement by direct extension
N2	Metastasis in ipsilateral mediastinal and/or subcarinal lymph node(s)
N3	Metastasis in contralateral mediastinal, contralateral hilar, ipsilateral or contralateral scalene, or supraclavicular lymph node(s)

Definition of distant metastasis (M)

M category	M criteria
M0	No distant metastasis
M1	Distant metastasis
M1a	Separate tumor nodule(s) in a contralateral lobe; tumor with pleural or pericardial nodules or malignant pleural or pericardial effusion. Most pleural (pericardial) effusions with lung cancer are a result of the tumor. In a few patients, however, multiple microscopic examinations of pleural (pericardial) fluid are negative for tumor, and the fluid is nonbloody and not an exudate. If these elements and clinical judgment dictate that the effusion is not related to the tumor, the effusion should be excluded as a staging descriptor
M1b	Single extrathoracic metastasis in a single organ (including involvement of a single nonregional node)
M1c	Multiple extrathoracic metastases in a single organ or in multiple organs

(*Continued*)

Table 1.2 (Continued)

AJCC prognostic stage groups

When T is...	And N is...	And M is...	Then the stage group is...
TX	N0	M0	Occult carcinoma
Tis	N0	M0	0
T1mi	N0	M0	IA1
T1a	N0	M0	IA1
T1a	N1	M0	IIB
T1a	N2	M0	IIIA
T1a	N3	M0	IIIB
T1b	N0	M0	IA2
T1b	N1	M0	IIB
T1b	N2	M0	IIIA
T1b	N3	M0	IIIB
T1c	N0	M0	IA3
T1c	N1	M0	IIB
T1c	N2	M0	IIIA
T1c	N3	M0	IIIB
T2a	N0	M0	IB
T2a	N1	M0	IIB
T2a	N2	M0	IIIA
T2a	N3	M0	IIIB
T2b	N0	M0	IIA
T2b	N1	M0	IIB
T2b	N2	M0	IIIA
T2b	N3	M0	IIIB
T3	N0	M0	IIB
T3	N1	M0	IIIA
T3	N2	M0	IIIB
T3	N3	M0	IIIC
T4	N0	M0	IIIA
T4	N1	M0	IIIA
T4	N2	M0	IIIB
T4	N3	M0	IIIC
Any T	Any N	M1a	IVA
Any T	Any N	M1b	IVA
Any T	Any N	M1c	IVB

Source: Amin MB, Edge SB, Greene FL, *et al.* (eds) AJCC Cancer Staging Manual, 8th edn. New York: Springer Nature, 2017. Reproduced with permission of Springer.

Treatment

The outcomes for patients with lung cancer have improved significantly in recent years. This is a result of improvements in staging, better surgical and radiation therapy techniques, availability of newer and more effective systemic therapeutic agents, understanding of molecular characteristics and the ability to individualize therapy, and improved supportive care measures. Improvement in survival has been noted for every stage of lung cancer in the past two decades. A team approach for the management of lung cancer including thoracic surgeons, radiation oncologists, medical oncologists, interventional pulmonologists, pathologists, radiologists, and nursing support is critical to develop and deliver appropriate treatments. Surgery, radiation therapy, and systemic therapy are all used for lung cancer.

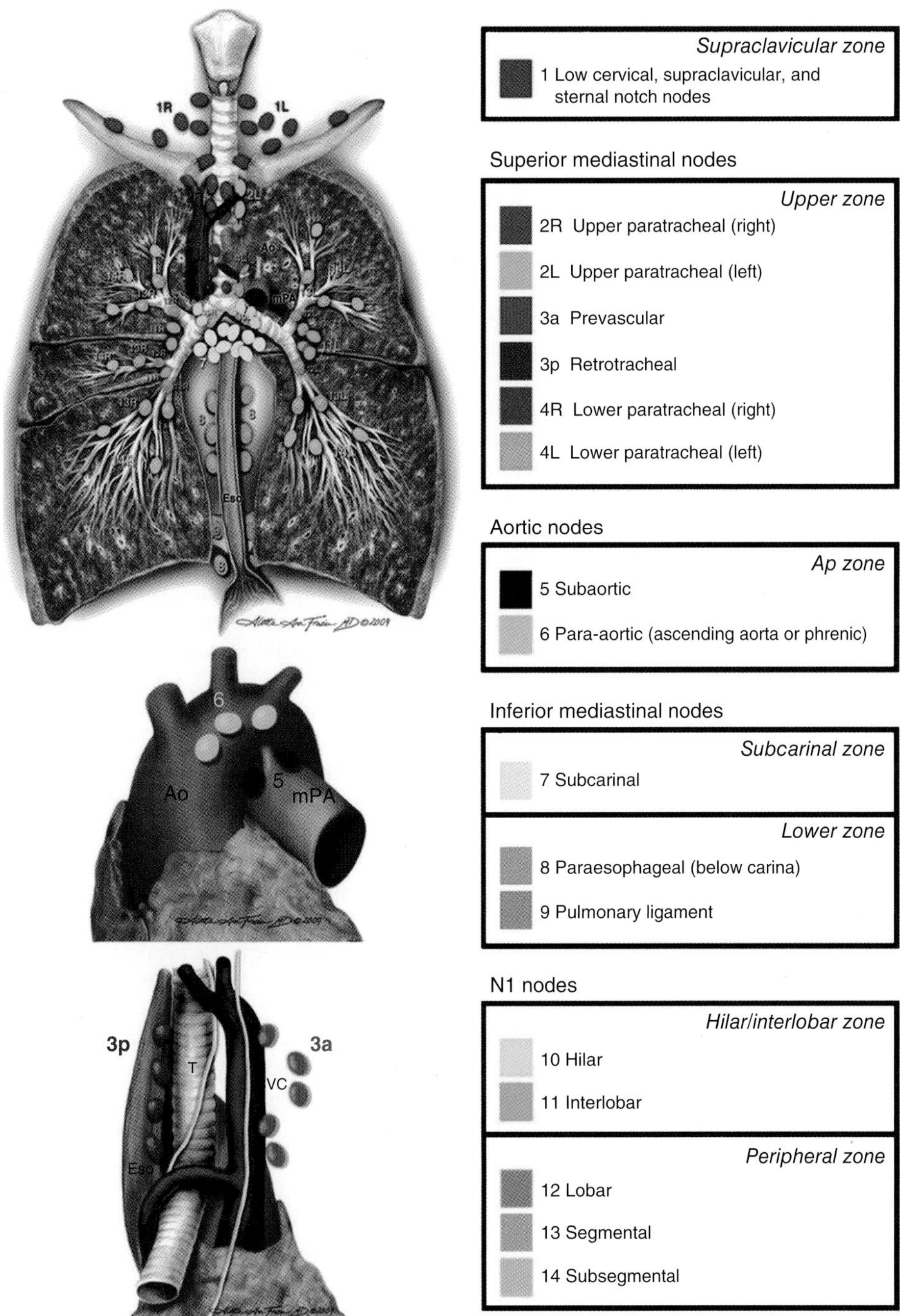

Figure 1.2 The International Association for the Study of Lung Cancer (IASLC) lymph node map, including the proposed grouping of lymph node stations into "zones" for the purposes of prognostic analyses. *Source:* Rusch *et al.* [30]. Reproduced with permission of Elsevier.

NSCLC

Surgery

Surgical management plays a major role in the treatment of early-stage lung cancer [31]. Patients with stages I, II, and selected stage III are considered potential candidates for surgical resection. Since most lung cancer patients suffer from smoking-related medical illness, nearly 40% of patients with early-stage lung cancer are not candidates for surgery due to limiting comorbid conditions. The commonly used parameters for inoperability include a baseline FEV_1 of <40%, a predicted postoperative FEV_1 of <30%, or a severely limited diffusion capacity. Such patients are referred to as 'medically inoperable' despite the presence of localized disease [32].

The first step in managing localized lung cancer is to stage the mediastinal lymph nodes. Cervical mediastinoscopy allows for staging of most relevant mediastinal lymph node stations with the exception of subaortic and para-aortic lymph nodes (levels 5 and 6). Cervical mediastinoscopy is associated with a mortality rate of <1%. Sampling of lymph nodes in levels 5 and 6 requires either a video-assisted thoracoscopy or anterior mediastinostomy. In recent years, endobronchial ultrasound-guided biopsy of mediastinal nodes has allowed for noninvasive staging, and to sample nodes in patients who have already undergone mediastinoscopy. With the advent of PET-CT scans, mediastinoscopy and endobronchial ultrasound are selectively utilized in the preoperative assessment based on the likelihood of nodal involvement. For peripheral tumors that are not associated with mediastinal adenopathy and do not have FDG uptake in the nodes, many surgeons advocate proceeding with surgical resection and sampling mediastinal nodes intraoperatively. However, for patients with nodes that are positive on the PET scan, sampling is strongly recommended before surgery. The false positivity rate for a PET scan in the mediastinum for patients with localized lung cancer is approximately 20%. The likelihood of nodal involvement in patients with a negative PET scan is approximately 5–15%.

Lobectomy is the standard surgical procedure of choice for patients with localized lung cancer. If anatomical resection cannot be achieved with lobectomy, either a bilobectomy or pneumonectomy might be necessary. Sleeve resection refers to removing the tumor along with the bronchus and anastomosing the remaining ends of the bronchial tree [33]. Surgical resection can be achieved by either performing a thoracotomy or by the video-assisted thoracic surgery approach. The latter is gaining wider use due to lower morbidity and a faster recovery from surgery. It also allows for better tolerance of postoperative systemic therapy. The ability to achieve an R0 resection is critical to surgical management of early-stage NSCLC. If this is not deemed feasible during preoperative workup, then surgery should not be attempted. For patients with positive surgical margins, a re-resection should be attempted whenever feasible. If not, postoperative radiotherapy should be administered.

Sublobar resections are not recommended due to the higher risk of local recurrence. An exception to this rule is for patients with peripheral tumors <2 cm in size, where studies have demonstrated excellent outcomes. An ongoing study is comparing sublobar resection to standard lobectomy and will likely provide definitive answers to this critical issue. Two important aspects of surgical management of lung cancers have been addressed in recent clinical trials. A randomized comparison of mediastinal lymph node dissection to nodal sampling demonstrated comparable outcomes for patients with NSCLC [34]. Another study compared sublobar resection followed by placement of I^{125} brachytherapy to the tumor bed to surgery alone in patients who are not candidates for standard lobectomy [35]. There was no difference in overall survival between the two groups and therefore, the brachytherapy approach is not recommended. Tumors involving the superior sulcus are managed with preoperative chemoradiotherapy. The decision to perform surgery for these tumors depends on extent of local invasion, involvement of the brachial plexus and mediastinal lymph node involvement.

The role of surgery in the management of stage III NSCLC with mediastinal nodal involvement continues to be controversial. Surgery alone is associated with poor outcome for stage III disease. In a randomized study, patients with N2-positive disease who underwent chemoradiotherapy followed by surgery did not have improved survival compared to chemoradiotherapy alone [36]. There was an especially high rate of postoperative mortality for patients who underwent pneumonectomy following chemoradiotherapy. Therefore, trimodality therapy is not recommended for patients who require a pneumonectomy. For patients with multistation N2 disease or bulky nodal disease, surgical resection is not recommended. It appears that clearance of the mediastinal node after induction therapy might be the most important predictor of benefit from surgical resection. This calls for restaging the mediastinum after induction therapy if surgery is contemplated.

The role of surgery in patients with oligometastatic disease can be considered under certain situations. Surgical resection of both the primary and a solitary brain metastasis has resulted in 5-year survival rates of approximately 20% [37]. However, this approach cannot be recommended for patients with mediastinal nodal involvement. Similar approaches to resect lung primary and solitary metastasis at other distant sites are not recommended for routine care.

Radiation Therapy

Radiotherapy is an important part of multimodality therapy for NSCLC. It is used in both the curative therapy setting for stage III disease and palliation of stage IV disease. In recent years, radiotherapy has been successfully tested for patients with medically unresectable stage I disease. There have been significant improvements in the delivery of radiotherapy over the past two decades. This allows for utilization of smaller radiation field size, thus reducing exposure of normal tissue to radiation and more effective treatment of tumor. Respiratory gating technique allows for the delivery of radiotherapy to the tumor regardless of the phase of respiration. Stereotactic body radiotherapy (SBRT) involves the delivery of high dose radiation to a limited tumor volume following stereotactic localization.

Stage I and II NSCLC

SBRT has emerged as an effective treatment option for patients with T1 and T2 node negative tumors that are not candidates for surgery due to medical comorbid illness. Delivery of SBRT over three to five fractions is associated with a nearly 90% local control rate [38]. SBRT is appropriate for peripheral tumors, whereas for centrally located tumors, studies are presently ongoing to determine the appropriate dose and the safety of this approach. The highly promising results with SBRT for localized NSCLC have prompted studies to compare SBRT to surgical resection even in medically fit patients. Studies are also underway to combine SBRT with systemic therapy for early-stage NSCLC.

Radiation therapy is indicated for patients with positive surgical margins following surgery for early-stage NSCLC. A dose of 60 Gy is administered for patients with microscopic margins, whereas for those with residual macroscopic disease doses of up to 66 Gy are administered in once daily fractions of 1.8–2 Gy each. For patients with negative surgical margins, there is no role for adjuvant radiotherapy. A meta-analysis published in 1998 reported a detrimental effect for patients treated with postoperative radiotherapy, especially for those with N0 and N1 disease [39]. Patients with N2 disease demonstrated a favorable survival trend with radiotherapy. This has also been observed in an analysis of the national Surveillance, Epidemiology and End Results database in the US [40]. Based on this, a prospective study is presently underway in Europe to compare postoperative radiation to observation in patients with surgically resected N2 disease. In this setting, radiotherapy is delivered to the bronchial stump, ipsilateral hilum, and involved mediastinal lymph node stations to a dose of approximately 50.4–54 Gy.

Stage III NSCLC

Radiation therapy is an essential component of multimodality therapy for management of stage III NSCLC. Surgery is appropriate for patients with T3N1 disease, but for patients with involvement of the mediastinal lymph nodes, administration of radiotherapy with chemotherapy results in improved outcomes. A subset of N2 positive patients might benefit from multimodality therapy that includes surgery. In such settings, radiation can be administered with chemotherapy as neoadjuvant therapy followed by surgical resection. Radiation therapy dose consists of 45 Gy of once daily fractions when given in the preoperative setting. More recently, a radiation dose of 60 Gy has been piloted with acceptable safety results. Potential candidates for the tri-modality therapy approach include stage IIIA patients who have single station or microscopic lymph node involvement and disease that is amenable to resection with lobectomy or bilobectomy.

For patients with stage III disease who are not appropriate for surgical resection, thoracic radiotherapy with concomitant chemotherapy is the recommended treatment. This category includes patients with bulky mediastinal disease, involvement of contralateral or supraclavicular nodes (N3) and direct invasion of major structures such as the vertebrae, trachea, major blood vessels, or esophagus by the primary tumor (T4). Radiotherapy is administered to a dose of 60–66 Gy in once daily fractions as part of definitive therapy for stage III disease. Five-year survival rates of approximately 20–25% have been reported with combined chemoradiotherapy in this setting [41]. The main adverse events associated with this approach include esophagitis and pneumonitis. The risk of pneumonitis depends on the extent of normal lung tissue and the dose of radiation received by the normal lung tissue in the radiation port. Radiation-related pneumonitis can occur in the acute setting immediately following the radiotherapy course or after 6–9 months.

Several efforts to improve upon standard chemoradiotherapy have been undertaken in the past two decades. Hyperfractionated radiotherapy with administration of two to three fractions/day has demonstrated favorable results over once-daily fractionation, particularly in squamous cell carcinoma [42, 43]. However, the logistical constraints associated with multiple daily fractions have limited the adoption of this approach. Another strategy studied in stage III disease involved utilization of higher doses of radiation of up to 74 Gy in once-daily fractions. A randomized study conducted by the RTOG comparing 74 Gy to 60 Gy demonstrated inferior survival with the higher dose [44]. Therefore, 60–66 Gy remains the standard radiation dose for stage III NSCLC.

Stage IV NSCLC

Radiotherapy is used for palliation of certain symptoms in patients with advanced-stage NSCLC. The main indications are for treatment of brain metastasis, relief of bronchial obstruction, hemoptysis and pain control. For brain metastasis, whole brain radiotherapy consists of 30–37.5 Gy given in 10–15 fractions. Stereotactic radiosurgery (SRS) is used instead of whole brain radiotherapy for patients with low volume brain metastasis that is limited to one to three lesions. SRS can also be given to lesions in the brain that progress following whole brain radiotherapy. The availability of SRS has greatly improved survival for patients with brain metastasis. Pain control in sites of bone metastasis or chest wall involvement can be achieved by a short course of radiotherapy. The dose and number of fractions is determined by the location and size of the lesion. Spinal cord compression is an emergency situation that is often managed with external beam radiotherapy. Surgical decompression is used in selected circumstances when neurological compromise is early and the patient has well-controlled systemic disease, and is followed by radiotherapy.

Systemic Therapy

Systemic therapy refers to the use of cytotoxic therapy, immunotherapy, or molecularly targeted agents. Systemic therapy was initially developed for patients with advanced-stage lung cancer. This has subsequently been extended to the treatment of earlier stages of lung cancer. The high propensity for metastasis of lung cancer cells provides the rationale for the use of systemic therapy even for patients with earlier stages of the disease who are treated with local therapies. A number of effective and well-tolerated cytotoxic agents have been developed over the past three decades that are utilized for routine care of patients with lung cancer (Table 1.3).

Advanced-Stage/Metastatic NSCLC

In patients with advanced-stage NSCLC, systemic chemotherapy improves both survival and quality of life. Platinum-based combination regimens were superior to supportive care alone in randomized trials and were associated with modest improvement in overall survival [45, 46]. Cisplatin was the first platinum compound developed in NSCLC. Subsequently carboplatin was studied as a better-tolerated alternative to cisplatin. The use of cisplatin is associated with adverse events such as nausea, emesis, nephrotoxicity, and neurotoxicity. The

Table 1.3 Commonly used chemotherapy agents for lung cancer.

Nonsmall cell lung cancer	Small cell lung cancer
Cisplatin	Cisplatin
Carboplatin	Carboplatin
Paclitaxel	Etoposide
Nab-Paclitaxel	Irinotecan
Docetaxel	Topotecan
Gemcitabine	
Pemetrexed (nonsquamous histology)	
Irinotecan	
Vinorelbine	

availability of highly effective antiemetic agents has greatly improved the tolerability of cisplatin. Carboplatin is associated with ease of administration in the outpatient setting. The dose-limiting toxicity of carboplatin is thrombocytopenia. Both compounds are efficacious in advanced NSCLC. In several randomized trials, the use of combination regimens was associated with a higher response rate and improved survival over cisplatin alone. Etoposide, vinblastine, vindesine, vinorelbine, taxanes, gemcitabine, irinotecan, and pemetrexed, have all been combined with cisplatin or carboplatin in the treatment of advanced NSCLC. The two-drug combination regimens have also been compared to monotherapy with a nonplatinum compound. For instance, a phase 3 study compared the combination of carboplatin and paclitaxel to paclitaxel alone for first-line therapy of advanced NSCLC [47]. The efficacy outcomes were all more favorable with the combination, though toxicity was also increased. This led to the adoption of combination chemotherapy as the recommended approach for the treatment of advanced NSCLC.

A meta-analysis of randomized trials to compare the efficacy of cisplatin to carboplatin in advanced-stage NSCLC demonstrated comparable survival [48]. When cisplatin was used in combination with a third-generation cytotoxic agent such as taxanes, gemcitabine, or vinorelbine, there was a statistically significant albeit modest improvement in survival. Cisplatin-based regimens were associated with a numerically higher incidence of treatment-related deaths. Taken together, though cisplatin-based regimens have a slight advantage in efficacy over carboplatin-based regimens in advanced NSCLC, the latter is associated with a favorable tolerability profile. With palliation being the goal of therapy in advanced NSCLC, carboplatin-based regimens have found wider adoption due to their favorable therapeutic index.

Several partner agents for platinum have demonstrated efficacy in advanced NSCLC. Paclitaxel, docetaxel, gemcitabine, irinotecan, pemetrexed, and vinorelbine have all demonstrated single-agent activity in advanced NSCLC with single-agent response rates of approximately 10–20%. Each of these agents can be given in combination with platinum with acceptable tolerability profile. In randomized trials, the efficacy across platinum-based combination regimens was similar. The ECOG 1594 trial randomized 1,206 advanced NSCLC patients to treatment with cisplatin–paclitaxel, cisplatin–docetaxel, cisplatin–gemcitabine or carboplatin–paclitaxel [49]. The median survival was comparable for all four regimens, and the differences were primarily in toxicity. The median survival was approximately 8 months and the median progression-free survival was 3.5–4.2 months for all four regimens. The 1-year survival rate was approximately 40%. The main toxicities associated with the paclitaxel–carboplatin regimen were neuropathy and myelosuppression. Thrombocytopenia was common with the cisplatin–gemcitabine regimen, while the cisplatin–docetaxel regimen was associated with myelosuppression. Based on E1594 and other contemporary studies, the choice of any one of these chemotherapy agents for front-line treatment is made upon consideration of toxicity, patient preference, schedule, and cost. Combinations of three cytotoxic agents are not recommended due to a higher toxicity burden and lack of incremental benefit.

Role of Histology in Choice of Chemotherapy

Until recently, chemotherapy regimens were considered to be suitable for all histological subtypes of NSCLC. This notion was dispelled in a phase 3 study of cisplatin–pemetrexed versus cisplatin–gemcitabine that was compared in patients with advanced-stage NSCLC [50]. The pemetrexed-based regimen was noninferior to the comparator for the overall patient population, but was associated with a superior survival for patients with nonsquamous histology. In patients with squamous histology, the gemcitabine-based regimen was superior. Consequently, the use of pemetrexed should be restricted to patients with nonsquamous histology only. The relative efficacy of taxanes versus pemetrexed in nonsquamous histology has not been compared directly. In a recent randomized study, patients were given either carboplatin and pemetrexed or carboplatin and paclitaxel. Patients on both treatment groups received bevacizumab, a monoclonal antibody against the vascular endothelial growth factor (VEGF) in addition to chemotherapy. There was no difference in overall survival between the two treatment groups [51]. Based on these observations, taxane-based and pemetrexed-based regimens are both appropriate for the treatment of patients with nonsquamous histology.

The US Food and Drug Administration (FDA) recently approved nanoparticle albumin-bound paclitaxel (nab-paclitaxel) for the treatment of advanced NSCLC. In contrast to the standard formulation, use of nab-paclitaxel does not require premedication and is not associated with hypersensitivity reactions. The incidence of neuropathy is also lower with the use of nab-paclitaxel. In a direct comparison to carboplatin and paclitaxel, the carboplatin-nab-paclitaxel regimen was associated with a favorable response rate, when given to patients with advanced NSCLC, though survival was not improved [52]. The improvement in response rate appeared to be restricted to squamous histology. The variable efficacy of pemetrexed and nab-paclitaxel based on histology should be considered when chemotherapy is selected for first-line treatment of advanced NSCLC.

Maintenance Therapy

The duration of chemotherapy for advanced-stage NSCLC has been debated and studied closely. Four to six cycles of combination therapy are considered optimal in the first-line setting. Continuation of combination treatment beyond this duration is associated with cumulative toxicities, but no tangible therapeutic benefit. More recently, a strategy of single-agent maintenance therapy has been successfully developed. In one approach referred to as 'switch maintenance', patients who derive clinical benefit with a platinum-based combination for four cycles are treated with an alternative cytotoxic or targeted agent that has not been previous administered. The 'continuation maintenance' strategy involves continuing the nonplatinum agent beyond the four cycles for patients who experience either an objective response or stable disease with combination therapy. Pemetrexed is the only cytotoxic agent that has demonstrated survival advantage as maintenance therapy in advanced NSCLC [53]. It has been tested both as continuation and switch maintenance therapies in advanced nonsquamous histology. The improvement in survival was of similar magnitude in randomized trials. Based on these observations, pemetrexed has been approved for maintenance therapy in the US and Europe. Erlotinib, an EGFR inhibitor, also extends survival when used as maintenance therapy in patients who received a platinum-based combination for four cycles [54]. The benefit was notable only for patients who experienced stable disease with combination chemotherapy. EGFR genotypic status was a significant determinant of efficacy of erlotinib, with a robust magnitude of progression-free survival benefit for patients with an activation mutation.

Pemetrexed and erlotinib are also efficacious when used as salvage therapy for patients with advanced NSCLC that experience disease progression during or after platinum-based chemotherapy. Therefore, the relative merits of using these agents as maintenance therapy versus after disease progression has been controversial. The benefits of maintenance therapy are counterbalanced by the toxicity, logistical, and cost factors. A 'wait and watch' approach after first-line therapy appears reasonable, though approximately 40% of the patients might never receive salvage therapy due to rapid disease progression or decline in performance status. For these reasons, careful discussion with the patients regarding the merits of maintenance therapy versus close observation is recommended.

Salvage Therapy

Nearly all patients with advanced NSCLC will experience disease progression regardless of the extent of benefit with first-line chemotherapy. Salvage therapy for such patients provides modest improvement in survival. Docetaxel, given at a dose of 75 mg/m^2 every 3 weeks, was the first proven agent in this setting. In randomized studies, docetaxel monotherapy was associated with improvements in survival when compared to best supportive care, and improved 1-year survival rate over first-generation cytotoxic agents [55]. Disease stabilization is observed in approximately 40% of patients, but objective response occurs in <10% with docetaxel in the salvage therapy setting. Pemetrexed is an alternative cytotoxic agent with proven efficacy as salvage therapy, but its use is restricted to patients with nonsquamous histology. In a randomized study, the overall survival associated with pemetrexed was noninferior to that with docetaxel [56]. However, the toxicity profile was better with pemetrexed as evidenced by lower incidence of fever with neutropenia and hospitalizations. EGFR inhibition with erlotinib, which was originally approved for salvage therapy of advanced NSCLC, is now only recommended for patients with EGFR sensitizing mutations [57].

The salvage therapy setting for advanced NSCLC has been substantially changed in the past year following the approval of three immune-check point inhibitors nivolumab, pembrolizumab, and atezolizumab. Nivolumab and pembrolizumab target the programmed death (PD-1) receptor, whereas atezolizumab targets PDL-1, a ligand for PD-1. Each one of these agents demonstrated superiority over docetaxel in improving survival when used as second-line therapy [58–61]. They were also associated with a favorable toxicity profile relative to chemotherapy. The salient efficacy data for these three agents are summarized in Table 1.4.

Targeted Therapy (Table 1.5)

Anti-Angiogenic Therapy

Approaches to inhibit angiogenesis as a therapeutic strategy have been extensively pursued in patients with advanced NSCLC. VEGF is a critical determinant of neoangiogenesis in the physiologic milieu and in cancer. Bevacizumab is a monoclonal antibody that binds and inhibits all active isoforms of VEGF. Building on strong preclinical observations, bevacizumab was studied in combination with standard chemotherapy for first-line therapy of advanced NSCLC [62]. The initial results were promising, though squamous histology was associated with a higher incidence of life-threatening hemoptysis. Further development of this agent was subsequently limited to nonsquamous histology. The ECOG 4599 study compared bevacizumab in combination with carboplatin and paclitaxel versus chemotherapy alone [63]. There was a significant improvement

Table 1.4 Immune checkpoint inhibitors as salvage therapy.

Agent	Response rate (%)	Median progression-free survival (months)	Median survival (months)
Nivolumab	20	3.5	9.2
vs			
Docetaxel (squamous histology)	9	2.8 (HR 0.62, P <0.001)	6.0 (HR 0.59, P <0.001)
Nivolumab	19	2.3	12. 2
vs			
Docetaxel (nonsquamous histology)	12	4.2 (HR 0.92, P = 0.39)	9.4 (HR 0.73, P = 0.002)
Pembrolizumab (2 mg/kg)[1]	18	3.9	12.7
vs			
Docetaxel	18	4.0 (HR 0.88, P = 0.07)	10.4 (HR 0.71, P = 0.0008)
Atezolizumab	14	2.8	13.8
vs			
Docetaxel	13	4.0 (HR 0.95, P = 0.49)	9.6 (HR 0.73, P = 0.0003)

[1] Study enrolled patients with PDL-1 expression >1%.

Table 1.5 Molecularly targeted agents with proven efficacy in lung cancer.

Epidermal growth factor receptor
Reversible inhibitors:
Erlotinib
Gefitinib
Irreversible inhibitors:
Afatinib
Osimertinib
Monoclonal antibody:
Cetuximab
Necitumumab
Anaplastic lymphoma kinase
Crizotinib
Ceritinib
Alectinib
Anti-angiogenic therapy
Bevacizumab
Ramucirumab

in overall survival (12.3 months vs 10.3 months) and progression-free survival (6.3 months vs 4.8 months) with the addition of bevacizumab. The notable adverse events included bleeding, hypertension, and proteinuria along with a higher risk of neutropenia. Another randomized study conducted in Europe failed to document a survival improvement with the addition of bevacizumab to cisplatin and gemcitabine, despite a modest improvement in progression-free survival [64]. In older individuals (age >70 years) bevacizumab appears to have a narrow therapeutic index due to higher risk of myelosuppression and bleeding [65]. All pivotal randomized trials performed with bevacizumab utilized it as maintenance therapy following six cycles of combination therapy. Therefore, the use of maintenance therapy with bevacizumab has been adopted in clinical practice for patients who receive it as part of the initial treatment regimen. The therapeutic value of maintenance bevacizumab has not been directly studied to date.

Ramucirumab, a monoclonal antibody against the VEGF receptor (R2), has proven efficacious as second-line therapy in combination with docetaxel [66]. A phase 3 study demonstrated modest gains in survival (10.5 months vs 9.5 months, HR 0.86) and progression-free survival (4.5 months vs 3.0 months, HR 0.76) for the combination compared to docetaxel alone. A small subset of patients in this study had received prior bevacizumab and appeared to derive benefit from a ramucirumab-based combination. The combination of docetaxel with ramucirumab has received approval from the US FDA for salvage therapy of advanced NSCLC. Other strategies to inhibit angiogenesis including small molecule inhibitors of VEGF tyrosine kinase and vascular disrupting agents have not been successful to date in advanced NSCLC. Efforts to identify biomarkers to predict benefit with bevacizumab and other antiangiogenic agents have been unsuccessful and have unquestionably restricted optimal utilization of these agents.

EGFR inhibition

Inhibition of EGFR is the first successful molecular treatment strategy in lung cancer. This has in no small measure contributed to the expanding role of targeted approaches and molecular classification of lung cancer. Initially, agents that target EGFR were evaluated based on preclinical observations of higher expression of the target protein in aggressive tumors. Objective response rates of 10–20% were noted with gefitinib and erlotinib, small molecule TKIs of EGFR. Subsequent studies demonstrated that patients with robust responses harbored an activation mutation in exons 19 or 21 of the EGFR [20, 21, 67, 68]. The mutations result in constitutive activation of the receptor and therefore the tumors are exquisitely sensitive to EGFR inhibition. EGFR activating mutations are exclusive to adenocarcinoma histology and occur at a higher frequency in women, never-smokers and patients with Asian ethnicity. In randomized studies of patients with an activating mutation, EGFR inhibition with either gefitinib or erlotinib was associated with an improvement in progression-free survival over platinum-based chemotherapy [69–71]. This has not translated into survival benefit, most likely due to most patients treated with chemotherapy subsequently receiving an EGFR inhibitor upon disease progression. Quality of life is also more favorable with EGFR inhibitors over chemotherapy in this setting. The importance of molecular testing before initiation of EGFR inhibitor therapy in first-line treatment is highlighted by the inferior outcomes in wild-type patients treated with targeted therapy. Afatinib, an irreversible EGFR TKI, has also demonstrated superiority over chemotherapy in patients with an activating mutation [72]. This agent is associated with a higher incidence of diarrhea relative to gefitinib and erlotinib. Another irreversible inhibitor, dacomitinib, is being compared to gefitinib in an ongoing phase 3 clinical trial.

The median progression-free survival with EGFR TKI in this setting is approximately 8–12 months. Mechanisms leading to resistance are increasingly being understood. A secondary mutation in exon 20 (T790) is responsible for resistance to EGFR TKI in nearly 60% of patients [22, 73]. Activation of alternate pathways such as MET signaling also contributes to resistance to EGFR inhibition.

Osimertinib, a third generation EGFR TKI, inhibits exon 19, 21, and T790M signaling. In early-phase clinical trials, osimertinib demonstrated a high response rate (65%) and median progression-free survival of 9–13 months for patients who developed acquired resistance through the T790M mechanism [74]. This agent has recently received accelerated approval from the US FDA and has emerged as the preferred agent for this patient subset. Osimertinib is under evaluation for front-line treatment of patients with EGFR mutations. The use of EGFR inhibitors in patients with earlier stages of the disease is not known, even for those with an activating mutation. Ongoing studies are evaluating the role of EGFR inhibition in patients with surgically resected NSCLC and those with locally advanced disease.

The use of combination chemotherapy with EGFR TKI cannot be recommended based on present experience. Cetuximab, a monoclonal antibody against EGFR, was associated with a modest improvement in overall survival when given in combination with cisplatin and vinorelbine for first-line treatment of advanced NSCLC [75]. Necitumumab, another monoclonal antibody against the EGFR, was recently approved for the treatment of patients with advanced-stage squamous cell lung cancer. A randomized study that compared the combination of cisplatin and gemcitabine given with or without necitumumab demonstrated modest improvements in survival and progression-free survival for the addition of the EGFR antibody [76]. The median overall survival with and without necitumumab were 11.5 months and 9.9 months respectively (HR 0.84, $P = 0.01$).

ALK Inhibitors

The oncogenic potential of gene rearrangement involving the anaplastic lymphoma kinase in lung cancer was described in 2007 [77]. The fusion gene results from inversion or translocation of portions of the echinoderm microtubule-associated protein-like 4 gene (*EML4*) with the *ALK* gene. Other fusion partners besides *EML4* have also been described for *ALK*. The *ALK* gene rearrangement is present in approximately 5–7% of patients with lung adenocarcinoma [78]. Clinical features associated with the *ALK* gene rearrangement include never-smokers, adenocarcinoma histology, signet ring features on histopathological evaluation, and younger age. Limited available data indicate that patients with *ALK* translocation respond poorly to conventional treatment options and might also be at higher risk of recurrent disease after surgical resection for early-stage NSCLC [79]. Crizotinib, an inhibitor of MET, ALK, and ROS1 tyrosine kinases has demonstrated a response rate of nearly 60% and a clinical benefit rate of 90% in ALK-positive NSCLC [23, 80, 81]. The median progression-free survival was 10 months in a phase 2 study for patients with ALK-positive advanced-stage NSCLC [82]. Based on these exciting data, the US FDA and the European Medicines Agency have both approved crizotinib for the treatment of patients with advanced-stage ALK-positive NSCLC. Crizotinib was compared to platinum-based chemotherapy in a phase 3 study which demonstrated higher response rate and median progression-free survival with crizotinib [83]. When compared to chemotherapy in the salvage therapy setting, critozinib was associated with a significant improvement in progression-free survival (7.7 months vs 3 months) and response rate (66% vs 20%) [81]. Interestingly, pemetrexed was associated with a favorable outcome compared to docetaxel in this patient population. Mechanisms of resistance to crizotinib include activation of either ALK-dependent or independent alternate pathways. A variety of secondary mutations have been described in patients who develop disease progression while on therapy with crizotinib. Ceritinib, a potent ALK inhibitor, has demonstrated a response rate of 60% in patients who developed disease progression during crizotinib therapy [84]. Alectinib, another second generation ALK inhibitor, is also effective for patients who progressed on crizotinib [85]. Both of these agents are also effective against brain metastasis. Other novel ALK inhibitors are also under development for management of crizotinib resistance or as primary therapy. The use of ALK inhibitors in the management of earlier stages of NSCLC is under investigation.

Other Targeted Subpopulations

The availability of advanced genomic technology has made it possible to identify new molecular 'drivers' in lung cancer. In lung adenocarcinoma, a fusion gene involving *ROS1*, observed in 1% of patients, also confers sensitivity to treatment with crizotinib [86, 87] Another fusion involving the *RET* gene has been identified in approximately 0.5–1% of patients [88–91]. Patients with mutations in *BRAF* appear to respond to therapy with dabrafenib, a BRAF inhibitor or the combination of dabrafenib and trametinib [92, 93]. These observations provide hope that the mutation status of patients can aid personalized treatment of patients with lung cancer. The Cancer Genome Atlas Project recently published results of gene sequencing studies in a cohort of patients with squamous cell lung carcinoma [25]. A number of potentially targetable mutations and other genetic abnormalities have been identified. Routine testing of patient tumor specimens for molecular targets is increasingly seen as a strategy to optimize treatment options for lung cancer.

Immune Checkpoint Inhibition

Recent progress in targeting the immune pathways that regulate cancer has resulted in major therapeutic gains for a number of malignancies, including lung cancer. Activation of the PD-1 pathway results in T-cell exhaustion, thereby blunting the ability of the host immune system to eliminate the cancer cell. Agents that target the PD-1 pathway have now demonstrated anticancer effects in lung cancer, both as salvage therapy and first-line therapy for a subset of patients. Nivolumab and pembrolizumab, monoclonal antibodies that target PD-1, demonstrated superiority over docetaxel for salvage therapy of advanced NSCLC (Table 1.4) [58, 59, 61]. Both agents improved overall survival and were associated with lower incidence of grades 3/4 toxicity relative to docetaxel. Atezolizumab, a monoclonal antibody against PDL-1, also demonstrated similar benefits against docetaxel. These agents have supplanted docetaxel and have become the preferred second-line therapy for advanced NSCLC.

A recent study in the front-line setting for advanced NSCLC demonstrated superior survival and progression-free survival with pembrolizumab over platinum-based chemotherapy for a subset of patients with advanced NSCLC [94]. Patients with tumor PDL-1 expression >50% were chosen for this study, which represents approximately 25–30% of advanced NSCLC. The median progression-free survival was 10.3 months with pembrolizumab compared to 6 months with chemotherapy (HR 0.50, $P < 0.001$). The overall survival hazard ratio was 0.60 favoring pembrolizumab. This has now led to the FDA approval of pembrolizumab for first-line therapy of advanced NSCLC for patients with tumors that have PDL1 expression >50%. This new paradigm shift in first-line therapy of NSCLC provides hope that the use of immune checkpoint inhibitors can be extended to other settings such as earlier stages of the disease to improve cure rates. Biomarkers to select patients for therapy are being studied. In addition, combination strategies to improve the efficacy of immune checkpoint inhibitors are also under development.

Management of Special Patient Populations

Elderly patients represent a growing subset of lung cancer patients. In the US, the median age at diagnosis of lung cancer is 70 years [95]. Aging is associated with decline in physiological and vital organ function that impact tolerance of systemic therapy. In addition, it is particularly more important to consider the implications of therapy on physical function and quality of life of older patients. A number of elderly-specific studies have been conducted in NSCLC patients. Initially, single-agent chemotherapy was compared to supportive care and demonstrated improved survival [96]. In subsequent studies, for elderly patients with a good performance status, platinum-based combinations were superior to single-agent therapy [47, 97]. The use of three-drug combinations of cytotoxic agents is not recommended for older patients. However, the appropriate use of targeted agents in older patients might be associated with clinical benefit.

A high percentage of NSCLC patients present with significant symptoms that are associated with a poor performance status. The median survival for advanced NSCLC patients with a performance status of 2 (ECOG scale) is dismal at less than 4 months. Poor performance status limits the ability of patients to tolerate combination chemotherapy. Studies conducted exclusively in patients with a poor performance status indicate a favorable role for chemotherapy. In at least one randomized study, platinum-based combination therapy was superior to single-agent therapy [98]. It is important to consider the underlying cause of poor performance status in making treatment plans for this patient population. For those with limiting comorbid conditions, a less aggressive approach with single-agent chemotherapy might be more appropriate. For those with targetable mutations, appropriate targeted therapy can be given regardless of the performance status given the greater potential for benefit.

Systemic Therapy in Early-Stage NSCLC

Despite optimal surgery, recurrence of disease continues to be common for early-stage NSCLC. This is attributed to the presence of micrometastasis in early-stage NSCLC. The use of systemic therapy following surgery was recently proven to be associated with an improvement in 5-year survival rate [99]. In randomized trials, cisplatin-based two-drug combination regimens were compared to observation following surgery for early-stage NSCLC [100–102]. For patients with stage II and IIIA NSCLC, there was an absolute improvement of survival of 5–15% at 5 years. This corresponds to a relative risk reduction of approximately 30% with adjuvant chemotherapy. The consistent survival benefit observed across multiple trials has resulted in the adoption of four cycles of cisplatin-based adjuvant therapy as the standard of care for early-stage NSCLC. In stage IA disease, however, potential benefits of chemotherapy are outweighed by the risks, and there is an overall detrimental effect. For patients with stage IB disease, post-hoc analysis from two randomized trials revealed that survival improvement with adjuvant therapy was restricted to patients with tumor size >4 cm [102, 103]. This observation is yet to be validated in prospective trials. The cisplatin–vinorelbine combination has been the regimen commonly utilized in clinical trials of adjuvant therapy. The availability of better tolerated newer agents that are effective in the treatment of advanced NSCLC such as taxanes, gemcitabine, and pemetrexed, have prompted physicians to use these agents with cisplatin in early-stage NSCLC. Presently there are no effective tools to predict the risk of recurrent disease beyond pathological stage. It is hoped that the use of adjuvant chemotherapy could be tailored to patients at high risk of recurrence, based on genomic or proteomic markers.

Locally Advanced NSCLC

Chemotherapy has a proven role in combination with radiotherapy in the management of stage III disease that is not amenable to surgical resection. Initially, chemotherapy was used sequentially with radiotherapy and resulted in an improved overall survival over radiotherapy alone. Both local and systemic control was improved with the combined modality approach. Subsequent studies demonstrated a modest superiority for concomitant administration of chemotherapy over sequential therapy [41, 104]. Both cisplatin and carboplatin-based regimens have been utilized for combined modality therapy and are associated with modest survival results. The relative merits of cisplatin versus carboplatin in this setting have not been studied. The regimen of cisplatin and etoposide allows for administration of full systemic dose of chemotherapy with radiotherapy. The widely used regimen of carboplatin and paclitaxel involves administration of lower 'radiosensitizing' doses of the two agents with radiotherapy followed by consolidation therapy with two cycles at regular doses. The latter approach has a favorable tolerability profile compared to cisplatin-based regimens. Esophagitis and pneumonitis are the most notable toxicities with the combined modality treatment of locally advanced NSCLC. The use of induction or consolidation chemotherapy in other settings has not resulted in improved survival. With modern combined chemoradiotherapy, cure rates of nearly 20–25% are achieved in locally advanced NSCLC.

SCLC

SCLC is characterized by initial sensitivity to systemic chemotherapy, though recurrence of disease is common regardless of the extent of initial response. Approximately two-thirds of the patients present with extensive-stage SCLC, defined as the presence of metastatic disease outside the chest or large volume thoracic disease that cannot be treated with radiotherapy. The overall goal of treatment of extensive-stage disease is palliation. The median survival of untreated extensive-stage SCLC is less than 2 months. The use of platinum-based chemotherapy results in a response rate of approximately 50–70% and a median survival of 9–11 months. Improvement in symptoms and functional status are commonly observed within a few days of initiation of systemic chemotherapy in SCLC. The regimen of cisplatin and etoposide is considered the standard approach for the treatment of SCLC. Carboplatin is considered an acceptable alternative in the treatment of extensive-stage disease. Four cycles of chemotherapy are considered optimal, though it can be extended for up to six cycles in responding patients. There is no proven role for maintenance therapy after combination chemotherapy. Despite the extent of initial response, disease recurrence develops in a median of 4–5 months. Disease that progresses either during or within 90 days of administration of cisplatin-based chemotherapy is referred to as "refractory" relapse. Disease recurrence outside this window of time represents a "sensitive" subgroup of patients who might benefit from subsequent salvage treatment options. The use of other approaches such as high-dose chemotherapy, alternating chemotherapy regimens, dose-dense therapy and three-drug combination regimens are not associated with improvement in survival [105]. In the Japanese patient population, the regimen of cisplatin and irinotecan has demonstrated superior results over cisplatin and etoposide. However, cisplatin–irinotecan was not superior to standard therapy in Western patients.

Salvage therapy has yielded modest results in relapsed SCLC, but the benefit is restricted to "sensitive" relapse. Topotecan is the only agent to demonstrate clinical benefit in relapsed SCLC. In a randomized study, topotecan was associated with favorable symptomatic parameters, but overall survival was not improved [106]. The response rate for topotecan in this setting is approximately 20%. Several novel agents are presently being studied in efforts to improve the outcomes for SCLC. Molecularly targeted agents against known targets appear rational and provide hope for improved outcomes.

Radiotherapy is utilized in patients with limited-stage SCLC. Cure can be achieved for approximately 30% of patients with limited-stage SCLC with combined modality therapy. Earlier initiation of radiotherapy appears to be superior to the delayed approach and has been adopted as the standard approach in fit patients. A randomized study demonstrated superior survival when 45 Gy of thoracic radiotherapy was given at twice daily fractions (BID) compared to the same dose given at one fraction per day along with cisplatin and etoposide chemotherapy [107]. An ongoing study will evaluate whether the 45 Gy of BID radiation is superior to 70 Gy of radiotherapy given once daily with concomitant chemotherapy for limited-stage SCLC.

Prophylactic cranial irradiation (PCI) is associated with a modest improvement in 5-year survival rate for patients with limited-stage SCLC that achieve a complete remission following combined modality therapy [108, 109]. This is due to the high risk of brain recurrence that is noted in patients with SCLC. Recent studies have demonstrated benefit with PCI even in patients with extensive-stage disease [110]. For patients who achieve a favorable response to combination chemotherapy, the use of PCI results in modest improvement in overall survival and reduced risk of recurrence in the brain. Based on this, PCI can be considered for appropriate patients with extensive-stage SCLC.

The role of surgery is limited to those with peripheral lung lesions without mediastinal nodal involvement. It is estimated that fewer than 5% of patients with SCLC are candidates for surgical resection. In 10–15% of patients with SCLC, a mixed histology with NSCLC features are observed. These patients might present with local progression following combined modality therapy resulting from the NSCLC component. These patients may be considered for surgical resection in selected situations.

Treatment advances in SCLC have lagged behind those for NSCLC in the past two decades. Consequently, the survival outcomes for SCLC have not changed considerably during this time. A concerted effort to develop appropriate preclinical models to test new agents, genomic subcategorization of SCLC, and discovery of new systemic anticancer agents are necessary to improve outcomes for this aggressive disease.

Follow-Up and Survivorship

Survivorship has emerged as an important area of research as outcomes for lung cancer have improved in recent years. Increasing numbers of survivors following surgery or chemoradiotherapy provide the impetus to investigate important topics such as optimal surveillance, follow-up for second primary disease, managing long-term consequences of chemoradiotherapy, etc. The importance of smoking cessation cannot be overemphasized given the high risk of second primary tumors in lung cancer survivors. Patients should be provided with appropriate opportunities to receive counseling, smoking cessation, and behavioral therapy.

There is presently no standard approach for optimal radiographic and clinical follow-up in patients who undergo surgical resection or chemoradiotherapy. CT scans are commonly used for follow-up of these patients. However, the relative merits of CT scan versus chest radiograph, frequency of evaluation, and the role of FDG-PET scans are all important questions that should be answered in prospective clinical trials. For patients with advanced-stage disease, CT scans are used to assess response to therapy and are often performed every two to three cycles of treatment. Given the proven role for salvage therapy, patients who are in follow-up after combination chemotherapy should be closely followed for development of new symptoms or clinical deterioration in addition to periodic radiographic studies.

Respiratory therapy should be offered to patients with dyspnea following surgery or chemoradiotherapy. Since a high proportion of these patients also have smoking-related pulmonary diseases, referral to a pulmonologist should be considered in symptomatic patients. Overall, a team approach that includes supportive care personnel, oncologists, and appropriate additional specialists, should be utilized to ensure the return of lung cancer survivors to normalcy to the fullest extent possible.

Acknowledgements

The authors would like to acknowledge Anthea Hammond, PhD, of Emory University, for providing editorial assistance.

References

1 Torre LA, Bray F, Siegel RL, *et al.* Global cancer statistics, 2012. *CA Cancer J Clin* 2015;65:87–108.

2 Kamangar F, Dores GM, Anderson WF. Patterns of cancer incidence, mortality, and prevalence across five continents: defining priorities to reduce cancer disparities in different geographic regions of the world. *J Clin Oncol* 2006;24:2137–50.

3 Siegel RL, Miller KD, Jemal A. *Cancer statistics*, 2017. CA Cancer J Clin, in press

4 International Agency for Research on Cancer GLOBOCAN 2008 cancer fact sheet: lung cancer incidence and mortality worldwide. Available from URL: http://globocan.iarc.fr (accessed December 2013).

5 Wang YC, Wei LJ, Liu JT, Li SX, Wang QS. Comparison of cancer incidence between china and the USA. *Cancer Biol Med* 2012;9:128–32.

6 Govindan R, Ding L, Griffith M, *et al.* Genomic landscape of non-small cell lung cancer in smokers and never-smokers. *Cell* 2012;150:1121–34.

7 Stayner L, Welch LS, Lemen R. The worldwide pandemic of asbestos-related diseases. *Annu Rev Public Health* 2013;34:205–16.

8 Doll R. Mortality from lung cancer in asbestos workers. *Br J Ind Med* 1955;12:81–6.

9 Balmes JR. Asbestos and lung cancer: what we know. *Am J Respir Crit Care Med* 2013;188:8–9.

10 Lantz PM, Mendez D, Philbert MA. Radon, smoking, and lung cancer: the need to refocus radon control policy. *Am J Public Health* 2013;103:443–7.

11 Pawel DJ, Puskin JS. The U.S. Environmental Protection Agency's assessment of risks from indoor radon. *Health Phys* 2004;87:68–74.

12 Travis WD, Brambilla E, Noguchi M, *et al.* International association for the study of lung cancer/american thoracic society/european respiratory society international multidisciplinary classification of lung adenocarcinoma. *J Thorac Oncol* 2011;6:244–85.

13 Kummar S, Fogarasi M, Canova A, Mota A, Ciesielski T. Cytokeratin 7 and 20 staining for the diagnosis of lung and colorectal adenocarcinoma. *Br J Cancer* 2002;86:1884–7.

14 Sterlacci W, Savic S, Schmid T, *et al.* Tissue-sparing application of the newly proposed IASLC/ATS/ERS classification of adenocarcinoma of the lung shows practical diagnostic and prognostic impact. *Am J Clin Pathol* 2012;137:946–56.

15 Travis WD. Advances in neuroendocrine lung tumors. *Ann Oncol* 2010;21(Suppl 7):vii65–71.

16 Paci M, Cavazza A, Annessi V, *et al.* Large cell neuroendocrine carcinoma of the lung: a 10-year clinicopathologic retrospective study. *Ann Thorac Surg* 2004;77:1163–7.

17 Nicholson SA, Beasley MB, Brambilla E, *et al.* Small cell lung carcinoma (SCLC): a clinicopathologic study of 100 cases with surgical specimens. *Am J Surg Pathol* 2002;26:1184–97.

18 Pao W, Hutchinson KE. Chipping away at the lung cancer genome. *Nat Med* 2012;18:349–51.

19 Riely GJ, Marks J, Pao W. KRAS mutations in non-small cell lung cancer. *Proc Am Thorac Soc* 2009;6:201–5.

20 Lynch TJ, Bell DW, Sordella R, *et al.* Activating mutations in the epidermal growth factor receptor underlying responsiveness of non-small-cell lung cancer to gefitinib. *N Engl J Med* 2004;350:2129–39.

21 Paez JG, Janne PA, Lee JC, *et al.* EGFR mutations in lung cancer: correlation with clinical response to gefitinib therapy. *Science* 2004;304:1497–500.

22 Kobayashi S, Boggon TJ, Dayaram T, *et al.* EGFR mutation and resistance of non-small-cell lung cancer to gefitinib. *N Engl J Med* 2005;352:786–92.

23 Kwak EL, Bang YJ, Camidge DR, *et al.* Anaplastic lymphoma kinase inhibition in non-small-cell lung cancer. *N Engl J Med* 2010;363:1693–703.

24 Cardarella S, Johnson BE. The impact of genomic changes on treatment of lung cancer. *Am J Respir Crit Care Med* 2013;188:770–5.

25 Aregbe AO, Sherer EA, Egorin MJ, *et al.* Population pharmacokinetic analysis of 17-dimethylaminoethylamino-17-demethoxygeldanamycin (17-DMAG) in adult patients with solid tumors. *Cancer Chemother Pharmacol* 2012;70:201–5.

26 Kaifi JT, Toth JW, Gusani NJ, *et al.* Multidisciplinary management of malignant pleural effusion. *J Surg Oncol* 2012;105:731–8.

27 National Lung Screening Trial Research T, Aberle DR, Adams AM, *et al.* Reduced lung-cancer mortality with low-dose computed tomographic screening. *N Engl J Med* 2011;365:395–409.

28 Goldstraw P, Crowley J, Chansky K, *et al.* The IASLC Lung Cancer Staging Project: proposals for the revision of the TNM stage groupings in the forthcoming (seventh) edition of the TNM Classification of malignant tumours. *J Thorac Oncol* 2007;2:706–14.

29 Amin M, Edge S, Greene R, Byrd D, Brookland R. *Cancer Staging Manual*, 8th edn. American Joint Committee on Cancer. New York: Springer, 2017.

30 Rusch VW, Asamura H, Watanabe H, *et al.* The IASLC lung cancer staging project: a proposal for a new international lymph node map in the forthcoming seventh edition of the TNM classification for lung cancer. *J Thorac Oncol* 2009;4:568–77.

31 Ginsberg RJ, Rubinstein LV. Randomized trial of lobectomy versus limited resection for T1 N0 non-small cell lung cancer Lung Cancer Study Group. *Ann Thorac Surg* 1995;60:615–22; discussion 622–3.

32 Brunelli A, Kim AW, Berger KI, Addrizzo-Harris DJ. Physiologic evaluation of the patient with lung cancer being considered for resectional surgery: diagnosis and management of lung cancer, 3rd edn. *American College of Chest Physicians evidence-based clinical practice guidelines. Chest* 2013;143:e166S–90S.

33 Predina JD, Kunkala M, Aliperti LA, Singhal AK, Singhal S. Sleeve lobectomy: current indications and future directions. *Ann Thorac Cardiovasc Surg* 2010;16:310–18.

34 Wu Y, Huang ZF, Wang SY, Yang XN, Ou W. A randomized trial of systematic nodal dissection in resectable non-small cell lung cancer. *Lung Cancer* 2002;36:1–6.

35 Fernando HC, Landreneau RL, Mandrekar S, *et al.* Impact of brachytherapy on local recurrence after sublobar resection: results from ACOSOG Z4032 (Alliance), a phase III randomized trial for high-risk operable non-small cell lung cancer (NSCLC). *J Clin Oncol* 2013;31:Abstract # 7502.

36 Albain KS, Swann RS, Rusch VW, *et al.* Radiotherapy plus chemotherapy with or without surgical resection for stage III non-small-cell lung cancer: a phase III randomised controlled trial. *Lancet* 2009;374:379–86.

37 Collaud S, Stahel R, Inci I, *et al.* Survival of patients treated surgically for synchronous single-organ metastatic NSCLC and advanced pathologic TN stage. *Lung Cancer* 2012;78:234–8.

38 Timmerman R, Paulus R, Galvin J, *et al.* Stereotactic body radiation therapy for inoperable early stage lung cancer. *JAMA* 2010;303:1070–6.

39 PORT Meta-analysis Trialists Group. Postoperative radiotherapy in non-small-cell lung cancer: systematic review and meta-analysis of individual patient data from nine randomised controlled trials. *Lancet* 1998;352:257–63.

40 Lally BE, Zelterman D, Colasanto JM, *et al.* Postoperative radiotherapy for stage II or III non-small-cell lung cancer using the surveillance, epidemiology, and end results database. *J Clin Oncol* 2006;24:2998–3006.

41 Curran WJ, Jr., Paulus R, Langer CJ, *et al.* Sequential vs. concurrent chemoradiation for stage III non-small cell lung cancer: randomized phase III trial RTOG 9410. *J Natl Cancer Inst* 2011;103:1452–60.

42 Saunders M, Dische S, Barrett A, *et al.* Continuous hyperfractionated accelerated radiotherapy (CHART) versus conventional radiotherapy in non-small-cell lung cancer: a randomised multicentre trial. *CHART Steering Committee. Lancet* 1997;350:161–5.

43 Belani CP, Wang W, Johnson DH, *et al.* Phase III study of the Eastern Cooperative Oncology Group (ECOG 2597): induction chemotherapy followed by either standard thoracic radiotherapy or hyperfractionated accelerated radiotherapy for patients with unresectable stage IIIA and B non-small-cell lung cancer. *J Clin Oncol* 2005;23:3760–7.

44 Bradley JD, Paulus R, Komaki R, *et al.* A randomized phase III comparison of standard-dose (60 Gy) versus high-dose (74 Gy) conformal chemoradiotherapy with or without cetuximab for stage III non-small cell lung cancer: results on radiation dose in RTOG 0617. *J Clin Oncol* 2013;31:S7501.

45 Spiro SG, Rudd RM, Souhami RL, *et al.* Chemotherapy versus supportive care in advanced non-small cell lung cancer: improved survival without detriment to quality of life. *Thorax* 2004;59:828–36.

46 Non-small Cell Lung cancer. Collaborative Group. Chemotherapy in non-small cell lung cancer: a meta-analysis using updated data on individual patients from 52 randomised clinical trials. *BMJ* 1995;311:899–909.

47 Lilenbaum RC, Herndon JE, 2nd, List MA, *et al.* Single-agent versus combination chemotherapy in advanced non-small-cell lung cancer: the cancer and leukemia group B (study 9730). *J Clin Oncol* 2005;23:190–6.

48 Ardizzoni A, Boni L, Tiseo M, *et al.* Cisplatin- versus carboplatin-based chemotherapy in first-line treatment of advanced non-small-cell lung cancer: an individual patient data meta-analysis. *J Natl Cancer Inst* 2007;99:847–57.

49 Schiller JH, Harrington D, Belani CP, *et al.* Comparison of four chemotherapy regimens for advanced non-small-cell lung cancer. *N Engl J Med* 2002;346:92–8.

50 Scagliotti GV, Parikh P, von Pawel J, *et al.* Phase III study comparing cisplatin plus gemcitabine with cisplatin plus pemetrexed in chemotherapy-naive patients with advanced-stage non-small-cell lung cancer. *J Clin Oncol* 2008;26:3543–51.

51 Patel JD, Socinski MA, Garon EB, *et al. A Randomized, Open-Label, Phase III, Superiority Study of Pemetrexed(Pem) + Carboplatin(Cb) + Bevacizumab(Bev) Followed by Maintenance Pem + Bev versus Paclitaxel (Pac)+Cb+Bev Followed by Maintenance Bev in Patients with Stage IIIB or IV Non-Squamous Non-Small Cell Lung cancer.* (NS-NSCLC). ASTRO. Chicago, 2012.

52 Socinski MA, Bondarenko I, Karaseva NA, *et al.* Weekly nab-paclitaxel in combination with carboplatin versus solvent-based paclitaxel plus carboplatin as first-line therapy in patients with advanced non-small-cell lung cancer: final results of a phase III trial. *J Clin Oncol* 2012;30:2055–62.

53 Ciuleanu T, Brodowicz T, Zielinski C, *et al.* Maintenance pemetrexed plus best supportive care versus placebo plus best supportive care for non-small-cell lung cancer: a randomised, double-blind, phase 3 study. *Lancet* 2009;374:1432–40.

54 Cappuzzo F, Ciuleanu T, Stelmakh L, *et al.* Erlotinib as maintenance treatment in advanced non-small-cell lung cancer: a multicentre, randomised, placebo-controlled phase 3 study. *Lancet Oncol* 2010;11:521–9.

55 Fossella FV, DeVore R, Kerr RN, *et al.* Randomized phase III trial of docetaxel versus vinorelbine or ifosfamide in patients with advanced non-small-cell lung cancer previously treated with platinum-containing chemotherapy regimens. The TAX 320 Non-Small Cell Lung Cancer Study Group. *J Clin Oncol* 2000;18:2354–62.

56 Hanna N, Shepherd FA, Fossella FV, *et al.* Randomized phase III trial of pemetrexed versus docetaxel in patients with non-small-cell lung cancer previously treated with chemotherapy. *J Clin Oncol* 2004;22:1589–97.

57 Shepherd FA, Rodrigues Pereira J, Ciuleanu T, *et al.* Erlotinib in previously treated non-small-cell lung cancer. *N Engl J Med* 2005;353:123–32.

58 Brahmer J, Reckamp KL, Baas P, *et al.* Nivolumab versus docetaxel in advanced squamous-cell non-small-cell lung cancer. *N Engl J Med* 2015;373:123–35.

59 Borghaei H, Paz-Ares L, Horn L, *et al.* Nivolumab versus docetaxel in advanced nonsquamous non-small-cell lung cancer. *N Engl J Med* 2015;373:1627–39.

60 Herbst RS, Baas P, Kim DW, *et al.* Pembrolizumab versus docetaxel for previously treated, PD-L1-positive, advanced non-small-cell lung cancer (KEYNOTE-010): a randomised controlled trial. *Lancet* 2016;387:1540–50.

61 Barlesi F, Park K, Ciardiello F, *et al.* Primary analysis from OAK, a randomized phase III study comparing atezolizumab with docetaxel in 2L/3L NSCLC Primary analysis from OAK, a randomized phase III study comparing atezolizumab with docetaxel in 2L/3L NSCLC. Proc ESMO, 2016.

62 Johnson DH, Fehrenbacher L, Novotny WF, *et al.* Randomized phase II trial comparing bevacizumab plus carboplatin and paclitaxel with carboplatin and paclitaxel alone in previously untreated locally advanced or metastatic non-small-cell lung cancer. *J Clin Oncol* 2004;22:2184–91.

63 Sandler A, Gray R, Perry MC, *et al.* Paclitaxel-carboplatin alone or with bevacizumab for non-small-cell lung cancer. *N Engl J Med* 2006;355:2542–50.

64 Manegold M, von Pawel J, Zatloukal P, *et al.* Randomised, double-blind multicentre phase III study of bevacizumab in combination with cisplatin and gemcitabine in chemotherapy-naïve patients with advanced or recurrent non-squamous non-small cell lung cancer (NSCLC): BO17704. *J Clin Oncol* 2007;25:LBA7514.

65 Ramalingam SS, Dahlberg SE, Langer CJ, *et al.* Outcomes for elderly, advanced-stage non small-cell lung cancer patients

treated with bevacizumab in combination with carboplatin and paclitaxel: analysis of Eastern Cooperative Oncology Group Trial 4599. *J Clin Oncol* 2008;26:60–5.

66 Garon EB, Ciuleanu TE, Arrieta O, *et al.* Ramucirumab plus docetaxel versus placebo plus docetaxel for second-line treatment of stage IV non-small-cell lung cancer after disease progression on platinum-based therapy (REVEL): a multicentre, double-blind, randomised phase 3 trial. *Lancet* 2014;384:665–73.

67 Huang SF, Liu HP, Li LH, *et al.* High frequency of epidermal growth factor receptor mutations with complex patterns in non-small cell lung cancers related to gefitinib responsiveness in Taiwan. *Clin Cancer Res* 2004;10:8195–203.

68 Pao W, Miller V, Zakowski M, *et al.* EGF receptor gene mutations are common in lung cancers from "never smokers" and are associated with sensitivity of tumors to gefitinib and erlotinib. *Proc Natl Acad Sci USA* 2004;101:13306–11.

69 Maemondo M, Inoue A, Kobayashi K, *et al.* Gefitinib or chemotherapy for non-small-cell lung cancer with mutated EGFR. *N Engl J Med* 2010;362:2380–8.

70 Rosell R, Carcereny E, Gervais R, *et al.* Erlotinib versus standard chemotherapy as first-line treatment for European patients with advanced EGFR mutation-positive non-small-cell lung cancer (EURTAC): a multicentre, open-label, randomised phase 3 trial. *Lancet Oncol* 2012;13:239–46.

71 Zhou C, Wu YL, Chen G, *et al.* Erlotinib versus chemotherapy as first-line treatment for patients with advanced EGFR mutation-positive non-small-cell lung cancer (OPTIMAL, CTONG-0802): a multicentre, open-label, randomised, phase 3 study. *Lancet Oncol* 2011;12:735–42.

72 Sequist LV, Yang JC, Yamamoto N, *et al.* Phase III Study of afatinib or cisplatin plus pemetrexed in patients with metastatic lung adenocarcinoma with EGFR mutations. *J Clin Oncol* 2013;31:3327–34.

73 Pao W, Miller VA, Politi KA, *et al.* Acquired resistance of lung adenocarcinomas to gefitinib or erlotinib is associated with a second mutation in the EGFR kinase domain. *PLoS Med* 2005;2:e73.

74 Janne PA, Yang JC, Kim DW, *et al.* AZD9291 in EGFR inhibitor-resistant non-small-cell lung cancer. *N Engl J Med* 2015;372:1689–99.

75 Rosell R, Robinet G, Szczesna A, *et al.* Randomized phase II study of cetuximab plus cisplatin/vinorelbine compared with cisplatin/vinorelbine alone as first-line therapy in EGFR-expressing advanced non-small-cell lung cancer. *Ann Oncol* 2008;19:362–9.

76 Thatcher N, Hirsch FR, Luft AV, *et al.* Necitumumab plus gemcitabine and cisplatin versus gemcitabine and cisplatin alone as first-line therapy in patients with stage IV squamous non-small-cell lung cancer (SQUIRE): an open-label, randomised, controlled phase 3 trial. *Lancet Oncol* 2015;16:763–74.

77 Soda M, Choi YL, Enomoto M, *et al.* Identification of the transforming EML4-ALK fusion gene in non-small-cell lung cancer. *Nature* 2007;448:561–6.

78 Rikova K, Guo A, Zeng Q, *et al.* Global survey of phosphotyrosine signaling identifies oncogenic kinases in lung cancer. *Cell* 2007;131:1190–203.

79 Shaw AT, Yeap BY, Solomon BJ, *et al.* Effect of crizotinib on overall survival in patients with advanced non-small-cell lung cancer harbouring ALK gene rearrangement: a retrospective analysis. *Lancet Oncol* 2011;12:1004–12.

80 Camidge DR, Bang YJ, Kwak EL, *et al.* Activity and safety of crizotinib in patients with ALK-positive non-small-cell lung cancer: updated results from a phase 1 study. *Lancet Oncol* 2012;13:1011–19.

81 Shaw AT, Kim DW, Nakagawa K, *et al.* Crizotinib versus chemotherapy in advanced ALK-positive lung cancer. *N Engl J Med* 2013;368:2385–94.

82 Kim D, Ahn M, Shi Y, *et al.* Results of a global phase II study with crizotinib in advanced ALK-positive non-small cell lung cancer (NSCLC). *J Clin Oncol* 2012;30:7533.

83 Solomon BJ, Mok T, Kim DW, *et al.* First-line crizotinib versus chemotherapy in ALK-positive lung cancer. *N Engl J Med* 2014;371:2167–77.

84 Mehra R, Camidge DR, Sharma S, *et al.* First-in-human phase I study of the ALK inhibitor LDK378 in advanced solid tumors. *J Clin Oncol* 2012;30:3007.

85 Shaw AT, Gandhi L, Gadgeel S, *et al.* Alectinib in ALK-positive, crizotinib-resistant, non-small-cell lung cancer: a single-group, multicentre, phase 2 trial. *Lancet Oncol* 2016;17:234–42.

86 Bergethon K, Shaw AT, Ou SH, *et al.* ROS1 rearrangements define a unique molecular class of lung cancers. *J Clin Oncol* 2012;30:863–70.

87 Davies KD, Le AT, Theodoro MF, *et al.* Identifying and targeting ROS1 gene fusions in non-small cell lung cancer. *Clin Cancer Res* 2012;18:4570–9.

88 Ju YS, Lee WC, Shin JY, *et al.* A transforming KIF5B and RET gene fusion in lung adenocarcinoma revealed from whole-genome and transcriptome sequencing. *Genome Res* 2012;22:436–45.

89 Kohno T, Ichikawa H, Totoki Y, *et al.* KIF5B-RET fusions in lung adenocarcinoma. *Nat Med* 2012;18:375–7.

90 Lipson D, Capelletti M, Yelensky R, *et al.* Identification of new ALK and RET gene fusions from colorectal and lung cancer biopsies. *Nat Med* 2012;18:382–4.

91 Takeuchi K, Soda M, Togashi Y, *et al.* RET, ROS1 and ALK fusions in lung cancer. *Nat Med* 2012;18:378–81.

92 Planchard D, Mazieres J, Riely GJ, *et al.* Interim results of phase II study BRF113928 of dabrafenib in BRAF V600E mutation–positive non-small cell lung cancer (NSCLC) patients. *J Clin Oncol* 2013;31:8009.

93 Planchard D, Besse B, Groen HJ, *et al.* Dabrafenib plus trametinib in patients with previously treated BRAF(V600E)-mutant metastatic non-small cell lung cancer: an open-label, multicentre phase 2 trial. *Lancet Oncol* 2016;17:984–93.

94 Reck M, Rodriguez-Abreu D, Robinson AG, *et al.* Pembrolizumab versus chemotherapy for PD-L1-positive non-small-cell lung cancer. *N Engl J Med* 2016;375:1823–33.

95 Owonikoko TK, Ragin CC, Belani CP, *et al.* Lung cancer in elderly patients: an analysis of the surveillance, epidemiology, and end results database. *J Clin Oncol* 2007;25:5570–7.

96 The Elderly Lung Cancer Vinorelbine Italian Study Group. Effects of vinorelbine on quality of life and survival of elderly patients with advanced non-small-cell lung cancer. *J Natl Cancer Inst* 1999;91:66–72.

97 Quoix E, Zalcman G, Oster JP, *et al.* Carboplatin and weekly paclitaxel doublet chemotherapy compared with monotherapy in elderly patients with advanced non-small-cell lung cancer: IFCT-0501 randomised, phase 3 trial. *Lancet* 2011;378:1079–88.

98 Lilenbaum R, Zukin M, Pereira JR, *et al.* A randomized phase III trial of single-agent pemetrexed (P) versus carboplatin and pemetrexed (CP) in patients with advanced non-small cell lung cancer (NSCLC) and performance status (PS) of 2. *J Clin Oncol* 2012;30:Abstract # 7506.

99 Pignon JP, Tribodet H, Scagliotti GV, *et al.* Lung adjuvant cisplatin evaluation: a pooled analysis by the LACE Collaborative Group. *J Clin Oncol* 2008;26:3552–9.

100 Arriagada R, Bergman B, Dunant A, *et al.* Cisplatin-based adjuvant chemotherapy in patients with completely resected non-small-cell lung cancer. *N Engl J Med* 2004;350:351–60.

101 Douillard JY, Rosell R, De Lena M, *et al.* Adjuvant vinorelbine plus cisplatin versus observation in patients with completely resected stage IB-IIIA non-small-cell lung cancer (Adjuvant Navelbine International Trialist Association [ANITA]): a randomised controlled trial. *Lancet Oncol* 2006;7:719–27.

102 Winton T, Livingston R, Johnson D, *et al.* Vinorelbine plus cisplatin vs. observation in resected non-small-cell lung cancer. *N Engl J Med* 2005;352:2589–97.

103 Strauss GM, Herndon JE, 2nd, Maddaus MA, *et al.* Adjuvant paclitaxel plus carboplatin compared with observation in stage IB non-small-cell lung cancer: CALGB 9633 with the Cancer and Leukemia Group B, Radiation Therapy Oncology Group, and North Central Cancer Treatment Group Study Groups. *J Clin Oncol* 2008;26:5043–51.

104 Furuse K, Fukuoka M, Kawahara M, *et al.* Phase III study of concurrent versus sequential thoracic radiotherapy in combination with mitomycin, vindesine, and cisplatin in unresectable stage III non-small-cell lung cancer. *J Clin Oncol* 1999;17:2692–9.

105 Kalemkerian GP, Akerley W, Bogner P, *et al.* Small cell lung cancer. *J Natl Compr Canc Netw* 2013;11:78–98.

106 O'Brien ME, Ciuleanu TE, Tsekov H, *et al.* Phase III trial comparing supportive care alone with supportive care with oral topotecan in patients with relapsed small-cell lung cancer. *J Clin Oncol* 2006;24:5441–7.

107 Turrisi AT, 3rd, Kim K, Blum R, *et al.* Twice-daily compared with once-daily thoracic radiotherapy in limited small-cell lung cancer treated concurrently with cisplatin and etoposide. *N Engl J Med* 1999;340:265–71.

108 Le Pechoux C, Dunant A, Senan S, *et al.* Standard-dose versus higher-dose prophylactic cranial irradiation (PCI) in patients with limited-stage small-cell lung cancer in complete remission after chemotherapy and thoracic radiotherapy (PCI 99-01, EORTC 22003–08004, RTOG 0212, and IFCT 99-01): a randomised clinical trial. *Lancet Oncol* 2009;10:467–74.

109 Auperin A, Arriagada R, Pignon JP, *et al.* Prophylactic cranial irradiation for patients with small-cell lung cancer in complete remission. Prophylactic Cranial Irradiation Overview Collaborative Group. *N Engl J Med* 1999;341:476–84.

110 Slotman BJ, Mauer ME, Bottomley A, *et al.* Prophylactic cranial irradiation in extensive disease small-cell lung cancer: short-term health-related quality of life and patient reported symptoms: results of an international Phase III randomized controlled trial by the EORTC Radiation Oncology and Lung Cancer Groups. *J Clin Oncol* 2009;27:78–84.

2

Other Thoracic Malignancies

Brandon H. Tieu[1], Mehee Choi[2], Kyle Robinson[3], and Charles R. Thomas, Jr[1]

[1] Knight Cancer Institute, Oregon Health & Science University, Portland, Oregon, USA
[2] Loyola University Chicago School of Medicine, Chicago, Illinois, USA
[3] Hospital of the University of Pennsylvania, Philadelphia, Pennsylvania, USA

Thymoma and Thymic Carcinoma

Incidence and Mortality

Thymic malignancies are rare, slow growing tumors of the anterior mediastinum. Thymomas can spread locally, metastasize, and recur decades after therapy and should not be considered "benign". They typically occur in the fourth to eighth decade with a peak in the seventh decade, and account for 50% of anterior mediastinal masses in patients older than 50 years of age. The ratio of males to females is essentially equal [1]. In the United States (US), incidence rates are highest among Asian/Pacific Islander populations and African Americans, and lowest among Hispanics and non-Hispanic Whites [2]. The incidence of thymomas is 0.13 per 100,000 person years in the US [2]. Five-year survival rates are approximately 93%, 85%, 65%, and 53% for Masaoka stages I–IVa, respectively. Ten-year survival rates are 90%, 75%, 56%, and 38% for stages I–IVa, respectively [1]. Thymic carcinomas are more aggressive and more likely to metastasize to lymph nodes and distant sites compared to thymomas. They have 5-year survival rates of approximately 30–50% [3, 4] and median survival of 6.6 years [5].

Etiology and Risk Factors

No known environmental or lifestyle risk factors are associated with incidence of thymoma or thymic carcinoma. The only consistent associations are age and ethnicity

Pathology

Thymomas are derived from the epithelial component (cortical and medullary) of the thymus. These neoplastic epithelial cells are mixed in various proportions with non-neoplastic lymphocytes, primarily T cells. The World Health Organization (WHO) histologic classification system includes several subtypes of thymomas (type A, AB, B1, B2, and B3), and thymic carcinomas (Type C) (Table 2.1). Thymic carcinomas can be distinguished from thymomas by their malignant cytologic and architectural features. Several subtypes of thymic carcinoma have been described including squamous cell, sarcomatoid, mucoepidermoid, papillary, basaloid, and undifferentiated carcinomas [6, 7].

Diagnosis and Staging

Approximately one-third of patients with thymic malignancies are asymptomatic with another one-third presenting with cough, dyspnea or chest pain [1]. A mass in the anterior mediastinum could represent other benign and malignant tumors such as lymphoma, thymic carcinoids, germ cell tumors, thyroid goiters, thymic cysts, or metastatic lung cancer, which should be considered during the patient's evaluation. Thymomas are relatively uncommon below the age of 20 but make up 15–40% of anterior mediastinal masses between the ages of 20 and 40 [1]. Beta-human chorionic gonadotropin and alpha-fetoprotein levels should be determined if germ cell tumors are suspected in young males. Thyroid-stimulating hormone, triiodothyronine, or thyroxine levels should be assessed in those suspected to have intrathoracic thyroid goiters.

Approximately 40–45% of patients with thymomas will present with myasthenia gravis (MG) [8]. Only 10–15% of patients with MG will have a thymoma [9]. Patients present with a fluctuating degree of ocular (diplopia, ptosis), bulbar (dysarthria, dysphagia), limb, and respiratory muscle weakness. The weakness is a result of autoantibodies against the acetylcholine receptors or against muscle receptor specific tyrosine kinase. Adequate medical control of MG should be achieved prior to surgical resection. Other paraneoplastic conditions such as red cell aplasia and hypogammaglobulinemia occur in 2–5% of patients [9].

If an anterior mediastinal mass is suspected on chest X-ray, a computed tomography (CT) scan of the chest with contrast should be obtained. Thymomas are usually well defined, round or oval masses in the thymus. Magnetic resonance imaging can be considered in patients with severe iodine contrast allergies [10]. Positron emission tomography (PET)/CT can be useful in

The American Cancer Society's Oncology in Practice: Clinical Management, First Edition. Edited by The American Cancer Society.

Table 2.1 World Health Organization (WHO) Histologic Classification.

Type	Histologic description
A	A tumor composed of a population of neoplastic thymic epithelial cells having spindle/oval shape, lacking nuclear atypia, and accompanied by few or no nonneoplastic lymphocytes
AB	A tumor in which foci having the features of type A thymoma are admixed with foci rich in lymphocytes
B1	A tumor that resembles the normal functional thymus in that it combines large expanses having an appearance practically indistinguishable from normal thymic cortex with areas resembling thymic medulla
B2	A tumor in which the neoplastic epithelial component appears as scattered plump cells with vesicular nuclei and distinct nucleoli among a heavy population of lymphocytes. Perivascular spaces are common and sometimes very prominent. A perivascular arrangement of tumor cells resulting in a palisading effect may be seen
B3	A type of thymoma predominantly composed of epithelial cells having a round or polygonal shape and exhibiting no or mild atypia. They are admixed with a mild component of lymphocytes, resulting in a sheet like growth of the neoplastic epithelial cells
C	A thymic tumor (thymic carcinoma) exhibiting clear-cut cytologic atypia and a set of cytoarchitectural features no longer specific to the thymus, but rather analogous to those seen in carcinomas of other organs. Type C thymomas lack immature lymphocytes; whatever lymphocytes may be present are mature and usually admixed with plasma cells

Table 2.2 Masaoka-Koga Clinical Staging of Thymoma [13, 14, 15].

Stage	Diagnostic criteria
I	Macroscopically and microscopically completely encapsulated tumor
IIA	Microscopic transcapsular invasion
IIB	Macroscopic invasion into thymic tissue or surrounding fatty tissue, or grossly adherent to but not through mediastinal pleura or pericardium
III	Macroscopic invasion into neighboring organ (i.e., pericardium, great vessels, or lung)
IVA	Pleural or pericardial dissemination
IVB	Lymphogenous or hematogenous metastasis

detecting metastatic disease [11]. Close attention should be made to vascular invasion or involvement of other mediastinal structures which can limit surgical resection and indicate the need for neoadjuvant therapy. If a thymic malignancy is suspected and deemed surgically resectable, patients should undergo resection without tissue biopsy. For locally advanced or unresectable lesions or in cases where lymphoma is suspected, fine-needle aspiration, core-needle biopsy, or open biopsy can be performed for tissue diagnosis [12].

The Masaoka-Koga staging system is the most commonly used classification system for thymic malignancies (Table 2.2), and was recommended by the International Thymic Malignancy Interest Group (ITMIG) [13]. Historically, no standardized staging system for thymic malignancies has been defined by the American Joint Commission on Cancer or the Union for International Cancer Control until the new eighth edition classification system [16] (Table 2.3). The primary extent of involvement (T) is classified by the level of tissue involvement that is determined by microscopic invasion. A node map was developed by ITMIG and the International Association for the Study of Lung Cancer and is used for the new nodal staging system. N1 nodes are in the anterior mediastinum and lower cervical regions, while N2 nodes are deep cervical, supraclavicular, and middle mediastinal nodes. Metastatic disease is subclassified between separate pleural (visceral or parietal) or pericardial nodules (M1a) and pulmonary intraparenchymal or distant organ metastasis (M1b).

Table 2.3 Thymic malignancy TNM staging.

Primary tumor (T)	
T0	No evidence of a primary tumor
T1	Tumor encapsulated or extending into the mediastinal fat; may involve the mediastinal pleura
T1a	No mediastinal pleura involvement
T1b	Direct invasion of mediastinal pleura
T2	Tumor with direct invasion of the pericardium (either partial or full thickness)
T3	Tumor with direct invasion into any of the following: lung, brachiocephalic vein (innominate vein), superior vena cava, phrenic nerve, chest wall, or extrapericardial pulmonary artery or veins
T4	Tumor with direct invasion into any of the following: aorta (ascending, arch or descending), arch vessels, intrapericardial pulmonary artery, myocardium, trachea, esophagus
Regional lymph nodes (N)	
NX	Regional lymph nodes not assessed
N0	No regional lymph node metastasis
N1	Metastases in anterior (perithymic) lymph nodes
N2	Metastases in deep intrathoracic or cervical lymph nodes
Distant metastasis (M)	
M0	No pleural, pericardial, or distant metastasis
M1a	Separate pleural or pericardial nodule(s)
M1b	Pulmonary intraparenchymal nodule or distant organ metastasis

Stage grouping

Stage	T	N	M
I	T1a, T1b	N0	M0
II	T2	N0	M0
IIIA	T3	N0	M0
IIIB	T4	N0	M0
IVA	Any T	N1	M0
	Any T	N0, N1	M1a
IVB	Any T	N2	M0, M1a
	Any T	Any N	M1b

Source: Detterbeck and Marom [16]. Used with permission of the American College of Surgeons, Chicago, Illinois. The original source for this information is the AJCC Cancer Staging Manual, 8th edn (2017), which is published by Springer Science + Business Media.

Treatment

Patients with thymic malignancies should be evaluated and managed by a multidisciplinary team that includes thoracic surgeons, medical oncologists, radiation oncologists, chest radiologists, surgical pathologists, and pulmonologists [17]. Surgery is the recommended treatment for all clinically resectable thymomas and thymic carcinomas. For locally advanced and metastatic disease, multimodality therapy with or without surgery is recommended [18].

Surgery

The goal of surgery is *en bloc* R0 resection (complete resection with no microscopic residual tumor) of the lesion with total thymectomy including contiguous and noncontiguous disease. The ability to achieve a complete macroscopic and microscopic resection varies with stage [1]. Locally advanced tumors may require resection of adjacent structures such as the pericardium, pleura, lung, phrenic nerve, and possibly vascular structures to achieve a R0 resection. Bilateral phrenic nerve resection results in respiratory morbidity and should be avoided. Routine evaluation of pleural surfaces should be performed for metastatic disease. For patients who develop a resectable recurrence, surgery is recommended and provides excellent long-term survival (72–77%, 5-year) if complete resection can be achieved [19, 20].

Thymectomy can be performed through a sternotomy, thoracotomy, or with minimally invasive approaches such as a transcervical approach, video-assisted, or robotic-assisted thoracoscopic surgery. Minimally invasive approaches lack robust long-term data on recurrence or survival, but can be considered if the standard oncologic principles are met [21]. The ITMIG has proposed a policy on the handling and reporting of surgical and pathological findings by surgeons and pathologists so future validation studies can be performed [22].

Radiotherapy

Thymomas are relatively radiosensitive. Neoadjuvant radiotherapy with or without chemotherapy is indicated in cases of marginally resectable tumors to enhance the ability to achieve complete resection [23].

Although surgery is the treatment of choice for stage I–III thymoma, many physicians advocate the use of adjuvant radiotherapy, particularly in cases of: incomplete resection; extension beyond the capsule; extensive pleural adherence; microscopic pleural invasion; macroscopic invasion of the pericardium, large vessels, or lung; or aggressive histology (WHO grade B3 or C) [24].

Completely resected stage I thymomas have an excellent prognosis and adjuvant therapy is not indicated [25]. Indications for postoperative radiotherapy for stage II thymoma are not well defined [24]. Postoperative radiotherapy is generally indicated in the setting of incomplete resection. For completely resected stage II thymoma, results in the literature regarding the benefits of radiotherapy are conflicting [19, 26, 27]. Patients with stage III thymomas or thymic carcinomas have a higher risk of recurrence and should receive adjuvant radiotherapy to aid in local control [28, 29].

For unresectable disease, radiation with or without chemotherapy remains the treatment of choice. Radiotherapy also can be an effective palliative treatment for symptomatic metastatic disease [25].

Radiotherapy Treatment Techniques

The planning target volume should include the surgical bed, any gross residual tumor, and areas suspected of harboring subclinical disease (including mediastinal nodes if high risk) with a 2 cm margin (Figure 2.1). Postoperative radiotherapy is delivered using standard fractionation with 1.8–2.0 Gy fractions to a total of 45–50 Gy for margin-negative resections, 54–60 Gy for microscopically positive margins, and 60–70 Gy for unresectable and macroscopically positive margins [30]. For patients with pleural disease, the risk of developing pleural dissemination is high (38%). In this group of patients, the use of hemithoracic irradiation of 10–17 Gy over 2–3 weeks in conjunction with a mediastinal dose of 40 Gy should be considered to improve locoregional control [31]. Neoadjuvant radiotherapy may be delivered using standard fractionation up to a total dose of 45 Gy [25, 32]. Palliative radiation courses such as 30 Gy in 10 fractions are administered for symptomatic local sites. Modern radiotherapy techniques such as intensity-modulated radiotherapy (IMRT) or image-guided radiotherapy may allow more sparing of adjacent organs and structures than standard 3D conformal techniques [24, 25].

Chemotherapy

Chemotherapy is active in thymic malignancies, and is utilized in the primary, postoperative, and locally advanced or metastatic settings [33]. Several different chemotherapy combinations have been used as the primary treatment modality in patients with stage III thymoma or in large tumors in an effort to improve the likelihood of a complete resection [34]. The regimens used in thymic malignancies are usually platinum based, including cisplatin, doxorubicin, and cyclophosphomide (PAC); cisplatin, doxorubicin, vincristine, and cyclophosphamide (ADOC); and cisplatin, etoposide, and ifosfamide (VIP) [35–37].

PAC is recommended as the frontline regimen by the National Cancer Care Network for advanced-staged thymomas, primarily based on treatment of 29 patients with metastatic, locally progressive, or recurrent thymoma [35, 38]. There was an overall response rate of 50% and a median survival of 37.7 months with this regimen [35]. For those patients unable to tolerate cisplatin- or anthracycline-based therapy, carboplatin and paclitaxel does have some activity on unresectable thymomas or thymic carcinomas [39].

Thymic carcinomas are more aggressive than thymomas, and are less responsive to chemotherapy. Although the ADOC regimen is active in thymic carcinoma, carboplatin and paclitaxel is a less toxic regimen and most commonly used [39, 40].

Targeted therapies have shown some promise in thymic malignancies, although in a very small number of patients. Thymomas have shown increased EGFR expression and thymic carcinomas have likewise shown high expression of c-KIT as well as programmed death 1 and programmed death ligand, which are potential therapeutic targets [34, 41, 42]. A recent phase II study indicated promising activity of sunitinib (a multi-targeted receptor tyrosine kinase inhibitor) in previously treated patients with thymic carcinoma [43].

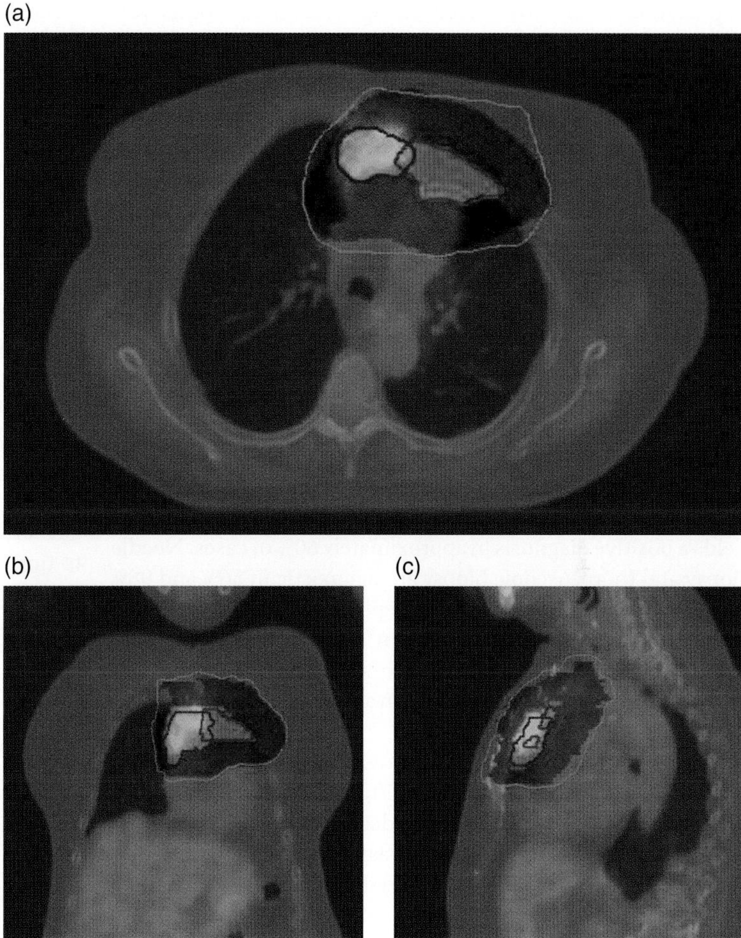

Figure 2.1 Three-dimensional intensity-modulated radiation therapy treatment plan for Masaoka stage IIB thymic carcinoma status post radical thymectomy with a positive margin in (a) axial, (b) coronal, and (c) sagittal planes. The preoperative PET scan has been fused to the computed tomography simulation scan for target delineation purposes. The *red* line delineates the preoperative gross tumor volume. The *pink* line delineates the postoperative tumor bed. The color-wash display demonstrates the clinical target volume in *green* and the planning target volume in *blue*. The *orange* line represents the 6000 cGy isodose line. Radiation was delivered with intensity-modulated radiation therapy using five fields of 6-MV photons to 6000 cGy over 30 fractions.

Follow-up

Local recurrence involving the pleural space, lung, or the mediastinum is more common than distant metastasis. The average time to recurrence for thymomas is 5 years [1, 19, 44]. A comprehensive review found recurrence rates of 3%, 11%, 30%, and 43% for Masaoka stage I–IVa thymomas, respectively [36]. The ITMIG has recommended annual CT scans of the chest for 5 years after surgical resection. Subsequently, chest radiographs and CT scans can be obtained in alternating years until year 11 followed by annual chest radiographs to 20 years. Resected stage III or IVA thymoma, thymic carcinoma, or incompletely resected tumors should have CT scans of the chest every 6 months for the first 3 years [46].

Malignant Pleural Mesothelioma

Incidence and Mortality

Malignant pleural mesothelioma (MPM) is an uncommon cancer with an approximate incidence of 2,000–3,000 cases per year in the US [47]. The mesothelioma incidence rate, based on cases diagnosed between 2009 and 2013, was approximately 1.8 per 100,000 men per year and 0.4 per 100,000 women per year [48].

The incidence in the US is leveling off [47], but is expected to rise in countries with increased utilization and fewer regulations on exposure and mining of asbestos [49]. Mesothelioma most commonly occurs in the pleura, but can occur on other serosal membranes (e.g., pericardium, peritoneum, tunica vaginalis testes).

Etiology and Risk Factors

The link between MPM and asbestos exposure was noted in a landmark study in 1960 [50] and is the biggest risk factor for MPM. A latency period between exposure to asbestos and development of mesothelioma has been reported by different investigators to be approximately 40 years, with shorter periods in heavily exposed individuals [51]. Previous radiation therapy also increases the risks of MPM [52]. The median age at the time of diagnosis is 63 years. Median survivals are 21, 19, 16 and 12 months for stage I–IV, respectively [53]. Recent studies indicate that germline mutations of the BAP1 tumor suppressor gene are responsible for a cancer predisposition syndrome that includes mesothelioma, cutaneous melanoma, uveal melanoma, and other cancers [54, 55].

Pathology

Histologic subtypes for MPM include epithelioid, sarcomatoid, biphasic (epithelioid and sarcomatoid), and desmoplastic. Epithelioid tumors are the most common, while desmoplastic MPM is extremely rare. Immunohistochemical staining can help to differentiate MPM from benign disease and other primary and secondary malignancies involving the pleura. Calretinin, cytokeratin, and vimentin are generally expressed in MPM [55, 57].

Diagnosis and Staging

Patients with MPM present with nonspecific symptoms. A thorough evaluation includes a detailed history of the patient's asbestos exposure. Early-stage patients may complain of dyspnea associated with a pleural effusion. As the disease progresses, patients may note pain due to chest wall invasion followed by worsening dyspnea due to lung entrapment, chest wall restriction, or contralateral effusion and ascites. Physical examination may demonstrate decreased breath sounds, dullness to percussion or a palpable chest wall mass.

For patients presenting with a pleural effusion, thoracentesis can be both diagnostic and therapeutic. Pleural fluid cytology yields a positive diagnosis in approximately 60% of cases. Needle biopsy and thoracoscopic biopsy are diagnostic in 86% and 98% of cases, respectively [58, 59]. If the pleural space is obliterated making thoracoscopy impossible, an open biopsy can be pursued. Incisions should be aligned to allow for resection at the time of surgery as MPM tends to invade in to the chest wall at these sites.

Staging workup should include a CT scan of the chest and abdomen with contrast and a PET-CT. Mediastinal lymph node staging can be done either with mediastinoscopy or endobronchial ultrasound with fine-needle aspiration. Magnetic resonance imaging should be considered to identify mediastinal invasion, chest wall involvement, or transdiaphragmatic extension [60]. PET-CT should be obtained before any pleurodesis procedure to lower the risk of a false-positive study [61, 62]. Video-assisted thoracoscopic surgery and laparoscopy can be performed if contralateral or peritoneal disease is suspected.

The TNM staging system for MPM was initially proposed by the International Mesothelioma Interest Group and in collaboration with the International Association for the Study of Lung Cancer has recently been updated for the eighth edition of the American Joint Commission on Cancer staging manual (Table 2.4) [63].

Treatment

Patients should be evaluated by a multidisciplinary team with experience in managing MPM. Select patients with a good performance status and clinical stage I–III disease are candidates for multimodality therapy. Most patients present with advanced-stage disease, making treatment difficult and cure rare. Surgery is recommended for medically operable patients with clinical stage I–III MPM as part of multimodality therapy where complete gross cytoreduction of the tumor can be achieved. Patients in the International Association for the Study of Lung Cancer mesothelioma database who had curative intent surgery plus either chemotherapy or radiation had better outcomes compared to surgery alone (median survival, 20 vs 11 months) [53]. To determine medical operability, patients should have pulmonary function tests with a carbon monoxide diffusion capacity, a ventilation perfusion scan (if $FEV_1 < 80\%$ predicted), and a cardiac stress test.

Surgery for MPM includes either extrapleural pneumonectomy (EPP) or a lung-sparing procedure with pleurectomy and decortication (P/D). EPP involves *en bloc* resection of the lung, pleura, pericardium, and ipsilateral diaphragm. Standard P/D removes the involved pleura and any gross disease. A radical or extended P/D includes the removal of the pericardium and ipsilateral diaphragm with the pleura. Mediastinal lymph node sampling should be performed with both EPP and P/D. Deciding which operation to offer a patient should take in to consideration the ability to provide a complete gross resection, the planned adjuvant therapy, and the patient's prognosis.

There is a lack of randomized controlled studies to prove a survival benefit of surgery. The Mesothelioma and Radical Surgery randomized feasibility study assessed the benefit of EPP after neoadjuvant chemotherapy compared to chemotherapy alone [64]. EPP had increased morbidity but did not improve survival. The study has been criticized for its small sample size, lack of standardized chemotherapy regimens, and data relating to time from chemotherapy to EPP [65]. A direct comparison of the effects of EPP versus P/D is hard to assess due to complex patient factors and clinical scenarios directing the type of surgical intervention. A retrospective review of 663 patients who had surgical resection for MPM noted a higher operative mortality for EPP (7%) compared to P/D (4%). P/D had a better survival (median survival, 12 vs 16 months: $P < 0.001$), but this difference was thought to be related to selection bias and a difference in patient characteristics [66]. The theoretical advantages of EPP are a more complete cytoreduction and allowing for higher doses of adjuvant radiation therapy resulting in lower rates of local recurrence (33% vs 65% compared to P/D) [66]. A recent meta-analysis of EPP (1391 patients) and P/D (1512 patients), reported a significantly higher mortality associated with EPP (4.5% vs 1.7%; $P < 0.05$). Median survivals favoring EPP were reported in 53% of the studies, but of those that reported at least a 2-year survival (seven of 24) the two cohorts had similar survivals [67].

EPP has been recommended for select patients with a good performance status, minimal comorbidities, stage II–III disease, epithelioid histology, and no N2 disease [68, 69]. P/D should be considered for stage I disease [66] or for patients who cannot tolerate EPP [70]. For patients who cannot tolerate any resection or have symptomatic effusions, palliative therapeutic options include pleurodesis or PleurX® catheter placement.

Radiotherapy

MPM has intermediate radiosensitivity, similar to nonsmall cell lung cancer. Radiotherapy alone is not curative, due to the large radiation doses needed for tumor sterilization, large target volumes, and proximity to radiosensitive normal structures.

High dose radiotherapy to the entire hemithorax after pleurectomy and decortication has been shown to improve local control compared to historical controls; however, it has not been shown to improve survival [71]. Significant radiation toxicities, primarily pneumonitis, pulmonary fibrosis, pericardial effusion, esophagitis, and esophageal stricture have been reported in patients treated with adjuvant radiotherapy following P/D [72–74]. Thus, adjuvant radiation in this setting should be considered with the goal of reducing locoregional failure, preferably on clinical trial.

Table 2.4 Malignant pleural mesothelioma TNM staging.

Primary tumor (T)	
TX	Primary tumor cannot be assessed
T0	No evidence of a primary tumor
T1	Tumor is limited to the ipsilateral parietal pleura with or without involvement of: • Visceral pleura • Mediastinal pleura • Diaphragmatic pleura
T2	Tumor involving each of the ipsilateral pleural surfaces (parietal, mediastinal, diaphragmatic, and visceral pleura) with at least one of the following: • Involvement of the diaphragmatic muscle • Extension of tumor from the visceral pleura into the underlying pulmonary parenchyma
T3	Locally advanced but *potentially resectable tumor*. Tumor involving all the ipsilateral pleural surfaces (parietal, mediastinal, diaphragmatic, and visceral pleura) with at least one of the following: • Involvement of the endothoracic fascia • Extension into the mediastinal fat • Solitary, completely resectable focus of tumor extending into the soft tissue of the chest wall • Nontransmural involvement of the pericardium
T4	Locally advanced *technically unresectable tumor*. Tumor involving all the ipsilateral pleural surfaces (parietal, mediastinal, diaphragmatic, and visceral pleura) with at least one of the following: • Diffuse extension or multifocal masses of tumor in the chest wall, with or without associated rib destruction • Direct diaphragmatic extension of the tumor to the peritoneum • Direct extension of the tumor to the contralateral pleura • Direct extension of the tumor to a mediastinal organ • Direct extension of the tumor into the spine • Tumor extending through to the internal surface of the pericardium with or without a pericardial effusion or tumor involving the myocardium
Regional lymph nodes (N)	
NX	Regional lymph nodes cannot be assessed
NO	No regional lymph node metastases
N1	Metastases in the ipsilateral bronchopulmonary, hilar, or mediastinal (including the internal mammary, peridiaphragmatic, pericardial fat pad, or intercostal) lymph nodes
N2	Metastases in the contralateral mediastinal, ipsilateral, or contralateral supraclavicular lymph nodes
Distant metastasis (M)	
M0	No distant metastasis
M1	Distant metastasis

Stage grouping

Stage	**T**	**N**	**M**
IA	T1	N0	M0
IB	T2, T3	N0	M0
II	T1, T2	N1	M0
IIIA	T3	N1	M0
IIIB	T1, T2, T3	N2	M0
	T4	Any N	M0
IV	Any T	Any N	M1

Source: adapted from AJCC Cancer Staging Manual, 8th edn [63]. Used with permission of the American College of Surgeons, Chicago, Illinois. The original source for this information is the AJCC Cancer Staging Manual, 8th edn (2017), which is published by Springer Science + Business Media.

Postoperative radiotherapy is given after EPP to improve local control and to prevent recurrence at the instrument-tract after pleural intervention. Adjuvant radiotherapy to 50–54 Gy reduces local recurrence rates after EPP in carefully selected patients [75]. IMRT has allowed safe delivery of higher doses of up to 60 Gy in the adjuvant setting after EPP [76, 77]. Prophylactic radiation to surgical tracts has been shown to prevent local recurrences at these sites [78, 79].

Radiotherapy Treatment Techniques

The target volume should include the entire hemithorax, thoracotomy incision, biopsy tracks, and sites of chest drains [75, 80]. Postoperative radiotherapy is delivered to this target volume using standard fractionation with 1.8–2.0 Gy fractions to total 50–54 Gy. A total dose of 54–60 Gy is recommended for microscopically positive margins. A total of 60 Gy or greater is recommended for macroscopic residual disease. Modern radiotherapy techniques such as IMRT or image-guided radiotherapy may allow more sparing of adjacent critical structures than 3D conformal techniques [71].

Prophylactic doses of 21 Gy in seven fractions help to prevent surgical tract recurrences [78, 79]. Palliative chest wall radiation to doses >40 Gy at doses of ≥4 Gy per fraction appear to be more effective in providing symptomatic relief than lower doses [79]. Palliation of bone or brain metastases is treated with standard courses such as 30 Gy in 10 fractions.

Chemotherapy and Trimodality Therapy

The benefit of chemotherapy in MPM was first demonstrated in the metastatic or inoperable setting. Prior to 2000, it was unclear whether chemotherapy provided a benefit over supportive care. In 2003, the combination of cisplatin with pemetrexed was studied in a large ($n = 456$) chemotherapy naive population [81]. Cisplatin plus pemetrexed produced a significantly superior response rate of 41.3%, and median survival of 12.1 months, compared to 16.7% and 9.3 months in the control group of single agent cisplatin. The National Cancer Care Network recommends four combination systemic therapy regimens that can be used either alone or as part of multimodality therapy for MPM. Cisplatin and pemetrexed is recommended as the first-line regimen (category I). Carboplatin can be substituted for patients with medical contraindications to cisplatin and gemcitabine is recommended for patients who are unable to receive pemetrexed. Cisplatin, pemetrexed, and bevacizumab can be used for patients with unresectable disease and are able to receive bevacizumab [82]. There is no current standard second-line agent for MPM. Although multiple targeted agents are now playing a role in nonsmall cell lung cancer, no agent has yet proven to be beneficial to patients with MPM. There are currently multiple pathways being investigated in early clinical studies in patients with MPM [83].

Even with the added benefits of local control with adjuvant radiation therapy after EPP, distant recurrence remains a problem and affects survival [75]. Multiple studies have investigated giving neoadjuvant cisplatin in the setting of trimodality therapy [56]. Patients in the largest study that completed all three forms of therapy achieved a median survival of 29 months and 62% were alive at 2 years [84].

Intrapleural therapies such as hyperthermic intracavitary chemotherapy [85, 86], hyperthermic povidone-iodine lavage [87], photodynamic therapy [88], and immunogenetic therapy [89] have been studied but clear benefits of their use are still lacking [90].

Follow-up

No well-established, defined follow-up guidelines are available for MPM. Similar follow-up for lung cancer, including clinic visits with CT scans of chest and abdomen every 4–6 months for the first 2–3 years followed by annual imaging thereafter, seems appropriate due to the aggressive nature of the disease and the high risk for recurrence.

References

1 Detterbeck FC. Evaluation and treatment of stage I and II thymoma. *J Thorac Oncol* 2010;5(10 Suppl 4):S318–22.

2 Engels EA. Epidemiology of thymoma and associated malignancies. *J Thorac Oncol* 2010;5(10 Suppl 4):S260–5.

3 Eng TY, Fuller CD, Jagirdar J, Bains Y, Thomas CR, Jr. Thymic carcinoma: state of the art review. *Int J Radiat Oncol Biol Phys* 2004;59(3):654–64.

4 Weksler B, Dhupar R, Parikh V, *et al.* Thymic carcinoma: a multivariate analysis of factors predictive of survival in 290 patients. *Ann Thorac Surg* 2013;95(1):299–303.

5 Ahmad U, Yao X, Detterbeck F, *et al.* Thymic carcinoma outcomes and prognosis: results of an international analysis. *J Thorac Cardiovasc Surg* 2015;149(1):95–101.

6 Kelly RJ. Thymoma versus thymic carcinoma: differences in biology impacting treatment. *J Natl Compr Canc Netw* 2013;11(5):577–83.

7 Marx A, Chan JK, Coindre JM, *et al.* The 2015 World Health Organization classification of tumors of the thymus: continuity and changes. *J Thorac Oncol* 2015;10(10):1383–95.

8 Muller-Hermelink HK, Marx A, Geuder K, Kirchner T. The pathological basis of thymoma-associated myasthenia gravis. *Ann NY Acad Sci* 1993;681:56–65.

9 Detterbeck FC, Parsons AM. Thymic tumors. *Ann Thorac Surg* 2004;77:1860–9.

10 Marom EM. Imaging thymoma. *J Thorac Oncol* 2010;5(10 Suppl 4):S296–303.

11 Sung YM, Lee KS, Kim BT, *et al.* 18F–FDG PET/CT of thymic epithelial tumors: usefulness for distinguishing and staging tumor subgroups. *J Nucl Med* 2006;47(10):1628–34.

12 Marchevsky A, Marx A, Strobel P, *et al.* Policies and reporting guidelines for small biopsy specimens of mediastinal masses. *J Thorac Oncol* 2011;6(Suppl 3):S1724–9.

13 Detterbeck FC, Nicholson AG, Kondo K, Van Schil P, Moran C. The Masaoka-Koga stage classification for thymic malignancies: clarification and definition of terms. *J Thorac Oncol* 2011;6(Suppl 3):S1710–6.

14 Masaoka A, Monden Y, Nakahara K, Tanioka T. Follow-up study of thymomas with special reference to their clinical stages. *Cancer* 1981;48(11):2485–92.

15 Koga K, Matsuno Y, Noguchi M, *et al.* A review of 79 thymomas: modification of staging system and reappraisal of conventional division into invasive and non-invasive thymoma. *Pathol Int* 1994;44(5):359–67.
16 Detterbeck FC, Marom E. Thymus. In: MB Amin, SB Edge, FL Greene, *et al.* (eds) *AJCC Cancer Staging Manual*, 8th edn. New York: Springer Nature, 2017.
17 Ruffini E, Van Raemdonck D, Detterbeck F, *et al.* Management of thymic tumors: a survey of current practice among members of the European Society of Thoracic Surgeons. *J Thorac Oncol* 2011;6(3):614–23.
18 Thymomas and Thymic Carcinomas. National Comprehensive Cancer Network, 2013.
19 Ruffini E, Mancuso M, Oliaro A, *et al.* Recurrence of thymoma: analysis of clinicopathologic features, treatment, and outcome. *J Thorac Cardiovasc Surg* 1997;113(1):55–63.
20 Margaritora S, Cesario A, Cusumano G, *et al.* Single-centre 40-year results of redo operation for recurrent thymomas. *Eur J Cardiothorac Surg* 2011;40(4):894–900.
21 Toker A, Sonett J, Zielinski M, *et al.* Standard terms, definitions, and policies for minimally invasive resection of thymoma. *J Thorac Oncol* 2011;6(Suppl 3):S1739–42.
22 Detterbeck FC, Moran C, Huang J, *et al.* Which way is up? Policies and procedures for surgeons and pathologists regarding resection specimens of thymic malignancy. *J Thorac Oncol* 2011;6(Suppl 3):S1730–8.
23 Yagi K, Hirata T, Fukuse T, *et al.* Surgical treatment for invasive thymoma, especially when the superior vena cava is invaded. *Ann Thorac Surg* 1996;61(2):521–4.
24 Gomez DR, Fuller CD, Chennupati S, Thomas CR, Jr. Mediastinal and tracheal cancer. In: EC Halperin, LW Brady, CA Perez, DE Wazer (eds) *Perez and Brady's Principles and Practice of Radiation Oncology* 6th edn. Baltimore: Lippincott Williams & Wilkins, 2013.
25 Rengan R, Bonner Millar LP, Thomas CR Jr. Uncommon thoracic tumours. In: L Gunderson, J Tepper (eds) *Clinical Radiation Oncology*, 3rd edn. Philadelphia: Elsevier, 2011:859–89.
26 Rena O, Papalia E, Oliaro A, *et al.* Does adjuvant radiation therapy improve disease-free survival in completely resected Masaoka stage II thymoma? *Eur J Cardiothorac Surg* 2007;31(1):109–13.
27 Ogawa K, Uno T, Toita T, *et al.* Postoperative radiotherapy for patients with completely resected thymoma: a multi-institutional, retrospective review of 103 patients. *Cancer* 2002;94(5):1405–13.
28 Thomas CR, Wright CD, Loehrer PJ. Thymoma: state of the art. *J Clin Oncol* 1999;17(7):2280–9.
29 Fuller CD, Housman DM, Thomas CR. Radiotherapy for thymoma and thymic carcinoma. *Hematol Oncol Clin North Am* 2008;22(3):489–507.
30 Eng TY, Thomas CR, Jr. Radiation therapy in the management of thymic tumors. *Semin Thorac Cardiovasc Surg* 2005;17(1):32–40.
31 Uematsu M, Yoshida H, Kondo M, *et al.* Entire hemithorax irradiation following complete resection in patients with stage II–III invasive thymoma. *Int J Radiat Oncol Biol Phys* 1996;35(2):357–60.
32 Fuller CD, Ramahi EH, Aherne N, Eng TY, Thomas CR, Jr. Radiotherapy for thymic neoplasms. *J Thorac Oncol* 2010;5(10 Suppl 4):S327–35.
33 Girard N, Lal R, Wakelee H, Riely GJ, Loehrer PJ. Chemotherapy definitions and policies for thymic malignancies. *J Thorac Oncol* 2011;6(Suppl 3):S1749–55.
34 Rajan A, Giaccone G. Treatment of advanced thymoma and thymic carcinoma. *Curr Treat Options Oncol* 2008;9(4–6):277–87.
35 Loehrer PJ, Sr., Kim K, Aisner SC, *et al.* Cisplatin plus doxorubicin plus cyclophosphamide in metastatic or recurrent thymoma: final results of an intergroup trial. The Eastern Cooperative Oncology Group, Southwest Oncology Group, and Southeastern Cancer Study Group. *J Clin Oncol* 1994;12(6):1164–8.
36 Fornasiero A, Daniele O, Ghiotto C, *et al.* Chemotherapy for invasive thymoma. A 13-year experience. *Cancer* 1991;68(1):30–3.
37 Loehrer PJ, Sr., Jiroutek M, Aisner S, *et al.* Combined etoposide, ifosfamide, and cisplatin in the treatment of patients with advanced thymoma and thymic carcinoma: an intergroup trial. *Cancer* 2001;91(11):2010–5.
38 Ettinger DS, Riely GJ, Akerley W, *et al.* Thymomas and thymic carcinomas. *J Natl Compr Canc Netw* 2013;11(5):562–76.
39 Lemma GL, Lee JW, Aisner SC, *et al.* Phase II study of carboplatin and paclitaxel in advanced thymoma and thymic carcinoma. *J Clin Oncol* 2011;29(15):2060–5.
40 Koizumi T, Takabayashi Y, Yamagishi S, *et al.* Chemotherapy for advanced thymic carcinoma: clinical response to cisplatin, doxorubicin, vincristine, and cyclophosphamide (ADOC chemotherapy). *Am J Clin Oncol* 2002 Jun;25(3):266–8.
41 Kelly RJ, Petrini I, Rajan A, Wang Y, Giaccone G. Thymic malignancies: from clinical management to targeted therapies. *J Clin Oncol* 2011;29(36):4820–7.
42 Yokoyama S, Miyoshi H, Nakashima K, *et al.* Prognostic value of programmed death ligand 1 and programmed death 1 expression in thymic carcinoma. *Clin Cancer Res* 2016; 22(18):4727–34.
43 Thomas A, Rajan A, Berman A, *et al.* Sunitinib in patients with chemotherapy-refractory thymoma and thymic carcinoma: an open-label phase 2 trial. *Lancet Oncol* 2015;16(2):177–86.
44 Blumberg D, Port JL, Weksler B, *et al.* Thymoma: a multivariate analysis of factors predicting survival. *Ann Thorac Surg* 1995;60(4):908–13; discussion 914.
45 Detterbeck F, Parsons AM. Thymic tumors: a review of current diagnosis, classification, and treatment. In: *Pearson's Thoracic and Esophageal Surgery*, 3rd edn. Philadelphia: Elsevier, 2008:1589–614.
46 Huang J, Detterbeck FC, Wang Z, Loehrer PJ, Sr. Standard outcome measures for thymic malignancies. *J Thorac Oncol* 2011;6(Suppl 3):S1691–7.
47 Price B, Ware A. Time trend of mesothelioma incidence in the United States and projection of future cases: an update based on SEER data for 1973 through 2005. *Crit Rev Toxicol* 2009;39(7):576–88.
48 Howlader N, Noone AM, Krapcho M, *et al.* (eds). SEER Cancer Statistics Review, 1975–2013, National Cancer Institute. Bethesda, MD, http://seer.cancer.gov/csr/1975_2013/ based on November 2015 SEER data submission, posted to the SEER web site, April 2016.

49 Park EK, Takahashi K, Hoshuyama T, *et al.* Global magnitude of reported and unreported mesothelioma. *Environ Health Perspect* 2011;119(4):514–8.
50 Wagner JC, Sleggs CA, Marchand P. Diffuse pleural mesothelioma and asbestos exposure in the North Western Cape Province. *Br J Ind Med* 1960;17:260–71.
51 Robinson B. Malignant pleural mesothelioma: an epidemiological perspective. *Ann Cardiothorac Surg* 2012;1(4):491–6.
52 De Bruin ML, Burgers JA, Baas P, *et al.* Malignant mesothelioma after radiation treatment for Hodgkin lymphoma. *Blood* 2009;113(16):3679–81.
53 Rusch VW, Giroux D, Kennedy C, *et al.* Initial analysis of the international association for the study of lung cancer mesothelioma database. *J Thorac Oncol* 2012;7(11):1631–9.
54 Ohar JA, Cheung M, Talarchek J, *et al.* Germline BAP1 mutational landscape of asbestos-exposed malignant mesothelioma patients with family history of cancer. *Cancer Res* 2016;76(2):206–15.
54 Betti M, Aspesi A, Biasi A, *et al.* CDKN2A and BAP1 germline mutations predispose to melanoma and mesothelioma. *Cancer Lett* 2016;378(2):120–30.
56 Yanagawa J, Rusch V. Surgical management of malignant pleural mesothelioma. *Thorac Surg Clin* 2013;23(1):73–87.
57 Galateau-Salle F, Churg A, Roggli V, Travis WD, for World Health Organization Committee for Tumors of the Pleura. The 2015 World Health Organization classification of tumors of the pleura: advances since the 2004 classification. *J Thorac Oncol* 2016;11(2):142–54.
58 Adams RF, Gleeson FV. Percutaneous image-guided cutting-needle biopsy of the pleura in the presence of a suspected malignant effusion. *Radiology* 2001;219(2):510–4.
59 Boutin C, Rey F. Thoracoscopy in pleural malignant mesothelioma: a prospective study of 188 consecutive patients. Part 1: Diagnosis. *Cancer* 1993;72(2):389–93.
60 Heelan RT, Rusch VW, Begg CB, *et al.* Staging of malignant pleural mesothelioma: comparison of CT and MR imaging. *Am J Roentgenol* 1999;172(4):1039–47.
61 Nguyen NC, Tran I, Hueser CN, *et al.* F-18 FDG PET/CT characterization of talc pleurodesis-induced pleural changes over time: a retrospective study. *Clin Nucl Med* 2009;34(12):886–90.
62 Ahmadzadehfar H, Palmedo H, Strunk H, *et al.* False positive 18F-FDG-PET/CT in a patient after talc pleurodesis. *Lung Cancer* 2007;58(3):418–21.
63 Rusch VW, Chansky K, Nowak AK, *et al.* Malignant pleural mesothelioma. In: MB Amin, SB Edge, FL Greene, *et al.* (eds) *AJCC Cancer Staging Manual*, 8th edn. New York: Springer Nature, 2017.
64 Treasure T, Lang-Lazdunski L, Waller D, *et al.* Extra-pleural pneumonectomy versus no extra-pleural pneumonectomy for patients with malignant pleural mesothelioma: clinical outcomes of the Mesothelioma and Radical Surgery (MARS) randomised feasibility study. *Lancet Oncol* 2011;12(8):763–72.
65 Weder W, Stahel RA, Baas P, *et al.* The MARS feasibility trial: conclusions not supported by data. *Lancet Oncol* 2011;12(12):1093–4; author reply 4–5.
66 Flores RM, Pass HI, Seshan VE, *et al.* Extrapleural pneumonectomy versus pleurectomy/decortication in the surgical management of malignant pleural mesothelioma: results in 663 patients. *J Thorac Cardiovasc Surg* 2008;135(3):620–6.
67 Taioli E, Wolf AS, Flores RM. Meta-analysis of survival after pleurectomy decortication versus extrapleural pneumonectomy in mesothelioma. *Ann Thorac Surg* 2015;99(2):472–80.
68 Zauderer MG, Krug LM. The evolution of multimodality therapy for malignant pleural mesothelioma. *Curr Treat Options Oncol* 2011;12(2):163–72.
69 Kaufman AJ, Flores RM. Surgical treatment of malignant pleural mesothelioma. *Curr Treat Options Oncol* 2011;12(2):201–16.
70 Nakas A, von Meyenfeldt E, Lau K, Muller S, Waller D. Long-term survival after lung-sparing total pleurectomy for locally advanced (International Mesothelioma Interest Group Stage T3-T4) non-sarcomatoid malignant pleural mesothelioma. *Eur J Cardiothorac Surg* 2012;41(5):1031–6.
71 Baldini EH. Radiation therapy options for malignant pleural mesothelioma. *Semin Thorac Cardiovasc Surg* 2009;21(2):159–63.
72 Rusch VW. Pleurectomy/decortication and adjuvant therapy for malignant mesothelioma. *Chest* 1993;103(4 Suppl):382S–4S.
73 Gupta V, Mychalczak B, Krug L, *et al.* Hemithoracic radiation therapy after pleurectomy/decortication for malignant pleural mesothelioma. *Int J Radiat Oncol Biol Phys* 2005;63(4):1045–52.
74 Lee TT, Everett DL, Shu HK, *et al.* Radical pleurectomy/decortication and intraoperative radiotherapy followed by conformal radiation with or without chemotherapy for malignant pleural mesothelioma. *J Thorac Cardiovasc Surg* 2002;124(6):1183–9.
75 Rusch VW, Rosenzweig K, Venkatraman E, *et al.* A phase II trial of surgical resection and adjuvant high-dose hemithoracic radiation for malignant pleural mesothelioma. *J Thorac Cardiovasc Surg* 2001;122(4):788–95.
76 Ahamad A, Stevens CW, Smythe WR, *et al.* Intensity-modulated radiation therapy: a novel approach to the management of malignant pleural mesothelioma. *Int J Radiat Oncol Biol Phys* 2003;55(3):768–75.
77 Forster KM, Smythe WR, Starkschall G, *et al.* Intensity-modulated radiotherapy following extrapleural pneumonectomy for the treatment of malignant mesothelioma: clinical implementation. *Int J Radiat Oncol Biol Phys* 2003;55(3):606–16.
78 Boutin C, Rey F, Viallat JR. Prevention of malignant seeding after invasive diagnostic procedures in patients with pleural mesothelioma. A randomized trial of local radiotherapy. *Chest* 1995;108(3):754–8.
79 Di Salvo M, Gambaro G, Pagella S, *et al.* Prevention of malignant seeding at drain sites after invasive procedures (surgery and/or thoracoscopy) by hypofractionated radiotherapy in patients with pleural mesothelioma. *Acta Oncol* 2008;47(6):1094–8.

80 Gupta V, Krug LM, Laser B, *et al.* Patterns of local and nodal failure in malignant pleural mesothelioma after extrapleural pneumonectomy and photon-electron radiotherapy. *J Thorac Oncol* 2009;4(6):746–50.

81 Vogelzang NJ, Rusthoven JJ, Symanowski J, *et al.* Phase III study of pemetrexed in combination with cisplatin versus cisplatin alone in patients with malignant pleural mesothelioma. *J Clin Oncol* 2003;21(14):2636–44.

82 Ettinger DS, Wood DE, Akerley W, *et al.* NCCN Guidelines Insights: Malignant Pleural Mesothelioma, Version 3.2016. *J Natl Comp Canc Netw* 2016;14(7):825–36.

83 Nowak A. Chemotherapy for malignant pleural mesothelioma: a review of current management and a look to the future. *Ann Cardiothorac Surg* 2012;1(4):508–15.

84 Krug LM, Pass HI, Rusch VW, *et al.* Multicenter phase II trial of neoadjuvant pemetrexed plus cisplatin followed by extrapleural pneumonectomy and radiation for malignant pleural mesothelioma. *J Clin Oncol* 2009;27(18):3007–13.

85 Chang MY, Sugarbaker DJ. Innovative therapies: intraoperative intracavitary chemotherapy. *Thorac Surg Clin* 2004;14(4):549–56.

86 Tilleman TR, Richards WG, Zellos L, *et al.* Extrapleural pneumonectomy followed by intracavitary intraoperative hyperthermic cisplatin with pharmacologic cytoprotection for treatment of malignant pleural mesothelioma: a phase II prospective study. *J Thorac Cardiovasc Surg* 2009;138(2):405–11.

87 Lang-Lazdunski L, Bille A, Belcher E, *et al.* Pleurectomy/decortication, hyperthermic pleural lavage with povidone-iodine followed by adjuvant chemotherapy in patients with malignant pleural mesothelioma. *J Thorac Oncol* 2011;6(10):1746–52.

88 Pass HI, Temeck BK, Kranda K, *et al.* Phase III randomized trial of surgery with or without intraoperative photodynamic therapy and postoperative immunochemotherapy for malignant pleural mesothelioma. *Ann Surg Oncol* 1997;4(8):628–33.

89 Haas AR, Sterman DH. Novel intrapleural therapies for malignant diseases. *Respiration* 2012;83(4):277–92.

90 Bronte G, Incorvaia L, Rizzo S, *et al.* The resistance related to targeted therapy in malignant pleural mesothelioma: Why has not the target been hit yet? *Crit Rev Oncol/Hematol* 2016;107:20–32.

Section 2

Digestive System Cancers

3

Esophageal Cancer

Ravi Shridhar, Khaldoun Almhanna, Sarah E. Hoffe, Matthew Biagioli, Domenico Coppola, and Kenneth L. Meredith

Moffitt Cancer Center, Tampa, Florida, USA

Introduction

There has been a marked shift in the management of esophageal or gastroesophageal junction (GEJ) cancers from surgery alone to multimodality approaches. Several clinical trials and meta-analyses have demonstrated a survival benefit to neoadjuvant treatment prior to surgery [1–3].

Incidence and Mortality

Approximately 16,940 new cases of esophageal cancer (13,360 in men and 3,580 in women) are diagnosed (1.0% of cancer diagnoses) and approximately 15,450 deaths from this disease occur (2.64% of cancer deaths) annually in the United States (US) [4]. The incidence rate of esophageal cancers, based on cases diagnosed in the US between 2009 and 2013, was approximately 4.3 per 100,000 persons per year. Approximately 61.79% of these esophageal cancers were adenocarcinomas (AC) and 32.8% were squamous cell carcinomas (SCC) [5]. The mortality rate during the same period was 4.1 per 100,000 persons per year.

Worldwide, approximately 455,800 cases of esophageal cancer are diagnosed and 400,200 deaths occur each year [6]. Incidence rates vary internationally by more than 21-fold, with the highest rates in southern and eastern Africa and eastern Asia, and the lowest in western America. The incidence of esophageal AC has been increasing in several western countries due to increases in obesity, while SCC rates are decreasing as a result of reductions in tobacco use and alcohol consumption. However, in certain Asian countries like Taiwan, SCC is increasing because of increases in tobacco and alcohol consumption [4].

Etiology

Age, Race, Ethnicity, and Gender

The median age at diagnosis in the US is 67 years and 30.1% of patients are at least 75 years of age at the time of diagnosis. The esophageal cancer (all histologies combined) incidence rates for males and females in the US are 7.4 and 1.7 per 100,000 persons per year, respectively. The overall esophageal cancer incidence rates (per 100,000 persons per year) in the US are highest among non-Hispanic Whites (4.8) and African Americans (4.4), and are lowest for Asian Americans/Pacific Islanders (2.0) and Hispanics (2.8). Among racial and ethnic groups in the US, the proportion of adenocarcinomas among esophageal cancers is highest among Whites (69.1%), American Indians/Alaska Natives (61.3%), and Hispanics (57.4), and lowest for African Americans (16.6%) and Asian Americans/Pacific Islanders (26.7%) [5].

Squamous Cell Carcinoma

In high incidence areas, there is no gender specificity for SCC, while it is more common in men in low incidence areas. Several risk factors have been identified to predict an increased risk of SCC. The most common risk factors are smoking and alcohol consumption. Dietary factors include foods containing N-nitroso compounds found in pickled vegetables, chewing areca nuts or betel quid, high temperature beverages, red meat intake, low selenium, and zinc deficiency, while intake of fruits, vegetables, and folate are associated with a reduced risk of SCC. Increased risk is associated with pre-existing esophageal disease such as achalasia and prior caustic injury. Prior gastrectomy, atrophic gastritis, human papillomavirus, tylosis, use of bisphosphonates, previous upper aerodigestive tract cancer, and poor oral hygiene are also associated with an increased risk of SCC [7]. SCC of the esophagus is associated with several hereditary cancer

The American Cancer Society's Oncology in Practice: Clinical Management, First Edition. Edited by The American Cancer Society.

predisposition syndromes, including tylosis (focal nonepidermolytic palmoplantar keratoderma, also known as Howel-Evans syndrome), Fanconi anemia, and Bloom syndrome [3].

Adenocarcinomas

The most significant risk factor for the development of esophageal AC is gastroesophageal reflux disease (GERD). Chronic reflux causes the squamous epithelium to undergo columnar metaplasia to Barrett esophagus (BE) which in turn may become increasingly dysplastic and eventually evolve into AC. Although most cases of BE are sporadic, several familial clusters have been reported [3]. Other risk factors include smoking (particularly in BE patients), obesity, *Helicobacter pylori* infections (inverse association) [8], use of drugs that decrease lower esophageal pressure (nitroglycerine, beta agonists, anticholinergics), prior cholecystectomy, and exposure to N-nitroso compounds. Alcohol is not associated with increased risk of AC, which may be lessened with wine consumption. COX2 inhibition with nonsteroidal anti-inflammatory drugs is not protective. There is also a suggestion that there might be a protective effect with cereal fiber and antioxidants [7].

Clinical Presentation

The most common presenting symptom is progressive dysphagia (90%) leading to weight loss. Other findings include odynophagia, chest pain, cough, and fever associated with possible tracheoesophageal fistulas, hoarseness associated with tumor involvement of the recurrent laryngeal nerve, and melena resulting from intraluminal bleeding. Patients with bleeding tumors may experience significant fatigue from anemia.

Anatomy, Pathology, and Pathways of Spread

The esophagus is broken down into three regions; cervical, thoracic, and gastroesophageal junction (GEJ). The cervical esophagus starts from the inferior aspect of the cricoid cartilage at the cricopharyngeus muscle to the thoracic inlet or sternal notch. These cancers tend to behave more like head and neck cancers. The thoracic esophagus starts at the thoracic inlet and continues to the diaphragmatic hiatus. The thoracic esophagus is further subdivided into upper, middle, and distal esophageal subsites. The upper esophagus starts at the thoracic inlet at 18–20 cm (location in the esophagus is measured from the incisors) and extends to the level of the tracheal bifurcation at 23–25 cm. The mid-thoracic esophagus starts at the tracheal bifurcation and extends midway down to the GEJ at 32 cm. The distal esophagus starts at 32 cm and extends down to the GEJ, roughly 40 cm from the incisors. GEJ cancers involve the squamocolumnar transition and are further subdivided by the Siewert classification into three classes [9]. Siewert type 1 AC start in the distal esophagus and usually arise from an area with specialized intestinal metaplasia and may infiltrate the GEJ from above. Siewert type 2 tumors arise immediately adjacent to the GEJ. Siewert type 3 tumors start subcardially and extend superiorly to or past the GEJ and distal esophagus. Typically, most SCC arise in the upper and middle esophagus, while AC mostly occur in the distal esophagus and GEJ [4].

Pathways of nodal spread are dictated by tumor location, but all cancers can spread locally to invade local structures and distantly to the lungs, liver, bones, abdomen, peritoneum, and less likely, brain. Regionally, cervical esophageal cancers spread regionally to cervical, scalene, supraclavicular nodes, and mediastinal nodes. Upper and middle esophageal cancers spread to supraclavicular, mediastinal, and periesophageal lymph nodes. Tumors above the carina have a higher incidence of involved supraclavicular lymph nodes. Tumors of the distal esophagus and GEJ, involve periesophageal, celiac, perigastric, and gastrohepatic ligament lymph nodes. Siewert type 3 tumors behave more like gastric cancers and spread to periportal, peripancreatic, periduodenal, perigastric, and paraaortic nodes.

Diagnostic Workup

Diagnosis of esophageal cancer is usually through direct visualization through esophagogastroduodenoscopy with biopsy of suspicious lesions. Endoscopic ultrasound (EUS) staging is done for staging of the primary tumor, to assess invasion of local structures, for determination of resectability (invasion of pleura, pericardium or diaphragm versus aorta, trachea, bronchus, and vertebral body), and regional lymph node status, unless other examinations have already identified distant metastases. Contrast-enhanced computed tomography (CT) of the thorax and abdomen alone and in conjunction with positron emission tomography (PET-CT), and EUS are used for staging [3]. PET utilizing [18 F]-fluorodeoxyglucose is more sensitive compared to CT alone or EUS for detecting the presence of metastatic disease [10–12]. PET-CT scans have been shown to affect the surgical management of up to 20% of patients [13]. While PET-CT scans are more sensitive and specific than CT, they complement each other in that a CT scan will further verify any false positives and negatives from PET-CT as most tumors have to be at least 1 cm for PET-CT detection. Finally, bronchoscopy should be performed in patients with upper or middle esophageal cancers to rule out airway invasion, tracheoesophageal fistula, and determine the need for tracheal stents. Restaging after chemoradiation with EUS, esophagogastroduodenoscopy with biopsy, and PET-CT has been examined to determine response. However, none of these techniques has a high accuracy for determining complete response pathologically. McLoughlin *et al.* reported that the accuracy of a negative PET-CT after chemoradiation was 56% for predicting a pathologic complete response [14]. A study of postchemoradiation EUS predicted for complete response in only 17% of patients [15]. Finally, a negative endoscopic biopsy after chemoradiation had a negative predictive value of only 31% [16].

Staging

The American Joint Committee on Cancer and 8th Edition Cancer Staging Manual for esophageal cancer includes separate staging for SCC and AC, and incorporation of tumor grade and location to the overall staging classification (Table 3.1) [17, 18].

Table 3.1 American Joint Committee on Cancer (AJCC) 8th edn. Esophageal cancer staging.

Definition of primary tumor (T)

Squamous cell carcinoma and adenocarcinoma

T category	T criteria
TX	Tumor cannot be assessed
T0	No evidence of primary tumor
Tis	High-grade dysplasia, defined as malignant cells confined to the epithelium by the basement membrane
T1	Tumor invades the lamina propria, muscularis mucosae, or submucosa
T1a	Tumor invades the lamina propria or muscularis mucosae
T1b	Tumor invades the submucosa
T2	Tumor invades the muscularis propria
T3	Tumor invades adventitia
T4	Tumor invades adjacent structures
T4a	Tumor invades the pleura, pericardium, azygos vein, diaphragm, or peritoneum
T4b	Tumor invades other adjacent structures, such as the aorta, vertebral body, or airway

Definition of regional lymph nodes (N)

Squamous cell carcinoma and adenocarcinoma

N category	N criteria
NX	Regional lymph nodes cannot be assessed
N0	No regional lymph node metastasis
N1	Metastasis in one or two regional lymph nodes
N2	Metastasis in three to six regional lymph nodes
N3	Metastasis in seven or more regional lymph nodes

Definition of distant metastasis (M)

Squamous cell carcinoma and adenocarcinoma

M category	M criteria
M0	No distant metastasis
M1	Distant metastasis

Definition of histologic grade (G)

Squamous cell carcinoma and adenocarcinoma

G	G definition
GX	Grade cannot be assessed
G1	Well differentiated
G2	Moderately differentiated
G3	Poorly differentiated, undifferentiated

(*Continued*)

Table 3.1 (Continued)

Definition of location (L)

Squamous cell carcinoma

Location plays a role in the stage grouping of esophageal squamous cancers

Location category	Location criteria
X	Location unknown
Upper	Cervical esophagus to lower border of azygos vein
Middle	Lower border of azygos vein to lower border of inferior pulmonary vein
Lower	Lower border of inferior pulmonary vein to stomach, including gastroesophageal junction

Note: location is defined by the position of the epicenter of the tumor in the esophagus

AJCC prognostic stage groups

Squamous cell carcinoma

Clinical (cTNM)

When cT is...	And cN is...	And M is...	Then the stage group is...
Tis	N0	M0	0
T1	N0–1	M0	I
T2	N0–1	M0	II
T3	N0	M0	II
T3	N1	M0	III
T1–3	N2	M0	III
T4	N0–2	M0	IVA
Any T	N3	M0	IVA
Any T	Any N	M1	IVB

Pathological (pTNM)

When pT is...	And pN is...	And M is	And G is...	And location is...	Then the stage group is...
Tis	N0	M0	N/A	Any	0
T1a	N0	M0	G1	Any	IA
T1a	N0	M0	G2–3	Any	IB
T1a	N0	M0	GX	Any	IA
T1b	N0	M0	G1–3	Any	IB
T1b	N0	M0	GX	Any	IB
T2	N0	M0	G1	Any	IB
T2	N0	M0	G2–3	Any	IIA
T2	N0	M0	GX	Any	IIA
T3	N0	M0	Any	Lower	IIA
T3	N0	M0	G1	Upper/middle	IIA
T3	N0	M0	G2–3	Upper/middle	IIB
T3	N0	M0	GX	Any	IIB
T3	N0	M0	Any	Location X	IIB
T1	N1	M0	Any	Any	IIB

Table 3.1 (Continued)

Pathological (pTNM)

When pT is...	And pN is...	And M is	And G is...	And location is...	Then the stage group is...
T1	N2	M0	Any	Any	IIIA
T2	N1	M0	Any	Any	IIIA
T2	N2	M0	Any	Any	IIIB
T3	N1–2	M0	Any	Any	IIIB
T4a	N0–1	M0	Any	Any	IIIB
T4a	N2	M0	Any	Any	IVA
T4b	N0–2	M0	Any	Any	IVA
Any T	N3	M0	Any	Any	IVA
Any T	Any N	M1	Any	Any	IVB

Postneoadjuvant therapy (ypTNM)

When yp T is...	And yp N is...	And M is...	Then the stage group is...
T0–2	N0	M0	I
T3	N0	M0	II
T0–2	N1	M0	IIIA
T3	N1	M0	IIIB
T0–3	N2	M0	IIIB
T4a	N0	M0	IIIB
T4a	N1–2	M0	IVA
T4a	NX	M0	IVA
T4b	N0–2	M0	IVA
Any T	N3	M0	IVA
Any T	Any N	M1	IVB

Adenocarcinoma

Clinical (cTNM)

When cT is...	And cN is...	And M is...	Then the stage group is...
Tis	N0	M0	0
T1	N0	M0	I
T1	N1	M0	IIA
T2	N0	M0	IIB
T2	N1	M0	III
T3	N0–1	M0	III
T4a	N0–1	M0	III
T1-T4a	N2	M0	IVA
T4b	N0–2	M0	IVA
Any T	N3	M0	IVA
Any T	Any N	M1	IVB

(*Continued*)

Table 3.1 (Continued)

Pathological (pTNM)

When pT is...	And pN is...	And M is...	And G is...	Then the stage group is...
Tis	N0	M0	N/A	0
T1a	N0	M0	G1	IA
T1a	N0	M0	GX	IA
T1a	N0	M0	G2	IB
T1b	N0	M0	G1–2	IB
T1b	N0	M0	GX	IB
T1	N0	M0	G3	IC
T2	N0	M0	G1–2	IC
T2	N0	M0	G3	IIA
T2	N0	M0	GX	IIA
T1	N1	M0	Any	IIB
T3	N0	M0	Any	IIB
T1	N2	M0	Any	IIIA
T2	N1	N0	Any	IIIA
T2	N2	M0	Any	IIIB
T3	N1–2	M0	Any	IIIB
T4a	N0–1	M0	Any	IIIB
T4a	N2	M0	Any	IVA
T4b	N0–2	M0	Any	IVA
Any T	N3	M0	Any	IVA
Any T	Any N	M1	Any	IVB

Postneoadjuvant therapy (ypTNM)

When yp T is...	And yp N is...	And M is...	Then the stage group is...
T0–2	N0	M0	I
T3	N0	M0	II
T0–2	N1	M0	IIIA
T3	N1	M0	IIIB
T0–3	N2	M0	IIIB
T4a	N0	M0	IIIB
T4a	N1–2	M0	IVA
T4a	NX	M0	IVA
T4b	N0–2	M0	IVA
Any T	N3	M0	IVA
Any T	Any N	M1	IVB

Source: Rice *et al.* [17]. Used with permission of the American College of Surgeons, Chicago, Illinois. The original source for this information is the AJCC Cancer Staging Manual, 8th edn (2017), which is published by Springer Science + Business Media.

Prevention and Screening

Barrett Esophagus

Barrett esophagus (BE) is the metaplastic replacement of the stratified squamous esophageal epithelium with columnar epithelium. It is thought to occur from chronic GERD [20]. BE is the most important identifiable risk factor for esophageal adenocarcinoma. The American College of Gastroenterology has defined BE as an endoscopically recognized change in the esophageal epithelium that is confirmed to have intestinal metaplasia by biopsy [21]. Prospective studies have documented the progression from BE to low-grade dysplasia (LGD), high-grade dysplasia (HGD), and eventually, invasive adenocarcinoma [22]. In addition, there is a gastric-type BE that has been described. In a series of patients with gastric-type dysplasia, it was noted that neoplastic progression occurred in 64% of patients with pure gastric and 26% of patients with mixed gastric-intestinal dysplasia [23]. While esophagectomy is a standard treatment for HGD and T1 tumors, locally ablative therapies like endoscopic mucosal resection, radiofrequency ablation, photodynamic therapy, and cryotherapy have now started to play a significant role in the management of these lesions [24]. However, the accuracy of EUS staging for T1 tumors has been called into question [25]. Tumor depth was correctly staged by EUS in only 39% of pT1a tumors and 51% of pT1b tumors. Of the EUS staged cT1a (lamina propria) cN0 lesions, there were positive lymph nodes in 15% of pathologic specimens. Patients with pT1a (muscularis mucosa) lesions had a 9% rate of pathologic lymph node involvement, and those with pT1b tumors had a 17% rate of lymph node spread. In addition, while AC can be successfully treated with chemoradiation, this treatment will not eradicate the BE, and any remaining dysplastic epithelium is prone to forming *de novo* cancers. Either surgical resection with negative BE margins or ablative therapies mentioned above must be performed after chemoradiation to eliminate this high risk dysplasia [3, 26, 27].

Treatment of GERD and Chemoprevention

The American Gastroenterological Association (AGA) supports the use of GERD therapy for symptom relief of reflux esophagitis in BE patients [28]. For patients without symptoms of GERD or signs of reflux esophagitis, proton pump inhibitors (PPIs) can be used to reduce the risk of neoplastic progression of dysplasia, regardless of the lack of prospective trials. PPIs have been shown to cause BE regression, while H2 blockers did not. In a randomized, double-blind study of ranitidine (an H2 blocker) versus omeprazole (a PPI), it was noted that omeprazole had a greater degree of acid suppression and that there was a statistically significant regression of BE compared to no change with ranitidine [29]. A large prospective study demonstrated that patients who used PPIs had a significantly reduced risk of developing HGD or AC, whereas there was no benefit seen with H2 blockers [30]. Epidemiologic studies suggested a BE prevention benefit to nonsteroidal anti-inflammatory drugs, specifically >325 mg aspirin [31]. A meta-analysis also confirmed that aspirin use was inversely associated with the incidence of AC in BE patients [32]. However, a chemoprevention trial with a COX-2 inhibitor, celecoxib, failed to prevent progression of BE to HGD and ultimately AC [33]. Finally, the combination of statins and aspirin appears to provide a synergistic protection against neoplastic progression of BE compared to aspirin [34].

Screening and Surveillance

The 2011 AGA guidelines for the management of BE suggest screening for BE if multiple risk factors associated with esophageal AC (age 50 years or older, male sex, white race, chronic GERD, hiatal hernia, elevated body mass index, or intra-abdominal distribution of body fat) are present [28]. The AGA recommended against screening the general population with GERD for BE. For patients with BE, GERD therapy to treat symptoms and to heal reflux esophagitis is clearly indicated, as it is for patients without BE. The diagnosis of dysplasia in BE should be confirmed by at least one additional pathologist, preferably one who is an expert in esophageal histopathology. Endoscopic surveillance is suggested for patients with BE every 3–5 years if there is no dysplasia, every 6–12 months for LGD, and every 3 months for HGD. Use of biomarkers to confirm histologic diagnosis of LGD or HGD is not recommended. Endoscopic eradication therapy with radiofrequency ablation, photodynamic therapy, or endoscopic resection rather than surveillance is recommended for treatment of patients with confirmed HGD within BE. Endoscopic resection is recommended for patients who have dysplasia in BE associated with a visible mucosal irregularity.

Treatment

The three treatment modalities involved in the treatment of esophageal carcinoma include surgery, chemotherapy, and radiation therapy. While the treatment sections have been organized into each specific modality, multimodality treatment is usually required and is strongly influenced by stage. Treatment recommendations by stage are displayed in Table 3.2.

Surgery

Single modality surgery was the mainstay of treatment for esophageal cancer prior to use of neoadjuvant multimodality techniques (see later sections). There is a direct correlation of outcome and institutional volume. Patients who undergo esophagectomy at high volume centers have lower treatment-related mortality rates, better survival, and significantly shorter hospital length of stay when compared to low volume institutions [35, 36]. This is likely related to many factors including surgeon experience [37], and the institution's ability to deal with complications that require multidisciplinary management, dedicated intensive care teams, skilled nursing, respiratory therapy, clinical care pathways, and availability of certain therapeutic equipment.

Technique

Transthoracic or Transhiatal Esophagectomy

Transhiatal esophagectomy (THE) and transthoracic esophagectomy (TTE Ivor-Lewis esophagectomy) are the two most common techniques performed. The choice of technique depends on a number of factors including extent of lymphadenectomy, tumor location, and surgeon's preference. THE involves a mobilization

Table 3.2 Treatment recommendations by stage.

Stage	Surgical status	Recommendation
T1aN0M0	-	1) Endoscopic mucosal resection followed by endoscopic ablation 2) Esophagectomy* (if flat or ulcerated lesion not amenable to endoscopic removal)
T1bN0M0	Medically operable	Esophagectomy*
	Medically inoperable	Definitive CRT**
T2N0M0	Medically operable	1) Esophagectomy* (well differentiated and <2 cm) 2) Preoperative CRT
	Medically inoperable	Definitive CRT**
T1-2 N1-3 M0 and T3-4aN0-3 M0	Medically operable	1) Preoperative CRT 2) Induction chemo, preoperative CRT (if radiation field would be excessively large) 3) Preoperative chemo (for adenocarcinoma and GEJ tumors)
	Medically inoperable	1) Definitive CRT** 2) Induction chemo, definitive CRT**
T4bN0-3 M0	Unresectable	1) Definitive CRT** 2) Induction chemo, definitive CRT**
TxNxM1	Inoperable by stage	Systemic chemotherapy +/- palliative stent, radiation, or brachytherapy

CRT, chemoradiotherapy; GEJ, gastroesophageal junction.
*Consider adjuvant chemotherapy or chemoradiation based on high risk pathologic features like positive margins or positive lymph nodes.
**Consider brachytherapy boost for local residual disease.

1. Radiation dose: (i) definitive is 45–50.4 Gy; (ii) preoperative is 41.4–50.4 Gy.
2. Concurrent chemotherapy regimens include: (i) cisplatin (75 mg/m^2 on week 1 and week 5) and weekly protracted venous infusion 5-FU (225 mg/m^2; over 5 days); (ii) weekly carboplatin and taxol (use lower range of radiation dose due to pneumonitis issues); (iii) biweekly oxaliplatin and protracted venous infusion 5-FU (225 mg/m^2; over 5 days); (iv) protracted venous infusion 5-FU (225 mg/m^2; over 5 days) in the adjuvant setting.
3. Brachytherapy boost dose is 9–15 Gy in three fractions prescribed to surface (brachytherapy should be avoided if there is involvement or close proximity to airway due to tracheoesophageal fistula).

of the stomach with sparing of the gastroepipolic artery, upper abdominal lymphadenectomy, blunt dissection of the thoracic esophagus, and a left cervical esophagogastric anastomosis [38]. TTE also requires mobilization of the stomach with an upper abdominal lymphadenectomy, but differs from the transhiatal approach in that a right thoracotomy with radial dissection around the thoracic esophagus with its surrounding mediastinal lymphatic tissue is performed. The anastomosis is created within the thoracic space. The theoretical advantage with the thoracic approach is the oncological resection of the mediastinal lymph nodes and wider radial margin of the primary tumor. There are modifications of both techniques that have been described [39]. The perioperative morbidity and mortality of the two techniques was compared in a randomized trial [40]. A total of 220 patients were assigned to either a THE or TTE approach. The trial concluded that perioperative morbidity was higher with the TTE with no significant difference in in-hospital mortality or overall survival. THE was associated with a shorter operative time, lower blood loss, fewer pulmonary complications, decreased chylous leaks, shorter duration of mechanical ventilation, and shorter stay in the intensive care unit and hospital. Similar results were confirmed in a meta-analysis involving 7,527 patients from 50 studies with either TTE or THE obtaining a 5-year survival of 20% [41]; however, THE showed an increased incidence of anastomotic leaks and recurrent laryngeal nerve injury.

Minimally Invasive Esophagectomy Techniques

Multiple transhiatal and transthoracic minimally invasive esophagectomy (MIE) approaches have been described combining thoracoscopic and/or laparoscopic procedures. The first attempts at MIE involved thoracoscopic esophageal mobilization, laparotomy for gastric mobilization, and a cervical anastomosis. The morbidity of a thoracotomy was avoided while allowing for complete mediastinal dissection. This technique has been reported by several groups with excellent results [39]. Relative contraindications to laparoscopy may include prior major abdominal resections. Contraindications to thoracoscopy include extensive pleural adhesions, prior pneumonectomy, bulky tumors, and locally infiltrative tumors, especially those with airway involvement. Finally, while it has been recommended that MIE should not be performed in patients treated with neoadjuvant therapy [42], others have found MIE can safely be performed after induction therapy [33, 43]. MIE is a technically advanced surgical procedure associated with a prolonged learning curve and it has been noted that at least 17 cases are required to gain technical expertise and 35 cases have to be performed to observe differences in blood loss, postoperative pulmonary infection, and number of lymph nodes retrieved [44, 45]. Major intraoperative complications include bleeding, tracheobronchial injury, and recurrent laryngeal nerve injury have been reported with MIE [39]. A randomized controlled trial was conducted in esophageal cancer comparing MIE (59 patients) versus open esophagectomy (56 patients) [46]. Pulmonary infection in the first 2 weeks was noted in 16 (29%) patients in the open esophagectomy group versus five (9%) patients in the MIE group (relative risk (RR) 0.30, 95% CI 0.12–0.76). In-hospital pulmonary infection was noted in 19 (34%) patients in the open esophagectomy group versus seven (12%) patients in the minimally invasive group (0.35, 0.16–0.78).

Robotic Esophagectomy

While laparoscopic THE is an ideal choice of procedure, several problems arise including the instrumentation, the narrow field of the mediastinum, and the two-dimensional view. Robotic systems may overcome some of these limitations. This technique provides magnified three-dimensional visualization and greater range of instrument motion allowing for diminished intraoperative complications which have been reported by several groups [39]. de la Fuente *et al.* reported on a large series of robotic-assisted Ivor-Lewis (RAIL) esophagectomies with a hand-assisted laparosopic abdominal approach [47]. In the first 50 patients that underwent RAIL [47], the median number of lymph nodes resected was 18.5 and all patients achieved an R0 resection. Postoperative complications occurred in 14 (28%) patients, including atrial fibrillation in five (10%), pneumonia in five (10%), anastomotic leak in one (2%), and chyle leak in two (4%). The median intensive care unit stay and length of hospitalization were 2 and 9 days respectively. Total mean operating time calculated from time of skin incision to wound closure was 445 minutes; however, operative times decreased over time. Similarly, there was a trend toward lower complications after the first 29 cases but this did not reach statistical significance. There were no in-hospital mortalities. Hernandez *et al.* reported that the learning curve to become proficient in performing RAIL was 20 cases [48]. Currently, TTE, THE, MIE, and RAIL are all considered appropriate surgical options, with optimal choices among these depending on the tumor location, patient preference, and the surgeon's preference and experience [3, 49].

PET-CT and Surgery

PET-CT may identify which patients might benefit from surgery [14, 50]. A series from Wake Forest showed that there was no benefit to surgery if patients had a negative PET-CT scan after induction therapy [50]. In contrast, a series from the Moffitt Cancer Center showed that in 81 patients, a negative and positive postchemoradiotherapy PET-CT scan had positive predictive values for predicting pathologic complete response and residual disease of 35% and 70%, respectively [14].

Role of Surgery

The role of surgery in the management of locally advanced esophageal cancer is controversial. Surgery alone is reserved for patients with HGD, or with T1N0, or T2N0 esophageal cancers. However, caution must be exercised when patients are staged as T2N0 by EUS as it has been shown that almost 50% are upstaged at the time of surgery [51]. While there are no data to address the role of surgery in AC, three randomized trials conducted by the Germans, French, and Chinese have addressed the role of esophagectomy in SCC [52–54]. All three trials showed no difference in overall survival comparing definitive versus preoperative treatment. In the German and French trials, while there was no difference in overall survival, there was a significant difference in local control and disease-free survival in favor of surgery; however, there was also higher treatment-related mortality associated with surgery. A meta-analysis of these three randomized trials of 512 patients comparing definitive chemoradiation versus preoperative chemoradiation followed by surgery or surgery alone revealed no difference in survival or morbidity but treatment-related mortality risk was lower in the definitive chemoradiation group (HR 7.6; 95% CI: 1.76–32.88) [55]. Based on these results, one may conclude that for SCC of the esophagus, patients undergoing surgery may benefit from local control and disease-free survival but are at significantly increased risk of treatment-related mortality. While prospective data and meta-analysis show no survival benefit to surgery after chemoradiation for SCC, there is a disease-free survival and local control benefit. It would seem reasonable to offer surgery for SCC patients who have biopsy-proven residual disease 6–12 weeks after treatment. For patients with AC, surgery should be part of a multimodality treatment regimen.

Radiation Without Chemotherapy

Radiation therapy alone is considered palliative. Local control and survival are poor despite combining with surgery either preoperatively or postoperatively [1, 2, 56]. Local recurrence rates have been reported as high as 77% with standard fractionation [56, 57]. In a retrospective review, radiation therapy alone resulted in a 5-year overall survival of 6% [58]. Several attempts were made to improve local control and survival by combining radiation and surgery. A meta-analysis of five randomized trials of 1147 patients was conducted to assess the benefit of neoadjuvant radiation versus surgery alone [59] but only showed a trend for increased survival with preoperative radiation ($P = 0.06$).

Chemotherapy

Preoperative Chemotherapy

There are several trials examining the benefit of preoperative chemotherapy in esophageal and GEJ cancers (Table 3.3). A survival benefit was reported in four trials [60–64]. A common finding in these trials is that response to therapy confers a survival benefit compared to nonresponse (Table 3.3). Responders are more likely to attain an R0 resection. While the MAGIC trial was conducted for gastric cancer, 25% of the patients had distal esophageal and GEJ cancer. In the MAGIC trial, 503 patients with gastric, distal esophageal, or gastroesophageal junction AC were randomized to surgery alone or three cycles of epirubicin, cisplatin, and 5-FU (ECF) given perioperatively [62]. There was a significant overall survival benefit associated with perioperative ECF (5 year overall survival 36% vs 23%, $P = 0.009$). In a trial similar to the MAGIC trial, Ychou *et al.* examined the role of perioperative cisplatin and 5-FU in gastric, distal esophageal, or gastroesophageal junction AC [64]; however, distal esophageal and GEJ adenocarcinomas comprised 75% of patients. There was a significant survival benefit associated with chemotherapy with a 5-year overall survival of 38% versus 24% ($P = 0.02$). In a trial by Boonstra *et al.*, 169 patients with esophageal SCC were randomized to surgery alone versus preoperative cisplatin and 5-FU [61]. Five-year survival in the combined modality group was 27% versus 17% for surgery alone ($P = 0.03$). While an Radiation Therapy Oncology Group (RTOG) trial failed to show a survival benefit with preoperative cisplatin and 5-FU [65], a similar trial by the Medical Research Council in Europe showed a significant survival benefit (5-year survival 23% vs 17%, $P = 0.03$) with the addition of cisplatin and 5-FU preoperatively for esophageal cancer [60, 63]. There were notable differences between the two trials including twice as many patients randomized, fewer cycles of chemotherapy delivered preoperatively, more adenocarcinomas, and more patients going to surgery in the Medical Research Council trial.

Table 3.3 Trials of neoadjuvant chemotherapy versus surgery alone.

Study	*n*	Histology	Chemotherapy	Response (%)	Responders' survival	Survival	*P*
Roth [104]	19	100% SCC	Cisplatin/vind/bleomycin	47	MS	MS 9 m	ns
	20		None		20 m vs 6 m		
Nygaard [105]	50	100% SCC	None	–	–	9% (3 y)	0.32
	58		Cisplatin/bleomycin			3%	
	56		None[1]			21%	
	53		Cisplatin/bleomycin[1]			17%	
Schlag [106]	22	100% SCC	Cisplatin/5-FU	50	MS	MS 10 m	ns
	24		None		13 m vs 5 m		
Maipang [107]	24	100% SCC	Cisplatin/vinb/bleomycin	53	–	31% (3 y)	ns
	22		None			36%	
Law [108]	74	100% SCC	Cisplatin/5-FU	58	MS	MS 17 m	ns
	73		None		42 m vs 8 m	MS 13 m	
Boonstra [61]	85	100% SCC	Cisplatin/etoposide	38	–	26%	0.03
	84		None			17%	
Kelsen [65]	216	52% AC	Cisplatin/5-FU	19	MS	23% (3 y)	ns
	227		None		3.3 y vs 1.1 y	26%	
Ancona [109]	48	100% SCC	Cisplatin/5-FU	40	5 y	42% (4 y)	ns
	48		None		60% vs 12%	28%	
Cunningham [62][2]	250	100% AC	Epirubicin/cisplatin/5-FU	–	–	36% (5 y)	0.009
	253		None			23%	
Allum [60, 63]	400	67% AC	Cisplatin/5-FU	–	–	23% (5 y)	0.03
	402		None			17%	
Ychou [64][3]	113	100% AC	Cisplatin/5-FU	–	–	38% (5y)	0.02
	111		None			24%	

[1] Radiation therapy to 35 Gy given sequentially.
[2] 25% distal esophagus and gastroesophageal junction.
[3] 75% distal esophagus and gastroesophageal junction.
vind, vindesin; vinb, vinblastine; 5-FU, fluorouracil; AC, adenocarcinoma; SCC, squamous cell carcinoma; MS, median survival; ns, not significant; m, months; y, years.

Several meta-analyses examining survival after chemotherapy or chemoradiotherapy and surgery compared to surgery alone for esophageal cancer have been performed (Table 3.4). With the exception of Greer *et al.* [66], all analyses [55, 67–71] show a significant reduction in mortality associated with neoadjuvant chemoradiation. However, some do show a significantly higher treatment-related mortality with chemoradiation [67, 69, 70]. The most recent meta-analysis of 12 randomized trials encompassing 1,854 patients demonstrated that the hazard ratio for all-cause mortality for neoadjuvant chemoradiotherapy was 0.78 (95% CI: 0.7–0.88; P <0.0001). In addition, the benefit was maintained for both SCC (HR 0.80; 95% CI: 0.68–0.93; P=0.004) and AC (HR 0.75; 95% CI: 0.59–0.95; P=0.02) [71]. The survival benefit of neoadjuvant chemotherapy for esophageal cancer has also been investigated [55, 68, 71] (Table 3.3). While two analyses show a significant reduction in mortality with preoperative chemotherapy [68, 71], the benefit is restricted to AC with no apparent benefit in SCC.

Adjuvant Chemotherapy

There are limited data to support adjuvant chemotherapy in esophageal cancer; however, it may be recommended in patients with pathologically positive lymph nodes. Adjuvant chemotherapy after chemoradiotherapy and/or surgery is poorly tolerated and only 50% of patients are able to complete the prescribed regimens [56, 62, 64, 72]. There is little prospective data to support adjuvant chemotherapy after neoadjuvant chemoradiotherapy. There are three trials of adjuvant chemotherapy after initial surgery and all were negative for a survival benefit [73–75]. However, a meta-analysis reported from China of seven trials encompassing 864 patients noted a 3-year survival benefit with adjuvant chemotherapy (RR 0.89; 95% CI: 0.71–0.95; P=0.009) [76].

PET-CT and Chemotherapy

One consistent finding is that the response to chemotherapy does confer a survival benefit and does increase the likelihood of an R0 resection. PET-CT has been used to monitor response to treatment as well [77–80]. A cut-off value of 35% change in PET standardized uptake value predicted for survival (P=0.04). This result led to the MUNICON trial [78], in which patients with distal esophageal or gastroesophageal cancer had a PET after one cycle of induction chemotherapy. Responders (defined as decrease in standardized uptake value by 35%) continued chemotherapy prior to resection and nonresponders went directly to surgery. While the median survival was not reached in responders, nonresponders had a median survival of 26 months (P=0.015). In a follow-up study, MUNICON II addressed the role of salvage chemoradiation in PET nonresponders in patients with GEJ cancer [81]. Two-year overall survival for responders and nonresponders was 71% versus 42%, respectively (P=0.1).

Chemoradiation

Definitive Chemoradiotherapy

Randomized controlled data show benefit to adding mitomycin C or cisplatin-based regimens concurrent with radiation [1, 2]. Bleomycin regimens concurrent with radiation showed no benefit [82]. An Eastern Cooperative Oncology Group randomized trial that utilized concurrent mitomycin C-5FU with radiation in 119 patients with esophageal SCC showed a statistically significant difference in median overall survival of 14.8 months with chemotherapy compared to 9.3 months without chemotherapy. A significant survival benefit was shown with cisplatin-5FU-radiation (50.4 Gy) compared to radiation alone to 64.8 Gy in the RTOG 85-01 trial [56]. Most of the patients had SCC. The trial was stopped after the first interim analysis showed a significant survival benefit, and additional patients were enrolled in the chemoradiation arm only. The 5-year updated survival for all patients receiving chemoradiation was 27% versus 0% for radiation alone patients [83]. Despite the survival benefit, almost 50% of patients had residual disease at 1 year. This result led to investigation of dose escalation concurrent with radiation. The intergroup 0123 trial randomized patients to chemoradiation to 50.4 Gy versus 64.8 Gy [84]. There was no benefit to dose escalation and even a suggestion of a survival detriment. A meta-analysis showed a significant survival benefit to concurrent chemoradiation while there was no benefit to sequential chemotherapy and radiation [85].

Neoadjuvant Chemoradiation

Several randomized trials have been conducted to determine the benefit from neoadjuvant chemoradiotherapy [1, 2] (Table 3.5). However, these trials were either underpowered, had poor performing control arms, or failed to show a significant survival benefit. Most recently, the CROSS trial showed a significant survival benefit to neoadjuvant chemoradiation [86]. In this trial, 368 patients were randomized to neoadjuvant chemoradiation with 41.4 Gy over 4.5 weeks concurrent with weekly carboplatin and paclitaxel followed by surgery versus surgery alone. An R0 resection was obtained in 92% of chemoradiation patients versus 69% in the surgery only patients (P <0.001). Pathologic complete response was documented in 29% of chemoradiation patients. With a median follow-up of 45 months, median and 5-year overall survival was 49.4 months and 47% for the chemoradiation group versus 24 months and 34% for the surgery only group (P=0.003). The benefit of neoadjuvant chemoradiation was noted in both SCC (univariate HR 0.453, P=0.011; multivariate HR 0.422, P=0.007) and AC (univariate HR 0.732, P=0.049; multivariate HR 0.741, P=0.07). Most importantly, the local and peritoneal recurrence rate was significantly lower with preoperative chemoradiation [87].

Several meta-analyses have been published to examine survival after chemoradiotherapy and surgery compared to surgery alone for esophageal cancer (Table 3.4). All analyses [55, 67–71] show a survival benefit to neoadjuvant chemoradiation with the exception of Greer *et al.* [66]. Three of the analyses do show a significantly higher treatment-related mortality with chemoradiation [67, 69, 70]. The most recent and largest meta-analysis identified 12 randomized trials of 1,854 patients comparing chemoradiation and surgery versus surgery alone. The hazard ratio for all-cause mortality for neoadjuvant chemoradiotherapy was 0.78 (P <0.0001) and the benefit was maintained for both SCC (HR 0.80; P=0.004) and AC (HR 0.75; P=0.02) [71]. The overall recurrence rate in the surgery arm was 58% versus 35% in the CRT plus surgery arm. Preoperative chemoradiation reduced locoregional recurrence from 34 to 14% (P <0.001) and

Table 3.4 Meta-analyses of preoperative chemotherapy or chemoradiation versus surgery.

Study (year)	Therapy	No. of Studies	*n*	RR/OR/HR (95% CI)	*P*-value
Urschel [70] 2003	CRT	9	1116	0.66 (0.47–0.92) (3 y survival)	0.016
				1.6 (0.99–2.68) (postop mortality)	0.053
Fiorica [67] 2004	CRT	6	764	0.53 (0.31–0.93) (survival)	0.03
				2.1 (1.18–3.73) (postop mortality)	0.01
Greer [66] 2005	CRT	6	738	0.86 (0.74–1.01)	0.07
Gebski [68] 2007	CRT	10	1209	0.81 (0.7–0.93)	0.002
	Chemo	8	1724	0.90 (0.81–1.00) (all) 0.78 (0.64–0.95) (AC) 0.88 (0.75–1.03) (SCC)	0.05 (all) 0.014 (AC) 0.12 (SCC)
Jin [69] 2009	CRT	11	1308	1.46 (1.07–1.99) (5 y survival)[1]	0.02
				1.7 (1.03–2.73) (postop mortality)	0.02
Kranzfelder [55] 2011 (100% SCC)	CRT	9	1099	0.81 (0.7–0.95)	0.008
	Chemo	8	1707	0.93 (0.81–1.08)	0.368
Sjoquist [71] 2011	CRT	12	1854	0.78 (0.7–0.88)	<0.0001
	Chemo	9	1981	0.87 (0.79–0.96) (all) 0.83 (0.71–0.95) (AC) 0.92 (0.81–1.04) (SCC)	0.05 (all) 0.01 (AC) 0.18 (SCC)

AC, adenocarcinoma; CI, confidence interval; CRT, chemoradiotherapy; HR, hazard ratio; OR, odds ratio; RR, relative risk; SCC, squamous cell carcinoma.

[1] No benefit in SCC.

peritoneal carcinomatosis from 14 to 4% (P <0.001). There was a small but significant effect on hematogenous dissemination in favor of the chemoradiation group (35% vs 29%; $P = 0.025$) [87].

Preoperative Chemotherapy Versus Chemoradiotherapy

The German POET study addressed whether neoadjuvant chemoradiation added to preoperative chemotherapy would benefit patients with GEJ cancers. This was a randomized trial of GEJ AC comparing preoperative chemotherapy and surgery versus preoperative chemotherapy followed by chemoradiation and surgery [88]. It was planned to enroll 354 patients; unfortunately, the trial was stopped due to poor accrual after 125 patients were enrolled. The induction chemotherapy regiment was cisplatin, leucovorin, and 5-FU. Radiation (30 Gy in 3 weeks) was delivered concurrently with cisplatin and etoposide. A trend for increased survival was observed in the chemoradiation arm where 3-year survival in the patients receiving radiation was 47% versus 27% for unirridiated patients ($P = 0.07$).

Adjuvant Chemoradiotherapy

Results for the INT0116 trial established adjuvant chemoradiotherapy as the standard of care in patients with node-positive adenocarcinoma of the stomach and GEJ [72]. A total of 556 patients with resected GEJ or stomach adenocarcinoma were randomized to surgery alone (control arm) or surgery plus adjuvant chemoradiotherapy (experimental arm). Chemoradiation was 45 Gy over 5 weeks with infusional 5-FU. Median and 3-year overall survival was increased from 27 months and 41% in the control group to 36 months and 50% in the chemoradiotherapy group ($P = 0.005$). In a three-arm Chinese study of stage II and III SCC of the esophagus, patients were randomized to surgery alone, preoperative chemoradiation, and postoperative chemoradiation [89]. Chemoradiation was 40 Gy in 4 weeks concurrent with cisplatin and taxol. There was a significant improvement in overall survival in patients treated with postoperative and preoperative chemoradiation.

Brachytherapy

Esophageal brachytherapy (BT) is an intraluminal treatment of radiation therapy applied directly to the tumor. It consists of the placement of a catheter down the esophagus with subsequent application of a tethered radioactive source administered down the tube to deliver a very high dose of radiation directly to the luminal component of the tumor. Treatments are short in duration and allow for better sparing of normal surrounding tissues such as the lungs, heart, and liver when compared to external beam radiation therapy. BT has been used primarily in two settings: as palliation for locally advanced obstructing or bleeding tumors and as a boost to external beam radiation therapy for definitive management of nonsurgical candidates. BT has been investigated for its use as a boost after external beam radiation therapy with or without chemotherapy. However, a trial by Calais *et al.* and RTOG 92-07 [90, 91] concluded that survival was no different with the addition of BT. Additionally, caution must be taken given the risk for fistulas. The high fistula rate in the RTOG trial was likely due to the high BT dose delivered concurrently with chemotherapy. In regards to palliation, metal stents have shown benefit in relieving dysphagia [24]. In a multicenter Dutch study [92], patients with dysphagia due to unresectable esophageal cancer were randomized to placement of a stent ($n = 108$) or single dose (12 Gy) BT ($n = 101$). Dysphagia improved more rapidly after stent placement compared to BT, but long-term relief of dysphagia was better with BT. Higher complication rates were noted with stent placement (33% versus 21%; $P = 0.02$). The groups did not differ with regard to the incidence of persistent or recurrent dysphagia or median survival (P >0.20). In the long term, quality-of-life scores were higher in the brachytherapy group.

Technique

Chemoradiation for esophageal cancers has resulted in increased survival over radiation or surgery alone; however, it is fraught with high rates of acute toxicity and long-term esophagitis, strictures, pneumonitis, and pericarditis. This necessitates hospital admissions, feeding tube placement, and stent placements. Historically, radiation to the esophagus was delivered with two-dimensional techniques (as in RTOG 8501) utilizing a barium esophagram approach that treated a large volume of normal tissue. This significantly changed with the advent of CT scans and computer software that allowed patients to be scanned in the treatment position and so that the intended dose could be shaped three-dimensionally by three-dimensional conformal radiotherapy (3DCRT), utilizing customized shaped blocks to maximize the dose to the intended target and minimize the dose to the surrounding healthy tissue. More recently, intensity modulated radiation therapy (IMRT) has been utilized in the clinical setting. IMRT requires advanced treatment planning software to deliver nonuniform radiation through a series of beamlets that vary the intensity of dose across tumor–normal tissue interfaces. The beamlets can be produced through multiple prechosen beam angles or through a volumetric 360° arc delivery of a continuously modulated photon beam [1]. However, IMRT requires precise delineation of target volumes which can be achieved with either fiducial marker placement or fusion of PET scans to the treatment planning CT [93]. In addition, respiratory motion of the target volume has to be considered and addressed with either creating a larger target volume or using abdominal compression to limit respiratory excursion. Finally, daily variation of gastric distention can dramatically affect dosing of target volumes which may require planning and treatment on empty stomachs. Finally, daily image guidance with cone-beam CTs will aid in better target localization [1, 94, 95].

Comparative outcomes of IMRT versus 3DCRT have been reported. A Chinese study compared the outcomes of 60 esophageal cancer patients treated with either IMRT or 3DCRT concurrent with cisplatin and docetaxel. A total dose of 64 Gy was delivered in 30 fractions [96]. Response rates were higher in the IMRT group, but there was no difference in survival. An MD Anderson study compared outcomes of 676 esophageal cancer patients treated between 1998 and 2008 with IMRT or 3DCRT, with concurrent chemotherapy [97]. The IMRT patients were less likely to receive induction chemotherapy, had better performance status, and were less likely to die but more likely to have first failure be distant. The IMRT group was superior with respect to overall survival (P <0.001) and locoregional recurrence ($P = 0.0038$). There were no differences seen in cancer-related mortality or distant metastasis between the two groups. Most

Table 3.5 Trials of neoadjuvant chemoradiation versus surgery alone.

Study	*n*	Histology	Chemoradiation regimen	Pathologic complete response (%)	Overall survival	*P*-value
Walsh [110]	58 55	100% AC	40 Gy (3 weeks)/cisplatin/5-FU None	25	MS 16 m vs 11 m 3 y 32% vs 6%	0.01
Urba [111]	50 50	75% AC	45 Gy (1.5 Gy BID)/cisplatin/5-FU/Vinb None	28	MS 17 m vs 18 m 3 y 30% vs 16%	0.15
Lee [112]	51 50	100% SCC	45.6 Gy (1.2 Gy BID)/cisplatin/5-FU None	43	MS 28 m vs 27 m	0.69
Burmeister [113]	128 128	62% AC	35 Gy (3 weeks)/cisplatin/5-FU None	14	MS 29 m vs 19 m	0.57
Tepper [114]	30 26	75% AC	50.4 Gy (5.5 weeks)/cisplatin/5-FU None	40	MS 4.5 y vs 1.8 y 5 y 39% vs 16%	0.002
Lv [89]	80 80	100% SCC	40 Gy (4 weeks)/cisplatin/taxol None	NR	MS 53 m vs 36 m 5 y 44% vs 34%	0.04
Mariette [115]	97 98	71% SCC	45 Gy (5 weeks)/cisplatin/5-FU None	NR	MS 32 m vs 45 m 3 y 49% vs 55%	0.68
van Hagen [116]	180 188	75% AC	41.4 Gy (4.5 weeks)/carboplatin/taxol None	29	MS 49 m vs 24 m 5 y 47% vs 34%	0.003

AC, adenocarcinoma; BID, twice daily; 5-FU, 5-fluorouracil; MS, median survival; m, months; NR, not reported; SCC, squamous cell carcinoma; Vinb, vinblastine; y, years.

recently, Freilich *et al.* reported on a series of 232 (138 IMRT, 94 3DCRT) patients with esophageal cancer treated with 3DCRT or IMRT [94]. Median dose was 50.4 Gy (range 44–64.8) to gross disease. There was no significant difference based on radiation technique with respect to overall survival, but IMRT was associated with a significant decrease in acute grade ≧3 toxicity on univariate and multivariate analysis.

Biologic Therapy

Epidermal Growth Factor Receptor

Epidermal growth factor receptor (EGFR) expression correlates with poor prognosis and radioresistance [98]. While several phase II studies showed promise in esophageal cancer in the phase II setting with the addition of anti-EGFR antibodies [98], randomized controlled trials failed to show a survival benefit. Two randomized controlled trials looked at the role of targeted therapy with an anti-EGFR antibody, cetuximab, in combination with chemoradiotherapy for definitive treatment of esophageal cancer. The SCOPE-1 trial was a randomized phase II/III trial where patients with esophageal carcinoma (73% SCC) were treated with capecitabine-cisplatin-50 Gy with or without cetuximab [99]. They unfortunately did not meet their phase II endpoint and the trial was stopped after 258 patients were enrolled. Overall results were detrimental with the addition of cetuximab. Not only was there increased toxicity leading to increased failure to complete treatment, median survival was significantly worse in patients receiving cetuximab. After the report of this trial, accrual to the ongoing RTOG 0436 trial addressing the role of cetuximab was halted. Results were presented at the 2014 GI ASCO meeting. This was a phase III trial for patients with esophageal carcinoma treated with cisplatin-paclitaxel-50.4 Gy with or without cetuximab [100]. There was no difference in survival, toxicity, or response rate.

Human Epidermal Growth Factor Receptor-2

Amplification of the human epidermal growth factor receptor-2 (*HER2*) gene and overexpression of its protein product is involved in a variety of malignancies including GEJ AC and correlates with a poor prognosis [101]. A large randomized phase III trial of HER2-positive metastatic gastric or GEJ adenocarcinoma, Trastuzumab for Gastric Cancer, was conducted to assess the benefit of adding trastuzamab to cisplatin-5FU or a cisplatin-capecitabine doublet [102]. On intent-to-treat analysis, there was a significant improvement in median survival in patients receiving trastuzamab (13.8 months versus 11.1 months; $P = 0.0046$). Response rate, time to progression, and duration of response were significantly higher in the trastuzumab plus chemotherapy group as well. RTOG 1010 is a randomized phase III trial of HER2-positive mid to distal esophageal and GEJ adenocarcinoma being randomized to concurrent chemoradiation with carboplatin-paclitaxel-50.4 Gy versus carboplatin-paclitaxel-trastuzamab-50.4 Gy, with the primary endpoint being disease-free survival. National Comprehensive Cancer Network guidelines recommend addition of trastuzumab to chemotherapy regimens for patients with HER2-overexpressing and/or *HER2*-amplified metastatic esophageal adenocarcinoma [3].

Other Targets and Agents

Ramucirumab is a recombinant monoclonal antibody to VEGFR-2 that is approved for second-line treatment of gastroesophageal adenocarcinoma. Several clinical trials of immune checkpoint inhibitors are in progress [103].

Follow-up and Survivorship

Guidelines for follow-up have been established by the National Comprehensive Cancer Network [3]. For patients with *in situ* or T1a disease amenable to ablative techniques, assessment with endoscopic surveillance should occur every 3 months for 1 year, then annually. For patients who undergo an R0 resection, observation is recommended. For R1 resections, adjuvant chemoradiation is recommended. If a patient received preoperative chemoradiation, then either observation or adjuvant chemotherapy is recommended. For patients with locally advanced disease treated with definitive chemoradiation, response assessment must be performed at 6–12 weeks after treatment. If there is no persistent disease, then history and physical examination, and nutritional counseling should be performed every 3–6 months for 1–2 years, then every 6–12 months for 3–5 years, then annually. Chemistry, complete blood counts, imaging, and endoscopy should be done only as clinically indicated.

Long-term side effects from chemoradiation include benign esophageal strictures requiring dilation or stent (12%), radiation pneumonitis (2%), pericardial and pleural effusions (2%), rehabilitation and hospitalization (16%), and requirement of feeding tube for nutrition (7%) [94]. Tracheoesophageal fistulas may occur after chemoradiation, but are most likely not due to treatment, but rather to progression of cancer. Aspiration and speech paralysis may occur after surgery due to recurrent laryngeal nerve injury.

References

1 Shridhar R, Almhanna K, Meredith KL, *et al.* Radiation therapy and esophageal cancer. *Cancer Control* 2013;20(2):97–110.

2 Shridhar R, Imani-Shikhabadi R, Davis B, Streeter OA, Thomas CR, Jr. Curative treatment of esophageal cancer; an evidenced based review. *J Gastrointest Cancer* 2013:44(4):375–84.

3 NCCN Clinical Practice Guidelines in Oncology. Esophageal and Esaophagogastric Junction Cancers, Version 2.2016. nccn.org (accessed 18 January 2017).

4 Siegel RL, Miller KD, Jemal A. Cancer statistics, 2017. *CA Cancer J Clin* 2017;67(1):7–30.

5 Howlader N, Noone AM, Krapcho M (eds). *SEER Cancer Statistics Review, 1975–2013, National Cancer Institute.* Bethesda, MD, http://seer.cancer.gov/csr/1975_2013/, based on November 2015 SEER data submission, posted to the SEER web site, April 2016.

6 Torre LA, Bray F, Siegel RL, *et al.* Global cancer statistics, 2012. *CA Cancer J Clin* 2015;65(2):87–108.
7 Gibson M. Epidemiology, Pathobiology, and Clinical Manifestations of Esophageal Cancer, *UpToDate Website. Updated February* 10, 2017. Accessed October 16, 2017. https://www.uptodate.com/contents/epidemiology-pathobiology-and-clinical-manifestations-of-esophageal-cancer?source=contentShare&csi=6fa9591b-6e41-45ce-94c9-bae062bfcd37.
8 Lagergren J, Lagergren P. Recent developments in esophageal adenocarcinoma. *CA Cancer J Clin* 2013:63(4):232–48.
9 Rüdiger Siewert J, Feith M, Werner M, Stein HJ. Adenocarcinoma of the esophagogastric junction: results of surgical therapy based on anatomical/topographic classification in 1,002 consecutive patients. *Ann Surg* 2000:232(3):353–61.
10 Flamen P, Lerut A, Van Cutsem E, *et al.* Utility of positron emission tomography for the staging of patients with potentially operable esophageal carcinoma. *J Clin Oncol* 2000;18(18):3202–10.
11 Meyers BF, Downey RJ, Decker PA, *et al.* The utility of positron emission tomography in staging of potentially operable carcinoma of the thoracic esophagus: results of the American College of Surgeons Oncology Group Z0060 trial. *J Thorac Cardiovasc Surg* 2007;133(3):738–45.
12 van Vliet EP, Heijenbrok-Kal MH, Hunink MG, Kuipers EJ, Siersema PD. Staging investigations for oesophageal cancer: a meta-analysis. *Br J Cancer* 2008;98(3):547–57.
13 Luketich JD, Friedman DM, Weigel TL, *et al.* Evaluation of distant metastases in esophageal cancer: 100 consecutive positron emission tomography scans. *Ann Thorac Surg* 1999;68(4):1133–6; discussion 1136–7.
14 McLoughlin JM, Melis M, Siegel EM, *et al.* Are patients with esophageal cancer who become PET negative after neoadjuvant chemoradiation free of cancer? *J Am Coll Surg* 2008;206(5):879–86; discussion 886–7.
15 Zuccaro G, Jr., Rice TW, Goldblum J, *et al.* Endoscopic ultrasound cannot determine suitability for esophagectomy after aggressive chemoradiotherapy for esophageal cancer. *Am J Gastroenterol* 1999;94(4):906–12.
16 Sarkaria IS, Rizk NP, Bains MS, *et al.* Post-treatment endoscopic biopsy is a poor-predictor of pathologic response in patients undergoing chemoradiation therapy for esophageal cancer. *Ann Surg* 2009;249(5):764–7.
17 Rice TW, Kelsen D, Blackstone EH, *et al.* Esophagus and esophagogastric junction. In: Amin MB, *et al.* (eds) *AJCC Cancer Staging Manual*, 8th edn. New York: Springer, 2017.
18 Rice TW, Ishwaran H, Kelsen DP, *et al.* Recommendations for neoadjuvant pathologic staging (ypTNM) of cancer of the esophagus and esophagogastric junction for the 8th edition AJCC/UICC staging manuals. *Dis Esophagus* 2016;29(8):906–12.
19 Talsma K, van Hagen P, Grotenhuis BA, *et al.* Comparison of the 6th and 7th Editions of the UICC-AJCC TNM Classification for Esophageal Cancer. *Ann Surg Oncol* 2012;19(7):2142–8.
20 Spechler SJ, Goyal RK. Barrett's esophagus. *N Engl J Med* 1986;315(6):362–71.
21 Sampliner RE and Practice Parameters Committee of the American College of Gastroenterology. Updated guidelines for the diagnosis, surveillance, and therapy of Barrett's esophagus. *Am J Gastroenterol* 2002;97(8):1888–95.
22 Hameeteman W, Tytgat GN, Houthoff HJ, van den Tweel JG. Barrett's esophagus: development of dysplasia and adenocarcinoma. *Gastroenterology* 1989;96(5 Pt 1):1249–56.
23 Mahajan D, Bennett AE, Liu X, Bena J, Bronner MP. Grading of gastric foveolar-type dysplasia in Barrett's esophagus. *Mod Pathol* 2010;23(1):1–11.
24 Vignesh S, Hoffe SE, Meredith KL, *et al.* Endoscopic therapy of neoplasia related to Barrett's esophagus and endoscopic palliation of esophageal cancer. *Cancer Control* 2013;20(2):117–29.
25 Bergeron EJ, Lin J, Chang AC, Orringer MB, Reddy RM. Endoscopic ultrasound is inadequate to determine which T1/T2 esophageal tumors are candidates for endoluminal therapies. *J Thorac Cardiovasc Surg* 2014;147(2):765–73.
26 Barthel JS, Kucera S, Harris C, *et al.* Cryoablation of persistent Barrett's epithelium after definitive chemoradiation therapy for esophageal adenocarcinoma. *Gastrointest Endosc* 2011;74(1):51–7.
27 Barthel JS, Kucera ST, Lin JL, *et al.* Does Barrett's esophagus respond to chemoradiation therapy for adenocarcinoma of the esophagus? *Gastrointest Endosc* 2010;71(2):235–40.
28 American Gastroenterological Association. American Gastroenterological Association medical position statement on the management of Barrett's esophagus. *Gastroenterology* 2011;140(3):1084–91.
29 Peters FT, Ganesh S, Kuipers EJ, *et al.* Endoscopic regression of Barrett's oesophagus during omeprazole treatment; a randomised double blind study. *Gut* 1999;45(4):489–94.
30 Kastelein F, Spaander MC, Steyerberg EW, *et al.* Proton pump inhibitors reduce the risk of neoplastic progression in patients with Barrett's esophagus. *Clin Gastroenterol Hepatol* 2013;11(4):382–8.
31 Omer ZB, Ananthakrishnan AN, Nattinger KJ, *et al.* Aspirin protects against Barrett's esophagus in a multivariate logistic regression analysis. *Clin Gastroenterol Hepatol* 2012;10(7):722–7.
32 Abnet CC, Freedman ND, Kamangar F, *et al.* Non-steroidal anti-inflammatory drugs and risk of gastric and oesophageal adenocarcinomas: results from a cohort study and a meta-analysis. *Br J Cancer* 2009;100(3):551–7.
33 Heath EI, Canto MI, Piantadosi S, *et al.* Secondary chemoprevention of Barrett's esophagus with celecoxib: results of a randomized trial. *J Natl Cancer Inst* 2007;99(7):545–57.
34 Kastelein F, Canto MI, Piantadosi S, *et al.* Nonsteroidal anti-inflammatory drugs and statins have chemopreventative effects in patients with Barrett's esophagus. *Gastroenterology* 2011;141(6):2000–8; quiz e13–4.
35 Markar SR, Karthikesalingam A, Thrumurthy S, Low DE. Volume-outcome relationship in surgery for esophageal malignancy: systematic review and meta-analysis 2000–2011. *J Gastrointest Surg* 2012;16(5):1055–63.
36 Birkmeyer JD, Siewers AE, Finlayson EV, *et al.* Hospital volume and surgical mortality in the United States. *N Engl J Med* 2002;346(15):1128–37.
37 Derogar M, Sadr-Azodi O, Johar A, Lagergren P, Lagergren J. Hospital and surgeon volume in relation to survival after esophageal cancer surgery in a population-based study. *J Clin Oncol* 2013;31(5):551–7.

38 Barreto JC, Posner MC. Transhiatal versus transthoracic esophagectomy for esophageal cancer. *World J Gastroenterol* 2010;16(30):3804–10.

39 Yamamoto M, Weber JM, Karl RC, Meredith KL. Minimally invasive surgery for esophageal cancer: review of the literature and institutional experience. *Cancer Control* 2013;20(2):130–7.

40 Hulscher JB, van Sandick JW, de Boer AG, *et al.* Extended transthoracic resection compared with limited transhiatal resection for adenocarcinoma of the esophagus. *N Engl J Med* 2002;347(21):1662–9.

41 Hulscher JB, Tijssen JG, Obertop H, van Lanschot JJ. Transthoracic versus transhiatal resection for carcinoma of the esophagus: a meta-analysis. *Ann Thorac Surg* 2001; 72(1):306–13.

42 Nakatsuchi T, Otani M, Osugi H, Ito Y, Koike T. The necessity of chest physical therapy for thoracoscopic oesophagectomy. *J Int Med Res* 2005;33(4):434–41.

43 Luketich JD, Alvelo-Rivera M, Buenaventura PO, *et al.* Minimally invasive esophagectomy: outcomes in 222 patients. *Ann Surg* 2003;238(4):486–94; discussion 494–5.

44 Osugi H, Takemura M, Higashino M, *et al.* Learning curve of video-assisted thoracoscopic esophagectomy and extensive lymphadenectomy for squamous cell cancer of the thoracic esophagus and results. *Surg Endosc* 2003;17(3):515–9.

45 Osugi H, Takemura M, Lee S, *et al.* Thoracoscopic esophagectomy for intrathoracic esophageal cancer. *Ann Thorac Cardiovasc Surg* 2005;11(4):221–7.

46 Biere SS, van Berge Henegouwen MI, Maas KW, *et al.* Minimally invasive versus open oesophagectomy for patients with oesophageal cancer: a multicentre, open-label, randomised controlled trial. *Lancet* 2012;379(9829):1887–92.

47 de la Fuente SG, Weber J, Hoffe SE, *et al.* Initial experience from a large referral center with robotic-assisted Ivor Lewis esophagogastrectomy for oncologic purposes. *Surg Endosc* 2013;27(9):3339–47.

48 Hernandez JM, Dimou F, Weber J, *et al.* Defining the learning curve for robotic-assisted esophagogastrectomy. *J Gastrointest Surg* 2013;17(8):1346–51.

49 Qureshi YA, Dawas KI, Mughal M, Mohammadi B. Minimally invasive and robotic esophagectomy: evolution and evidence. *J Surg Oncol* 2016;114(6):731–5.

50 Monjazeb AM, Dawas KI, Mughal M, Mohammadi B. Outcomes of patients with esophageal cancer staged with [(1) F]fluorodeoxyglucose positron emission tomography (FDG-PET): can postchemoradiotherapy FDG-PET predict the utility of resection? *J Clin Oncol* 2010;28(31):4714–21.

51 Crabtree TD, Kosinski AS, Puri V, *et al.* Evaluation of the reliability of clinical staging of T2 N0 esophageal cancer: a review of the Society of Thoracic Surgeons database. *Ann Thorac Surg* 2013;96(2):382–90.

52 Bedenne L, Michel P, Bouché O, *et al.* Chemoradiation followed by surgery compared with chemoradiation alone in squamous cancer of the esophagus: FFCD 9102. *J Clin Oncol* 2007;25(10):1160–8.

53 Chiu PW, Chan AC, Leung SF, *et al.* Multicenter prospective randomized trial comparing standard esophagectomy with chemoradiotherapy for treatment of squamous esophageal cancer: early results from the Chinese University Research Group for Esophageal Cancer (CURE). *J Gastrointest Surg* 2005;9(6):794–802.

54 Stahl M, Stuschke M, Lehmann N, *et al.* Chemoradiation with and without surgery in patients with locally advanced squamous cell carcinoma of the esophagus. *J Clin Oncol* 2005;23(10):2310–7.

55 Kranzfelder M, Schuster T, Geinitz H, Friess H, Büchler P. Meta-analysis of neoadjuvant treatment modalities and definitive non-surgical therapy for oesophageal squamous cell cancer. *Br J Surg* 2011;98(6):768–83.

56 Herskovic A, Martz K, al-Sarraf M, *et al.* Combined chemotherapy and radiotherapy compared with radiotherapy alone in patients with cancer of the esophagus. *N Engl J Med* 1992;326(24):1593–8.

57 John MJ, Flam MS, Mowry PA, *et al.* Radiotherapy alone and chemoradiation for nonmetastatic esophageal carcinoma. A critical review of chemoradiation. *Cancer* 1989;63(12):2397–403.

58 Earlam R, Cunha-Melo JR. Oesophogeal squamous cell carcinoms: II. A critical view of radiotherapy. *Br J Surg* 1980;67(7):457–61.

59 Arnott SJ, Duncan W, Gignoux M, *et al.* Preoperative radiotherapy for esophageal carcinoma. *Cochrane Database Syst Rev* 2005(4):CD001799.

60 Allum WH, Stenning SP, Bancewicz J, Clark PI, Langley RE. Long-term results of a randomized trial of surgery with or without preoperative chemotherapy in esophageal cancer. *J Clin Oncol* 2009;27(30):5062–7.

61 Boonstra JJ, Kok TC, Wijnhoven BP, *et al.* Chemotherapy followed by surgery versus surgery alone in patients with resectable oesophageal squamous cell carcinoma: long-term results of a randomized controlled trial. *BMC Cancer* 2011;11:181.

62 Cunningham D, Allum WH, Stenning SP, *et al.* Perioperative chemotherapy versus surgery alone for resectable gastroesophageal cancer. *N Engl J Med* 2006;355(1):11–20.

63 Medical Research Council Oesophageal Cancer Working Group. Surgical resection with or without preoperative chemotherapy in oesophageal cancer: a randomised controlled trial. *Lancet* 2002;359(9319):1727–33.

64 Ychou M, Boige V, Pignon JP, *et al.* Perioperative chemotherapy compared with surgery alone for resectable gastroesophageal adenocarcinoma: an FNCLCC and FFCD multicenter phase III trial. *J Clin Oncol* 2011;29(13):1715–21.

65 Kelsen DP, Winter KA, Gunderson LL, *et al.* Long-term results of RTOG trial 8911 (USA Intergroup 113): a random assignment trial comparison of chemotherapy followed by surgery compared with surgery alone for esophageal cancer. *J Clin Oncol* 2007;25(24):3719–25.

66 Greer SE, Goodney PP, Sutton JE, Birkmeyer JD. Neoadjuvant chemoradiotherapy for esophageal carcinoma: a meta-analysis. *Surgery* 2005;137(2):172–7.

67 Fiorica F, Di Bona D, Schepis F, *et al.* Preoperative chemoradiotherapy for o esophageal cancer: a systematic review and meta-analysis. *Gut* 2004;53(7):925–30.

68 Gebski V, Burmeister B, Smithers BM, *et al.* Survival benefits from neoadjuvant chemoradiotherapy or chemotherapy in oesophageal carcinoma: a meta-analysis. *Lancet Oncol* 2007;8(3):226–34.

69 Jin HL, Zhu H, Ling TS, Zhang HJ, Shi RH. Neoadjuvant chemoradiotherapy for resectable esophageal carcinoma: a meta-analysis. *World J Gastroenterol* 2009; 15(47):5983–91.

70 Urschel JD, Vasan H. A meta-analysis of randomized controlled trials that compared neoadjuvant chemoradiation and surgery to surgery alone for resectable esophageal cancer. *Am J Surg* 2003;185(6):538–43.

71 Sjoquist KM, Burmeister BH, Smithers BM, *et al.* Survival after neoadjuvant chemotherapy or chemoradiotherapy for resectable oesophageal carcinoma: an updated meta-analysis. *Lancet Oncol* 2011;12(7):681–92.

72 Macdonald JS, Smalley SR, Benedetti J, *et al.* Chemoradiotherapy after surgery compared with surgery alone for adenocarcinoma of the stomach or gastroesophageal junction. *N Engl J Med* 2001;345(10):725–30.

73 Ando N, Iizuka T, Kakegawa T, *et al.* A randomized trial of surgery with and without chemotherapy for localized squamous carcinoma of the thoracic esophagus: the Japan Clinical Oncology Group Study. *J Thorac Cardiovasc Surg* 1997;114(2):205–9.

74 Ando N, Iizuka T, Ide H, *et al.* Surgery plus chemotherapy compared with surgery alone for localized squamous cell carcinoma of the thoracic esophagus: a Japan Clinical Oncology Group Study–JCOG9204. *J Clin Oncol* 2003;21(24):4592–6.

75 Pouliquen X, Levard H, Hay JM. 5-Fluorouracil and cisplatin therapy after palliative surgical resection of squamous cell carcinoma of the esophagus. A multicenter randomized trial. French Associations for Surgical Research. *Ann Surg* 1996;223(2):127–33.

76 Huang WZ, Fu JH, Hu Y, Zhang X, Yang H. [Meta-analysis of postoperative adjuvant chemotherapy for localized esophageal carcinoma]. *Ai Zheng* 2006;25(10):1303–6.

77 Downey RJ, Akhurst T, Ilson D, *et al.* Whole body 18FDG-PET and the response of esophageal cancer to induction therapy: results of a prospective trial. *J Clin Oncol* 2003;21(3):428–32.

78 Lordick F, Ott K, Krause BJ, *et al.* PET to assess early metabolic response and to guide treatment of adenocarcinoma of the oesophagogastric junction: the MUNICON phase II trial. *Lancet Oncol* 2007;8(9):797–805.

79 Weber WA, Ott K, Becker K, *et al.* Prediction of response to preoperative chemotherapy in adenocarcinomas of the esophagogastric junction by metabolic imaging. *J Clin Oncol* 2001;19(12):3058–65.

80 Wieder HA, Brücher BL, Zimmermann F, *et al.* Time course of tumor metabolic activity during chemoradiotherapy of esophageal squamous cell carcinoma and response to treatment. *J Clin Oncol* 2004;22(5):900–8.

81 zum Buschenfelde CM, Herrmann K, Schuster T, *et al.* (18) F-FDG PET-guided salvage neoadjuvant radiochemotherapy of adenocarcinoma of the esophagogastric junction: the MUNICON II trial. *J Nucl Med* 2011;52(8):1189–96.

82 Araujo CM, Souhami L, Gil RA, *et al.* A randomized trial comparing radiation therapy versus concomitant radiation therapy and chemotherapy in carcinoma of the thoracic esophagus. *Cancer* 1991;67(9):2258–61.

83 Cooper JS, Guo MD, Herskovic A, *et al.* Chemoradiotherapy of locally advanced esophageal cancer: long-term follow-up of a prospective randomized trial (RTOG 85-01). *Radiation Therapy Oncology Group. JAMA* 1999;281(17):1623–7.

84 Minsky BD, Pajak TF, Ginsberg RJ, *et al.* INT 0123 (Radiation Therapy Oncology Group 94-05) phase III trial of combined-modality therapy for esophageal cancer: high-dose versus standard-dose radiation therapy. *J Clin Oncol* 2002;20(5):1167–74.

85 Wong R, Malthaner R. Combined chemotherapy and radiotherapy (without surgery) compared with radiotherapy alone in localized carcinoma of the esophagus. *Cochrane Database Syst Rev* 2006(1):CD002092.

86 van Hagen P, Hulshof MC, van Lanschot JJ, *et al.* Preoperative chemoradiotherapy for esophageal or junctional cancer. *N Engl J Med* 2013;366(22):2074–84.

87 Oppedijk V, van der Gaast A, van Lanschot JJ, *et al.* Patterns of recurrence after surgery alone versus preoperative chemoradiotherapy and surgery in the CROSS Trials. *J Clin Oncol* 2014;32(5):385–91.

88 Stahl M, Walz MK, Stuschke M, *et al.* Phase III comparison of preoperative chemotherapy compared with chemoradiotherapy in patients with locally advanced adenocarcinoma of the esophagogastric junction. *J Clin Oncol* 2009;27(6):851–6.

89 Lv J, Cao XF, Zhu B, *et al.* Long-term efficacy of perioperative chemoradiotherapy on esophageal squamous cell carcinoma. *World J Gastroenterol* 2010;16(13):1649–54.

90 Calais G, Dorval E, Louisot P, *et al.* Radiotherapy with high dose rate brachytherapy boost and concomitant chemotherapy for Stages IIB and III esophageal carcinoma: results of a pilot study. *Int J Radiat Oncol Biol Phys* 1997;38(4):769–75.

91 Gaspar LE, Qian C, Kocha WI, *et al.* A phase I/II study of external beam radiation, brachytherapy and concurrent chemotherapy in localized cancer of the esophagus (RTOG 92-07): preliminary toxicity report. *Int J Radiat Oncol Biol Phys* 1997; 37(3):593–9.

92 Homs MY, Steyerberg EW, Eijkenboom WM, *et al.* [Palliative treatment of esophageal cancer with dysphagia: more favourable outcome from single-dose internal brachytherapy than from the placement of a self-expanding stent; a multicenter randomised study]. *Ned Tijdschr Geneeskd* 2005;149(50):2800–6.

93 Fernandez D, Hoffe SE, Barthel JS, *et al.* Stability of endoscopic ultrasound-guided fiducial marker placement for esophageal cancer target delineation and image-guided radiation therapy. *Pract Radiat Oncol* 2013;3:32–39.

94 Freilich J, Hoffe SE, Almhanna K, *et al.* Comparative outcomes for 3d conformal versus intensity modulated radiation therapy for esophageal cancer. *Dis Esophagus,* 2015;28(4):352–7.

95 Shridhar R, *et al.* Outcomes of definitive or preoperative IMRT chemoradiation for esophageal cancer. *J Radiat Oncol* 2012;1(4):347–54.

96 Lin XD, Shi XY, Zhou TC, Zhang WJ. [Intensity-modulated or 3-D conformal radiotherapy combined with chemotherapy with docetaxel and cisplatin for locally advanced esophageal carcinoma]. *Nan Fang Yi Ke Da Xue Xue Bao* 2011;31(7):1264–7.

97 Lin SH, Wang L, Myles B, *et al.* propensity score-based comparison of long-term outcomes with 3-dimensional conformal radiotherapy vs intensity-modulated radiotherapy for esophageal cancer. *Int J Radiat Oncol Biol Phys* 2012;84(5):1078–85.

98 Ayyappan S, Prabhakar D, Sharma N. Epidermal growth factor receptor (EGFR)-targeted therapies in esophagogastric cancer. *Anticancer Res* 2013;33(10):4139–55.

99 Crosby T, *et al.* SCOPE 1: A phase II/III trial of chemoradiotherapy in esophageal cancer plus or minus cetuximab. *J Clin Oncol* 2012. 30 (suppl 34; abstr LBA3).

100 Suntharalingam M, *et al.* The initial report of RTOG 0436: a phase III trial evaluating the addition of cetuximab to paclitaxel, cisplatin, and radiation for patients with esophageal cancer treated without surgery. *J Clin Oncol* 2014;32(suppl 3; abstr LBA6).

101 Yonemura Y, Ninomiya I, Yamaguchi A, *et al.* Evaluation of immunoreactivity for erbB-2 protein as a marker of poor short term prognosis in gastric cancer. *Cancer Res* 1991;51(3):1034–8.

102 Bang YJ, Van Cutsem E, Feyereislova A, *et al.* Trastuzumab in combination with chemotherapy versus chemotherapy alone for treatment of HER2-positive advanced gastric or gastro-oesophageal junction cancer (ToGA): a phase 3, open-label, randomised controlled trial. *Lancet* 2010;376(9742):687–97.

103 Wang VE, Grandis JR, Ko AH. New strategies in esophageal carcinoma: Translational insights from signaling pathways and immune checkpoints. *Clin Cancer Res* 2016;22(17):4283–90.

104 Roth JA, Pass HI, Flanagan MM, *et al.* Randomized clinical trial of preoperative and postoperative adjuvant chemotherapy with cisplatin, vindesine, and bleomycin for carcinoma of the esophagus. *J Thorac Cardiovasc Surg* 1988;96(2):242–8.

105 Nygaard K, Hagen S, Hansen HS, *et al.* Pre-operative radiotherapy prolongs survival in operable esophageal carcinoma: a randomized, multicenter study of pre-operative radiotherapy and chemotherapy. The second Scandinavian trial in esophageal cancer. *World J Surg* 1992;16(6):1104–9; discussion 1110.

106 Schlag PM. Randomized trial of preoperative chemotherapy for squamous cell cancer of the esophagus. The Chirurgische Arbeitsgemeinschaft Fuer Onkologie der Deutschen Gesellschaft Fuer Chirurgie Study Group. *Arch Surg* 1992;127(12):1446–50.

107 Maipang T, Vasinanukorn P, Petpichetchian C, *et al.* Induction chemotherapy in the treatment of patients with carcinoma of the esophagus. *J Surg Oncol* 1994;56(3):191–7.

108 Law S, Fok M, Chow S, Chu KM, Wong J. Preoperative chemotherapy versus surgical therapy alone for squamous cell carcinoma of the esophagus: a prospective randomized trial. *J Thorac Cardiovasc Surg* 1997;114(2):210–7.

109 Ancona E, Ruol A, Santi S, *et al.* Only pathologic complete response to neoadjuvant chemotherapy improves significantly the long term survival of patients with resectable esophageal squamous cell carcinoma: final report of a randomized, controlled trial of preoperative chemotherapy versus surgery alone. *Cancer* 2001;91(11):2165–74.

110 Walsh TN, Noonan N, Hollywood D, *et al.* A comparison of multimodal therapy and surgery for esophageal adenocarcinoma. *N Engl J Med* 1996;335(7):462–7.

111 Urba SG, Orringer MB, Turrisi A, *et al.* Randomized trial of preoperative chemoradiation versus surgery alone in patients with locoregional esophageal carcinoma. *J Clin Oncol* 2001;19(2):305–13.

112 Lee JL, Park SI, Kim SB, *et al.* A single institutional phase III trial of preoperative chemotherapy with hyperfractionation radiotherapy plus surgery versus surgery alone for resectable esophageal squamous cell carcinoma. *Ann Oncol* 2004;15(6):947–54.

113 Burmeister BH, Smithers BM, Gebski V, *et al.* Surgery alone versus chemoradiotherapy followed by surgery for resectable cancer of the oesophagus: a randomised controlled phase III trial. *Lancet Oncol* 2005;6(9):659–68.

114 Tepper J, Krasna MJ, Niedzwiecki D, *et al.* Phase III trial of trimodality therapy with cisplatin, fluorouracil, radiotherapy, and surgery compared with surgery alone for esophageal cancer: CALGB 9781. *J Clin Oncol* 2008;26(7):1086–92.

115 Mariette C, *et al.* Surgery alone versus chemoradiotherapy followed by surgery for localized esophageal cancer: Analysis of a randomized controlled phase III trial FFCD 9901. *J Clin Oncol* 2010;28(15 s):4005.

116 van Hagen P, Hulshof MC, van Lanschot JJ, *et al.* Preoperative chemoradiotherapy for esophageal or junctional cancer. *N Engl J Med*, 2012. 366(22):2074–84.

4

Gastric Adenocarcinoma

Roger H. Kim[1], *Quyen D. Chu*[2], *and Benjamin D. Li*[3]

[1] Southern Illinois University of Medicine, Springfield, Illinois, USA
[2] Louisiana State University Health Sciences Center, Shreveport, Louisiana, USA
[3] MetroHealth Cancer Center, Cleveland, Ohio, USA

Incidence and Mortality

Gastric cancer is the fifth most common malignancy of the digestive system in the United States (US), with approximately 28,000 new cases and 10,960 deaths expected during 2017 [1]. Globally, gastric adenocarcinoma is the fifth most common malignancy overall, accounting for 951,600 estimated new cases in 2012 and representing 6.8% of all cancers [2]. Gastric cancer is the third leading cause of global cancer-related death, accounting for 723,100 estimated deaths in 2012 [2]. More than 73% of global gastric cancer cases occur in Asia [3].

While the 5-year survival rate for gastric cancer in the US remained low at 31% from 2006 to 2012, this represented an improvement over the 15% 5-year survival rate from 1975 to 1977 [4, 5]. Over the decade spanning 2004–2013, the incidence and mortality rates for gastric cancer in the US declined by 1.5% and 2.6%, respectively [5]. The incidence and mortality rates for gastric cancer are nearly twice as high in Asian Americans/Pacific Islanders, Hispanics, and African Americans as in non-Hispanic Whites [5]. The higher incidences in these ethnic groups may reflect higher rates of *Helicobacter pylori* (*H. pylori*) infection and poorer dietary patterns.

Risk Factors and Prevention

Many risk factors for gastric adenocarcinoma have been described and investigated. Table 4.1 lists the factors that have been shown to have an association with increased or decreased incidence of gastric cancer.

A higher incidence rate for gastric cancer is seen in males compared to females, at about a 2:1 ratio [5]. This ratio is relatively consistent, regardless of ethnicity. Gastric cancer incidence also increases steadily with age, with incidence rates at ages 20–24 years, 50–54 years, and 80–84 years of 0.2, 8.0, and 49.7 per 100,000 per year, respectively [5].

Dietary habits have been shown to have an influence on the risk of gastric cancer. In particular, diets high in salted foods have been shown to be associated with an increased risk of gastric cancer and gastric cancer mortality [6–9]. Conversely, fruits and vegetables have been found to have a significant protective effect, with a significant reduction in gastric cancer incidence among subjects with an intake of two to five servings of fruits and vegetables per day compared to those with less than one serving per day [10, 11]. Low vitamin C levels have been linked to increased gastric cancer incidence and some studies have shown a decreased risk of gastric cancer with higher vitamin C dietary intake [12, 13]. However, more recent therapeutic studies have failed to demonstrate a significant decrease in risk with vitamin C supplementation [14].

Other lifestyle factors have been shown to be risk factors for gastric cancer. As in many other types of malignancies, smoking increases the risk of developing gastric cancer. A recent meta-analysis revealed the relative risk of gastric cancer in smokers to be 1.53 [15]. In addition, smoking is an independent risk factor for decreased disease free survival and overall survival among gastric cancer patients [16]. Heavy alcohol intake (more than four drinks per day) was shown to have a relative risk of 1.2 for development of gastric cancer; moderate levels of alcohol intake had no apparent association with gastric cancer [17]. Overweight patients, as defined by a body mass index (BMI) greater than 25, have a higher risk of gastric cancer [18]. This association appears to strengthen with increasing BMI [18].

H. pylori infection has been repeatedly implicated as a risk factor for gastric adenocarcinoma, with one meta-analysis identifying a twofold increase in risk [19]. *H. pylori* infection appears to be particularly associated with the development of intestinal-type gastric cancer and is more commonly associated with distal gastric cancers [20]. In addition, *H. pylori* infection may have a synergistic effect with other risk factors, such as a smoking, alcohol consumption, and high salt intake [12, 21, 22]. Epstein–Barr virus has also been associated with gastric cancer [23].

The American Cancer Society's Oncology in Practice: Clinical Management, First Edition. Edited by The American Cancer Society.

Table 4.1 Risk factors and preventative factors for gastric adenocarcinoma.

Risk factors
Smoking
Salt intake
Alcohol
Helicobacter pylori infection
Epstein-Barr virus infection
Hereditary diffuse gastric cancer
Lynch syndrome
Preventative factors
Fruits/vegetables
Vitamin C

A germline mutation in CDH1 on chromosome 16, which encodes for E-cadherin, causes hereditary diffuse gastric cancer. This autosomal dominant genetic predisposition syndrome is characterized by the development of diffuse gastric cancer before the age of 40 and an increased risk of breast cancer and colon cancer [24, 25]. The risk of developing gastric cancer with known E-cadherin mutations is 70–80% [25, 26]; prophylactic gastrectomies are performed for these patients, and approximately 90% of cases reveal occult gastric carcinoma in the resected specimens [12]. Gastric cancer incidence has also been shown to be increased in patients with Lynch syndrome, or hereditary nonpolyposis colorectal cancer syndrome [27], although it appears that the natural history of gastric cancer in this syndrome is not significantly different than that of sporadic gastric cancer [28].

Pathology

Many classification systems have been proposed for the histopathologic characterization of gastric adenocarcinoma [29]. The two most widely accepted are the Lauren classification and the World Health Organization classification [29]. There are two distinct histological subtypes of gastric adenocarcinoma according to the Lauren classification: intestinal and diffuse [30]. The intestinal type is characterized by the tendency of the cells to form tubular gland-like structures, while the diffuse type demonstrates an absence of cell-to-cell interactions and is characterized by a pattern of scattered tumor cells [30]. The intestinal type occurs more frequently in male patients and in the elderly [31–35]. It has been associated with atrophic gastritis and with the aforementioned high-risk dietary habits. The diffuse subtype of gastric adenocarcinoma is more common in younger patients and in female patients; it has been demonstrated to carry a worse prognosis than the intestinal subtype [36–38]. Together, these two subtypes represent approximately 85% of gastric adenocarcinomas, with the remainder being comprised of mixed histology and other less common subtypes. In contrast to the two subtypes of the Lauren classification system, the World Health Organization classification categorizes gastric cancer into four subtypes: papillary, tubular, mucinous, and signet ring cell [39, 40].

Amplification of the human epidermal growth factor 2 gene (*HER2/neu*) and overexpression of the HER 2 protein has been demonstrated to be associated with the development of gastric and gastroesophageal junction adenocarcinomas [41, 42]. *HER2/neu* is a proto-oncogene, located on chromosome 17 and encodes a tyrosine kinase receptor, which is a member of the epidermal growth factor receptor family. *HER2/neu* gene amplification in gastric cancer occurs at a rate of 9–18%; HER2 protein overexpression occurs at rate of 8–53% [43]. HER2 overexpression is more common in the intestinal subtype of gastric cancer than the diffuse subtype [44]. The clinical significance of *HER2/neu* amplification is unclear: some studies have demonstrated that HER2-positivity is associated with poor prognosis [45–47], while others have shown that it is not an independent predictor of patient outcomes [48, 49]. In spite of this discrepancy, targeted therapy towards HER2-positive gastric adenocarcinomas has shown clinical benefit, as demonstrated in the Trastuzumab for Gastric Cancer (ToGA) study [50]. Because of this, HER2 testing is recommended for all patients with metastatic gastric cancer. Immunohistochemistry (IHC) is generally the first method used for HER2 testing. IHC scores range from 0 to 3+, based on the intensity and extent of immunostaining of tumor cells, as well as the percentage of immunoreactive tumor cells. IHC scores of 0 and 1+ are considered negative; 3+ is considered positive. An IHC score of 2+ is considered equivocal and generally followed up with fluorescence *in situ* hybridization to determine *HER2*-positivity [43].

Diagnosis

Among the reasons for the generally poor clinical outcomes for patients with gastric adenocarcinoma is that it lacks specific symptoms at an early stage. The majority of patients with early gastric cancer are either asymptomatic or have nonspecific upper abdominal pain that is usually classified as dyspepsia. Because up to 40% of the general population has dyspeptic symptoms, the utility of this symptom as a predictor of early gastric cancer is severely limited [51]. The most common presenting symptoms of early gastric cancer are epigastric pain, weight loss, and nausea/vomiting [52]. Other symptoms of gastric cancer include anorexia, gastrointestinal bleeding, and anemia [53]. Early satiety may occur due to decreased distensibility of the stomach due to diffuse involvement of the tumor, as in linitis plastica. Dysphagia can occur due to mechanical obstruction from proximal gastric tumors. Distal gastric adenocarcinomas can result in gastric outlet obstruction.

Likewise, physical signs of gastric cancer often only present in later stages. A palpable abdominal mass from either the primary tumor or a liver metastasis may be present in advanced disease. Abdominal swelling from ascites can occur either due to metastatic liver involvement or due to peritoneal carcinomatosis. Occasionally, palpable lymphadenopathy can be found, either in the left supraclavicular region (Virchow node) [54] or the periumbilical area (Sister Mary Joseph node) [55]. Additionally, a palpable ovarian mass (Krukenberg tumor) or a mass in the cul-de-sac palpable on rectal examination (Blumer shelf) may represent peritoneal spread from gastric cancer [56].

Once the diagnosis of gastric adenocarcinoma is suspected, flexible esophagogastroduodenoscopy (EGD) is the first diagnostic modality that should be employed. Although barium contrast upper gastrointestinal series radiography can identify malignant lesions, it has lower sensitivity (54% vs 92%) and specificity (91% vs 100%) than EGD [57]. This is particularly an issue in early gastric cancer, where the sensitivity of an upper gastrointestinal series can be as low as 14% [58]. In addition, EGD allows for tissue diagnosis by endoscopic biopsy of any visualized abnormality. When multiple biopsies are taken around the craters of gastric ulcers, diagnostic accuracy of EGD approaches 98% [59]. Once the histopathologic diagnosis of gastric cancer has been confirmed, a clinical staging workup can be performed.

Staging

Historically, gastric cancer has been somewhat unique among malignancies in that there were two major staging classifications in use. The American Joint Committee on Cancer (AJCC) and the Union for International Cancer Control (UICC) jointly developed the TNM staging system that is used by western hemisphere countries. This system was revised in 2016 for the 8th edition of the AJCC Staging Manual and is described in Table 4.2 [60]. The Japanese Classification of Gastric Carcinoma (JC) was developed by the Japanese Gastric Cancer Association (JGCA), formerly known as the Japanese Research Society of Gastric Carcinoma [61]. This system traditionally differed from the AJCC/UICC system in the classification of regional lymph node metastases by anatomic location, rather than number. Fortunately, the JGCA decided to comply with the AJCC/UICC system for its most recent revision of the JC, published in 2011, to allow for a unified worldwide staging system. One difference between the two staging systems was the handling of tumors of the esophagogastric junction (EGJ). The 7th edition of the AJCC had designated tumors arising in the stomach 5 cm or less from the EGJ to be staged using the TNM system for esophageal cancer rather than the staging system for gastric cancer. Fortunately, this has been revised in the 8th edition of the AJCC [60] to mirror the definition used by the JC: EGJ tumors as those arising 2 cm above to 2 cm below the EGJ, and tumors in the subcardia of the stomach as gastric adenocarcinomas [62]. The staging for gastric cancer has been markedly simplified by the agreement of the two staging systems.

The primary purpose in staging for gastric cancer is to determine the extent of disease for treatment planning. The goal of the initial workup is to classify patients into one of three groups: localized cancer (Tis or T1a), locoregional cancer, or metastatic cancer (M1). Following initial tissue diagnosis, usually obtained through upper endoscopy, a number of diagnostic modalities can be utilized: computed tomography (CT) scan, positron emission tomography (PET), magnetic resonance imaging, endoscopic ultrasound (EUS), and laparoscopic staging.

CT scan is often the first staging modality utilized in gastric cancer. If evidence of distant metastases is discovered on CT scan, it may be the only modality utilized, as further studies are unlikely to change the management. CT accuracy in identifying the presence or absence of metastatic disease ranges from 70 to

Table 4.2 American Joint Committee on Cancer (AJCC) TNM Staging Classification for Carcinoma of the Stomach (8th edn, 2017).

Primary Tumor (T)	
TX	Primary tumor cannot be assessed
T0	No evidence of primary tumor
Tis	Carcinoma *in situ*: intraepithelial tumor without invasion of the lamina propria, high grade dysplasia
T1a	Tumor invades lamina propria or muscularis mucosae
T1b	Tumor invades submucosa
T2	Tumor invades muscularis propria
T3	Tumor penetrates subserosal connective tissue without invasion of visceral peritoneum or adjacent structures
T4a	Tumor invades serosa (visceral peritoneum)
T4b	Tumor invades adjacent structures/organs
Regional Lymph Nodes (N)	
NX	Regional lymph nodes cannot be assessed
N0	No regional lymph node metastasis
N1	Metastasis in 1–2 regional lymph nodes
N2	Metastasis in 3–6 regional lymph nodes
N3a	Metastasis in 7–15 regional lymph nodes
N3b	Metastasis in 16 or more regional lymph nodes
Distant Metastasis (M)	
M0	No distant metastasis
M1	Distant metastasis

Anatomic Stage/ Prognostic Groups				5-year Overall Survival
Stage 0	Tis	N0	M0	
Stage IA	T1	N0	M0	56.7%
Stage IB	T2 T1	N0 N1	M0 M0	
Stage IIA	T3 T2 T1	N0 N1 N2	M0 M0 M0	47.3%
Stage IIB	T4a T3 T2 T1	N0 N1 N2 N3a	M0 M0 M0 M0	33.1%
Stage IIIA	T4b T4a T3 T2	N0 N1 or N2 N2 N3a	M0 M0 M0 M0	25.9%
Stage IIIB	T4b T4a T3 T2 T1	N1 or N2 N3 N3a N3b N3b	M0 M0 M0 M0 M0	
Stage IIIC	T4b T4a T3	N3a or N3b N3b N3b	M0 M0 M0	
Stage IV	Any T	Any N	M1	5.0%

Source: Used with permission of the American College of Surgeons, Chicago, Illinois. The original source for this information is the AJCC Cancer Staging Manual, 8th edn (2017), which is published by Springer Science + Business Media.

80% [63, 64]. Although CT is generally accurate at identifying hepatic metastasis, in 20–30% of patients with negative CTs, peritoneal metastases are found on exploration, whether by laparoscopy or laparotomy [65, 66]. This is because many peritoneal metastases are smaller than 5 mm, which is generally beyond the resolution of even modern CT scanners. CT is generally less accurate in determining the T (50–70%) and N-classification (50–70%) [64, 67, 68].

The use of PET scanning, often combined with CT imaging, has the limitation of decreased sensitivity due to low tracer uptake in certain gastric cancer subtypes, in particular diffuse or mucinous types [69]. PET has similar accuracy to CT scanning in terms of the T and N classifications [70]. PET scan is most useful as an adjunct to CT imaging for the detection of occult metastatic disease, as PET/CT identifies otherwise radiographically silent metastases in 10% of cases [71].

EUS is a good staging modality for gastric cancer; EUS has been found to be superior to CT in terms of determining the T classification [72]. However, improved resolution of modern CT scanners is narrowing the gap between CT and EUS [73, 74]. EUS is especially useful in determining if patients have localized disease who may be candidates for limited resection techniques. EUS has a sensitivity of 86% and a specificity of 91% in differentiating between T1/T2 and T3/T4 lesions and a sensitivity of 86% and a specificity of 91% in differentiating between T1 and T3/T4 lesions [75]. EUS is less reliable in assessing the nodal status, primarily due to the distance of certain LN stations from the ultrasound probe. However, it is important to point out that determining the N classification for gastric cancer appears to be difficult in any imaging modality. EUS is generally unreliable in detecting distant metastases, although some liver metastases are visible by EUS.

Diagnostic laparoscopy has a role in the staging of gastric cancer, because 20–30% of patients with negative preoperative imaging will have occult peritoneal metastases detected on exploration [65, 76]. Staging laparoscopy prior to definitive curative resection can allow visualization of radiographically occult, small (<5 mm) peritoneal metastases. The use of diagnostic laparoscopy in gastric cancer has been shown to alter treatment plans in 8–59% of cases, and allows an avoidance of unnecessary laparotomy in up to 40% of cases [77]. However, there remains some uncertainty about whether diagnostic laparoscopy is still useful in the era of multidetector CT scanners and whether these rates are reflective of current practice patterns. In order to increase the yield of diagnostic laparoscopy, some experts recommend limiting its application to patient with T3/T4 disease, as determined by EUS [66]. The addition of peritoneal lavage cytology to diagnostic laparoscopy may allow the further selection of patients who will not benefit from curative resection, as the presence of free cancer cells in the peritoneal cavity predicts poor prognosis similar to that of stage IV patients, even in the absence of macroscopic peritoneal disease [78, 79].

Treatment

As with most other malignancies, the modern treatment of gastric cancer is multidisciplinary in nature. Surgical resection remains the mainstay of curative treatment strategies, although endoscopic resection techniques are being developed, and laparoscopy is being investigated as a possible alternative approach to gastrectomy. The use of chemotherapy or radiation, given in the preoperative or postoperative settings, has shown an improvement in patient outcomes. Treatment decisions for patients with gastric cancer should be made based on both the initial staging and an assessment of their ability to tolerate major surgery.

Surgery

Localized gastric cancer is defined as tumors that are either *in situ* or without submucosal invasion (Tis or T1a) and without evidence of nodal involvement (N0) on preoperative staging. In patients with localized gastric cancer who are medically fit, endoscopic mucosal resection (EMR) or endoscopic submucosal dissection (ESD) are being investigated as possible alternatives to traditional gastrectomy. The rationale for endoscopic resection techniques is based on the observation that, in a series of over 5000 patients undergoing gastrectomy, no nodal involvement was present in patients with certain tumor characteristics: intestinal-type adenocarcinoma that is well-differentiated, confined to the mucosa, and either <30 mm diameter with ulceration, or any tumor size without ulceration [80]. Both EMR and ESD require specialized equipment and experienced personnel. In addition, it is important to note that EMR and ESD have not yet been compared to traditional surgical techniques for gastric cancer in a prospective trial. Furthermore, because localized gastric cancer has a low incidence in the US, the applicability of these techniques that were developed and popularized in Japan may be limited. As a general rule, the use of endoscopic techniques for the treatment of localized gastric cancer should be considered investigational at this time.

Locoregional gastric cancer is defined as tumors that are T1b or higher and have no evidence of metastatic disease (M0). For these patients who are medically fit, surgical resection with lymphadenectomy is the primary treatment option. There are two major considerations regarding the approach to surgical resection: the extent of gastrectomy and the extent of lymph node dissection.

The surgical principle guiding the decision of how much of the stomach to resect is the need to achieve adequate surgical margins, generally at least 5 cm. For tumors located in the proximal stomach, total gastrectomy is recommended. Figure 4.1 depicts a total gastrectomy with Roux-en-Y reconstruction to restore gastrointestinal tract continuity as well as provide for biliary and pancreatic drainage from the duodenum. As indicated, the proximal jejunal "Y" limb should be anastomosed to the distal jejunal "Roux" limb about 40–60 cm from the esophagojejunal anastomosis, to avoid bile reflux. Proximal subtotal gastrectomy has largely been abandoned because of significantly poorer quality of life postoperatively, in part due to a higher incidence of reflux esophagitis [81]. For tumors located in the distal stomach, a distal subtotal gastrectomy is recommended. This is based on two multicenter randomized clinical trials from France and Italy that demonstrated no difference in 5-year survival for subtotal versus total gastrectomy for distal gastric adenocarcinomas [82, 83]. Table 4.3 summarizes the results of these trials. A distal gastrectomy with Billroth II

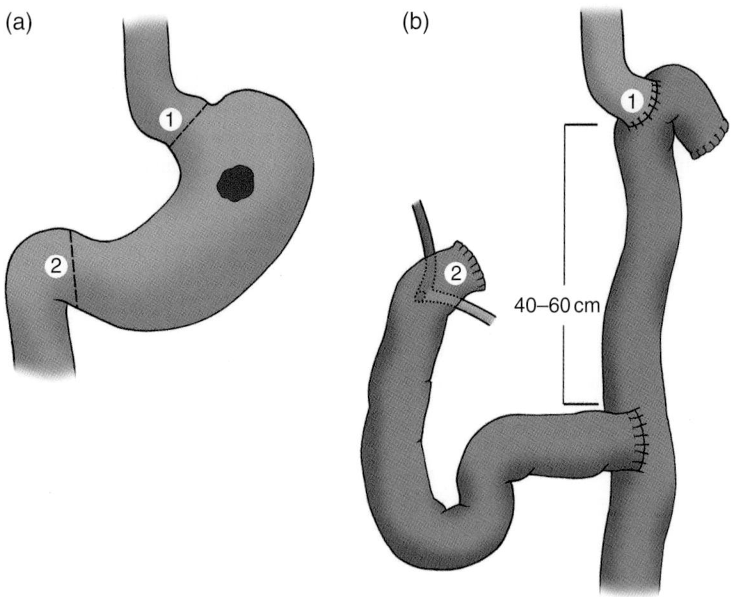

Figure 4.1 (a) Total gastrectomy for gastric cancer. (b) Roux-en-Y reconstruction after total gastrectomy. *Source:* Modified from and reproduced with permission from Chu *et al.* [142].

Table 4.3 Randomized clinical trials comparing total versus subtotal gastrectomy for distal gastric cancers.

Trial	Number of patients	Perioperative mortality (%)	Complications (%)	Five-year survival (%)
Gouzi *et al.* 1989 [82]	SG: 76 TG: 93	3.2 1.3 (*P* = ns)	34 32 (*P* = ns)	48 48 (*P* = ns)
Bozzetti *et al.* 1999 [83]	SG: 315 TG: 303	1.3 2.3	NR	65 62 (*P* = ns)

SG, subtotal gastrectomy; TG, total gastrectomy; ns, not significant; NR, not reported.

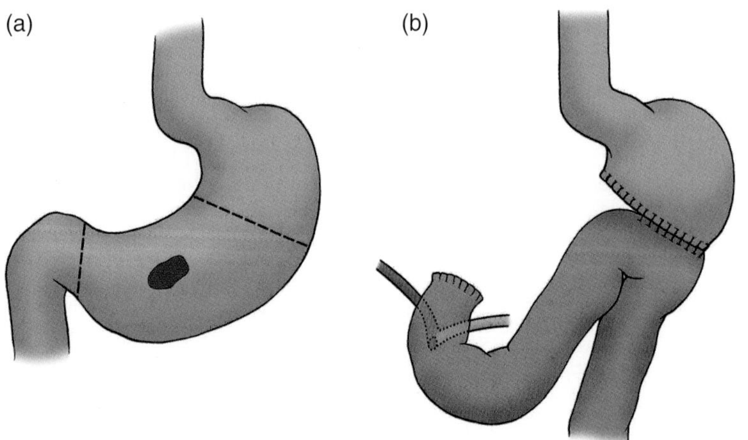

Figure 4.2 (a) Distal gastrectomy for gastric cancer. (b) Billroth II reconstruction after distal gastrectomy. *Source:* Modified from and reproduced with permission from Chu *et al.* [142].

gastrojejunostomy for reconstruction is illustrated in Figure 4.2. For a Billroth II reconstruction, the recommended length of the afferent limb is 25 cm, to minimize the risk of afferent loop syndrome that can occur if this limb is too long [84]. Some surgeons advocate a Roux-en-Y reconstruction after distal gastrectomy.

The extent of lymph node dissection that is optimal for gastric cancer has been an area of significant debate over the years. The nodal stations around the stomach are anatomically defined by the JGCA and are indicated in Figure 4.3 and Table 4.4 [85]. Removal of the perigastric lymph nodes (stations 1–6) is generally defined as a D1 lymphadenectomy. Removal of the regional lymph nodes (stations 7–11) is generally defined as a D2 lymphadenectomy, although in Japan, station 7 is included in a D1 lymph node dissection, and station 12 is included in a D2 lymph node dissection [85]. A D3 lymphadenectomy, which consists of a D2 lymphadenectomy with the addition of para-aortic nodal dissection, is associated with a higher complication rate and does not improve overall or recurrence-free survival [86]. As a result, D3 lymphadenectomy is not recommended and has

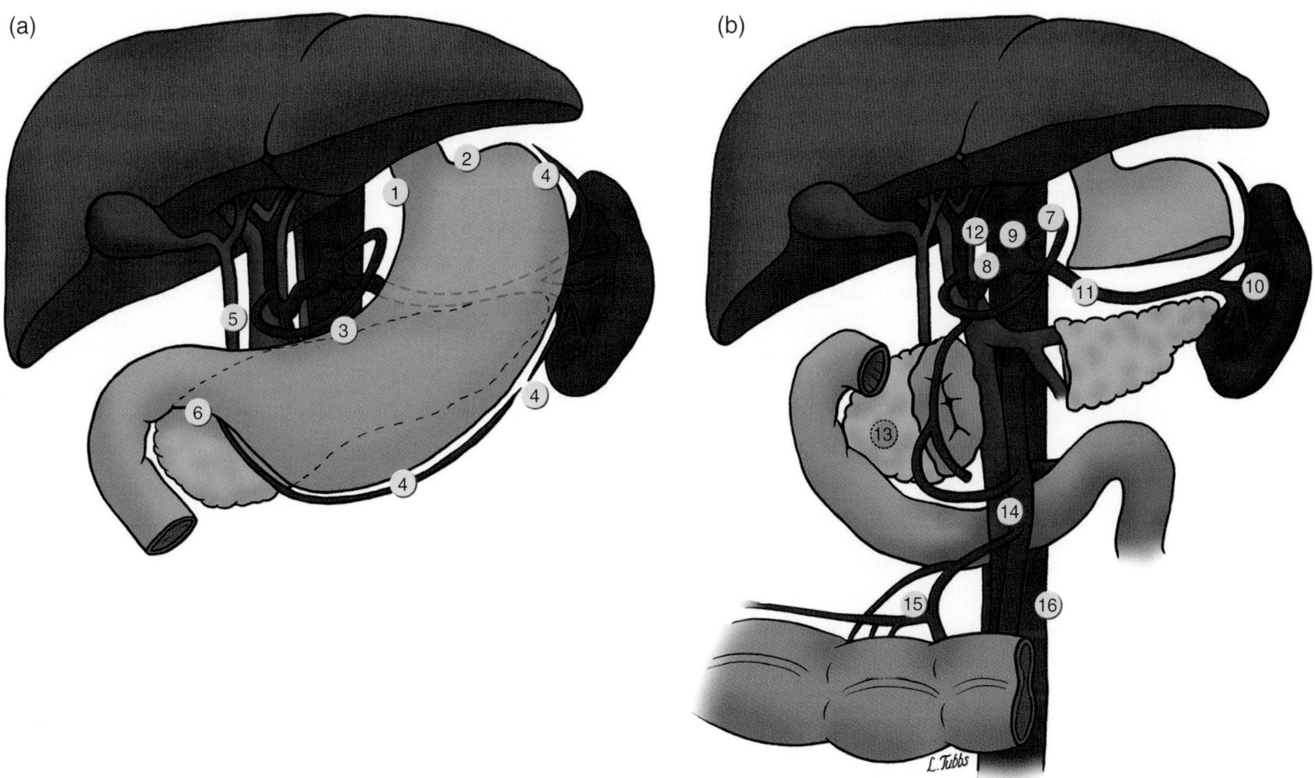

Figure 4.3 Anatomic location of lymph node stations relevant to gastric cancer surgery. (a) Nodal stations 1–6. (b) Nodal stations 7–16. *Source:* Modified from and reproduced with permission from Chu *et al.* [142].

Table 4.4 Anatomic definitions of lymph node stations for gastric cancer.

Number	Anatomic location	Included in D1/D2 lymphadenectomy
1	Right paracardial	D1
2	Left paracardial	D1
3	Lesser curvature of stomach, along left and right gastric arteries	D1
4	Greater curvature of stomach, along left and right gastroepiploic arteries and short gastric arteries	D1
5	Suprapyloric, along right gastric artery	D1
6	Infrapyloric, along right gastroepiploic artery	D1
7	Trunk of left gastric artery	D1/D2
8	Common hepatic artery	D2
9	Celiac artery	D2
10	Splenic hilum	D2
11	Splenic artery	D2
12	Hepatoduodenal ligament, along proper hepatic artery, common bile duct and portal vein	D2
13	Posterior surface of pancreatic head	
14	Superior mesenteric vein	
15	Middle colic vessels	
16	Para-aortic	

largely been abandoned in practice [61]. However, some controversy remains about whether D1 or D2 lymph node dissection is the recommended treatment option for gastric cancer. Although multiple retrospective series have shown that D2 lymphadenectomy improves survival, the results are less clear in randomized trials. The results of these trials are summarized in Table 4.5. The Cape Town South Africa trial was the first randomized trial to compare D1 and D2 lymph node dissection [87]. This trial found no significant difference in 3-year survival between the two groups. A significant criticism of this trial is the small sample size; only 43 patients were eligible for inclusion.

The British Medical Research Council (MRC) Gastric Cancer Surgical Trial and the Dutch Gastric Cancer Group Trial both failed to demonstrate a difference in 5-year survival between D1 and D2 lymphadenectomy [88–91]. Both trials had a higher perioperative mortality and morbidity in the D2 group, primarily associated with the higher frequency of concurrent splenectomy or pancreatectomy. The practice of routine pancreatectomy or splenectomy during gastrectomy for gastric cancer has been largely abandoned and is currently recommended only when there is direct tumor extension into these organs and resection is necessary to achieve negative margins [92, 93]. The MRC trial is also criticized for the inadequate training of participating surgeons in D2 lymphadenectomy [94]. The Dutch trial was slightly better in this regard, but still had a high noncompliance rate [90]. The long-term follow-up of the Dutch trial reported no difference in 15-year survival rates between the D1 and D2 groups (21% vs 29%, $P=0.34$) [95].

The Taiwan trial was a single institution randomized trial [96, 97]. Although the term D3 lymphadenectomy is used in their manuscript, this trial compared what is currently defined as D1 and D2 lymph node dissections. The surgical quality control was more meticulous than in the MRC and Dutch trials. There was no difference in perioperative mortality or morbidity. Patients receiving D2 lymphadenectomy had a higher 5-year survival than the group receiving D1 lymph node dissection (60% vs 54%, $P=0.041$).

Preliminary results from the Italian Gastric Cancer Study Group Trial were published in 2010 [98]. In this trial, splenectomy and pancreatectomy were performed only in selected cases. Surgical quality control was excellent. There were no differences in perioperative mortality or morbidity. Unfortunately, this study did not reach its accrual target. Five-year survival data has not yet been reported.

Because of the results of these trials, the debate over the recommended extent of lymph node dissection continues. Some authors assert that the Dutch trial results have ended the debate in favor of D1 lymphadenectomy [99]. Others insist that D2 lymphadenectomy may have some benefit over D1 lymphadenectomy, but this benefit can only be realized if the procedure can be performed with minimal added morbidity and mortality [100, 101]. The minimum lymph node dissection for gastric cancer should be at least a D1; a D2 lymph node dissection should be performed by experienced surgeons in high volume centers [96, 97].

An area of development in the surgical treatment of gastric cancer is the utilization of minimally-invasive surgical techniques, namely, laparoscopic approaches to gastrectomy. At this time, laparoscopic total gastrectomy has not been compared to open total gastrectomy in a randomized prospective study. To date, six randomized clinical trials have been performed comparing laparoscopic-assisted distal gastrectomy (LADG) to open distal gastrectomy (ODG) for gastric cancer [102–107]. Of these, only one has reported on the long-term oncologic outcomes, with no significant difference in 5-year overall survival (58.9% for LADG vs 55.7% for ODG) [104]. A recent meta-analysis that grouped both randomized and high quality nonrandomized controlled trials concluded that LADG was associated with longer operative times, but fewer complications, lower estimated blood loss and shorter hospital stay when compared to ODG [108]. Operative mortality was similar, but patients undergoing ODG had a higher number of lymph nodes harvested, although this difference was relatively small (weighted mean difference of 3.9 nodes). The clinical significance of this difference and whether LADG has similar long-term oncologic outcomes to ODG will depend on the final reports of ongoing clinical trials. The largest of these is the Korea Laparoscopic Gastrointestinal Surgery Study Group (KLASS trial), which randomized a total of 1,415 patients; long-term oncologic outcomes from this trial are pending [109].

Table 4.5 Randomized clinical trials comparing D1 and D2 lymphadenectomy for gastric cancer. Note that survival is 5-year survival unless otherwise specified.

Trial	Number of patients	Perioperative mortality (%)	Complications (%)	Overall survival (%)	Note
Cape Town South Africa trial [87]	D1: 22 D2: 21	0 0 (P = ns)	NR	78 76 (P = ns)	3-year survival
British MRC trial [89]	D1: 200 D2: 200	6.5 13 ($P=0.04$)	28 46 ($P<0.001$)	35 33 (P = ns)	
Dutch trial [91]	D1: 380 D2: 331	4 10 ($P=0.004$)	25 43 ($P<0.001$)	45 47 (P = ns)	
Taiwan trial [97]	D1: 110 D2: 111	0 0 (P = ns)	7.3 17 ($P=0.012$)	54 60 ($P=0.041$)	
Italian trial [98]	D1: 133 D2: 134	3.0 2.2 (P = ns)	12 18 (P = ns)	NR	Prelim results only

ns, not significant; NR, not reported.

Adjuvant Therapy

Due to the high rates of recurrence after curative surgical resection, multiple investigators have studied various strategies of adjuvant therapy, with either chemotherapy, radiation, or a combined approach. A summary of the major randomized clinical trials of adjuvant therapy for gastric cancer is presented in Table 4.6. The use of adjuvant external beam radiation therapy (XRT) after surgery was compared to surgery alone in the British Stomach Cancer Group; no difference in overall survival was observed [110].

The landmark trial for adjuvant therapy for gastric cancer was the Intergroup 0116 trial, which compared surgery alone to surgery and postoperative chemoradiation [111, 112]. The adjuvant therapy arm was administered fluorouracil (5-FU), leucovorin (LV), and a total of 45 Gy XRT. The 3-year overall survival for the chemoradiation group was 50% vs 41% for the surgery-only group ($P = 0.005$). The median survival for the chemoradiation and surgery-only groups were 35 and 27 months, respectively ($P = 0.0046$), with more than 10 years of follow-up. The findings of the Intergroup 0116 trial changed the standard of care in the US from observation alone after surgery to adjuvant chemoradiation. However, this trial was not without criticism: although the design of the trial had recommended D2 lymphadenectomy, it was only performed in 10% of patients. D1 lymphadenectomy was performed in 36% of patients; 54% of patients in Intergroup 0116 did not even receive a D1 lymph node dissection. Because of this, some critics of this trial have asserted that the primary benefit of chemoradiation is to mask the effect of suboptimal surgical quality.

The Intergroup trial Cancer and Leukemia Group B (CALGB) 80101 compared the Intergroup 0116 regimen (bolus 5-FU and LV with 5-FU plus concurrent XRT) with adjuvant epirubicin, cisplatin and 5-FU (ECF) given before and after 5-FU plus concurrent XRT. Final analysis has not been published, but preliminary data presented at the 2011 American Society of Clinical Oncology Annual Meeting showed no difference in 3-year overall survival between the two arms (50% vs 52%, $P = 0.80$) [113].

The Adjuvant Chemoradiation Therapy in Stomach Cancer (ARTIST) Trial was designed primarily to examine the impact of postoperative chemoradiation in gastric cancer after curative surgical resection and D2 lymphadenectomy [114]. Patients were randomized to receive chemotherapy consisting of capecitabine and cisplatin (XP) or chemoradiation with XP and 45 Gy XRT (XP/XRT). Five-year overall survival was not significantly different between the XP and XP/XRT arms (73% vs 75%, $P = 0.0484$) [115]. Subset analysis did reveal improved disease-free survival with XP/XRT among patients with node-positive disease. In light of this finding, the ARTIST-II trial has been designed to examine chemotherapy vs chemoradiation in node-positive patients following gastrectomy.

The ChemoRadiotherapy after Induction Chemotherapy in Cancer of the Stomach (CRITICS) study in the Netherlands compared adjuvant chemotherapy with adjuvant chemoradiation in patients who received neoadjuvant chemotherapy, gastrectomy, and D2 lymphadenectomy. Although final results have not yet been published, findings presented at the 2016 American Society of Clinical Oncology Annual Meeting demonstrated no difference in overall survival for the chemotherapy and chemoradiation arms (41.3% vs 40.9%, $P = 0.99$) [116].

There have been a multitude of randomized clinical trials comparing adjuvant chemotherapy to surgery alone for gastric cancer. Many of these were underpowered and had variable, mostly negative, results. Recently, two large randomized trials in

Table 4.6 Randomized clinical trials on adjuvant therapy for gastric cancer. Note that survival is 5-year survival unless otherwise specified.

Trial	Intervention	Number of patients	Overall survival (%)	Note
British 2nd Adjuvant Trial [110]	Surgery Surgery + XRT Surgery + chemotherapy (MAF)	145 153 138	20 12 19 ($P = 0.14$)	
Intergroup 0116 [111]	Surgery Surgery + chemoradiation (5-FU/LV + XRT)	277 282	41 50 ($P = 0.005$)	3-year survival
CALGB 80101 [113]	Surgery + chemoradiation (5-FU/LV + XRT) Surgery + chemoradiation (ECF + XRT)	267 279	50 52 ($P = 0.80$)	3-year survival
ARTIST trial [115]	Surgery + chemotherapy (XP) Surgery + chemoradiation (XP + XRT)	228 230	73 75 ($P = 0.484$)	
CRITICS study [116]	Neoadjuvant chemotherapy (ECC/EOC) + surgery + chemotherapy (ECC/EOC) Neoadjuvant chemotherapy + surgery + chemoradiation (XP + XRT)	393 395	41 41 ($P = 0.99$)	
CLASSIC trial [118]	Surgery Surgery + chemotherapy (XELOX)	515 520	69 78 ($P = 0.0015$)	
ACTS-GC [119]	Surgery Surgery + chemotherapy (S-1)	530 529	61 (HR = 0.67) 72 (CI = 0.54–0.83)	

CI, 95% confidence interval; ECC/EOC, epirubicin, cisplatin or oxaliplatin, and capecitabine; ECF, epirubicin, cisplatin, and fluorouracil; 5-FU, fluorouracil; HR, hazard ratio; LV, leucovorin; MAF, mitomycin, doxorubicin, and fluorouracil; XELOX, capecitabine and oxaliplatin; XP, capecitabine and cisplatin; XRT, external beam radiation therapy.

Asia have demonstrated the benefit of adjuvant chemotherapy. The Capecitabine and Oxaliplatin Adjuvant Study in Stomach Cancer (CLASSIC) trial compared adjuvant capecitabine and oxaliplatin (XELOX) after curative gastrectomy and D2 lymphadenectomy with surgery alone [117]. Final results demonstrated an improved 5-year overall survival for adjuvant XELOX compared to surgery alone (78% vs 69%, $P = 0.0015$) [118].

The Adjuvant Chemotherapy Trial of S-1 for Gastric Cancer (ACTS-GC) compared adjuvant S-1, a novel combination of tegafur (a 5-FU prodrug), gimeracil, and oteracil, with surgery alone, in patients who had undergone D2 lymphadenectomy. Five-year overall survival for the S-1 arm was 71.7%, compared to 61.1% for the surgery alone group, with a hazard ratio for death of 0.669 (95% CI 0.540–0.828) [119]. As a result, S-1 has become standard therapy in Japan. However, S-1 is not yet available in the US and it remains unclear if these results will be reproducible outside of East Asian patient populations.

Neoadjuvant Therapy

For locoregional gastric cancer, neoadjuvant treatment can be administered prior to an attempt at curative surgical resection. This can be applied both to patients with resectable as well as those with disease initially deemed unresectable, but without metastatic disease. The theoretical benefit of this approach is twofold: it may permit curative resection in patients who present initially with unresectable disease, and it may spare unnecessary gastrectomy in patients who have development of metastatic disease during neoadjuvant treatment, therefore selecting out patients with aggressive tumor biology for whom upfront surgery may have been futile. The findings of the three major randomized clinical trials that examined neoadjuvant therapy in gastric cancer is presented in Table 4.7.

The Medical Research Council Adjuvant Gastric Infusional Chemotherapy (MAGIC) trial was conducted in the United Kingdom and compared perioperative chemotherapy, consisting of three cycles of ECF, given before and after surgery, with surgery alone. This trial included patients with lower esophageal or EGJ tumors (26%), which complicates interpretation of the results. In addition, the extent of the lymph node dissection was at the discretion of the surgeon. Because of this, only 43% of the perioperative ECF group and 40% of the surgery only group underwent D2 lymphadenectomy. Despite these limitations and the fact that only 42% of the ECF arm were able to complete the entire treatment protocol, the 5-year overall survival for the ECF arm was 36% compared to 23% for the surgery only arm ($P = 0.009$) [120]. The MAGIC trial regimen has been widely adopted as standard therapy in Europe. Capecitabine has generally replaced 5-FU in the regimen, due to ease of administration

The Fédération Nationale des Centres de Lutte contre le Cancer (FNCLCC) and the Fédération Francophone de Cancérologie Digestive (FFCD) trial compared perioperative chemotherapy, consisting of 5-FU and cisplatin (CF), with surgery alone. Similar to the MAGIC trial, the extent of lymphadenectomy was left to the discretion of the surgeon. The FNCLCC/FFCD trial had an even greater proportion of esophageal and EGJ tumors, with only 25% of patients having true gastric cancer. However, similar results to the MAGIC trial were reported, with 5-year overall survivals for the chemotherapy and surgery only groups at 38% and 24%, respectively ($P = 0.02$) [121].

In contrast to the MAGIC and FNCLCC/FFCD trials, the European Organisation for Research and Treatment of Cancer (EORTC) trial 40594 did not demonstrate a survival benefit for neoadjuvant chemotherapy consisting of cisplatin, LV, and 5-FU when compared with surgery alone. The EORTC trial was closed early due to poor accrual, with only 144 of the planned 360 patients enrolled. Two-year overall survival was 73% for the neoadjuvant group and 70% for the surgery only group ($P = 0.466$) [122]. However, due to the poor accrual, this trial was underpowered to demonstrate a survival advantage.

Although neoadjuvant chemoradiation is commonly used for esophageal and EGJ tumors, there have been no randomized trials that have examined this strategy in noncardia gastric adenocarcinomas. There have also been no trials directly comparing the neoadjuvant approach with the adjuvant approach. In particular, it is unclear if the perioperative chemotherapy regimens of the MAGIC and FNCLCC/FFCD trials are superior to the postoperative chemoradiation strategy of the Intergroup 0116 trial. The aforementioned CRITICS trial did compare postoperative chemotherapy to postoperative chemoradiation, but only in patients who had all received preoperative chemotherapy and therefore did not adequately address this question [116]. The ongoing Trial of Preoperative Therapy for Gastric and Esophageal Junction Adenocarcinoma (TOPGEAR) will compare perioperative chemotherapy to perioperative chemotherapy plus preoperative chemoradiation [123]. Currently,

Table 4.7 Randomized clinical trials on neoadjuvant therapy for gastric cancer. Note that survival is 5-year survival unless otherwise specified.

Trial	Intervention	Number of patients	Overall survival (%)	Note
MAGIC trial [120]	Surgery	253	23	
	ECF + surgery + ECF	250	36 ($P = 0.009$)	
FNCLCC/FFCD trial [121]	Surgery	111	24	
	CF + surgery + CF	113	38 ($P = 0.02$)	
EORTC trial 40954 [122]	Surgery	72	70	2-year survival, poor accrual
	CLF + surgery	72	73 ($P = 0.466$)	

CF, cisplatin and fluorouracil; CLF, cisplatin, leucovorin and fluorouracil; ECF, epirubicin, cisplatin and fluorouracil.

postoperative chemoradiation should be considered the standard of care for patients with node positive disease or T3–4 disease who have already undergone gastrectomy and did not receive any preoperative therapy. For patients being evaluated prior to gastrectomy, perioperative chemotherapy is recommended for patients with T2 or higher disease.

Palliative Therapy

The goals of therapy in patients with unresectable or metastatic gastric cancer are to palliate symptoms, improve survival and improve quality of life. Various chemotherapy regimens have been studied in a larger number of randomized trials, yet there remains no consensus as to which regimen should be the standard of care. Combination therapy has been associated with improved response rates when compared to single agent therapy, but no survival differences have been demonstrated [124–127].

Various combinations of 5-FU-based regimens have been compared. ECF was compared with 5-FU, doxorubicin, and methotrexate (FAMTX) and demonstrated to have a higher 1-year survival (36% vs 21%) and longer median survival times (8.9 months vs 5.7 months, $P = 0.0009$) [128]. ECF was compared to mitomycin, cisplatin, and 5-FU (MCF) in another randomized trial; 1-year survival was similar for the two regimens (40% vs 33%) as was median survival (9.4 months vs 8.7 months, $P = 0.315$), but quality-of-life measures favored ECF [129].

Because of the need for central venous access for the administration of 5-FU and the toxicity profile of cisplatin, the Randomized ECF for Advanced and Locally Advanced Esophagogastric Cancer 2 (REAL-2) trial compared with ECF and three regimens using substitute agents: oral capecitabine replacing 5-FU (ECX), oxaliplatin replacing cisplatin (EOF), or both replacements (EOX). Median survival times for the four regimens were similar: 9.9 months, 9.9 months, 9.3 months, and 11.2 months, respectively. One-year survival rates were also similar: 37.7%, 40.8%, 40.4%, and 46.8%, respectively [130]. These results suggest that the substitutions of capecitabine for 5-FU and oxaliplatin for cisplatin do not affect efficacy of the regimens. Furthermore, a direct comparison of EOX to ECF in the subgroup analysis showed a modest survival advantage for EOX, leading some to prefer EOX over ECF for first-line therapy.

The combination of docetaxel, cisplatin, and 5-FU (DCF) was compared to CF in the V325 study group trial. DCF had a higher 1-year overall survival than CF (40% vs 32%) and also had longer median survival (9.2 months vs 8.6 months, $P = 0.02$) [131]. DCF has not been compared to ECF in any phase III randomized trials. A trend towards improved outcomes for DCF over ECF was observed in a phase II trial, but DCF was also associated with increased myelosuppression and infectious complications [132]. Modified dosing schedules of DCF have been demonstrated to have equivalent efficacy with improved tolerability [133].

Irinotecan has also been utilized for treatment of advanced gastric cancer, both as a single agent or in combination regimens, with similar efficacy to non-irinotecan regimens [134, 135]. A French intergroup trial demonstrated no difference in median overall survival for FOLFIRI vs ECX (9.5 vs 9.7 months, $P = 0.95$), but did show longer median time to failure for FOLFIRI (5.1 vs 4.2 months, $P = 0.008$) [136]. FOLFIRI was better tolerated than ECX in this study. However, because irinotecan-based combinations have never demonstrated superiority over platinum-based regimens in any phase III trials, it is generally reserved as a second-line agent.

Targeted therapies have been examined for treatment of advanced gastric cancer. For patients with HER2-positive gastric adenocarcinomas, the aforementioned ToGA trial demonstrated that the addition of trastuzumab to chemotherapy with CF or cisplatin and capecitabine (CX) resulted in improved survival, with median survival of 13.8 months for the trastuzumab group compared to 11.1 months for the chemotherapy only group ($P = 0.0046$) [50]. However, the Avastin in Gastric Cancer (AVAGAST) trial failed to show a similar benefit for bevacizumab, an anti-VEGF monoclonal antibody, with a median survival of 12.1 months when compared to 10.1 months for CF or CX ($P = 0.1002$) [137]. Ramucirumab, a monoclonal VEGFR-2 antibody, demonstrated improved medial overall survival for patients who failed first-line therapy (5.2 vs 3.8 months, $P = 0.047$) in comparison to placebo in the REGARD trial [138]. The RAINBOW trial similarly showed improved median overall survival for ramucirumab when given in combination with paclitaxel as second-line therapy. However, a survival benefit was not shown when it was combined with FOLFOX as first-line therapy [139].

Follow-up

There have been randomized trials conducted regarding the optimal surveillance strategy for patients with gastric cancer. The National Comprehensive Cancer Network guidelines recommends a complete history and physical examination every 3–6 months for 1–2 years, every 6–12 months for 3–5 years, and then annually thereafter [140]. Laboratory evaluation, radiologic imaging studies, and endoscopic examinations should be performed when clinically indicated. Routine imaging surveillance does not appear to have a benefit in gastric adenocarcinoma [141].

References

1 Siegel RL, Miller KD, Jemal A. Cancer statistics, 2017. *CA Cancer J Clin* 2017;67:7–30.

2 Torre LA, Bray F, Siegel RL, *et al.* Global cancer statistics, 2012. *CA Cancer J Clin* 2015 Mar 1;65:87–108.

3 de Martel C, Forman D, Plummer M. Gastric cancer: epidemiology and risk factors. *Gastroenterol Clin North Am* 2013;42:219–40

4 American Cancer Society. *Cancer Facts & Figures 2017.* Atlanta: American Cancer Society, 2017.

5 Howlader N, Noone AM, Krapcho M, *et al.* (eds). *SEER Cancer Statistics Review, 1975–2013*, National Cancer Institute. Bethesda, MD. http://seer.cancer.gov/csr/1975_2013/, based on November 2015 SEER data submission, posted to the SEER web site, April 2016.

6 Shikata K, Kiyohara Y, Kubo M, *et al.* A prospective study of dietary salt intake and gastric cancer incidence in a defined Japanese population: the Hisayama study. *Int J Cancer* 2006;119:196–201.

7 Tsugane S. Salt, salted food intake, and risk of gastric cancer: epidemiologic evidence. *Cancer Sci* 2005;96:1–6.

8 Tsugane S, Sasazuki S. Diet and the risk of gastric cancer: review of epidemiological evidence. *Gastric Cancer* 2007;10:75–83.

9 Joossens JV, Hill MJ, Elliott P, *et al.* Dietary salt, nitrate and stomach cancer mortality in 24 countries. European Cancer Prevention (ECP) and the INTERSALT Cooperative Research Group. *Int J Epidemiol* 1996;25:494–504.

10 Larsson SC, Bergkvist L, Wolk A. Fruit and vegetable consumption and incidence of gastric cancer: a prospective study. *Cancer Epidemiol Biomarkers Prev* 2006;15:1998–2001.

11 Riboli E, Norat T. Epidemiologic evidence of the protective effect of fruit and vegetables on cancer risk. *Am J Clin Nutr* 2003;78:569.

12 Guggenheim DE, Shah MA. Gastric cancer epidemiology and risk factors. *J Surg Oncol* 2013;107:230–6.

13 You WC, Blot WJ, Chang YS, *et al.* Diet and high risk of stomach cancer in Shandong, China. *Cancer Res* 1988;48:3518–23.

14 Ma J-L, Zhang L, Brown LM, *et al.* Fifteen-year effects of Helicobacter pylori, garlic, and vitamin treatments on gastric cancer incidence and mortality. *J Natl Cancer Inst* 2012;104:488–92.

15 Ladeiras-Lopes R, Pereira AK, Nogueira A, *et al.* Smoking and gastric cancer: systematic review and meta-analysis of cohort studies. *Cancer Causes Control* 2008;19:689–701.

16 Smyth EC, Capanu M, Janjigian YY, *et al.* Tobacco use is associated with increased recurrence and death from gastric cancer. *Ann Surg Oncol* 2012;19:2088–94.

17 Tramacere I, Negri E, Pelucchi C, *et al.* A meta-analysis on alcohol drinking and gastric cancer risk. *Ann Oncol* 2012;23:28–36.

18 Yang P, Zhou Y, Chen B, *et al.* Overweight, obesity and gastric cancer risk: results from a meta-analysis of cohort studies. *Eur J Cancer* 2009;45:2867–73.

19 Eslick GD, Lim LL, Byles JE, *et al.* Association of Helicobacter pylori infection with gastric carcinoma: a meta-analysis. *Am J Gastroenterol* 1999;94:2373–9.

20 Uemura N, Okamoto S, Yamamoto S, *et al.* Helicobacter pylori infection and the development of gastric cancer. *N Engl J Med* 2001;345:784–9.

21 Fox JG, Dangler CA, Taylor NS, *et al.* High-salt diet induces gastric epithelial hyperplasia and parietal cell loss, and enhances Helicobacter pylori colonization in C57BL/6 mice. *Cancer Res* 1999;59:4823–8.

22 Loh JT, Torres VJ, Cover TL. Regulation of Helicobacter pylori cagA expression in response to salt. *Cancer Res* 2007;67:4709–15.

23 Murphy G, Pfeiffer R, Camargo MC, Rabkin CS. Meta-analysis shows that prevalence of Epstein-Barr virus-positive gastric cancer differs based on sex and anatomic location. *Gastroenterology* 2009;137:824–33.

24 Guilford P, Hopkins J, Harraway J, *et al.* E-cadherin germline mutations in familial gastric cancer. *Nature* 1998;392:402–5.

25 Fitzgerald RC, Hardwick R, Huntsman D, *et al.* Hereditary diffuse gastric cancer: updated consensus guidelines for clinical management and directions for future research. *J Med Genet* 2010;47:436–44.

26 Guilford P, Humar B, Blair V. Hereditary diffuse gastric cancer: translation of CDH1 germline mutations into clinical practice. *Gastric Cancer* 2010;13:1–10.

27 Lynch HT, Grady W, Suriano G, Huntsman D. Gastric cancer: new genetic developments. *J Surg Oncol* 2005;90:114–33.

28 Aarnio M, Salovaara R, Aaltonen LA, *et al.* Features of gastric cancer in hereditary non-polyposis colorectal cancer syndrome. *Int J Cancer* 1997;74:551–5.

29 Luebke T, Baldus SE, Grass G, *et al.* Histological grading in gastric cancer by Ming classification: correlation with histopathological subtypes, metastasis, and prognosis. *World J Surg* 2005;29:1422–7.

30 Lauren P. The two histological main types of gastric carcinoma: diffuse and so-called intestinal-type carcinoma. An attempt at a histo-clinical classification. *Acta Pathol Microbiol Scand* 1965;64:31–49.

31 Correa P, Cuello C, Duque E. Carcinoma and intestinal metaplasia of the stomach in Colombian migrants. *J Natl Cancer Inst* 1970;44:297–306.

32 Munoz N, Correa P, Cuello C, Duque E. Histologic types of gastric carcinoma in high- and low-risk areas. *Int J Cancer* 1968;3:809–18.

33 Stalsberg H. Histological typing of gastric carcinoma. A comparison of surgical and autopsy materials, and of primary tumours and metastases. *Acta Pathol Microbiol Scand A* 1972;80:509–14.

34 Kim KH, Chi CH, Lee SK, *et al.* Histologic types of gastric carcinoma among Koreans. *Cancer* 1972;29:1261–3.

35 Qiu MZ, Cai MY, Zhang DS, *et al.* Clinicopathological characteristics and prognostic analysis of Lauren classification in gastric adenocarcinoma in China. *J Transl Med* 2013;11:58.

36 Yamashita K, Sakuramoto S, Katada N, *et al.* Diffuse type advanced gastric cancer showing dismal prognosis is characterized by deeper invasion and emerging peritoneal cancer cell: the latest comparative study to intestinal advanced gastric cancer. *Hepatogastroenterology* 2009;56:276–81.

37 Miyahara R, Niwa Y, Matsuura T, *et al.* Prevalence and prognosis of gastric cancer detected by screening in a large Japanese population: data from a single institute over 30 years. *J Gastroenterol Hepatol* 2007;22:1435–42.

38 Zheng H, Takahashi H, Murai Y, *et al.* Pathobiological characteristics of intestinal and diffuse-type gastric carcinoma in Japan: an immunostaining study on the tissue microarray. *J Clin Pathol* 2007;60:273–7.

39 Watanabe H, Nishimaki T. [Factors affecting the growth and extension of gastric cancer–analysis of retrospective observation]. *Gan To Kagaku Ryoho* 1983;10:482–8.

40 Hamilton SR, Aaltonen LA. *World Health Organization Classification of Tumours. Pathology and Genetics of Tumours of the Digestive System*. Lyon, France: IARC Press, 2000.

41 Fukushige S, Matsubara K, Yoshida M, *et al.* Localization of a novel v-erbB-related gene, c-erbB-2, on human chromosome 17 and its amplification in a gastric cancer cell line. *Mol Cell Biol* 1986;6:955–8.

42 Sakai K, Mori S, Kawamoto T, *et al.* Expression of epidermal growth factor receptors on normal human gastric epithelia and gastric carcinomas. *J Natl Cancer Inst* 1986;77:1047–52.
43 Hechtman JF, Polydorides AD. HER2/neu gene amplification and protein overexpression in gastric and gastroesophageal junction adenocarcinoma: a review of histopathology, diagnostic testing, and clinical implications. *Arch Pathol Lab Med* 2012;136:691–7.
44 Yan B, Yau EX, Bte Omar SS, *et al.* A study of HER2 gene amplification and protein expression in gastric cancer. *J Clin Pathol* 2010;63:839–42.
45 Tanner M, Hollmen M, Junttila TT, *et al.* Amplification of HER-2 in gastric carcinoma: association with Topoisomerase IIalpha gene amplification, intestinal type, poor prognosis and sensitivity to trastuzumab. *Ann Oncol* 2005;16:273–8.
46 Jorgensen JT, Hersom M. HER2 as a prognostic marker in gastric cancer – a systematic analysis of data from the literature. *J Cancer* 2012;3:137–44.
47 Chua TC, Merrett ND. Clinicopathologic factors associated with HER2-positive gastric cancer and its impact on survival outcomes–a systematic review. *Int J Cancer* 2012;130:2845–56.
48 Janjigian YY, Werner D, Pauligk C, *et al.* Prognosis of metastatic gastric and gastroesophageal junction cancer by HER2 status: a European and USA International collaborative analysis. *Ann Oncol* 2012;23:2656–62.
49 Grabsch H, Sivakumar S, Gray S, *et al.* HER2 expression in gastric cancer: rare, heterogeneous and of no prognostic value – conclusions from 924 cases of two independent series. *Cell Oncol* 2010;32:57–65.
50 Bang Y-J, Van Cutsem E, Feyereislova A, *et al.* Trastuzumab in combination with chemotherapy versus chemotherapy alone for treatment of HER2-positive advanced gastric or gastro-oesophageal junction cancer (ToGA): a phase 3, open-label, randomised controlled trial. *Lancet* 2010;376:687–97.
51 Axon A. Symptoms and diagnosis of gastric cancer at early curable stage. *Best Pract Res Clin Gastroenterol* 2006;20:697–708.
52 Everett SM, Axon AT. Early gastric cancer in Europe. *Gut* 1997;41:142–50.
53 Wanebo HJ, Kennedy BJ, Chmiel J, *et al.* Cancer of the stomach. A patient care study by the American College of Surgeons. *Ann Surg* 1993;218:583–92.
54 Morgenstern L. The Virchow-Troisier node: a historical note. *Am J Surg* 1979;138:703.
55 Benson JR, Singh S, Thomas JM. Sister Joseph's nodule: a case report and review. *Eur J Surg Oncol* 1997;23:451–4.
56 Gilliland R, Gill PJ. Incidence and prognosis of Krukenberg tumour in Northern Ireland. *Br J Surg* 1992;79:1364–6.
57 Dooley CP, Larson AW, Stace NH, *et al.* Double-contrast barium meal and upper gastrointestinal endoscopy. A comparative study. *Ann Intern Med* 1984;101:538–45.
58 Longo WE, Zucker KA, Zdon MJ, Modlin IM. Detection of early gastric cancer in an aggressive endoscopy unit. *Am Surg* 1989;55:100–4.
59 Graham DY, Schwartz JT, Cain GD, Gyorkey F. Prospective evaluation of biopsy number in the diagnosis of esophageal and gastric carcinoma. *Gastroenterology* 1982;82:228–31.
60 Amin MB. *AJCC Cancer Staging Manual*, Eighth Edition. New York: Springer, 2017.
61 Sano T, Aiko T. New Japanese classifications and treatment guidelines for gastric cancer: revision concepts and major revised points. *Gastric Cancer* 2011;14:97–100.
62 Japanese Gastric Cancer Association. Japanese classification of gastric carcinoma: 3rd English edition. *Gastric Cancer* 2011;14:101–12.
63 Davies J, Chalmers AG, Sue-Ling HM, *et al.* Spiral computed tomography and operative staging of gastric carcinoma: a comparison with histopathological staging. *Gut* 1997;41:314–19.
64 Dux M, Richter GM, Hansmann J, *et al.* Helical hydro-CT for diagnosis and staging of gastric carcinoma. *J Comput Assist Tomogr* 1999;23:913–22.
65 Lowy AM, Mansfield PF, Leach SD, Ajani J. Laparoscopic staging for gastric cancer. *Surgery* 1996;119:611–14.
66 Power DG, Schattner MA, Gerdes H, *et al.* Endoscopic ultrasound can improve the selection for laparoscopy in patients with localized gastric cancer. *J Am Coll Surg* 2009;208:173–8.
67 Lee IJ, Lee JM, Kim SH, *et al.* Diagnostic performance of 64-channel multidetector CT in the evaluation of gastric cancer: differentiation of mucosal cancer (T1a) from submucosal involvement (T1b and T2). *Radiology* 2010;255:805–14.
68 Rossi M, Broglia L, Maccioni F, *et al.* Hydro-CT in patients with gastric cancer: preoperative radiologic staging. *Eur Radiol* 1997;7:659–64.
69 Mukai K, Ishida Y, Okajima K, *et al.* Usefulness of preoperative FDG-PET for detection of gastric cancer. *Gastric Cancer* 2006;9:192–6.
70 Chen J, Cheong J-H, Yun MJ, *et al.* Improvement in preoperative staging of gastric adenocarcinoma with positron emission tomography. *Cancer* 2005;103:2383–90.
71 Smyth E, Schoder H, Strong VE, *et al.* A prospective evaluation of the utility of 2-deoxy-2-[(18) F]fluoro-D-glucose positron emission tomography and computed tomography in staging locally advanced gastric cancer. *Cancer* 2012;118:5481–8.
72 Polkowski M, Palucki J, Wronska E, *et al.* Endosonography versus helical computed tomography for locoregional staging of gastric cancer. *Endoscopy* 2004;36:617–23.
73 Bhandari S, Shim CS, Kim JH, *et al.* Usefulness of three-dimensional, multidetector row CT (virtual gastroscopy and multiplanar reconstruction) in the evaluation of gastric cancer: a comparison with conventional endoscopy, EUS, and histopathology. *Gastrointest Endosc* 2004;59:619–26.
74 Hwang SW, Lee DH, Lee SH, *et al.* Preoperative staging of gastric cancer by endoscopic ultrasonography and multidetector-row computed tomography. *J Gastroenterol Hepatol* 2010;25:512–18.
75 Mocellin S, Marchet A, Nitti D. EUS for the staging of gastric cancer: a meta-analysis. *Gastrointest Endosc* 2011;73:1122–34.
76 Sarela AI, Lefkowitz R, Brennan MF, Karpeh MS. Selection of patients with gastric adenocarcinoma for laparoscopic staging. *Am J Surg* 2006;191:134–8.
77 Leake P-A, Cardoso R, Seevaratnam R, *et al.* A systematic review of the accuracy and indications for diagnostic laparoscopy prior to curative-intent resection of gastric cancer. *Gastric Cancer* 2012;15 Suppl 1:38–47.

78 Burke EC, Karpeh MS, Conlon KC, Brennan MF. Peritoneal lavage cytology in gastric cancer: an independent predictor of outcome. *Ann Surg Oncol* 1998;5:411–15.

79 Leake P-A, Cardoso R, Seevaratnam R, *et al.* A systematic review of the accuracy and utility of peritoneal cytology in patients with gastric cancer. *Gastric Cancer* 2012;15 Suppl 1:27–37.

80 Gotoda T, Yanagisawa A, Sasako M, *et al.* Incidence of lymph node metastasis from early gastric cancer: estimation with a large number of cases at two large centers. *Gastric Cancer* 2000;3:219–25.

81 Buhl K, Schlag P, Herfarth C. Quality of life and functional results following different types of resection for gastric carcinoma. *Eur J Surg Oncol* 1990;16:404–9.

82 Gouzi JL, Huguier M, Fagniez PL, *et al.* Total versus subtotal gastrectomy for adenocarcinoma of the gastric antrum. A French prospective controlled study. *Ann Surg* 1989;209:162–6.

83 Bozzetti F, Marubini E, Bonfanti G, *et al.* Subtotal versus total gastrectomy for gastric cancer: five-year survival rates in a multicenter randomized Italian trial. Italian Gastrointestinal Tumor Study Group. *Ann Surg* 1999;230:170–8.

84 Eagon JC, Miedema BW, Kelly KA. Postgastrectomy syndromes. *Surg Clin North Am* 1992;72:445–65.

85 Japanese Gastric Cancer Association. Japanese gastric cancer treatment guidelines 2010 (ver. 3). *Gastric Cancer* 2011;14:113–23.

86 Sasako M, Sano T, Yamamoto S, *et al.* D2 lymphadenectomy alone or with para-aortic nodal dissection for gastric cancer. *N Engl J Med* 2008;359:453–62.

87 Dent DM, Madden MV, Price SK. Randomized comparison of R1 and R2 gastrectomy for gastric carcinoma. *Br J Surg* 1988;75:110–12.

88 Cuschieri A, Fayers P, Fielding J, *et al.* Postoperative morbidity and mortality after D1 and D2 resections for gastric cancer: preliminary results of the MRC randomised controlled surgical trial. *The Surgical Cooperative Group. Lancet* 1996;347:995–9.

89 Cuschieri A, Weeden S, Fielding J, *et al.* Patient survival after D1 and D2 resections for gastric cancer: long-term results of the MRC randomized surgical trial. *Surgical Co-operative Group. Br J Cancer* 1999;79:1522–30.

90 Bonenkamp JJ, Hermans J, Sasako M, *et al.* Extended lymph-node dissection for gastric cancer. *N Engl J Med* 1999;340:908–14.

91 Hartgrink HH, van de Velde CJH, Putter H, *et al.* Extended lymph node dissection for gastric cancer: who may benefit? Final results of the randomized Dutch gastric cancer group trial. *J Clin Oncol* 2004;22:2069–77.

92 Csendes A, Burdiles P, Rojas J, *et al.* A prospective randomized study comparing D2 total gastrectomy versus D2 total gastrectomy plus splenectomy in 187 patients with gastric carcinoma. *Surgery* 2002;131:401–7.

93 Yu W, Choi GS, Chung HY. Randomized clinical trial of splenectomy versus splenic preservation in patients with proximal gastric cancer. *Br J Surg* 2006;93:559–63.

94 McCulloch P, Nita ME, Kazi H, Gama-Rodrigues J. Extended versus limited lymph nodes dissection technique for adenocarcinoma of the stomach. Cochrane Database Syst Rev 2004.

95 Songun I, Putter H, Kranenbarg EM-K, *et al.* Surgical treatment of gastric cancer: 15-year follow-up results of the randomised nationwide Dutch D1D2 trial. *Lancet Oncol* 2010;11:439–49.

96 Wu CW, Hsiung CA, Lo SS, *et al.* Randomized clinical trial of morbidity after D1 and D3 surgery for gastric cancer. *Br J Surg* 2004;91:283–7.

97 Wu C-W, Hsiung CA, Lo S-S, *et al.* Nodal dissection for patients with gastric cancer: a randomised controlled trial. *Lancet Oncol* 2006;7:309–15.

98 Degiuli M, Sasako M, Ponti A. Morbidity and mortality in the Italian Gastric Cancer Study Group randomized clinical trial of D1 versus D2 resection for gastric cancer. *Br J Surg* 2010;97:643–9.

99 Petrelli NJ. The debate is over; it's time to move on. *J Clin Oncol* 2004;22:2041–2.

100 de Bree E, Charalampakis V, Melissas J, Tsiftsis DD. The extent of lymph node dissection for gastric cancer: a critical appraisal. *J Surg Oncol* 2010;102:552–62.

101 Schmidt B, Yoon SS. D1 versus D2 lymphadenectomy for gastric cancer. *J Surg Oncol* 2013;107:259–64.

102 Kitano S, Shiraishi N, Fujii K, *et al.* A randomized controlled trial comparing open vs laparoscopy-assisted distal gastrectomy for the treatment of early gastric cancer: an interim report. *Surgery* 2002;131:306–11.

103 Lee JH, Han HS. A prospective randomized study comparing open vs laparoscopy-assisted distal gastrectomy in early gastric cancer: early results. *Surg Endosc* 2005;19:168–73.

104 Huscher CGS, Mingoli A, Sgarzini G, *et al.* Laparoscopic versus open subtotal gastrectomy for distal gastric cancer: five-year results of a randomized prospective trial. *Ann Surg* 2005;241:232–7.

105 Hayashi H, Ochiai T, Shimada H, Gunji Y. Prospective randomized study of open versus laparoscopy-assisted distal gastrectomy with extraperigastric lymph node dissection for early gastric cancer. *Surg Endosc* 2005;19:1172–6.

106 Kim Y-W, Baik YH, Yun YH, *et al.* Improved quality of life outcomes after laparoscopy-assisted distal gastrectomy for early gastric cancer: results of a prospective randomized clinical trial. *Ann Surg* 2008;248:721–7.

107 Kim H-H, Hyung WJ, Cho GS, *et al.* Morbidity and mortality of laparoscopic gastrectomy versus open gastrectomy for gastric cancer: an interim report–a phase III multicenter, prospective, randomized Trial (KLASS Trial). *Ann Surg* 2010;251:417–20.

108 Vinuela EF, Gonen M, Brennan MF, *et al.* Laparoscopic versus open distal gastrectomy for gastric cancer: a meta-analysis of randomized controlled trials and high-quality nonrandomized studies. *Ann Surg* 2012;255:446–56.

109 Kim H-H, Han S-U, Kim M-C, *et al.* Prospective randomized controlled trial (phase III) to comparing laparoscopic distal gastrectomy with open distal gastrectomy for gastric adenocarcinoma (KLASS 01). *J Korean Surg Soc* 2013;84:123–30.

110 Hallissey MT, Dunn JA, Ward LC, Allum WH. The second British Stomach Cancer Group trial of adjuvant radiotherapy or chemotherapy in resectable gastric cancer: five-year follow-up. *Lancet* 1994;343:1309–12.

111 Macdonald JS, Smalley SR, Benedetti J, *et al.* Chemoradiotherapy after surgery compared with surgery alone for adenocarcinoma of the stomach or gastroesophageal junction. *N Engl J Med* 2001;345:725–30.

112 Smalley SR, Benedetti JK, Haller DG, *et al.* Updated analysis of SWOG-directed intergroup study 0116: a phase III trial of adjuvant radiochemotherapy versus observation after curative gastric cancer resection. *J Clin Oncol* 2012;30:2327–33.

113 Fuchs CS, Tepper JE, Niedzwiecki D, *et al.* Postoperative adjuvant chemoradiation for gastric or gastroesophageal junction (GEJ) adenocarcinoma using epirubicin, cisplatin, and infusional (CI) 5-FU (ECF) before and after CI 5-FU and radiotherapy (CRT) compared with bolus 5-FU/LV before and after CRT: Intergroup trial CALGB 80101. *Abstract. J Clin Oncol* 2011;29:4003.

114 Lee J, Lim DH, Kim S, *et al.* Phase III trial comparing capecitabine plus cisplatin versus capecitabine plus cisplatin with concurrent capecitabine radiotherapy in completely resected gastric cancer with D2 lymph node dissection: the ARTIST trial. *J Clin Oncol* 2012;30:268–73.

115 Park SH, Sohn TS, Lee J, *et al.* Phase III Trial to Compare Adjuvant Chemotherapy With Capecitabine and Cisplatin Versus Concurrent Chemoradiotherapy in Gastric Cancer: Final Report of the Adjuvant Chemoradiotherapy in Stomach Tumors Trial, Including Survival and Subset Analyses. *J Clin Oncol* 2015;33:3130–6.

116 Verheij M, Jansen EP, Cats A, *et al.* A multicenter randomized phase III trial of neo-adjuvant chemotherapy followed by surgery and chemotherapy or by surgery and chemoradiotherapy in resectable gastric cancer: first results from the CRITICS study. *Abstract. J Clin Oncol* 2016;34:4000.

117 Bang Y-J, Kim Y-W, Yang H-K, *et al.* Adjuvant capecitabine and oxaliplatin for gastric cancer after D2 gastrectomy (CLASSIC): a phase 3 open-label, randomised controlled trial. *Lancet* 2012;379:315–21.

118 Noh SH, Park SR, Yang HK, *et al.* Adjuvant capecitabine plus oxaliplatin for gastric cancer after D2 gastrectomy (CLASSIC): 5-year follow-up of an open-label, randomised phase 3 trial. *Lancet Oncol* 2014;15:1389–96.

119 Sasako M, Sakuramoto S, Katai H, *et al.* Five-year outcomes of a randomized phase III trial comparing adjuvant chemotherapy with S-1 versus surgery alone in stage II or III gastric cancer. *J Clin Oncol* 2011;29:4387–93.

120 Cunningham D, Allum WH, Stenning SP, *et al.* Perioperative chemotherapy versus surgery alone for resectable gastroesophageal cancer. *N Engl J Med* 2006;355:11–20.

121 Ychou M, Boige V, Pignon J-P, *et al.* Perioperative chemotherapy compared with surgery alone for resectable gastroesophageal adenocarcinoma: an FNCLCC and FFCD multicenter phase III trial. *J Clin Oncol* 2011;29:1715–21.

122 Schuhmacher C, Gretschel S, Lordick F, *et al.* Neoadjuvant chemotherapy compared with surgery alone for locally advanced cancer of the stomach and cardia: European Organisation for Research and Treatment of Cancer randomized trial 40954. *J Clin Oncol* 2010;28:5210–18.

123 Leong T, Smithers BM, Michael M, *et al.* *TOPGEAR: a randomised phase III trial of perioperative ECF chemotherapy versus preoperative chemoradiation plus perioperative ECF chemotherapy for resectable gastric cancer (an international, intergroup trial of the AGITG/TROG/EORTC/NCIC CTG).* BMC Cancer 2015;15:532.

124 Bleiberg H, Conroy T, Paillot B, *et al.* Randomised phase II study of cisplatin and 5-fluorouracil (5-FU) versus cisplatin alone in advanced squamous cell oesophageal cancer. *Eur J Cancer* 1997;33:1216–20.

125 Ohtsu A, Shimada Y, Shirao K, *et al.* Randomized phase III trial of fluorouracil alone versus fluorouracil plus cisplatin versus uracil and tegafur plus mitomycin in patients with unresectable, advanced gastric cancer: The Japan Clinical Oncology Group Study (JCOG9205). *J Clin Oncol* 2003;21:54–9.

126 Koizumi W, Narahara H, Hara T, *et al.* S-1 plus cisplatin versus S-1 alone for first-line treatment of advanced gastric cancer (SPIRITS trial): a phase III trial. *Lancet Oncol* 2008;9:215–21.

127 Cullinan SA, Moertel CG, Fleming TR, *et al.* A comparison of three chemotherapeutic regimens in the treatment of advanced pancreatic and gastric carcinoma. Fluorouracil vs fluorouracil and doxorubicin vs fluorouracil, doxorubicin, and mitomycin. *JAMA* 1985;253:2061–7.

128 Webb A, Cunningham D, Scarffe JH, *et al.* Randomized trial comparing epirubicin, cisplatin, and fluorouracil versus fluorouracil, doxorubicin, and methotrexate in advanced esophagogastric cancer. *J Clin Oncol* 1997;15:261–7.

129 Ross P, Nicolson M, Cunningham D, *et al.* Prospective randomized trial comparing mitomycin, cisplatin, and protracted venous-infusion fluorouracil (PVI 5-FU) With epirubicin, cisplatin, and PVI 5-FU in advanced esophagogastric cancer. *J Clin Oncol* 2002;20:1996–2004.

130 Cunningham D, Starling N, Rao S, *et al.* Capecitabine and oxaliplatin for advanced esophagogastric cancer. *N Engl J Med* 2008;358:36–46.

131 Van Cutsem E, Moiseyenko VM, Tjulandin S, *et al.* Phase III study of docetaxel and cisplatin plus fluorouracil compared with cisplatin and fluorouracil as first-line therapy for advanced gastric cancer: a report of the V325 Study Group. *J Clin Oncol* 2006;24:4991–7.

132 Roth AD, Fazio N, Stupp R, *et al.* Docetaxel, cisplatin, and fluorouracil; docetaxel and cisplatin; and epirubicin, cisplatin, and fluorouracil as systemic treatment for advanced gastric carcinoma: a randomized phase II trial of the Swiss Group for Clinical Cancer Research. *J Clin Oncol* 2007;25:3217–23.

133 Shah MA, Jhawer M, Ilson DH, *et al.* Phase II study of modified docetaxel, cisplatin, and fluorouracil with bevacizumab in patients with metastatic gastroesophageal adenocarcinoma. *J Clin Oncol* 2011;29:868–74.

134 Bouche O, Raoul JL, Bonnetain F, *et al.* Randomized multicenter phase II trial of a biweekly regimen of fluorouracil and leucovorin (LV5FU2), LV5FU2 plus cisplatin, or LV5FU2 plus irinotecan in patients with previously untreated metastatic gastric cancer: a Federation Francophone de Cancerologie Digestive Group Study–FFCD 9803. *J Clin Oncol* 2004;22:4319–28.

135 Enzinger PC, Ryan DP, Clark JW, *et al.* Weekly docetaxel, cisplatin, and irinotecan (TPC): results of a multicenter phase

II trial in patients with metastatic esophagogastric cancer. *Ann Oncol* 2009;20:475–80.

136 Guimbaud R, Louvet C, Ries P, *et al.* Prospective, randomized, multicenter, phase III study of fluorouracil, leucovorin, and irinotecan versus epirubicin, cisplatin, and capecitabine in advanced gastric adenocarcinoma: a French intergroup (Fédération Francophone de Cancérologie Digestive, Fédération Nationale des Centres de Lutte Contre le Cancer, and Groupe Coopérateur Multidisciplinaire en Oncologie) study. *J Clin Oncol* 2014;32:3520–6.

137 Ohtsu A, Shah MA, Van Cutsem E, *et al.* Bevacizumab in combination with chemotherapy as first-line therapy in advanced gastric cancer: a randomized, double-blind, placebo-controlled phase III study. *J Clin Oncol* 2011;29:3968–76.

138 Fuchs CS, Tomasek J, Yong CJ, *et al.* Ramucirumab monotherapy for previously treated advanced gastric or gastro-oesophageal junction adenocarcinoma (REGARD): an international, randomised, multicentre, placebo-controlled, phase 3 trial. *Lancet* 2014;383:31–9.

139 Yoon HH, Bendell JC, Braiteh FS, *et al.* Ramucirumab combined with FOLFOX as front-line therapy for advanced esophageal, gastroesophageal junction, or gastric adenocarcinoma: a randomized, double-blind, multicenter Phase II trial. *Ann Oncol* 2016;27:2196–203.

140 National Comprehensive Cancer Network: Gastric Cancer, version 3.2016. In NCCN Clinical Practice Guidelines in Oncology, 2016.

141 Jensen EH, Tuttle TM. Preoperative staging and postoperative surveillance for gastric cancer. *Surg Oncol Clin N Am* 2007;16:329–42.

142 Chu QD, Gibbs JF, Zibari GB, eds. *Surgical Oncology: A Practical and Comprehensive Approach*. New York: Springer-Verlag 2015;195–216.

5

Small Bowel Cancer (Excluding Gastrointestinal Stromal Tumors and Carcinoid)

Alireza Hamidian Jahromi[1], Roger H. Kim[2], Quyen D. Chu[1], and Benjamin D. Li[3]

[1] *Louisiana State University Health Sciences Center, Shreveport, Louisiana, USA*
[2] *Southern Illinois University School of Medicine, Springfield, Illinois, USA*
[3] *MetroHealth Cancer Center, Cleveland, Ohio, USA*

Introduction

The four most common subtypes of small bowel cancer in the United States (US) are: (i) neuroendocrine cancer (40.4%); (ii) adenocarcinoma (23.9%); (iii) lymphoma (16.9%); and (iv) sarcoma, including gastrointestinal stromal tumor (GIST) (8.6%) [1]. Carcinoid tumors of the digestive system and GISTs will be discussed in separate chapters. This chapter will be devoted to adenocarcinoma and lymphoma of the small bowel.

The rarity of small bowel cancer and the vague and nonspecific nature of its presentation make the diagnosis of small bowel malignancy challenging. Delay in diagnosis is generally the rule; early stage disease is infrequent unless incidentally found. Much of our current knowledge of small bowel cancer comes from retrospective studies, reported case series, and data derived from large cancer registries.

Incidence and Mortality

The American Cancer Society estimates that 10,190 people living in the US (5,380 male and 4,810 female) will be diagnosed with, and 1,390 (770 male, 620 female) will die of, small intestine cancers in 2017 [2]. Although the small intestine constitutes 75% of the gastrointestinal (GI) tract length, small bowel cancer accounts for about 5% of all malignancies of the GI tract (from the esophagus to the anus). Proposed explanations for this low rate of malignant transformation of the small bowel include: (i) fast transit time (thus decreased carcinogen exposure); (ii) alkaline to neutral content (decreased carcinogen activity); (iii) low bacterial content; (iv) high folate content (protective against carcinogens); (v) high level of lymphoid tissue activity (immune-protective against cancer cells); and (vi) presence of fewer stem cells [3].

A small bowel malignancy is often a second primary malignancy. In a review of two tumor registries in Canada, there was a greater than eightfold increase in the risk for another malignancy in patients with small bowel cancer. In more than 70% of these patients, the small bowel malignancy represented the second primary malignancy, with colorectal cancer being the most common initial primary malignancy [4].

The most frequent sites of small bowel cancer are the duodenum and proximal jejunum [5]. In population-based cancer registries for Canada, 54.7% of small bowel adenocarcinomas occurred in the duodenum, 29.9% in the jejunum, and 16.0% in the ileum. In contrast, small bowel lymphoma was more frequent in the ileum (50%) compared with the jejunum (30%) and the duodenum (20%). The mean and median ages of patients with lymphoma (mean age = 59.6 years) was significantly lower compared to adenocarcinoma (mean age = 65.2 years) and carcinoid (mean age = 64.7 years) cases ($P < 0.05$) [6].

Based on the National Cancer Institute's Surveillance, Epidemiology, and End Results (SEER) database, the median age of the patients with a small bowel cancer diagnosis is 65 years [7]. There is a slight preponderance of male (2.6 per 100,000) over female (1.9 per 100,000) cases [7]. Data from SEER indicate higher incidence and mortality rates for small bowel cancers (all histologies combined) among African Americans compared with the Whites, American Indians/Alaska Natives, Hispanics, and Asian/Pacific Islanders [7].

Risk Factors

Lifestyle Factors

Cigarette smoking has consistently been shown to be a strong risk factor for small bowel cancers [8, 9]. For example, Chen *et al.* estimated a 6.2-fold increase in the risk of adenocarcinoma of the small bowel in cigarette smokers compared with nonsmokers [10].

Alcohol consumption has also been proposed as an independent risk factor for small bowel cancer [8, 9]. In the same study by Chen *et al.*, alcohol consumption was associated with an increased risk for adenocarcinoma (odds ratio = 5.5)

The American Cancer Society's Oncology in Practice: Clinical Management, First Edition. Edited by The American Cancer Society.

compared to nondrinkers. Even after adjustment for cigarette smoking, alcohol consumption was associated with an increased risk of small bowel adenocarcinoma (odds ratio = 4) [10].

Dietary consumption of red meat may also be associated with an increased risk for small bowel cancers although the reports are not consistent [5, 8]. In a small case-control study, Negri *et al.* concluded that red meat consumption may be an important risk factor for the cancer (odds ratio = 4.6) [11]. Chow *et al.* performed a case-control study comparing deceased subjects with small bowel cancers with a control group and found that weekly or more frequent consumption of red meat and monthly or more frequent intake of salt-cured/smoked foods is associated with a two- to threefold increase in the risk of small bowel cancer [12]. However, a prospective study following 494,000 subjects for up to 8 years did not show any clear relationship between red/processed meat consumption and small bowel adenocarcinoma [8].

A recent meta-analysis indicated significantly increased risk associated with heavy alcohol consumption and nonsignificant associations with smoking and consumption of processed meats [13].

Underlying Conditions

Previous Cholecystectomy

In a longitudinal study using the Swedish Inpatient Register, Lagergren *et al.* evaluated 278,460 patients who had a cholecystectomy between 1965 and 1997 and found a possible positive association between cholecystectomy and small bowel cancer [14]. They reported a standardized incidence ratio of 1.77X in both male and female patients for adenocarcinoma of the small bowel after cholecystectomy. This risk remained elevated 33 years after surgery [14].

Celiac Disease

Patients with celiac disease appear to have an increased risk for small intestine cancer. One study of 381 celiac disease patients reported a standardized morbidity ratio (SMR) (ratio of observed to expected) of 34 for small bowel adenocarcinoma and a SMR of 9.1 for non-Hodgkin lymphoma (NHL). The NHL included both T-cell and B-cell types, which occurred in both GI as well as extraintestinal sites. Staying on a gluten-free diet seems to lower the risk of small bowel cancer development in celiac disease patients [15]. More recent studies confirm this effect but indicate a smaller magnitude. A population-based study of 32,439 Finnish adult celiac patients found standardized incidence ratios (SIRs) for small bowel cancer and for NHL (any site) of 4.29 and 1.94, respectively [1613a]. A recent meta-analysis found a pooled odds ratio for small intestine cancer incidence of 14.41 [1713b].

Crohn Disease

Patients with Crohn disease appear to have an increased risk of small bowel cancer and lymphoma [18]. Laukoetter *et al.* performed a meta-analysis and reviewed 20 clinical studies that were published between 1965 and 2008 and evaluated 40,547 patients with Crohn disease. Laukoetter reported the risk for small bowel cancer in these patients as 18.8 times more than in an age-matched standard population. The incidence of small bowel cancer in the Crohn disease population was 0.3/1,000 person years' duration. Duration of Crohn disease, age at diagnosis, and anatomical area of the disease had no significant correlation to the cancer risk [19].

Another meta-analysis published by Canavan *et al.* assessed the relative risk for small bowel cancer in Crohn patients to be 33.2 (15.9–60.9) times higher compared to the general population. This relative risk has not been significantly reduced for the last 30 years despite improved management of Crohn disease [20]. In another study of a cohort of 374 patients with Crohn disease, with a minimum of 10 years' follow-up, the risk of colorectal cancers was found to be stable, which the authors attributed to maintenance treatment with 5-aminosalisylic acid preparations and surgery in case of treatment failure. In contrast, the risk of small bowel cancers was found to be increased by more than 60-fold even in the presence of maintenance treatments [21]. Male gender, chronic fistulous disease, surgically excluded small bowel loops, proximal small bowel disease, and 6-mercaptopurine use were all correlated with small bowel cancer [22]. Small bowel cancer in Crohn patients is most often seen in the ileum.

In a population-based cohort study that included nearly 50,000 Swedish patients with inflammatory bowel disease, Askling *et al.* compared the SIR of inflammatory bowel disease patients with the Swedish population. While there was no statistically significant increased risk of lymphoma for ulcerative colitis patients (SIR 1.0, 0.8–1.3), the overall rate of lymphoma for Crohn patients was slightly increased (SIR 1.3, 1.0–1.6) and there was a significantly higher rate of NHL (SIR 1.55, 1.2–2.0) but not Hodgkin disease (SIR 1.03, 0.4–2.2) [23]. Following a review of the literature, Siegel suggested that the increased risk of lymphoma in the Crohn population may be attributable to the immune-modulator and anti-TNF treatments [24].

Inherited Conditions

MUTYH-Associated Polyposis

MUTYH-associated polyposis is caused by bi-allelic mutations in the *MUTYH* gene. People with this syndrome are predisposed to develop colon polyps, colon cancer (100% in the absence of surveillance), small intestine polyps (17–25% of the patients), small intestine cancer (lifetime risk of duodenal cancer is estimated at 4%), as well as ovary, skin, thyroid, and bladder cancers [25].

Cystic Fibrosis

Patients with cystic fibrosis have two involved copies of the *CFTR* gene. Sheldon *et al.* reported on a cohort of 412 patients with cystic fibrosis. The number of malignancies observed in this cohort was compared with the expected number of malignancies based on the age, gender, and calendar-year-specific cancer registration rates of the area. They concluded that the risk for adenocarcinoma of the terminal ileum was associated with cystic fibrosis [26]. Large population-based studies in Europe, the US, and Canada have also confirmed the increased risk of digestive tract (esophagus, small, and large intestine) cancers, with an observed to expected cancer ratio of 11.5 (4.2–25.4) for small bowel cancers in the cystic fibrosis patients [27, 28].

Familial Adenomatous Polyposis

Small bowel manifestations of familial adenomatous polyposis (FAP) include adenomas and adenocarcinomas, most commonly involving the duodenum. Prophylactic pan-colectomy has reduced the mortality due to colorectal cancer, but has resulted in small bowel cancer (periampulary adenocarcinoma) becoming the current leading cause of death in FAP patients [29].

Hereditary Non-Polyposis Colorectal Cancer (Lynch Syndrome)

This disorder is caused by a defect in genes involved in DNA mismatch repair. An abnormal copy of these genes leads to defective DNA damage repair and microsatellite instability, resulting in an increased risk for colon, small intestine, endometrial, stomach, renal pelvis, ureter, and ovarian cancers [30]. The mutation carriers have a 4% estimated risk of developing small bowel cancers during their lifetime (relative risk of 100 compared to the general population) [31]. Patients with Lynch syndrome also tend to develop small bowel cancers at a much younger age, on average 10–20 years earlier than in the general population [231].

Peutz-Jeghers Syndrome

Peutz-Jeghers syndrome (PJS) is a rare autosomal dominant inherited condition and is associated with formation of hamartomatous polyps in the stomach, small and large intestines, bladder, nose, upper airways, and the lungs. Patients with PJS have hyperpigmentation of the skin and mucous membranes, and very often present with complications of the polyps including bleeding, bowel obstruction, and intussusceptions (50% chance of developing intussusceptions before the age of 20). People with PJS have an increased risk of many types of cancer, including small intestine adenocarcinoma. The lifetime cumulative risk of small bowel cancers is estimated to be 13%, with a relative risk of 520-fold compared to the general population [32].

Screening/Surveillance for Small Bowel Cancer

In patients with conditions known to be associated with increased risk for small bowel cancer, some authors have suggested a small bowel screening/surveillance program. The recommendations apply specifically for patients with Crohn disease, celiac disease, and inherited risk for small bowel adenocarcinoma (FAP, hereditary non-polyposis colorectal cancer, and PJS patients) [2, 31]. This has included the use of esophagogastroduodenoscopy, small bowel enteroclysis, capsule endoscopy, and double balloon enteroscopy. These modalities will be discussed in detail later in this chapter.

Pathology

Adenocarcinoma

Adenocarcinoma of the small bowel develops either as a polypoid fungating mass or in a napkin-ring pattern. Due to late presentation, penetration of the bowel, invasion of the mesentery, regional nodal involvement, invasion to other bowel segments, and distant metastasis to the liver, for example, are quite common. An adenoma to carcinoma sequence has been proposed for small bowel adenocarcinoma [33].

Lymphoma of the Small Bowel

The small bowel is a common site for GI lymphoma, second only to the stomach. Major subtypes of the small intestinal lymphoma include: (i) diffuse large B-cell lymphoma; (ii) mucosal-associated lymphoid tissue lymphoma; and (iii) peripheral T-cell lymphoma and Burkitt lymphoma [3].

Diagnosis

The clinical presentation of small bowel cancers can be very subtle, often leading to a delay in diagnosis. Abdominal pain, nausea, vomiting and signs of bowel obstruction, weight loss, anorexia, GI bleed, and bowel perforation can all be presenting symptoms. Weight loss is more commonly associated with small bowel lymphoma, GI bleeding is more frequently associated with GIST and sarcoma, and obstructive symptoms are more common presenting symptoms in the adenocarcinoma and carcinoid tumors [3]. Significant numbers of patients are diagnosed only after surgery [34].

Maglinte *et al.* performed a root cause analysis on the factors attributed to the late diagnosis of the small intestine tumors. Physicians not ordering the appropriate diagnostic test and radiologists failing to make the diagnosis were the two most important causes for the delay in diagnosis, on average resulting in a 20-month delay in diagnosis. In contrast, patients' delay in seeking medical consultation was on average responsible for 2.5 months of delay [35, 36]. Improvement in the current armamentarium of radiologic studies and emergence of new endoscopic diagnostic tools may improve the diagnostic yield of a patient's workup; however, having a high index of suspicion for small bowel malignancy in patients presenting repeatedly with vague abdominal symptoms is necessary for an early and accurate diagnosis.

Radiologic Assessment

Radiologic studies that are used in the diagnosis and staging of small bowel cancers include: abdominal CT scan, enteroclysis using plain X-ray or fluoroscopy, CT-enteroclysis, magnetic resonance (MR)-enteroclysis and positron emission tomography (PET-CT).

Abdominal CT

CT scan is widely used for the initial assessment of patients presenting with vague abdominal and/or GI-related symptoms. The sensitivity and specificity of abdominal CT in diagnosing small bowel malignancy ranges from 17 to 100% and 80 to 98% respectively, depending on the stage of the disease [37, 38]. CT scan is also helpful for disease staging as well as postoperative surveillance (staging accuracy of 47%). Neoplastic lesions should be suspected when small bowel wall thickening (≥1.5 cm) or a discrete mesenteric mass is present [38]. Annular narrowing of the small bowel lumen with irregular edges, eccentric thickening of the bowel wall, mesenteric fat stranding, target

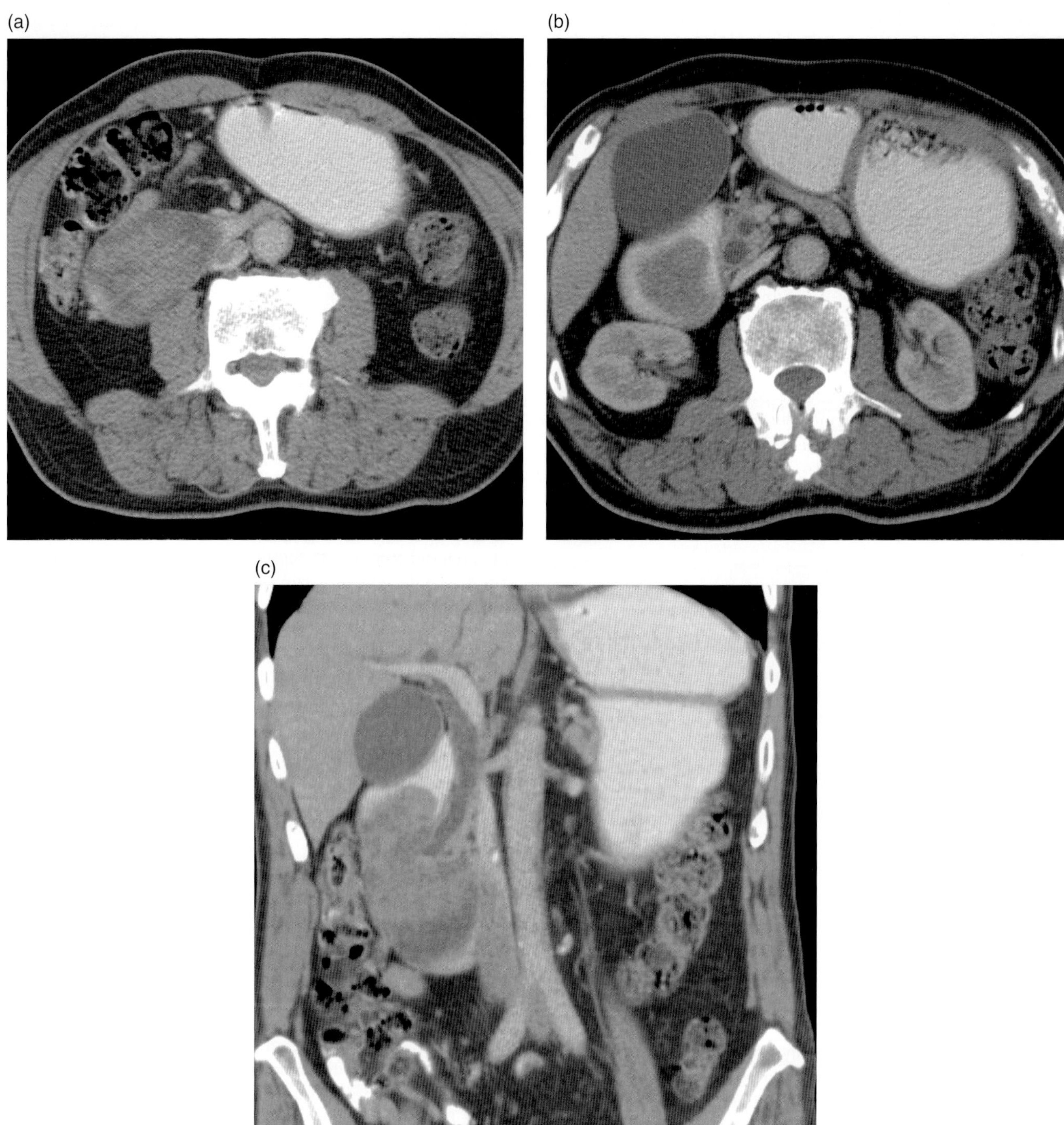

Figure 5.1 (a–c) Representative images of an abdominal CT scan in a patient with adenocarcinoma of small bowel.

lesions, discrete mass as the leading point of intussusceptions, aneurysmal dilatation of the small bowel, and overt lymphadenopathy are some of the common CT findings associated with adenocarcinoma of small bowel (Figure 5.1) [3].

Dudiak *et al.*, in a retrospective study, found that abdominal CT scan was helpful in predicting the type of pathology for small bowel cancers in 33–60% of cases depending on the tumor type [39]. Characteristic radiologic appearance for lymphoma was annular shape, large tumor (mean size = 9.5 cm), with aneurysmal ulceration (larger luminal diameter than the adjacent unaffected bowel) and bulky mesenteric/retroperitoneal lymphadenopathy (Figure 5.2). In contrast, presence of small (mean size = 6.5 cm), solitary, proximal small bowel masses with nonbulky lymphadenopathy were characteristics of adenocarcinoma [39].

Enteroclysis

Due to multiple overlaps of the small bowel loops in the center of the abdomen and active peristalsis, detailed evaluation of the

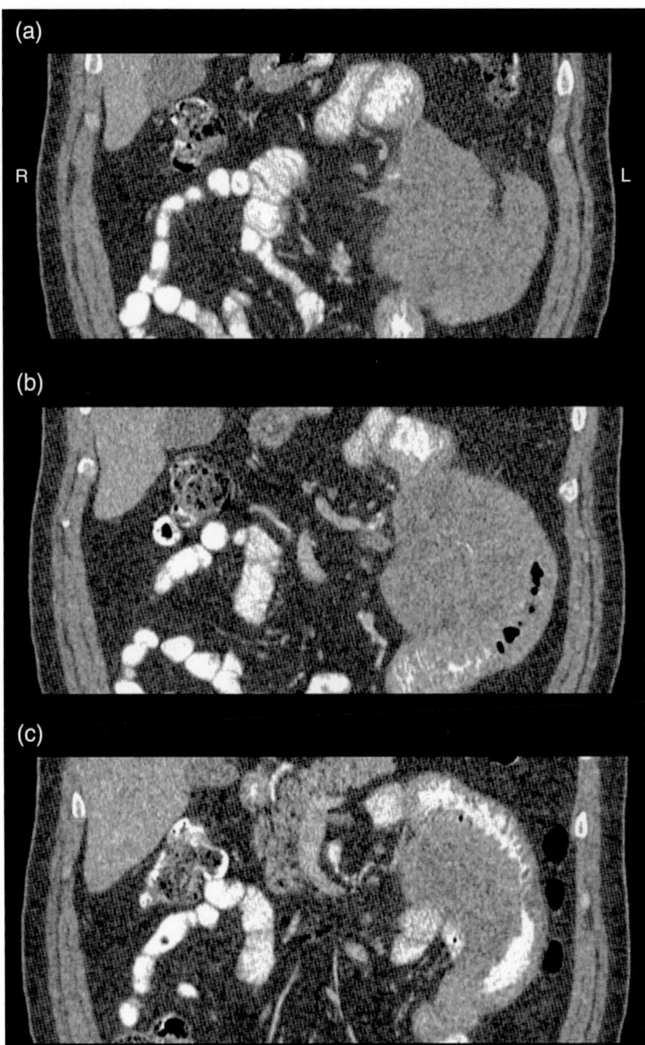

Figure 5.2 (a–c) Representative images of an abdominal CT scan in a patient with lymphoma of small bowel.

small bowel using barium is more difficult than in the colon and stomach [37]. Additionally, while barium is helpful in visualizing intraluminal lesions, it is not as helpful in demonstrating mesentery invasion by a small bowel cancer.

Enteroclysis, the use of real-time fluoroscopic X-ray evaluation of the small bowel using infusion of the contrast through upper GI tubes, has been shown to be superior to the conventional small bowel follow-through (sensitivity of 95% vs 60%) in the detection of the small bowel malignancies [40, 41]. Visualization of the actual tumor was also significantly higher using enteroclysis compared with small bowel follow-through (90% vs 33%) [40]. Specificity of the double-contrast barium evaluation has ranged from 53 to 83% in different studies [38]. Punched-out lesions, filling defects, blank spaces or mass effects, focal aneurysmal dilatation, aperistaltic segments, ballooned and thickened segments, crowding of folds, kinking of the bowel wall, and broad-based ulcerations are some of the radiologic findings [3]. Due to its high negative predictive value, a detailed contrast enteroclysis was once considered as the consensus primary radiologic investigation for the initial diagnostic workup for small bowel cancer [41]. The use of hypotonic agents, glucagon, as well as per-oral pneumocolic techniques have been shown to increase the accuracy of the barium studies, especially for the distal ileal lesions [37, 42].

CT-Enteroclysis

Recent improvements in CT scan quality and the introduction of the multidetector CT scanners (MDCT) have improved the ability of the CT scans to assess accurately the small bowel mesentery. Merging MDCT and enteroclysis has improved the specificity of each test alone; the reported CT-enteroclysis sensitivity, specificity, and diagnostic accuracy are 83%, 100%, and 89%, respectively [1, 43]. By performing a water/contrast enhanced MDCT-enteroclysis, the ability to visualize intraluminal small bowel lesions is further enhanced [44–47]. CT-enteroclysis has been shown to be superior to conventional CT and contrast enteroclysis alone in detecting small bowel pathologies [43, 48]. Some reports have calculated the overall accuracy of the contrast- and water-enhanced MDCT-enteroclysis for depiction of small-bowel neoplasms to be as high as 85% [46].

MR-Enteroclysis

The role of MRI of the small bowel was once thought to be limited to inflammatory diseases (e.g. Crohn patient) [37]. With the introduction of MR-enteroclysis (MR-enterography), there are reports on its high-yield ability to predict accurately the site and stage of small bowel cancer [49]. This technique utilizes real-time MR fluoroscopy following infusion of contrast through upper GI tubes. Different contrast agents, including negative iron-based, positive gadolinium-based, and methylcellulose in water as the enteric contrast together with intravenous gadopentetate dimeglumine, could have been used.

In a recent study, Pappalardo *et al.* retrospectively assessed the role of MR-enterography in the preoperative surgical planning of patients with suspected small bowel cancer. The authors reported concordance rate of 100% for localization, 87%, 80%, and 96.8% for the T, N, M stage prediction and 62% for histology prediction between the preoperative MR-enterography and the postoperative findings. The accuracy of MR-enterography prediction of final histology was not different in various tumor types. This accuracy (62%, 42–78%) was not sufficiently high to determine the correct therapeutic management [49].

PET-CT

This combined morphologic and functional imaging modality has been shown to have a high sensitivity for detection of colorectal cancers and is superior to a CT scan in staging of local and metastatic colorectal cancers [50]. The role of the PET-CT in the diagnosis and staging of small bowel cancers are not as well explored. PET-CT is useful in the initial diagnosis (showing mural thickening and increased fludeoxyglucose uptake), staging, restaging, and evaluation of response to treatment in small bowel adenocarcinomas (Figure 5.3) [51]. The value of PET-CT to detect local and distant metastasis has not been formally evaluated for small bowel adenocarcinomas as for colorectal cancers [51].

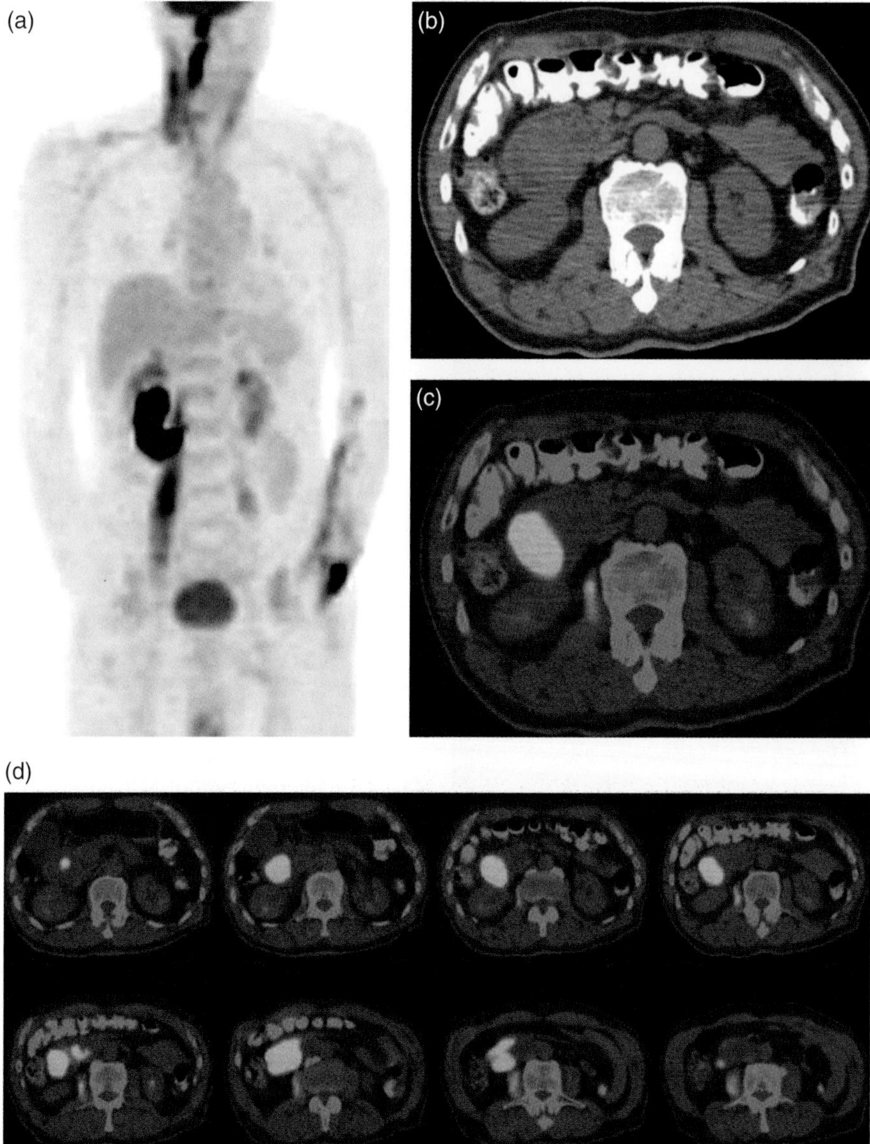

Figure 5.3 PET-CT image in a patient with duodenal adenocarcinoma. A very intensely fludeoxyglucose-avid heterogenous mass lesion involving the second and third portion of duodenum is seen in (c, d). A few not prominent but not particularly enlarged (a, b) modestly fludeoxyglucose-avid lymph nodes are seen in the vicinity of the primary lesion in the right upper abdomen and are suspicious for early nodal metastatic involvement (c, d SUV max = 39.0, SUV average = 22.6).

PET-CT is accurate for baseline staging and provides important prognostic information in the systemic lymphoma [51, 52]; the value of PET-CT in the evaluation of small bowel lymphoma as a distinctive entity is not well documented. In a study on 19 patients with GI tract lymphoma (four gastric, 13 small bowel, two small and large bowel), Kumar *et al.* compared the accuracy of PET and CT in evaluation of treatment response based on the post-treatment clinical and biopsy results. The sensitivity, specificity, positive, and negative predictive values, and accuracy of post-therapy PET were 86%, 100%, 100%, 92%, and 95%, respectively. The corresponding values for CT scan were 67%, 75%, 75%, 90%, and 79%, respectively. Patients with positive post-treatment PET had statistically significant lower disease free survival proportion (0%) than patients with positive post-treatment CT (33%) ($P = 0.04$) [53]. Despite the mild physiologic fludeoxyglucose tracer uptake of the GI tract, PET appears to be useful in determining response to treatment in patients with GI tract lymphomas in cases with a positive pretreatment PET [53].

Endoscopic Assessment

The adoption of the newer endoscopic techniques, such as wireless capsule endoscopy and double balloon enteroscopy (DBE), has for the first time allowed endoscopists to directly visualize the entire surface area of the small intestine. Wireless capsule endoscopy is emerging as a new standard of care for diagnosis of small bowel cancers [54–57]. This method uses capsules equipped with a small camera (the size and shape of a pill) that continuously record images from the internal bowel lumen following ingestion by the patient. In a meta-analysis of 24 studies, the overall diagnostic yield of capsule endoscopy alone was 87% for the small bowel pathologies with a missed rate of 10% [57].

The emergence of DBE has greatly enhanced the management of small bowel pathologies. Since its introduction in 2001 by Yamamoto *et al.*, it has rapidly gained widespread acceptance for its therapeutic as well as diagnostic role in the management of small bowel cancer [58–60]. In DBE, the enteroscope is equipped with an overtube (a tube which fits over the enteroscope) and two balloons that are located at the end of the enteroscope camera and the overtube. In DBE (also called push-and-pull enteroscopy), following advancement of the scope from the proximal small bowel for a short distance in front of the overtube, the distal balloon is inflated and the scope is pulled back. Alternating inflation of the two balloons and interval pulling, along with the friction between the balloons and small bowel lumen, accordion the small bowel back to the overtube and allows for visualization of the entire length of the small intestine.

In a prospective study, May *et al.* evaluated 137 patients with suspected small bowel pathologies (mainly chronic GI bleeding) using DBE. An oral and anal route for DBE visualized on average 240 ± 100 cm and 140 ± 90 cm of the small bowel lumen respectively. The average investigation time was 73.5 ± 25 min. The overall diagnostic yield was 80%. They reported that DBE is a feasible and safe diagnostic/therapeutic procedure [61].

The complication rate for DBE appears to be very low (1% risk of major complications including pancreatitis, bleeding, and perforation in some reported series) compared with a 5% complications rate for other therapeutic procedures [62]. A prospective multicenter trial in three European medical centers showed that DBE was diagnostic in 72% of the cases studied and there were no major procedure-associated complications, such as perforation, bleeding, or injury to the small bowel tissue or mesentery noted [63].

Staging

Small bowel adenocarcinoma is staged according to the TNM classification designated by the American Joint Committee on Cancer (Table 5.1) [64].

Lymphoma of the small bowel is most commonly staged using the "Paris" staging system, first proposed (2003) by the European Gastro-Intestinal Lymphoma Study Group. This is a modified specific version of the TNM system for staging of GI lymphomas, which is based on the depth of tumor infiltration, extent of nodal involvement, specific lymphoma spreading, and their histopathological characteristics as shown in Table 5.2 [65].

Treatment

Treatment options for the small bowel adenocarcinoma depend on the tumor location (duodenum vs jejunum/ileum), T-category (extent of bowel and adjacent structure involvement),

Table 5.1 TNM staging of small bowel adenocarcinoma.

Definition of Primary Tumor (T)

T Category	T Criteria
TX	Primary tumor cannot be assessed
T0	No evidence of primary tumor
Tis	High-grade dysplasia/carcinoma *in situ*
T1	Tumor invades the lamina propria or submucosa
T1a	Tumor invades the lamina propria
T1b	Tumor invades the submucosa
T2	Tumor invades the muscularis propria
T3	Tumor invades through the muscularis propria into the subserosa, or extends into nonperitonealized perimuscular tissue (mesentery or retroperitoneum) without serosal penetration[1]
T4	Tumor perforates the visceral peritoneum or directly invades other organs or structures (e.g., other loops of small intestine, mesentery of adjacent loops of bowel, and abdominal wall by way of serosa; for duodenum only, invasion of pancreas or bile duct)

[1] Note: For T3 tumors, the nonperitonealized perimuscular tissue is, for the jejunum and ileum, part of the mesentery and, for the duodenum in areas where serosa is lacking, part of the interface with the pancreas.

Definition of Regional Lymph Node (N)

N Category	N Criteria
NX	Regional lymph nodes cannot be assessed
N0	No regional lymph node metastasis
N1	Metastasis in one or two regional lymph nodes
N2	Metastasis in three or more regional lymph nodes

Definition of Distant Metastasis (M)

M Category	M Criteria
M0	No distant metastasis
M1	Distant metastasis present

AJCC Prognostic Stage Groups

Adenocarcinoma

When T is...	And N is...	And M is...	Then the stage group is...
Tis	N0	M0	0
T1–2	N0	M0	I
T3	N0	M0	IIA
T4	N0	M0	IIB
Any T	N1	M0	IIIA
Any T	N2	M0	IIIB
Any T	Any N	M1	IV

Table 5.2 Paris staging system for primary gastrointestinal lymphomas.[1,2]

TX	Lymphoma extent not specified
TO	No evidence of lymphoma
T1	Lymphoma confined to the mucosa/submucosa
T1m	Lymphoma confined to mucosa
T1sm	Lymphoma confined to submucosa
T2	Lymphoma infiltrates muscularis propria or subserosa
T3	Lymphoma penetrates serosa (visceral peritoneum) without invasion of adjacent structures
T4	Lymphoma invades adjacent structures or organs
NX	Involvement of lymph nodes not assessed
NO	No evidence of lymph node involvement
N1[3]	Involvement of regional lymph nodes
N2	Involvement of intra-abdominal lymph nodes beyond the regional area
N3	Spread to extra-abdominal lymph nodes
MX	Dissemination of lymphoma not assessed
MO	No evidence of extranodal dissemination
M1	Non-continuous involvement of separate site in gastrointestinal tract (e.g., stomach, rectum)
M2	Non-continuous involvement of other tissues (e.g., peritoneum, pleura) or organs (e.g., tonsils,.parotid gland, ocular adnexa, lung, liver, spleen, kidney, breast, etc.)
BX	Involvement of bone marrow not assessed
B0	No evidence of bone marrow involvement
B1	Lymphomatous infiltration of bone marrow
TNM	Clinical staging: status of tumor, node, metastasis, bone marrow
pTNMB	Histopathological staging: status of tumor, node, metastasis, bone marrow
pN	The histological examination will ordinarily include 6 or more lymph nodes

Source: Ruskoné-Fourmestraux, *et al.* [65]. Reproduced with permission of BMJ Publishing Group Ltd.

[1] Valid for lymphomas originating from the gastro-oesophageal junction to the anus (as defined by identical histomorphological structure).

[2] In case of more than one visible lesion synchronously originating in the gastrointestinal tract, give the characteristics of the more advanced lesion.

[3] Anatomical designation of lymph nodes as "regional" according to site:
(a) Stomach: perigastric nodes and those located along the ramifications of the coeliac artery (that is, left gastric artery, common hepatic artery, splenic artery) in accordance with compartments I and II of the Japanese Research Society for Gastric Cancer (1995); (b) Duodenum: pancreaticoduodenal, pyloric, hepatic, and superior mesenteric nodes; (c) Jejunum/ileum: mesenteric nodes and, for the terminal ileum only, the ileocolic as well as the posterior caecal nodes; (d) Colorectum: pericolic and perirectal nodes and those located along the ileocolic, right, middle, and left colic, inferior mesenteric, superior rectal, and internal iliac arteries.

N-category (degree and extent of lymph node involvement and whether they are within the scope of resection), and M-category (extraintestinal disease vs distant metastasis). Curative surgery, palliative surgery, and/or chemoradiation are the possible treatment options.

Complete surgical resection is the single best potentially curative treatment. En bloc resection of the ileal/jejunal tumors, along with draining regional lymph nodes and nonvital adjacent organs/structures when there is invasion, with the goal of tumor-free resection margins, is the mainstay for surgical therapy [66]. Tumors of the terminal ileum may require ileocecectomy for a complete resection.

Adenocarcinomas arising from the duodenum and periampullary cancers require a nuanced approach. Resection options include endoscopic resection, transduodenal local excision, segmental duodenectomy, pancreas-preserving duodenal resection, and pancreaticoduodenectomy [66]. Endoscopic resection using the submucosal saline infiltration technique and transduodenal local resection, are reserved for early (stage-I) or small size (<5 cm) duodenal cancers and polypoid/protruded lesions [66, 67]. Due to the possible risk of distant lymph node metastasis, this technique is not recommended in depressed tumors with or without marginal elevation [67].

The objective for limited resection remains a tumor-free surgical resection. If this is not achievable with limited resection, consideration must be given to the more radical resection if a reasonable chance for a tumor-free resection margin can be achieved. In locally advanced disease, there are some suggestions that pancreaticoduodenectomy or pancreas-preserving duodenal resection yields better survival rates compared with a segmental duodenal resection if the tumor-free resection margins can be achieved with the larger resection [68–71].

Although curative resection in the absence of distant metastasis is associated with the best survival outcome in the patient with a small bowel adenocarcinoma, systemic recurrence is a common outcome and is associated with mortality. In a multivariate analysis, Agrawal *et al.* reported that curative resection was an independent predictor of survival, and that the median survival time for patients treated with curative resection of small bowel adenocarcinoma was 56.4 months [72]. However, their analysis showed that even following curative resection, 66.7% of recurrences were at distant sites (liver and lung) and that the median time to recurrence was 17 months. This would suggest the potential use of adjuvant systemic therapy after curative surgery.

Unfortunately, there is a lack of data to recommend a definitive role for postoperative adjuvant systemic therapy. In a Cochrane Central Register of Controlled Trials report by Singhal *et al.*, no phase-III randomized controlled trial was present comparing postoperative adjuvant chemotherapy regimens versus placebo or demonstrating benefits for systemic adjuvant therapy [73].

In a report by Agrawal *et al.*, 23.8% of recurrences occurred locally as peritoneal carcinomatosis [72]. Small bowel cancers are considered to be relatively radio-resistant, thus the role of postoperative or intraoperative radiotherapy in the prevention of local recurrence in locally advanced disease is yet to be defined [62]. For patients with noncurative resection, the progression of disease to death is within a median period of 10 months (range 2–18 months) [72].

Patients with locally advanced tumors who are not candidates for operation/resection, or in cases where the tumor has a distant metastasis, are generally treated with chemoradiation. Different chemotherapy regimens have been used for neoadjuvant or adjuvant therapy. These include 5-fluorouracil alone or in combination with other agents including cyclophosphamide, adriamycin, vincristine, doxorubicin, cisplatin, mytomycin-C, capecitabine, irinotecan, methotrexate, epirubicin, oxaliplatin, and prednisone [1, 66, 74]. Table 5.3 summarizes some of the

Table 5.3 A summary of some of the studies evaluating the outcome of patients with small bowel adenocarcinoma receiving neoadjuvant/adjuvant chemoradiation.

Study (reference)	Study detail	Chemotherapy regimens	Results
Duke University study by Kelsey *et al.* [75]	Surgery ($n = 16$) versus surgery + CR ($n = 16$) in patients with adenocarcinoma of duodenum	Surgery + CR patients (neoadjuvant ($n = 11$), adjuvant ($n = 5$) CR) received radiotherapy (median dose = 50.4 Gy) and 5-FU-based chemotherapy.	5-year survival (57% vs 44%, $P = 0.42$) DFS (54% vs 44%, $P = 0.55$) Local control (70% vs 49%, $P = 0.84$)
MD Anderson Cancer Center study by Overman *et al.* [74]	Adjuvant therapy (chemotherapy/ chemotherapy + radiation/CR/radiation) in patients with small bowel adenocarcinoma following curative (margin-negative) surgical resection	Chemotherapy (5-FU/5-FU + platinum/capecitabine/ CAPOX/5-FU-irinotecan) ($n = 18$);CR ($n = 3$);radiation ($n = 2$);chemotherapy + radiation(CAPOX + capecitabine + radiation/5-FU + cisplatin + 5-FU + radiation/5-FU + cisplatin + capecitabine + radiation) ($n = 7$).	Adjuvant chemotherapy offered improved DFS (HR = 0.27; 95% CI = 0.07-0.98, $P = 0.05$), but not OS (HR = 0.47; 95% CI = 0.13-1.62, $P = 0.23$)
London Royal Marsden Hospital study by Crawley *et al.* [76]	Protracted 5-FU infusion in patients with advanced (unresectable) small bowel adenocarcinoma	Epirubicin (50 mg m^{-2})/cisplatin (60 mg m^{-2}) /5-FU (200 mg m^{-2}) ($n = 8$)	Overall response rate = 37.5%. Median OS = 13 months (range 1–28) PFS = 7.8 months (range 0–15)
Multicenter retrospective study by Tsushima *et al.* [77]	Patients with unresectable or recurrent small bowel adenocarcinoma treated only with chemotherapy ($n = 132$)	(A) Fluoropyrimidine monotherapy ($n = 60$) (B) fluoropyrimidine-cisplatin ($n = 17$) (C) Fluoro-pyrimidine-oxaliplatin combination ($n = 22$) (D) fluoropyrimidine-irinotecan ($n = 11$)	Median PFS for group A,B,C,D were 5.4, 3.8, 8.2,5.6 months respectively Increase in PFS for group C patients (receiving fluoro-pyrimidine-oxaliplatin) compared to groups A,B,D (HR 0.45, 95% CI = 0.23-0.88, $P = 0.02$)
Phase II study by Xiang *et al.* [78]	Safety and efficacy of modified FOLFOX chemotherapy in metastatic or advanced (unresectable) small bowel adenocarcinoma	FOLFOX chemotherapy regimen (biweekly oxaliplatin (85 mg m^{-2}) in combination with continuous infusion of 5-FU (2600 mg m^{-2}) and leucovorin (400 mg m^{-2}) ($n = 33$)	Objective response rate = 48.5% Median OS = 15.2 months Median time to progression = 7.8 months
Phase II study by Overman *et al.* [79]	Chemotherapy in patients with metastatic or advanced (unresectable) small bowel adenocarcinoma	CAPOX (21-day cycle with oxaliplatin (130 mg m^{-2}) on day one and capecitabine (750 mg m^{-2}) on days 1 through 14) ($n = 30$)	Overall response rate = 50% Median time to progression = 11.3 months Median OS = 20.4 months Subset analysis of metastatic disease patients ($n = 25$): Median time to progression = 9.4 months Median OS = 15.5 months
Chinese study group by Zhang *et al.* [80]	Chemotherapy in patients with advanced (unresectable)/metastatic small bowel adenocarcinoma	FOLFOX (5-FU (400 mg m^{-2}) + leucovorin (400 mg m^{-2}) + oxaliplatin (85 mg m^{-2}) repeated every 2 weeks) ($n = 28$) CAPOX (capecitabine (1000 mg m^{-2}) plus oxaliplatin (130 mg m^{-2}) repeated every 21 days) ($n = 6$)	Partial response = 32.3% Stable disease = 29.4% Objective response = 32.3% Disease control rate = 61.7%

5-FU, 5-fluorouracil; DFS, disease free survival; CR, chemoradiation; OS, overall survival; CAPOX, capecitabine and oxaliplatin; PFS, progression free survival.

studies evaluating the outcome of patients with small bowel adenocarcinoma receiving neoadjuvant/adjuvant chemoradiation.

In a retrospective study, Onkendi *et al.* assessed the role of neoadjuvant chemoradiation in the management of initially unresectable or recurrent duodenal adenocarcinoma in a small group of patients ($n = 10$). Nine patients (90%) became resectable after neoadjuvant chemoradiation: three had complete/near complete (<1 mm of residual disease) pathologic responses [81].

In patients with unresectable tumors, palliative surgeries include GI bypass to treat ongoing or prevent future bowel obstructions. Resection of a tumor for GI bleeding can be considered [66]. Radiologic or endoscopic interventions (stent placement) are considered alternatives for open and laparoscopic bypass procedures.

Palliative chemotherapy has been shown to be helpful in some studies [82]. In a retrospective study on 91 patients with advanced small bowel cancer, 40 patients received fluoropyrimidine-based palliative chemotherapy (median four cycles). The median overall survival and progression-free survival (PFS) were 11.8 and 5.7 months respectively, compared to 4.1 months and 1.3 months in untreated patients [82].

Lymphoma

The treatment options for patients with small bowel lymphoma are determined by the subtype of the lymphoma and the sites of cancer involvement. While the majority of the lymphoma subtypes respond well to chemotherapeutic regimens, certain lymphomas (anaplastic type) may be resistant to most chemotherapeutic agents.

The majority of the available evidence on management of small bowel lymphoma is driven from retrospective reviews concerning GI lymphomas as a complete entity where data on the subgroup of small bowel lymphoma should be extracted from the presented data whenever possible [83].

Systemic chemotherapy is the treatment of choice for small bowel lymphoma. This is in part due to the likely systemic nature of lymphoma of the GI tract even when localized, as well as the difficulty of complete resection in certain anatomic locations, such as duodenal lymphoma requiring pancreaticoduodenectomy. Thus, surgery is reserved for patients who present with complications from lymphoma, such as complete bowel obstruction, perforation with peritoneal soilage, and/or life-threatening hemorrhage [83].

Patients with T-cell small bowel lymphoma generally have more advanced disease on presentation (compared with B-cell lymphoma) and more often require emergent surgery at the time of presentation [83]. In a review article by Beaton *et al.*, the authors proposed that in treating small bowel lymphoma, chemotherapy has overall survival benefit compared with surgery alone. Their proposed strategy was to preserve surgery for control of local complications of the tumor [83].

Treatment of patients with diffuse large B-cell lymphoma of the small intestine are mainly surgical resection (palliative resection for localized disease) plus adjuvant radiation or chemotherapy using a CHOP (cyclophosphamide, doxorubicin, vincristine, and prednisone) regimen. As immunodeficiency and human immunodeficiency virus infection are considered risk factors for this type of lymphoma [3], treating the underlying immunosuppressant, such as the underlying human immunodeficiency virus infection should also be considered.

Treatment of mucosal-associated lymphoid tissue lymphoma includes antibiotics for the early stages (tetracycline), surgical resection and/or chemoradiation. In Burkitt lymphoma, the management consists primarily of chemotherapy (vincristine, cyclophosphamide, doxorubicin, and methotrexate) [84]. High dose chemotherapy with autologous stem cell transplantation in localized T-cell lymphoma of the small bowel has been shown to improve the prognosis [85].While the 5-year PFS for the enteropathy-associated T-cell lymphoma in the large series are reported to range from 3.2 to 18% with an overall survival of 19.7 to 20%, the results of a novel chemotherapy regimen with ifosfamide, etoposide, and epirubicin alternating with methotrexate followed by autologous stem cell transplantation is more promising, with a 5-year PFS of 52% and OS of 60% [86].

Follow-Up and Survivorship

The 5-year observed survival for patients with small bowel adenocarcinomas is approximately 30–50%, with a median survival of 20–56 months [66, 72, 87]. Factors negatively affecting survival include gender (male), higher age (>55 years), tumor location (duodenum or ileum), grade and stage of the tumors, lack of surgical resection and the presence of distant metastases [66, 87]. The 5-year observed survival across small bowel lymphoma subtypes is approximately 50%. Factors that negatively affect patient survival include gender (male) and age (>75 years) [87].

Data supporting the efficacy of routine endoscopic/radiologic imaging for small bowel cancer surveillance to improve survival is at best sparse. Additionally, re-resection of an isolated recurrence, like an anastomotic recurrence, may or may not be feasible (e.g., ileal vs duodenal), and isolated recurrence amenable to complete resection is a rare event. Thus, routine use of surveillance endoscopy and intensive radiologic imaging cannot be justified at this time.

Instead, imaging and workup should be directed by symptoms (e.g., new onset nausea/vomiting, colicky abdominal pain) or by physical findings. Isolated focal recurrent disease and second primary small carcinoma should be considered for resection after careful weighing of the risks and long-term sequelae (such as short gut syndrome), if the benefit includes potential for a prolonged disease-free period and/or cure. There may also be a role for cytoreductive surgery plus hyperthermic intraoperative chemotherapy in carefully selected patients with recurrence confined to the peritoneal cavity [88]. Finally, surgery may also be considered for palliation, such as enteroenterostomy for bowel obstruction, in the setting of unresectable disease.

Acknowledgements

The authors would like to thank: Dr Guillermo Sangster, MD; Dr Amol Takalkar, MD; and Dr Maureen Heldmann, MD who helped with preparation of the radiology slides; Ms Lory Tubs who helped with preparation of the figures; and Mr John Cyrus who provided us with editorial assistance.

References

1 Goodman MT, Matsuno RK, Shvetsov YB. racial and ethnic variation in the incidence of small bowel cancer subtypes in the United States, 1995–2008. *Dis Colon Rectum* 2013;56(4):441.
2 Siegel R, Miller KD, Jemal A. Cancer Statistics, 2017. *CA Cancer J Clin* 2017;67(1):7–30.
3 Zeh HJ, Federle M. Cancer of the small intestine. In: VT DeVita, TS Lawrence, SA Rosenberg (eds) *Cancer: Principles and Practice of Oncology*, 8th edn. Philadelphia: Lippincott Williams & Wilkins, 2008:1186–204.
4 Ripley D, Weinerman BH. Increased incidence of second malignancies associated with small bowel adenocarcinoma. *Can J Gastroenterol* 1997;11(1):65–8.
5 Lowenfels AB, Sonni A. Distribution of small bowel tumors. *Cancer Lett* 1977;3(1–2:83–6.
6 Gabos S, Berkel J, Band P, *et al.* Small bowel cancer in western Canada. *Int J Epidemiol* 1993;22(2):198–206.
7 *SEER Cancer Stat Facts: Small Intestine Cancer.* Bethesda: National Cancer Institute. http://seer.cancer.gov/statfacts/html/smint.html (accessed 20 September 2017).
8 Pan SY, Morrison H. Epidemiology of cancer of the small intestine. *World J Gastrointest Oncol* 2011;3(3):33–42.
9 Schottenfeld D, Beebe-Dimmer JL, Vigneau FD. The epidemiology and pathogenesis of neoplasia in the small intestine. *Ann Epidemiol* 2009;19(1):58–69.
10 Chen CC, Neugut AI, Rotterdam H. Risk factors for adenocarcinomas and malignant carcinoids of the small intestine: preliminary findings. *Cancer Epidemiol Biomarkers Prev* 1994;3(3):205–7.
11 Negri E, Bosetti C, La Vecchia C, *et al.* Risk factors for adenocarcinoma of the small intestine. *Int J Cancer* 1999;82(2):171–4.
12 Chow WH, Linet MS, McLaughlin JK, *et al.* Risk factors for small intestine cancer. *Cancer Causes Control* 1993;4(2):163–9.
13 Bennett CM, Coleman HG, Veal PG, *et al.* Lifestyle factors and small intestine adenocarcinoma risk: a systematic review and meta-analysis. *Cancer Epidemiol* 2015;39(3):265–73.
14 Lagergren J, Ye W, Ekbom A. Intestinal cancer after cholecystectomy: is bile involved in carcinogenesis? *Gastroenterology* 2001;121(3):542–7.
15 Green PH, Fleischauer AT, Bhagat G, *et al.* Risk of malignancy in patients with celiac disease. *Am J Med* 2003;115(3):191–5.
16 Ilus T, Kaukinen K, Virta LJ, Pukkala E, Collin P. Incidence of malignancies in diagnosed celiac patients: a population-based estimate. *American J Gastroenterol* 2014;109(9):1471–7.
17 Han Y, Chen W, Li P, Ye J. Association between coeliac disease and risk of any malignancy and gastrointestinal malignancy: a meta-analysis. *Medicine* 2015;94(38):e1612.
18 Von Roon AC, Reese G, Teare J, *et al.* The risk of cancer in patients with Crohn's disease. *Dis Colon Rectum* 2007;50(6):839–55.
19 Laukoetter MG, Mennigen R, Hannig CM, *et al.* Intestinal cancer risk in Crohn's disease: a meta-analysis. *J Gastrointest Surg* 2011;15(4):576–83.
20 Canavan C, Abrams KR, Mayberry J. Meta-analysis: colorectal and small bowel cancer risk in patients with Crohn's disease. *Aliment Pharmacol Ther* 2006;23(8):1097–104.
21 Jess T, Winther KV, Munkholm P, *et al.* Intestinal and extraintestinal cancer in Crohn's disease: follow-up of a population-based cohort in Copenhagen County, *Denmark. Aliment Pharmacol Ther* 2004;19(3):287–93.
22 Lashner BA. Risk factors for small bowel cancer in Crohn's disease. *Dig Dis Sci* 1992;37(8):1179–84.
23 Askling J, Brandt L, Lapidus A, *et al.* Risk of haematopoietic cancer in patients with inflammatory bowel disease. *Gut* 2005;54(5):617–22.
24 Siegel CA. Risk of lymphoma in inflammatory bowel disease. *Gastroenterol Hepatol* 2009;5(11):784–90.
25 Nielsen M, Lynch H, Infante E, Brand R. *MUTYH*-Associated Polyposis. GeneReviews™ https://www.ncbi.nlm.nih.gov/books/NBK107219/. Seattle (WA); Initial Posting: October 4, 2012; Last Update: September 24, 2015 (accessed 20 September 2017).
26 Sheldon CD, Hodson ME, Carpenter LM, *et al.* A cohort study of cystic fibrosis and malignancy. *Br J Cancer* 1993;68(5):1025–8.
27 Neglia JP, FitzSimmons SC, Maisonneuve P, *et al.* The risk of cancer among patients with cystic fibrosis. Cystic Fibrosis and Cancer Study Group. *N Engl J Med* 1995;332(8):494–9.
28 Maisonneuve P, Marshall BC, Knapp EA, Lowenfels AB. Cancer risk in cystic fibrosis: a 20-year nationwide study from the United States. *J Natl Cancer Inst* 2012;105(2):122–9.
29 Nugent KP, Spigelman AD, Phillips RK. Life expectancy after colectomy and ileorectal anastomosis for familial adenomatous polyposis. *Dis Colon Rectum* 1993;36(11):1059–62.
30 Schulmann K, Brasch FE, Kunstmann E, *et al.* HNPCC-associated small bowel cancer: clinical and molecular characteristics. *Gastroenterology* 2005;128(3):590–9.
31 Koornstra JJ, Kleibeuker JH, Vasen HF. Small-bowel cancer in Lynch syndrome: is it time for surveillance? *Lancet Oncol* 2008;9(9):901–5.
32 Korsse SE, Dewint P, Kuipers EJ, *et al.* Small bowel endoscopy and Peutz-Jeghers syndrome. *Best Pract Res Clin Gastroenterol* 2012;26(3):263–78.
33 Sellner F. Investigations on the significance of the adenoma-carcinoma sequence in the small bowel. *Cancer* 1990;66(4):702–15.
34 Ciresi DL, Scholten DJ. The continuing clinical dilemma of primary tumors of the small intestine. *Am Surg* 1995;61(8):698–703.
35 Maglinte DD, O'Connor K, Bessette J, *et al.* The role of the physician in the late diagnosis of primary malignant tumors of the small intestine. *Am J Gastroenterol* 1991;86(3):304–8.
36 Maglinte DD, Chernish SM, Bessette J, *et al.* Factors in the diagnostic delays of small bowel malignancy. *Indiana Med* 1991;84(6):392–6.
37 Maglinte DT, Reyes BL. Small bowel cancer. *Radiologic diagnosis. Radiol Clin North Am* 1997;35(2):361–80.
38 Buckley JA, Jones B, Fishman EK. Small bowel cancer. Imaging features and staging. *Radiol Clin North Am* 1997;35(2):381–402.
39 Dudiak KM, Johnson CD, Stephens DH. Primary tumors of the small intestine: CT evaluation. *Am J Roentgenol* 1989;152(5):995–8.

40 Bessette JR, Maglinte DD, Kelvin FM, *et al.* Primary malignant tumors in the small bowel: a comparison of the small-bowel enema and conventional follow-through examination. *Am J Roentgenol* 1989;153(4):741–4.

41 Maglinte DD, Kelvin FM, O'Connor K, *et al.* Current status of small bowel radiography. *Abdom Imaging* 1996;21(3):247–57.

42 Violon D, Steppe R, Potvliege R. Improved retrograde ileography with glucagon. *Am J Roentgenol* 1981;136(4):833–4.

43 Minordi LM, Vecchioli A, Guidi L, *et al.* Multidetector CT enteroclysis versus barium enteroclysis with methylcellulose in patients with suspected small bowel disease. *Eur Radiol* 2006;16(7):1527–36.

44 Maglinte DD, Sandrasegaran K, Lappas JC, *et al.* CT enteroclysis. *Radiology* 2007;245(3):661–71.

45 Maglinte DD, Sandrasegaran K, Lappas JC. CT enteroclysis: techniques and applications. *Radiol Clin North Am* 2007;45(2):289–301.

46 Pilleul F, Penigaud M, Milot L, *et al.* Possible small-bowel neoplasms: contrast-enhanced and water-enhanced multidetector CT enteroclysis. *Radiology* 2006;241(3):796–801.

47 Bender GN, Maglinte DD, Klöppel VR, *et al.* CT enteroclysis: a superfluous diagnostic procedure or valuable when investigating small-bowel disease? *Am J Roentgenol* 1999;172(2):373–8.

48 Bender GN, Timmons JH, Williard WC, *et al.* Computed tomographic enteroclysis: one methodology. *Invest Radiol* 1996;31(1):43–9.

49 Pappalardo G, Gualdi G, Nunziale A, *et al.* The impact of magnetic resonance in the preoperative staging and the surgical planning for treating small bowel neoplasms. *Surg Today* 2013;43(6):613–9.

50 Dasari BV, Gardiner KR. Management of adenocarcinoma of the small intestine. *Gastrointest Cancer Res* 2009;3(3):121–2.

51 Cronin CG, Scott J, Kambadakone A, *et al.* Utility of positron emission tomography/CT in the evaluation of small bowel pathology. *Br J Radiol* 2012;85(1017):1211–21.

52 Cronin CG, Swords R, Truong MT, *et al.* Clinical utility of PET/CT in lymphoma. *Am J Roentgenol* 2010;194(1):W91–W103.

53 Kumar R, Xiu Y, Potenta S, *et al.* 18 F-FDG PET for evaluation of the treatment response in patients with gastrointestinal tract lymphomas. *J Nucl Med* 2004;45(11):1796–803.

54 Ell C, Remke S, May A, *et al.* The first prospective controlled trial comparing wireless capsule endoscopy with push enteroscopy in chronic gastrointestinal bleeding. *Endoscopy* 2002;34(9):685–9.

55 Adler SN, Bjarnason I. What we have learned and what to expect from capsule endoscopy. *World J Gastrointest Endosc* 2012;4(10):448–52.

56 Marmo R, Rotondano G, Piscopo R, *et al.* Meta-analysis: capsule enteroscopy vs. conventional modalities in diagnosis of small bowel diseases. *Aliment Pharmacol Ther* 2005;22(7):595–604.

57 Lewis BS, Eisen GM, Friedman S. A pooled analysis to evaluate results of capsule endoscopy trials. *Endoscopy* 2005;37(10):960–5.

58 Cangemi DJ, Patel MK, Gomez V, *et al.* Small bowel tumors discovered during double-balloon enteroscopy: analysis of a large prospectively collected single-center database. *J Clin Gastroenterol* 2013;47(9):769–72.

59 Yamamoto H, Sekine Y, Sato Y, *et al.* Total enteroscopy with a nonsurgical steerable double-balloon method. *Gastrointest Endosc* 2001;53(2):216–20.

60 Jovanovic I, Vormbrock K, Zimmermann L, *et al.* Therapeutic double-balloon enteroscopy: a binational, three-center experience. *Dig Dis* 2011;1:27–31.

61 May A, Nachbar L, Ell C. Double-balloon enteroscopy (push-and-pull enteroscopy) of the small bowel: feasibility and diagnostic and therapeutic yield in patients with suspected small bowel disease. *Gastrointest Endosc* 2005;62(1):62–70.

62 Rondonotti E, Sunada K, Yano T, *et al.* Double-balloon endoscopy in clinical practice: where are we now? *Dig Endosc* 2012;24(4):209–19.

63 Ell C, May A, Nachbar L, *et al.* Push-and-pull enteroscopy in the small bowel using the double-balloon technique: results of a prospective European multicenter study. *Endoscopy* 2005;37(7):613–6.

64 Coit DG, Kelsen D, Tang LH, *et al.* Small intestine. In: M Amin, S Edge, R Greene, D Byrd, R Brookland (eds) *Cancer Staging Manual*, 8th Edition. American Joint Committee on Cancer. New York: Springer, 2017.

65 Ruskoné-Fourmestraux A, Dragosics B, Morgner A, *et al.* Paris staging system for primary gastrointestinal lymphomas. *Gut* 2003;52(6):912–3.

66 Hutchins RR, Bani Hani A, Kojodjojo P, *et al.* Adenocarcinoma of the small bowel. *ANZ J Surg* 2001;71(7):428–37.

67 Hirasawa R, Iishi H, Tatsuta M, *et al.* Clinicopathologic features and endoscopic resection of duodenal adenocarcinomas and adenomas with the submucosal saline injection technique. *Gastrointest Endosc* 1997;46(6):507–13.

68 Rose DM, Hochwald SN, Klimstra DS, *et al.* Primary duodenal adenocarcinoma: a ten-year experience with 79 patients. *J Am Coll Surg* 1996;183(2):89–96.

69 Santoro E, Sacchi M, Scutari F, *et al.* Primary adenocarcinoma of the duodenum: treatment and survival in 89 patients. *Hepatogastroenterology* 1997;44(16):1157–63.

70 Sohn TA, Lillemoe KD, Cameron JL, *et al.* Adenocarcinoma of the duodenum: factors influencing long-term survival. *J Gastrointest Surg* 1998;2(1):79–87.

71 Han SL, Cheng J, Zhou HZ, *et al.* The surgical treatment and outcome for primary duodenal adenocarcinoma. *J Gastrointest Cancer* 2010;41(4):243–7.

72 Agrawal S, McCarron EC, Gibbs JF, *et al.* Surgical management and outcome in primary adenocarcinoma of the small bowel. *Ann Surg Oncol* 2007;14(8):2263–9.

73 Singhal N, Singhal D. Adjuvant chemotherapy for small intestine adenocarcinoma. *Cochrane Database Syst Rev* 2007;(3):CD005202.

74 Overman MJ, Kopetz S, Lin E, Abbruzzese JL, Wolff RA. Is there a role for adjuvant therapy in resected adenocarcinoma of the small intestine. *Acta Oncol* 2010;49(4):474–9.

75 Kelsey CR, Nelson JW, Willett CG, *et al.* Duodenal adenocarcinoma: patterns of failure after resection and the role of chemoradiotherapy. *Int J Radiat Oncol Biol Phys* 2007;69(5):1436–41.

76 Crawley C, Ross P, Norman A, *et al.* The Royal Marsden experience of a small bowel adenocarcinoma treated with protracted venous infusion 5-fluorouracil. *Br J Cancer* 1998;78(4):508–10.

77 Tsushima T, Taguri M, Honma Y, *et al.* Multicenter retrospective study of 132 patients with unresectable small bowel adenocarcinoma treated with chemotherapy. *Oncologist* 2012;17(9):1163–70.

78 Xiang XJ, Liu YW, Zhang L, *et al.* A phase II study of modified FOLFOX as first-line chemotherapy in advanced small bowel adenocarcinoma. *Anticancer Drugs* 2012;23(5):561–6.

79 Overman MJ, Varadhachary GR, Kopetz S, *et al.* Phase II study of capecitabine and oxaliplatin for advanced adenocarcinoma of the small bowel and ampulla of Vater. *J Clin Oncol* 2009;27(16):2598–603.

80 Zhang L, Wang LY, Deng YM, *et al.* Efficacy of the FOLFOX/CAPOX regimen for advanced small bowel adenocarcinoma: a three-center study from China. *J BUON* 2011;16(4):689–96.

81 Onkendi EO, Boostrom SY, Sarr MG, *et al.* Neoadjuvant treatment of duodenal adenocarcinoma: a rescue strategy. *J Gastrointest Surg* 2012;16(2):320–4.

82 Koo DH, Yun SC, Hong YS, *et al.* Systemic chemotherapy for treatment of advanced small bowel adenocarcinoma with prognostic factor analysis: retrospective study. *BMC Cancer* 2011;11:205.

83 Beaton C, Davies M, Beynon J. The management of primary small bowel and colon lymphoma – a review. *Int J Colorectal Dis* 2012;27(5):555–63.

84 Blum KA, Lozanski G, Byrd JC. Adult Burkitt leukemia and lymphoma. *Blood* 2004;104(10):3009–20.

85 Chandesris MO, Malamut G, Verkarre V, *et al.* Enteropathy-associated T-cell lymphoma: a review on clinical presentation, diagnosis, therapeutic strategies and perspectives. *Gastroenterol Clin Biol* 2010;34(11):590–605.

86 Sieniawski MK, Lennard AL. Enteropathy-associated T-cell lymphoma: epidemiology, clinical features, and current treatment strategies. *Curr Hematol Malig Rep* 2011;6(4):231–40.

87 Hrabe JE, Cullen JJ. Management of the small bowel tumors. In: JL Cameron, AM Cameron (eds) *Current Surgical Therapy*, 10th edn. Philadelphia: Mosby Elsevier, 2011:106–110.

88 Jacks SP, Hundley JC, Shen P, Russell GB, Levine EA. Cytoreductive surgery and intraperitoneal hyperthermic chemotherapy for peritoneal carcinomatosis from small bowel adenocarcinoma. *J Surg Oncol* 2005;91(2):112–9.

6

Adenocarcinoma of the Pancreas

Quyen D. Chu[1], Erkut Borazanci[1], Roger H. Kim[2], and Guillermo Sangster[1]

[1] Louisiana State University Health Sciences Center, Shreveport, Louisiana, USA
[2] Southern Illinois University School of Medicine, Springfield, Illinois, USA

Introduction

Pancreatic adenocarcinoma is one of the most aggressive cancers and despite advances in perioperative care, surgical techniques, and modern chemotherapy, significant improvement in prolonging survival has been marginal [1–3]. Surgery remains the only treatment for potential cure, but despite successful resection, only a minority of patients can be considered to be truly cured [4]. Whether patients receive chemotherapy and/or radiation therapy before or after surgery, outcome remains dismal. It is likely that the majority of pancreatic cancers are chemo- and radioresistant. Significant impact on this disease will therefore require novel therapeutics and better understanding of its biology.

Incidence and Mortality

Cancer of the pancreas ranks third (exceeded only by lung and colorectal cancers) as a leading cause of cancer-related deaths in the United States (US) and seventh worldwide [1, 2]. It is estimated that in 2017, there will be 53,670 new cases of pancreatic cancer diagnosed in the US, and 43,090 deaths from this disease. The majority of these pancreatic cancers (97%) are of exocrine histology, of which 90% are adenocarcinoma [5]. There are other rare exocrine histologies, some of which include acinar cell carcinoma, adenosquamous carcinoma, serous cystoadenocarcinoma, mucinous cystoadenocarcinoma, and solid and pseudopapillary tumors [6]. Pancreatic endocrine cancers are considered in Chapter 39 (Gastroenteropancreatic Neuroendocrine Tumors).

The incidence rate of cancers of the pancreas, overall, based on cases diagnosed in in the US from 2009 to 2013, was approximately 14.1 per 100,000 men and 11.0 per 100,000 women per year. During the same time period, the age-adjusted death rates were 12.5 and 9.5 per 100,000 men and women, respectively, per year. Incidence rates and death rates in the US are highest among African Americans, lowest for Asian/Pacific Islanders, and intermediate for other racial and ethnic groups. The lifetime risk of developing cancer of the pancreas is approximately 1.54% [7].

The 5-year relative survival rate for all cancers combined increased from 35% (1950–1954) to 70% (2006–2012). In contrast, the absolute increase in relative survival for pancreatic cancer was much less, improving from 1% (1950–1954) to 9% (2006–20012) [7] (Table 6.1).

Etiology and Risk Factors

To date, several risk factors have been implicated in the development of pancreatic cancer such as tobacco use, alcohol use, diabetes, male sex, obesity, people who have blood types A, B, or AB compared to O, high fat diet, occupational exposures, family history, chronic pancreatitis, and *Helicobacter pylori* infection [8, 9]. Tobacco users have a 2.5–3.6-fold increase risk of developing pancreatic cancer compared to nontobacco users [10]. Pancreatic cancer specimens from people who smoke possess more mutations than those who do not [11].

Pancreatitis, peptic ulcers, gastrectomy, cholelithiasis, cholecystectomy, and appendectomy have been associated with the development of pancreatic cancer [12]. Hereditary pancreatitis is a rare form of pancreatitis and patients with this disorder generally present with repeat bouts of acute pancreatitis. Mutations in the cationic trypsinogen gene (*PRSS1*) or in the serine protease inhibitor gene (*SPINK1*) have been identified [6]. Patients with hereditary pancreatitis have a 58-fold increased risk of developing pancreatic cancer and a 30–40% lifetime risk of developing pancreatic cancer by the age of 70 [6, 13].

A familial form of pancreatic cancer is seen in approximately 7–10% of patients with pancreatic cancer [14]. This is defined as having at least two first-degree relatives with the disease. There is a 32-fold increased risk of developing pancreatic cancer when three or more first-degree relatives are diagnosed with

The American Cancer Society's Oncology in Practice: Clinical Management, First Edition. Edited by The American Cancer Society.

Table 6.1 Trends in 5-year survival by diagnosis in US.

Sites	1950–1954 (%)	2006–2012 (%)
All sites combined	35	70
Breast (females)	60	92
Colorectal	37	67
Esophagus	4	22
Testis	57	97
Pancreas	1	9

Source: Howlader *et al.* [7].

pancreatic cancer [15], and a 57-fold increased risk when four or more first-degree relatives are affected [16]. Several germline gene mutations have been implicated in the development of pancreatic cancer [9]. These include *BRCA2* (involved in DNA repair), *PALPB2* (helps localize *BRCA2*), *CDKN2A* (a cell cycle regulator), *ATM* (ataxia telangiectasia mutated gene, involved in DNA repair), *STK11* (a serine threonine kinase that regulates cell proliferation and associated with Peutz-Jehers Syndrome), *PRSS1* (involved in hereditary pancreatitis), and *MLH1*, *MSH2*, *MSH6*, *PMS2* (mismatch repair genes associated with Lynch syndrome) [8, 12]. Recent genome-wide sequencing or genome-wide association studies have found several potential significant genetic polymorphisms, including the gene *HNF1A*. This gene is involved in the differentiation of pancreatic cells [17]. Currently, there are no recommendations regarding genetic screening for those with a family history of pancreatic cancer outside of a clinical trial [18]. A recent expert panel concluded that while screening for pancreatic cancer has identified pancreatic neoplasms in asymptomatic patients with strong family histories of pancreatic cancer, there is still more work to be done regarding the management of these patients [19].

A pooled analysis of 14 cohort studies evaluating anthropometric factors and the risk of developing pancreatic cancer found a 47% increase pancreatic cancer risk among individuals with a body mass index ≥30 kg/m^2 (obese) at baseline versus body mass index between 21 and 22.9 kg/m^2 [20].

Diabetes mellitus is also related to the development of pancreatic cancer. While diabetes mellitus can develop secondary to pancreatic damage by the malignancy itself, those with diabetes mellitus for over 10 years have a 30– 40% risk of developing pancreatic cancer [21]. Metformin appears to be protective, decreasing the risk of the developing pancreatic cancer [12].

Biology

Pancreatic adenocarcinoma develops through a series of noninvasive precursor lesions called pancreatic intraepithelial neoplasm (PanIN) [9]. The lesion initially begins as minimally dysplastic epithelium and then progresses to PanIN grades 1A and 1B, severe dysplasia, PanIN grades 2 and 3, and finally invasive carcinoma [8]. Less frequently, intraductal papillary mucinous neoplasms and mucinous cystic neoplasms can also give rise to pancreatic cancer. Early PanIN1 lesions frequently have *KRAS* mutations and then progress to develop mutated *p16/CDKN2A*, *p53*, and *SMAD4* [22].

The most commonly identified somatic mutation involves the activation of the *KRAS* oncogene [9]. This mutation appears to be involved in nearly all cases of pancreatic adenocarcinoma [23]. The constitutive activity of *KRAS* causes an increase of cellular proliferation, survival, and invasion of pancreatic cancer cells. *KRAS* activation also appears to suppress T-cell immunity, which helps tumor proliferation [24]. An experiment published in 2012 looked at a mouse model of pancreatic cancer and found that expression of *KRAS* increased the infiltration of myeloid-derived suppressor cells, which are also known as GR1 + CD11b + [24]. These cells suppress T-cell-mediated antitumor immune response that helps drive tumor growth. When these cells' activity levels decrease, tumor growth also decreases [24, 25]. Other major driver mutations are the inactivation of the tumor suppressor gene *CDKN2A*, which encodes the inhibitor of cyclin-dependent kinase 4 (INK4A), and inactivation of the tumor suppressor genes *TP53* and *SMAD4* [8]. *CDKN2A* has been found to be mutated in 95% of pancreatic cancer. Mutations in this gene lead to inactivation of *CDKN2A*, which in turn results in the loss of the p16 protein, itself a regulator of the cell cycle during the G1 to S transition, resulting in an increase in cell proliferation [8]. *SMAD4* or deleted in pancreatic cancer 4 (*DPC4*) is mutated in 50% of pancreatic cancers, again resulting in a loss of activity of that gene. This loss leads to dysregulation of signaling control pathways involved with transforming growth factor β (TGF-β) [8].

Epigenetic changes have also been implicated in the pathogenesis of pancreatic cancer. Epigenetic changes are those involving alterations in DNA methylation, histone modification, and non-coding RNA leading to alterations in gene expression. These changes appear to play a role in the aggressiveness of the disease along with resistance to traditional treatment [9].

Tumor-stromal interactions involving pancreatic cancer contributes to oncogenic signaling and the stroma itself can become a physical barrier that prevents chemotherapeutic drugs from reaching the pancreatic cancer cells. Cancer-associated fibroblasts are widely recognized as promoters of tumorigenesis as they can promote the transformation of epithelium to immortalization along with enhancing tumor growth [22].

The Hedgehog pathway, which is involved in normal embryonic development, can help drive the fibroblast-driven stromal growth of pancreatic cancer [26]. Through stimulation from various growth factors, pancreatic stellate cells or myofibroblasts secrete collagen and other components of the extracellular matrix that compromise the pancreatic stroma. This microenvironment is responsible for the poor vasculature in pancreatic cancer that inhibits drug delivery, along with driving the process of tumor growth, progression, invasion, and metastasis. Targeting the stromal environment may help with delivery of chemotherapeutic agents to pancreatic cancer [26].

Clinical Presentation

Most patients with pancreatic cancer present with regional or distant disease (80%) [27]. There is no screening test for pancreatic cancer. Although 15–20% of patients with adenocarcinoma of the pancreas present with resectable disease, 80% of them will relapse within 2 years following resection [28]. The presenting signs and symptoms will depend on the location of the disease within the pancreas; for patients with cancer of the head of the pancreas, evidence of obstruction such as jaundice or gastric outlet obstruction may be the initial sign and symptom. Abdominal pain may be due to pancreatitis secondary to pancreatic duct obstruction. For those with cancer in the body of the pancreas, pain may be the initial symptom due to infiltration of the celiac nerve plexus. In such a situation, the tumor is generally unresectable because of its invasion into major blood supply such as the superior mesenteric artery.

The most frequent presenting symptoms are asthenia, weight loss, anorexia, and abdominal pain. Note that about 13% of the patients present with Courvoisier's sign (nontender, enlarged, palpable gallbladder in a jaundiced patient) and 3% present with the Armand Trousseau sign of malignancies (thrombophlebitis) [29]. Jaundice, hepatomegaly, right upper quadrant mass, and cachexia are the most common signs of pancreatic cancer. Choluria (dark urine) occurs in almost 60% of patients and hypocholia (clay-colored stool) occurs in 54% of patients with pancreatic cancer [29]. A patient who presents with jaundice, choluria, and/or hypocholia should be considered to have biliary obstruction until proven otherwise. In such a patient, pancreatic cancer should be on top of the list of differential diagnoses.

Approximately 25% of patients with pancreatic cancer have diabetes mellitus at diagnosis and 40% have glucose intolerance [30]. Ascites can occur in up to 20% of patients and this generally portends advanced disease [31].

Evaluation and Management

Management of patients with pancreatic cancer requires a multidisciplinary approach [32]. A patient who presents with a pancreatic mass will require an in-depth evaluation, which includes a complete history and physical examination and review of laboratory and radiologic studies. From a surgical perspective, the following questions are mentally noted: (i) does the patient have a surgical disease; (ii) is the disease resectable; and finally (iii) is the patient a surgical candidate. All three criteria must be met before offering the patient the surgical option. For example, patients who have a mass in the head of the pancreas may have a surgical disease, but should they present with multiple comorbidities, extensive disease, and/or a mass in the umbilicus (Sister Joseph Mary Node) or in the supraclavicular region (Virchow's node), this would preclude them from having a surgical resection. A complete history and physical examination will assist with determining whether the patient is a surgical candidate, while a review of the patient's computed tomography (CT) scan and/or magnetic resonance imaging (MRI) will help answer the first two questions.

Imaging

Most patients with pancreatic carcinoma show advanced regional or distant disease at the time of diagnosis. Over recent years, the advent of many new techniques has assisted clinicians to detect, diagnose, and stage patients with pancreatic cancer better. The main goal of imaging is to identify suspicious lesions and determine whether or not the tumor is resectable, and to correctly identify patients who would benefit from surgery, thereby avoiding unnecessary surgical interventions for others [33].

Multidetector Computed Tomography

Because of the widespread availability of multidetector computed tomography (MDCT) and its capacity to image the entire body in a single breathhold acquisition, this modality is considered the gold standard when pancreatic cancer is suspected [34, 35]. MDCT is the most cost-effective diagnostic imaging modality to evaluate patients with suspected pancreatic cancer. Although it provides excellent anatomic detail, it may not depict small tumors or peritoneal metastasis.

The creation of isotropic volume rendering and multiplanar reconstructions assist accurate preoperative staging and planning (Figure 6.1) [36]. The reported predictive values of MDCT to determine whether tumors are resectable or not are 73–91%

(a)

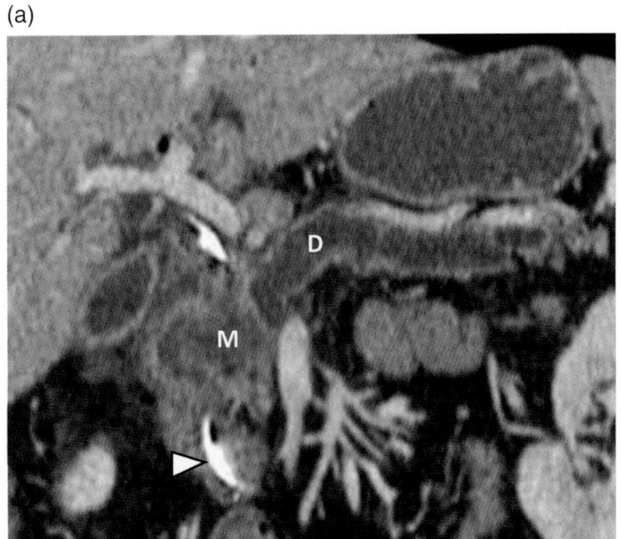

(b)

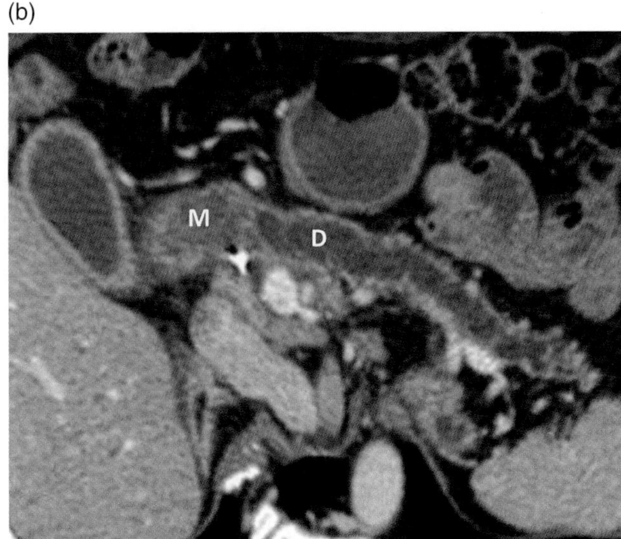

Figure 6.1 (a) Coronal and (b) curved multiplanar MDCT reconstructions of a patient with a path-proven adenocarcinoma showing a hypoattenuating mass M, with ductal dilatation D, and parenchymal atrophy. A biliary stent (arrowhead) is also present to relieve CBD obstruction. *Source:* Quyen D. Chu, MD, MBA, FACS. Reproduced with permission of Dr Chu.

and 95–100%, respectively, with a sensitivity of 95–100% and a specificity of 72–100% tumor detection [34, 35, 37, 38]. Despite recent technical advances, MDCT has still limitations in distinguishing mass-forming pancreatitis from adenocarcinomas [35]. Likewise, it is often challenging to detect small (<2 cm) tumors, which are the most likely to be resectable [39]. Criteria of unresectability include: celiac or para-aortic nodal involvement, distant metastases, and invasion of adjacent organs such as stomach and colon. Resection of pancreatic cancer is rarely appropriate in patients with evidence of vascular encasement (Figure 6.2), although portal vein resection may be technically possible. In some centers such as ours, the need for vascular reconstruction has not been considered a contraindication for attempting radical pancreatectomy. Limited sensitivity in detecting liver and peritoneal metastases still remain important pitfalls in the preoperative evaluation process [40].

Figure 6.2 Axial abdominal contrast enhanced CT shows an unresectable pancreatic adenocarcinoma arising from the pancreatic body (M) with cystic necrosis and encasement of the celiac trunk (arrow). *Source:* Quyen D. Chu, MD, MBA, FACS. Reproduced with permission of Dr Chu.

MRI

MRI is potentially as accurate as CT in detecting and staging pancreatic cancer, with the benefit of avoiding the radiation exposure, and should be considered as a problem-solving modality if a diagnostic dilemma persists after MDCT. A substantial benefit with MRI is the possibility to perform cholangiopancreatography, thereby providing detailed information on the pancreatic and biliary ducts and sparing many patients from undergoing invasive procedures such as endoscopic retrograde cholangiopancreatography [41]. An MRI may also be a useful diagnostic tool for those patients with a history of iodine contrast allergy.

Endoscopic Ultrasonography

This operator-dependent and time-consuming modality improves accuracy in staging pancreatic carcinoma by providing a detailed demonstration of local vascular invasion of the portal vein and/or arterial vessels. Endoscopic ultrasonography-guided fine-needle aspiration biopsy is also useful for determining nodal status. Although helpful, endoscopic ultrasonography is less accurate than MDCT in determining portal vein and/or arterial involvement [41].

Positron Emission Tomography

The role of positron emission tomography (PET)/CT in pancreatic imaging is still evolving. PET/CT may be useful in the initial diagnosis (Figure 6.3), staging, or restaging of pancreatic adenocarcinomas, as well as in evaluating the response to treatment.

Diagnostic Laparoscopy

Diagnostic laparoscopy (DL) may be a useful modality in selected patients, although its use is not a standard of care. DL can identify occult metastatic disease in up to 30% of patients

(a)

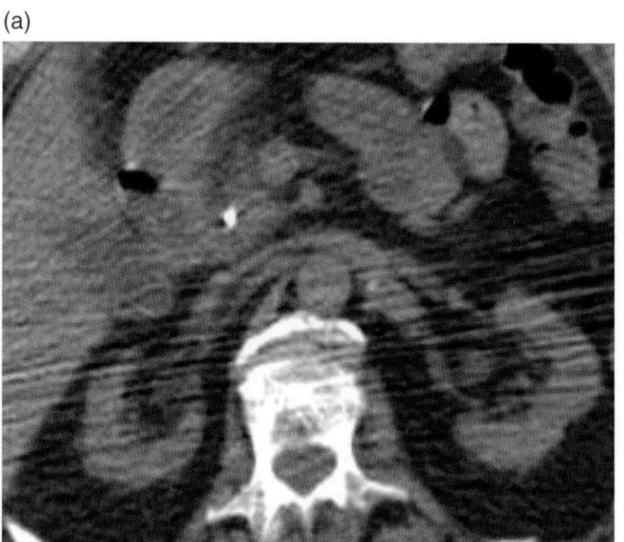

(b)

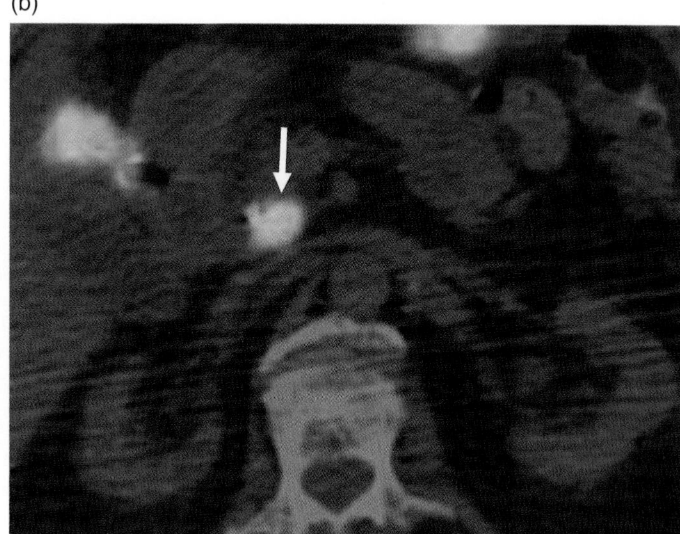

Figure 6.3 A poorly delineated hypodense mass in the head of the pancreas is identified on CT (a) shows intense FDG uptake on PET/CT (b, arrow). Surgical resection yielded pancreatic adenocarcinoma. *Source:* Quyen D. Chu, MD, MBA, FACS. Reproduced with permission of Dr Chu.

[42], disease that may not otherwise be detected by imaging modalities such as transabdominal ultrasound, CT, MRI, or PET [43]. Evidence of stage 4 disease includes peritoneal studding, serosal implants, and/or subcentimeter liver implants.

Improvement of CT scanners over time has decreased the utility of routine DL [33, 44, 45]. However, DL should be considered for the following situations: (i) patients with a high CA 19-9 level; (ii) cancer in the body or tail of the pancreas (almost 50% of such patients have peritoneal disease); (iii) large tumor; and/or (iv) imaging suggestive of metastatic disease [45–47].

Staging

There are two well-recognized staging systems for pancreatic adenocarcinoma: (i) the American Joint Committee on Cancer, also vernacularly referred to as the TNM systems (Table 6.2), and (ii) the National Comprehensive Cancer Network (NCCN) [48, 49].The former staging system is also used by the Union for International Cancer Control and is useful following resection while the latter, although it does incorporate the American Joint Committee on Cancer system, is useful as a pretreatment staging system and includes an expert consensus statement spearheaded by societies such as the Americas Hepato-Pancreato-Biliary Association, the Society for the Surgery of the Alimentary Tract, and the Society of Surgical Oncology [50, 51] (Table 6.3).

The NCCN criteria classify patients based on whether surgical resection is an option. This is an important point to consider because surgery is the only known modality that offers a potential cure for these patients. NCCN groups patients into four groups: (i) localized and resectable disease; (ii) borderline resectable; (iii) unresectable; and (iv) metastatic. Such classification is predicated on radiologic studies such as abdominal CT scans. Readers should be cognizant that the borderline resectable category was not introduced until 2006 [52]. As such, any interpretation, comparison, and extrapolation of results from older studies should be done with caution.

Table 6.2 TNM staging system for pancreatic adenocarcinoma.

Primary tumor (T)	Regional lymph nodes (N)	Distant metastasis (M)
Tx: primary tumor cannot be assessed	Nx: regional lymph nodes cannot be assessed	M0: no distant metastasis
T0: no evidence of primary tumor	N0: no regional lymph node metastasis	M1: distant metastasis
Tis: carcinoma *in situ* (this includes high-grade pancreatic intraepithelial neoplasia (PanIn-3), intraductal papillary mucinous neoplasm with high-grade dysplasia, intraductal tubulopapillary neoplasm with high-grade dysplasia, and mucinous cystic neoplasm with high-grade dysplasia)	N1: metastasis in one to three regional lymph nodes	
T1: ≤2 cm in greatest dimension	N2: metastasis in four or more regional lymph nodes	
T1a: tumor ≤0.5 cm in greatest dimension		
T1b: tumor >0.5 cm and <1 cm in greatest dimension		
T1c: tumor 1–2 cm in greatest dimension		
T2: >2 cm and ≤4 cm in greatest dimension		
T3: tumor >4 cm in greatest dimension		
T4: tumor involves the celiac axis, superior mesenteric artery, and/or common hepatic artery, regardless of size		

Group staging

Stage 0	Tis	N0	M0
Stage IA	T1	N0	M0
Stage IB	T2	N0	M0
Stage IIA	T3	N0	M0
Stage IIB	T1 T2 T3	N1 N1 N1	M0 M0 M0
Stage III	T1 T2 T3 T4	N2 N2 N2 Any N	M0 M0 M0 M0
Stage IV	Any T	Any N	M1

Source: Amin *et al.* [49]. Used with permission of the American College of Surgeons, Chicago, Illinois. The original source for this information is the AJCC Cancer Staging Manual, 8th edn (2017), which is published by Springer Science + Business Media.

Treatment: Overview

For patients with metastatic disease, elective surgical resection is generally contraindicated. Although borderline resectable and unresectable are defined as separate groups, for all practical purposes, their therapeutic approach is similar; both are offered neoadjuvant therapy instead of upfront surgical resection. Therefore, most of the debate regarding whether to offer upfront surgery or neoadjuvant therapy centers on the group with localized/resectable disease. Again, the readers are reminded of the limitations of the literature when reading about diseases that are defined as resectable, borderline resectable, or unresectable since these definitions were not standardized until recently. For example, a loss of a fat plane between the tumor in the head of the pancreas and the superior mesenteric vein (SMV), or clear involvement of a short segment of the portal vein as seen on a CT scan, might be considered as borderline by one surgeon but resectable by another. In such instance, should the tumor be deemed clearly resectable or borderline resectable? If it is clearly resectable, then upfront surgery is a viable option whereas if it is deemed borderline resectable, then a neoadjuvant approach might be the preferred option. Despite these limitations, it is still worthwhile to have a thorough working knowledge about the subject.

Regardless of the initial approach to treatment, it is critical to be cognizant that the surgeon should strive to achieve a negative

Table 6.3 The National Comprehensive Cancer Network (NCCN) and the American Hepato-Pancreato-Biliary Association (AHPBA)/Society of Surgical Oncology (SSO)/Society of the Alimentary Tract (SSAT) Pretreatment Staging System of Pancreatic Adenocarcinoma.

Classification	Presurgical imaging criteria	Recommended treatment
Localized and clearly resectable	• Absence of distant metastases • Clear fat planes around the CA, HA, and SMA • No SMV/PV distortion	Surgery followed by adjuvant chemoradiation or Preoperative chemoradiation followed by surgery
Borderline resectable	• Absence of distant metastases • SMV/PV: – Distortion or narrowing – Occlusion but with suitable vessel proximal and distal, allowing for safe resection and replacement • CHA: – Abutment or short segment encasement • CA: – No abutment or encasement • SMA: – Abutment ≤1800 of artery circumference • GDA: – Encasement up to HA	Neoadjuvant therapy
Locally advanced or unresectable	• Absence of distant metastases • Head: – SMA encasement exceeding >1800 – CA abutment – Unreconstructable SMV/PV occlusion – Aortic or IVC invasion or encasement • Body: – SMA or CA encasement >1800 – Unreconstructable SMV/PV occlusion – Aortic invasion • Tail: – SMA or CA encasement >1800 – Nodal status: metastases to lymph node beyond the field of resection	Chemoradiation
Metastatic	• Any evidence of distant metastases	Palliative treatment: nonoperative, if possible

Source: [48, 50, 51].
CA, coronary artery; CHA, common hepatic artery; GDA, gastroduodenal artery; HA, hepatic artery; IVC, inferior vena cava; SMA, superior mesenteric artery; SMV/PV, superior mesenteric vein/portal vein.

margin (R0) status since the survival for an R0 resection is 18–23 months as compared to 14–15 months for microscopically positive margins (R1) and 10–11 months for macroscopically involved disease [53].

Localized and Resectable Pancreatic Cancer

Adjuvant Therapy

Localized or resectable pancreatic cancer implies that there is no evidence of metastatic disease and that the tumor can be completely resected without vascular involvement. On CT scans, one looks for a nice fat plane between the pancreatic head mass and the SMV (Figure 6.4).

For patients with localized and resectable pancreatic cancer, options include surgery followed by adjuvant therapy (adjuvant approach) or chemoradiotherapy followed by surgery (neoadjuvant approach). As of September 2016, there were eleven phase 3 clinical trials to support the adjuvant therapy approach [54–65] (Table 6.4). In contrast, there are only phase 1 or 2 trials supporting the neoadjuvant approach [66–71] (Table 6.5). Despite the difference in the numbers of clinical trials and lack of a direct comparison between the neoadjuvant and adjuvant approach, limited available evidence suggests comparable outcomes between the two.

Notwithstanding the ample evidence from phase 3 clinical trials supporting the role of adjuvant therapy, there is no consensus on what the optimal adjuvant regimen should be. Each study is fraught with its own limitations [3]. The European Organization for Research and Treatment of Cancer Trial assessed the efficacy of adjuvant radiation therapy and 5-FU for both pancreatic head and periampullary adenocarcinomas, although the latter has a better prognosis than the former [3, 55]. Although the regimen was well tolerated, there was a lack of a survival advantage with the adjuvant group over the surgery alone group; the median survivals for the treatment and the observation arms were 24 and 19 months, respectively, and the

5-year survivals for the treatment and observation arms were 28% and 22%, respectively ($P = 0.208$) [3, 55]. The study may have been underpowered and by including periampullary tumors, outcomes favoring adjuvant therapy may have been overshadowed.

The European Study Group for Pancreatic Cancer Trial (ESPAC-1) study was the largest randomized trial on adjuvant therapy for pancreatic cancer at the time and found that 5-FU/leucovorin was superior to observation and that the addition of radiotherapy had a deleterious effect. However, ESPAC-1 had some weaknesses, some of which include complex study design and suboptimal radiotherapy quality control [3].

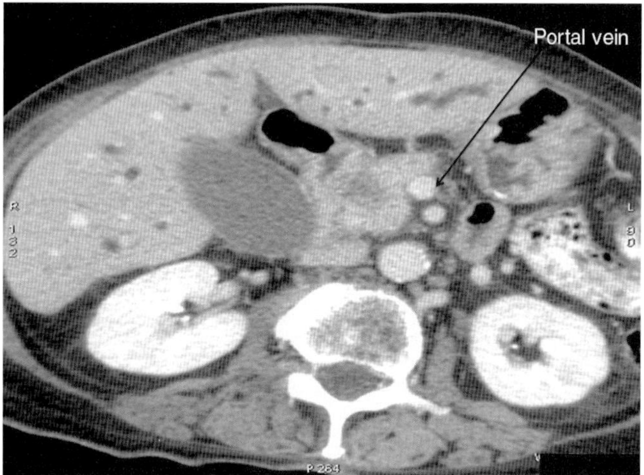

Figure 6.4 CT scan of a patient with a mass in the head of the pancreas that is localized and easily resectable. Note a nice fat plane between the mass and the portal vein. A Whipple procedure demonstrated an adenocarcinoma of the head of the pancreas. *Source:* Chu *et al.* [116]. Reproduced with permission of Quyen D. Chu, MD, MBA, FACS.

The Charité Onkologie (CONKO-001) trial was a phase 3 randomized control trial that enrolled 368 patients with at least a macroscopic complete resection (R1 or R0) without any prior chemotherapy or radiation therapy treatment [57]. Patients were randomized to observation only following surgery or receive gemcitabine for 24 weeks. The median disease-free survival was significantly higher in the gemcitabine group compared to the observation group (13.4 months vs 6.9 months; $P < 0.001$). The final results of CONKO-001 demonstrated a significantly higher median overall survival (OS) for the gemcitabine group compared to the observation group (22.8 months vs 20.2 months; $P = 0.01$) [72].

The Radiation Therapy Oncology Group (RTOG) 9704 was a phase 3 trial that examined the role of adding gemcitabine to adjuvant fluorouracil (5-FU) and radiation therapy in patients with resected pancreatic cancer patients [59]. Although adding gemcitabine improved survival, such observation was not statistically significant, regardless of the location of the primary tumor (i.e., head vs body/tail) [73]. The median survival for the 5-FU and gemcitabine group was 17.1 months and 22 months, respectively, and the 5-year survival was 18% in the 5-FU group and 22% in gemcitabine group ($P = 0.12$) for those with cancer in the head of the pancreas [73].

Another adjuvant trial that also showed no survival advantage with using gemcitabine was the ESPAC-3 trial [60]. This phase 3 study randomized patients to receive either folinic acid (i.e., leucovorin) and 5-FU or gemcitabine; both were given over a 24-week period. Postoperative radiation was not used in either arm. The median survival for the 5-FU group and gemcitabine group was 23.0 months and 23.6 months, respectively ($P = 0.39$). One and 2-year survival figures were 79.3% and 48.6%,

Table 6.4 Randomized phase 3 trials of adjuvant therapy for resectable pancreatic cancer.

Trials, year (reference)	Patients (*n*)	Treatment regimen	5 year (%)	Median survival (months) (*P*-value)
GITSG, 1985 [54]	43	Obs –vs- ChemoXRT	NA	11 vs 20 (0.03)
Bakkevold, 1993 [61]	61	Obs –vs- Chemo	8 vs 4	11 vs 23 (0.02)
EORTC, 1999 [55]	114	Obs –vs- ChemoXRT	10 vs 20	12.6 vs 17.1 (0.099)
ESPAC-1, 2001 [56]	289	No chemo –vs- Chemo	8 vs 21	15.5 vs 20.1 (0.009)
RTOG-9704, 2004 [59, 73]	538	Gem-5-FU-XRT –vs- 5-FU-5-FU-XRT	20.5 vs 22	17.1 vs 18 (0.12)[1]
CONKO-001 [57, 72]	354	Obs –vs- Gem	10.4 vs 20.7	20.2 vs 22.8 (0.01)
Ueno, 2009 [62]	119	Obs-vs-Chemo	11 vs 24 (NS)	5 vs 11.4 (0.01) (DFS)
ESPAC-3, 2010 [60]	1088	5-FU –vs- Gem	NA	23.0 vs 23.6 (0.39)
Von Hoff [63]	861	Gem-vs- Gem + nab-paclitaxel	4% vs 9%[2]	6.7 vs 8.5 (<0.001)
CONKO-005, 2015 [64]	436	Gem-vs- Gem + Erlo	10 % vs 28%	26.5 vs 24.6 (NS)
ESPAC-4, 2016 [65]	732	Gem –vs- Gem + CAP	NA	25.5 vs 28.0 (0.032)

Source: Chu *et al.* [116]. Reproduced with permission of Quyen D. Chu, MD, MBA, FACS.
CAP, capecitabine; Chemo, chemotherapy; CONKO, Charité Onkologie; DFS, disease-free survival; ESPAC, European Study Group for Pancreatic Cancer; EORTC, European Organization for Research and Treatment of Cancer; Erlo, erlotinib; Gem, gemcitabine; GITSG, Gastrointestinal Tumor Study Group;
NA, not available; NS, not significant; Obs, observation; RTOG, Radiation Therapy Oncology Group.
[1] Cancer in head of pancreas.
[2] 2-year survival rate.

Table 6.5 Phase 1 and 2 trials of neoadjuvant therapy for resectable pancreatic cancer.

Trials (author), year (reference)	Patients (*n*)	Treatment regimen	Median survival (months)
Desai, 2007 [68]	12	Gem/Ox/XRT/Gem/Ox	12.5
Varadhachary, 2008 [69]	79	Gem/Cis/Gem/XRT	17.4
Evans, 2008 [70]	86	Gem/XRT	23
Heinrich, 2008 [117]	28	Gem/Cis	26.5
Le Scodan, 2008 [71]	41	5-FU/Cis/XRT	9.4
Gillen, 2010 [67]	4,394	Meta-analysis of 111 studies	20

Source: Chu *et al.* [116]. Reproduced with permission of Quyen D. Chu, MD, MBA, FACS.
5-FU, 5-Fluorouracil; Gem, gemcitabine; Ox, oxalaplatin; Cis, cisplatin.

respectively for 5-FU and 78.5% and 48.1% for patients treated with gemcitabine [60].

Despite no differences in OS between 5-FU and gemcitabine, gemcitabine had a more favorable toxicity profile than 5-FU. Two of the three subsequent trials comparing gemcitabine alone versus gemcitabine combined with other therapy demonstrated OS benefits [63, 65]. Von Hoff *et al.* randomized 861 patients to receive either gemcitabine alone or combined with nab-paclitaxel found that the median survival was significantly higher in the nab-paclitaxel group (8.5 months vs 6.7 months; P <0.001) [63]. ESPAC-4 recently reported a significant increase in median survival when gemcitabine was combined with capecitabine (28 months) compared to gemcitabine alone (25.5 months; P = 0.032) [65]. However, the addition of erlotinib to gemcitabine (24.6 months) did not appear to have any survival advantage when compared to gemcitabine alone (26.5 months; not significant) [64].

Whether radiation is used as adjuvant therapy depends on which side of the Atlantic Ocean one practices. The results of RTOG 9704, ESPAC-1, and ESPAC-3 suggest that adjuvant chemotherapy is beneficial while the addition of radiation is deleterious. Most patients in Europe are treated with chemotherapy alone, while those in the US are still given radiation.

NCCN currently recommends that for those with a complete resection without evidence of recurrent or metastatic disease, enrollment into a clinical trial is the preferred choice. Acceptable options include chemotherapy alone (either gemcitabine, 5-FU/leucovorin, continuous 5-FU infusion, capecitabine), or systemic gemcitabine or 5-FU given before or after chemoradiation [48].

Neoadjuvant Therapy

Proponents of the neoadjuvant approach argue that upfront chemotherapy provides early treatment of occult disease. This is especially important considering that up to 80% of patients with pancreatic cancer develop distant disease. An additional advantage with the neoadjuvant approach is that almost all qualified patients receive the benefit of chemotherapy, whereas up to 25% of eligible patients who had upfront surgery do not receive the intended adjuvant treatment because of a prolonged surgical recovery period [74].

Another theoretical advantage with the neoadjuvant approach is that it downstages the tumor, although it can be argued that such benefit is negligible in those who already have a resectable tumor at presentation. Finally, neoadjuvant therapy can be used as a biologic gauge, identifying those patients with undetected occult disease who rapidly develop progressive disease during treatment and, therefore, would not have benefitted from upfront surgery; such a scenario can occur in up to 25% of the patients [74].

Opponents of the neoadjuvant approach argue that such an approach delays surgery, the only known modality that can potentially cure the patient. Other concerns include worsening of the patient's condition following neoadjuvant therapy (which may preclude surgical resection), cancer spread due to delay of surgical resection, inaccurate surgical pathologic staging, and the patient's refusal to undergo surgery following complications from neoadjuvant therapy.

Given the clinical equipoise, the ideal clinical trial is a head-to-head comparison of adjuvant therapy versus neoadjuvant therapy for patients with resectable pancreatic cancer. Currently, such a multicenter phase 3 trial (NEOPAC) is being conducted. This trial compares adjuvant gemcitabine with neoadjuvant gemcitabine/oxaliplatin plus adjuvant gemcitabine [66].

Until further data are available, adjuvant therapy remains the standard of care for patients with localized/resectable pancreatic cancer. NCCN currently recommends that neoadjuvant therapy should be reserved for special situations such as those who appear to have resectable disease but have poor prognostic features (i.e., markedly elevated CA 19-9, large primary tumor, large regional lymph nodes, excessive weight loss, extreme pain) or those who qualify for a clinical trial [48].

Borderline Resectable Pancreatic Cancer

Borderline resectable pancreatic cancers are generally those that involve the mesenteric vessels for which a resection might result in a compromised surgical margin (Figure 6.5). Although the term borderline resectable pancreatic cancer first appeared in an article in 1999 [75], it was not until 2008 that it became a distinct category following a consensus conference sponsored by the Americas Hepato-Pancreato-Biliary Association, the Society for the Surgery of the Alimentary Tract, and the Society of Surgical Oncology [50, 51]. NCCN has recognized borderline resectable pancreatic cancer as a separate entity [48]. Despite such recognition, there remains a general lack of agreement on several details such as the degree of venous and arterial involvement and whether abutment of the veins should be included in this category [75]. Because borderline resectable pancreatic cancer was

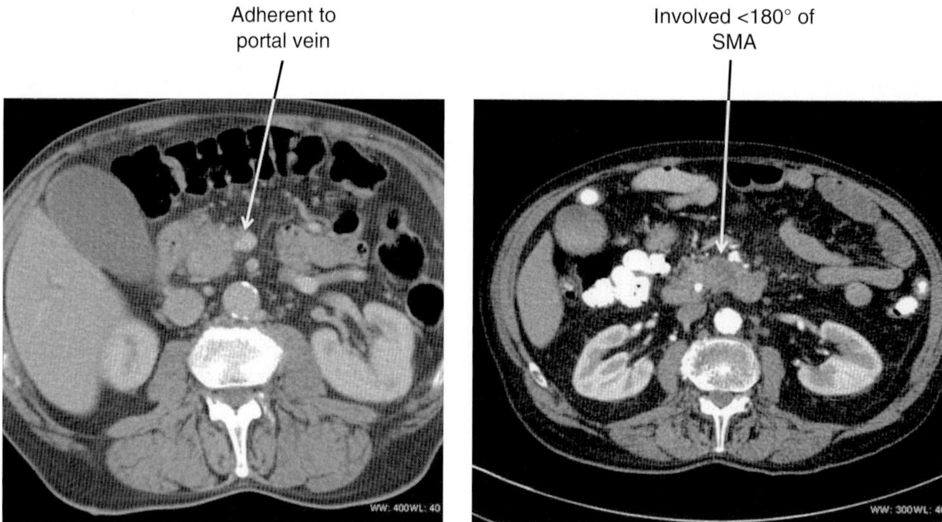

Figure 6.5 CT scans of patients with borderline resectable pancreatic cancer. Both patients underwent neoadjuvant therapy prior to a successful Whipple operation *Source:* Chu *et al.* [116]. Reproduced with permission of Quyen D. Chu, MD, MBA, FACS.

only recently recognized as a separate entity, there is a lack of sufficient data to determine the optimal regimen for treating these patients. Regardless, the preferred approach is similar to those with locally advanced or unresectable pancreatic cancer (LAPC), mainly neoadjuvant therapy followed by evaluation for surgical resection, with the understanding that there is no clear evidence to either support or refute chemoradiation therapy or induction chemotherapy followed by chemoradiation therapy. Approximately 30–60% are surgical candidates following multimodality therapy and in those patients, 80–90% can achieve negative margin status [76–78] For those who successfully completed the neoadjuvant regimen and surgical resection, the median OS ranges from 34 to 40 months, a figure that is comparable to those with resectable pancreatic cancer who had undergone the neoadjuvant approach [76, 78, 79].

The Alliance for Clinical Trials in Oncology (Alliance), in cooperation with the Southwest Oncology Group, the Eastern Cooperative Oncology Group (ECOG), and the RTOG recently received National Cancer Institute approval to conduct a multi-institutional prospective trial (Alliance A021101) to assess the feasibility of using preoperative chemotherapy (FOLFIRINOX – folinic acid, fluorouracil, irinotecan, oxaliplatin) and capecitabine-based chemoradiation for patients with borderline resectable pancreatic cancer [80–82].

Radiographic criteria include [82]:

- An interface between the primary tumor and superior mesenteric vein/portal vein (SMV/PV) exists that measures 180° or greater of the circumference of the vessel wall
- Short segment occlusion of the SMV/PV exists with normal vein above and below the level of obstruction that is amenable to resection and venous reconstruction
- Short segment interface (of any degree) between tumor and hepatic artery exists with normal artery proximal and distal to the interface that is amenable to resection and arterial reconstruction
- An interface between the tumor and superior mesenteric artery exists that measures less than 180° of the circumference of the vessel wall.

Other Considerations

Portal Vein Resection

On occasions, the tumor may be adherent to or involve the SMV, PV or both. In such cases, an SMV/PV resection may be required to achieve an R0 (microscopically negative margin) or R1 (grossly negative, but microscopically positive margin) status. However, such a formidable task should only be attempted by experienced surgeons. Recommended criteria for vascular resection/reconstruction include adequate inflow and outflow of the reconstructed veins, lack of involvement of the superior mesenteric artery or hepatic artery, and achieving an R0/R1 resection [50]. Recent data suggest that a Whipple procedure for patients with vascular involvement who needed vascular resection/reconstruction do just as well as those who underwent a Whipple procedure and did not have vascular involvement [83, 84].

Extended Lymphadenectomy

There is no evidence that an extended lymphadenectomy improves survival [85]. With rare exceptions (i.e., part of a clinical trial, large tumor requiring lymphadenectomy as part of the *en bloc* resection), a routine extended lymphadenectomy should not be performed as part of the definite operation [86].

Preoperative Biliary Drainage

It is not uncommon for patients with pancreatic cancer to present with obstructive jaundice. This is especially true for those with tumors in the ampullary region since up to 70% of patients with cancer in this area present with obstructive jaundice [87, 88]. Symptoms from obstructive jaundice can range from mild to severe and sequelae include hepatic dysfunction, coagulation abnormalities, and cholangitis [89, 90]. Decompression of the biliary system may be required, which can successfully be accomplished with either endoscopic or percutaneous biliary stent placement. However, the routine use of such procedures in the preoperative setting remains controversial.

The rationale for preoperative biliary decompression stemmed from early clinical experience that revealed that jaundiced patients undergoing surgical resection were at risk for developing postoperative complications such as infection, bleeding, and renal failure [91]. However, a multicenter, randomized trial comparing preoperative biliary drainage with surgery alone for patients with cancer of the head of the pancreas found that the preoperative biliary drainage group had a significantly higher complication rate (74%) than the surgery-only group (39%; P <0.001) [92].

Consideration for preoperative biliary drainage include patients who have cholangitis, severe intractable pruritus, coagulation disorders, and those who will not undergo immediate surgical resection (i.e., neoadjuvant therapy group and those who require correction of their poor nutritional status) [89, 90]. In such situations, a self-expanding metallic stent is preferable over plastic stents [93].

Classic Whipple versus Pylorus-Sparing Whipple

Pancreaticoduodenectomy, often referred to as the Whipple procedure, is performed for patients with cancer confined to the head of the pancreas, which includes those in the periampullary region. For cancers located at the body or tail of the pancreas, the procedure of choice is a distal pancreatectomy and splenectomy.

The conventional Whipple or "classic Whipple" involves resection of organs such as the head of the pancreas, the duodenum, the distal stomach, and the distal bile duct (Figure 6.6). Gastrointestinal continuity requires the use of the jejunum to connect to the pancreas (pancreaticojejunostomy), the bile duct (hepatojejunostomy), and stomach (gastrojejunostomy) (Figure 6.7). A jejunostomy feeding tube is often performed just in case the patient has a significant delay in tolerating oral intake.

Another alternative to the classic Whipple is the pylorus-sparing Whipple. Here, the distal stomach and the pylorus are preserved while the very proximal portion of the duodenum is resected. The jejunum is then anastomosed to the duodenum (duodenojejunostomy) rather than to the stomach as would be the case with the classic Whipple (Figure 6.8).

The decision to perform either the classic Whipple or the pylorus-preserving Whipple rests upon the surgeon's preference. In a prospective, randomized, multicenter analysis comparing the classic Whipple procedure to the pylorus-preserving Whipple for patients with suspected pancreatic or periampullary cancer, Tran *et al.* found no significant difference in median blood loss, duration of the operation, incidence of delayed gastric emptying, or survival between the two groups [94].

Whether it is necessary to place an intraoperative drain as part of the surgical procedure is currently debated [95, 96]. However, we believe that such a decision should be based on the surgeon's preference and level of comfort.

LAPC

Patients with unresectable locoregional disease (i.e., locally advanced) are those that have no distant disease but whose tumors encase major vessels for which surgical resection is prohibitive (Figures 6.2 and 6.9). Although patients with LAPC are at a high risk of developing metastatic disease, approximately 30% of them died of localized progressive disease without having apparent distant disease [78]. This suggests that perhaps a proportion of these patients might benefit from a surgical resection, the only known modality that has a potential for cure, after multimodality therapy. Without treatment, these patients may develop intestinal obstruction, intestinal ischemia, and bleeding from progression of their disease.

For patients with LAPC, upfront neoadjuvant therapy is the preferred approach. The goal is to shrink the tumor so that it can be resectable. Approximately 30% of the patients are resectable after such a regimen [48] and the median OS following resection ranges between 13.4 and 16.5 months [97, 98].

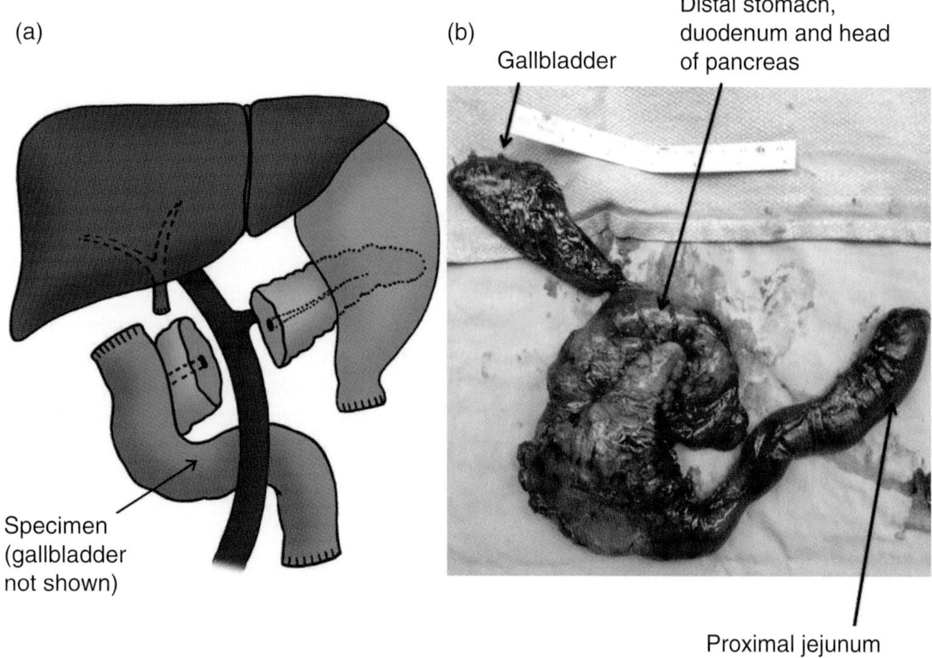

Figure 6.6 Organs removed in a Whipple procedure.

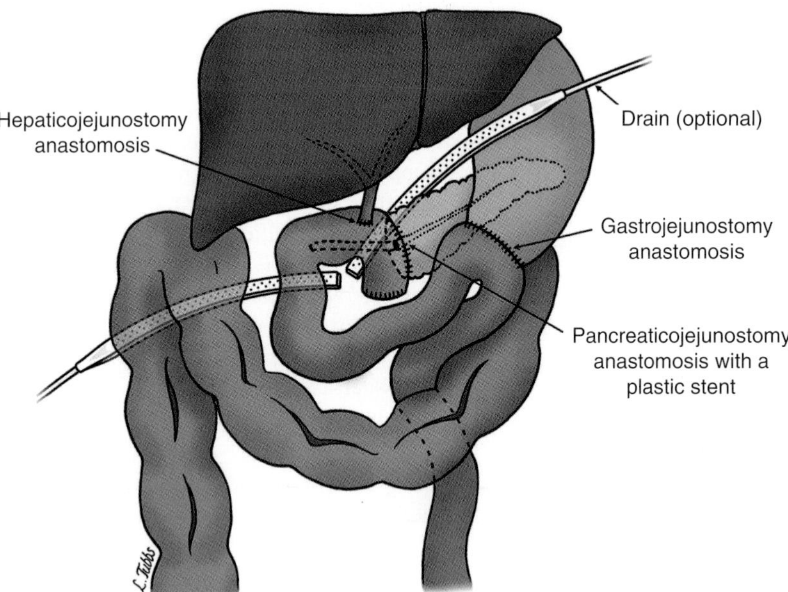

Figure 6.7 "Classic" Whipple.

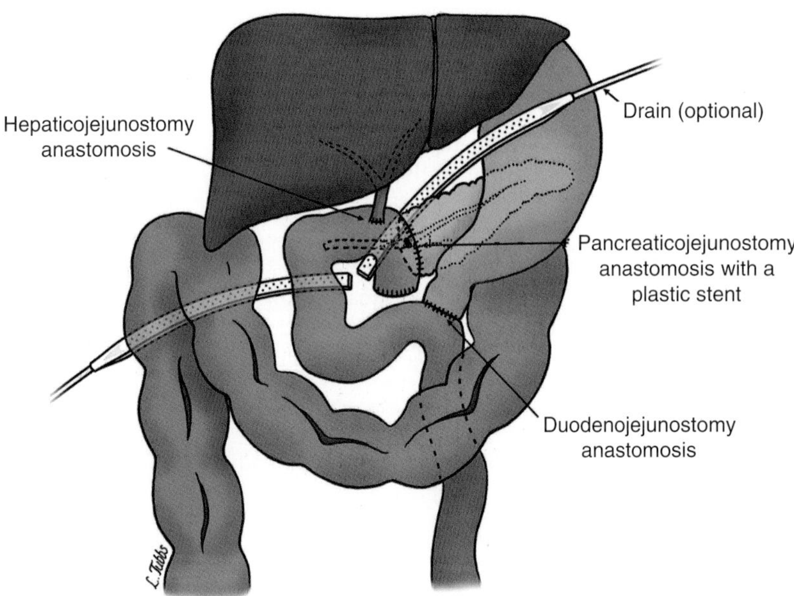

Figure 6.8 Pylorus-sparing Whipple.

Treatment options include four to six cycles of systemic therapy followed by chemoradiotherapy for those who continued to have localized disease (Table 6.6). The objective of chemoradiotherapy is to prevent local disease progression and is based on older clinical trials that demonstrated superior outcome with chemoradiotherapy over chemotherapy [99, 100]. However, recent trials demonstrated no survival benefit with chemoradiotherapy as compared with chemotherapy alone [97, 98]. The GERCOR-LAP-07 multi-institutional phase 3 trial was a two-phase study for which patients were randomly assigned to receive either gemcitabine alone or gemcitabine/erlotinib in the initial phase. Following 4 months of chemotherapy, patients with stable disease are again randomly assigned to either continue chemotherapy or to receive chemoradiation (up to 54 Gy of radiation with concurrent capecitabine) [97]. Although there was a significant decrease in local progression in the chemoradiation group (32% vs 46%; P = 0.03), there was no significant difference in OS when compared to chemotherapy alone [97].

The conflicting results of these trials reveal the complexity of this recalcitrant disease. Nonetheless, they offer the opportunity to individualize treatment regimens. For instance, a clinician may choose to offer chemotherapy only for a frail patient, or induction chemotherapy followed by chemoradiation therapy for a patient with a bulky tumor who has no evidence of distant disease

Metastatic Pancreatic Cancer

Approximately 53% of patients diagnosed with pancreatic cancer will present with metastatic disease [27]. OS in patients with metastatic pancreatic cancer is very poor. Untreated, the median survival is approximately 2–3 months [28]. According

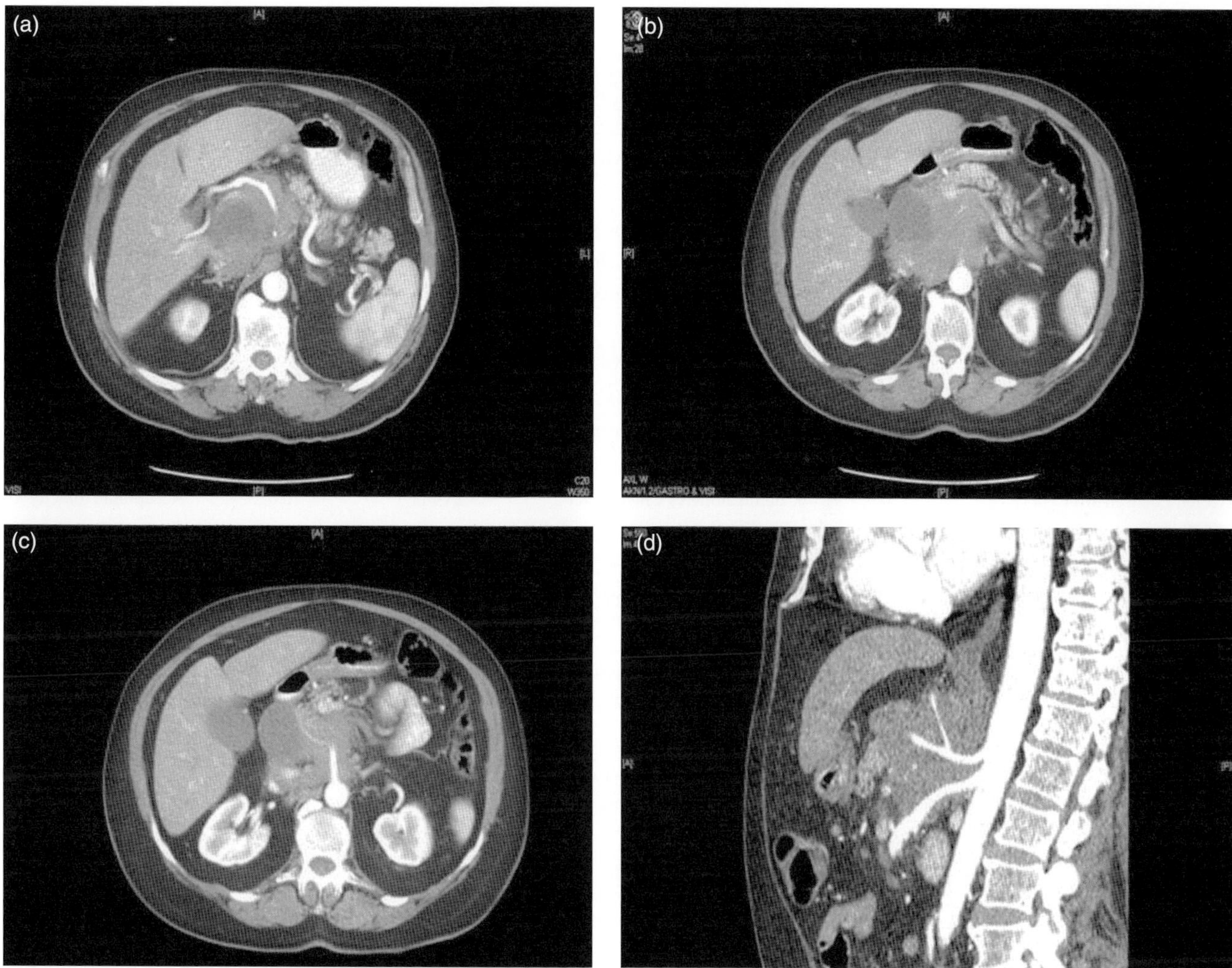

Figure 6.9 CT scans of a patient with locally advanced or unresectable pancreatic cancer. Note the encasement of major arterial blood vessels (i.e., hepatic artery, celiac artery). This patient remained unresectable despite having completed chemoradiation therapy. *Source:* Chu *et al.* [116]. Reproduced with permission of Quyen D. Chu, MD, MBA, FACS.

to current NCCN guidelines, treatment of metastatic pancreatic cancer is stratified by performance status as defined as by ECOG. Good performance status is defined as those with an ECOG of 0 or 1, having a patent biliary system/stent, good pain control, and adequate nutritional status [48]. For those with a poor performance status, either gemcitabine or best supportive care is recommended. For those with good performance status, there are several options available.

The backbone that forms current therapy recommendations is based upon trials examining gemcitabine and fluorouracil (5-FU). A landmark study published in 1997 showed that among patients with advanced pancreatic cancer randomized to either gemcitabine 1000 mg/m^2 weekly for 7 weeks with 1 week of rest then weekly for 3 weeks in a 4 week cycle or to 5-FU 600 mg/m^2 weekly, OS was 5.65 months in the gemcitabine group versus 4.41 months in the 5-FU group. More significantly the survival rate was 18% at 1 year for the gemcitabine-treated group versus 2% for the 5-FU group [101].

A phase III study comparing erlotinib/gemcitabine to gemcitabine alone showed an improvement in OS of 6.24 months vs 5.91 months. One-year survival was also greater with the combination having a 23% survival rate at 1 year compared to 17% in the gemcitabine alone arm. In a secondary analysis, patients with a grade 2 or greater rash treated with erlotnib/gemcitabine also had a median survival of 10.5 months and 1-year survival of 43%, versus those with a grade 0 or 1 rash of 5.3, 5.8 months and 16%, 9% respectively [102]. One issue with this study was the significant increase in grade 3/4 toxicity including diarrhea, fatigue, and infection. This treatment combination is a category 1 recommendation in NCCN guidelines, but it has not been widely practiced in the clinical setting [8].

In another recent trial, the MPACT (Metastatic Pancreatic Adenocarcinoma Clinical Trial) study, the combination of gemcitabine and abraxane (which is paclitaxel albumin bound) versus gemcitabine alone in advanced pancreatic cancer showed an OS of 8.5 months vs 6.7 months, respectively [103]. Furthermore, 1-year survival was 35% in the combination arm versus 22% in the single agent arm. There have been several other studies testing gemcitabine-based combinations such as gemcitabine/cetuximab [104] and gemcitabine/erlotinib/bevacizumab [105], but these have not shown improvement in response or survival compared to single agent gemcitabine.

Table 6.6 Selected studies of locally advanced pancreatic cancer.

Trial, author, year (reference)	Patients (*n*)	Treatment regimen	Median survival (months)	*P*-value	Comments
GITSG, Moertel, 1981 [118]	194	XRT alone vs ChemoXRT (Chemo = 5-FU)	5.7 vs 10.1	<0.01	Favored ChemoXRT
GITSG, 1985 [54]	43	Chemo alone vs ChemoXRT (Chemo = 5-FU, MMC, Strep)	8 vs 10.5	<0.02	Favored ChemoXRT
ECOG, Klaassen, 1985 [100]	91	Chemo alone vs ChemoXRT (Chemo = 5-FU)	8.2 vs 8.3	NS	Retrospective study
ECOG, Cohen, 2005 [119]	114	XRT alone vs ChemoXRT (Chemo = 5-FU, MMC)	7.1 vs 8.4	NS	Toxicity higher in ChemoXRT group
FFCD/SFRO, Chauffert, 2008 [120]	119	Chemo alone vs ChemoXRT (Chemo = 5-FU, GEM, Cis)	13 vs 8.6	0.03	Toxicity higser in ChemoXRT group
ECOG, Loehrer, 2011 [121]	74	Chemo alone vs ChemoXRT (Chemo = GEM)	9.2 vs 11.1	0.017	Acceptable toxicity in ChemoXRT group
GERCOR, Huguet, 2007 [99]	181	Chemo alone vs induction chemo followed by ChemoXRT (Chemo = GEM)	11.7 vs 15	0.0009	Retrospective study
MDACC, Krishnan, 2007 [122]	323	ChemoXRT vs induction chemo followed by ChemoXRT (Chemo = GEM)	8.5 vs 11.9	<0.001	Retrospective study

Source: Chu *et al.* [116]. Reproduced with permission of Quyen D. Chu, MD, MBA, FACS.
Chemo, chemotherapy; ChemoXRT, chemoradiotherapy; Cis, cisplatin; GEM, gemcitabine; 5-FU, 5-Fluorouracil; MMC, mitomycin C; NS, not significant; Strep, streptozocin; XRT, radiation therapy.

Another recent study was a multicenter randomized phase 2–3 trial that randomizes newly diagnosed patients with metastatic pancreatic cancer to receive either a combination chemotherapy of oxaliplatin, irinotecan, fluorouracil, and leucovorin (FOLFIRINOX) versus gemcitabine [106]. The primary end point of the study was OS, which was found to be 11.1 months in the FOLFIRINOX group as opposed to 6.8 months in the gemcitabine group. Overall survivals at 1 year and 18 months were 48.4% and 18.6% in the FOLFIRINOX group as opposed to 20.6% and 6.0% in the gemcitabine group. Regarding adverse events, there was a 45.7% incidence of grade 3 or 4 neutropenia in the combination group versus 21% in the gemcitabine group; several other adverse events were more common in the former including febrile neutropenia, thrombocytopenia, anemia, diarrhea, sensory neuropathy, and elevated level of transaminases [106]. Because of the intensity of this regimen and concerns regarding tolerability, a number of clinicians have considered dropping the bolus 5-FU [107].

Recommendations for second-line therapy in the setting of advanced/metastatic pancreatic cancer are 5-FU or capecitabine with oxaliplatin, which are based on a phase 2 trial with patients already treated with gemcitabine [108]. Patients who were given capecitabine and oxaliplatin had a progression-free survival of 9.9 weeks with 6 month and 1 year survival rates of 44% and 21% respectively [108].

The CONKO-003 trial studied patients who had been given gemcitabine for advanced pancreatic cancer initially [109, 110], and were then randomized to either best supportive care (BSC) or a regimen consisting of oxaliplatin, folinic acid, and 5-FU (OFF). Median second-line survival time after randomization was 4.82 months in the OFF group versus 2.3 months in the BSC alone. OS for the patients receiving gemcitabine followed by OFF was 9.09 months, and was 7.90 months for the gemcitabine and BSC [110]. Thus, despite studies of several different combinations, current treatment options appear limited and only mildly effective for advanced pancreatic cancer. The future for pancreatic cancer therapy lies in the continued drive for understanding the biology of the disease and using more specific targeted therapies.

Palliative and Supportive Care

For patients with advanced or metastatic cancer and poor performance status who are unable to tolerate chemotherapy, early palliative care is an appropriate option [9, 111]. Depression, pain, and malnutrition are common with these patients and palliative care is essential in addressing these and other issues. Pain management is important and if the cause is identified, patients can undergo nerve ablation through endoscopic ultrasound or CT-guided procedures [9, 111]. Radiation therapy can relieve pain from locally advanced disease [9, 111]. Other concerns include biliary obstruction, which can be relieved with the endoscopic placement of a biliary stent, preferably a bare metal one as they last longer than plastic [112]. Other options for addressing biliary obstruction include percutaneous biliary drainage with subsequent internalization or open biliary–enteric bypass.

Gastric outlet obstruction is another complication of pancreatic cancer. Patients with good performance status may undergo an open or laparoscopic gastrojejunostomy with a J-tube and even a placement of an enteral stent. In poor performance status patients with gastric outlet obstruction an enteral stent placement or placement of a percutaneous endoscopic gastrostomy tube can be done [113]. Patients with pancreatic cancer frequently develop venous thromboembolism, so prophylaxis with low-molecular-weight heparin is preferred over warfarin. [114]. Another intervention with major impact on quality of life is the use of pancreatic enzyme replacement, as deficiency is common in patients with advanced disease. A recent study from Australia revealed a significant amount of distress in patients whose dietary problems were not addressed [115]. There are several resources such as the Pancreatic Cancer Action Network (www.pancan.org) and the American Cancer Society (www.cancer.org) that assist patients and their families. This may also be found in Chapter 27 of *The American Cancer Society's Principles of Oncology: Prevention to Survivorship.*

Conclusion

Pancreatic adenocarcinoma remains a formidable disease that requires a multidisciplinary approach. Surgery remains the only modality that offers a potential cure, although chemoradiation also plays a pivotal role in improving the OS of patients with pancreatic adenocarcinoma. As we continue to gain a better understanding of the biology of pancreatic cancer, it is foreseeable that in the near future, newer target-specific agents will be developed against this lethal disease.

References

1 Siegel RL, Miller KD, Jemal A. Cancer statistics, 2017. *CA Cancer J Clin* 2017;67(1):7–30.

2 Torre LA, Bray F, Siegel RL, *et al.* Global cancer statistics, 2012. *Ca Cancer J Clin* 2015;65(2):87–108.

3 Chu QD, Khushalani N, Javle MM, Douglass HO, Gibbs JF. Should adjuvant therapy remain the standard of care for patients with resected adenocarcinoma of the pancreas? *Ann Surg Oncol* 2003;10(5):539–45.

4 Gibbs J, Smith J. Surgical treatment of pancreatic carcinoma. In: AK Rustgi JM Crawford (eds) *Gastrointestinal Cancers: Biology and Clinical Management*. Philadelphia: Saunders, 2003:541–7.

5 Ries LAG YJ, Keel GE, Eisner MP, Lin YD, Horner M-J. SEER Survival Monograph: Cancer Survival Among Adults: U.S. SEER Program, 1988–2001. Patient and Tumor Characteristics. In: National Cancer Institute SP, NIH, ed. Vol Pub. No. 07-6215. Bethesda, MD2007.

6 Wolfgang CL, Herman JM, Laheru DA, *et al.* Recent progress in pancreatic cancer. *CA Cancer J Clin* 2013;63(5):318–48.

7 Howlader N, Noone AM, Krapcho M, *et al.* (eds) *SEER Cancer Statistics Review, 1975–2013, National Cancer Institute.* Bethesda, MD. http://seer.cancer.gov/csr/1975_2013/, based on November 2015 SEER data submission, posted to the SEER web site, April 2016.

8 Hidalgo M. Pancreatic cancer. *N Engl J Med* 2010;362(17): 1605–17.

9 Vincent A, Herman J, Schulick R, Hruban RH, Goggins M. Pancreatic cancer. *Lancet* 2011;378(9791):607–20.

10 Hassan MM, Bondy ML, Wolff RA, *et al.* Risk factors for pancreatic cancer: case-control study. *Am J Gastroenterol* 2007;102(12):2696–707.

11 Blackford A, Parmigiani G, Kensler TW, *et al.* Genetic mutations associated with cigarette smoking in pancreatic cancer. *Cancer Res* 2009;69(8):3681–8.

12 Olson SH. Selected medical conditions and risk of pancreatic cancer. *Mol Carcinog* 2012;51(1):75–97.

13 Lowenfels AB, Maisonneuve P, DiMagno EP, *et al.* Hereditary pancreatitis and the risk of pancreatic cancer. International Hereditary Pancreatitis Study Group. *J Natl Cancer Inst* 1997;89(6):442–6.

14 Petersen GM, de Andrade M, Goggins M, *et al.* Pancreatic cancer genetic epidemiology consortium. *Cancer Epidemiol Biomarkers Prev* 2006;15(4):704–10.

15 Klein AP, Brune KA, Petersen GM, *et al.* Prospective risk of pancreatic cancer in familial pancreatic cancer kindreds. *Cancer Res* 2004;64(7):2634–8.

16 Tersmette AC, Petersen GM, Offerhaus GJ, *et al.* Increased risk of incident pancreatic cancer among first-degree relatives of patients with familial pancreatic cancer. *Clin Cancer Res* 2001;7(3):738–44.

17 Pierce BL, Ahsan H. Genome-wide "pleiotropy scan" identifies HNF1A region as a novel pancreatic cancer susceptibility locus. *Cancer Res* 2011;71(13):4352–8.

18 Brand RE, Lerch MM, Rubinstein WS, *et al.* Advances in counselling and surveillance of patients at risk for pancreatic cancer. *Gut* 2007;56(10):1460–9.

19 Canto MI, Harinck F, Hruban RH, *et al.* International Cancer of the Pancreas Screening (CAPS) Consortium summit on the management of patients with increased risk for familial pancreatic cancer. *Gut* 2013;62(3):339–47.

20 Genkinger JM, Spiegelman D, Anderson KE, *et al.* A pooled analysis of 14 cohort studies of anthropometric factors and pancreatic cancer risk. *Int J Cancer* 2011;129(7):1708–17.

21 Li D, Tang H, Hassan MM, *et al.* Diabetes and risk of pancreatic cancer: a pooled analysis of three large case-control studies. *Cancer Causes Control* 2011;22(2):189–97.

22 Morris JP, Wang SC, Hebrok M. KRAS, Hedgehog, Wnt and the twisted developmental biology of pancreatic ductal adenocarcinoma. *Nat Rev Cancer* 2010;10(10):683–95.

23 Bardeesy N, DePinho RA. Pancreatic cancer biology and genetics. *Nat Rev Cancer* 2002;2(12):897–909.

24 Pylayeva-Gupta Y, Lee KE, Hajdu CH, Miller G, Bar-Sagi D. Oncogenic Kras-induced GM-CSF production promotes the development of pancreatic neoplasia. *Cancer Cell* 2012;21(6):836–47.

25 Bayne LJ, Beatty GL, Jhala N, *et al.* Tumor-derived granulocyte-macrophage colony-stimulating factor regulates myeloid inflammation and T cell immunity in pancreatic cancer. *Cancer Cell* 2012;21(6):822–35.
26 Olive KP, Jacobetz MA, Davidson CJ, *et al.* Inhibition of Hedgehog signaling enhances delivery of chemotherapy in a mouse model of pancreatic cancer. *Science* 2009;324(5933): 1457–61.
27 Siegel R, Naishadham D, Jemal A. Cancer statistics, 2013. *CA Cancer J Clin* 2013;63(1):11–30.
28 Stathis A, Moore MJ. Advanced pancreatic carcinoma: current treatment and future challenges. *Nat Rev Clin Oncol* 2010;7(3):163–72.
29 Porta M, Fabregat X, Malats N, *et al.* Exocrine pancreatic cancer: symptoms at presentation and their relation to tumour site and stage. *Clin Transl Oncol* 2005;7(5):189–97.
30 Chari ST, Leibson CL, Rabe KG, *et al.* Pancreatic cancer-associated diabetes mellitus: prevalence and temporal association with diagnosis of cancer. *Gastroenterology* 2008;134(1):95–101.
31 Adam RA, Adam YG. Malignant ascites: past, present, and future. *J Am Coll Surg* 2004;198(6):999–1011.
32 Pawlik TM, Laheru D, Hruban RH, *et al.* Evaluating the impact of a single-day multidisciplinary clinic on the management of pancreatic cancer. *Ann Surg Oncol* 2008;15(8):2081–8.
33 Zamboni GA, Kruskal JB, Vollmer CM, *et al.* Pancreatic adenocarcinoma: value of multidetector CT angiography in preoperative evaluation. *Radiology* 2007;245(3):770–8.
34 Sahani DV, Bonaffini PA, Catalano OA, Guimaraes AR, Blake MA. State-of-the-art PET/CT of the pancreas: current role and emerging indications. *Radiographics* 2012;32(4):1133–58; discussion 1158–60.
35 Vargas R, Nino-Murcia M, Trueblood W, Jeffrey RB. MDCT in Pancreatic adenocarcinoma: prediction of vascular invasion and resectability using a multiphasic technique with curved planar reformations. *Am J Roentgenol* 2004;182(2):419–25.
36 Fukushima H, Itoh S, Takada A, *et al.* Diagnostic value of curved multiplanar reformatted images in multislice CT for the detection of resectable pancreatic ductal adenocarcinoma. *Eur Radiol* 2006;16(8):1709–18.
37 Manak E, Merkel S, Klein P, *et al.* Resectability of pancreatic adenocarcinoma: assessment using multidetector-row computed tomography with multiplanar reformations. *Abdom Imaging* 2009;34(1):75–80.
38 Valls C, Andía E, Sanchez A, *et al.* Dual-phase helical CT of pancreatic adenocarcinoma: assessment of resectability before surgery. *Am J Roentgenol* 2002;178(4):821–6.
39 Bronstein YL, Loyer EM, Kaur H, *et al.* Detection of small pancreatic tumors with multiphasic helical CT. *Am J Roentgenol* 2004;182(3):619–23.
40 Kaneko OF, Lee DM, Wong J, *et al.* Performance of multidetector computed tomographic angiography in determining surgical resectability of pancreatic head adenocarcinoma. *J Comput Assist Tomogr* 2010;34(5):732–8.
41 Andersson R, Vagianos CE, Williamson RC. Preoperative staging and evaluation of resectability in pancreatic ductal adenocarcinoma. *HPB (Oxford)* 2004;6(1):5–12.
42 Mayo SC, Austin DF, Sheppard BC, *et al.* Evolving preoperative evaluation of patients with pancreatic cancer: does laparoscopy have a role in the current era? *J Am Coll Surg* 2009;208(1):87–95.
43 Ahmed SI, Bochkarev V, Oleynikov D, Sasson AR. Patients with pancreatic adenocarcinoma benefit from staging laparoscopy. *J Laparoendosc Adv Surg Tech A* 2006;16(5):458–63.
44 Camacho D, Reichenbach D, Duerr GD, *et al.* Value of laparoscopy in the staging of pancreatic cancer. *JOP* 2005;6(6):552–61.
45 Pisters PW, Lee JE, Vauthey JN, Charnsangavej C, Evans DB. Laparoscopy in the staging of pancreatic cancer. *Br J Surg* 2001;88(3):325–37.
46 Karachristos A, Scarmeas N, Hoffman JP. CA 19-9 levels predict results of staging laparoscopy in pancreatic cancer. *J Gastrointest Surg* 2005;9(9):1286–92.
47 del Castillo CF, Warshaw L. Peritoneal metastases in pancreatic carcinoma. *Hepatogastroenterology* 1993;40(5):430–2.
48 National Comprehensive Cancer Network (NCCN) Guidelines. Available at: www.nccn.org (accessed 21 September 2017).
49 Amin M, Edge S, Greene F, *et al.* *American Joint Committee on Cancer (AJCC) Cancer Staging Manual*, 8th edn. New York: Springer, 2017.
50 Evans DB, Farnell MB, Lillemoe KD, *et al.* Surgical treatment of resectable and borderline resectable pancreas cancer: expert consensus statement. *Ann Surg Oncol* 2009;16(7):1736–44.
51 Callery MP, Chang KJ, Fishman EK, *et al.*Pretreatment assessment of resectable and borderline resectable pancreatic cancer: expert consensus statement. *Ann Surg Oncol* 2009;16(7):1727–33.
52 Varadhachary GR, Tamm EP, Abbruzzese JL, *et al.* Borderline resectable pancreatic cancer: definitions, management, and role of preoperative therapy. *Ann Surg Oncol* 2006;13(8):1035–46.
53 Winter JM, Cameron JL, Campbell KA, *et al.* 1423 pancreaticoduodenectomies for pancreatic cancer: A single-institution experience. *J Gastrointest Surg* 2006;10(9):1199–210; discussion 1210–11.
54 Kalser MH, Ellenberg SS. Pancreatic cancer. Adjuvant combined radiation and chemotherapy following curative resection. *Arch Surg* 1985;120(8):899–903.
55 Klinkenbijl JH, Jeekel J, Sahmoud T, *et al.* Adjuvant radiotherapy and 5-fluorouracil after curative resection of cancer of the pancreas and periampullary region: phase III trial of the EORTC gastrointestinal tract cancer cooperative group. *Ann Surg* 1999;230(6):776–82; discussion 782–4.
56 Neoptolemos JP, Dunn JA, Stocken DD, *et al.* Adjuvant chemoradiotherapy and chemotherapy in resectable pancreatic cancer: a randomised controlled trial. *Lancet* 2001;358(9293):1576–85.
57 Oettle H, Post S, Neuhaus P, *et al.* Adjuvant chemotherapy with gemcitabine vs observation in patients undergoing curative-intent resection of pancreatic cancer: a randomized controlled trial. *JAMA* 2007;297(3):267–77.

58 Neuhaus P, Riess H, Post S, *et al.* CONKO-001: Final results of the randomized, prospective, multicenter phase III trial of adjuvant chemotherapy with gemcitabine versus observation in patients with resected pancreatic cancer (PC). *J Clin Oncol* 2008;26 Suppl 1(Abstract LBA 4504).

59 Regine WF, Winter KA, Abrams RA, *et al.* Fluorouracil vs gemcitabine chemotherapy before and after fluorouracil-based chemoradiation following resection of pancreatic adenocarcinoma: a randomized controlled trial. *JAMA* 2008;299(9):1019–26.

60 Neoptolemos JP, Stocken DD, Bassi C, *et al.* Adjuvant chemotherapy with fluorouracil plus folinic acid vs gemcitabine following pancreatic cancer resection: a randomized controlled trial. *JAMA* 2010;304(10):1073–81.

61 Bakkevold KE, Arnesjø B, Dahl O, Kambestad B. Adjuvant combination chemotherapy (AMF) following radical resection of carcinoma of the pancreas and papilla of Vater–results of a controlled, prospective, randomised multicentre study. *Eur J Cancer* 1993;29A(5):698–703.

62 Ueno H, Kosuge T, Matsuyama Y, *et al.* A randomised phase III trial comparing gemcitabine with surgery-only in patients with resected pancreatic cancer: Japanese Study Group of Adjuvant Therapy for Pancreatic Cancer. *Br J Cancer* 2009;101(6):908–15.

63 Von Hoff DD, Ervin T, Arena FP, *et al.* Increased survival in pancreatic cancer with nab-paclitaxel plus gemcitabine. *N Engl J Med* 2013;369(18):1691–703.

64 Sinn M, Liersch T, Gellert K, *et al.* CONKO-005. Adjuvant therapy in R0 resected pancreatic cancer patients with gemcitabine plus erlotinib versus gemcitabine for 24 weeks – a prospective randomized phase III study. *J Clin Oncol* 2015:33(suppl; abstr 4007).

65 Neoptolemos J, Palmer D, Ghaneh P, *et al.* ESPAC-4: a multicenter, international, open-label randomized controlled phase III trial of adjuvant combination chemotherapy of gemcitabine (GEM) and capecitabine (CAP) versus monotherapy gemcitabine in patients with resected pancreatic ductal adenocarcinoma. *J Clin Oncol* 34;2016 (Supple;abstr LBA4006).

66 Heinrich S, Pestalozzi B, Lesurtel M, *et al.* Adjuvant gemcitabine versus NEOadjuvant gemcitabine/oxaliplatin plus adjuvant gemcitabine in resectable pancreatic cancer: a randomized multicenter phase III study (NEOPAC study). *BMC Cancer* 2011;11:346.

67 Gillen S, Schuster T, Meyer Zum Büschenfelde C, Friess H, Kleeff J. Preoperative/neoadjuvant therapy in pancreatic cancer: a systematic review and meta-analysis of response and resection percentages. *PLoS Med* 2010;7(4):e1000267.

68 Desai SP, Ben-Josef E, Normolle DP, *et al.* Phase I study of oxaliplatin, full-dose gemcitabine, and concurrent radiation therapy in pancreatic cancer. *J Clin Oncol* 2007;25(29): 4587–92.

69 Varadhachary GR, Wolff RA, Crane CH, *et al.* Preoperative gemcitabine and cisplatin followed by gemcitabine-based chemoradiation for resectable adenocarcinoma of the pancreatic head. *J Clin Oncol* 2008;26(21):3487–95.

70 Evans DB, Varadhachary GR, Crane CH, *et al.* Preoperative gemcitabine-based chemoradiation for patients with resectable adenocarcinoma of the pancreatic head. *J Clin Oncol* 2008;26(21):3496–502.

71 Le Scodan R, Mornex F, Partensky C, *et al.* Histopathological response to preoperative chemoradiation for resectable pancreatic adenocarcinoma: the French Phase II FFCD 9704-SFRO Trial. *Am J Clin Oncol* 2008;31(6):545–52.

72 Oettle H, Neuhaus P, Hochhaus A, *et al.* Adjuvant chemotherapy with gemcitabine and long-term outcomes among patients with resected pancreatic cancer: the CONKO-001 randomized trial. *JAMA* 2013;310(14):1473–81.

73 Regine WF, Winter KA, Abrams R, *et al.* Fluorouracil-based chemoradiation with either gemcitabine or fluorouracil chemotherapy after resection of pancreatic adenocarcinoma: 5-year analysis of the U.S. Intergroup/RTOG 9704 phase III trial. *Ann Surg Oncol* 2011;18(5):1319–26.

74 Breslin TM, Hess KR, Harbison DB, *et al.* Neoadjuvant chemoradiotherapy for adenocarcinoma of the pancreas: treatment variables and survival duration. *Ann Surg Oncol* 2001;8(2):123–32.

75 Papavasiliou P, Chun YS, Hoffman JP. How to define and manage borderline resectable pancreatic cancer. *Surg Clin North Am* 2013;93(3):663–74.

76 Katz MH, Pisters PW, Evans DB, *et al.* Borderline resectable pancreatic cancer: the importance of this emerging stage of disease. *J Am Coll Surg* 2008;206(5):833–46; discussion 846–8.

77 Abrams RA, Lowy AM, O'Reilly EM, *et al.* Combined modality treatment of resectable and borderline resectable pancreas cancer: expert consensus statement. *Ann Surg Oncol* 2009;16(7):1751–6.

78 Tsai S, Christians K, Ritch P, *et al.* Multimodality therapy in patients with borderline resectable or locally advanced pancreatic cancer: importance of locoregional therapies for a systemic disease. *JOP* 2016;12:915–27.

79 Ferrone CR, Marchegiani G, Hong TS, *et al.* Radiological and surgical implications of neoadjuvant treatment with FOLFIRINOX for locally advanced and borderline resectable pancreatic cancer. *Ann Surg* 2015;261(1):12–17.

80 Katz MH, Pisters PW, Lee JE, Fleming JB. Borderline resectable pancreatic cancer: what have we learned and where do we go from here? *Ann Surg Oncol* 2011;18(3):608–10.

81 Katz MH, Marsh R, Herman JM, *et al.* Borderline resectable pancreatic cancer: need for standardization and methods for optimal clinical trial design. *Ann Surg Oncol* 2013;20(8):2787–95.

82 Katz MH, Ahmad S, Nelson H. Borderline resectable pancreatic cancer: pushing the technical limits of surgery. *Bull Am Coll Surg* 2013;98(1):61–3.

83 Tseng JF, Raut CP, Lee JE, *et al.* Pancreaticoduodenectomy with vascular resection: margin status and survival duration. *J Gastrointest Surg* 2004;8(8):935–49; discussion 949–50.

84 Raut CP, Tseng JF, Sun CC, *et al.* Impact of resection status on pattern of failure and survival after pancreaticoduodenectomy for pancreatic adenocarcinoma. *Ann Surg* 2007;246(1):52–60.

85 Yeo CJ, Cameron JL, Lillemoe KD, *et al.* Pancreaticoduodenectomy with or without distal gastrectomy and extended retroperitoneal lymphadenectomy for periampullary adenocarcinoma, part 2: randomized controlled trial evaluating survival, morbidity, and mortality. *Ann Surg* 2002;236(3):355–66; discussion 366–8.

86 Tempero MA, Arnoletti JP, Behrman S, *et al.* Pancreatic adenocarcinoma. *J Natl Compr Canc Netw* 2010;8(9): 972–1017.

87 Uchida H, Shibata K, Iwaki K, *et al.* Ampullary cancer and preoperative jaundice: possible indication of the minimal surgery. *Hepatogastroenterology* 2009;56(93):1194–8.
88 Hatzaras I, George N, Muscarella P, *et al.* Predictors of survival in periampullary cancers following pancreaticoduodenectomy. *Ann Surg Oncol* 2010;17(4): 991–7.
89 Kloek JJ, Heger M, van der Gaag NA, *et al.* Effect of preoperative biliary drainage on coagulation and fibrinolysis in severe obstructive cholestasis. *J Clin Gastroenterol* 2010;44(9):646–52.
90 Bonin EA, Baron TH. Preoperative biliary stents in pancreatic cancer. *J Hepatobiliary Pancreat Sci* 2011;18(5): 621–9.
91 Dixon JM, Armstrong CP, Duffy SW, Davies GC. Factors affecting morbidity and mortality after surgery for obstructive jaundice: a review of 373 patients. *Gut* 1983; 24(9):845–52.
92 van der Gaag NA, Rauws EA, van Eijck CH, *et al.* Preoperative biliary drainage for cancer of the head of the pancreas. *N Engl J Med* 2010;362(2):129–37.
93 Decker C, Christein JD, Phadnis MA, Wilcox CM, Varadarajulu S. Biliary metal stents are superior to plastic stents for preoperative biliary decompression in pancreatic cancer. *Surg Endosc* 2011;25(7):2364–7.
94 Tran KT, Smeenk HG, van Eijck CH, *et al.* Pylorus preserving pancreaticoduodenectomy versus standard Whipple procedure: a prospective, randomized, multicenter analysis of 170 patients with pancreatic and periampullary tumors. *Ann Surg* 2004;240(5):738–45.
95 Fisher WE, Hodges SE, Silberfein EJ, *et al.* Pancreatic resection without routine intraperitoneal drainage. *HPB (Oxford)* 2011;13(7):503–10.
96 Mehta VV, Fisher SB, Maithel SK, *et al.* Is it time to abandon routine operative drain use? A single institution assessment of 709 consecutive pancreaticoduodenectomies. *J Am Coll Surg* 2013;216(4):635–42; discussion 642–4.
97 Hammel P, Huguet F, van Laethem J, *et al.* Effect of chemoradiotherapy vs chemotherapy on survival in patients with locally advanced pancreatic cancer controlled after 4 months of gemcitabine with or without erlotinib: the LAP07 randomized clinical trial. *JAMA* 2016;315:1844–53.
98 Mukherjee S, Hurt CN, Bridgewater J, *et al.* Gemcitabine-based or capecitabine-based chemoradiotherapy for locally advanced pancreatic cancer (SCALOP): a multicentre, randomised, phase 2 trial. *Lancet Oncol* 2013;14(4):317–26.
99 Huguet F, André T, Hammel P, *et al.* Impact of chemoradiotherapy after disease control with chemotherapy in locally advanced pancreatic adenocarcinoma in GERCOR phase II and III studies. *J Clin Oncol* 2007;25(3):326–31.
100 Klaassen DJ, MacIntyre JM, Catton GE, Engstrom PF, Moertel CG. Treatment of locally unresectable cancer of the stomach and pancreas: a randomized comparison of 5-fluorouracil alone with radiation plus concurrent and maintenance 5-fluorouracil–an Eastern Cooperative Oncology Group study. *J Clin Oncol* 1985;3(3):373–8.
101 Burris HA, Moore MJ, Andersen J, *et al.* Improvements in survival and clinical benefit with gemcitabine as first-line therapy for patients with advanced pancreas cancer: a randomized trial. *J Clin Oncol* 1997;15(6):2403–13.
102 Moore MJ, Goldstein D, Hamm J, *et al.* Erlotinib plus gemcitabine compared with gemcitabine alone in patients with advanced pancreatic cancer: a phase III trial of the National Cancer Institute of Canada Clinical Trials Group. *J Clin Oncol* 2007;25(15):1960–6.
103 von Hoff D. *Randomized phase 3 study of weekly nab-paclitaxel plus gemcitabine versus gemcitabine alone in patients with metastatic adenocarcinoma of the pancreas* (MPACT). Phase 3 metastatic pancreatic cancer (late breaking abstract). January 24–26, 2013. San Francisco: American Society of Clinical Oncology (GI), 2013.
104 Philip PA, Benedetti J, Corless CL, *et al.* Phase III study comparing gemcitabine plus cetuximab versus gemcitabine in patients with advanced pancreatic adenocarcinoma: Southwest Oncology Group-directed intergroup trial S0205. *J Clin Oncol* 2010;28(22):3605–10.
105 Van Cutsem E, Vervenne WL, Bennouna J, *et al.* Phase III trial of bevacizumab in combination with gemcitabine and erlotinib in patients with metastatic pancreatic cancer. *J Clin Oncol* 2009;27(13):2231–7.
106 Conroy T, Desseigne F, Ychou M, *et al.* FOLFIRINOX versus gemcitabine for metastatic pancreatic cancer. *N Engl J Med* 2011;364(19):1817–25.
107 Conroy T, Gavoille C, Samalin E, Ychou M, Ducreux M. The role of the FOLFIRINOX regimen for advanced pancreatic cancer. *Curr Oncol Rep* 2013;15(2):182–9.
108 Xiong HQ, Varadhachary GR, Blais JC, *et al.* Phase 2 trial of oxaliplatin plus capecitabine (XELOX) as second-line therapy for patients with advanced pancreatic cancer. *Cancer* 2008;113(8):2046–52.
109 Pelzer U, Kubica K, Stieler J, *et al.* A randomized trial in patients with gemcitabine refractory pancreatic cancer. Final results of the CONKO 003 study. *J Clin Oncol* 2008;26(Suppl) (Abstr 4508).
110 Pelzer U, Schwaner I, Stieler J, *et al.* Best supportive care (BSC) versus oxaliplatin, folinic acid and 5-fluorouracil (OFF) plus BSC in patients for second–line advanced pancreatic cancer: a phase III-study from the German CONKO-study group. *Eur J Cancer* 2011;47(11):1676–81.
111 Greer JA, Jackson VA, Meier DE, Temel JS. Early integration of palliative care services with standard oncology care for patients with advanced cancer. *CA Cancer J Clin* 2013;63(5):349–63.
112 Moss A, Morris E, MacMathuna P. Palliatie biliary stents for obstructing pancreatic carcinoma. *Cochrane Database Syst Rev* 2006;2(CD004200).
113 Temel JS, Greer JA, Muzikansky A, *et al.* Early palliative care for patients with metastatic non-small-cell lung cancer. *N Engl J Med* 2010;363(8):733–42.
114 Khorana AA, Fine RL. Pancreatic cancer and thromboembolic disease. *Lancet Oncol* 2004;5(11):655–63.
115 Gooden HM, White KJ. Pancreatic cancer and supportive care–pancreatic exocrine insufficiency negatively impacts on quality of life. *Support Care Cancer* 2013;21(7): 1835–41.
116 Smith J, Chu Q, Tseng J. Pancreatic Adenocarcinoma. In: QD Chu, J Gibbs, G Zibari (eds) *Surgical Oncology: A Practical*

and Comprehensive Approach. New York: Springer, 2014:283–313.

117 Heinrich S, Schäfer M, Weber A, *et al.* Neoadjuvant chemotherapy generates a significant tumor response in resectable pancreatic cancer without increasing morbidity: results of a prospective phase II trial. *Ann Surg* 2008;248(6):1014–22.

118 Moertel CG, Frytak S, Hahn RG, *et al.* Therapy of locally unresectable pancreatic carcinoma: a randomized comparison of high dose (6000 rads) radiation alone, moderate dose radiation (4000 rads + 5-fluorouracil), and high dose radiation + 5-fluorouracil: The Gastrointestinal Tumor Study Group. *Cancer* 1981;48(8):1705–10.

119 Cohen SJ, Dobelbower R, Lipsitz S, *et al.* A randomized phase III study of radiotherapy alone or with 5-fluorouracil and mitomycin-C in patients with locally advanced adenocarcinoma of the pancreas: Eastern Cooperative Oncology Group study E8282. *Int J Radiat Oncol Biol Phys* 2005;62(5):1345–50.

120 Chauffert B, Mornex F, Bonnetain F, *et al.* Phase III trial comparing intensive induction chemoradiotherapy (60 Gy, infusional 5-FU and intermittent cisplatin) followed by maintenance gemcitabine with gemcitabine alone for locally advanced unresectable pancreatic cancer. Definitive results of the 2000-01 FFCD/SFRO study. *Ann Oncol* 2008;19(9): 1592–9.

121 Loehrer PJ, Feng Y, Cardenes H, *et al.* Gemcitabine alone versus gemcitabine plus radiotherapy in patients with locally advanced pancreatic cancer: an Eastern Cooperative Oncology Group trial. *J Clin Oncol* 2011;29(31):4105–12.

122 Krishnan S, Rana V, Janjan NA, *et al.* Induction chemotherapy selects patients with locally advanced, unresectable pancreatic cancer for optimal benefit from consolidative chemoradiation therapy. *Cancer* 2007;110(1):47–55.

7

Liver Cancers

Celina Ang, Sonia Reichert, and Randall F. Holcombe

Mount Sinai Medical Center, New York, New York, USA

Incidence and Mortality

Liver cancer is the sixth most common cancer and the second leading cause of cancer mortality worldwide [1]. Incidence rates are highest in east and south-east Asia and in northern and western Africa. Worldwide, hepatocellular carcinoma (HCC) represents 70–90% of liver cancers [1]. Statistical data are compiled by the National Cancer Institute's Surveillance, Epidemiology, and End Results (SEER) Program for the category of "liver and intrahepatic bile duct cancer" [2].

According to the American Cancer Society, approximately 40,710 new cases of liver and intrahepatic bile duct cancers (29,200 men and 11,510 women) are diagnosed and approximately 28,920 deaths (19,610 men and 9,310 women) from these cancers occur annually in the United States [3]. The incidence rate of cancers of the liver and intrahepatic bile ducts, overall, based on cases diagnosed between 2009 and 2013, was approximately 8.4 per 100,000 persons per year. During the same time period, the age-adjusted death rate was 6.1 per 100,000 persons per year. The lifetime risk of developing cancer of the liver and intrahepatic bile ducts is approximately 0.95%. These overall statistics largely reflect those of HCC, which in the United States accounts for 73.8% of cancers of the liver and intrahepatic bile duct [2].

Etiology and Risk Factors

Viral Hepatitis

Infection with viral hepatitis B (HBV) and C (HCV) are collectively responsible for 74.3% of HCC cases worldwide [4]. A member of the Hepadnaviridae family of DNA viruses, HBV integrates itself into the host genome and initiates viral replication through reverse transcription. Hepatocarcinogenesis occurs as a result of genomic instability caused by insertional mutagenesis, viral protein oncogenesis, and by inflammation and fibrosis elicited by the host immune response [5]. The degree of HBV replicative activity has been shown to correlate with increased HCC risk [6]. HCV is an RNA Flavivirus that induces chronic liver inflammation, oxidative stress, and cycles of regeneration, proliferation, and fibrosis. These events cause genomic, proteomic, and transcriptomic aberrations that ultimately lead to HCC. Unlike HBV, HCC that arises in the context of HCV infection is virtually always preceded by cirrhosis [7]. Treatment of viral hepatitis has been shown to reduce, but not eliminate, the risk of HCC [8].

Alcohol

Alcohol metabolism by alcohol dehydrogenase produces acetaldehyde, a recognized hepatocarcinogen. Chronic alcohol consumption is immunosuppressive and often coexists with nutritional deficiencies in folate and vitamin B12 which are essential for DNA synthesis and antioxidant production [9]. Alcohol strongly potentiates the carcinogenic effects of viral hepatitis, diabetes, and other hepatotoxins [9, 10]. Long-term (>10 years) alcohol cessation can decrease the risk of HCC [11].

Nonalcoholic Fatty Liver Disease

Obesity, hyperlipidemia and insulin resistance comprise the metabolic syndrome which is a risk factor for nonalcoholic fatty liver disease (NAFLD), the most common cause of liver disease in developed countries. NAFLD spans a continuum of progressive hepatic steatosis and dysfunction occurring over decades, leading to nonalcoholic steatohepatitis (NASH) and cirrhosis. HCC arises in 4–27% of patients with NASH following the onset of cirrhosis, although HCC can also occur in the absence of steatohepatitis and fibrosis [12]. NAFLD HCC is typically diagnosed at a more advanced age (median 65–70 years) than HCC due to other causes of liver disease [12, 13]. NASH-induced hepatocarcinogenesis is thought to be driven by the upregulation of insulin-like growth factor signaling, increased oxidative stress, the release of inflammatory cytokines and proangiogenic factors, and the downregulation of anti-inflammatory and antiproliferative tumor suppressors [12–14].

The American Cancer Society's Oncology in Practice: Clinical Management, First Edition. Edited by The American Cancer Society.

Iron Overload Disorders and Hereditary Hemochromatosis

Hereditary hemochromatosis (HH) is caused by C282Y and/or H63D mutations in the *HFE* gene. Patients with HH have a 100–200-fold increased risk of developing HCC, and the overall prevalence is approximately 10% with higher rates reported among those with cirrhosis. Iron overload is strongly associated with HCC, even in the absence of an *HFE* mutation or cirrhosis. The mechanisms of iron-induced hepatocarcinogenesis include direct mitogenic effects, structural DNA damage, and mutagenesis as a result of oxidative stress, lipid peroxidation, and immunosuppression [15].

Aflatoxins

Aflatoxins are produced by the *Aspergillus* fungi which grow in the hot, humid climates of south-east Asia and sub-Saharan Africa and are consumed in the form of infected peanuts, grains, and legumes. The main carcinogenic aflatoxin – B1 – induces the formation of DNA adducts leading to missense mutations in p53 and oxidative hepatocytic damage [16]. It is estimated that aflatoxin exposure contributes to 4.6–28.2% of all HCC cases worldwide [17].

Betel Quid

Chewing of betel quid, derived from the areca nut of the *Areca catechu* palm tree, is a popular practice in southern Asian countries like Taiwan. Chronic betel quid chewing has been implicated in the development of HCC and aerodigestive tract neoplasms. The principal carcinogenic ingredients are nitrosamines and safrole which cause impairments in hepatic detoxification and metabolism, chronic inflammation and oxidative damage, and genetic instability [18, 19].

Alpha-1 Antitrypsin Deficiency

The liver glycoprotein alpha-1 antitrypsin (A1AT) is a key mediator in the host response to tissue inflammation and injury. Plasma A1AT deficiency is most commonly caused by Z and/or S mutations in the Pi locus, giving rise to panlobular emphysema, childhood liver disease, cirrhosis and HCC in adults [20, 21]. A1AT deficiency may also potentiate the hepatocarcinogenic effects of infection with HBV or HCV [21]. In addition to HCC, cholangiocarcinoma and mixed HCC-cholangiocarcioma have been reported in association with A1AT deficiency in PiZ heterozygotes [22].

Cigarette Smoking

The relationship between cigarette smoking, HCC risk, and mortality is controversial and difficult to ascertain given that smoking is often associated with other behaviors that increase HCC and cancer risk in general such as alcohol consumption [11, 23].

Microcystins

The high incidence of HCC in certain parts of rural China has been linked to the consumption of pond or ditch water contaminated with microcystins, a hepatotoxin produced by blue–green algae [24].

Pathogenesis

The pathogenesis of HCC is complicated and is the byproduct of intersecting risk factors with diverse mechanisms of hepatocytotoxicity. Hepatocellular injury due to chronic inflammation, oxidative damage, and other stressors causes DNA damage and instability, leading to altered gene expression, dysregulation of metabolic and homeostatic processes, and loss of the normal equilibrium between tumor suppressors and oncogenes, culminating in a final common pathway of carcinogenesis. Key alterations in HCC include *TERT* promoter mutations or amplification, mutation or deletion of cell cycle regulators including *TP53* and *CDKN2A*, oxidative stress regulators, vascular endothelial growth factor (VEGF) and other angiogenic mediators, MAP kinase and PI3K/Akt/mTOR cascades, and the Wnt/ß-catenin axes [25]. The complex molecular taxonomy of HCC has led to challenges in therapeutic targeting, given the myriad interactions between cascades as part of a much larger signaling network.

Prevention, Screening, and Surveillance

Primary prevention of HCC consists of a combination of lifestyle and risk factor modifications, and treatment of treatable predisposing conditions. Weight loss and smoking and alcohol cessation have known health benefits that extend beyond reducing HCC incidence and death. Avoidance of hepatotoxins should be encouraged where applicable. Phlebotomy for patients with HH and the use of metformin or thiazolidenediones in diabetic patients have been associated with a decreased risk for HCC, although these have not been officially endorsed as preventive measures [14, 15]. HBV and the subsequent development of HCC can be effectively prevented through adherence to universal vaccination guidelines [26]. Clearance of HBV and HCV as a result of antiviral therapy has been shown to decrease but not completely eliminate the risk of HCC, although its preventive impact in the context of established cirrhosis is uncertain [8].

Surveillance and screening programs for patients with risk factors for HCC can help to decrease mortality (Table 7.1). A study conducted in China randomized approximately 19,000 patients with HBV or chronic hepatitis to screening with ultrasonography and serum AFP every 6 months versus no screening. Despite a compliance rate of only 60% in the screening group, HCC mortality was reduced by 38% [27].

Semiannual monitoring of cirrhotic individuals with a ≥1.5%/year risk of developing HCC is considered cost effective and is endorsed by the American and European Associations for the Study of Liver Disease (AASLD, EASL), Asia–Pacific Association for the Study of the Liver and National Comprehensive Cancer Network [28–31]. "At risk" populations who should be screened include patients with HBV or HCV, including those without cirrhosis and who seroconverted or had a sustained virologic response to antivirals. Among HBV patients, there are gender and ethnogeographic differences in predisposition which influence the age at which screening should commence. Native Asian and African carriers of HBV tend to develop HCC at a younger age and earlier screening is therefore recommended

Table 7.1 Hepatocellular carcinoma screening/surveillance recommendations.

Who should undergo screening/surveillance
Chronic liver disease with cirrhosis: • HCV • HBV • Stage 4 primary biliary cirrhosis • Hemochromatosis • Alpha-1-antitrypsin deficiency • NAFLD
HBV carriers +/− cirrhosis: • With family history of HCC • Asian males ≥40 years old, Asian females ≥50 years old • African/North American Blacks
Benefit of screening/surveillance unclear: • HCV without cirrhosis • NAFLD without cirrhosis • Autoimmune hepatitis with cirrhosis
Screening modalities and recall policies
Abdominal ultrasound at 6 months
AFP not recommended by AASLD or EASL
If abnormal ultrasound: • Nodule <1 cm – close follow-up at 3–6 months then at 6 months if stable for a year • Nodule 1–2 cm – contrast-enhanced multiphasic cross-sectional imaging or biopsy • Nodule >2 cm – contrast-enhanced multiphasic cross-sectional imaging; diagnose as HCC if "radiographic hallmark" present[1]

Source: adapted from [28, 32].
[1] See Diagnosis section. AASLD, American Association for the Study of Liver Disease; EASL, European Association for the study of Liver Disease; AHBV, hepatitis B virus; HCC, hepatocellular carcinoma; HCV, hepatitis C virus; NAFLD, nonalcoholic fatty liver disease.

[30, 32]. Patients coinfected with HIV and viral hepatitis, and cirrhosis from nonviral etiologies including alcoholic liver disease, NASH, HH, and primary biliary cirrhosis, should also undergo surveillance [28–30]. Screening recommendations for cirrhosis due to autoimmune hepatitis or A1AT deficiency have not been universally endorsed [28–31].

Diagnosis

HCC represents an exception to the typical oncologic diagnostic algorithm that mandates histopathologic confirmation of the diagnosis before proceeding with treatment. Imaging has assumed a pivotal role in diagnosing HCC, in some instances obviating the need for a biopsy or tumor marker assessments. The strengths and pitfalls of the noninvasive diagnostic approach, reasons for pursuing a histopathologic diagnosis, and the various imaging and laboratory diagnostic tests in current use are discussed below.

Imaging

Advances in dynamic contrast-enhanced imaging technology led to the characterization of the "HCC radiologic hallmark" – arterial hyperenhancement followed by venous/delayed phase washout – which is the cornerstone of noninvasive diagnostic criteria for HCC in patients with cirrhosis [28]. The acquisition of high-quality, multiphase contrast-enhanced images via either helical computed tomography (CT) or magnetic resonance imaging (MRI) is key for making an accurate diagnosis.

CT

Multidetector CT (MDCT) scans obtain high-quality, thin-sliced images at a rapid pace and can generate three-dimensional images of tumor vascular anatomy for treatment planning [33]. Triphasic CT scans capturing hepatic arterial, portal venous, and delayed phases have a diagnostic sensitivity and specificity of 89% and 99%, respectively [34].

MRI

On MRI, HCC most commonly appears as a hypointense lesion on T1 that becomes hyperintense on T2, with arterial enhancement and venous washout during dynamic gadolinium-enhanced imaging. Additional features suggestive of HCC include the presence of a fibrous capsule and rapid interval growth [33].

To Biopsy or Not to Biopsy?

Making the Diagnosis Noninvasively

Guidelines for noninvasive diagnosis were developed to avoid the risks of bleeding and needle tract seeding associated with biopsy. Proponents of the noninvasive approach also cite the difficulty of distinguishing between high-grade dysplastic nodules and early, well-differentiated HCCs pathologically. In the most recent iteration of the AASLD and EASL guidelines, presence of the radiologic hallmark on a single multiphasic cross-sectional imaging modality (helical CT or gadolinium MRI) is sufficient to diagnose tumors >2 cm, and may also be enough to diagnose tumors 1–2 cm in diameter if performed at high-volume tertiary care centers with access to advanced imaging technology [28, 30]. Adherence to these criteria permits the diagnosis of HCC in cirrhotic patients with an overall sensitivity and specificity of approximately 80% and ≥90%, respectively, with gadolinium-MRI being the most sensitive technique [35].

A biopsy is still indicated for nodules arising in noncirrhotic livers and nodules in cirrhotic livers that display an atypical enhancement pattern [28, 30].

Rationale for Biopsy

The yield and accuracy of noninvasive diagnostic criteria are predicated upon the sensitivity and specificity of the imaging modalities used. Even with improved imaging technologies, the accurate distinction of HCC from other malignant or benign lesions remains challenging, especially for small tumors measuring 1–2 cm which are less likely to be hypervascular [36]. Other disease entities (e.g., cholangiocarcinoma, mixed HCC-cholangiocarcinoma) can also display the "HCC radiologic hallmark" [37, 38]. Since the treatment and prognosis of these differ significantly from HCC, knowledge of the correct diagnosis is critical and would not otherwise be possible to distinguish without a biopsy. The incidence of needle tract seeding following a liver biopsy for HCC is estimated at 2.7% overall [39], although it is unclear if this is affected by the size of lesion being biopsied [30]. Though not specifically reported, the risks of needle tract seeding and hemorrhage are likely to be low for tumors <2 cm [30]. Thus, clinicians should not be dissuaded from pursuing a biopsy if deemed necessary to make the diagnosis, especially if it might potentially spare patients from exposure to unnecessary invasive or noxious procedures.

Beyond diagnostic purposes, tissue procurement has become increasingly important for the advancement of personalized medicine in oncology. Tumor specimens provide material for genetic and molecular profiling which can facilitate biomarker and therapeutic target discovery, and the elucidation of drug resistance mechanisms.

Tumor Markers

Serum α-fetoprotein (AFP) is a 70 kDa glycoprotein produced by endodermal yolk sac cells and hepatocytes during embryogenesis. It functions as a carrier/transport molecule that binds to fatty acids, bilirubin, steroids, and xenobiotics, and may also harbor growth regulatory and immunosuppressive properties. As AFP production is normally suppressed in adults, rising serum levels reflect pathologic synthetic reactivation due to liver regeneration and/or hepatocarcinogenesis [40]. Serum AFP levels have prognostic value in HCC [41] and may be used to monitor the disease course and response to therapy [41, 42]. AFP is less useful as a diagnostic tool because of its limited specificity for HCC; although an AFP cutoff of ≥100 mg/L is associated with 99% specificity, this comes at the expense of decreased sensitivity ranging from 17 to 31% [40]. As a result, serum AFP is no longer a part of the AASLD and EASL diagnostic algorithms.

Lectin-bound AFP variants such as lens culinaris agglutinin A-reactive AFP (AFP-L3) and erythroagglutinating phytohemagglutinin (AFP P4 + P5) may have greater sensitivity and specificity than AFP for the detection of HCC amongst cirrhotic patients [43], but requires further study. Des-γ-carboxyprothrombin (DCP) is an abnormal prothrombin variant synthesized in the absence of vitamin K. DCP levels have been shown to discriminate HCC from chronic viral hepatitis, liver metastases, and normal subjects, and may have utility in monitoring responses to therapy [44]. Functionally, DCP demonstrates proproliferative and proangiogenic properties [45, 46]. DCP is reportedly more sensitive and specific than AFP, although HCC detection can be further enhanced when the two markers are combined [40].

Other biomarkers: the heparin sulfate proteoglycan, glypican-3 (GPC-3), osteopontin (OPN), golgi protein 73, squamous cell carcinoma antigen (SCCA), and microRNAs are other emerging biomarkers that have shown promising sensitivity and specificity either alone or in combination with more established markers in diagnosing HCC [40].

Pathology

Macroscopic Appearance

Grossly, HCCs appear as heterogeneous masses of variable size with focal areas of hemorrhage and/or necrosis. Unlike other cancers, HCC tumors tend to be soft due to the paucity of desmoplastic stroma [47]. Three major growth patterns have been identified: (i) nodular expanding consisting of a dominant lesion with satellitosis; (ii) a large, solitary infiltrative mass with poorly demarcated edges, which is typically seen in noncirrhotic livers; (iii) diffuse pattern characterized by small nodules occupying the entire liver in a miliary-like distribution. The presence of macroscopic vascular invasion and an infiltrative type growth pattern are associated with a poor prognosis [48, 49].

Microscopic Appearance

HCC cells are morphologically similar to normal hepatocytes though this varies depending on the degree of differentiation. Cells are polygonal, contain finely granular eosinophilic cytoplasm, large nuclei with prominent nucleoli, and a high nuclear:cytoplasmic ratio. Tumor cells may contain biliary pigments, fat and/or glycogen deposits, and Mallory Denk bodies which are typically associated with alcoholic liver disease. Biliary canaliculi are typically present and are interspersed between cells [47].

Various growth patterns have been documented; the most common is the trabecular pattern consisting of cells arranged in thick cords separated by venous sinusoids. Dilation of biliary canaliculi within the trabeculae or central degeneration of the trabeculae produces the pseudoglandular or acinar pattern. The compact or solid pattern consists of thickened, compressed trabeculae forming a mass [47, 48].

Histological subtypes of HCC include the clear cell variant, characterized by abundant intracellular fat and/or glycogen. Scirrhous HCC is an extremely rare subtype containing abundant fibrous stroma. Sarcomatoid HCC contains spindle-shaped or giant tumor cells. Sclerosing HCC also contains abundant fibrous stroma with densely packed tumor cells [47, 48].

Immunohistochemistry

Immunostains for HepPar-1 and AFP are positive in up to 90% and 50% of HCCs, respectively. Fibrinogen, α-1-antitrypsin, and albumin may also stain positive in well- differentiated tumors [47, 48]. Newer markers including glypican-3, heat shock protein 70 (hsp70), and glutamine synthase have a high sensitivity and specificity, especially when used in combination. Distinguishing well-differentiated HCC from dysplastic nodules is challenging. Positivity for any two of these three markers has a sensitivity and specificity of 72% and 100%, respectively, for differentiating early, low grade HCCs from dysplastic nodules [50]. Cytokeratin stains including AE1/AE3, CK7 and CK20 have variable to weak expression and are considered less useful for diagnosing HCC.

Polyclonal antiserum to CEA (pCEA) can help to identify bile canaliculi present in normal liver and HCC but not liver metastases [51]. Complete, homogeneous staining for the endothelial marker CD34 across all sinusoidal spaces is also typical for HCC, whereas negative and incomplete staining patterns are more typically seen in normal or cirrhotic liver and benign hepatic lesions, respectively [52].

Molecular Pathology

There is an emerging body of work demonstrating that HCC can be diagnosed using gene expression profiling. Investigators have characterized gene signatures that distinguish between normal and cirrhotic liver, cirrhosis and dysplasia, dysplasia and early HCC, and early and late HCC arising in the context of HCV [53]. The same group has also identified a signature that can predict the presence of vascular invasion with an accuracy rate of 69% [54] which may help to improve prognostication of patients using biopsy material alone. Furthermore, molecular-based subgroups of HCC driven by different biological processes and associated with distinct clinicopathologic phenotypes have been identified [55, 56].

Staging

Seven different HCC staging systems have been developed, reflecting the challenge of capturing the biologic, etiologic, ethnic, and geographic factors that influence disease behavior and prognosis.

American Joint Committee on Cancer Tumor Node Metastases System

The American Joint Committee on Cancer Tumor Node Metastases (TNM) system for hepatocellular carcinoma is a purely anatomical staging system. T, N, and M definitions and stage groupings for the current (8th) edition of this system are shown in Table 7.2 [57].

Table 7.2 American Joint Committee on Cancer (AJCC) TNM staging system for hepatocellular carcinoma.

Tumor category	Nodal (regional) category	Distant metastasis category
TxNxMx = tumor, nodes, distant metastases cannot be assessed		
T0 = none	N0 = no involvement	M0 = none
T1 = solitary tumor, no vascular invasion T1a = solitary tumor ≤2 cm T1b = solitary tumor >2 cm without vascular invasion	N1 = regional nodal metastases	M1 = distant metastases
T2 = multiple tumors ≤5 cm *or* solitary tumor >2 cm with vascular invasion		
T3 = multiple tumors, at least one measuring > 5 cm		
T4 = ≥1 tumor with major branch portal or hepatic vein invasion		
T4 = single or multiple tumors of any size involving major branch of portal or hepatic vein or tumor(s) with direct invasion of adjacent organs other than the gallbladder or with perforation of the visceral peritoneum.		

Source: adapted from AJCC Prognostic Stage Groups [57]. Used with permission of the American College of Surgeons, Chicago, Illinois. The original source for this information is the AJCC Cancer Staging Manual, 8th edn (2017), which is published by Springer Science+Business Media. Stage I, T1N0M0; Stage II, T2N0M0; Stage IIIA, T3aN0M0; Stage IIIB, T3bN0M0; Stage IIIC, T4N0M0; Stage IVA, TanyN1M0; Stage IVB, TanyNanyM1.

An important limitation of the TNM system is that it does not consider hepatic synthetic function which, as will be discussed later, is a critical determinant of prognosis and treatment options. In addition, the presence of microvascular invasion can only be determined in resected lesions, which may not be an appropriate treatment for some patients [30].

Okuda

The Okuda system assigns patients to one of three stages using four variables: ascites, albumin, bilirubin and tumor size [58]. The Okuda system has been criticized for omitting important tumor-related variables such as size, multiplicity, and portal vein thrombosis (PVT) which limit its prognostic potential in early stage disease [59].

Barcelona Clinic Liver Cancer Staging and Treatment Algorithm

The Barcelona Clinic Liver Cancer (BCLC) classification assigns patients to one of five stages (0, A, B, C and D) based on performance status, Child–Pugh score, and tumor extent (Figure 7.1). Prognostic information and treatment recommendations are provided for each stage based on the best available evidence. The BCLC system has been validated in several western cohorts in which HCV is the predominant risk factor [60–62], and has been shown to outperform the Union for International Cancer Control TNM 6th edition and other staging systems to be discussed below. Several limitations of the BCLC system should be noted. First, it has not been validated in Asian populations among whom HBV is endemic and differences in the culture of clinical practice must be considered. Second, the "advanced" or "stage C" category encompasses both portal vein invasion and extrahepatic metastases and may be less discriminatory than other systems which separate these entities [63, 64]. Third, the BCLC system stages patients radiographically but does not provide guidance regarding the management of indeterminate lesions which, depending on how they are interpreted, could impact management and outcome [65]. The prognostic power of the BCLC system may be improved by the integration of molecular biomarkers. Stratification of each BCLC stage by serum VEGF and IGF-1 levels further subdivides patients into better or worse prognostic groups, with the worst outcomes observed amongst those with high VEGF/low IGF-1 levels. In particular, significant survival differences were noted within the BCLC stage C group [66].

Groupe d'Etude et de Traitement du Carcinome Hepatocellulaire (GETCH)

The GETCH considers five variables: performance status, bilirubin, alkaline phosphatase, AFP, portal vein occlusion, which are assigned a weighted score based on Cox regression coefficients. Patients in group A have a score of 0 and are at low risk of death; scores of 1–5 fall within group B intermediate risk; group C includes scores ≥6 and indicate a high risk of death from HCC [67]. The GETCH has not been externally validated, but did appear to have good predictive ability for the outcomes of patients with advanced HCC in a North American series [64].

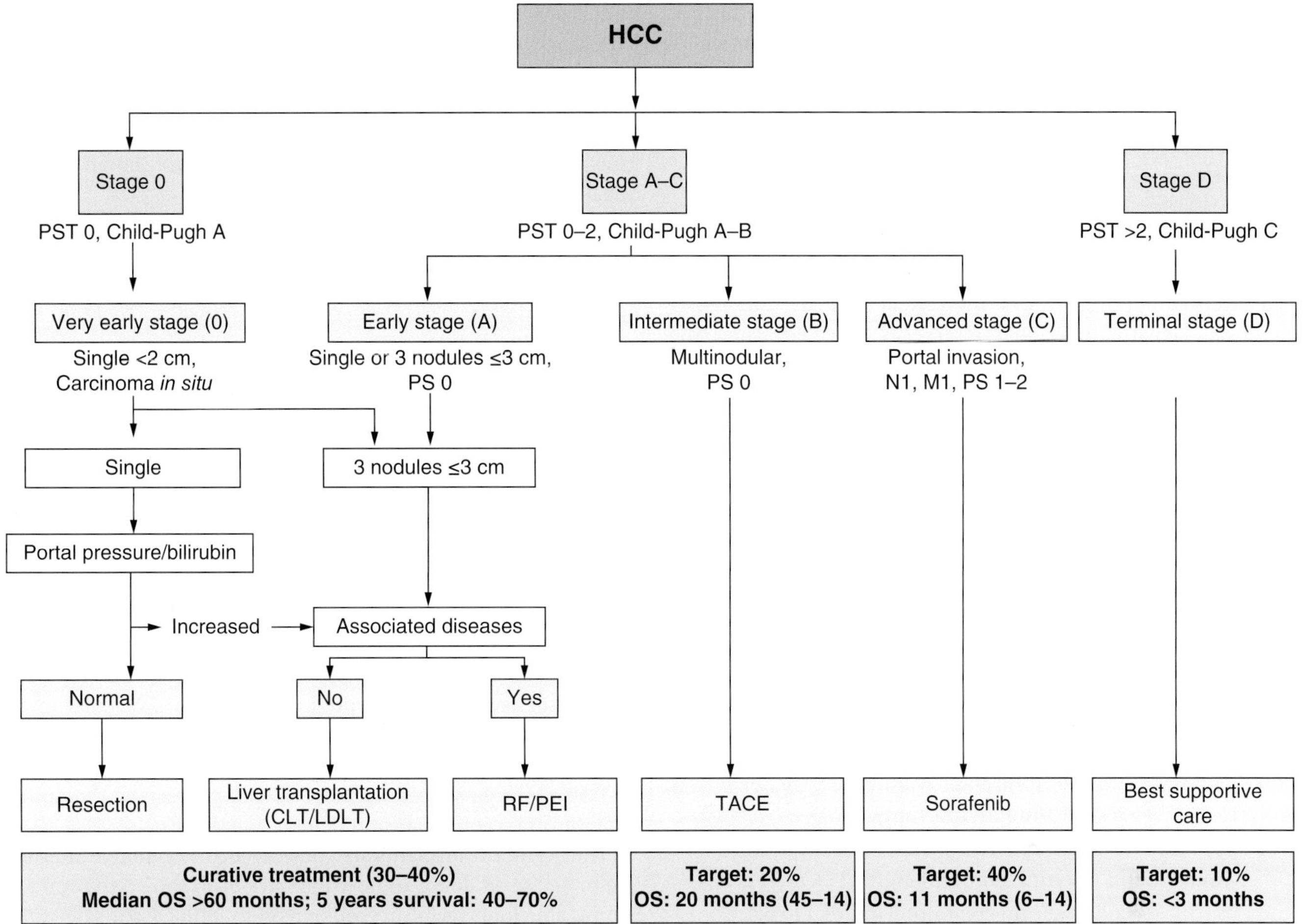

Figure 7.1 The Barcelona Clinic Liver Cancer (BCLC) staging and treatment algorithm. *Source:* European Association for the Study of the Liver 2012 [28]. Reproduced with permission of Elsevier.

Cancer of the Liver Italian Program

The Cancer of the Liver Italian Program (CLIP) score incorporates serum AFP, tumor morphology (uni vs multinodular and tumor occupying ≤50% vs >50% of liver volume), the presence or absence of PVT, and Child–Pugh score. Each variable is assigned a score of 0, 1, or 2 based on severity and the values are summated. Higher scores reflect more advanced disease and a poorer prognosis [68].

Chinese University Prognostic Index

The Chinese University Prognostic Index (CUPI) was developed and validated in a cohort of 926 patients from a single center in Hong Kong, 80% of whom had HBV. It includes six variables: symptoms, ascites, AFP, total bilirubin, alkaline phosphatase, and TNM 5th edition stage, each of which is given a weighted value. The sum of the scores classifies patients into low-risk (CUPI score ≤1), intermediate risk (CUPI 2–7) or high risk (CUPI ≥8) groups. Comparison of the CUPI with the Okuda, CLIP, and TNM systems within this population showed that the CUPI was more sensitive and predictive of survival, showing significant discrimination throughout the follow-up period [69]. The CUPI was among the staging systems most predictive of survival in a North American patient cohort with advanced HCC [64].

Japanese Integrated Staging System

The Japanese Integrated Staging System (JIS) system combines the Child–Pugh score with the Liver Cancer Study Group of Japan (LCSGJ) TNM classification which is determined by how many of the following criteria are present: solitary tumor, <2 cm in diameter, no vascular invasion (stage I = all three present; stage II = two present; stage III = one present; stage IV = none present). Each category within the Child–Pugh and LCSGJ TNM systems is given a numerical value, and the sum of these generates the JIS score which ranges from 0 to 5. The JIS system has been validated and compared to the CLIP was found to provide superior stratification and prognostication among Japanese patients [70].

There is no single staging system that has been uniformly adopted for the global management and prognostication of HCC. Although the BCLC algorithm has been endorsed by the AASLD and EASL as the reference tool for guiding clinical practice and framing clinical trial design, it has not been validated in nonwestern populations that account for a significant proportion of the global HCC burden. Efforts to improve the prognostic utility of the BCLC and other staging systems by incorporating emerging molecular data remain a work in progress.

Therapy

Assessing Patient Appropriateness for Therapy

The management of HCC must consider two equally important and often competing factors: the cancer and the underlying cirrhosis. Hepatic functional reserve is assessed using the Child–Pugh classification system and Model for End Stage Liver Disease (MELD) score.

The Child–Pugh classification measures cirrhosis severity using a composite of three laboratory and two clinical variables. Each variable is assigned a numerical value and the sum of these is used to assign patients to one of three groups: A/well-compensated, B/functional compromise and C/decompensated [71] (see Table 7.3). A strong correlation between Child–Pugh score and survival in cirrhotics has been demonstrated; 2-year survival is approximately 90%, 50%, and 35% for patients in the A, B, and C groups, respectively [72].

The MELD score is calculated using a natural logarithmic equation incorporating international normalized ratio (INR), serum creatinine, and bilirubin [73]. It is primarily used for prioritizing patients on the transplant waiting list; higher scores indicate a higher risk of 3-month mortality.

$$\text{MELD} = 3.8\left[\text{Ln serum bilirubin}(\text{mg/dL})\right] + 11.2(\text{Ln INR}) + 9.6\left[\text{Ln serum creatinine}(\text{mg/dL})\right] + 6.4.$$

Although objective by virtue of its reliance on laboratory values, the MELD score needs to be interpreted within the clinical context since other factors that could legitimately impact transplant priority may not be reflected by serum markers. Patients with HCC, cholestatic and polycystic liver diseases, cystic fibrosis, and metabolic disorders are granted exception scores that allow them to receive higher priority beyond their native MELD scores [74, 75].

Transplant

Orthotopic liver transplantation (OLT) is the only potentially curative option for HCC, treating both the malignancy and underlying cirrhosis. Patients are selected for OLT based on liver function and anatomical parameters. The most commonly used tool for determining patient eligibility based on disease extent is the Milan criteria: solitary tumor ≤5 cm *or* up to three tumors ≤3 cm without portal invasion, nodal or distant metastases [76]. Adherence to these criteria has been shown to produce post-OLT 10-year survival rates exceeding 70% [77]. The Milan criteria have been adopted by the United Network for Organ Sharing for liver allocation.

Expanded criteria have been explored in an effort to increase patient eligibility. The University of California San Francisco criteria (solitary tumor ≤6.5 cm *or* up to three tumors with a maximum diameter of ≤4.5 cm, and a summed total tumor diameter ≤8 cm) and "Up to Seven" rule (meet Milan criteria and sum of largest tumor plus tumor number equals 7) have reported outcomes comparable to the Milan criteria which remains the "gold standard" [78, 79].

"Bridging" therapies such as locoregional ablative measures or resection can help to overcome anatomical and waiting time barriers to OLT via tumor downstaging and/or temporization without compromising outcomes [80, 81]. Tumor resection in individuals with well-compensated cirrhosis may permit the more selective use of OLT; those with high-risk histopathologic features for recurrence (i.e., poor differentiation, vascular invasion, nonencapsulation) may undergo a subsequent pre-emptive transplant while those with low-risk features may reserve OLT as a salvage procedure [80, 81], thus preserving the donor pool for other potential candidates.

Living donor transplants are considered an acceptable alternative to deceased donor organs and have been shown to produce comparable long-term survival outcomes [80]. Donor safety is a key consideration; perioperative morbidity and mortality are reportedly 30–40% and 0.15–0.5%, respectively [82]. Although OLT is potentially curative, patients are committed to lifelong immunosuppression and its attendant risks including secondary malignancies and recurrences which occur in 10–20% of patients [80]. Studies suggest that the commonly used calcineurin inhibitors (e.g., tacrolimus, cyclosporine) may be tumorigenic. mTOR-based immunosuppressive regimens may be associated with fewer recurrences and better outcomes [83].

Table 7.3 Child–Pugh score.

Points	1	2	3
Albumin	>3.5 g/dL	2.8-3.5 g/dL	<2.8 g/dL
Total bilirubin	<2.0 mg/dL	2.0–3.0 mg/dL	>3.0 mg/dL
INR	<1.7	1.7–2.3	>2.3
Clinical ascites	None	Mild	Moderate
Encephalopathy	None	Grade 1–2	Grade 3–4

Source: adapted from Pugh *et al.* [71].
Child–Pugh A, 5–6; Child–Pugh B, 7–9; Child–Pugh C ≥10.

Resection

Surgery is the cornerstone of care for patients with limited volume HCC and adequate hepatic functional reserve. With modern surgical techniques, 5-year survival ranges from 30–50% and perioperative mortality is 3–5% in cirrhotic patients undergoing hepatectomy [84]. In patients who fall within Milan criteria, 5-year survival outcomes are comparable to those achieved by OLT, approaching 50–70% in some series [85, 86].

In selecting candidates for resection, both tumor and hepatic functional parameters are considered. The presence of portal hypertension (i.e., portal venous gradient >10 mmHg, varices or splenomegaly with platelets <100,000/mm^3, varices) is a major predictor of postoperative hepatic decompensation, and is compounded by the presence of hyperbilirubinemia [86]. Recurrence rates are high following resection with up to 70% of patients relapsing by 5 years [86]. A distinction is made between "early" and "late" recurrences occurring ≤2 years or >2 years after surgery, respectively. While the former entity typically arises from pre-existing intrahepatic micrometastases, the latter entity represents *de novo* tumors. This hypothesis is supported by gene-expression profiling data from peritumoral liver parenchyma which was shown to be significantly predictive of HCC recurrences >2 years after surgery, but not earlier recurrences [87]. Major clinicopathologic predictors of recurrence include the presence of vascular invasion, tumor multinodularity, and poor differentiation [86]. Where appropriate, recurrent HCC should be aggressively treated using a multimodality approach of repeated resection and/or nonsurgical ablative therapies because long-term survival can still be achieved. Median postrecurrence survival times measured in years have been reported [88, 89].

Adjuvant Therapy For Patients Undergoing OLT or Resection

Adjuvant transarterial I131-labelled lipiodol and peretinoin – an oral vitamin A derivative – were both shown to decrease the risk of recurrence and prolong survival in randomized studies, but these effects were not durable or borne out in subsequent studies [90–93]. In the post-OLT setting, the I131-labelled monoclonal antibody against the HCC-specific molecule HAb18G/CD147 has shown promise as an adjuvant therapy in a randomized prospective study, though long-term follow-up results are needed [80, 94].

Adjuvant sorafenib was not shown to be effective in the STORM trial which randomized 1114 patients to placebo or sorafenib at standard doses following curative resection or local ablation [95]. Recurrence-free survival was virtually identical in both the sorafenib and placebo arms (33.3 months vs 33.7 months, HR 0.94, $P = 0.26$). The higher than anticipated proportion of patients on sorafenib who required dose modifications (~90%) and who had discontinued therapy at one year (~50%) may have contributed to the negative results. Sorafenib is currently being evaluated post-OLT in both phase I and II studies (www.clinicaltrials.gov, NCT00844168, NCT01624285). Sorafenib is discussed further later in the chapter.

Taken together, in the absence of data supporting an effective adjuvant strategy, the current standard of care following OLT or resection is expectant management or participation in a clinical trial.

Locoregional Ablative Therapies

A variety of locoregional ablative therapies have been shown to be effective alternatives to resection for patients are medically unfit for surgery and/or have technically unresectable disease.

Percutaneous Ethanol Ablation

Percutaneous ethanol ablation (PEI) with 95% ethanol causes cell death via ischemic and cytotoxic injury. Favored for its low-cost, accessibility, and safety, PEI is highly effective (complete tumor ablation achieved in 98% of cases) and potentially curative with 5, 10, and even 20-year survival rates of 49%, 18%, and 7%, respectively. The best outcomes are achieved in Child–Pugh A or B patients who have one to three tumors with a maximum diameter of ≤3 cm. Although durable local control can be achieved, distant recurrences occur in >50% by 5 years [96].

Radiofrequency Ablation

Radiofrequency ablation (RFA) utilizes microwaves to generate thermal energy, resulting in coagulative necrosis. Complete tumor responses are achievable in >90% of cases with a single session of RFA, whereas multiple PEI sessions may be needed to achieve similar results [100]. RFA has replaced PEI as the preferred treatment modality for early stage HCCs at many centers, having been shown to produce superior tumor control and survival [97–99].

The question of whether the results achieved with RFA can rival those of surgery is an active subject of debate [100]. Randomized controlled trials comparing RFA versus resection in patients with limited volume disease (i.e., one to two nodules, maximum diameter <4–5 cm) have arrived at different conclusions [101–103]. RFA efficacy is dependent on tumor size, number, and location. Tumors >4–5 cm are less likely to be adequately contained with the ablation field, and perivascular lesions may be undertreated as a result of thermal dilution by the "heat sink" effect. Superficial tumors may also be suboptimally treated because they can be difficult to visualize, their depth may not be adequately assessed, and there is a risk of damaging adjacent structures. Some of these limitations may be overcome by performing an open as opposed to percutaneous RFA [101]. At the present time, EASL/AASLD guidelines still list surgery as the reference treatment strategy for early stage HCC [28, 30].

Microwave Ablation

Microwave ablation uses electromagnetic energy to cause thermal ablation. Microwave ablation generates larger heat zones, faster ablation times, and higher intratumoral temperatures which may be able to overcome the heat sink effect associated with perivascular tumors [104, 105]. Retrospective data suggest that microwave ablation and RFA are similarly efficacious in patients with limited disease [106].

Transarterial Embolic Therapies

Transarterial tumor embolization with chemotherapy-loaded or radiolabelled particles capitalizes on the differences in blood supply to hepatic tumors and normal parenchyma. Because hepatic tumors are primarily supplied by the hepatic artery whereas normal liver is 75% perfused by portal venous circulation, selective tumor targeting can be achieved with relative sparing of the surrounding parenchyma.

Transarterial Chemoembolization

Conventional transarterial chemoembolization (cTACE) involves the delivery of a chemotherapy–lipiodol (a viscous poppy-seed oil derivative) emulsion followed by embolic particles into the tumor-feeding artery, causing cell death by ischemic and cytotoxic injury. Treatments are delivered every 2–4 months as indicated by tumor response and volume [106]. Doxorubicin, cisplatin, and mitomycin-C are the most commonly employed therapeutic agents, and no particular drug alone or combination has been shown to be superior to the others [107]. cTACE was adopted for the treatment of BCLC stage B HCC on the basis of two randomized, placebo-controlled trials which demonstrated a survival benefit in treatment-naïve patients with good hepatic function, no extrahepatic metastases, or main portal vein involvement [28, 30, 108, 109]. Objective responses are observed in 15–55% of patients, resulting in delayed time to tumor progression and vascular invasion [28, 109]. Recent cohort studies have reported median survival times exceeding 3 years in highly selected patients with Child–Pugh A disease and one to three tumors each ≤3 cm in diameter [110, 111] – a population that would also be eligible for resection. The presence of more extensive disease and advanced liver dysfunction has been shown to impact outcomes negatively. The main side effects associated with cTACE include postembolization syndrome characterized by pain, nausea, vomiting, fever, and hypertension as well as the potential for liver abscesses, biliary or vascular injury, and tumor rupture in <1% of patients [106].

Drug-Eluting Bead TACE

TACE using chemotherapy loaded microspheres – also known as drug-eluting bead (DEB)-TACE – offers several advantages over cTACE including: (i) more precise and accurate drug loading and delivery; (ii) controlled and sustained drug release; and (iii) reduced systemic bioavailability despite high drug doses resulting in decreased systemic toxicities [106, 112]. Doxorubicin-based DEB-TACE and cTACE were compared in the randomized phase II PRECISION V trial [113]. Patients with Child–Pugh C cirrhosis, tumor volume >50%, vascular invasion and/or extrahepatic metastases were excluded. Although DEB-TACE was not superior to cTACE with respect to the primary endpoint of tumor response at 6 months, objective response and disease control rates were higher, and safety and tolerability were significantly improved on the DEB-TACE arm. Disease control rates were significantly better in Child–Pugh B patients with bulkier disease treated with DEB-TACE instead of cTACE [113]. In a recent series which included BCLC A/B patients with an excellent performance status and Child–Pugh ≤ B7 cirrhosis, median survival was 48.5 months and median time to untreatable disease progression was nearly 2 years with DEB-TACE [114]. Although the question of whether survival with DEB-TACE is superior to cTACE has yet to be answered prospectively, a retrospective study of 71 patients reported a significantly longer median survival time in patients treated with DEB-TACE compared to cTACE (610 days and 284 days, $P = 0.03$) [115].

Bland Transarterial Embolization

Whether chemotherapy is necessary to achieve optimal efficacy and durability of outcomes with TACE is unclear. In a retrospective review which included patients with portal vein occlusion and extrahepatic disease treated with transarterial embolization (TAE), median and 3-year survival were 21 months and 33%, respectively. When patients with these characteristics were excluded from the analysis, median and 3-year survival were 40 months and 51%, respectively, similar to those achieved with cTACE [116]. A randomized study reported better local control, time to progression and recurrence-free survival with DEB-TACE compared to TAE, but 1-year survival was similar between the arms [117]. Another randomized study reported no differences between DEB-TACE and TAE with respect to objective response rate, to progression, progression-free and overall survival, safety, and tolerability [118].

Transarterial Radioembolization

Transarterial radioembolization (TARE) replaces chemotherapy-loaded beads with yttrium-90 labelled microparticles, selectively delivering radiation at significantly higher doses than can be attained with external beam radiation (i.e., 222–390 Gy vs 30–50 Gy) [119]. Unlike cTACE and DEB-TACE, TARE can be performed on an outpatient basis and complete ablation can be achieved in a single session. Since vessel occlusion is not necessary for therapeutic efficacy, TARE may be considered for patients with portal vein occlusion who would otherwise be excluded from receiving TACE due to concerns about inducing ischemic hepatitis and hepatic failure [106, 120]. Response rates range from 30 to 50% with TARE, and median survival is approximately 17 months and 10 months in patients with BCLC stage B and C disease, respectively [106]. Although there are no head to head comparisons, several retrospective reviews report favorable outcomes with TARE compared to cTACE/DEB-TACE [106]. The most common side effects associated with TARE include fatigue, ulcer formation due to nontarget microsphere deposition, liver fibrosis, cholecystitis, and radiation pneumonitis especially if pulmonary shunting is present [106, 120].

Taken together, the strongest data demonstrating the efficacy and survival benefit of transarterial embolic therapies come from studies conducted in highly selected patient populations with excellent performance status and liver function, without portal vein involvement or extrahepatic disease. The introduction of newer techniques such as superselective TACE and TARE has made it feasible to treat patients with portal vein involvement, but safety remains a concern.

External Beam Radiation

Although TARE can overcome the sensitivity of the hepatic parenchyma that has limited the ability to deliver radiation in tumoricidal doses, it is an invasive procedure that may not be appropriate for some patients. Advances in external beam radiation (EBRT) techniques demonstrate feasibility for treating HCC. Retrospective series and uncontrolled studies suggest that EBRT is effective in palliating pain from metastases, can induce meaningful responses in 40–90% of patients including those with PVT, and may be potentially curative in some patients [121, 122]. Prospective studies are examining the role of EBRT as an adjunct to other locoregional as well as systemic therapies.

Systemic Therapy

Until recent years, there were no effective systemic therapies for HCC not amenable to surgery or nonsurgical locoregional therapies and patients were relegated to best supportive care. "Traditional" cytotoxic as well as endocrine therapies have been extensively explored and are generally considered ineffective in HCC [123–126]. The limited activity of chemotherapy in HCC may be due in part to expression levels of drug-resistance genes [127] as well as the underlying cirrhosis which limits chemotolerance.

Sorafenib

Advances in our understanding of cancer molecular biology and the advent of "targeted" agents which intercept the aberrations that generate and sustain malignant behavior have revolutionized the practice of oncology, and have provided options for malignancies such as HCC that were once considered untreatable. The small molecule multikinase inhibitor – sorafenib – is the prototype targeted agent for HCC, and still remains the only systemic agent known to be effective for this disease.

Sorafenib inhibits Raf, Flt-3, c-Kit, RET, VEGFR and PDGFR-associated kinases though its primary mechanism of action is believed to be antiangiogenic [128]. Following promising results in a single arm phase II trial [129], the multicenter phase III SHARP and Asia–Pacific trials showed that sorafenib significantly improved time to progression and overall survival in advanced HCC patients compared to placebo [130, 131], ultimately leading to its approval for HCC by the FDA. Notably, although the hazard ratios for survival were virtually identical in both trials (0.69 and 0.68), the median survival times with sorafenib were 10.7 months and 6.5 months in the SHARP and Asia–Pacific trials, respectively [130, 131]. The disparity in survival may be attributable to differences in liver disease etiology; in the SHARP study, approximately 30% and 20% of patients had HCV and HBV as their underlying risk factor whereas 70% of patients on the Asia–Pacific trial had HBV [130, 131]. A pattern of improved outcomes with sorafenib in HCV compared to HBV patients has been reported in several retrospective series, and in a subgroup analysis from a phase III trial of sorafenib versus sunitinib [132–134]. A potential explanation for the apparent differences in sensitivity based on viral etiology may relate to the activation of Raf-1 – a target of sorafenib – by HCV core protein, thus sensitizing infected cells [135].

The most common grade 3–4 side effects associated with sorafenib are hypertension, fatigue, abdominal pain, diarrhea, hand–foot skin reaction, and liver dysfunction which occur in 2–11% of patients [130, 131]. It should be noted that in both trials, >95% of patients had Child–Pugh A disease. Since sorafenib is hepatically metabolized, tolerance in individuals with liver dysfunction is a concern, with shorter survival times and a higher risk of hepatic decompensation in Child–Pugh B compared to A patients [136]. Similar findings were reported in the phase IV GIDEON study [137]. A phase I study of sorafenib in patients with renal and hepatic dysfunction has shown serum total bilirubin and albumin levels to be key variables in determining sorafenib tolerance; dose reductions are needed in those with a bilirubin >1.5 × the upper limit of normal and/or albumin <2.5 mg/dL [138].

Sorafenib Combinations

The combination of sorafenib and doxorubicin showed promising activity in a randomized phase II study [139]. Patients on the combination arm experienced a significant improvement in median time to progression (6.4 months vs 2.8 months, $P = 0.02$), and median survival compared to doxorubicin alone (13.7 months vs 6.5 months, $P = 0.006$). Sorafenib +/− doxorubicin is currently being assessed in a multicenter phase III trial (www.clinicaltrials.gov, NCT01272557).

Combined modality therapy with cTACE or DEB-TACE and sorafenib has been evaluated in several studies. TACE-induced hypoxia and ischemia generate a rise in VEGF that peaks 24 h postprocedure before progressively declining over subsequent days [140]. Post-TACE VEGF peaks have been associated with the development of distant metastases [141]. It was hypothesized that sorafenib might abrogate the rise in VEGF, translating into delayed time to progression and longer survival. Although feasible and safe [142], the combination of TACE and sorafenib has not been shown to improve outcomes in two randomized studies conducted in patients with BCLC stage B disease [143, 144]. TACE +/− sorafenib continues to be evaluated in a phase III cooperative group trial that will include patients with branch/lobar but not main portal vein involvement (www.clinicaltrials.gov, NCT01004978).

Clinical trials combining sorafenib with newer locoregional modalities such as TARE (www.clinicaltrials.gov, NCT01135056, NCT01126645) and external beam radiation techniques (www.clinicaltrials.gov, NCT01328223, NCT01618253, NCT01141478, NCT01319942) are currently underway at several centers worldwide.

Second-Line Therapy

In the phase III RESORCE trial, regorafenib, a multikinase inhibitor of KIT, RET, PDGFR, RAF kinases, VEGFR1-3 and TIE-2, increased overall survival compared to placebo (10.6 months vs 7.8 months, HR 0.62, $P < 0.001$) in patients who had progressed on sorafenib [145]. Progression-free survival, as well as objective response and disease control rates were also improved on regorafenib. Although grade ≥3 adverse events such as hand–foot skin reaction, fatigue, diarrhea, and hypertension were more frequent with regorafenib, patient-reported quality of life was similar to that reported with placebo [146].

Other Agents

Anti-Epidermal Growth Factor Receptor

Anti-epidermal growth factor receptor (EGFR) small molecule tyrosine kinase inhibitors (TKIs) and monoclonal antibodies (mAbs) including gefitnib, erlotinib, lapatinib, and cetuximab have each been studied in single arm phase II trials [147–153]. While erlotinib appeared to have a disease stabilizing effect in 40–50% of patients [147, 148], as a group these agents do not appear to have clinically relevant activity. The phase III SEARCH study comparing sorafenib plus erlotinib versus sorafenib did not demonstrate any statistically significant differences in survival or time to progression [154]. Predictive biomarkers characterized in colorectal and lung malignancies such as activating KRAS and EGFR mutations have not been robustly explored in HCC.

Insulin-Like Growth Factor-1 Receptor

The insulin-like growth factor-1 receptor mAb cixutumumab was inactive in HCC and caused grade 3/4 hyperglycemia in 46% of patients in a phase II study [155]. Results from phase I and II studies of other anti-insulin-like growth factor-1 receptor antibodies are pending (www.clinicaltrials.gov, NCT00956436, NCT01334710).

c-Met and Hepatocyte Growth Factor

Anti c-Met agents have shown promising activity in sorafenib-refractory HCC. A randomized phase II study of the c-Met TKI tivantinib reported a statistically significant improvement in median time to progression over placebo in sorafenib-refractory HCC, particularly in patients with high as opposed to low tumor c-Met expression by immunohistochemistry [156]. A randomized phase II discontinuation study of the dual c-Met/VEGFR-2 antibody cabozantinib reported a tumor regression rate and median progression-free and overall survival times of 78%, 4.4 months and 15.1 months, respectively [157].

MAP Kinase Pathway

Data on the activity of agents targeting Ras, Raf, and Mek in HCC are sparse and have not shown any compelling signals of activity [158]. A phase II study of selumetinib, a Mek 1/2 inhibitor, was terminated for inefficacy [159] but a phase I/II combination study with sorafenib is ongoing (www.clinicaltrials.gov, NCT01029418).

PI3K/Akt/mTOR Pathway

mTOR inhibitors have garnered interest in HCC as immunosuppressants post-OLT and for the treatment of established HCC. Several retrospective series indicate that mTOR-based immunosuppressive agents are associated with lower recurrence rates and better survival post-OLT [82]. However, a recent phase III trial of second-line everolimus failed to improve outcomes over placebo in sorafenib-refractory HCC [160].

Anti-Angiogenic Agents

Agents targeting VEGF or its receptor include bevacizumab, ramucirumab, and cediranib. Bevacizumab showed promising single agent activity, but 11% of patients had a grade ≥3 hemorrhagic event including one fatal variceal bleed [161]. A phase II study of first-line bevacizumab and erlotinib reported an objective response rate of 24% and median progression-free and overall survival were 7.2 months and 13.7 months, respectively [162]. A phase III trial of bevacizumab/erlotinib versus sorafenib has been launched (www.clinicaltrials.gov, NCT00881751).

Ramucirumab, an anti-VEGFR2 mAb, was evaluated in second-line post-sorafenib patients in the phase III REACH study [163]. In the overall study population, ramucirumab did not significantly improve overall survival compared to placebo (9.2 months vs 7.6 months, HR 0.87, $P=0.14$). However, among patients with a baseline AFP >400 ng/mL, survival was significantly improved with ramucirumab versus placebo (7.8 months vs 4.2 months, HR 0.67, $P=0.006$). The relationship between baseline elevated AFP and response to ramucirumab in second-line post-sorafenib progression is currently being studied in the ongoing phase III REACH-2 study (www.clinicaltrials.gov, NCT02435433).

The bFGF inhibitor brivanib was evaluated in two phase III studies as first-line therapy versus sorafenib and in sorafenib-refractory HCC – both were negative [164, 165]. Linifanib is a dual VEGFR/PDGFR TKI that was evaluated against sorafenib in a phase III trial. Although survival outcomes were comparable, the predefined superiority and noninferiority thresholds for linifanib were not met [166].

Sunitinib is a multikinase inhibitor with a spectrum similar to sorafenib. Based on several phase II trials showing modest activity [167–169], a phase III Asian trial of sunitinib versus sorafenib was launched. Compared to sorafenib, sunitinib was more toxic and survival outcomes were inferior [170].

Immunotherapy

The immune checkpoint inhibitor, nivolumab, has shown promising activity in a phase I/II study conducted in patients with advanced HCC, approximately 70% of whom had previously received sorafenib [171]. Objective responses were observed in 19% of patients including two complete responses, and occurred in both hepatitis-infected and uninfected patients. An interim analysis of the study reported a median response duration of nearly 2 years, median survival was 15 months, and 48% of patients were still alive at 18 months [172]. Antiviral responses in hepatitis C infected patients were also reported. A phase III trial of first-line nivolumab versus sorafenib in advanced HCC is currently recruiting (www.clinicaltrials.gov, NCT02576509).

Therapeutic Response Evaluation in HCC

The RECIST (Response Evaluation Criteria in Solid Tumors) guidelines are the most commonly used metric for assessing the effects of antineoplastic therapy on malignant diseases. RECIST guidelines use changes in unidimensional measurements to determine whether patients are responding to or progressing on therapy [173].

Conventional RECIST guidelines are considered inadequate for capturing responses to therapies with antiangiogenic properties (i.e., sorafenib, transarterial therapies) in HCC. In the phase II and III studies of sorafenib, only 2–3% of patients had partial responses by RECIST – seemingly incongruous with the reported survival benefit [129–131]. Modified response assessment tools evaluate changes in tumor vascularity and/or necrosis which may be more sensitive markers of therapeutic activity. In the initial phase II study of sorafenib, the ratio of central necrosis to tumor volume was associated with clinical benefit [129, 174]. Modified RECIST guidelines, endorsed by EASL and the AASLD, measure changes in the size of arterially enhancing (i.e., viable) areas within a tumor instead of the entire tumor [175]. These novel techniques require validation.

Follow-Up and Survivorship

Given the high propensity for HCC to return post-treatment and the rarity of true "cures" even after radical therapies like OLT and surgery, all patients need to be closely monitored for recurrences. The NCCN guidelines recommend serial imaging and AFP levels every 3–6 months during the first 2 years following surgery or transplant, then every 6–12 months thereafter [31].

Conclusion

HCC is a heterogeneous and complex disease entity that, in its advanced stages, remains recalcitrant to the ongoing endeavor to develop effective therapies beyond sorafenib. Therapies tailored to specific biomarker-enriched populations may hold the best promise for the next breakthrough. In addition to continued research efforts, prevention and early detection are key measures for combating HCC.

References

1 Torre LA, Bray F, Siegel RL, *et al.* Global cancer statistics, 2012. *Ca Cancer J Clin* 2015;65(2):87–108.
2 Howlader N, Noone AM, Krapcho M, *et al.* (eds). SEER Cancer Statistics Review, 1975–2013, National Cancer Institute. Bethesda, MD, http://seer.cancer.gov/csr/1975_2013/, based on November 2015 SEER data submission, posted to the SEER web site, April 2016.
3 Siegel RL, Miller KD, Jemal A. Cancer statistics, 2017. *CA Cancer J Clin* 2017;67(1):7–30.
4 Plummer M, de Martel C, Vignat J, *et al.* Global burden of cancers attributable to infections in 2012: a synthetic analysis. *Lancet Global Health* 2016;4(9):e609–16.
5 Pollicino T, Saitta C, Raimondo G. Hepatocellular carcinoma: the point of view of the hepatitis B virus. *Carcinogenesis* 2011;32(8):1122–32.
6 Chen CJ, Yang HI, Su J. Risk of hepatocellular carcinoma across a biological gradient of serum hepatitis B virus DNA level. *JAMA* 2006;295(1):65–73.
7 Yamashita T, Honda M, Kaneko S. Molecular mechanisms of hepatocarcinogenesis in chronic hepatitis C virus infection. *J Gastroenterol Hepatol* 2011;26(6):960–4.
8 Shen YC, Hsu C, Cheng CC, *et al.* A critical evaluation of the preventive effect of antiviral therapy on the development of hepatocellular carcinoma in patients with chronic hepatitis C or B: a novel approach by using meta-regression. *Oncology* 2012;82(5):275–89.
9 Voigt MD. Alcohol in hepatocellular carcinoma. *Clin Liver Dis* 2005;9(1):151–69.
10 Hassan MM, Hwang LY, Hatten CJ, *et al.* Risk factors for hepatocellular carcinoma: synergism of alcohol with viral hepatitis and diabetes mellitus. *Hepatology* 2002;36(5):1206–13.
11 Shih WL, Chang HC, Liaw YF, *et al.* Influences of tobacco and alcohol use on hepatocellular carcinoma survival. *Int J Cancer* 2012;131(11):2612–21.
12 Starley BQ, Calcagno CJ, Harrison SA. Nonalcoholic fatty liver disease and hepatocellular carcinoma: a weighty connection. *Hepatology* 2010;51(5):1820–32.
13 Siegel AB, Zhu AX. Metabolic syndrome and hepatocellular carcinoma: two growing epidemics with a potential link. *Cancer* 2009:115:5651–61.
14 Baffy G, Brunt EM, Caldwell SH. Hepatocellular carcinoma in non-alcoholic fatty liver disease: an emerging menace. *J Hepatol* 2012;56(6):1384–91.
15 Kowdley KV. Iron, hemochromatosis, and hepatocellular carcinoma. *Gastroenterology* 2004;127(5 Suppl 1):S79–86.
16 Wu HC, Santella R. The role of aflatoxins in hepatocellular carcinoma. *Hepat Mon* 2012;12(10 HCC):e723.
17 Liu Y, Wu F. Global burden of aflatoxin-induced hepatocellular carcinoma: a risk assessment. *Environ Health Perspect* 2010;118(6):818–24.
18 Tsai JF, Jeng JE, Chuang LY, *et al.* Habitual betel quid chewing and risk for hepatocellular carcinoma complicating cirrhosis. *Medicine (Baltimore)* 2004;83(3):176–87.
19 Chung Y-T, Chan C-L, Wu C-C, *et al.* Safrole-DNA adduct in hepatocellular carcinoma associated with betel quid chewing. *Toxicol Lett* 2008;183:21–7.
20 Topic A, Ljujic Am, Radojkovic D. Alpha-1-antitrypsin in pathogenesis of hepatocellular carcinoma. *Hepat Mon* 2012;12(10 HCC):e7042.
21 Carrell RW, Lomas DA. Alpha-1-antitrypsin deficiency – a model for conformational diseases. *N Engl J Med* 2002;346(1):45–53.
22 Zhou H, Fischer HP. Liver carcinoma in PiZ alpha-1-antitrypsin deficiency. *Am J Surg Pathol* 1998;22(6):742–8.
23 Siegel AB, Conner K, Wang S, *et al.* Smoking and hepatocellular carcinoma mortality. *Exp Ther Med* 2012;3(1):124–8.
24 Ueno Y, Nagata S, Tsutsumi T, *et al.* Detection of microcystins, a blue-green algal hepatotoxin, in drinking water sampled in Haimen and Fusui, endemic areas of primary liver cancer in China, by highly sensitive immunoassay. *Carcinogenesis* 1996;17:1317–21.
25 Llovet JM, Zucman-Rossi J, Pikarsky E, *et al.* Hepatocellular carcinoma. *Nat Rev Dis Primers* 2016;2:16018.
26 Chang MH, You SL, Chen CJ, *et al.* Decreased incidence of hepatocellular carcinoma in hepatitis B vaccines: a 20 year follow-up study. *J Natl Cancer Inst* 2009;101:1348–55.
27 Zhang BH, Yang BH, Tang ZY. Randomized controlled trial of screening for hepatocellular carcinoma. *J Cancer Res Clin Oncol* 2004;130(7):417–22.
28 European Association for the Study of the Liver, European Organization for Research and Treatment of Cancer. EASL-EORTC clinical practice guidelines: management of hepatocellular carcinoma. *J Hepatol* 2012;56(4):908–43.
29 Della Corte C, Colombo M. Surveillance for hepatocellular carcinoma. *Semin Oncol* 2012;39(4):384–98.
30 Bruix J, Sherman M. Management of hepatocellular carcinoma: an update. *Hepatology* 2011;53(3):1020–2.
31 Hepatobiliary Cancers Version 1.2013. NCCN Guidelines. National Comprehensive Cancer Network. 21 May 2013. Accessed 22 May 2013.
32 Kew MC, Macerollo P. Effect of age on the etiologic role of the hepatitis B virus in hepatocellular carcinoma in blacks. *Gastroenterology* 1988;94(2):439–42.
33 Ayyappan AP, Jhaveri KS. CT and MRI of hepatocellular carcinoma: an update. *Expert Rev Anticancer Ther* 2010;10(4):507–19.
34 Lim JH, Choi D, Kim SH. Detection of hepatocellular carcinoma: value of adding delayed phase imaging to dual-phase helical CT. *Am J Roentgenol* 2002;179:67–73.
35 Leoni S, Piscaglia F, Golfieri R, *et al.* The impact of vascular and nonvascular findings on the invasive diagnosis of small hepatocellular carcinoma based on the EASL and AASLD criteria. *Am J Gastroenterol* 2010;105(3):599–609.
36 Bolondi L, Gaiani S, Celli N, *et al.* Characterization of small nodules in cirrhosis by assessment of vascularity: the problem of hypovascular hepatocellular carcinoma. *Hepatology* 2005;42(1):27–34.
37 Sanada Y, Shiozaki S, Aoki H, *et al.* A clinical study of 11 cases of combined hepatocellular-cholangiocarcinoma assessment of enhancement patterns on dynamic computed tomography before resection. *Hepatol Res* 2005;32:185–95.

38 Rimola J, Forner A, Reig M, *et al.* Cholangiocarcinoma in cirrhosis; absence of contrast washout in delayed phases by magnetic resonance imaging avoids misdiagnosis of hepatocellular carcinoma. *Hepatology* 2009;50:791–8.

39 Silva MA, Hegab B, Hyde C, *et al.* Needle track seeding following biopsy of liver lesions in the diagnosis of hepatocellular cancer: a systematic review and meta-analysis. *Gut* 2008;57:1592–6.

40 El Makarem MA. An overview of biomarkers for the diagnosis of hepatocellular carcinoma. *Hepat Mon* 2012;12(10 HCC):e6122.

41 Tyson GL, Duan Z, Kramer JR, *et al.* Level of alpha-fetoprotein predicts mortality among patients with hepatitis C-related hepatocellular carcinoma. *Clin Gastroenterol Hepatol* 2011;9(11):989–94.

42 Yau T, Yao TJ, Chan P, *et al.* The significance of early alpha-fetoprotein level changes in predicting clinical and survival benefits in advanced hepatocellular carcinoma patients receiving sorafenib. *Oncologist* 2011;16(9):1270–9.

43 Sterling RK, Jeffers L, Gordon F, *et al.* Clinical utility of AFP-L3% measurement in North American patients with HCV-related cirrhosis. *Am J Gastroenterol* 2007;102(10):2196–205.

44 Liebman HA, Furie BC, Tong MJ, *et al.* Des-gamma-carboxy (abnormal) prothrombin as a serum marker of primary hepatocellular carcinoma. *N Engl J Med* 1984;310(22):1427–31.

45 Suzuki M, Shiraha H, Fujikawa T, *et al.* Des–gamma-carboxyprothrombin is a potential autologous growth factor for hepatocellular carcinoma. *J Biol Chem* 2005;280(8):6409–15.

46 Fujikawa T, Shiraha H, Ueda N, *et al.* Des-gamma-carboxyl prothrombin-promoted vascular endoethelial cell proliferation and migration. *J Biol Chem* 2007;282(12):8741–8.

47 Goodman ZD. Neoplasms of the liver. *Mod Pathol* 2007;20 Suppl 1:S49–60.

48 Paradis V. Histopathology of hepatocellular carcinoma. *Recent Results Cancer Res* 2013;190:21–32.

49 Okuda K, Peters RL, Simson IW. Gross anatomic features of hepatocellular carcinoma from three disparate geographic areas: proposal of new classification. *Cancer* 1983;54:2165–73.

50 Tremosini S, Forner A, Boix L, *et al.* Prospective validation of an immunohistochemical panel (glypican 3, heat shock protein 70 and glutamine synthetase) in liver biopsies for diagnosis of very early hepatocellular carcinoma. *Gut* 2012;61(10):1481–7.

51 Wolber RA, Greene CA, Dupuis BA. Polyclonal carcinoembryonic antigen staining in the cytologic differential diagnosis of primary and metastatic hepatic malignancies. *Acta Cytol* 1991;35(2):215–20.

52 Coston WM, Leora S, Lau SK, *et al.* Distinction of hepatocellular carcinoma from benign hepatic mimickers using glypican-3 and CD34 immunohistochemistry. *Am J Surg Pathol* 2008;32(3):433–44.

53 Wurmbach E, Chen YB, Khitrov G, *et al.* Genome-wide molecular profiles of HCV-induced dysplasia and hepatocellular carcinoma. *Hepatology* 2007;45(4):938–47.

54 Minguez B, Hoshida Y, Villanueva A, *et al.* Gene-expression signature of vascular invasion in hepatocellular carcinoma. *J Hepatol* 2011;55(6):1325–31.

55 Hoshida Y, Nijman SMB, Kobayashi M, *et al.* Integrative transcriptome analysis reveals common molecular subclasses of human hepatocellular carcinoma. *Cancer Res* 2009;69(18):7385–92.

56 Toffanin S, Hoshida Y, Lachenmayer A, *et al.* MicroRNA-based classification of hepatocellular carcinoma and oncogenic role of miR-517a. *Gastroenterology* 2011;140(5):1618–28.

57 Abou-Alfa GK, Pawlik TM, Shindoh J, Vauthey JN. *Liver. In: MB Amin, SB Edge, FL Greene, et al. (eds) AJCC Cancer Staging Manual, Eighth Edition.* New York: Springer Nature, 2017.

58 Okuda K, Ohtsuki T, Obata H, *et al.* Natural history of hepatocellular carcinoma and prognosis in relation to treatment. Study of 850 patients. *Cancer* 1985;56(4):918–28.

59 Kudo M, Chung H, Osaki Y. Prognostic staging system for hepatocellular carcinoma (CLIP): its value and limitations, and a proposal for a new staging system, the Japan Integrated Staging Score (JIS score). *J Gastroenterol* 2003;38(3):207–15.

60 Marrero JA, Fontana RJ, Barrat A, *et al.* Prognosis of hepatocellular carcinoma: comparison of 7 staging systems in an American cohort. *Hepatology* 2005;41(4):707–16.

61 Cillo U, Vitale A, Grigoletto F, *et al.* Prospective validation of the Barcelona Clinic Liver Cancer staging system. *J Hepatol* 2006;44(4):723–31.

62 Guglielmi A, Ruzzenente A, Pachera S, *et al.* Comparison of seven staging systems in cirrhotic patients with hepatocellular carcinoma in a cohort of patients who underwent radiofrequency ablation with complete response. *Am J Gastroenterol* 2008;103(3):597–604

63 Han KH, Kudo M, Ye SL, *et al.* Asian consensus workshop report: expert consensus guideline for the management of intermediate and advanced hepatocellular carcinoma in Asia. *Oncology* 2011;81(Suppl 1):158–64.

64 Huitzil-Melendez FD, Capanu M, O'Reilly EM, *et al.* Advanced hepatocellular carcinoma: which staging systems best predict prognosis? *J Clin Oncol* 2010;28(17):2889–95.

65 Kim SE, Lee HC, Kim KM, *et al.* Applicability of the BCLC staging system to patients with hepatocellular carcinoma in Korea: analysis at a single center with a liver transplant center. *Korean J Hepatol* 2011;17(2):113–119.

66 Kaseb AO, Morris JS, Hassan MM, *et al.* Clinical and prognostic implications of plasma insulin-like growth factor-1 and vascular endothelial growth factor in patients with hepatocellular carcinoma. *J Clin Oncol* 2011;29(29):3892–9.

67 Chevret S, Trinchet JC, Mathieu D, *et al.* A new prognostic classification for predicting survival in patients with hepatocellular carcinoma. Groupe d'Etude et de Traitement du Carcinoma Hepatocellulaire. *J Hepatol* 1999;31(1):133–41.

68 A new prognostic system for hepatocellular carcinoma: a retrospective study of 435 patients: the Cancer of the Liver Italian Program (CLIP) investigators. Hepatology 1998;28(3):751–5.

69 Leung TW, Tang AM, Zee B, *et al.* Construction of the Chinese University Prognostic Index for hepatocellular carcinoma and comparison with the TNM staging system, the Okuda staging system, and the Cancer of the Liver Italian Program staging system: a study based on 926 patients. *Cancer* 2002;94(6):1760–9.

70 Kudo M, Chung H, Haji S, *et al.* Validation of a new prognostic staging system for hepatocellular carcinoma: the JIS score compared with the CLIP score. *Hepatology* 2004;40(6):1396–405.
71 Pugh RN, Murray-Lyon IM, Dawson JL, *et al.* Transection of the oesophagus for bleeding oesophageal varices. *Br J Surg* 1973;60(8):646–9.
72 Albers I, Hartmann H, Bircher J, Creutzfeldt W. Superiority of the Child-Pugh classification to quantitative liver function tests for assessing prognosis of liver cirrhosis. *Scand J Gastroenterol* 1989;24(3):269–76.
73 Malinchoc M, Kamath PS, Gordon FD, *et al.* A model to predict poor survival in patients undergoing transjugular intrahepatic portosystemic hunts. *Hepatology* 2000;31(4):864–71.
74 Quante M, Benckert C, Thelen A, Jonas S. Experience since MELD implementation: how does the new system deliver? *Int J Hepatol* 2012;2012:264015.
75 Asrani SK, Kim WR. Model for end stage liver disease: end of the first decade. *Clin Liver Dis* 2011;15(4):685–98.
76 Mazzaferro V, Regalia E, Doci R, *et al.* Liver transplantation for the treatment of small hepatocellular carcinomas in patients with cirrhosis. *N Engl J Med* 1996;334(11):693–9.
77 Mazzaferro V, Chun YS, Poon RTP, *et al.* Liver transplantation for hepatocellular carcinoma. *Ann Surg Oncol* 2008;15(4):1001–7.
78 Yao FY, Ferrell L, Bass NM, *et al.* Liver transplantation for hepatocellular carcinoma: expansion of the tumor size limits does not adversely impact survival. *Hepatology* 2001;6:1394–403.
79 Mazzaferro V, Llovet JM, Miceli R, *et al.* Predicting survival after liver transplantation in patients with hepatocellular carcinoma beyond the Milan criteria: a retrospective, exploratory analysis. *Lancet Oncol* 2009;10(1):35–43.
80 Melloul E, Lesurtel M, Carr BI, Clavien PA. Developments in liver transplantation for hepatocellular carcinoma. *Semin Oncol* 2012;39(4):510–21.
81 Fuks D, Dokmak S, Paradis V, *et al.* Benefit of initial resection of hepatocellular carcinoma followed by transplantation in case of recurrence: an intention-to-treat analysis. *Hepatology* 2012;55:132–40.
82 Trotter JF, Adam R, Lo CM, Kenison J. Documented deaths of hepatic lobe donors for living donor liver transplantation. *Liver Transpl* 2006;12:1485–8.
83 Treiber G. mTOR inhibitors for hepatocellular carcinoma: a forward-moving target. *Expert Rev Anticancer Ther* 2009;9(2):247–61.
84 Song T, Ip E, Fong Y. Hepatocellular carcinoma: current surgical management. *Gastroenterology* 2004;127: S248–60.
85 Dhir M, Lyden ER, Smith LM, Are C. Comparison of outcomes of transplantation and resection in patients with early hepatocellular carcinoma: a meta-analysis. *HPB (Oxford)* 2012;14(9):635–45.
86 Llovet JM, Schwartz M, Mazzaferro M. Resection and liver transplantation for hepatocellular carcinoma. *Semin Liver Dis* 2005;25(2):181–200.
87 Hoshida Y, Villanueva A, Kobayashi M, *et al.* Gene expression in fixed tissues and outcome in hepatocellular carcinoma. *N Engl J Med* 2008;359(19):1995–2004.
88 Shrager B, Jibara GA, Schwartz M, Roayaie S. Resection of hepatocellular carcinoma without cirrhosis. *Ann Surg* 2012;255(6):1135–43.
89 Roayaie S, Schwartz JD, Sung MW, *et al.* Recurrence of hepatocellular carcinoma after liver transplant: patterns and prognosis. *Liver Transpl* 2004;10(4):534–40.
90 Lau WY, Lai EC, Leung TW, Yu SC. Adjuvant intra-arterial iodine-131-labeled lipiodol for resectable hepatocellular carcinoma: a prospective randomized trial – update on 5-year and 10-year survival. *Ann Surg* 2008;247(1):43–8.
91 Muto Y, Moriwaki H, Ninomiya M, *et al.* Prevention of second primary tumors by an acyclic retinoid, polyprenoic acid, in patients with hepatocellular carcinoma. Hepatoma Prevention Study Group. *N Engl J Med* 1996;334(24):1561–7.
92 Muto Y, Moriwaki H, Saito A. Prevention of second primary tumors by an acyclic retinoid in patients with hepatocellular carcinoma. *N Engl J Med* 1999;340(13):1046–7.
93 Okita K, Matsui O, Kumada K, *et al.* Effect of peretinoin on recurrence of hepatocellular carcinoma (HCC): results of a phase II/III randomized placebo-controlled trial. *J Clin Oncol* 2010;28(suppl; abstr 4024):15s.
94 Xu J, Shen ZY, Chen XG, *et al.* A randomized controlled trial of Licartin for preventing hepatoma recurrence after liver transplantation. *Hepatology* 2007;45(2):269–76.
95 Bruix J, Takayama T, Mazzaferro V, *et al.* Adjuvant sorafenib for hepatocellular carcinoma after resection or ablation (STORM): a phase 3, randomized, double-blind, placebo-controlled trial. *Lancet Oncol* 2015:16(13):1344–54.
96 Shiina S, Tateishi R, Imamura M, *et al.* Percutaneous ethanol injection for hepatocellular carcinoma: 20-year outcome and prognostic factors. *Liver Int* 2012;32(9):1434–42.
97 Lencioni RA, Allgaier HP, Cioni D, *et al.* Small hepatocellular carcinoma in cirrhosis: randomized comparison of radio-frequency thermal ablation versus percutaneous ethanol injection. *Radiology* 2003;228(1):235–40.
98 Bouza C, Lopez-Cuadrado T, Alcazar R, *et al.* Meta-analysis of percutaneous radiofrequency ablation versus ethanol injection in hepatocellular carcinoma. *BMC Gastroenterol* 2009;9:31.
99 Orlando A, Leandro G, Olivo M, *et al.* Radiofrequency thermal ablation vs. percutaneous ethanol injection for small hepatocellular carcinoma in cirrhosis: meta-analysis of randomized controlled trials. *Am J Gastroenterol* 2009;104(2):514–24.
100 Livraghi T, Meloni F, Di Stasi M, *et al.* Sustained complete response and complications rates after radiofrequency ablation of very early hepatocellular carcinoma in cirrhosis: is resection still the treatment of choice? *Hepatology* 2008;47:82–9.
101 Feng K, Yan J, Li X, *et al.* A randomized controlled trial of radiofrequency ablation and surgical resection in the treatment of small hepatocellular carcinoma. *J Hepatol* 2012;57(4):794–802.
102 Chen MS, Li JQ, Zheng Y, *et al.* A prospective randomized trial comparing percutaneous local ablative therapy and partial hepatectomy for small hepatocellular carcinoma. *Ann Surg* 2006;243:321–8.

103 Huang J, Yan L, Cheng Z, *et al.* A randomized trial comparing radiofrequency ablation and surgical resection for HCC conforming to the Milan criteria. *Ann Surg* 2010;252(6):903–12.

104 Bhardwaj N, Strickland AD, Ahmad F, *et al.* Liver ablation techniques: a review. *Surgical Endoscopy* 2010;24(2):254–65.

105 Ding J, Jin X, Liu J, *et al.* Comparison of two different thermal techniques for the treatment of hepatocellular carcinoma. *Eur J Radiol* 2013;82(9):1379–84.

106 Salem R, Lewandowski RJ. Chemoembolization and radioembolization for hepatocellular carcinoma. *Clin Gastroenterol Hepatol* 2013;11(6):604–11.

107 Marelli L, Stigliano R, Triantos C, *et al.* Transarterial therapy for hepatocellular carcinoma: which technique is more effective? A systematic review of cohort and randomized studies. *Cardiovasc Intervent Radiol* 2007;30(1):6–25.

108 Lo C-M, Ngan H, Tso W-K, *et al.* Randomized controlled trial of transarterial lipiodol chemoembolization for unresectable hepatocellular carcinoma. *Hepatology* 2002;35:1164–71.

109 Llovet JM, Real MI, Montana X, *et al.* Arterial embolization or chemoembolization versus symptomatic treatment in patients with unresectable hepatocellular carcinoma: a randomized controlled trial. *Lancet* 2002;359:1734–9.

110 Lewandowski RJ, Mulcahy MF, Kulik LM, *et al.* Chemoembolization for hepatocellular carcinoma: comprehensive imaging and survival analysis in a 172 patient cohort. *Radiology* 2010;255(3):955–65.

111 Takayasu K, Arii S, Kudo M, *et al.* Superselective transarterial chemoembolization for hepatocellular carcinoma. Validation of treatment algorithm proposed by Japanese guidelines. *J Hepatol* 2012;56(4):886–92.

112 Lewis AL, Gonzalez, MV, Lloyd AW, *et al.* DC bead: in vitro characterization of a drug-delivery device for transarterial chemoembolization. *J Vasc Interv Radiol* 2006;17(2 Pt 1):335–42.

113 Lammer J, Malagari K, Vogl T, *et al.* Prospective randomized study of doxorubicin-eluting-bead embolization in the treatment of hepatocellular carcinoma: results of the PRECISION V study. *Cardiovasc Intervent Radiol* 2010;33(1):41–52.

114 Burrel M, Reig M, Forner A, *et al.* Survival of patients with hepatocellular carcinoma treated by transarterial chemoembolisation (TACE) using Drug Eluting Beads. Implications for clinical practice and trial design. *J Hepatol* 2012;56(6):1330–5.

115 Dhanasekaran R, Kooby DA, Staley CA, *et al.* Comparison of conventional transarterial chemoembolization (TACE) and chemoembolization with doxorubicin drug eluting beads (DEB) for unresectable hepatocellular carcinoma (HCC). *J Surg Oncol* 2010;101(6):476–80.

116 Maluccio MA, Covey AM, Porat LB, *et al.* Transcatheter arterial embolization with only particles for the treatment of unresectable hepatocellular carcinoma. *J Vasc Interv Radiol* 2008;19(6):862–9.

117 Malagari K, Pomoni M, Kelekis A, *et al.* Prospective randomized comparison of chemoembolization with doxorubicin-eluting beads and bland embolization with BeadBlock for hepatocellular carcinoma. *Cardiovasc Intervent Radiol* 2010;33(3):541–51.

118 Brown KT, Gonen M, Do KG, *et al.* A randomized single blind controlled trial of beads versus doxorubicin-eluting beads for arterial embolization of hepatocellular carcinoma (HCC). 2013 Gastrointestinal Cancers Symposium. *J Clin Oncol* 2012;30 (suppl 34; abstr 143).

119 Young JY, Rhee TK, Atassi B, *et al.* Radiation dose limits and liver toxicities resulting from multiple yttrium-90 radioembolization treatments for hepatocellular carcinoma. *J Vasc Interv Radiol* 2007;18(11):1375–82.

120 Kulik LM, Carr BI, Mulcahy MF, *et al.* Safety and efficacy of 90Y radiotherapy for hepatocellular carcinoma with and without portal thrombosis. *Hepatology* 2008;47(1):71–81.

121 Hawkins MS, Dawson LA. Radiation therapy for hepatocellular carcinoma: from palliation to cure. *Cancer* 2006;106(8):1653–63.

122 Kim YJ, Chung SM, Choi BO, Kay CS. Hepatocellular carcinoma with portal vein tumor thrombosis: improved treatment outcomes with external beam radiation therapy. *Hepatol Res* 2011;41(9):813–24.

123 Olweny CL, Toya T, Katongole-Mbedde E, *et al.* Treatment of hepatocellular carcinoma with adriamycin. *Cancer* 1975;36:1250–7.

124 Yeo W, Lam KC, Zee B, *et al.* A randomized phase III study of doxorubicin versus cisplatin/interferon-alpha2B/doxorubicin/fluorouracil (PIAF) combination chemotherapy for unresectable hepatocellular carcinoma. *J Natl Cancer Inst* 2005;97(20):1532–8.

125 Nowak A, Findlay M, Culjak G, Stockler M. Tamoxifen for hepatocellular carcinoma. *Cochrane Database Syst Rev* 2004;(3):CD001024.

126 Guo TK, Hao XY, Ma B, *et al.* Octreotide for advanced hepatocellular carcinoma: a meta-analysis of randomized controlled trials. *J Cancer Res Clin Oncol* 2009;135(12):1685–92.

127 Huang CC, Wu MC, Xu GW, *et al.* Overexpression of the MDR1 gene and p-glycoprotein in human hepatocellular carcinoma. *J Natl Cancer Inst* 1992;84(4):262–4.

128 Wilhelm SM, Carter C, Tang L, *et al.* BAY 43-9006 exhibits broad spectrum oral antitumor activity and targets the RAF/MEK/ERK pathway and receptor tyrosine kinases involved in tumor progression and angiogenesis. *Cancer Res* 2004;64(19):7099–109.

129 Abou-Alfa GK, Schwartz L, Ricci S, *et al.* Phase II study of sorafenib in patients with advanced hepatocellular carcinoma. *J Clin Oncol* 2006;24(26):4293–300.

130 Llovet JM, Ricci S, Mazzaferro V, *et al.* Sorafenib in advanced hepatocellular carcinoma. *N Engl J Med* 2008;359(4):378–90.

131 Cheng AL, Kang YK, Chen Z, *et al.* Efficacy and safety of sorafenib in patients in the Asia-Pacific region with advanced hepatocellular carcinoma: a phase III randomised, double-blind, placebo-controlled trial. *Lancet Oncol* 2009;10(1):25–34.

132 Huitzil-Melendez FD, Saltz LB, Song J, *et al.* Retrospective analysis of outcome in hepatocellular carcinoma patients with hepatitis C versus B treated with sorafenib. 2007 Gastrointestinal Cancers Symposium, abstract 173.

133 Bruix J, Raoul JL, Sherman M, *et al.* Efficacy and safety of sorafenib in patients with advanced hepatocellular carcinoma: subanalyses of a phase III trial. *J Hepatol* 2012;57(4):821–9.

134 Cheng AL, Kang Y, Lin D, *et al.* Phase III study of sunitinib versus sorafenib in advanced hepatocellular carcinoma. *J Clin Oncol* 2011;29(suppl; abstr 4000).

135 Aoki H, Hayashi J, Moriyama M, *et al.* Hepatitis C virus core protein interacts with 14-3-3 protein and activates the kinase Raf-1. *J Virol* 2000;74(4):1736–41.

136 Abou-Alfa GK, Amadori D, Santoro A, *et al.* Safety and efficacy of sorafenib in patients with hepatocellular carcinoma (HCC) and Child-Pugh A versus B cirrhosis. *Gastrointest Cancer Res* 2011;4(2):40–4.

137 Marrero JA, Lencioni R, Kudo M, *et al.* Global investigation of therapeutic decisions in hepatocellular carcinoma and of its treatment with sorafenib (GIDEON): clinical findings in patients with liver dysfunction. *J Clin Oncol* 29:2011(suppl; abstr 4001).

138 Miller AA, Murry DJ, Owzar K, *et al.* Phase I and pharmacokinetic study of sorafenib in patients with hepatic or renal dysfunction: CALGB 60301. *J Clin Oncol* 2009;27(11):1800–5.

139 Abou-Alfa GK, Johnson P, Knox JJ, *et al.* Doxorubicin plus sorafenib vs doxorubicin alone in patients with advanced hepatocellular carcinoma: a randomized trial. *JAMA* 2010;304(19):2154–60.

140 Li X, Feng GS, Zheng CS, *et al.* Expression of plasma vascular endothelial growth factor in patients with hepatocellular carcinoma and effect of transcatheter arterial chemoembolization therapy on plasma vascular endothelial growth factor level. *World J Gastroenterol* 2004;10:2878–82.

141 Xiong ZP, Yang SR, Liang ZY, *et al.* Association between vascular endothelial growth factor and metastasis after transcatheter arterial chemoembolization in patients with hepatocellular carcinoma. *Hepatobiliary Pancreat Dis Int* 2004;3(3):386–90.

142 Pawlik TM, Reyes DK, Cosgrove D, *et al.* Phase II trial of sorafenib combined with concurrent trans-arterial embolization with doxorubicin-eluting beads for hepatocellular carcinoma. *J Clin Oncol* 2011;29(30):3960–7.

143 Kudo M, Imanaka K, Chida N, *et al.* Phase III study of sorafenib after transarterial chemoembolization in Japanese and Korean patients with unresectable hepatocellular carcinoma. *Eur J Cancer* 2011;47(14):2117–27.

144 Lencioni R, Llovet JM, Han G, *et al.* Sorafenib or placebo in combination with transarterial chemoembolization (TACE) with doxorubicin-eluting beads (DEBDOX) for intermediate-stage hepatocellular carcinoma (HCC): phase II, randomized, double-blind SPACE trial. *J Clin Oncol* 2012;30(suppl 4; abstr LBA154).

145 Bruix J, Merle P, Granito A, *et al.* Efficacy and safety of regorafenib versus placebo in patients with hepatocellular carcinoma (HCC) progressing on sorafenib: results of the international, randomized phase 3 RESORCE trial. 2016 World Congress on GI Cancer, Barcelona, Spain, abstract LBA03.

146 Bruix J, Merle P, Granito A, *et al.* Efficacy, safety, and health-related quality of life (HRQoL) of regorafenib in patients with hepatocellular carcinoma (HCC) progressing on sorafenib: Results of the international double-blind phase 3 RESORCE trial. 2016 ESMO Congress, Copenhagen, Denmark, abstract LBA28.

147 Philip PA, Mahoney MR, Allmer C, *et al.* Phase II study of Erlotinib (OSI-774) in patients with advanced hepatocellular cancer. *J Clin Oncol* 2005;23:6657–63.

148 Thomas MB, Chadha R, Glover K, *et al.* Phase 2 study of erlotinib in patients with unresectable hepatocellular carcinoma. *Cancer* 2007;110:1059–67.

149 O'Dwyer PJ, Biantonio BJ, Levy DE, *et al.* Gefitinib in advanced unresectable hepatocellular carcinoma: results from the Eastern Cooperative Oncology Group's Study E1203. 2006 ASCO Annual Meeting Proceedings Part I. J Clin Oncol 2006;24(18S, June 20 Supplement):4143.

150 Ramanathan RK, Belani CP, Singh DA, *et al.* A phase II study of lapatinib in patients with advanced biliary tree and hepatocellular cancer. *Cancer Chemother Pharmacol* 2009;64(4):777–83.

151 Bekaii-Saab T, Markowitz J, Prescott N, *et al.* A multi-institutional phase II study of the efficacy and tolerability of lapatinib in patients with advanced hepatocellular carcinoma. *Clin Cancer Res* 2009;15:5895–901.

152 Zhu AX, Stuart K, Blaszkowsky LS, *et al.* Phase 2 study of cetuximab in patients with advanced hepatocellular carcinoma. *Cancer* 2007;110(3):581–9.

153 Gruenwald V, Wilkens L, Gebel M, *et al.* A phase II open-label study of cetuximab in unresectable hepatocellular carcinoma: final results. 2007 ASCO Annual Meeting Proceedings Part I. J Clin Oncol 2007;25(18S June 20 Supplement):4598.

154 Zhu A, Rosmorduc O, Evans J, *et al.* SEARCH: a phase III, randomized, double-blind, placebo-controlled trial of sorafenib plus erlotinib in patients with hepatocellular carcinoma (HCC). *Ann Oncol* 2012;23(Suppl. 9).

155 Abou-Alfa GK, Gansukh B, Chou JF, *et al.* Phase II study of cixutumumab (IMC-A12, NSC742460; C) in hepatocellular carcinoma (HCC). *J Clin Oncol* 2011;29(suppl; abstr 4043).

156 Santoro A, Rimassa L, Borbath I, *et al.* Tivantinib for second-line treatment of advanced hepatocellular carcinoma: a randomized, placebo-controlled phase 2 study. *Lancet Oncol* 2013;14(1):55–63.

157 Verslype C, Cohn AL, Kelley RK, *et al.* Activity of cabozantinib (XL184) in hepatocellular carcinoma: results from a randomized phase II discontinuation study. *J Clin Oncol* 2012;30(suppl; abstr 4007).

158 Ang C, Owen D, Abou-Alfa GK. Systemic therapy in advanced HCC. In: *Clinical Interventional Radiology.* Elsevier. In press.

159 O'Neil BH, Goff LW, Kauh JS, *et al.* Phase II study of the mitogen-activated protein kinase 1/2 inhibitor selumetinib in patients with advanced hepatocellular carcinoma. *J Clin Oncol* 2011;29(17):2350–6.

160 Novartis study of Afinitor in advanced liver cancer does not meet primary endpoint of overall survival. Novartis media release 2013 August 7. http://www.novartis.com/newsroom/media-releases/en/2013/1721562.shtml (accessed 27 August 2013).

161 Siegel AB, Cohen EL, Ocean A, *et al.* Phase II trial evaluating clinical and biologic effects of bevacizumab in advanced, unresectable hepatocellular carcinoma. *J Clin Oncol* 2008;26(18):2992–8.

162 Kaseb AO, Garrett Mayer E, Morris JS, *et al.* Efficacy of bevacizumab and erlotinib for advanced hepatocellular carcinoma and predictors of outcome: final results of a phase II trial. *Oncology* 2012;82(2):67–74.

163 Zhu AX, Park JO, Ryoo BY, *et al.* Ramucirumab versus placebo as second-line treatment in patients with advanced hepatocellular carcinoma following first-line therapy with sorafenib (REACH): a randomized, double-blind, multicenter, phase 3 trial. *Lancet Oncol* 2015;16(7):859–70.

164 Johnson PJ, Qin S, Park J-W, *et al.* Brivanib vs. sorafenib as first-line therapy in patients with unresectable, advanced hepatocellular carcinoma: results from the randomized phase III BRISK-FL study. *J Clin Oncol* 2013;31(28):2517–24.

165 Llovet J, Decaens T, Raoul J, *et al.* Brivanib in patients with advanced hepatocellular carcinoma who were intolerant to sorafenib or for whom sorafenib failed: results from the randomized phase III BRISK-PS study. *J Clin Oncol* 2013;31(28):3509–16.

166 Cainap C, Qin S, Huang W-T, *et al.* Phase III trial of linifanib versus sorafenib in patients with advanced hepatocellular carcinoma (HCC). *J Clin Oncol* 30:2012(suppl 34; abstr 249).

167 Zhu AX, Sahani DV, Duda DG, *et al.* Efficacy, safety, and potential biomarkers of sunitinib monotherapy in advanced hepatocellular carcinoma: a phase II study. *J Clin Oncol* 2009;27(18):3027–35.

168 Faivre S, Raymond E, Boucher E, *et al.* Safety and efficacy of sunitinib in patients with advanced hepatocellular carcinoma: an open-label, multicentre phase II study. *Lancet Oncol* 2009;10(8):794–800.

169 Koeberle D, Montemurro M, Samaras P, *et al.* Continuous sunitinib treatment in patients with advanced hepatocellular carcinoma: a Swiss Group for Clinical Cancer Research (SAKK) and Swiss Association for the Study of the Liver (SASL) multicenter phase II trial (SAKK 77/06). *Oncologist* 2010;15(3):285–92.

170 Cheng AL, Kang Y, Lin D, *et al.* Phase III study of sunitinib versus sorafenib in advanced hepatocellular carcinoma. *J Clin Oncol* 2011;29(suppl; abstr 4000).

171 El-Khoueiry AB, Melero I, Crocenzi TS, *et al.* Phase I/II safety and antitumor activity of nivolumab in patients with advanced hepatocellular carcinoma (HCC): CA209-040. J Clin Oncol 2015;33(suppl;abstr LBA101).

172 El-Khoueiry AB, Sangro B, Yau TC, *et al.* Phase I/II safety and antitumor activity of nivolumab in pateints with advanced hepatocellular carcinoma: interim analysis of the CheckMate-040 dose escalation study. *J Clin Oncol* 2016;34(suppl; abstr 4012).

173 Eisenhauer EA, Therasse P, Bogaerts J, *et al.* New response evaluation criteria in solid tumours: revised RECIST guidelines (version 1.1) *Eur J Cancer* 2009;45(2):228–47.

174 Abou-Alfa GK, Zhao B, Capanu M, *et al.* Tumor Necrosis as a Correlate for Response in Subgroup of Patients with Advanced Hepatocellular Carcinoma (HCC) Treated with Sorafenib. ESMO 2008, Stockholm, Sweden, abstract 547P.

175 Lencioni R, Llovet JM. Modified RECIST (mRECIST) assessment for hepatocellular carcinoma. *Semin Liver Dis* 2010;30(1):52–60.

8

Biliary Tract Cancers/Cholangiocarcinomas

Celina Ang, Sonia Reichert, and Randall F. Holcombe

Mount Sinai Medical Center, New York, New York, USA

Introduction

Biliary tract cancers originate from malignant transformation of cholangiocytes, the epithelial cells lining the biliary ducts and includes the gallbladder. Gallbladder carcinoma is the most common subtype of bile duct cancers. In the literature the term cholangiocarcinoma (CCA) and bile duct cancers are used interchangeably. In this chapter, we will refer to all bile duct cancers as CCA. Since CCA may arise from every portion of the biliary tree, they are classified anatomically as intrahepatic (within the hepatic parenchyma) or extrahepatic (hepatic ducts and common bile duct including the intrapancreatic portion of the common bile duct) [1]. Perihilar (the junction of the right and left hepatic ducts), or Klatskin tumors are included in the classification as extrahepatic bile duct cancers. Intrahepatic CCA is the second most common primary liver tumor after hepatocellular carcinoma and represents 15% of liver cancers [2].

Incidence and Mortality

The incidence of biliary tract cancers has marked variation worldwide with highest incidence rates in regions where liver flukes are endemic. In south-east Asia (South Korea, south-east China, and Thailand) the incidence rates for intrahepatic CCA are four per 100,000 with the highest reported rate in Khon Kaen, Thailand (incidence of liver cancers up to 118 per 100,000 with 85% histologically confirmed as CCA) [2]. The overall incidence rate for intrahepatic CCA in the United States (US) is 1.6 cases per 100,000 individuals per year [3]. Incidence rates for gallbladder and for other biliary tract cancers (extrahepatic CCA and ampullary cancer) incidence rates are 1.2 per 100,000 and 1.9 per 100,000 per year, respectively [4].

The American Cancer Society estimates that 40,710 cancers of the liver and intrahepatic bile ducts (mostly hepatocellular carcinoma (HCC)) and 11,740 cancers of the gallbladder and other biliary sites will be diagnosed in the US during 2017. The American Cancer Society estimates deaths from cancers of the liver and intrahepatic bile ducts, and from cancers of the gallbladder and other biliary sites are 28,920 and 3,830, respectively [5].

An increase in incidence in western countries of intrahepatic CCA has been observed but there is debate as to whether this is a true increase or as some studies have suggested, reflects a misclassification of perihilar tumors as intrahepatic instead of extrahepatic [6]. In the US, the highest incidence rates for intrahepatic CCA are among Asians and Pacific Islanders, American Indians, and Hispanics (1.8-fold), and rates are lower among African Americans and whites [3,7].

Risk Factors

There is a strong association between chronic biliary tract infection and inflammation and the development of CCA. Identified risk factors includes: liver flukes (*Clonorchis sinesis*, *Opistorchis viverrini*), primary sclerosing cholangitis, choledochal cysts, viral hepatitis B and C, HIV, obesity, diabetes, fatty liver disease and cirrhosis, toxins (alcohol, thorotrast (thorium dioxide), vinyl chloride, nitrosamines), and hepatolithiasis [1,8–11]. Gallstones are present in about 80% of patients with gallbladder carcinoma. Chronic cholecystitis has also been closely linked to the development of gallbladder carcinoma [12]. In contrast, cholelithiasis is not closely linked with the etiology of other subtypes of CCA. Approximately 90% of patients diagnosed with CCA in western countries have no identifiable risk factors [13].

Pathogenesis

Molecular and genetic aberrations include the activation of growth signaling pathways such as hepatocyte growth factor (HGF), interleukin-6 (IL-6), ErbB-2, K-ras, BRAF and COX-2. The IL-6 growth factor cytokine has been implicated to play a

The American Cancer Society's Oncology in Practice: Clinical Management, First Edition. Edited by The American Cancer Society.

central role in cholangiocarcinogenesis [1,14]. IL-6, a proinflammatory cytokine, is produced by normal biliary epithelial cells and cholangiocytes in response to inflammatory mediators [15]. Constitutive production of IL-6 occurs in neoplastic transformed biliary cells, which is further enhanced by tumor necrosis factor (TNF)-alpha and interleukin-1 [16]. IL-6 increases proliferation in malignant cholangiocytes and activates cell survival pathways via JAK2-STAT3 activation [17].

Screening

Although early detection is needed for improved survival rates, there have been no proven effective screening tests for CCA or gallbladder cancer. Serum and stool tests for liver flukes may be promising approaches for endemic areas. Several tumor markers have been studied to support a diagnosis of CCA in high risk patients, including carbohydrate antigen (CA 19-9) and carcinoembryonic antigen (CEA). However these are also elevated in other malignant diseases (HCC, pancreatic cancer) as well as benign diseases (alcoholic liver disease, chronic viral hepatitis) and in conditions where screening would be helpful in diagnosing CCA including primary sclerosing cholangitis [18]. Cut-off values of 100 U/mL and 129 U/mL have been proposed by two different series published by the Mayo clinic [19,20]. However, the positive predictive value was only 56.6%. To date, both CA 19-9 and CEA have not been shown to be sensitive markers for screening purposes and are not currently recommended for routine use in high risk patients [21].

Diagnosis

Clinical Presentation

Intrahepatic CCA is typically asymptomatic in the early stages and is seen as an incidental intrahepatic mass on imaging. Imaging often reveals a liver tumor frequently associated with satellite nodules in the periphery. In most cases it presents in advanced disease with weight loss, fever, and/or abdominal pain.

Extrahepatic CCA typically presents with jaundice due to biliary obstruction. Extrahepatic CCA often grow longitudinally along the bile duct rather than in a radial direction from the bile duct. For this reason, ultrasound, computed tomography (CT), and magnetic resonance imaging (MRI) have a lower diagnostic yield in this subtype.

Gallbladder carcinoma may be diagnosed at advanced stage as most gallbladder carcinomas mimic biliary colic or chronic cholecystitis. Often, however, it is identified as an incidental finding at surgery or during pathologic review of a cholecystectomy specimen.

Diagnostic Studies

Imaging

Despite their low diagnostic yield, delayed contrast CT or MRI are recommended in the workup of CCA primarily to identify patients who are potentially resectable. Imaging may identify the extent of disease, involvement of major vessels, nearby lymph nodes, and distant sites. Unlike hepatocellular carcinoma, CCA lacks a characteristic imaging appearance. Biliary imaging such as magnetic resonance cholangiography, endoscopic retrograde cholangiopancreatography, or percutaneous transhepatic cholangiography may be helpful to evaluate the extent of invasion. Positron emission tomography has been increasingly used to detect lymph node involvement or distant metastatic disease in potentially resectable patients [22,23].

Biopsy

Cell or tissue samples via brush cytology or forceps biopsy obtained in patients undergoing endoscopic and percutaneous transhepatic procedures for biliary strictures is the most common technique for definitive diagnosis. The sensitivity of brush cytology for cancer diagnosis ranges from 30 to 60%. The cancer detection rate with forceps biopsy is higher ranging from 43 to 81%. Fine-needle aspiration via endoscopic ultrasound has a diagnostic yield of 45–86% [24].

Markers

Obstructive jaundice is accompanied by nonspecific increases in serum bilirubin, alkaline phosphatase, and gamma glutamyl transpeptidase. The most widely studied biomarkers in CCA are CA 19-9 and CEA but their use remains limited because of low specificity. However, they can be useful in following the effect of treatment and detecting disease recurrence.

Pathology

Cholangiocarcinomas lack extensive necrosis and are most commonly "mass forming" [25]. Extrahepatic CCA typically displays a periductal infiltrating growth pattern, growing in sheets of cells along the biliary tree, which helps to explain the apparent discrepancy between imaging findings and extent of disease upon resection.

Microscopically, CCAs are adenocarcinomas consisting of tubules, acini, solid nests, or trabeculae embedded in a desmoplastic stroma [25]. They typically express cytokeratin 7 and 19 and have cytoplasmic positivity for CEA. Intrahepatic CCAs can be distinguished from metastatic colon cancer by their negative cytokeratin 20 and CDX-2 [26].

Lymphatic, venous, and/or perineural invasion by CCA are associated with an increased rate of relapse and worse prognosis [27]. Extrahepatic CCAs frequently spread by direct extension into surrounding soft tissues and along the walls of bile ducts. Lymph node involvement in resected patients is more common in distal extrahepatic CCA compared to perihilar and intrahepatic CCA [28].

Staging

The AJCC Cancer Staging Manual 8th edition includes separate staging for intrahepatic bile duct tumors, perihilar (extrahepatic) bile duct tumors, distal bile duct tumors, and gallbladder carcinoma [29].

Management

Resectable Disease

Complete resection is the only potentially curative therapy for both intrahepatic and extrahepatic CCA. However, less than one-third of patients are deemed resectable at presentation. Even with resection, the 5-year survival rates following resection for intrahepatic, hilar, and distal tumors are 20–32%, 30–42%, and 18–54% respectively [30].

Intrahepatic CCA

Major hepatectomy removing more than three liver segments and removal of the common bile duct and vascular structures is often necessary to achieve complete resection. The main complications are liver failure and sepsis. Approximately 20–30% of resected patients are found to have incidental peritoneal deposits.

Extrahepatic CCA

Biliary tree, lymphatic resection, and partial liver resection may be required for complete (R0) resection. Major hepatectomy for hilar CCAs carries a large risk of hepatic insufficiency which often limits the number of patients who may be resectable. More distal lesions are managed by Whipple's pancreaticoduodenectomy. Portal vein embolization has reduced the rates of liver failure in cases of extended hepatectomy resection from 20 to 6% [31]. A recent study showed that preoperative cholangitis is the most important preoperative factor related to inhospital mortality [32].

Gallbladder Carcinoma

Surgical resection ranges from simple cholecystectomy to more complex surgery, which may involve liver, bile duct, and pancreatic resections. While many gallbladder cancers are found incidentally following laparoscopic cholecystectomy, the only role for laparascopic surgery in known disease is to determine resectability [33]. Lymph node metastasis in the celiac, superior mesenteric and para-aortic lymph nodes (N2) represents unresectable disease [10].

Liver Transplantation

Although hepatic resection is the primary curative treatment for CCA, the location, extent of disease, and vascular encasement frequently precludes potential complete resection. In addition, extensive surgical resection is not tolerated in some patients because of underlying liver dysfunction. Initial studies with orthotopic liver transplantation (OLT) for unresectable CCA were disappointing because of high rates of recurrence (53–84%) and a poor 5-year survival rate less than 15% [34]. This is especially true for intrahepatic CCAs which are generally recognized to be contraindicated to receive OLT. However, prompted by long-term survivors in patients with negative surgical margins and negative lymph nodes, studies were performed first at the University of Nebraska and later at the Mayo Clinic using neoadjuvant chemoradiation followed by OLT in highly selected patients with early stage, unresectable hilar CCA [35]. Patients found to have metastasis at operative staging did not undergo OLT. A report of 90 patients who underwent OLT had a 71% 5-year survival [36]. Recently, a multicenter retrospective study involving 12 transplant programs in the US showed that for those patients who have undergone OLT with neoadjuvant therapy had a recurrence-free survival of 78%, 65%, and 59% at 2, 5, and 10 years respectively [35]. These studies suggest that liver transplantation with neoadjuvant chemoradiotherapy is a curative option in carefully selected early stage hilar CCA.

Palliation of Symptoms for Unresectable Disease

There are a limited number of therapeutic options available to patients with unresectable CCA and gallbladder cancer. The median survival for unresectable disease is only 6–10 months. The therapeutic strategy of choice in these patients is to prevent cholestasis which is crucial in preventing pruritis, cholangitis, and death [37]. This is achieved by endoscopic and percutaneous stenting, biliary bypass, or photodynamic therapy.

Locoregional Therapies

Most CCA patients only develop distant metastases at late stages of the disease and in principle, locoregional therapies for disease control is a promising approach. Therapies such as radiofrequency ablation, transarterial chemoembolization, and photodynamic therapy have been shown to be safe and effective in small series of patients. Locoregional therapies may be considered as primary treatment of disease in selected patients, or may be used to consolidate favorable responses to systemic therapy. Randomized clinical trials are unfortunately lacking to prove a survival benefit with these strategies.

Radiofrequency Ablation

Percutaneous radiofrequency ablation is a minimally invasive technique using high-frequency alternating current to cause tissue coagulation and tumor destruction. Small case series suggest a benefit of local tumor control in patients with intermediate (3–5 cm) or small (<3 cm) intrahepatic CCAs who are not eligible for surgical resection [38,39].

Photodynamic Therapy

Photodynamic therapy (PDT) is a minimally invasive palliative strategy that entails the administration of a photosensitive molecule that accumulates in proliferating tissues such as malignancies. The use of a light at a specific wavelength targeted at the local tumor generates reactive oxygen species leading to selective tumor-cell death. It can reach peripheral lesions in the biliary tree. A recent meta-analysis of six studies suggests a promising benefit on survival, biliary drainage, and quality of life with PDT compared to biliary stent placement in the palliative setting [40]. In one randomized prospective study, the combination of stenting and subsequent PDT prolonged survival over stenting alone (498 vs 98 days, P <0.0001) [41].

Chemoembolization

Trans-arterial chemoembolization involves the application of a chemotherapeutic agent combined with hepatic artery embolization to interfere with nutrient delivery and simultaneously deliver local concentration of chemotherapeutic agents. While it is a proven strategy in HCC, data to support its use in CCA is limited to case series and retrospective studies. Local disease control (75%) was shown in a series of 62 patients with intrahepatic CCA and adenocarcinoma of unknown origin with the use of mitomycin C, doxorubicin, and cisplatin [42]. A retrospective study of 155 therapy-naive patients with intrahepatic CCA treated with cisplatin-based trans-arterial chemoembolization showed a significantly increased overall survival (OS) compared to best supportive care (12.2 vs 3.3 months, P <0.001). Disease control (stable disease or partial response) was achieved in 89% of patients.

Radiation Therapy

The use of external beam radiation therapy has been limited because of hepatic toxicity with doses exceeding 40 Gy. There are limited data beyond small case series regarding stereotactic body radiotherapy. However, this approach has promising results with a low toxicity profile [43].

Chemotherapy and Chemoradiotherapy

Adjuvant Chemotherapy

Adjuvant chemotherapy/chemoradiotherapy is often recommended given the high risk of disease recurrence and locoregional spread, though its benefit has been debated. A meta-analysis of 6712 patients with biliary tract cancers reported a significant improvement in survival with adjuvant therapy in patients with lymph node or margin-positive disease [44]. Chemotherapy or chemoradiotherapy yielded superior outcomes compared to adjuvant radiotherapy alone. The use of adjuvant gemcitabine or 5-fluorouracil (5-FU)-based chemotherapy is supported by several prospective studies. In the ESPAC-3 study, adjuvant gemcitabine or 5-FU significantly improved outcomes compared to observation in patients with resected periampullary cancers with high risk features including poor differentiation, nodal involvement, and bile duct primaries [45]. A phase III study in resected pancreaticobiliary cancer patients showed a 5-year overall and disease-free survival benefit for noncuratively resected gallbladder carcinoma with the use of mitomycin C and 5-FU [46]. A recent single arm phase II study of adjuvant capecitabine and gemcitabine followed by chemoradiation reported promising results in patients with resected extrahepatic cholangiocarcinoma and gallbladder cancer compared to historical data [47]. A nomogram has also been developed to help clinicians determine which patients with resected gallbladder cancer should receive adjuvant chemoradiation [48]. In this model, patients with > T2 tumors and node positive disease appear to derive a survival benefit from adjuvant therapy.

Unresectable or Metastatic Disease

At the time of recurrence, or for most patients that present with unresectable disease at presentation, systemic chemotherapy is used for disease control and palliation of symptoms. Prognosis is measured in months and is characterized by rapid decline with symptoms of progressive biliary obstruction. The most active agents are 5-FU, gemcitabine, cisplatin, and oxaliplatin. Single-agent 5-FU-based chemotherapy has shown a response rate of approximately 10–20% [49].

The largest randomized phase IIII prospective study to show a survival benefit in locally advanced and metastatic CCA and gallbladder carcinoma patients was with the combination of gemcitabine and cisplatin [50]. Median OS was 11.7 versus 8.1 months (P <0.001) and median progression-free survival (PFS) was 8.0 versus 5.0 months (P <0.001) in favor of combination therapy versus gemcitabine alone. Although there are no standard second-line therapies at the time of progression on this regimen, various combinations of gemcitabine, cisplatin, capecitabine, oxaliplatin, epirubicin, and 5-FU have shown activity and can be considered on disease progression [51].

Several therapeutic approaches targeting molecular alterations in biliary tract cancers have been evaluated [52,53]:

- Epidermal growth factor receptor (EGFR) is expressed in 81–100% of intrahepatic CCA, but in a lower rate in extrahepatic and gallbladder carcinomas (53–79% and 39–83% respectively) [54]. Erlotinib, an anti-EGFR tyrosine kinase inhibitor, has been tested alone, in combination with bevacizumab, and with chemotherapy [55–57]. Objective response and stable disease rates range from 7 to 16% and 43 to 51%, respectively. Median OS with erlotinib alone is 7.5 months, and in combination with bevacizumab or GEMOX (gemcitabine) is 9.5–9.9 months. In a randomized phase III study, GEMOX + erlotinib significantly improved PFS (5.9 vs 3.0 months, P = 0.049) compared to GEMOX alone in the subgroup of patients with cholangiocarcinoma, but not OS [57]. The anti-EGFR antibodies cetuximab and panitumumab have also been studied in randomized phase II studies with GEMOX [58,59]. In contrast to the cetuximab study which enrolled all-comers, all patients enrolled in the panitumumab study were KRAS wild-type. Objective response and disease control rates were not significantly improved in the combination arms of both studies compared to GEMOX alone. Median PFS and OS in the combination arms of both studies were 5.5 months and 5.3 months, respectively, and 12.4 months and 9.9 months, respectively. In the phase II study with cetuximab, outcomes did not appear to differ according to tumor KRAS, BRAF or EGFR status [58].
- Vascular endothelial growth factor (VEGF) is expressed in approximately 50% of intrahepatic CCAs and 32–59% of extrahepatic CCAs [60]. Bevacizumab has been studied in a phase II trial in combination with GEMOX with a response rate of 40%, median PFS was 7.6 months, and OS was 14.2 months [61]. In another single-arm phase II study, the anti-VEGFR, PDGFR, FLT-3, RET tyrosine kinase inhibitor sorafenib plus gemcitabine and cisplatin. Bevacizumab combined with gemcitabine and cisplatin yielded partial responses in 12% of patients, stable disease in 76% and a median PFS and OS of 6.5 months and 14.4 months, respectively [62].

Additional studies of agents targeting the fibroblast growth factor receptor, isocitrate dehydrogenase 1 and 2, BRAF, and ALK in molecularly enriched populations are currently underway [63]. The immune checkpoint inhibitor, pembrolizumab, has also shown promising preliminary activity in advanced biliary tract cancers [64].

Follow-Up and Survivorship

For patients achieving remission following surgical resection, there are no standard guidelines for surveillance imaging. Because of the high risk of relapse for most patients, CT and MRI imaging is often performed frequently, though a survival advantage for early detection of relapse has not been demonstrated. If surveillance scans are performed, they should include imaging of the thorax because of the possibility of lung metastases. Patients with relapse may be candidates for re-resection, stereotactic body radiotherapy, or palliative chemotherapy.

Patients remaining in remission should be followed closely for signs of hepatic decompensation due to reduced hepatic reserve following surgery. Appropriate hepatitis vaccinations, avoidance of hepatotoxic medications, and excessive alcohol ingestion are recommended.

References

1 Braconi C, Patel T. Cholangiocarcinoma: new insights into disease pathogenesis and biology. *Infect Dis Clin North Am* 2010:24(4):871–84, vii.

2 de Martel C, Plummer M, Franceschi S. Cholangiocarcinoma: descriptive epidemiology and risk factors. *Gastroenterol Clin Biol* 2010;34(3):173–80.

3 Mosadeghi S, Liu B, Bhuket T, Wong RJ. Sex-specific and race/ethnicity-specific disparities in cholangiocarcinoma incidence and prevalence in the USA: an updated analysis of the 2000–2011 Surveillance, Epidemiology and End Results registry. *Hepatol Res* 2016;46(7):669–77.

4 Howlader N, Noone AM, Krapcho M, *et al.* (eds). SEER Cancer Statistics Review, 1975–2013, National Cancer Institute. Bethesda, MD, http://seer.cancer.gov/csr/1975_2013/, based on November 2015 SEER data submission, posted to the SEER web site, April 2016

5 Siegel RL, Miller KD, Jemal A. Cancer statistics, 2017. *CA Cancer J Clin* 2017;67(1):7–30.

6 Khan SA, *et al.* Rising trends in cholangiocarcinoma: is the ICD classification system misleading us? *J Hepatol* 2012;56(4):848–54.

7 McLean L, Patel T. Racial and ethnic variations in the epidemiology of intrahepatic cholangiocarcinoma in the United States. *Liver Int* 2006;26(9):1047–53.

8 Tyson GL, El-Serag HB. Risk factors for cholangiocarcinoma. *Hepatology* 2011;54(1):173–84.

9 Welzel TM, Graubard BI, El-Serag HB, *et al.* Risk factors for intrahepatic and extrahepatic cholangiocarcinoma in the United States: a population-based case-control study. *Clin Gastroenterol Hepatol* 2007:5(10):1221–8.

10 Torbenson, M, Yeh MM, Abraham SC. Bile duct dysplasia in the setting of chronic hepatitis C and alcohol cirrhosis. *Am J Surg Pathol* 2007;31(9):1410–3.

11 Shaib YH, El-Serag HB, Nooka AK, *et al.* Risk factors for intrahepatic and extrahepatic cholangiocarcinoma: a hospital-based case-control study. *Am J Gastroenterol* 2007;102(5):1016–21.

12 Boutros C, *et al.* Gallbladder cancer: past, present and an uncertain future. *Surg Oncol* 2012;21(4):e183–91.

13 Ben-Menachem T. Risk factors for cholangiocarcinoma. *Eur J Gastroenterol Hepatol* 2007;19(8):615–7.

14 Smirnova OV, Ostroukhova TY, Bogorad RL. JAK-STAT pathway in carcinogenesis: is it relevant to cholangiocarcinoma progression? *World J Gastroenterol* 2007; 13(48):6478–91.

15 Sugawara, H., Yasoshima M, Katayanagi K, *et al.* Relationship between interleukin-6 and proliferation and differentiation in cholangiocarcinoma. *Histopathology* 1998; 33(2):145–53.

16 Park J, Tadlock L, Gores GJ, Patel T. Inhibition of interleukin 6-mediated mitogen-activated protein kinase activation attenuates growth of a cholangiocarcinoma cell line. *Hepatology* 1999;30(5):1128–33.

17 Meng F, Yamagiwa Y, Ueno Y, Patel T. Over-expression of interleukin-6 enhances cell survival and transformed cell growth in human malignant cholangiocytes. *J Hepatol* 2006;44(6):1055–65.

18 Yachimski PD, Pratt S. Cholangiocarcinoma: natural history, treatment, and strategies for surveillance in high-risk patients. *J Clin Gastroenterol* 2008;42(2):178–90.

19 Chalasani N, Baluyut A, Ismail A., *et al.* Cholangiocarcinoma in patients with primary sclerosing cholangitis: a multicenter case-control study. *Hepatology* 2000;31(1):7–11.

20 Nichols JC, Gores GJ, LaRusso NF, *et al.* Diagnostic role of serum CA 19-9 for cholangiocarcinoma in patients with primary sclerosing cholangitis. *Mayo Clin Proc* 1993;68(9):874–9.

21 Bjornsson E, Kilander A, Olsson R. CA 19-9 and CEA are unreliable markers for cholangiocarcinoma in patients with primary sclerosing cholangitis. *Liver* 1999; 19(6):501–8.

22 Petrowsky H, Wildbrett P, Husarik DB, *et al.* Impact of integrated positron emission tomography and computed tomography on staging and management of gallbladder cancer and cholangiocarcinoma. *J Hepatol* 2006;45(1):43–50.

23 Corvera CU, Blumgart LH, Akhurst T, *et al.* 18F-fluorodeoxyglucose positron emission tomography influences management decisions in patients with biliary cancer. *J Am Coll Surg* 2008;206(1):57–65.

24 Weber A, Schmid RM, Prinz C. Diagnostic approaches for cholangiocarcinoma. *World J Gastroenterol* 2008;4(26):4131–6.

25 Esposito IP. Schirmacher P. Pathological aspects of cholangiocarcinoma. *HPB (Oxford)* 2008;10(2):83–6.

26 Rullier A, Le Bail B, Fawaz R, *et al.* Cytokeratin 7 and 20 expression in cholangiocarcinomas varies along the biliary tract but still differs from that in colorectal carcinoma metastasis. *Am J Surg Pathol* 2000;24(6):870–6.

27 Hanazaki, K., Kajikawa S, Shimozawa N, *et al.* Prognostic factors of intrahepatic cholangiocarcinoma after hepatic resection: univariate and multivariate analysis. *Hepatogastroenterology* 2002;49(44):311–6.

28 DeOliveira ML, Cunningham SC, Cameron JL, *et al.* Cholangiocarcinoma: thirty-one-year experience with 564 patients at a single institution. *Ann Surg* 2007;245(5):755–62.

29 Amin M, Edge S, Greene R, Byrd D, Brookland R (eds). *Cancer Staging Manual 8th Edition. American Joint Committee on Cancer*. New York: Springer, 2017.

30 Murakami Y, Uemura K, Sudo T, *et al.* Prognostic factors after surgical resection for intrahepatic, hilar, and distal cholangiocarcinoma. *Ann Surg Oncol* 2011;18(3):651–8.

31 Igami T, Nishio H, Ebata T, *et al.* Surgical treatment of hilar cholangiocarcinoma in the "new era": the Nagoya University experience. *J Hepatobiliary Pancreat Sci* 2010; 17(4):449–54.

32 Sakata J, Shirai Y, Tsuchiya Y, *et al.* Preoperative cholangitis independently increases in-hospital mortality after combined major hepatic and bile duct resection for hilar cholangiocarcinoma. *Langenbecks Arch Surg* 2009;394(6):1065–72.

33 Huang CS, Lien HH, Jeng JY, Huang SH. Role of laparoscopic cholecystectomy in the management of polypoid lesions of the gallbladder. *Surg Laparosc Endosc Percutan Tech* 2001;11(4):242–7.

34 Masuoka HC, Rosen CB. Transplantation for cholangiocarcinoma. *Clin Liver Dis* 2011; 15(4):699–715.

35 Darwish Murad S, Kim WR, Harnois DM, *et al.* Efficacy of neoadjuvant chemoradiation, followed by liver transplantation, for perihilar cholangiocarcinoma at 12 US centers. *Gastroenterology* 2012;143(1):88–98 e3; quiz e14.

36 Rosen CB, Heimbach JK, Gores GJ. Surgery for cholangiocarcinoma: the role of liver transplantation. *HPB (Oxford)* 2008;10(3):186–9.

37 Cheon YK, Lee TY, Lee SM, Yoon JY, Shim CS. Longterm outcome of photodynamic therapy compared with biliary stenting alone in patients with advanced hilar cholangiocarcinoma. *HPB (Oxford)* 2012;14(3):185–93.

38 Kim JH, Won HJ, Shin YM, Kim KA, Kim PN. Radiofrequency ablation for the treatment of primary intrahepatic cholangiocarcinoma. *Am J Roentgenol* 2011; 196(2):W205–9.

39 Xu HX, Wang Y, Lu MD, Liu LN. Percutaneous ultrasound-guided thermal ablation for intrahepatic cholangiocarcinoma. *Br J Radiol* 2012;85(1016):1078–84.

40 Leggett CL, Gorospe EC, Murad MH, *et al.* Photodynamic therapy for unresectable cholangiocarcinoma: a comparative effectiveness systematic review and meta-analyses. *Photodiagnosis Photodyn Ther* 2012;9(3):189–95.

41 Ortner ME, Caca K, Berr F, *et al.* Successful photodynamic therapy for nonresectable cholangiocarcinoma: a randomized prospective study. *Gastroenterology* 2003; 125(5):1355–63.

42 Kiefer MV, Albert M, McNally M, *et al.* Chemoembolization of intrahepatic cholangiocarcinoma with cisplatinum, doxorubicin, mitomycin C, ethiodol, and polyvinyl alcohol: a 2-center study. *Cancer* 2011;117(7):1498–505.

43 Ibarra RA, Rojas D, Snyder L, *et al.* Multicenter results of stereotactic body radiotherapy (SBRT) for non-resectable primary liver tumors. *Acta Oncol* 2012;51(5):575–83.

44 Horgan AM Amir E, Walter T, Knox JJ. Adjuvant therapy in the treatment of biliary tract cancer: a systematic review and meta-analysis. *J Clin Oncol* 2012;30:1934–40.

45 Neoptolemos JP, Moore MJ, Cox TF, *et al.* Effect of adjuvant chemotherapy with fluorouracil plus folinic acid or gemcitabine vs observation on survival in patients with resected periampullary adenocarcinoma: the ESPAC-3 periampullary cancer randomized trial. *JAMA* 2012;308(2):147–56.

46 Takada T, Amano H, Yasuda H, *et al.* Is postoperative adjuvant chemotherapy useful for gallbladder carcinoma? A phase III multicenter prospective randomized controlled trial in patients with resected pancreaticobiliary carcinoma. *Cancer* 2002;95(8):1685–95.

47 Ben-Josef E, Guthrie KA, El-Khoueiry AB, *et al.* SWOG S0809: A phase II intergroup trial of adjuvant capecitabine and gemcitabine followed by radiotherapy and concurrent capecitabine in extrahepatic cholangiocarcinoma and gallbladder carcinoma. *J Clin Oncol* 2015:33(24):2617–22.

48 Wang SJ, Lemieux A, Kalpathy-Cramer J, *et al.* Nomogram for predicting the benefit of adjuvant chemoradiotherapy for resected gallbladder cancer. *J Clin Oncol* 2011;29(35):4627–32.

49 Glimelius, B., Hoffman K, Sjödén PO, *et al.* Chemotherapy improves survival and quality of life in advanced pancreatic and biliary cancer. *Ann Oncol* 1996;7(6):593–600.

50 Valle J, Wasan H, Palmer DH, *et al.* Cisplatin plus gemcitabine versus gemcitabine for biliary tract cancer. *N Engl J Med* 2010;362(14):1273–81.

51 Hezel AF, Zhu AX. Systemic therapy for biliary tract cancers. *Oncologist* 2008; 13(4):415–23.

52 Faris JE, Zhu AX. Targeted therapy for biliary tract cancers. *J Hepatobiliary Pancreat Sci* 2012;19(4):326–36.

53 Marino D, Leone F, Cavalloni G, Cagnazzo C, Aglietta M, *et al.* Biliary tract carcinomas: from chemotherapy to targeted therapy. *Crit Rev Oncol Hematol* 2013;85(2):136–48.

54 Pignochino Y, Sarotto I, Peraldo-Neia C, *et al.* Targeting EGFR/HER2 pathways enhances the antiproliferative effect of gemcitabine in biliary tract and gallbladder carcinomas. *BMC Cancer* 2010;10:631.

55 Philip PA, Mahoney MR, Allmer C, *et al.* Phase II study of erlotinib in patients with advanced biliary cancer. *J Clin Oncol* 2006;24(19):3069–74.

56 Lubner SJ, Mahoney MR, Kolesar JL, *et al.* Report of a multicenter phase II trial testing a combination of biweekly bevacizumab and daily erlotinib in patients with unresectable biliary cancer: a phase II Consortium study. *J Clin Oncol* 2010:28(21):3491–7.

57 Lee J, Park SH, Chang HM, *et al.* Gemcitabine and oxaliplatin with or without erlotinib in advanced biliary tract cancer: a multicentre, open-label, radomised, phase 3 study. *Lancet Oncol* 2012;13(2):181–8.

58 Malka D, Cervera P, Foulon S, *et al.* Gemcitabine and oxaliplatin with or without cetuximab in advanced biliary tract cancer (BINGO): a randomised, open-label, non-comparative phase 2 trial. *Lancet Oncol* 2014;15(8):819–28.

59 Leone F, Marino D, Cereda S, *et al.* Panitumumab in combination with gemcitabine and oxaliplatin does not prolong survival in wild-type KRAS advanced biliary tract cancer: a randomized phase 2 trial (Vecti-BIL study). *Cancer* 2016;122(4):574–81.

60 Yoshikawa D, Ojima H, Iwasaki M, *et al.* Clinicopathological and prognostic significance of EGFR, VEGF, and HER2 expression in cholangiocarcinoma. *Br J Cancer* 2008;98(2):418–25.

61 Zhu AX, Meyerhardt JA, Blaszkowsky LS, *et al.* Efficacy and safety of gemcitabine, oxaliplatin, and bevacizumab in advanced biliary-tract cancers and correlation of changes in 18-fluorodeoxyglucose PET with clinical outcome: a phase 2 study. *Lancet Oncol* 2010:11(1): 48–54.

62 Lee JK, Capanu M, O'Reilly EM, *et al.* A phase II study of gemcitabine and cisplatin plus sorafenib in patients with advanced biliary adenocarcinomas. *Br J Cancer* 2013;109(4):915–9.

63 Kelley RK, Bardeesy N. Biliary tract cancers: finding better ways to lump and split. *J Clin Oncol* 2015;33(24):2588–90.

64 Bang YJ, *et al.* Safety and efficacy of pembrolizumab (MK-3475) in patients with advanced biliary tract cancer: interim results of KEYNOTE-028. *Eur J Cancer* 2015;51: Suppl 3:S112, Abstract #525.

9

Colon and Rectal Cancer

Lauren Kosinski[1], Ben George[2], Kiran K. Turaga[3], Candice A. Johnstone[2], and Mohammad Mahmoud[3]

[1] The Seed House, Chestertown, Maryland, USA
[2] Medical College of Wisconsin, Milwaukee, Wisconsin, USA
[3] University of Chicago, Chicago, Illinois, USA

Introduction

The goals of this chapter are to introduce all aspects of colorectal cancer (CRC) from epidemiology, staging, treatment modalities and planning, sequencing of treatment in locoregional and metastatic disease to surveillance, palliative care, survivorship, and prevention. The role of multidisciplinary involvement at all phases of diagnosis and treatment has been emphasized as has recognition that, despite the importance of utilizing evidence-based, stage-related treatment guidelines, treatment plans are necessarily individualized. Understanding the logic of how plans are rationally individualized will equip the reader with the tools to participate more meaningfully in multidisciplinary conferences to plan patient care. Finally, we distinguish cancer cure versus cancer control, noting how improved therapies are leading to longer survival even with persistent disease, and how this trend challenges some of our thinking about survivorship.

Incidence and Mortality

Despite the steady decrease in incidence and mortality rates over the last three decades, CRC is still the fourth most commonly diagnosed cancer and the second leading cause of cancer death in the United States (US) [1, 2]. Five-year relative survival has increased from 48.5% in 1975 to 66.1% in 2005. More than one million Americans are living as CRC survivors [3].

Approximately 71,420 men and 64,010 women are diagnosed with CRC (accounting for 8% of all malignancies) and approximately 27,150 men and 23,110 women die of CRC each year in the US. [1]. The colorectal cancer incidence rate was 41.0 per 100,000 people per year between 2009 and 2013. During the same period, the annual age-adjusted death rate due to colorectal cancer was 15.1 per 100,000 [3].

Adenocarcinoma is not only the predominant histologic type of CRC, it is also the most common GI tract malignancy overall [1, 3]. The National Cancer Data Base (NCDB) has information about 913,415 colon cancer patients diagnosed between 2000 and 2011. Of these cases, subtypes including mucinous adenocarcinoma (8%) and adenocarcinoma arising in an adenomatous polyp (14%) were distinguished [4].

Gastroenteropancreatic neuroendocrine tumors (NETs), commonly known as carcinoid tumors, occur more frequently in the small bowel than the hindgut except among African Americans in whom the rectum is the most common gastrointestinal site. In the hindgut, rectal NETs are more common than colonic (0.86 vs 0.20 per 100,000). The 5-year survival rate for rectal (74–88%) and appendiceal (70–79%) NETs is better than in other colon segments (41–61%) [5, 6] (see Chapter 39 for more information about NETs).

Malignant lymphomas of the colon and rectum are rare, accounting for about 0.6% of all CRCs with diffuse large B-cell lymphoma being the most common histological subtype [7, 8]. Most colorectal lymphomas occur in the right colon [7, 9]. The incidence rate was 3.5 per million in the year 2000. The 5-year relative survival is 53% [7].

Squamous cell carcinoma represents 0.3% of all large intestine malignancies, predominantly affecting the rectum (93.4%), and has a 5-year relative survival of 48.9% [7].

Gastrointestinal stromal tumors are rare and constitute 0.1% of all colon and rectum tumors [10], and are discussed in greater detail in Chapter 11.

Risk Factors

Several risk factors have been associated with colon and rectal cancer, but some of these (family history and physical inactivity) are more strongly associated with colon than rectal cancer [11].

Age

More than 94% of CRC patients are over 44 years of age. The median age at the time of CRC diagnosis is 68 years [3].

The American Cancer Society's Oncology in Practice: Clinical Management, First Edition. Edited by The American Cancer Society.

Race and Gender

Incidence and mortality rates of CRC are approximately 30% and 40% higher, respectively in men than in women in the US. The lifetime risk of developing cancer of the colon or rectum is approximately 4.4% [3]. Among African Americans, the incidence rates are approximately 25% higher and mortality rates are 50% higher than among whites [2].

Familial History of CRC

About 20% of all CRC have a familial association. The number and younger age of CRC onset among first degree relatives (parent, sibling, or offspring) increase the risk of developing CRC. Having just one first degree relative with CRC increases an individual's risk two- to threefold compared to the general population. Having two first degree relatives with CRC or a young first-degree relative (diagnosed before the age of 45) increases the risk of CRC three to six times compared to people with no family history [12].

Polyps

Precursor polyps increasingly are diagnosed at the time of screening in people over 50 years of age (see Chapter 11 in *The American Cancer Society's Principles of Oncology: Prevention to Survivorship*).

Hereditary Risk Factors

Hereditary cases of CRC (≤10%) are associated with a particular genotype (see Pathophysiology). However, the prevalence of cancer susceptibility gene mutations is higher among individuals diagnosed with CRC prior to age 50 [13]. For more information, refer to Chapter 5 in *The American Cancer Society's Principles of Oncology: Prevention to Survivorship*. Two hereditary CRC syndromes are described.

Hereditary Non-Polyposis Colorectal Cancer (HNPCC) or Lynch Syndrome

This autosomal dominant syndrome due to mutations in mismatch repair (MMR) genes is associated with younger age of CRC diagnosis than sporadic CRC (42–61 years), predominance of right-sided cancer, and associated cancers at other sites [14]. The lifetime risk of developing CRC is 54–74% for men and 30–52% for women. Women with HNPCC have a 50% risk of developing endometrial carcinoma. The combined risk of developing a cancer at another site, principally ovarian, gastric, small bowel, pancreatic, hepatobiliary, brain, and urothelial neoplasms is ≤15% [15–17]. Amsterdam criteria and Bethesda guidelines define clinical criteria for diagnosing Lynch syndrome (see Table 9.1) [18, 19].

Familial Adenomatous Polyposis (FAP)

A germline mutation in the *APC* gene causes this autosomal dominant syndrome, and its variants accounts for approximately 1% of new CRC [20, 21]. There is nearly complete penetrance of colonic manifestations, and CRC occurs by the age of 40–50 years in the majority of patients [14, 22]. Penetrance of extracolonic manifestations (fundic gland polyps, duodenal polyps, thyroid cancers, central nervous system tumors, and childhood hepatoblastoma) is more variable. Duodenal adenomas have a 4–12% risk of malignant transformation [23, 24]. In contrast to classic FAP which is characterized by ≥100 adenomatous polyps, the attenuated form has fewer polyps (10–20 polyps) and lower risk of CRC (80% lifetime risk) that usually occurs later (fifth decade) [22, 25, 26].

Table 9.1 Amsterdam and Bethesda Criteria.

	Amsterdam II Criteria: 3-2-1 Rule	**Revised Bethesda Guidelines: Any one of the following**
Family members diagnosed with HNPCC-associated cancer[1]	3 relatives affected 2 or more successive generations affected	≥1 first degree relative, ≥1 diagnosed at age <50 >2 first or second degree relatives, diagnosed at any age
Age of diagnosis	1 diagnosis before age 50	CRC diagnosed at age <50
MSI-H histology[2]		At age <60
HNPCC-associated cancers		Synchronous or metachronous cancers diagnosed at any age
Sensitivity	77–81%	86–92%
Specificity	46–68%	49–58%

Source: Adapted from Kievit *et al.* [18] and Umar *et al.* [19].

[1] CRC, endometrial, stomach, ovarian, pancreas, ureter and renal pelvis, biliary tract, and brain tumors, sebaceous gland adenomas and keratoacanthomas, and carcinoma of the small bowel.

[2] Tumor-infiltrating lymphocytes, Crohn-like lymphocytic reaction, mucinous/signet-ring differentiation, or medullary growth pattern.

Inflammatory Bowel Disease

Ulcerative colitis and Crohn disease increase the risk of CRC 2.4-fold compared to the general population [27, 28]. CRC risk is proportional to the anatomic extent of active disease such that pancolitis poses a greater risk than segmental colitis [27, 29]. Duration of inflammatory bowel disease (IBD) also plays a major role increasing the cumulative risk of CRC. Patients with 10, 20, and 30-year history of ulcerative colitis have 1.6%, 8.3%, and 18.4% cumulative risk for CRC respectively [29]. Concurrent diagnosis of primary sclerosing cholangitis also increases the risk of CRC in IBD patients [30].

Prevention

There is a large body of literature reporting investigation of agents that have a potential role in primary and/or secondary prevention of CRC. The majority of these data are from observational studies and the evidence is not strong enough to recommend application to routine clinical practice. While there is more compelling data indicating that aspirin (ASA) and possibly other nonsteroidal anti-inflammatory drugs provides CRC risk reduction in average risk individuals, the balance of benefit and harm is not sufficiently favorable to recommend routine use. The US Preventive Services Task Force recently issued a grade B recommendation for "initiating low-dose aspirin use for the primary prevention of cardiovascular disease (CVD) and CRC in adults aged 50 to 59 years who have a 10% or greater 10-year CVD risk, are not at increased risk for bleeding, have a life expectancy of at least 10 years, and are willing to take low-dose aspirin daily for at least 10 years" [31].

Screening

Screening to detect colorectal cancer precursor lesions and early invasive disease has been demonstrated to reduce incidence of and mortality from this disease. Methods for colorectal cancer screening include fecal occult blood tests (which include guaiac-based and immunochemical-based tests), a multitarget test that combines an immunochemical-based test for occult blood with a stool DNA test, colonoscopy, flexible sigmoidoscopy, and computed tomography colonography [2, 32]. Guidelines for use of these tests are described in Chapter 11 of *The American Cancer Society's Principles of Oncology: Prevention to Survivorship.*

Signs and Symptoms

Most late stage tumors are symptomatic (63–92%), but the onset of symptoms is often indolent and results in delayed diagnosis [33].

Pain

While abdominal pain is a common presentation of malignancy, it is nonspecific. Steady pain may result from local invasion by the tumor into neighboring structures including the abdominal wall. Tenesmus or incontinence can occur when the pelvic floor or anal sphincter is involved. Alternatively, incontinence can also result from diarrhea caused by tumor mucus production (more often right colon or rectum) [34] or hypermotility due to partial obstruction.

Bleeding

Bleeding can be occult (anemia) or frank (melena or hematochezia). Bright red bleeding from rectal tumors leads to early diagnosis more often than for proximal tumors [35]. Because bleeding is the most common symptom and occurs in nearly two-thirds of all CRC cases, it must be taken seriously in all patients, even young ones [34, 36]. Although bleeding is typically a late sign of colon cancer, bleeding from rectal tumors can lead to earlier detection [35].

Change of Bowel Habit, Obstruction, Other Problems

Altered bowel habit such as decreased stool caliber or constipation occurs in 27% of patients and is more common with left-sided tumors [34]. Tumors of the right colon where the effluent is still fairly liquid rarely present with constipation unless the ileocecal valve is narrowed by tumor.

When early symptoms are ignored, progression to acute obstruction occurs in 15% of cases which results in catastrophic perforation in another 12–19% of cases. Often the perforation occurs in the thin-walled cecum proximal to the point of obstruction. Perforation causes feculent peritonitis, and intra-abdominal abscess formation and can be confused with diverticulitis or IBD. Colocutaneous or perirectal fistulae may develop. Colovesical fistulae are associated with urinary tract infections or pneumaturia. Except in cases of obstruction and perforation, overall prognosis is more strongly associated with the tumor's histopathological features than with specific symptoms or their duration. Perforation is associated with increased risk of peritoneal recurrence, and thus worse survival [37, 38]. An unusual presentation is sepsis from Group D streptococcus (*Streptococcus bovis*).

Pathophysiology

The pathophysiology of CRC can broadly be categorized as sporadic (~70%), familial (~25%), or hereditary (<10%). The multistep adenoma–carcinoma sequence involves the accumulation of genetic changes which confer a selective growth advantage to colonic epithelial cells [39]. Three distinct CRC tumorigenesis pathways have been elucidated:

1) The chromosomal instability (CIN) pathway or the adenomatous polyposis coli (APC) pathway characterized by chromosomal abnormalities including deletions, insertions, and loss of heterozygosity (LOH)
2) The DNA mismatch repair pathway associated with germline mutations in one of several DNA MMR genes
3) The hypermethylation (CIMP+) pathway associated with epigenetic alterations such as promoter methylation of certain genes including MMR genes.

CIN (APC) Pathway

One of the most crucial and early events in CRC tumorigenesis is loss of the *APC* gene [40]. A somatic mutation in both alleles of the *APC* gene is present in approximately 80% of patients with sporadic CRC, and the germline mutation of this gene is responsible for FAP [26].

Other well described gene alterations in the CIN pathway include *RAS* mutations, *TP53* gene mutations, 18q LOH, and abnormalities in the transforming growth factor-beta (TGF-β) signaling pathway.

DNA MMR Pathway (Microsatellite Instability)

Germline mutations in the DNA MMR genes are responsible for Lynch syndrome, and accounts for 3–5% of CRC. These tumors are microsatellite unstable (MSI-H) as a result of these mutations.

MSI-H status can also be seen in sporadic CRC, but this is usually due to epigenetic silencing of the MMR genes (usually *MLH1*) by promoter hypermethylation. In either case, since mutations in the MMR genes lead to a truncated or lost protein product, immunohistochemistry can be used for screening and has a predictive value virtually identical to that of polymerase chain reaction-based MSI testing [41].

Hypermethylation (CIMP+) Pathway

Epigenetic silencing of MMR genes results from promoter hypermethylation and gives rise to an MSI-H phenotype [42]. These tumors usually harbor a *BRAF* mutation [43, 44], which abrogates the favorable prognosis associated with MSI-H tumors [45]. Biologically, these tumors tend to arise from serrated polyps in the right side of the colon [46].

Staging

Staging of tumors not only provides a common language for studying cancers and treatment outcomes, it forms the starting place for rational treatment planning and enables us to forecast outcomes for patients considering treatment options.

TNM Staging System

The TNM staging system [47] is summarized in Table 9.2, but several features specific to CRC should be highlighted. Although the staging parameters are the same for colon and rectal cancers, the actual practice of staging tumors at the two sites is quite different. Preoperative staging is much more refined for rectal than colon cancer and more directly influences treatment planning. In contrast to the rectum, the T and N category cannot be reliably established for colon tumors preoperatively [48] except that computed tomography (CT) scans may distinguish T4 from other T status in 86% of cases [49, 50].

Physical examination findings such as distant or perirectal adenopathy, carcinomatosis settled in the Pouch of Douglas ("Blumer shelf"), or tumor fixation associated with invasion of neighboring structures appreciated by digital rectal examination or abdominal palpation contribute to staging. Most staging, however, depends on imaging: ultrasound, CT, magnetic resonance imaging (MRI), and positron emission tomography (PET) scan.

M Category

In the US, 19% of colon and 13% of rectal cancers are metastatic at the time of diagnosis [51], with liver and lung as the most common metastatic sites [48]. The American College of Radiology Appropriateness Criteria recommend a CT scan of the abdomen and pelvis and standard chest X-ray for initial staging of colon cancer. Although it is uncommon for lung metastases to develop before liver metastases, this does occur more often with rectal primary tumors than colon and underlies the American College of Radiology preference for chest CT over X-ray for initial staging of rectal cancer [48]. In colon cancer, the preoperative detection rate of liver metastases is as high as 99%, but detection of carcinomatosis by CT is poor (33%). Triple contrast CT of the liver, MRI, or PET are often necessary to discriminate metastatic from benign liver lesions. The sensitivity and specificity of PET identification of liver metastases or carcinomatosis is 89% and 64% respectively [48]. Especially when PET is negative, biopsy will be needed to confirm suspected metastasis.

T Category

In the absence of metastasis or locally advanced tumors, treatment of colon cancer typically commences with surgical resection. Rectal cancer therapy, on the other hand, depends on the T and N category and other tumor features. Ultrasound and MRI have proven more accurate than CT for estimating depth of rectal tumor penetration [52]. Each has limitations, and neither is reliable following neoadjuvant radiation therapy (RT). Not surprisingly, the accuracy depends on interpreter experience and use of rectal cancer specific protocols [53]. Ultrasound is difficult for tumors that are either very low or high in the rectum or near-obstructing. Despite the expense of MRI, it can provide valuable information for treatment planning that will be discussed later.

Table 9.2 Classification of colon and rectum cancer according to the AJCC 8th edition (2017).

Definitions of AJCC TNM	
Definition of Primary Tumor (T)	
T category	**T criteria**
TX	Primary tumor cannot be assessed
T0	No evidence of primary tumor
Tis	Carcinoma *in situ*, intramucosal carcinoma (involvement of lamina propria with no extension through muscularis mucosae)
T1	Tumor invades the submucosa (through the muscularis mucosa but not into the muscularis propria)
T2	Tumor invades the muscularis propria
T3	Tumor invades through the muscularis propria into pericolorectal tissues
T4	Tumor invades the visceral peritoneum or invades or adheres to adjacent organ or structure
T4a	Tumor invades through the visceral peritoneum (including gross perforation of the bowel through tumor and continuous invasion of tumor through areas of inflammation to the surface of the visceral peritoneum)
T4b	Tumor directly invades or adheres to adjacent organs or structures
Definition of Regional Lymph Node (N)	
N category	**N criteria**
NX	Regional lymph nodes cannot be assessed
N0	No regional lymph node metastasis
N1	One to three regional lymph nodes are positive (tumor in lymph nodes measuring ≥0.2 mm), or any number of tumor deposits are present and all identifiable lymph nodes are negative
N1a	One regional lymph node is positive
N1b	Two or three regional lymph nodes are positive
N1c	No regional lymph nodes are positive, but there are tumor deposits in the: • subserosa • mesentery • or nonperitonealized pericolic, or perirectal/mesorectal tissues.
N2	Four or more regional nodes are positive
N2a	Four to six regional lymph nodes are positive
N2b	Seven or more regional lymph nodes are positive

(*Continued*)

Table 9.2 (Continued)

Definition of Distant Metastasis (M)

M category	M criteria
M0	No distant metastasis by imaging, etc.; no evidence of tumor in distant sites or organs (This category is not assigned by pathologists.)
M1	Metastasis to one or more distant sites or organs or peritoneal metastasis is identified
M1a	Metastasis to one site or organ is identified without peritoneal metastastis
M1b	Metastasis to two or more sites or organs is identified without peritoneal metastasis
M1c	Metastasis to the peritoneal surface is identified alone or with other site or organ metastases

AJCC Prognostic Stage Groups

When T is...	And N is...	And M is...	Then the stage group is...
Tis	N0	M0	0
T1, T2	N0	M0	I
T3	N0	M0	IIA
T4a	N0	M0	IIB
T4b	N0	M0	IIC
T1–T2	N1/N1c	M0	IIIA
T1	N2a	M0	IIIA
T3–T4a	N1/N1c	M0	IIIB
T2–T3	N2a	M0	IIIB
T1–T2	N2b	M0	IIIB
T4a	N2a	M0	IIIC
T3–T4a	N2b	M0	IIIC
T4b	N1–N2	M0	IIIC
Any T	Any N	M1a	IVA
Any T	Any N	M1b	IVB
Any T	Any N	M1c	IVC

Source: Amin *et al.* [47]. Used with permission of the American College of Surgeons, Chicago, Illinois. The original source for this information is the AJCC Cancer Staging Manual, 8th Edition (2017), which is published by Springer Science+Business Media.

N Category

Regardless of imaging modality, there is always a trade-off between sensitivity and specificity identifying involved regional lymph nodes (LN). Again, both ultrasound and MRI appear to be more accurate than CT [54]. Size, morphology, inhomogeneity, and contour help to characterize LNs (Table 9.3).

Beyond TNM

Response to Neoadjuvant Chemoradiation

The TNM system is a powerful tool but fails to capture some very important prognostic features. Anatomic TNM categories recapitulate the behavior of typical solid organ tumor progression from primary site to regional lymph nodes to metastasis (see Chapter 11 in *The American Cancer Society's Principles of Oncology: Prevention to Survivorship*). Stage at different time points can be distinguished as clinical (prefix c) versus pathological (p) stage, post-treatment stage (y), or recurrence stage (r). Still, it is a static system that records status at two time points but does not grade treatment response. Thus, rectal tumor response to neoadjuvant chemoradiation (neoadjuvant CRT) which is emerging as perhaps the strongest predictor of outcome and may be a de facto bioassay of tumor virulence, is not reflected in the tumor stage [55].

Substratification of Depth of Penetration

Substratification of T1 and T3 categories may influence rectal cancer treatment planning. For T1, three levels of submucosa encroachment have been delineated: SM1 (most superficial) to SM3. SM1 tumors are less likely than SM2/SM3 tumors to involve regional LNs and may therefore be more suitable for full-thickness local excision (FTLE) alone than either radical resection or neoadjuvant CRT and FTLE [56]. For T3 rectal tumors, spread 5 mm beyond the muscularis propria has been associated with increased risk of both local and distant failure and has been proposed as a more reliable prognostic indicator of metastatic risk than regional LN positivity [57]. Also, T3 tumor proximity to the mesorectal fascia (MRF) may be a better indicator of need for neoadjuvant CRT than either node-positive status or T3 status since even excellent surgical technique can result in an involved circumferential resection margin (CRM) when the tumor abuts the MRF [58].

Lymphovascular Invasion

Lymphovascular invasion (LVI) also has been reported as a stronger negative prognostic factor than LN status [59]. Perhaps clinical nodal status and depth of tumor penetration beyond the muscularis propria are more easily determined with current technology and inadvertently serve as proxies for LVI [60].

Genetic Factors

Biologic and genetic factors such as MSI and MMR, *KRAS* and *BRAF* mutations are prognostic and predictive factors relevant to treatment planning but are not integral to TNM staging. Gene microarray studies have not yet matured but hold promise for more reliably predicting tumor behavior and enhancing stage grouping.

Pretreatment Assessment

When there are equivocal or contradictory staging studies and examinations, it can be helpful to determine the clinical stage at the multidisciplinary treatment conference where specialists can provide more nuanced interpretations of the studies and their relative accuracy.

Colon Cancer

Except when bleeding, obstruction, or perforation demands emergency resection, the preoperative assessment of colon cancer should include colonoscopy to complete evaluation of the colon, biopsy of the tumor, and staging imaging. The site should be tattooed in a way that is clearly stated in the colonoscopy report.

Table 9.3 Pretreatment radiologic staging parameters for endorectal ultrasound (ERUS) and magnetic resonance imaging (MRI).

	Rectal wall invasion [82, 168, 169]	Lymph node involvement [169–173]	Threatened circumferential margin (mesorectal fascia involvement) [52, 174]
ERUS	T1: Break in submucosa T2: Penetration through submucosa, thickening of muscularis propria T3: Extension into perirectal fat T4: Penetration into adjacent structure	Round shape, irregular contour, proximity to primary tumor, size >5 mm	Mesorectal fascia not imaged with ERUS
MRI	T1: Smooth muscularis propria margin T2: Tumor penetrates muscularis propria; spiculation in mesorectal fat can be fibrosis, not tumor T3: Nodular bulge or projection into mesorectum T4: Abnormal signal extends into adjacent organ (loss of fat plane not sufficient) or into peritoneal space	Irregular contour and heterogenous signal intensity are more accurate than size. Over 50% of pN-positive lymph nodes are <5 mm on MRI	Tumor <1 mm from mesorectal fascia on MRI. High correlation between pathologic CRM >1 mm if 5 mm separation of tumor from mesorectal fascia on MRI. Note: threat of proximity of suspicious lymph node to mesorectal fascia has not specifically been defined. Authors conservatively apply same measures to lymph node as tumor proximity.

Source: Kosinski *et al.* [54].
CRM, circumferential (radial) resection margin.

For patients under 50 or those who meet Amsterdam or Bethesda criteria (see Table 9.1), MSI should be assessed preoperatively on the biopsy specimen since HNPCC diagnosis may dictate extended resection. Digital rectal examination and anoscopy should be performed by the consulting surgeon to assess continence and exclude the presence of a second lesion which can be overlooked by colonoscopy. Sigmoid or rectosigmoid tumors are often found to be upper rectal when assessed by the consulting surgeon with flexible or rigid sigmoidoscopy. The laparoscopic surgeon should also consider repeating the colonoscopy to confirm tumor location even if previously tattooed, especially for tumors at the splenic flexure. The resection limits differ for distal transverse versus proximal descending colon tumors, and with laparoscopic resection, the tumor cannot be palpated, and port site placement differs [61, 62].

Rectal Cancer

Staging priorities are the same as outlined for colon cancer with a couple of notable exceptions. First, it is imperative that the rectal tumor be precisely localized by the consulting surgeon to help determine which operation will be performed and whether sphincter preservation is possible; flexible endoscopy can be misleading regarding tumor level. The pretreatment assessment determines the need for and response to neoadjuvant CRT. T and N category are assessed by either MRI or ultrasound. There has been a gradual migration towards using MRI for T status because of its superior evaluation of MRF involvement and LVI [54]. Note that "T stage" criteria developed for MRI do not precisely parallel TNM criteria (Table 9.4).

Treatment Modalities

Treatment is often thought of as local (or locoregional) or systemic, but in practical terms, there is an interplay that does not follow such neat divisions.

Surgery for Colon Cancer

Limits of Resection: Margins, Lymph Nodes, Technical Issues

The limits of resection of colon tumors are defined by the risk of microscopic longitudinal intramural spread, radial clearance of tumor, and sufficient LN harvest for accurate staging and treatment planning and removal of involved nodes. A 5 cm longitudinal margin is standard and is generally easily obtained in the colon in contrast to the rectum where a centimeter or two can make the difference between sphincter preservation and permanent colostomy. Close evaluation of microscopic longitudinal spread in rectal cancers has shown that 2 cm is safe [63]. Achieving a tumor-free radial margin can require *en bloc* resection of adherent neighboring structures. In a recent retrospective review, 16% of patients with pT3 or pT4 tumors underwent multivisceral resection. Of those tumors adherent to adjacent, resected structures, just 53% were pT4. Despite having a poorer prognosis T category and increased perioperative complications associated with more extensive resection, the disease-free survival was equivalent to pT3 patients undergoing standard resection [64]. Traversing tumor may contribute to seeding peritoneal tumor implants [65].

The standard that a minimum of 12 LNs be recovered from CRC resection specimens was adopted in 1999 by the College of American Pathologists as a Category 1 CRC prognostic factor based on studies reporting a correlation between increased number of LNs harvested and improved survival [66]. Failure to identify a minimum of 12 LNs can be a function of compromised surgical technique, incomplete evaluation of the specimen by the pathologist, or patient habitus. Above a certain threshold of LN harvest, however, stage does not change to account for improved survival, suggesting that LN retrieval may, beyond a minimum number, be a marker of other dimensions of quality care [67, 68]. Extended lymphadenectomy has not been shown to improve local recurrence (LR) or reduce distant failure in colon cancer in North America or Europe.

Table 9.4 AJCC/UICC T categories versus MERCURY Trial "T-Staging" criteria.[1]

	AJCC T category criteria	Mercury Trial "T staging" criteria [52, 175]
Tis	*In situ* carcinoma	No corresponding value
T0	No evidence of viable tumor cells	No evidence of primary tumor
T1	Tumor invades submucosa	Tumor invades submucosa. Low signal in submucosal layer or replacement of submucosal layer by abnormal signal not extending into circular muscle layer
T2	Tumor invades into but not through muscularis propria	Tumor invades into but not through muscularis propria. Intermediate signal intensity (higher signal than muscle, lower signal than submucosa) in muscularis propria; outer muscle coat replaced by tumor of intermediate signal intensity that does not extend beyond outer muscle into perirectal fat.
T3	Tumor invades through muscularis propria into mesorectal/subserosal fat	Tumor invades through muscularis propria into mesorectal/subserosal fat. Broad-based bulge or nodular projection (not fine spiculation) of intermediate signal intensity projecting beyond outer muscular coat
T3a	No corresponding category	Tumor extends <1 mm beyond muscularis propria
T3b	No corresponding category	Tumor extends 1–5 mm beyond muscularis propria
T3c	No corresponding category	Tumor extends >5–15 mm beyond muscularis propria
T3d	No corresponding category	Tumor extends >15 mm beyond muscularis propria
T4	Tumor invades the visceral peritoneum or invades or adheres to adjacent organ or structure	Tumor invades other organs. Extension of abnormal signal into adjacent organ; extension of tumor signal through peritoneal reflection
T4a	Tumor involves the visceral peritoneum	No corresponding category
T4b	Tumor invades adjacent structures/organs	See T4 above

Source: Kosinski *et al.* [54].
AJCC, American Joint Committee on Cancer; UICC, International Union Against Cancer.
[1] Mesorectal fascia involvement has not specifically been incorporated into magnetic resonance imaging (MRI) "T staging" schema, but a distance of >6 mm between the tumor or involved lymph node and the mesorectal fascia on MRI corresponds to a pathologic margin of ≥2 mm and a distance of >5 mm on MRI corresponds to a pathologic margin of ≥1 mm).
Adapted from [52] and [174]

However, retrospective analysis of colon cancer resection specimens found overall survival improved by 15% when the mesocolon was intact with a long vascular pedicle. In a comparison of Japanese D3 resections (high arterial ligation and extended lymphadenectomy) with German complete mesocolic excision and central (high) vascular ligation, the LN harvest was actually greater in the complete mesocolic excision specimens [69].

Technical issues also influence colon cancer resection limits. Figure 9.1 illustrates colon resection limits based on tumor site. Note that synchronous colon cancers can be managed with simultaneous segmental resections or subtotal colectomy; the rectum can usually be spared, but close observation will be required [70]. Total proctocolectomy is recommended for patients with CRC in the setting of ulcerative colitis. Extended resection should also be considered in patients with HNPC [71].

Operative Approach

Large tumor size or other adverse features such as extensive intra-abdominal adhesions may require that an open operation be performed, but laparoscopic colon resection for cancer has been shown to be safe and with at least comparable oncologic outcomes compared to conventional open surgery [72]. Robotic colon resections for cancer have been reported and appear to be safe; there is still debate about the value of this technology for colon resections given increased operating time and expense [73, 74].

Surgery for Rectal Cancer

Total Mesorectal Excision

To date, the greatest contribution to improved oncologic and functional rectal cancer surgery outcomes has been identification of the correct dissection plane: the MRF or "holy plane" of proctectomy [75] resulting in a total mesorectal excision (TME) (Figure 9.2). Specimen integrity can be graded by pathologists, and the interchange between pathologist and surgeon has led to quantifiable improvement in rectal cancer outcomes (see Table 9.5) [76]. Treatment outcomes have been achieved at the national level by implementing training programs for surgeons, radiologists, and pathologists in the TME technique, preoperative radiologic assessment of the cancer, and pathologic evaluation of the TME specimen [77, 78].

Adequate surgery alone (without neoadjuvant CRT or neoadjuvant RT) achieved the same LR reduction (~10%) as neoadjuvant RT without TME [75, 79–81]. Subsequent studies that paired neoadjuvant RT with TME showed a further reduction of LR to 5% [82–84]. Currently, work is underway to discriminate which features might spare costly neoadjuvant RT and its attendant sequelae even for T3 and node-positive rectal cancer; some of these were discussed in the previous section on staging.

Margins

Attainment of negative CRM for proctectomy corresponds with improved LR rates more strongly than longitudinal margin status. Current standards for the longitudinal margin are 2 cm

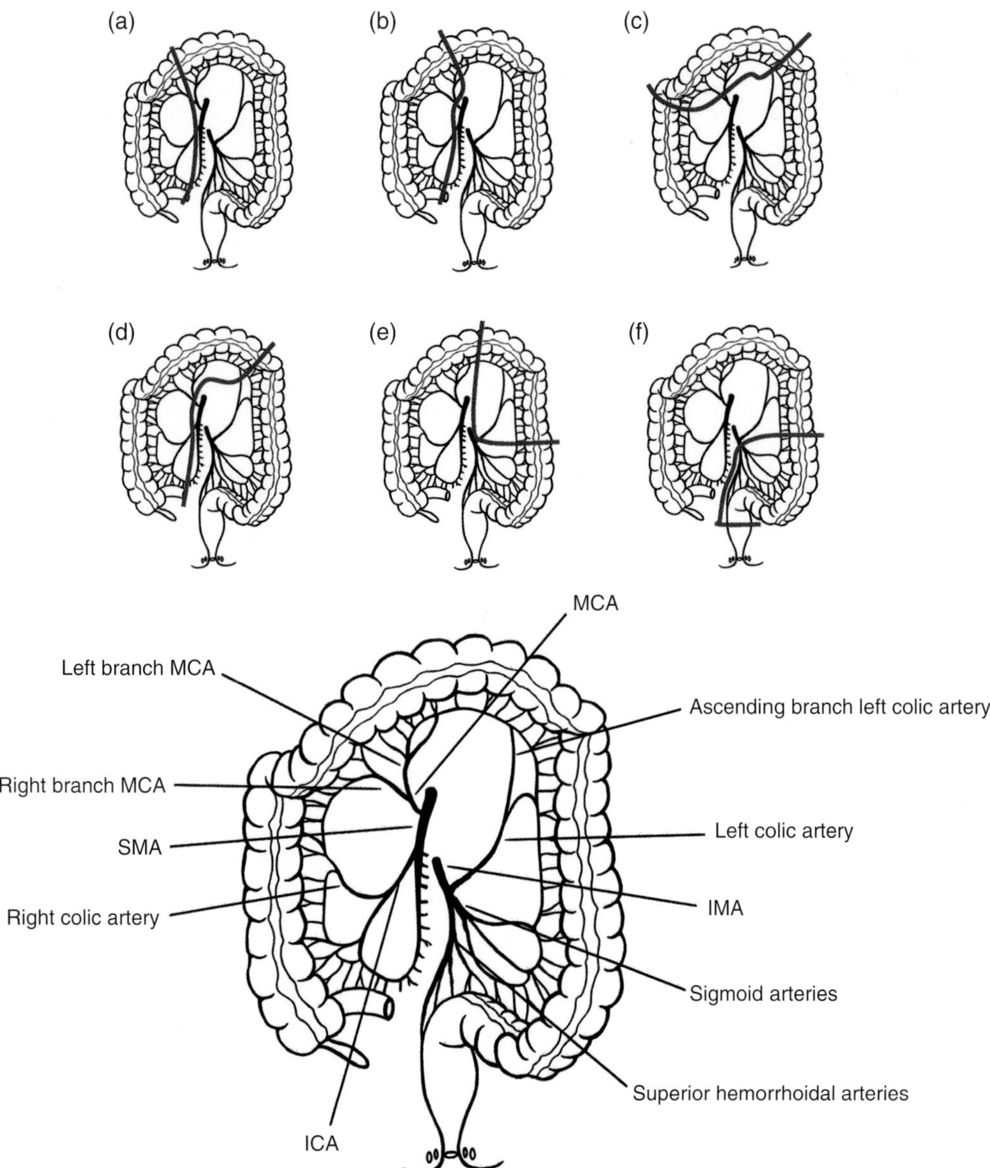

Figure 9.1 Colon cancer resections limits based on tumor location. (a) Right hemicolectomy. (b) Extended right hemicolectomy. (c) Transverse colectomy. (d) Extended right colectomy. (e) Left colectomy. (f) Sigmoid colectomy. ICA, ileocoloic artery; IMA, inferior mesenteric artery; MCA, middle coloic artery; SMA, superior mesenteric artery. *Source:* Sang W. Lee, MD, FACS, FASCRS. Reproduced with permission of Dr Lee.

of normal tissue distal to the tumor in the nonirradiated patient and 1 cm after neoadjuvant RT. The CRM must have a clearance of 1 mm to be considered negative. It is important to realize that a negative CRM can be achieved even if the TME is poor. In other words, there can be a satisfactory margin of normal tissue around the tumor even if the MRF is not intact. Likewise, a good quality TME can still result in an involved CRM if the tumor is very close to the MRF [54].

Rectal Cancer Operative Procedures

Operations for rectal cancer are broadly categorized as sphincter-sparing and nonsphincter-sparing (see Table 9.6 and Figure 9.3). An abdominoperineal resection which involves removal of the anus, rectum, and sometimes additional bowel results in a permanent colostomy and is the definitive nonsphincter-sparing procedure. Even when the anus is retained after removal of the rectum ("proctectomy" or "low anterior resection" (LAR)), an operation is still considered nonsphincter sparing if a permanent colostomy is constructed, a temporary colostomy is never reversed, or a diverting loop stoma is created as definitive (usually palliative) management of a rectal cancer. Sphincter-sparing operations can be further divided into radical resections (the rectum is removed) or FTLE. Three kinds of radical resections are performed: LAR, LAR with coloanal anastomosis, and intersphincteric resection. In this order, each is a strategy for sphincter preservation for increasingly more caudal tumors. A temporary diverting ileostomy or colostomy is usually created with resections that are either very low or intersphincteric when neoadjuvant CRT was given. Diverting stomas do not decrease leak rates but can reduce the morbidity of a leaking colorectal or coloanal anastomosis [85, 86].

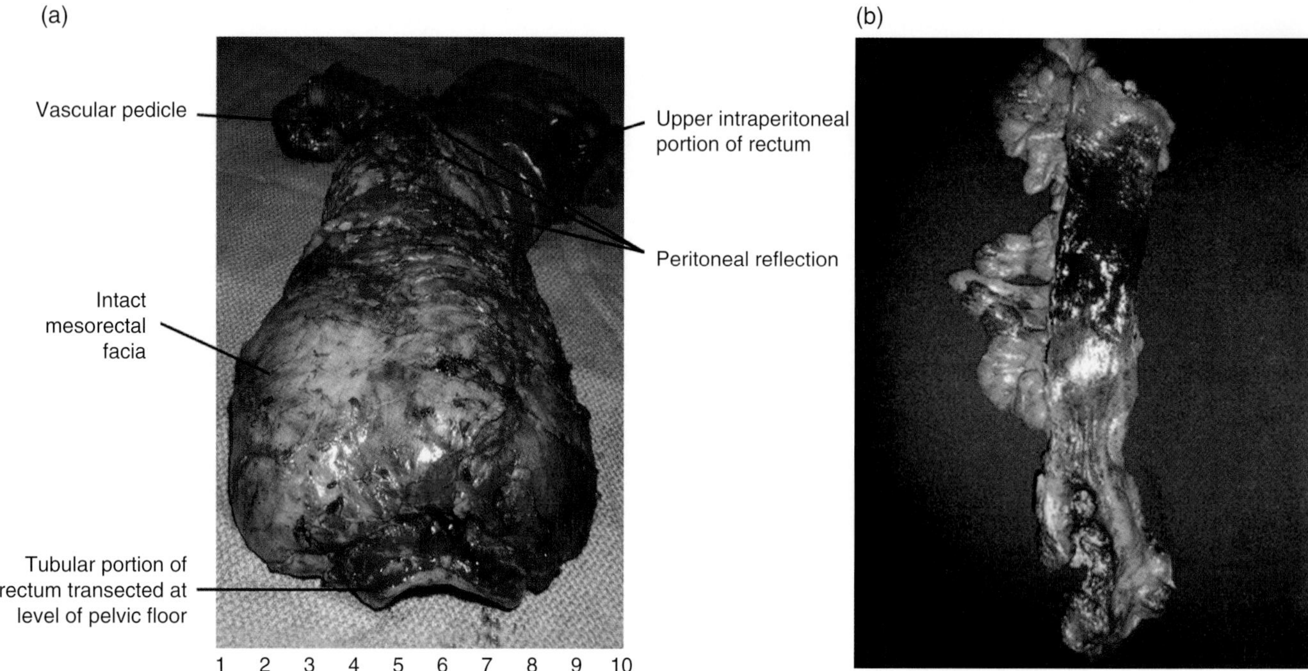

Figure 9.2 Total mesorectal excision (TME). (a) Good quality TME shows vascular pedicle and glistening mesorectal fascia without defects. (b) Poor quality TME with numerous defects noted not just through the mesorectal fascia but violating the muscularis propria. *Source:* Kosinski *et al.* [54].

Table 9.5 Total mesorectal excision quality grading and relationship to negative circumferential resection margin [76].

Negative circumferential resection margin (>1 mm) (%)	Mesorectal dissection grade	Features defining mesorectal dissection grade
75.9	Complete	Intact mesorectum
		Minor irregularities (<5 mm deep)
		No coning in toward distal margin
13.0	Nearly complete	Moderate bulk of mesorectum
		Moderate coning
		No muscularis propria visible except at levators
11.1	Incomplete	Little bulk to mesorectum with defects down to muscularis propria and/or very irregular surface

Source: Kosinski *et al.* [54].

Prospective randomized trials evaluating laparoscopic and robotic minimally invasive rectal cancer operations are underway [87]. There are numerous nonrandomized trials suggesting that, just as with minimally invasive colon cancer resections, these are safe alternatives to open operations [54].

Construction of Neorectum

Although a straight anastomosis between the colon and anal or rectal remnant can be performed and is still the best technical choice in many cases, data show better function in the first 6 months after surgery if the neorectal reservoir is enlarged by making a colon J-pouch or by performing a side-to-end (colon to rectum) anastomosis or coloplasty (Figure 9.4) [88–90].

Radiation Therapy

Radiation therapy (RT) has broader application for rectal than for colon cancer. Table 9.7 summarizes RT modalities. Chemotherapy administered concurrently with neoadjuvant RT sensitizes tumor cells to radiation [91]. RT can be given preoperatively (neoadjuvant RT), intra- or postoperatively (adjuvant RT). It can be administered externally (external beam RT) or internally (brachytherapy). When given via external beam, different techniques can be employed including 3D conformal RT, intensity-modulated RT, stereotactic body RT, or contact RT (Papillon technique). Used preoperatively, it can reduce tumor bulk and render tumors more resectable, enhance sphincter preservation rates, potentially "sterilize" contained perforations so that tumor cells are less likely to be dispersed throughout the abdominal cavity or pelvis during resection, and augment technically optimal surgical resection to reduce LR rates and improve overall survival [82–84]. Intraoperatively, it can reduce LR when resection margins are expected to be positive [92]. In rectal cancer neoadjuvant RT has better local control and less toxicity than adjuvant RT, so the need for adjuvant RT should generally be regarded as an indication of staging or operative failure [82]. There are fewer applications of RT in colon cancer treatment. Intraoperative RT or adjuvant RT can be delivered to the resection field following *en bloc* resection of the colon tumor invasion of the abdominal wall. Several retrospective series demonstrate a benefit of RT in the setting of perforation or invasion of an adjacent organ.

Table 9.6 Operations for rectal cancer.

	Radical resection (TME)[1]		No radical resection	
Sphincter-preserving	LAR with colorectal anastomosis	Proctectomy with transection below the peritoneal reflection (midrectum or lower) leaving a cuff of rectum; sigmoid colectomy; and colon J-pouch or straight anastomosis	TEM	Full-thickness local excision
	Ultra-LAR with coloanal anastomosis	Proctectomy with transection at the pelvic floor below the mesorectum at the rectal muscular tube, leaving rectal mucosa within the functional anal canal; sigmoid colectomy; and colon J-pouch or straight anastomosis	Transanal excision	Full-thickness local excision
	ISR or TATA	Proctectomy with transection of the rectum within the functional anal canal (at or just above dentate line, across the rectal mucosa and superior internal anal sphincter), sigmoid colectomy. Incision can be at the anal verge, in which case the entire internal anal sphincter is removed. Colon J-pouch or straight anastomosis		
	Total abdominoproctocolectomy with ileal J-pouch anastomosis	Proctectomy as for ultra-LAR or ISR, total colectomy, ileal J-pouch anal anastomosis		
Nonsphincter-preserving	APR	Anal canal removed (either intersphincteric dissection which preserves external anal sphincter, or extralevator or ischioanal dissection, which includes ischiorectal fat and entire sphincter muscle); proctectomy; sigmoidectomy; and permanent end stoma		
	Total abdominal proctocolectomy	Same as APR but the entire colon is removed and end ileostomy created		
Functionally nonsphincter-preserving	LAR with permanent colostomy	Same as LAR but no anastomosis is created. Anus is left in place and end stoma is created. May remove entire colon.	Permanent diverting colostomy	No resection, loop or end stoma

Source: Kosinski *et al.* [54].

APR, abdominoperineal resection; ISR, intersphincteric resection; LAR, low anterior resection; TATA, transabdominal transanal resection; TEM, transanal endoscopic microsurgery; TME, total mesorectal excision.

[1] Approach can be open, laparoscopic, hand-assisted laparoscopic, laparoscopic hybrid, or robotic.

External Beam RT

The two dominant external beam RT regimens for rectal cancer are:

- Short course ("5 × 5 therapy"): 5 Gy daily for 5 days without chemotherapy, less than 1 week delay to surgery.
- Long course: typically 1.8–2 Gy daily for 20–30 days, often with a boost to the tumor bed in the final days to achieve a total dose of 4500–5400 cGy, 6–12 week delay to surgery.

The goals of RT are to achieve or augment regional control while minimizing damage to normal tissue. This was enhanced by 3D conformal planning in the late 1980s and early 1990s [93, 94]. Intensity-modulated RT is a radiation technique that can be extremely useful to minimize collateral injury such as when a significant amount of small bowel would be exposed in the standard 3D plan. Nonetheless, the majority of patients with rectal cancer are treated with a 3D conformal approach. In the US, long course neoadjuvant CRT is the predominant regimen [95, 96]. This is also the only treatment regimen that sets the stage for potential nonoperative management of rectal cancer [97]. Elsewhere, short course therapy is often preferred and may be given only when the MRF is threatened or T3 tumor penetration is greater than 5 mm beyond the muscularis propria [80, 83]. RT is expensive and is associated with higher anastomotic leak rates, possibly poorer function of the neorectum (especially when given postoperatively), insufficiency fractures of the pelvis and femur, delayed microvascular disease and stricture of exposed bowel, bladder, and vagina, and potentially secondary tumors [82, 98–100]. The best use of RT is currently an active subject of debate among rectal cancer specialists.

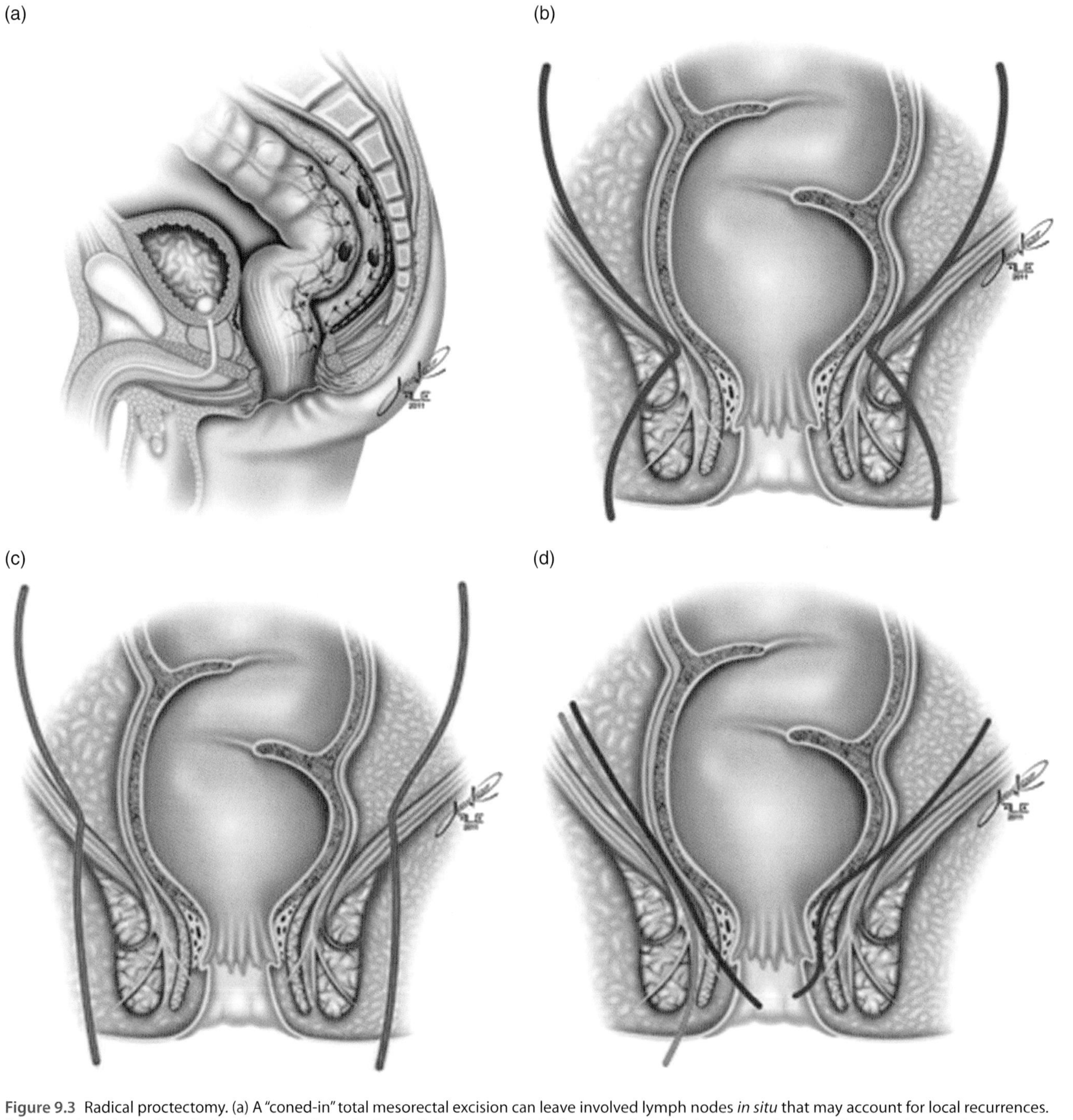

(a)

(b)

(c)

(d)

Figure 9.3 Radical proctectomy. (a) A "coned-in" total mesorectal excision can leave involved lymph nodes *in situ* that may account for local recurrences. (b) Dissection (shown in red) that leaves a waist at the level of the levators, which is appropriate for a low or ultralow anterior resection, can leave tumor behind during an abdominoperineal resection that is typically performed for suspected involvement of the levators. (c) An abdominoperineal resection with cylindrical excision (shown in green) that does not taper along the mesorectal fascia as it approaches the pelvic floor and more widely incorporates the levators which may result in lower positive circumferential margin rates. (d) Intersphincteric resections maintain gastrointestinal continuity but sacrifice some (or all) of the internal anal sphincter to achieve a full-thickness resection and negative circumferential resection margin in the very low rectum (green indicates standard resection beginning at or just above the dentate line; blue, complete removal of internal anal sphincter (not commonly performed)). Mucosectomy (indicated by the red line) does not achieve a full-thickness resection and is therefore not recommended for rectal cancer. *Source:* Kosinski *et al.* [54].

Particle Radiotherapy

Traditional RT uses photons to treat tumors. Expense has been a hurdle to introducing particle RT which uses protons or other charged particles to deliver energy to tumors. The appeal of proton therapy is the narrow range of high energy delivery to tissue. The relatively low dose delivery of energy to tissues before the peak dose (Bragg peak) delivery and the lack of exit dose beyond the target lesion may result in less collateral tissue damage. This is an active area of investigation.

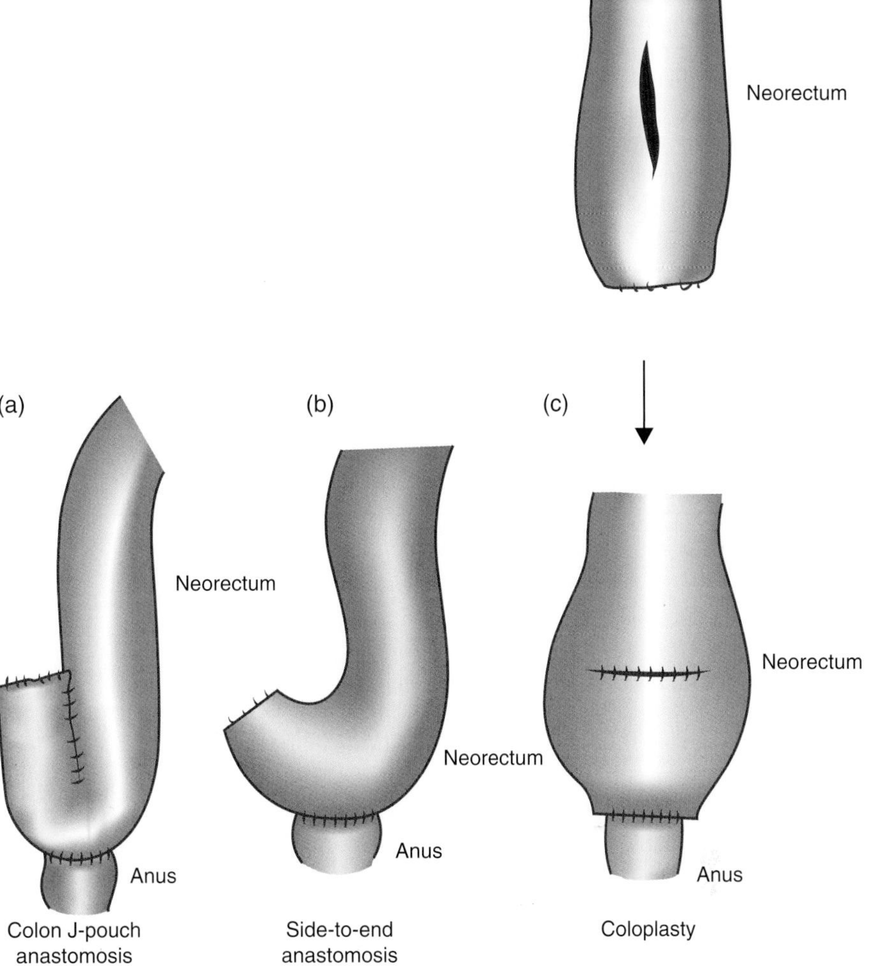

Figure 9.4 Neorectal construction. (a) Colon J-pouch anastomosis. (b) Side-to-end anastomosis. (c) Coloplasty.

Table 9.7 Radiotherapy treatment modalities.

Modality	Type		Energy source	Description
External beam (EBRT)	3-dimensional conformal radiation therapy (3DCRT)		Photons (linear accelerator)	Fractionated therapy delivered regionally
	Intensity modulated radiation therapy (IMRT)		Photons (linear accelerator)	Allows for nonuniform dose (dose painting)
	Particle radiotherapy		Protons (cyclotron)	Narrow range of energy delivery
	Stereotactic radiotherapy	Stereotactic body radiation therapy (SBRT)	Photons (linear accelerator)	Multiple conformal beams delivering the highest dose to area overlapped
		Gamma knife	Gamma rays (photons)	Single treatment; a type of stereotactic radiation therapy
		Cyber Knife™		
	Intraoperative radiotherapy (IORT)		Photons (IORT) or Electrons(IOERT)	
	Contact therapy (Papillon)		Photons or X-rays	
Brachytherapy	Interstitial implant		Photons (HDR= iridium, LDR= iodine)	Low-dose rate (LDR) or High-dose date (HDR)
	Endorectal or intracavitary brachytherapy (Vuong)		Photons (HDR = iridium 194, LDR = cesium 137)	
	Intra-arterial		Beta-emitter (Yittrium 90)	Theraspheres for liver metastasis
	Intravenous		Beta and gamma emitter (strontium or samarium)	For bone metastasis

Chemotherapy

Chemotherapy is usually classified as systemic therapy, but it also plays a role in local control of solid organ tumors and is utilized to achieve different goals in three settings: (i) neoadjuvant chemotherapy given preoperatively; (ii) adjuvant chemotherapy given after curative-intent surgery when there is locally advanced primary tumor, +/− positive regional LNs; (iii) chemotherapy for metastatic CRC given either with intent to convert unresectable metastases to resectable disease or as palliative therapy. Despite these differences, the regimens share some guiding principles:

- Fluoropyrimidines (5-fluorouracil (5-FU) or capecitabine) form the backbone of chemotherapy regimens
- Various cytotoxic and/or targeted agents are utilized concurrently or sequentially based on the goal of therapy, response, and toxicity associated with treatment
- When treatment is administered with a palliative intent, cancer cells often develop resistance to therapy largely due to emergence/selection advantage of chemotherapy resistant clones.

Common chemotherapy agents used in CRC are listed in Table 9.8. Chemotherapy is sometimes administered with a goal to "downstage" unresectable metastatic CRC to resectable status ("conversion therapy") to exploit the response (shrinkage) seen in both the primary tumor as well as the metastases. Response to chemotherapy, or lack thereof, in such situations may be a surrogate for tumor biology/tumor virulence.

Table 9.8 Common chemotherapy agents in colorectal cancer management.[1]

Class	Generic	Trade	Route	Mechanism
Cytotoxic therapies				
Antimetabolite (fluoropyrimidines)	5-fluorouracil (5-FU)	EFUDEX®	IV bolus, IV infusion, or continuous IV infusion	Interfere with DNA or RNA synthesis by substituting for normal building blocks
	capecitabine	Xeloda®	Oral tablet	
	floxuridine	FUDR®	Hepatic artery infusion	
Alkylating (platinum-based)	oxaliplatin	Eloxatin®	IV infusion	Directly damage DNA
Antitumor antibiotics	None currently used in CRC			Interfere with DNA production inside cancer cells
Topoisomerase inhibitors	irinotecan	Camptosar®	IV infusion	Interfere with topoisomerase separation of DNA strands necessary for replication
Thymidine phosphorylase inhibitor	trifluridine and tipiracil	Lonsurf®	Oral tablet	Inhibits DNA synthesis and inhibits cell proliferation
Mitotic inhibitors	None currently used in CRC			Naturally derived products that interfere with cell division and prevent production of proteins needed for cell division
Corticosteroids				Help treat symptoms of chemotherapy and prevent severe allergic reactions
Targeted therapies				Attack cancer cells more specifically than normal cells, usually targeting mutant genes or cells that make too many copies of a gene
Anti-VEGF antibody	bevacizumab	Avastin®	IV infusion	Block VEGF
Anti-VEGF and antiplacental growth factor	ziv-aflibercept	Zaltrap®	IV infusion	Block VEGF and PGF
Anti-EFGR	cetuximab	Erbitux®	IV infusion	Block receptor for EGF; chimeric monoclonal antibody
Anti-EFGR	panitumumab	Vectibix®	IV infusion	Block receptor for EGF; fully humanized monoclonal antibody
Anti-VEGFR and antityrosine kinase	regorafenib	Stivarga®	Oral tablets	Block VEGF receptor and tyrosine kinase
Anti-VEGFR2	ramucirumab	Cyramza®	IV infusion	Block VEGFR2
Differentiating agents	None currently used in CRC			Cause cancer cells to differentiate into normal cells
Hormone therapy	None currently used in CRC			Prevent production or cancer cell use of sex hormones needed for cancer cell proliferation
Immunotherapy	None currently used in CRC			Stimulate natural immune system to recognize and attack cancer cells
Other	Leucovorin (LV) (folinic acid)	Welcovorin®	IV infusion or oral tablet	Potentiates the effects of 5-FU by inhibiting thymidylate synthase

[1] www.cancer.org/treatment/treatmentsandsideeffects/guidetocancerdrugs. CRC, colorectal cancer; IV, intravenous.

Neoadjuvant Chemotherapy

Chemotherapy has been used in the neoadjuvant setting both to downsize tumors as well as to sensitize tumors to RT. While neoadjuvant chemoradiation is utilized very commonly in rectal cancers with the goal of sphincter preservation, there is emerging data to support the delivery of all intended therapy (chemotherapy and chemoradiation) in patients with locally advanced rectal cancer [101].While chemoradiation is considered a key component of neoadjuvant therapy in low rectal cancers, the role of radiotherapy is being reinvestigated in high rectal cancers, particularly in the context of robust responses associated with modern chemotherapy regimens and the long-term toxicity associated with radiotherapy. The currently ongoing North Central Cancer Treatment Group NCCTG-N1048 trial is designed to evaluate the role of radiotherapy in high rectal cancer [101, 102].

Adjuvant Chemotherapy

Surgical resection is the only curative-intent treatment for locoregional CRC. However, a minority of patients subsequently develop metastases, due to occult micrometastases that were present at the time of surgical resection. Although adjuvant chemotherapy is clearly beneficial in stage III CRC (reduces recurrence risk and improves overall survival), its role in earlier stage CRC is controversial. The 5-year survival benefit in stage II colon cancer is ≤5%. Features indicating potential benefit from adjuvant chemotherapy in stage II CRC include low LN recovery in surgical specimen (<12), perforated or obstructing tumor, lymphovascular invasion, poor differentiation, or perineural invasion [103]. Genetic profiles may soon help identify which stage II CRCs are likely to benefit from adjuvant chemotherapy [104].

The backbone of chemotherapy for adjuvant therapy in resected CRC is an intravenous or oral fluoropyrimidine (Table 9.9). A recurrence-free survival benefit has been shown in multiple trials by the addition of oxaliplatin (FOLFOX) to 5-FU in stage III CRC [105]. Since the benefit and safety of using oxaliplatin in elderly patients (>70) is controversial, its incorporation for adjuvant therapy in this population is individualized [106, 107].

The duration of adjuvant chemotherapy is 6 months. The optimal interval between surgery and initiation of adjuvant chemotherapy has not been established, but most adjuvant chemotherapy trials mandate initiation of treatment no later than 8 weeks from the date of surgery, and this has become the accepted clinical practice. One meta-analysis suggested that delay beyond 12 weeks was associated with increased mortality and disease relapse [108].

Chemotherapy for Metastatic CRC

Chemotherapy for metastatic CRC is administered primarily with palliative intent except in the subset of patients with oligometastatic disease confined to liver, lung, and in some cases peritoneum in whom cure is entertained as a possibility. In this subset, chemotherapy is administered as a prelude to surgical resection and is therefore neoadjuvant therapy. Deleterious effects of chemotherapy such as hepatotoxicity, splenomegaly, thrombocytopenia, and wound-healing problems that can compromise surgical outcomes must be carefully weighed by a multidisciplinary team. Currently, conversion therapy is administered for 3 months before metastasectomy followed by 'pseudo-adjuvant' therapy for 3 months after surgery [109].

Building on the fluoropyrimidine (5-FU or capecitabine) backbone, cytotoxic and/or targeted therapies are utilized in combination or sequentially based on the specific context in which chemotherapy is administered [110, 111]. FOLFOXIRI may be used in patients with good performance status, especially when planning conversion therapy [112]. The optimal combinations and sequences of these drugs have not been established, but the principle of palliative intent therapy is to ensure that patients get exposure to all active classes of drugs. Some drugs, including oxaliplatin and bevacizumab, are ineffective as single agents. Synergy occurs with some combinations, for example fluoropyrimidine + oxaliplatin. Besides capitalizing on synergy, another rationale for combination therapy is to ensure maximum exposure since there appears to be substantial decline in the efficacy of second-line regimens compared to front-line therapy. The desire to choose a combination that maximizes response rate is particularly strong when planning conversion therapy.

Table 9.9 Common chemotherapy regimens in colorectal cancer management.

Regimen	Agents	Agent class	Predictive biomarker[1]
FOLFOX	FOLinic acid, Fluorouracil, OXaliplatin	Other, cytotoxic, cytotoxic	None
CAPEOX (XELOX)	CAPEcitabine, OXaliplatin (XEloda, Oxaliplatin)	Cytotoxic, cytotoxic	None
FOLFIRI	FOLinic acid, Fluorouracil, IRInotecan	Other, cytotoxic, Cytotoxic	None
FOLFOXIRI	FOLinic acid, Fluorouracil, Oxaliplatin, IRInotecan	Other, cytotoxic, cytotoxic, cytotoxic	None
FOLFOX + panitumumab	FOLinic acid, Fluorouracil, OXaliplatin + Panitumumab	Cytotoxic, cytotoxic, cytotoxic, biologic	KRAS/BRAF
FOLFIRI + cetuximab	FOLinic acid, Fluorouracil, IRInotecan + Cetuximab	Cytotoxic, cytotoxic, cytotoxic, biologic	KRAS/BRAF
5-FU/LV + bevacizumab	5-Fluorouracil, Leucovorin + Bevacizumab	Cytotoxic, cytotoxic biologic	None

Source: Kosinski *et al.* [54].

[1] Biomarker currently used in clinical practice.

The optimal duration of front-line therapy in responding patients is unclear but requires balancing oncologic benefit and toxicities that accrue over time. The risk of oxaliplatin-related neuropathy increases at about 4 months. Fluoropyrimidine maintenance can then be continued +/− the addition of bevacizumab. Oxaliplatin can be reintroduced where there is disease progression [113, 114]. The intermittent addition of oxaliplatin to fluoropyrimidine maintenance appears to improve tolerance without compromising outcomes [115], whereas complete treatment breaks may be detrimental except in carefully selected cases [113]. When disease progresses, salvage regimens are introduced.

Interventional Radiology and Other Regional Therapies

The liver is the predominant site of metastases for patients with CRC [116], and almost a third of patients die of hepatic predominant metastatic disease due to the inability to control disease with systemic chemotherapy alone. Increasing hepatic toxicity from chemotherapy (steatohepatitis from irinotecan, steatohepatitis and sinusoidal dilatation from oxaliplatin) contributes further to hepatic failure [117]. While it is believed that liver metastases circulate from CRC primary tumors via the portal vein, hepatic metastases are actually supplied by the hepatic artery. Based on these observations and the unique dual blood supply of the liver, hepatic artery infusional therapies have been used for patients whose metastases are limited to the liver.

Hepatic Artery Infusion Pumps

Hepatic artery infusion pumps delivering floxuridine have been surgically implanted in both the unresectable and adjuvant settings leading to dramatic response rate and improved progression-free survival (PFS) in randomized trials [118–121]. However, improved overall survival has not been seen in meta-analyses which show a median-weighted overall survival of 15.9 versus 12.4 months ($P = 0.24$) [122]. Toxicity from hepatic artery infusion pumps also led to poor incorporation of this treatment strategy into current treatment paradigms which are constantly evolving as the number of systemic chemotherapy regimens increases [123].

Hepatic Artery Embolization Therapy

Interventional radiology has played an increasing role in catheter-based therapies that can be used for patients with hepatic metastases, by either selectively embolizing the hepatic artery with or without chemotherapy or by delivering a high concentration of beta-emitter particles that deliver high dose RT in a limited territory. Embolization can be undertaken with either resin or glass beads loaded with chemotherapeutic agents. Chemoembolization can also be achieved with lipiodol, a viscous, radio-opaque carrier substance. Radioembolization is a form of intravascular brachytherapy. Embolization of beads loaded with beta-emitter particles can deliver extremely high concentration RT to the liver, but since the hepatic arterial flow is not occluded completely, the recovery is fairly mild.

The percutaneous approach in regional therapies offers patients limited toxicity. Grade 3–5 toxicity in the first-line setting is less than 20% but increases significantly when given in conjunction with systemic chemotherapy [124–126]. Despite the very high response rate seen with regional therapies (90% at 3 months from radioembolization), benefits on overall survival and the durability of response are yet to be proven [126, 128]. Phase II/III trials and numerous retrospective studies have shown a PFS benefit in patients previously treated with systemic chemotherapy [127, 128]. Phase III trials are currently underway to investigate a role for first-line treatment with regional therapies.

Radiofrequency Ablation

Radiofrequency ablation can be performed percutaneously or intraoperatively by either laparoscopic or open approaches. For lesions less than 3 cm, it achieves significant cytoreduction of hepatic metastases [129]. In a randomized trial, radiofrequency ablation provided in conjunction with systemic chemotherapy showed improvement in PFS even in the presence of numerous unresectable liver lesions [130]. Although not currently adopted widely in practice due to the superior results of hepatic resection, this approach is certainly suitable for further studies.

Therapeutic Goals and Treatment Planning Strategies

The ideal CRC treatment is curative, but secondary goals are cancer control to prolong survival and optimize quality of life.

Multimodal Therapy and Multidisciplinary Treatment Planning Conferences

All CRC should be considered for multimodal therapy with the possible exception of nonrecurrent, early stage colon cancers. The cooperative effort of specialists is to fine tune stage-directed treatment guidelines [131, 132].

Tiered Treatment Planning [54]

Stage-directed treatment guidelines such as those published by the National Comprehensive Cancer Network are based on expert analysis of best evidence and form the foundation of CRC treatment [96, 133]. In truth, the process of rendering and then delivering a treatment plan for an individual patient is more complex and can appear chaotic. Complex decision-making tools have been proposed but are cumbersome and often require computer analysis [134], and they do not account for all the tiers of analysis that typically generate a plan, including:

- Conventional (Stage-Directed) Therapy based on consensus treatment guidelines
- Qualified Therapy accounts for specific tumor features that constitute technical or oncologic challenges such as low rectal level, large size, or LVI
- Tailored Therapy weighs patient factors such as comorbidities, genetic status, age, sphincter function, and patient preference
- Actual Therapy can be affected by things like adverse reaction to chemotherapy or RT, disease progression during the course of neoadjuvant therapy, or nonmedical issues such as patient financial hardship.

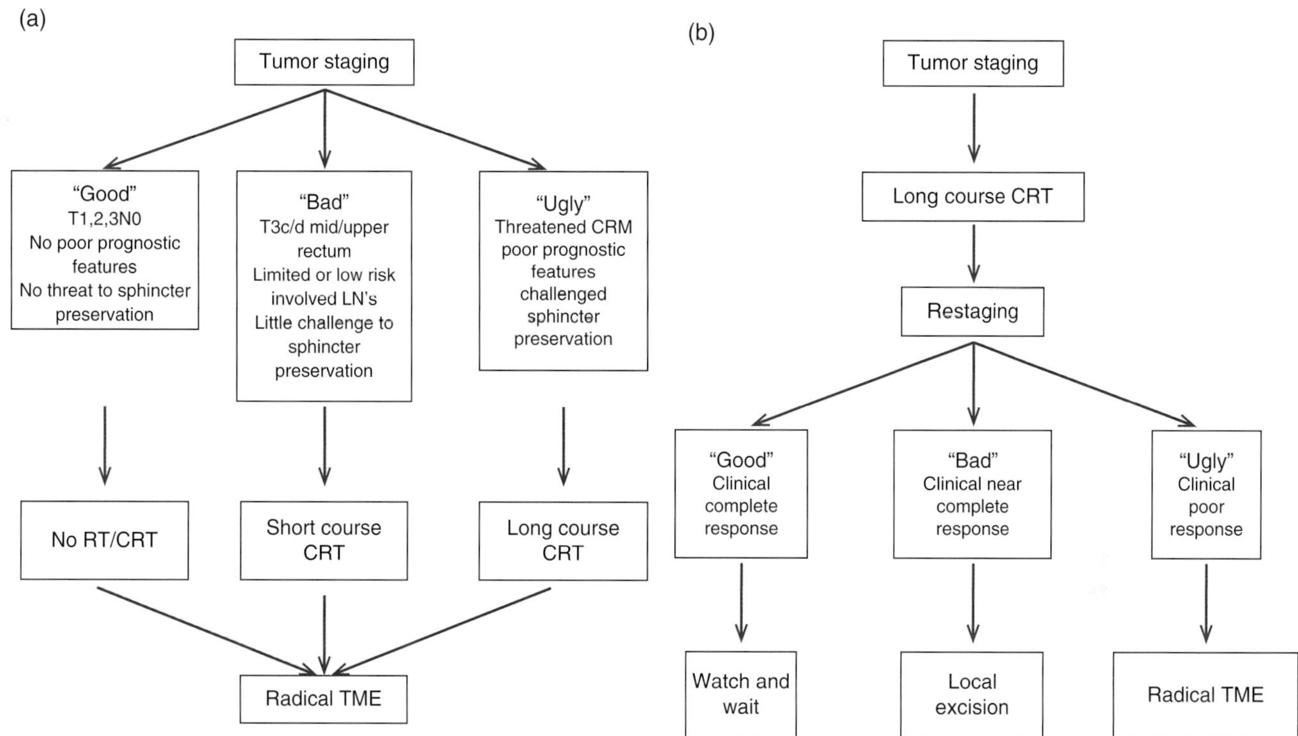

Figure 9.5 "The Good, the Bad, and the Ugly". (a) Selection of neoadjuvant regimen. (b) Selection of the surgical approach. CRM, circumferential (radial) resection margins; CRT, chemoradiation therapy; LNs, lymph nodes; RT, radiation therapy; TME, total mesorectal excision. *Source:* Kosinski *et al.* [54].

For rectal cancer, the prescribed therapy usually reflects favoring either radical surgery or RT. The treatment schemas differ as illustrated in Figure 9.5.

Nonmetastatic (Locoregional) Disease

The mainstay of nonmetastatic CRC treatment is still surgical resection. In general, tumors with higher risk of either occult nodal involvement or metastases, or increased LR risk are treated neoadjuvantly. Examples include very low rectal tumors [135] and threatened MRF. While FTLE alone is acceptable for cT1N0M0 rectal tumors, LR has been reported as ≥10–20% or more [135]. An unacceptably high LR rate of 35% is reported with FTLE alone for cT2N0M0 tumors. In either case, undetected recurrences may not be salvageable [136]. Neoadjuvant CRT may be useful in FTLE of T1- or T2-node negative rectal cancers [137].

Metastatic Disease and Sequencing Therapy

Sequencing Therapy – Common Issues

In stage IV CRC, it is often difficult to know whether to treat sites individually or simultaneously. While surgery and radiation remain at the forefront, chemotherapy is folded into treatment schema, and the ideal sequencing of these interventions unresolved. Chemotherapy is typically interrupted or delayed for elective invasive procedures to minimize effects of chemotherapy and associated immunosuppression. Consequently, resection of locoregional disease delays systemic therapy during the peri- and postoperative period, especially if there are complications of surgery (Table 9.10).

Chemotherapy for Hepatic Metastases

For *resectable hepatic metastases,* perioperative chemotherapy yields a better overall survival compared to surgery alone [109], but it can also increase the risk of surgical complications such as irinotecan-induced steatohepatitis associated with a 15% 90-day mortality following major hepatic resection [138] or increased blood loss due to hepatic sinusoidal dilatation from oxaliplatin therapy [139]. It can also make it difficult to localize the treated metastasis. The systemic clinical complete response rate is low (<10%), and microscopic disease is found in 83% of these resection specimens [140]. *Unresectable hepatic metastases* treated with conversion intent are usually reassessed after 6 months of chemotherapy.

Hepatic Metastasectomy

The focus of hepatic metastasectomy has shifted in the last decade from the extent of the resection to the extent of functional liver left behind. With margin-negative hepatic metastasectomy, the 5-year survival has improved to 60% while the 10-year survival remains at approximately 30% [141]. There are no randomized data comparing three resection strategies (primary tumor resection first, synchronous resections, or metastasectomy first), so how do we choose? The extent of resection required at both sites, patient vitality, and need for neoadjuvant RT often determine the approach. In robust individuals with low-risk resections, simultaneous resections are preferred [142]. Rectal resections, which are typically more challenging than colon resections, are often performed sequentially with mestastasectomies [143]. For low-risk rectal primaries that do not require neoadjuvant RT, the plan is more straightforward

Table 9.10 Metastatic colorectal cancer treatment planning grid.

	Metastases		
Primary tumor	**Resectable**	**Potentially resectable**	**Unresectable**
Resectable	CRx versus synchronous resection/ablation[1]	CRx → metastasis resected/ablated → consider primary resection	Trial CRx versus palliation/hospice
Potentially resectable	Induction CRx versus nCRT with CRx in rest period	CRx → metastasis resected/ablated → consider primary resection	Trial CRx versus palliation/hospice
Unresectable	CRx, add locoregional therapy (e.g., RT) for palliation as needed	CRx, add locoregional therapy (e.g., RT) for palliation as needed	Trial CRx versus palliation/hospice, add locoregional therapy (e.g., RT) for palliation as needed

CRx chemotherapy; nCRT, neoadjuvant chemoradiation; RT, radiation therapy; SBRT, stereotactic body radiation therapy.
[1] Examples of ablation techniques include SBRT or microwave ablation performed percutaneously or open.

and can be based on patient factors alone. When neoadjuvant RT is required for a rectal cancer, sequencing is more difficult.

Management of the Primary Tumor with Unresectable Metastases

Primary tumors do not need to be resected because they have a very low rate of complications (7%) [144]. Maintenance chemotherapy is the preferred treatment.

Pulmonary Metastases

Pulmonary metastatases are typically treated with surgery. The ideal operation is wedge resection or segmentectomy to preserve as much lung as possible. Stereotactic body RT is also an option. Local control rates are in the 80–>95% range depending on the size of the lesion.

Peritoneal Metastases

Peritoneal malignancy is discussed in Chapter 46.

Emergency Interventions

Some clinical emergencies derail ideal treatment plans for CRC. Fortunately, these are not so common, and it is still often possible to temporize the problem and apply the principles of staging and treatment described above.

Bleeding

Hemodynamically insignificant anemia can be supported medically with iron supplementation (intravenous or oral), erythropoietin, and blood transfusion. Brisk bleeding may prompt surgical resection if that is feasible. Arterial embolization by interventional radiology techniques can be useful when resection is not likely to be successful.

Obstruction

Surgical resection can be the best first step when it is feasible and there is concern for ischemia or perforation. or when the staging is complete and no neoadjuvant therapy is required. Self-expanding metal stents (SEMs) are an alternative to surgical diversion by means of a stoma, and they are more acceptable conceptually to patients. Problems with stent occlusion by fecal matter require careful attention to bowel care. Occlusion can also result from tumor ingrowth. Stent migration and perforation can also complicate their use. SEMs have little role in the rectum (and sometimes the rectosigmoid) because they often seat on the levators which can cause disabling tenesmus. Their placement can also preclude adequate clinical staging of rectal cancers; they interfere with ultrasound and cause artifact on CT and MRI. SEMs are best reserved as short-term bridges to surgery or as palliation in near-terminal patients or those unfit for surgery of any kind. A laparoscopic loop colostomy or open transverse loop colostomy rarely delays chemotherapy. Short-course palliative RT can also palliate obstruction, pain, and hematochezia.

Bowel Perforation

Free perforation mandates surgical exploration and resection if possible. Fecal diversion and washout may be the only option, and even if resection is performed, diverting colostomy is advisable. Besides the obvious problems of fecal contamination and sepsis, tumor dissemination in the abdominal cavity occurs with free perforation and compromises oncologic outcomes. Occasionally, a patient presents with a contained perforation. In this case, there is anecdotal success avoiding immediate resection and inevitable dissemination of tumor cells by creating a diverting stoma and treating with antibiotics. Subsequently, neoadjuvant CRT to kill viable tumor cells in the perforation cavity may reduce viable tumor cell spillage at the time of subsequent resection. Percutaneous drainage potentially seeds the drain tract with tumor cells.

Follow-Up and Surveillance

Outcomes

The three strongest prognostic factors for rectal cancer are: (i) magnitude of response to neoadjuvant therapy (especially complete response); (ii) negative CRM; and (iii) correct plane of dissection (TME). Even excellent surgical technique – which is critical to reducing LR and distant failure – can be enhanced by neoadjuvant RT. Hospital volumes and surgeon experience also appear to contribute [54].

Survival

The 5-year relative survival for colon cancer is 63% regardless of stage at time of diagnosis and 68.7% for rectal cancer [145]. Exclusive of M status, the relative survival rate for colon cancer ranges from 97.4% for T1N0 cancers to 15.7% for T4bN2b [146]. The relative 5-year survival rate for rectal cancer exclusive of M status ranges from 96.6% for T1N0 cancers to 14.1% for T4bN2b tumors [49]. Figure 9.6 illustrates observed survival as a function of both T and N category and is similar for rectal and colon cancer [146]. The American Joint Committee on Cancer Cancer Staging Manual documents 5-year survival as a function of stage (including M status) [47].

Local Recurrence

Historically, LR has been a much greater concern for rectal cancer than colon cancer, but modern treatment has dramatically reduced the incidence of recurrences in the pelvis. The rate of colon cancer LR at 10-year follow-up is approximately 11%. The rectal cancer LR rates are approximately 10% after sphincter-sparing proctectomy and 15% after abdominoperineal resection [147]. These rates are higher than those reported from the Dutch Rectal Cancer Trial 12-year follow-up in which 11% LR was observed in patients treated with surgery alone versus 5% for those who had neoadjuvant RT and TME [148].

Follow-up and Surveillance

Colon Cancer

Intensive surveillance is important because early detection of asymptomatic recurrences may lead to a curative intent surgery and improve survival [149, 150]. Table 9.11 shows the American Society of Clinical Oncology and National Comprehensive Cancer Network surveillance guidelines for stage II/III colon cancer. For stage I disease, surveillance includes colonoscopy at 1 and 4 years after surgery then every 5 years unless adenomas are found.

Surveillance of patients who had synchronous oligometastatic disease, have completed perioperative chemotherapy, and undergone R0 resection at all sites, is very similar to resected stage III colon cancer with the exception of more frequent CT imaging [96].

Rectal Cancer

Surveillance in rectal cancer patients is identical to colon cancer except that stage I disease is followed identically to colon stage II/III. Digital rectal examination and office endoscopy are important; early rectal cancer recurrence within reach of an examining finger is often first detected on physical examination.

Recurrent Disease

Routine surveillance and targeted investigation to evaluate patient complaints are fundamental to detecting local and distant treatment failures. In rectal cancer survivors, complaints of pelvic pain should be presumed to be a LR until proven otherwise. If PET fails to show fludeoxyglucose-uptake in a pelvic lesion seen by MRI or CT, biopsy, and even surgical exploration should be considered. After abdominoperineal resection, the diagnosis of pelvic recurrence is more challenging because of loss of access for palpation and endoscopic inspection. The carcinoembryonic antigen test is neither sensitive nor specific, yet remains part of CRC surveillance since it is a relatively inexpensive and uncomplicated test.

Treatment Failure, Salvage, Palliative Care, End of Life

Treatment Failure

In patients treated with a *curative intent*, treatment failure is defined as recurrent or metastatic disease. Salvage is possible in some of these patients, and intense surveillance is mandated to achieve early detection of treatment failures that can be retreated with curative intent. Since almost all failures develop within 5 years of resection and nearly 80% within the first 24 months, the surveillance schedule reflects this. Even so, following neoadjuvant CRT there appears to be a slight shift toward later recurrences (in the 5–10-year postresection period) indicating a need for ongoing follow-up beyond 5 years. In stage IV CRC patients treated with a *palliative intent*, treatment failure is defined as progression of local or metastatic disease.

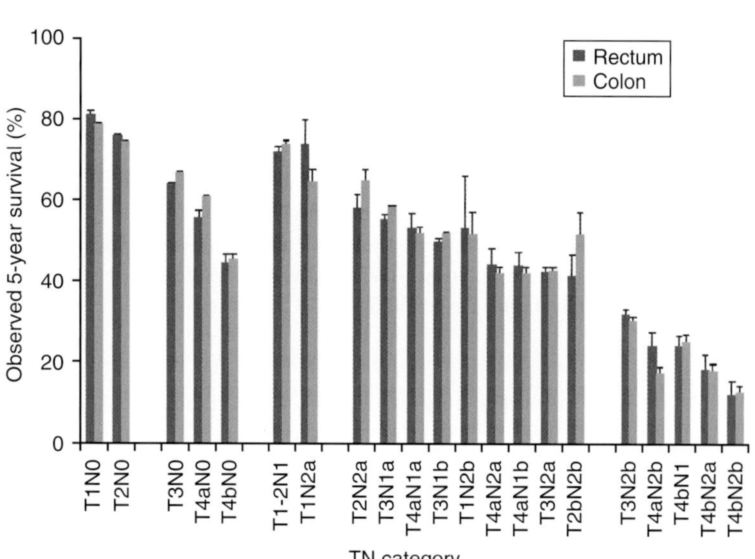

Figure 9.6 Observed 5-year survival by TN category. In the current Surveillance, Epidemiology, and End Results (SEER) colon cancer analysis and the previously reported SEER rectal cancer analysis, 5-year survival is strikingly similar by TN category of disease for patients with rectal or colon cancers. *Source:* Gunderson *et al.* [146].

Table 9.11 Surveillance for stage II/III colorectal cancer: comparison of American Society of Clinical Oncology (ASCO) and National Comprehensive Cancer Network (NCCN) [96, 133].

	ASCO	NCCN
History & physical examination	Every 3–6 months first 3 years then every 6 months during years 4 and 5.	Every 3–6 months for the first 2 years then every 6 months in years 3, 4 and 5.
Carcinoembryonic antigen	Every 3 months for 3 years (Stage II or III) but not during fluoruracial treatment (false positive rate).	Every 3–6 months for the first 2 years then every 6 months in years 3, 4 and 5.
Computed tomography scan	Chest and abdomen every year first 3 years if candidate for curative-intent surgery. Add pelvic CT for rectal cancer only.	Chest/abdomen/pelvis every 3–6 months in first 2 years then every 6–12 months in years 3, 4 and .5
Flexible sigmoidoscopy or rigid proctoscopy	For rectal cancer patients who did not receive pelvic radiation, every 6 months for 5 years.	If treated by local excision, perform with MRI or ERUS every 3–6 months for first 2 years then every 6 months in years 3, 4 and 5.
Colonoscopy	If no preoperative colonoscopy, full colonoscopy perioperatively, otherwise at 3 years then at 5 years if normal. More frequent exams if high-risk genetic syndrome.	If no preoperative colonoscopy, full colonoscopy within 3–6 months of surgery, otherwise at 1 year. If advanced adenoma, repeat in 1 year, otherwise repeat at year 3 and year 5.

Source: adapted from Desch *et al.* [177] and www.nccn.org.

Palliative Care and End of Life

One-fifth of CRC patients present with metastatic disease. A subset have oligometastatic disease and successfully undergo curative intent surgery and achieve a cure, but the majority die from their disease. Patients with refractory metastatic disease or LR will require palliation of symptoms.

Primary Tumor Symptoms

Management strategies for primary tumor symptoms such as obstruction, bleeding, and perforation in the palliative setting are similar to those discussed previously except that patient goals might guide supportive care rather than corrective interventions.

Intra-Abdominal, Pelvic, and Extra-Abdominal Spread

Palliation of patients with peritoneal carcinomatosis is by far one of the most challenging oncology problems. However, aggressive surgical cytoreduction followed by hyperthermic intraperitoneal chemotherapy is an option for some patients (see Chapter 46). Surgical resection of symptomatic bulky ovarian metastases may improve quality of life and prolong survival even when there are other visceral metastases [151]. Small bowel obstructions from carcinomatosis can sometimes be managed with resection, bypass, or proximal diversion with loop small bowel stomas. The risk of anastomotic leak is not trivial, especially when antiangiogenic agents have been used. When carcinomatosis cakes the bowel and precludes resection or diversion, a gastrostomy tube decompression is usually more comfortable than a long-standing nasogastric tube placement. Disabling pain or paralysis can result from nerve or spinal cord involvement; nerve blocks and RT are can help.

Malnutrition

Weight loss and malnutrition occur in 40–80% of patients with metastatic CRC resulting from cancer cachexia, mucositis, malabsorption, inability to ingest adequate calories, and metabolic perturbations. Early in the history of total parenteral nutrition (TPN), it was often withheld from advanced cancer patients due to concerns that it might "feed the tumor but not the patient". While these concerns have been largely laid to rest, there is still controversy about the efficacy of TPN in cancer patients preparing for surgery or at the end of life. Even though nutritional repletion by either the enteral or parenteral route holds intuitive appeal, not all patients with malignancy or cancer treatment-associated weight loss benefit from nutritional support. In fact, routine institution of nutritional support in patients with advanced incurable cancer is associated with a higher risk of treatment-related complications. Parenteral nutrition may be justified in patients with defined intestinal failure (e.g., short bowel syndrome or unresectable obstruction) whose prognosis can be measured in many months or years. TPN is generally not recommended in advanced cancer patients who are terminally ill and have an estimated life span of a few weeks to a few months [152–156].

Survivorship

As mortality from CRC has steadily declined in the US for the past three decades, the number of long-term survivors has increased. Survivorship care covers a broad range of issues including surveillance for CRC recurrence, prevention and recurrence of new or secondary malignancies, and a spectrum of medical and psychosocial issues consequent to cancer and its treatment [157].

Cancer-related fatigue, cumulative side effects of chemotherapy (such as oxaliplatin-induced peripheral neuropathy), RT-induced complications such as chronic proctitis and pelvic insufficiency fractures are all issues faced by CRC survivors, and awareness of these will help healthcare providers provide appropriate counseling and guidance. It is important to screen CRC as well as other cancer survivors for debilitating psychosocial distress [158], depression [158, 159], unemployment [160], and difficulty reintegrating into social relationships.

Some survivorship issues specific to CRC are relatively common. Proctectomy and pelvic RT can cause postproctectomy syndrome. Nerve injury, disruption of the sensitive transition zone in the anal canal, and reconstruction of the rectum with a smaller, less compliant neorectum contribute to symptoms such as chronic diarrhea, clustering of bowel movements, difficulty distinguishing stool from flatus, and incomplete evacuation [151, 159]. Many of these symptoms resolve 18–24 months after surgery. Manipulation of bowel consistency with high fiber regimens and antidiarrheal medications as well as dietary adjustments (elimination of lactose and raw fruits and vegetables, low-fat diets, probiotics) and antispasmodic prescription can help achieve acceptable bowel function [162, 163]. Patience and support typically lead to satisfactory function. On the horizon, sacral nerve stimulator implantation may improve pelvic floor function in this patient population.

Both urinary retention and incontinence are common among rectal cancer survivors. Abdominoperineal resection is more likely than LAR to cause long-term urinary incontinence. Treatment involves lifestyle changes (weight loss), bladder training and pelvic floor therapy, pessaries, and antimuscarinic therapy. As with defecation disorders, a sacral nerve stimulator may have a role. Sexual dysfunction, particularly in rectal cancer patients who received RT in addition to proctectomy, is common in both men (23–69%) and women (19–62%) [164], and unfortunately is not adequately addressed either during treatment or surveillance [165, 166]. Erectile dysfunction, decreased libido, and ejaculatory disorders are common male problems. Women usually suffer from dyspareunia, altered genital lubrication, decreased libido, and altered orgasms [167]. Treatment options for men include testosterone therapy to improve libido and erection, and phosphodiesterase-5 inhibition [168] or intracavernous pharmacologic injection for erectile dysfunction. Treatment options for women, however, are limited to water/silicon-based lubricants, vaginal moisturizers, and low-dose vaginal estrogen preparations to help with vaginal dryness and dyspareunia. Pelvic floor muscle training and vaginal dilators may be recommended for patients to prevent vaginal stenosis after RT [169] and pelvic floor manual therapies may be beneficial.

Most importantly, all CRC survivors should be encouraged to pursue a healthy lifestyle and follow age-appropriate screening recommendations.

Conclusion

The care of colon and rectal cancer patients is increasingly rewarding because of the inroads being made in staging and therapeutic options, the clear benefits of teamwork, our deepening understanding of the biology of these cancers that comes from careful reflection on their clinical behavior, and the opportunity to improve not just the oncologic but also the functional outcomes of our patients.

References

1 Siegel R, Miller KD, Jemal A. Cancer statistics, 2017. *CA Cancer J Clin* 2017;67:7–30.
2 American Cancer Society. *Colorectal Cancer Facts and Figures 2014–2016*. Atlanta: American Cancer Society, 2014. Available online from: http://www.cancer.org/research/cancerfactsstatistics/colorectal-cancer-facts-figures (accessed September 26 2017).
3 Howlader N, Noone AM, Krapcho M, *et al.* (eds). *SEER Cancer Statistics Review, 1975–2013*, National Cancer Institute. Bethesda, MD, http://seer.cancer.gov/csr/1975_2013/, based on November 2015 SEER data submission, posted to the SEER web site, April 2016.
4 The National Cancer Data Base (NCDB). NCDB: Histology of Colon Cancer Diagnosed in 2000 to 2011. [Online] Available from: http://cromwell.facs.org/BMarks/BMPub/Ver10/BMR_report_1st2.cfm?CFID=386597&CFTOKEN=23071079 (accessed 20 December 2013).
5 Hauso O, Gustafsson BI, Kidd M, *et al.* Neuroendocrine tumor epidemiology. *Cancer* 2008;113(10):2655–64.
6 Yao JC, Hassan M, Phan A, *et al.* One hundred years after "carcinoid": epidemiology of and prognostic factors for neuroendocrine tumors in 35,825 cases in the United States. *J Clin Oncol* 2008;26:3063–72.
7 Kang H, O'Connell JB, Leonardi MJ, *et al.* Rare tumors of the colon and rectum: a national review. *Int J Colorectal Dis* 2006;22(2):183–9.
8 Stanojevic GZ. Primary colorectal lymphoma: an overview. *World J Gastrointest Oncol* 2011;3(1):14.
9 Drolet S, Maclean AR, Stewart DA, *et al.* Primary colorectal lymphoma—clinical outcomes in a population-based series. *J Gastrointest Surg* 2011;15(10):1851–7.
10 Reddy R, Fleshman J. Colorectal gastrointestinal stromal tumors: a brief review. *Clin Colon Rectal Surg* 2006;19(2):69–77.
11 Wei EK, Giovannucci E, Wu K, *et al.* Comparison of risk factors for colon and rectal cancer. *Int J Cancer* 2004;108(3):433–42.
12 Johns LE, Houlston RS. A systematic review and meta-analysis of familial colorectal cancer risk. *Am J Gastroenterol* 2001;96(10):2992–3003.
13 Pearlman R, Frankel WL, Swanson B, *et al.* Prevalence and spectrum of germline cancer susceptibility gene mutations among patients with early-onset colorectal cancer. *JAMA Oncol* 2017;3(4):464–71.
14 Lynch HT, La Chapelle de A. Hereditary colorectal cancer. *N Engl J Med* 2003;348(10):919–32.
15 Barrow E, Hill J, Evans DG. Cancer risk in Lynch Syndrome. *Fam Cancer* 2013;12(2):229–40.
16 Lynch HT, Lynch JF, Lynch PM. Toward a consensus in molecular diagnosis of hereditary nonpolyposis colorectal cancer (Lynch syndrome). *J Natl Cancer Inst* 2007;99(4):261–3.
17 Erdman S, Holter S, Jasperson K. World Health Organization classification of tumors. *Cancer* 2000;88(12):126–9.
18 Kievit W, de Bruin JH, Adang EM, *et al.* Current clinical selection strategies for identification of hereditary non-polyposis colorectal cancer families are inadequate: a meta-analysis. *Clin Genet* 2005;65(4):308–16.
19 Umar A, Boland CR, Terdiman JP, *et al.* Revised Bethesda Guidelines for hereditary nonpolyposis colorectal cancer (Lynch syndrome) and microsatellite instability. *J Natl Cancer Inst* 2004;96(4):261–8.
20 Evans DG, Howard E, Giblin C, *et al.* Birth incidence and prevalence of tumor-prone syndromes: Estimates from a UK family genetic register service. *Am J Med Genet A* 2010;152A(2):327–32.
21 Talbot IC, Burt R, Järvinen H, Thomas G. World Health Organization classification of tumors. *Cancer* 2000;88(12):120–5.

22 Wennstrom J, Pierce ER, McKusick VA. Hereditary benign and malignant lesions of the large bowel. *Cancer* 1974;34(S3):850–7.
23 Jagelman DG, DeCosse JJ, Bussey HJ. Upper gastrointestinal cancer in familial adenomatous polyposis. *Lancet* 1988;1(8595):1149–51.
24 Wallace MH, Phillips RK. Upper gastrointestinal disease in patients with familial adenomatous polyposis. *Br J Surg* 1998;85(6):742–50.
25 Burt R, DiSario J, Cannon-Albright L. Genetics of colon cancer: impact of inheritance on colon cancer risk. *Annu Rev Med* 1996;46:371–9.
26 Sieber OM, Segditsas S, Knudsen AL, *et al.* Disease severity and genetic pathways in attenuated familial adenomatous polyposis vary greatly but depend on the site of the germline mutation. *Gut* 2006;55(10):1440–8.
27 Jess T, Rungoe C, Peyrin–Biroulet L. Risk of colorectal cancer in patients with ulcerative colitis: a meta-analysis of population-based cohort studies. *Clin Gastroenterol Hepatol* 2012;10(6):639–45.
28 Bernstein CN, Blanchard JF, Kliewer E, Wajda A. Cancer risk in patients with inflammatory bowel disease. *Cancer* 2001;91(4):854–62.
29 Eaden JA. The risk of colorectal cancer in ulcerative colitis: a meta-analysis. *Gut* 2001;48(4):526–35.
30 Brentnall T, Haggitt R, Rabinovitch P, *et al.* Risk and natural history of colonic neoplasia in patients with primary sclerosing cholangitis and ulcerative colitis. *Gastroenterology* 1996;110(2):331–8.
31 Bibbins-Domingo K. Aspirin use for the primary prevention of cardiovascular disease and colorectal cancer: US Preventive Services Task Force Recommendation Statement Aspirin Use for the Primary Prevention of CVD and CRC. *Ann Intern Med* 2016;164(12):836–45.
32 Smith RA, Andrews K, Brooks D, *et al.* Cancer screening in the United States, 2016: a review of current American Cancer Society guidelines and current issues in cancer screening. *CA Cancer J Clin* 2016;66(2):95–114.
33 Amri R, Bordeianou LG, Sylla P, Berger DL. Impact of screening colonoscopy on outcomes in colon cancer surgery. *JAMA Surg* 2013;148:747–54.
34 Majumdar SR, Fletcher RH, Evans AT. How does colorectal cancer present? Symptoms, duration, and clues to location. *Am J Gastroenterol* 1999;94:3039–45.
35 Polissar L, Sim D, Francis A. Survival of colorectal cancer patients in relation to duration of symptoms and other prognostic factors. *Dis Colon Rectum* 1981;24:364–9.
36 Myers EA, Feingold DL, Forde KA, *et al.* Colorectal cancer in patients under 50 years of age: a retrospective analysis of two institutions' experience. *World J Gastroenterol* 2013;19:5651–7.
37 Wolmark N, Wieand HS, Rockette HE, *et al.* The prognostic significance of tumor location and bowel obstruction in Dukes B and C colorectal cancer. Findings from the NSABP clinical trials. *Ann Surg* 1983;198:743–52.
38 Elias D, Honore C, Dumont F, *et al.* Results of systematic second-look surgery plus HIPEC in asymptomatic patients presenting a high risk of developing colorectal peritoneal carcinomatosis. *Ann Surg* 2011;254:289–93.
39 Fearon ER, Vogelstein B. A genetic model for colorectal tumorigenesis. *Cell* 1990;61(5):759–67.
40 Spirio LN, Samowitz W, Robertson J, *et al.* Alleles of APC modulate the frequency and classes of mutations that lead to colon polyps. *Nature Genet* 1998;20(4):385–8.
41 Hampel H, Frankel WL, Martin E, *et al.* Feasibility of screening for Lynch syndrome among patients with colorectal cancer. *J Clin Oncol* 2008;26(35):5783–8.
42 Veigl ML, Kasturi L, Olechnowicz J, *et al.* Biallelic inactivation of hMLH1 by epigenetic gene silencing, a novel mechanism causing human MSI cancers. *Proc Natl Acad Sci USA* 1998;95(15):8698–702.
43 Rajagopalan H, Bardelli A, Lengauer C, *et al.* Tumorigenesis: RAF/RAS oncogenes and mismatch-repair status. *Nature* 2002;418(6901):934.
44 Fang M, Hutchinson L, Deng A, Green MR. Common BRAF (V600E)-directed pathway mediates widespread epigenetic silencing in colorectal cancer and melanoma. *Proc Natl Acad Sci* 2016;113(5):1250–5.
45 Ogino S, Nosho K, Kirkner GJ, *et al.* CpG island methylator phenotype, microsatellite instability, BRAF mutation and clinical outcome in colon cancer. *Gut* 2009;58(1):90–6.
46 Noffsinger AE. Serrated polyps and colorectal cancer: new pathway to malignancy. *Ann Rev Pathol* 2009;4:343–64.
47 Jessup JM, Goldberg RM, Asare EA, *et al.* Colon and rectum. In: Amin M, Edge S, Greene R, Byrd D, Brookland R (eds) *Cancer Staging Manual 8th Edition, American Joint Committee on Cancer.* New York: Springer, 2017.
48 Dewhurst C, Rosen MP, Blake MA, *et al.* ACR Appropriateness Criteria® Pretreatment Staging of Colorectal Cancer. *J Am Coll Radiol* 2012;9(11):775–81.
49 Gunderson LL, Jessup JM, Sargent DJ, Greene FL, Stewart A. Revised tumor and node categorization for rectal cancer based on surveillance, epidemiology, and end results and rectal pooled analysis outcomes. *J Clin Oncol* 2010;28(2):256–63.
50 Grossmann I, Klaase J, Avenarius J, *et al.* The strengths and limitations of routine staging before treatment with abdominal CT in colorectal cancer. *BMC Cancer* 2011;11(1):433.
51 The National Cancer Data Base (NCDB). NCDB Public Benchmarks – Site by Stage of Top 11 (out of 11) Sites Cancers Diagnosed in 2000 to 2011. [Online] Available from: https://cromwell.facs.org/BMarks/BMPub/ver10/Docs/ https://cromwell.facs.org/BMarks/BMPub/ver10/Docs/ (accessed 20 December 2013).
52 Beets-Tan R, Beets G, Vliegen R, *et al.* Accuracy of magnetic resonance imaging in prediction of tumour-free resection margin in rectal cancer surgery. *Lancet* 2001;357(9255):497–504.
53 Al-Sukhni E, Milot L, Fruitman M, *et al.* Diagnostic accuracy of MRI for assessment of T Category, lymph node metastases, and circumferential resection margin involvement in patients with rectal cancer: a systematic review and meta-analysis. *Ann Surg Oncol* 2012;19(7):2212–23.
54 Kosinski L, Habr-Gama A, Ludwig K, Perez R. Shifting concepts in rectal cancer management. *CA Cancer J Clin* 2012;62(3):173–202.

55 Ryan R, Gibbons D, Hyland JM, *et al.* Pathological response following long-course neoadjuvant chemoradiotherapy for locally advanced rectal cancer. *Histopathology* 2005;47(2):141–6.
56 Kitajima K, Fujimori T, Fujii S, *et al.* Correlations between lymph node metastasis and depth of submucosal invasion in submucosal invasive colorectal carcinoma: a Japanese collaborative study. *J Gastroenterol* 2004;39(6):534–43.
57 Merkel S, Mansmann U, Siassi M, *et al.* The prognostic inhomogeneity in pT3 rectal carcinomas. *Int J Colorectal Dis* 2001;16(5):298–304.
58 Smith NJ, Shihab O, Arnaout A, Swift RI, Brown G. MRI for detection of extramural vascular invasion in rectal cancer. *Am J Roentgenol* 2014;191(5):1517–22.
59 Smith NJ, Barbachano Y, Norman AR, *et al.* Prognostic significance of magnetic resonance imaging-detected extramural vascular invasion in rectal cancer. *Br J Surg* 2008;95(2):229–36.
60 Tong T, Yao Z, Xu L, *et al.* Extramural depth of tumor invasion at thin-section MR in rectal cancer: associating with prognostic factors and ADC value. *J Magn Reson Imaging* 2014;40(3):738–44.
61 Feingold D, Addona T, Forde K, *et al.* Safety and reliability of tattooing colorectal neoplasms prior to laparoscopic resection. *J Gastrointest Surg* 2004;8(5):543–6.
62 Yeung JM, Maxwell-Armstrong C, Acheson AG. Colonic tattooing in laparoscopic surgery – making the mark? *Colorect Dis*;2009;11(5):527–30.
63 Williams NS, Dixon MF, Johnston D. Reappraisal of the 5 centimetre rule of distal excision for carcinoma of the rectum: A study of distal intramural spread and of patients' survival. *Br J Surg* 1983;70(3):150–4.
64 Nakafusa Y, Tanaka T, Tanaka M, *et al.* Comparison of multivisceral resection and standard operation for locally advanced colorectal cancer: analysis of prognostic factors for short-term and long-term outcome. *Dis Colon Rectum* 2004;47(12):2055–63.
65 Gricouroff G. Pathogenesis of recurrences on the suture line following surgical resection for carcinoma of the colon. *Cancer* 1967;20(5):673–6.
66 Compton CC, Fielding LP, Burgart LJ, *et al.* Prognostic Factors in Colorectal Cancer. College of American Pathologists Consensus Statement 1999. [Online] Available from: http://www.cap.org/apps/docs/pathology_reporting/Prognostic_Factors_in_Colorectal_Cancer_article.pdf (accessed 15 December 2013).
67 Washington K, Berlin J, Branton P, *et al.* Protocol for the examination of specimens from patients with primary carcinoma of the colon and rectum. [Online] Available from: http://www.cap.org/apps/docs/committees/cancer/cancer_protocols/2012/Colon_12protocol_3200.pdf; 2012 (accessed 15 December 2013).
68 Desch CE, McNiff KK, Schneider EC, *et al.* American Society of Clinical Oncology/National Comprehensive Cancer Network Quality Measures. *J Clin Oncol* 2008;26(21):3631–7.
69 West NP, Kobayashi H, Takahashi K, *et al.* Understanding optimal colonic cancer surgery: comparison of Japanese D3 resection and European complete mesocolic excision with central vascular ligation. *J Clin Oncol* 2012;30(15):1763–9.
70 Chang GJ, Kaiser AM, Mills S, Rafferty JF, Buie WD. Practice parameters for the management of colon cancer. *Dis Colon Rectum* 2012;55(8):831–43.
71 Church J, Simmang C. Practice parameters for the treatment of patients with dominantly inherited colorectal cancer (familial adenomatous polyposis and hereditary nonpolyposis colorectal cancer). *Dis Colon Rectum* 2003;46(8):1001–12.
72 Nelson H, Sargent DJ, Wieand HS, *et al.* A comparison of laparoscopically assisted and open colectomy for colon cancer. *N Engl J Med* 2004;350(20):2050–9.
73 D'Annibale A, Morpurgo E, Fiscon V, *et al.* Robotic and laparoscopic surgery for treatment of colorectal diseases. *Dis Colon Rectum* 2004;47(12):2162–8.
74 Lim D, Min B, Kim M, *et al.* Robotic versus laparoscopic anterior resection of sigmoid colon cancer: comparative study of long-term oncologic outcomes. *Surg Endosc* 2013;27(4):1379–85.
75 Heald RJ, Ryall R. Recurrent cancer after restorative resection of the rectum. *Br Med J* 1982;284:826–7.
76 Nagtegaal ID, van de Velde CJ, van der Worp E, *et al.* Macroscopic evaluation of rectal cancer resection specimen: clinical significance of the pathologist in quality control. *J Clin Oncol* 2002;20(7):1729–34.
77 Wibe A, Eriksen MT, Syse A, *et al.* Total mesorectal excision for rectal cancer – what can be achieved by a national audit? *Colorect Dis* 2003;5(5):471–7.
78 Martling A, Holm T, Rutqvist LE, *et al.* Impact of a surgical training programme on rectal cancer outcomes in Stockholm. *Br J Surg* 2005;92(2):225–9.
79 Cedermark B, Johansson H, Rutqvist LE. The Stockholm I trial of preoperative short term radiotherapy in operable rectal carcinoma. *Cancer*;1995;75(9):2269–75.
80 Trial SRC. Improved survival with preoperative radiotherapy in resectable rectal cancer. *N Engl J Med* 2000;336(14):980–7.
81 Martling A, Holm T, Johansson H, *et al.* The Stockholm II trial on preoperative radiotherapy in rectal carcinoma. *Cancer* 2001;92(4):896–902.
82 Sauer R, Becker H, Hohenberger W, *et al.* Preoperative versus postoperative chemoradiotherapy for rectal cancer. *N Engl J Med* 2004;351(17):1731–40.
83 Kapiteijn E, Marijnen CA, Nagtegaal ID, *et al.* Preoperative radiotherapy combined with total mesorectal excision for resectable rectal cancer. *N Engl J Med* 2001;345(9):638–46.
84 Bujko K, Nowacki MP, Nasierowska-Guttmejer A, *et al.* Long-term results of a randomized trial comparing preoperative short-course radiotherapy with preoperative conventionally fractionated chemoradiation for rectal cancer. *Br J Surg* 2006;93(10):1215–23.
85 ACOSOG. American College of Surgeons Oncology Group. ACOSOG Z6051. [Online] Available from: http://www.cancer.gov/clinicaltrials/search/view?cdrid=601816&version=patient&protocolsearchid=5787787 (accessed 30 December 2013).
86 Nastro P, Beral D, Hartley J, Monson JR. Local excision of rectal cancer: review of literature. *Digest Surg* 2005;22(1):6–15.
87 Collinson F, Jayne D, Pigazzi A, *et al.* An international, multicentre, prospective, randomised, controlled, unblinded, parallel-group trial of robotic-assisted versus standard laparoscopic surgery for the curative treatment of rectal cancer. *Int J Colorectal Dis* 2012;27(2):233–41.

88 Brown CJ, Fenech DS, McLeod RS. Reconstructive techniques after rectal resection for rectal cancer. *Cochrane Database Syst Rev* 2008;(2)CD006040.

89 Fazio WV, Zutshi M, Remzi FH, *et al.* A randomized multicenter trial to compare long-term functional outcome, quality of life, and complications of surgical procedures for low rectal cancers. *Ann Surg* 2007;246(3):481–8; discussion 488–90.

90 Ulrich AB, Seiler CM, Z'graggen K, *et al.* Early results from a randomized clinical trial of colon J pouch versus transverse coloplasty pouch after low anterior resection for rectal cancer. *Br J Surg* 2008;95(10):1257–63.

91 Bosset J, Calais G, Mineur L, *et al.* Enhanced tumorocidal effect of CRx with preoperative radiotherapy for rectal cancer: preliminary results—EORTC 22921. *J Clin Oncol* 2005;23(24):5620–7.

92 Willett CG, Czito BG, Tyler DS. Intraoperative radiation therapy. *J Clin Oncol* 2007;25(8):971–7.

93 Meyer J, Czito B, Yin F, Willett C. Advanced radiation therapy technologies in the treatment of rectal and anal cancer: intensity-modulated photon therapy and proton therapy. *Clin Colorect Cancer* 2007;6(5):348–56.

94 Marijnen CA, Glimelius B. The role of radiotherapy in rectal cancer. *Eur J Cancer* 2002;38(7):943–52.

95 Monson JR, Weiser MR, Buie WD, *et al.* Practice parameters for the management of rectal cancer (revised). *Dis Colon Rectum* 2013;56(5):535–50.

96 Benson AB, Venook AP, Cederquist L, Chan E, Chen Y-J, *et al.* NCCN Clinical Practice Guidelines in Oncology. Rectal Cancer 3. 2017. Available at: http://www.nccn.org Accessed December 8, 2018.

97 Habrgama A, Perez R, Nadalin W, *et al.* Long-term results of preoperative chemoradiation for distal rectal cancer correlation between final stage and survival. *J Gastrointest Surg* 2005;9(1):90–101.

98 Ooi B, Tjandra J, Green M. Morbidities of adjuvant chemotherapy and radiotherapy for resectable rectal cancer. *Dis Colon Rectum* 1999;42(3):403–18.

99 Folkesson J, Birgisson H, Pahlman L, *et al.* Swedish Rectal Cancer Trial: long lasting benefits from radiotherapy on survival and local recurrence rate. *J Clin Oncol* 2005;23(24):5644–50.

100 Peeters KC, van de Velde CJ, Leer JW, *et al.* Late side effects of short-course preoperative radiotherapy combined with total mesorectal excision for rectal cancer: increased bowel dysfunction in irradiated patients—A Dutch Colorectal Cancer Group Study. *J Clin Oncol* 2005;23(25):6199–206.

101 Chau I, Brown G, Cunningham D, *et al.* Neoadjuvant capecitabine and oxaliplatin followed by synchronous chemoradiation and total mesorectal excision in magnetic resonance imaging-defined poor-risk rectal cancer. *J Clin Oncol* 2006;24(4):668–74.

102 NCCTG-N1048 trial: Chemotherapy Alone or Chemotherapy Plus Radiation Therapy in Treating Patients with Locally Advanced Rectal Cancer Undergoing Surgery. Sponsored by the North Central Cancer Treatment Group and the National Cancer Institute. Website: http://www.cancer.gov/clinicaltrials/search/view?cdrid=715321&version=patient (Accessed 20 December 2013).

103 Andre T, Boni C, Navarro M, *et al.* Improved overall survival with oxaliplatin, fluorouracil, and leucovorin as adjuvant treatment in stage II or III colon cancer in the MOSAIC trial. *J Clin Oncol* 2009;27(19):3109–16.

104 Ribic CM, Sargent DJ, Moore MJ, *et al.* Tumor microsatellite-instability status as a predictor of benefit from fluorouracil-based adjuvant chemotherapy for colon cancer. *N Engl J Med* 2003;349:247–57.

105 Andre T, Boni C, Mounedji-Boudiaf L, *et al.* Oxaliplatin, fluorouracil, and leucovorin as adjuvant treatment for colon cancer. *N Engl J Med* 2004;350(23):2343–51.

106 McCleary NJ, Meyerhardt JA, Green E, *et al.* Impact of age on the efficacy of newer adjuvant therapies in patients with stage ii/iii colon cancer: findings from the ACCENT Database. *J Clin Oncol* 2013;31 (20):2600–6.

107 Sanoff HK, Carpenter WR, Martin CF, *et al.* Comparative effectiveness of oxaliplatin vs non-oxaliplatin-containing adjuvant chemotherapy for stage III colon cancer. *J Natl Cancer Inst* 2012;104(3):211–27.

108 Biagi JJ, Raphael MJ, Mackillop WJ, *et al.* Association between time to initiation of adjuvant chemotherapy and survival in colorectal cancer: a systematic review and meta-analysis. *JAMA* 2011;305(22):2335–42.

109 Nordlinger B, Sorbye H, Glimelius B, *et al.* Perioperative chemotherapy with FOLFOX4 and surgery versus surgery alone for resectable liver metastases from colorectal cancer (EORTC Intergroup trial 40983): a randomised controlled trial. *Lancet* 2008;371(9617):1007–16.

110 Hochster HS, Hart LL, Ramanathan RK, *et al.* Safety and efficacy of oxaliplatin and fluoropyrimidine regimens with or without bevacizumab as first-line treatment of metastatic colorectal cancer: results of the TREE Study. *J Clin Oncol* 2008;26(21):3523–9.

111 Tournigand C, Andre T, Achille E, *et al.* FOLFIRI followed by FOLFOX6 or the reverse sequence in advanced colorectal cancer: a randomized GERCOR study. *J Clin Oncol* 2004;22(2):229–37.

112 Falcone A, Ricci S, Brunetti I, *et al.* Phase III trial of infusional fluorouracil, leucovorin, oxaliplatin, and irinotecan (FOLFOXIRI) compared with infusional fluorouracil, leucovorin, and irinotecan (FOLFIRI) as first-line treatment for metastatic colorectal cancer: the Gruppo Oncologico Nord Ovest. *J Clin Oncol* 2007; 25(13):1670–6.

113 Chibaudel B, Maindrault-Goebel F, Lledo G, *et al.* Can chemotherapy be discontinued in unresectable metastatic colorectal cancer? The GERCOR OPTIMOX2 Study. *J Clin Oncol* 2009;27(34):5727–33.

114 Tournigand C, Cervantes A, Figer A, *et al.* OPTIMOX1: a randomized study of FOLFOX4 or FOLFOX7 with oxaliplatin in a stop-and-Go fashion in advanced colorectal cancer–a GERCOR study. *J Clin Oncol* 2006; 24(3):394–400.

115 Grothey A. Reintroduction of oxaliplatin: a viable approach to the long-term management of metastatic colorectal cancer. *Oncology* 2010;79(5-6):389–99.

116 McMillan DC, McArdle CS. Epidemiology of colorectal liver metastases. *Surg Oncol* 2007;16:3–5.

117 Vauthey JN, Pawlik TM, Ribero D, *et al.* Chemotherapy regimen predicts steatohepatitis and an increase in 90-day mortality after surgery for hepatic colorectal metastases. *J Clin Oncol* 2006;24:2065–72.

118 Kemeny N, Capanu M, D'Angelica M, *et al.* Phase I trial of adjuvant hepatic arterial infusion (HAI) with floxuridine (FUDR) and dexamethasone plus systemic oxaliplatin, 5-fluorouracil and leucovorin in patients with resected liver metastases from colorectal cancer. *Ann Oncol* 2009;20:1236–41.

119 Sigurdson ER, Ridge JA, Kemeny N, Daly JM. Tumor and liver drug uptake following hepatic artery and portal vein infusion. *J Clin Oncol* 1987;5:1836–40.

120 Kemeny NE, Melendez FD, Capanu M, *et al.* Conversion to resectability using hepatic artery infusion plus systemic chemotherapy for the treatment of unresectable liver metastases from colorectal carcinoma. *J Clin Oncol* 2009;27:3465–71.

121 Kemeny N, Daly J, Oderman P, *et al.* Hepatic artery pump infusion: toxicity and results in patients with metastatic colorectal carcinoma. *J Clin Oncol* 1984;2:595–600.

122 Mocellin S, Pilati P, Lise M, Nitti D. Meta-analysis of hepatic arterial infusion for unresectable liver metastases from colorectal cancer: the end of an era? *J Clin Oncol* 2007;25:5649–54.

123 Kemeny MM, Battifora H, Blayney DW, *et al.* Sclerosing cholangitis after continuous hepatic artery infusion of FUDR. *Ann Surg* 1985;202:176–81.

124 Sharma RA, van Hazel GA, Morgan B, *et al.* Radioembolization of liver metastases from colorectal cancer using yttrium-90 microspheres with concomitant systemic oxaliplatin, fluorouracil, and leucovorin chemotherapy. *J Clin Oncol* 2007;25:1099–106.

125 Richardson AJ, Laurence JM, Lam WV. Transarterial chemoembolization with irinotecan beads in the treatment of colorectal liver metastases: systematic review. *J Vasc Interv Radiol* 2013;24:1209–17.

126 Clark TW. Chemoembolization for colorectal liver metastases after FOLFOX failure. *J Vasc Interv Radiol* 2013;24:66–7.

127 Salman HS, Cynamon J, Jagust M, *et al.* Randomized phase II trial of embolization therapy versus chemoembolization therapy in previously treated patients with colorectal carcinoma metastatic to the liver. *Clin Colorectal Cancer* 2002;2:173–9.

128 Guadagni S. Hepatic arterial chemoembolization adopting dc bead, drug-eluting bead loaded with irinotecan (debiri) versus systemic therapy for hepatic metastases from colorectal cancer: a randomized study of efficacy and quality of life. *Ann Gastroenterol Hepatol* 2012;3:39–47.

129 Cirocchi R, Trastulli S, Boselli C, *et al.* Radiofrequency ablation in the treatment of liver metastases from colorectal cancer. *Cochrane Database Syst Rev* 2012;6:CD006317.

130 Final results of the EORTC intergroup randomized study 40004 (CLOCC) evaluating the benefit of radiofrequency ablation (RFA) combined with chemotherapy for unresectable colorectal liver metastases (CRC LM). ASCO Annual Meeting Proceedings (Post-Meeting Edition), 2010. *J Clin Oncol* 2010;28:3526.

131 Burton S, Brown G, Daniels IR, *et al.* MRI directed multidisciplinary team preoperative treatment strategy: the way to eliminate positive circumferential margins? *Br J Cancer* 2006;94(3):351–7.

132 Palmer G, Martling A, Cedermark B, Holm T. Preoperative tumour staging with multidisciplinary team assessment improves the outcome in locally advanced primary rectal cancer. *Colorect Dis* 2011;13(12):1361–9.

133 Benson AB, Venook AP, Cederquist L, Chan E, Chen Y-J, *et al.* NCCN Clinical Practice Guidelines in Oncology. Colon Cancer 2. 2017. Available at: http://www.nccn.org Accessed December 8, 2018.

134 Neuman HB, Elkin EB, Guillem JG, *et al.* Treatment for patients with rectal cancer and a clinical complete response to neoadjuvant therapy: a decision analysis. *Dis Colon Rectum* 2009;52(5):863–71.

135 Faerden AE, Naimy N, Wiik P, *et al.* Total mesorectal excision for rectal cancer: difference in outcome for low and high rectal cancer. *Dis Colon Rectum* 2005;48(12):2224–31.

136 Madbouly KM, Remzi FH, Erkek BA, *et al.* Recurrence after transanal excision of t1 rectal cancer: should we be concerned? *Dis Colon Rectum* 2005;48(4):711–21.

137 Garcia-Aguilar J, Shi Q, Chan E, *et al.* A Phase II trial of neoadjuvant chemoradiation and local excision for T2N0 rectal cancer: preliminary results of the ACOSOG Z6041 Trial. *Ann Surg Oncol* 2012;19(2):384–91.

138 Abdalla EK, Vauthey JN. Steatosis as a risk factor in liver surgery. *Ann Surg* 2007;246:340–1; author reply 341.

139 Aloia T, Sebagh M, Plasse M, *et al.* Liver histology and surgical outcomes after preoperative chemotherapy with fluorouracil plus oxaliplatin in colorectal cancer liver metastases. *J Clin Oncol* 2006;24:4983–90.

140 Kemeny N. Presurgical chemotherapy in patients being considered for liver resection. *Oncologist* 2007;12:825–39.

141 de Jong MC, Pulitano C, Ribero D, *et al.* Rates and patterns of recurrence following curative intent surgery for colorectal liver metastasis: an international multi-institutional analysis of 1669 patients. *Ann Surg* 2009;250:440–8.

142 Weber JC, Bachellier P, Oussoultzoglou E, Jaeck D. Simultaneous resection of colorectal primary tumour and synchronous liver metastases. *Br J Surg* 2003;90:956–62.

143 Hao CY, Ji JF. Surgical treatment of liver metastases of colorectal cancer: strategies and controversies in 2006. *Eur J Surg Oncol* 2006;32:473–83.

144 Cirocchi R, Trastulli S, Abraha I, *et al.* Non-resection versus resection for an asymptomatic primary tumour in patients with unresectable stage IV colorectal cancer. *Cochrane Database Syst Rev* 2012;8:CD008997.

145 SEER: The Surveillance, Epidemiology, and End Results (SEER) Stat Fact Sheets: Colon and Rectum Cancer (Online). Available from: http://seer.cancer.gov/statfacts/html/colorect.html (accessed 15 December 2013).

146 Gunderson LL, Jessup JM, Sargent DJ, Greene FL, Stewart AK. Revised TN categorization for colon cancer based on national survival outcomes data. *J Clin Oncol* 2010;28(2):264–71.

147 Green BL, Marshall HC, Collinson F, *et al.* Long-term follow-up of the Medical Research Council CLASICC trial of conventional versus laparoscopically assisted resection in colorectal cancer. *Br J Surg* 2013;100(1):75–82.

148 van Gijn W, Marijnen CA, Nagtegaal ID, *et al.* Preoperative radiotherapy combined with total mesorectal excision for resectable rectal cancer: 12-year follow-up of the multicentre, randomised controlled TME trial. *Lancet Oncol* 2011;12(6):575–582.

149 Jeffery GM, Hickey BE, Hider P. Follow-up strategies for patients treated for non-metastatic colorectal cancer. *Cochrane Database Syst Rev* 2002;(1):CD002200.

150 Renehan AG, Egger M, Saunders MP, O'Dwyer ST. Impact on survival of intensive follow up after curative resection for colorectal cancer: systematic review and meta-analysis of randomised trials. *BMJ* 2002;324(7341):813.

151 McCormick CC, Gardner GJ, Schulick RD, *et al.* The role of cytoreductive surgery for colon cancer metastatic to the ovary. *Gynecol Oncol* 2007;105(3):791–5.

152 Koretz RL, Avenell A, Lipman TO, Braunschweig CL, Milne AC. Does enteral nutrition affect clinical outcome? A systematic review of the randomized trials. *Am J Gastroenterol* 2007;102(2):412–29.

153 Koretz R, Lipman T, Klein S. AGA technical review on parenteral nutrition. *Gastroenterology* 2001;121(4): 970–1001.

154 Bozzetti F, Gavazzi C, Mariani L, Crippa F. Glucose-based total parenteral nutrition does not stimulate glucose uptake by humans tumours. *Clin Nutr* 2004;23(3):417–21.

155 Hoda D, Jatoi A, Burnes J, Loprinzi C, Kelly D. Should patients with advanced, incurable cancers ever be sent home with total parenteral nutrition? *Cancer* 2005;103(4):863–8.

156 Senesse P, Assenat E, Schneider S, *et al.* Nutritional support during oncologic treatment of patients with gastrointestinal cancer: who could benefit? *Cancer Treat Rev* 2008;34(6):568–75.

157 El-Shami K, Oeffinger KC, Erb NL, *et al.* American Cancer Society colorectal cancer survivorship care guidelines. *CA Cancer J Clin* 2015;65(6):427–55.

158 Lynch BM, Steginga SK, Hawkes AL, Pakenham KI, Dunn J. Describing and predicting psychological distress after colorectal cancer. *Cancer* 2008;112(6):1363–70.

159 Ramsey SD, Berry K, Moinpour C, Giedzinska A, Andersen MR. Quality of life in long term survivors of colorectal cancer. *Am J Gastroenterol* 2002;97(5):1228–34.

160 Taskila-Brandt T, Martikainen R, Virtanen SV, *et al.* The impact of education and occupation on the employment status of cancer survivors. *Eur J Cancer* 2004;40(16):2488–93.

161 Guren MG, Eriksen MT, Wiig JN, *et al.* Quality of life and functional outcome following anterior or abdominoperineal resection for rectal cancer. *Eur J Surg Oncol* 2005;31(7):735–42.

162 Gami B, Harrington K, Blake P, *et al.* How patients manage gastrointestinal symptoms after pelvic radiotherapy. *Aliment Pharmacol Ther* 2003;18(10):987–94.

163 McGough C, Baldwin C, Frost G, Andreyev HJ. Role of nutritional intervention in patients treated with radiotherapy for pelvic malignancy. *Br J Cancer* 2004;90(12):2278–87.

164 Ho PV, Lee Y, Stein SL, Temple LK. Sexual function after treatment for rectal cancer: a review. *Dis Colon Rectum* 2011;54(1):113–25.

165 Dowswell G, Ismail T, Greenfield S, *et al.* Men's experience of erectile dysfunction after treatment for colorectal cancer: qualitative interview study. *BMJ* 2011;343:d5824.

166 Park ER, Bober SL, Campbell EG, *et al.* General internist communication about sexual function with cancer survivors. *J Gen Intern Med* 2009;24 Suppl 2:S407–11.

167 Donovan KA, Thompson LM, Hoffe SE. Sexual function in colorectal cancer survivors. *Cancer Control* 2010;17(1):44–51.

168 Lindsey I, George B, Kettlewell M, Mortensen N. Randomized, double-blind, placebo-controlled trial of sildenafil (Viagra) for erectile dysfunction after rectal excision for cancer and inflammatory bowel disease. *Dis Colon Rectum* 2002;45(6):727–32.

169 Denton AS, Maher EJ. Interventions for the physical aspects of sexual dysfunction in women following pelvic radiotherapy. *Cochrane Database Syst Rev* 2003;(1):CD003750.

170 Kwok H, Bissett IP, Hill GL. Preoperative staging of rectal cancer. *Int J Colorect Dis* 15(1):9–20.

171 Muthusamy RV, Chang KJ. Optimal methods for staging rectal cancer. Clin Cancer Res 2007;13(22):6877s–84s.

172 Brown G, Richards CJ, Bourne MW, *et al.* Morphologic predictors of lymph node status in rectal cancer with use of high-spatial-resolution MR imaging with histopathologic comparison. *Radiology* 2003;227(2):371-7.

173 Kim JH, Beets GL, Kim M, Kessels AG, Beets-Tan RG. High-resolution MRI imaging for nodal staging in rectal cancer: are there any criteria in addition to the size? *Eur J Radiol* 2004;52(1):78–83.

174 Landmann RG, Wong DW, Hoepfl J, *et al.* Limitations of early rectal cancer nodal staging may explain failure after local excision. *Dis Colon Rectum* 2007;50(10):1520–5.

175 Guillem JG, Díaz-González JA, Minsky BD, *et al.* cT3N0 rectal cancer: potential overtreatment with preoperative chemoradiotherapy is warranted. *J Clin Oncol* 2008;26(3):368–73.

176 Sizer BF, Arulampalam T, Austin R, *et al.* MRI in predicting curative resection of rectal cancer: Defining a "window of opportunity" for laparoscopic surgery. *BMJ* 2006;333: 808–9.

177 Desch CE, Somerfield MR, Flynn PJ, *et al.* Colorectal cancer surveillance: 2005 update of an American Society of Clinical Oncology practice guideline. *J Clin Oncol* 2005;23(33):8512–9.

10

Anal Cancer

Cathy Eng[1], Ravi Shridhar[2], Emily Chan[3], Nataly Silva[1], Liana Tsikitis[4], Susan Hedlund[4], Michael D. Chuong[5], and Charles R. Thomas, Jr[4]

[1] MD Anderson Cancer Center, Houston, Texas, USA
[2] Moffitt Cancer Center, Tampa, Florida, USA
[3] Vanderbilt University, Nashville, Tennessee, USA
[4] Knight Cancer Institute, Oregon Health and Science University, Portland, Oregon, USA
[5] University of Maryland, Baltimore, Maryland, USA

Incidence and Mortality

It is expected that approximately 8,200 cases of anal cancer will be diagnosed in the United States in 2017 with an estimated 1,100 deaths. Of the 8,200 cases of anal cancer, 2,950 will be male and 5,250 will be female [1]. While it is an uncommon cancer accounting for <3% of all gastrointestinal malignancies, incidence increased almost twofold in men and 1.5-fold in women from the period 1973–1979 to 1994–2000 [2].

Risk Factors Screening and Prevention

Several well-known risk factors have been identified including various subtypes of the human papillomavirus (HPV), receptive anal intercourse, history of cervical, vulvar, or vaginal cancer, immunosuppression, and smoking [3–5]. High grade anal intraepithelial neoplasia (AIN) is a precursor to anal cancer and treatment of AIN may prevent the development of anal cancer. Screening of high-risk individuals like HIV-positive homosexual men with cytology, digital rectal examination, and HPV testing may significantly reduce the incidence of anal cancer. However, randomized studies are lacking [2,6–8].

Vaccination targeting the most common HPV types associated with cervical and anal cancer has been well studied. In a randomized trial of 4,065 males aged 16–26 years, use of a quadravalent vaccine compared to placebo showed a significant reduction in external genital lesions. In a planned subset analysis of this trial, it was shown that the incidence of AIN decreased by 50% with the quadravalent vaccine [2]. This led to FDA approval for the use of a quadravalent vaccine (Gardasil) to prevent anal cancer. Recently, in December 2014, the FDA approved the nine-valent HPV vaccine to cover five additional subtypes of HPV inclusive of 16, 18, 31, 33, 45, 52 and 58, and for the prevention of genital warts caused by subtypes 6 or 11 preventing up to 90% of all HPV-associated malignancies [9]. The recommended routine HPV vaccination age ranges for girls and boys are 9–26 years and ages 9–15 years, respectively, to prevent HPV-associated cancers.

Clinical Presentation

Rectal bleeding is the most common presenting sign of anal cancer, occurring in 45% of patients. However, this symptom is often attributed incorrectly to hemorrhoids since it is often associated with pain and/or discomfort, often resulting in prolonged delays in diagnosis. Rectal pain and/or fullness are reported by 30% of patients, and 20% of patients are asymptomatic at diagnosis. Other signs and symptoms include changes in bowel movements such as thin caliber stools and tenesmus. Condyloma are found in 50% of homosexual men with anal cancer. Pruritis is more common in tumors of the perianal skin, as well as anal Bowen disease and Paget disease. Most patients present with early-stage disease; only 10–20% present with American Joint Committee on Cancer (AJCC) stage IV [10].

Anatomy and Histology

The location of anal cancer is important because patients with cancers of the anal canal are treated differently from those with anal margin malignancies. The anal canal is the terminal part of the large intestine, and extends from the anorectal junction of the upper part of the pelvic floor to the anal verge (the hair-bearing skin around the anus). This area includes the mucosal dentate line as well as the anorectal ring, a palpable ring that defines the level of the puborectalis muscle of the pelvic floor. Anal margin tumors are tumors of the perianal skin (defined as a zone of the skin with a 5 cm radius centered at the anal verge; these cancers have high cure rates with wide local excision alone, particularly when small (<3 cm in diameter) and well

The American Cancer Society's Oncology in Practice: Clinical Management, First Edition. Edited by The American Cancer Society.

differentiated [11]). Local excision is only indicated for anal margin squamous cell cancer, and not for anal canal squamous cell cancer.

Squamous cell carcinoma (SCCA) is the most common histology of anal cancer, followed by adenocarcinoma and melanoma [12]. Rare histologic subtypes (representing, in aggregate, <3% of anal cancers), include carcinoid tumors, sarcomas, gastrointestinal stromal tumors, and lymphomas. Those SCCAs occurring above the dentate line are nonkeratinizing, whereas those at or below the dentate line are keratinizing.

Staging

Since radical surgery is no longer the first option in the primary treatment of anal SCCA, tumors are staged clinically by physical examination and radiographic imaging. SCCAs are currently staged according to the tumor, node, metastasis (TNM) staging system of the AJCC and the Union for International Cancer Control (UICC) 8th edition (Table 10.1) [13]. Tumor (T) category is determined by size and invasion of adjacent structures like vagina and prostate. Nodal (N) category is based on location of involved nodes including perirectal, pelvic, and inguinal lymph nodes. Tumors of the perianal skin are staged as skin cancers excluding melanoma.

Evaluation

Suspected anal SCCA patients require a detailed history to assess for known risk factors. The degree of rectal bleeding and sphincter incontinence should be ascertained. A complete physical examination with a thorough digital rectal examination to assess for circumferential involvement, sphincter tone, and tumor size (and prostate involvement in men) is essential. In women, a pelvic examination should also be performed to rule out concurrent cervical cancer and to determine any vaginal involvement. Examination of the inguinal region should be completed in all patients. Anoscopy, proctoscopy, and/or flexible sigmoidoscopy are required to determine the extent of anorectal involvement. Laboratory studies should include a complete blood count, renal and hepatic function, hepatitis, and HIV status.

Radiographic imaging should include computed tomography (CT) of the abdomen and pelvis to assess for metastatic disease to the liver, retroperitoneal lymph nodes, pelvic, and inguinal lymph nodes. Magnetic resonance imaging of the pelvis will provide better anatomic detail to determine invasion of local structures, especially the sphincter-related musculature, and to evaluate mesorectal lymph nodes. Positron emission tomography (PET)/CT has provided utility in identifying the primary tumor, spread to inguinal lymph nodes, and response to therapy. HIV-positive patients had a higher incidence of PET-positive inguinal lymphadenopathy. All suspicious inguinal adenopathy should be biopsied as reactive lymph nodes are not unusual given the proximity of the tumor and would be informative for accuracy of staging and radiation simulation.

Prognosis and Patterns of Spread

Anal SCCA can spread through direct extension and invasion of adjacent structures, lymphatic dissemination through perirectal, pelvic, and inguinal lymph nodes, and hematogenously to distant organs such as the liver and lungs. Tumors arising above the dentate line tend to spread to perirectal (N1) nodes and those at or below the dentate line spread to inguinofemoral (N2) nodes. The likelihood of spread to lymph nodes is directly related to the size and extent of invasion of the primary tumor. Nodal metastases are identified in 0–10% of T1–2 and 40–50% of T3–4 tumors [14,15]. Factors predicting worse overall and disease-free survival among subjects in the Radiation Therapy Oncology Group (RTOG) 9811 and the European Organisation for Research and Treatment of Cancer (EORTC) 22861 trials are male gender, larger tumor diameter, and positive lymph nodes [16,17].

Treatment

Anal Margin Cancer

Patients with T1 anal margin cancer should undergo wide local excision. In the event of a positive margin, re-excision should be attempted. If re-excision is not feasible, then radiation alone to a dose of 60 Gy is recommended. Patients with T2 or greater lesions should receive chemoradiation regimens similar to those used for anal canal cancers.

Anal Canal Cancer

Surgery

Prior to development of sphincter-preservation treatments, abdominoperineal resection (APR) was the standard of care for the primary treatment of anal carcinoma, with 5-year overall survival in the range of 25–75% [18–20]. Locoregional and distant relapse occurred in up to 35% and 10%, respectively, with higher rates of relapse among patients with positive pelvic or inguinal lymph nodes. APR is reserved for salvage therapy for residual or recurrent disease. Transanal excision is only indicated for AIN without invasion.

Chemoradiation

Nigro *et al.* established that complete response of anal SCCA was possible for patients treated with low dose radiotherapy (30 Gy) concurrent with 5-fluorouracil (5-FU) and mitomycin C (MMC) [21]. In a larger phase II study of patients treated preoperatively with the same chemoradiation regimen, 84% were rendered free of cancer. No recurrence of tumor was noted in those patients achieving a complete response. However, patients with residual cancer after preoperative therapy (15%) had recurrence at distant sites and died of disease [22]. Several randomized trials addressing the role of concurrent chemotherapy, induction chemotherapy, maintenance chemotherapy, and biologic therapy are summarized in Table 10.2.

Chemoradiation vs Radiation

While chemoradiation had been shown to be efficacious in patients with anal SCCA, some clinicians questioned the necessity of chemotherapy, as some early studies had demonstrated efficacy of high-dose radiation alone. Further, there was a concern about late toxicities with the radiation-potentiating effects of chemotherapy.

The United Kingdom Coordinating Committee on Cancer Research (UKCCCR) Anal Cancer Trial (ACT I) addressed this

Table 10.1 American Joint Committee on Cancer (AJCC) anal carcinoma staging, 8th edn (excluding melanoma, carcinoid, and sarcomas).

Definition of primary tumor (T)

T category	T criteria
TX	Primary tumor not assessed
T0	No evidence of primary tumor
Tis	High-grade squamous intraepithelial lesion (previously termed carcinoma *in situ*, Bowen disease, anal intraepithelial neoplasia II–III, high-grade anal intraepithelial neoplasia)
T1	Tumor ≤2 cm
T2	Tumor >2 cm but ≤5 cm
T3	Tumor >5 cm
T4	Tumor of any size invading adjacent organ(s), such as the vagina, urethra, or bladder

Definition of regional lymph node (N)

N category	N criteria
NX	Regional lymph nodes cannot be assessed
N0	No regional lymph node metastasis
N1	Metastasis in inguinal, mesorectal, internal iliac, or external iliac nodes
N1a	Metastasis in inguinal, mesorectal, or internal iliac lymph nodes
N1b	Metastasis in external iliac lymph nodes
N1c	Metastasis in external iliac with any N1a nodes

Definition of distant metastasis (M)

M category	M criteria
M0	No distant metastasis
M1	Distant metastasis

AJCC prognostic stage groups

When T is...	And N is...	And M is...	Then the stage group is...
Tis	N0	M0	0
T1	N0	M0	I
T1	N1	M0	IIIA
T2	N0	M0	IIA
T2	N1	M0	IIIA
T3	N0	M0	IIB
T3	N1	M0	IIIC
T4	N0	M0	IIIB
T4	N1	M0	IIIC
Any T	Any N	M1	IV

Source: used with permission of the American College of Surgeons, Chicago, Illinois. The original source for this information is the AJCC Cancer Staging Manual, 8th Edition (2017), which is published by Springer Science + Business Media.

question by randomizing 585 patients to either radiation monotherapy (45 Gy over 5 weeks) or the same radiation regimen combined with bolus 5-FU chemotherapy during the first and last week of radiation and MMC on day 1 [23]. Patients with a good response 6 weeks after treatment received a radiotherapy boost, and poor responders underwent salvage surgery. After a median follow-up of 42 months, the local failure occurred less often in the chemoradiation arm than to the radiation monotherapy arm (36% vs 59%; P <0.0001). Chemoradiation resulted in more early morbidity than radiation monotherapy (48% vs 39%, P = 0.03) but late morbidity rates (42% vs 38%, P = 0.39) were similar. Updated results after 13 years of follow-up showed median overall survival (OS) was 7.6 years for the chemoradiation arm and 5.4 years for the radiation alone arm. Although this difference was not statistically significant, the risk of dying from SCCA was significantly (P <0.004) lower (by 33%) with chemoradiation [24].

The EORTC also conducted a phase III randomized trial of radiation versus chemoradiation in 110 patients with anal SCCA [25]. Surgical resection was performed if patients had not

Table 10.2 Randomized trials of chemoradiation for anal cancer.

Trial	*n*	Treatment arms	Median follow-up (months)	Timepoint (years)	LC (%)	CFS (%)	Colostomy rate (%)	PFS (%)	DFS (%)	OS (%)
UKCCCR [23,24] **(ACT I)**	585	RT +/− 5-FU/MMC RT alone	157	10	66* 43	36* 26			36** 24	42** 36
EORTC [25]	110	RT +5-FU/MMC RT alone	42	5	69* 55					69** 64
RTOG 87-04 [31]	310	RT + 5-FU RT + 5-FU/MMC	36	4		59* 71	22* 9		51* 73	
RTOG 98-11 [34,35]	644	RT + 5-FU/MCC Induction CDDP → RT + 5-FU/CDDP	156	5	80** 74	72* 65	12** 17		68* 58	78* 71
ACT II [37]	940	RT + 5-FU/MMC RT + 5-FU/CDDP RT + 5-FU/MMC → adjuvant 5-FU/CDDP RT + 5-FU/CDDP → adjuvant 5-FU/CDDP	61	3	89** 87 88 88		(CDDP vs MMC) 11** 14	73** 72 73 74		
ACCORD-03 [36]	307	Induction 5-FU/CDDP → RT (standard boost) + 5-FU/MMC Induction 5-FU/CDDP → RT (high dose boost) + 5-FU/MMC RT (standard boost) + 5-FU/CDDP RT (high dose boost) + 5-FU/CDDP	50	5		70** 82 77 73				

CDDP, cisplatin; CFS, colostomy free survival; DFS, disease free survival; 5-FU, 5-fluorouracil; LC, local control; MMC, mitomycin C; OS, overall survival; PFS, progression free survival; RT, radiotherapy; *statistically significant; **not statistically significant.

responded 6 weeks after 45 Gy or if palpable residual disease persisted after therapy completion. Subjects in the chemoradiation arm received bolus 5-FU chemotherapy during the first and last week of radiation and MMC on day 1. Patients in the chemoradiation arm had a higher complete response rate (80% vs 54%), as well as fewer locoregional recurrences and higher colostomy-free rates ($P=0.002$). Unlike the results of ACT I, acute toxicities were not significantly different in the two groups. Late toxicities were also similar, with the exception of an increased incidence of anal canal ulcers in the combined modality group. The chemoradiation arm had an improved progression-free survival (PFS) ($P=0.05$). There was no difference in OS between the two groups, although it should be noted that the median survival time had not been reached at the time of the study report.

ACT I and the EORTC trials confirmed the superiority of chemoradiation over radiation alone in the treatment of anal SCCA. Both trials showed an improvement in locoregional control and PFS with the addition of chemotherapy. The ACT I trial further showed that the addition of chemotherapy increased OS, but this benefit was evident only after long-term follow-up, possibly due to the increase in nonanal cancer deaths in the chemoradiation arm during the first 10 years.

Role of Mitomycin C

While ACT I and the EORTC study established the role of chemotherapy in combination with radiation in the treatment of SCCA, concern regarding the toxicity of MMC led to subsequent studies to determine the benefit of adding MMC to 5-FU. Although MMC is among the most active cytotoxic antineoplastic agents [26], its toxicity is significant and can include life-threatening hemolytic uremic syndrome and thrombotic thrombocytopenic purpura [27–29]. The benefit of using MMC as part of a combined-modality approach for SCCA was initially reported before widespread recognition of the antitumor activity and radiosensitizing properties of cisplatin in the treatment of aerodigestive tract carcinomas [30].

RTOG 87-04/ECOG 1289 was a phase III intergroup study in which 310 patients with anal SCCA were randomized to chemoradiation with either 5-FU or 5-FU/MMC [31]. The MMC arm had a lower colostomy rate at 4 years (9% vs 23%, $P=0.002$), and although the addition of MMC improved 4-year PFS (73% vs 51%, $P=0.0003$), there was no statistically significant difference in 4-year OS. The addition of MMC did result in more acute toxicities ($P<0.001$). This trial confirmed the benefit of the adding MMC to 5-FU and radiation for SCCA but also suggested that it should not be used routinely in immunosuppressed individuals given the neutropenia rate and toxic deaths seen in the MMC arm.

Role of Cisplatin

Based on the encouraging results of phase II studies incorporating cisplatin [32,33] compared to historical results of chemoradiation with 5-FU and MMC, RTOG 98-11 was designed to evaluate whether cisplatin was superior to MMC.

Induction or Maintenance Chemotherapy

RTOG 98-11 was an intergroup phase III trial that randomized 682 patients with SCCA to chemoradiation with either bolus 5-FU/MMC or induction cisplatin and 5-FU followed by chemoradiation with cisplatin and 5-FU during radiation. [34]. Chemoradiation with 5-FU/MMC resulted in superior 5-year disease-free survival (DFS) (67.8% vs 57.8%, $P=0.006$) and 5-year OS (78.3% vs 70.7%, $P=0.026$) compared to chemoradiation with 5-FU and cisplatin [35]. Hence, chemoradiation with 5-FU/MMC remained the standard of care.

The cisplatin arm of RTOG 98-11 included two cycles of induction chemotherapy before chemoradiation was initiated, based on the hypothesis that induction chemotherapy could reduce the burden of disease and make the chemoradiation more effective, thereby improving DFS. As noted above, results for the cisplatin and 5-FU arm were inferior, suggesting no benefit for induction chemotherapy or for the use of cisplatin when MMC is an option.

The UNICANCER ACCORD 03 phase III trial sought to improve the efficacy of chemoradiation by either adding induction chemotherapy with 5-FU/cisplatin or dose escalation of the radiation boost [36]. Patients ($n=307$) with SCCA >4 cm or <4 cm and N1-3 M0 were randomized to one of four treatment arms: (i) arm A: two cycles of induction chemotherapy with 5-FU/cisplatin followed by chemoradiation with 45 Gy radiation over 5 weeks, plus standard dose boost (15 Gy); (ii) arm B: two cycles of induction chemotherapy with 5-FU/cisplatin followed by chemoradiation with 45 Gy radiation over 5 weeks plus high dose boost (20–25 Gy); (iii) arm C: chemoradiation with 45 Gy radiation over 5 weeks, 5-FU/cisplatin on weeks 1 and 5, and standard dose boost (15 Gy); and (iv) arm D: chemoradiation with 45 Gy radiation over 5 weeks, 5-FU/cisplatin on weeks 1 and 5, and high-dose boost (20–25 Gy). There was no statistically significant benefit in 5-year colostomy-free survival to either induction chemotherapy ($P=0.37$) or high-dose radiation boost ($P=0.067$). None of the secondary endpoints, including 5-year local control, 5-year disease-specific survival, and 5-year tumor-free survival, showed a statistically significant benefit with the addition of either induction chemotherapy or high-dose radiation boost.

To date, ACT II is the only large phase III trial to be completed in the locally advanced patient population which also evaluated the role of cisplatin in the treatment of SCCA [37]. This 2×2 factorial trial randomly assigned 940 subjects to one of four groups to receive radiation (50.4 Gy) and bolus 5-FU on the first and last week of radiation with either MMC or cisplatin, with or without two cycles of maintenance chemotherapy (5-FU/cisplatin). The primary endpoint was to establish superiority of 5-FU/cisplatin versus that of MMC for DFS. With regards to the cisplatin arm, there was no difference in complete response at 26 weeks (90.5% for MMC and 89.6% for cisplatin, $P=$ NS) or toxicity (71% for MMC and 72% for cisplatin, $P=$ NS). There was also no difference in 3-year PFS with regards to maintenance or no maintenance (74% vs 73% respectively, $P=$ NS). As expected, addition of MMC resulted in nonhematologic toxicities. Given these equivocal results, chemoradiation with 5-FU and MMC remain the standard of care for the treatment of SCCA.

Tumor Regression

Anal SCCA may respond to chemoradiotherapy immediately or slowly, over several months. Cummings *et al.* demonstrated that the rate of regression over time is not a good measure of the effectiveness of treatment. [38]. In a French study, patients with T3 or T4 tumors who achieved a >80% response after the initial phase of radiotherapy had 5-year colostomy-free survival of 65%, versus 25% of patients who had <80% response ($P = 0.002$). The ACT-II trial showed a pivotal finding. In 29% of patients who did not achieve a complete response at 11 weeks, complete response may still be achieved at 26 weeks. Hence, these results suggest it may be appropriate to follow patients with persistent disease conservatively for up to 26 weeks as there is no evidence of disease progression [37].

Intensity-Modulated Radiation Therapy

Intensity-modulated radiation therapy (IMRT) allows for safe tumor dose escalation while reducing dose to surrounding normal tissues like skin, small bowel, bladder, femoral heads, external genitalia, and bone marrow. IMRT has been evaluated in several dosimetric studies and shown to be superior compared to 3D conformal therapy planning [39–46]. Dermatologic and small bowel toxicity can necessitate treatment breaks which could potentially negatively affect outcomes. By reducing dose to surrounding normal tissues, acute toxicity will be minimized resulting in fewer treatment breaks and shorter overall treatment time [47–50]. Several small retrospective series with patient numbers ranging from 17 to 78 and median follow-up ranging from 16 to 24 months have demonstrated the safety and feasibility of IMRT chemoradiation (Table 10.3) [51–60]. Two to three year locoregional control, colostomy free survival, and overall survival range from 77 to 95%, 81 to 93%, and 87 to 100%, respectively. Acute grade 3 or greater gastrointestinal (GI) toxicity was reported in the range of 0–28%. Acute grade 3 or greater dermatologic toxicity was reported in the range of 0–38%. In RTOG 9811 where all patients were treated with conventional radiotherapy, acute grade 3+ GI and dermatologic toxicity were 36% and 49%, respectively [34,35]. RTOG 0529 is a completed prospective phase II trial to determine if dose-painted IMRT could reduce toxicity compared to RTOG 9811 [55]. The primary endpoint was a 15% reduction in combined grade 2+ genitourinary and gastrointestinal toxicity. Of 63 patients enrolled, 52 were evaluable. While the trial failed to meet its primary endpoint, there was a significant reduction in acute grade 2+ hematologic, grade 3+ dermatologic, and gastrointestinal toxicity. As such, IMRT has evolved as a *de facto* standard of care in the administration of radiotherapy for SCCA patients undergoing combined modality therapy [61].

Several retrospective studies comparing toxicity and outcomes of 3D conformal radiation to IMRT [47,49,50,62,63] are presented in Table 10.4. Four studies [47,49,50,63] report on toxicity with three studies showing significant reduction in acute grade 3+ GI and dermatologic toxicity [47,49,63] and one study by Chuong *et al.* showing a reduction in late grade 3+ GI toxicity in favor of IMRT (24.3% vs 5.8%; $P = 0.012$) [47]. All but one study [49] show equivalent outcomes with regard to locoregional control, colostomy-free survival, and overall survival. Bazan *et al.* do show that IMRT confers a survival and local control benefit over conventional radiation; however, the outcomes of their 3D conformal group are inferior to those reported in RTOG9811 and the other comparative studies.

Management of Inguinal Lymph Nodes

Inguinal metastases are present at diagnosis in 0–33% of patients with anal SCCA; prevalence is even higher among those with AJCC T-categories T3–4 [64]. Prophylactic inguinal irradiation can reduce the inguinal recurrence rate among clinically node-negative patients from a range of 7.5–13% (without treatment), to approximately 1.3–3% [31,65–70]. Patients with T3–4 tumors and clinically uninvolved inguinal lymph nodes should have chemoradiation that includes inguinal irradiation [70,71]. The role of inguinal radiation in T1–2 tumors is still controversial. A phase II study by Matthews *et al.* revealed that the overall inguinal recurrence rate in 44 patients with T1–2 N0 tumors without inguinal radiation was 22.5% [72]. In a retrospective study from Zilli *et al.*, they reported outcomes of T2N0 patients treated with chemoradiotherapy versus radiotherapy with or without inguinal radiation in 116 patients [73]. Overall 5-year inguinal relapse-free survival was 92.3%. Inguinal recurrence occurred in two patients (4.7%) treated without inguinal radiation. There were no groin relapses in patients treated with groin radiation. The 5-year locoregional control rates for patients treated with and without groin radiation and with radiotherapy alone versus chemoradiotherapy were 80.1% versus 77.8% ($P = 0.967$) and 71.0% versus 85.4% ($P = 0.147$), respectively. A trend toward a higher rate of grade 3+ acute toxicity was observed in patients treated with groin radiation (53% vs 31%, $P = 0.076$). Determination of who should be treated with groin radiation prophylactically will depend on increasing reliance of PET-CT. The study also showed that groin radiation was associated with increased grade toxicity [73]. However, lower doses of 36–42 Gy in 1.5–1.8 Gy fractions with IMRT to clinically uninvolved nodal regions has resulted in equivalent oncological outcomes with an associated decrease in dermal toxicity [47,51,52,54,55].

Immunocompromised Patients

Chemoradiation therapy is not contraindicated for HIV-positive patients with anal SCCA. While acute treatment-related toxicity and relapse rates may be higher in patients with HIV-AIDS treated with chemoradiotherapy, their response to therapy and survival is comparable to those of HIV-negative patients [74–77]. However, dosage reduction of MMC may be necessary for patients with HIV-related complications given the high degree of myelosuppression that increases the chance of opportunistic infections [2].

Metastatic Disease

Chemotherapeutic Regimens in the Treatment of Metastatic Anal SCCA

Several challenges remain in the treatment of metastatic anal SCCA. Most of the published evidence regarding metastatic anal canal cancer consists of small case series. Most chemotherapeutic regimens, mainly 5-FU and platinum-based therapy, have been adapted from studies of SCCA of other primary tumor sites. The optimal duration of chemotherapy remains unestablished. Based on our preliminary findings, systemic chemotherapy should be considered in any anal SCCA patients with good performance status and should be continued indefinitely for maximal outcome if tolerated well.

Table 10.3 Summary of studies evaluating intensity-modulated radiation therapy-based chemoradiation for anal cancer.

Study	*n*	Median tumor dose (Gy) (range)	Median Follow-up (months)	Timepoint (years)	LRC (%)	CFS (%)	OS (%)	Acute G3+ GI toxicity (%)	Acute G3+ skin toxicity (%)
Retrospective studies									
Milano *et al.* [56]	17	54 (45–59.4)	20.3	2	82	82	91	0	0
Salama *et al.* [59]	53	51.5 (32–60.9)	14.5	1.5	84	84	93.4	15.1	37.7
Pepek *et al.* [58]	29	54 (37.8–64)	19	2	95	91	100	9	0
Call *et al.* [51]	34	50.4 (48.6–57.6)	22	3	88	NR	87	NA	NA
Chuong *et al.* [52]	52	56 (50–62.5)	21	3	94	93	100	9.6	11.5
Kachnic *et al.* [54]	43	54	24	2	95	90	94	7	10
DeFoe *et al.* [53]	78	55.8	16	2	84	81	87	28	29
Vieillot *et al.* [60]	39	63 (40–65)	24	2	77	85	89	10	0
Mitchell et *al.* [57]	65	54 (50–58.8)	19	2	93	NR	96	9	17
Prospective studies (RTOG 9811 3DCRT included for comparison)									
RTOG 0529 Ph II [55]	52	50.4 (T2); 54 (T3–4)	27	2	NA[1]	NA[1]	86	21	23
RTOG 9811 Ph III 34, 35]	649	(45–59)	NR	5	80[2]	72[2]	78.3[2]	36[3]	49[3]

[1] 2-year outcomes similar to RTOG 9811.
[2] mitomycin C arm.
[3] all patients.
CFS, colostomy free survival; IMRT, intensity-modulated radiation therapy; LRC, locoregional control; NA, not available; OS, overall survival; RTOG, Radiation Therapy Oncology Group; 3DCRT, conventional radiation therapy.

Table 10.4 Retrospective studies comparing 3D conformal radiotherapy versus intensity-modulated radiation therapy for anal cancer.

Study	Technique	*n*	Median dose (Gy) (range)	Median follow-up (months)	Median RT days	Timepoint (years)	LRC (%)	CFS (%)	OS (%)	Acute G3+ GI toxicity (%)	Acute G3+ skin toxicity (%)
Saarilathi *et al.* [63]	3DCRT	39	NR	81	NA	NA	92.3	NR	NR	12	32
	IMRT	20	NR	19	NA	NA	85	NR	NR	0	16
	P-value						0.54			0.004	NS
Bazan *et al.* [49]	3DCRT	17	54 (45–62.4)	26	57	3	57	NR	52	29	41
	IMRT	29	54 (45–59.4)	32	40	3	92	91	88	7	21
	P-value				<0.0001		<0.01		<0.01	0.003	0.003
Dewas *et al.* [50]	3DCRT	27	59.4 (30.6–66.6)	60	59	2	88	81.1	81.1	3.7	33.3
	IMRT	24	59.4 (30.6–66.6)	23	47	2	65.8	60.3	88.5	20.8	37.5
	P-value				0.0007		NS	0.12	0.58	0.088	0.756
Dasgupta *et al.* [62]	3DCRT	178	45 (45–50.4)	73.2	39	2	82	91	90	NA	NA
	IMRT	45	54 (50–56)	27.6	40	2	87	97	93	NA	NA
	P-value		<0.01		0.62		0.2	0.1	0.91		
Chuong *et al.* [47]	3DCRT	37	59.4 (45–63)	62	49	3	92	94	86	30[1]	65
	IMRT	52	56 (50–62.5)	20	39	3	91	91.3	91	9.6[1]	11.5
	P-value		0.038		<0.0001		>0.1	>0.1	>0.1	0.061	<0.0001

[1] Chronic grade 3+ gastrointestinal toxicity for 3DCRT versus IMRT is 24.3% vs 5.8% ($P = 0.012$); CFS, colostomy free survival; IMRT, intensity modulated radiation therapy; LRC, locoregional control; NA, not available; NS, not significant; OS, overall survival; RT, radiotherapy; 3DCRT, 3D conformal radiation therapy;

The Gold Standard: 5-Fluorouracil (5-FU) and Cisplatin

The most commonly reported regimen is continuous infusion of 5-FU (1 g/m^2/day × 5 days) plus an infusion of cisplatin (100 mg/m^2) on day 2, every 4 weeks which, in a series of 18 patients, demonstrated a partial response rate of up to 50% and a complete response rate of 15% [34,78–82]. All patients received a median of four cycles and all had acceptable toxicities. The most common toxicities included mucositis, nausea, vomiting, diarrhea, neutropenia, electrolyte imbalances, peripheral neuropathy, and tinnitus. Although typically providing some degree of response, long-term control or cure has not been reported in patients with metastatic SCCA receiving this regimen.

Carboplatin/Paclitaxel/Continuous Infusion 5-FU (TPF)

Hainsworth *et al.* conducted a phase II study of 60 patients with metastatic SCCA of any nonpulmonary primary site of which only four patients had SCCA of the anal canal. The chemotherapy regimen consisted of paclitaxel 200 mg/m^2, 1-h intravenous infusion, days 1 and 22; carboplatin (AUC = 6, days 1 and 22); 5-FU 225 mg/m^2/day, by 24-h continuous intravenous infusion, days 1–36; repeated every 6 weeks. In this study, all patients received a maximum of four cycles of therapy, which caused a high incidence of grade 3/4 toxicities including myelosuppression (48%), diarrhea (17%), and mucositis (28%). The overall and complete response rates were 65% and 25%, respectively. Two patients with a primary anal SCCA had complete responses. The median duration of response for the anal SCCA patients was 26 months [83].

Novel Approaches

Treatment-naïve patients: the InterAACT trial (EA 2133; NCT02560298) is the first randomized phase II of 5-FU/cisplatin versus carboplatin/paclitaxel in newly diagnosed metastatic patients. This international trial has completed enrollment with final results pending.

Previously treated patients: a phase I expanded cohort study of the single agent immune checkpoint kinase inhibitor LY2606368 was conducted in heavily pretreated patients ($n = 26$) [84]. Single agent LY260636 resulted in a response rate of 16% (one complete response; three partial response as per RECIST criteria 1.1).

The role of immune checkpoint (PD-1) inhibitors against the programmed death ligand have also been evaluated. A phase IB expanded cohort study of pembrolizumab was conducted in previously treated SCCA tumors overexpressing PD-1 resulting in a response rate of 13% [85,86]. NCI9673 was the first phase II study completed to evaluate the role of immune checkpoint inhibitors of single agent nivolumab resulting in a response rate of 24% (two complete responses; seven partial responses) [87]. NCI9673 is undergoing an amendment to allow additional patient enrollment. Additional studies are currently being proposed to evaluate the role of immune checkpoint inhibitors in locally advanced anal cancer.

Other novel approaches include a live attenuated *Listeria monocytogenes* (Lm-)-based immunotherapy (ADXS11-001) which was developed for the treatment of HPV-associated diseases. ADXS11-001 secretes an antigen-adjuvant fusion (Lm-LLO) protein consisting of a truncated fragment of the Lm protein listeriolysin O (LLO) fused to HPV-16/E7. A pilot trial led by Safran *et al.* (NCT02399813) suggests there may be a role for ADXS11-001 in early stage anal cancer [88]. FAWCETT (NCT02399813) is a phase II single agent trial that is currently ongoing in previously treated metastatic anal cancer.

Salvage Therapy

Locoregional Recurrence

Locoregional recurrence occurs after chemoradiation in approximately 10–30% of patients with anal SCCA [89,90]. Patients with recurrence after chemoradiation who undergo salvage APR surgery have a 5-year survival of 40–60% compared to a 3-year overall survival of 5% for patients who are unsuitable for surgery [91]. In a study from MD Anderson Cancer Center of 31 patients with locoregional recurrence [89], the 5-year survival rate following salvage APR was 64%; the most significant prognostic factor was a negative resection margin [92]. Median survival for patients with negative and positive margins after salvage surgery was 33.0 versus 14.3 months, respectively.

Patients with inguinal recurrence who did not receive groin radiation were salvaged with chemoradiation. However, if there is inguinal recurrence after groin radiation, an inguinal lymph node dissection should be performed. APR can be avoided if there is no recurrence in the anus in patients with inguinal recurrence.

Radiation Techniques

Target Volume and Radiation Field Design

With the increased utilization of multifield techniques for 3D conformal radiotherapy (3DCRT) and IMRT, proper delineation of tumor and nodal volumes is required. The gross tumor volume (GTV) is representative of the tumor and grossly involved lymph nodes. The extent of GTV can be determined by information from physical examination and endoscopic findings. In addition, GTV can be more accurately delineated by fusion of the treatment planning CT scan to a treatment planning magnetic resonance image or PET-CT scan obtained at the time of simulation. The clinical target volume (CTV) includes microscopic extension of the GTV in addition to the high-risk nodal areas including perirectal and mesorectal nodes, pelvic lymph nodes including bilateral internal and external iliac chains, bilateral inguinal lymphatics, and presacral nodes. The superior extent of the CTV is at the level of the sacral promontory or the iliac bifurcation. The inferior extent of the CTV is 3 cm below the GTV of the anal canal.

NCCN recommends following the multifield technique per RTOG 9811 [34], although IMRT-based treatment is being more commonly used [61]. PET-CT should be performed for treatment planning purposes for accurate delineation of the GTV and involved lymphatics. For node-negative patients, field reduction off the superior border and groins is recommended after 30.6 and 36 Gy, respectively. Attempts should be made to reduce dose to the femoral heads. In patients treated with an AP (anteroposterior)–PA (posteroanterior) approach, lateral inguinal lymphatics should be brought to a minimum dose of 36 Gy using an anterior *en face* electron boost matched to the PA field exit dose. IMRT can be used in place of 3DCRT but requires precise contouring of normal tissues, GTV, and CTV to reduce marginal miss. In RTOG 0529, 81% of patients required IMRT replanning with three cases of major deviations of normal tissues [55]. Atlases for precise contouring of SCCA targets and normal tissues are available at the RTOG (http://atc.wustl.edu/protocols/rtog-closed/0529/ANAL_Ca_CTVs_5-21-07_Final.pdf, accessed 28 September 2017) and from the Australasian Gastrointestinal Trials Group [93].

Treatment Breaks

ECOG 4292, a phase II trial of chemoradiation with 5-FU and cisplatin in SCCA, enrolled 33 subjects [32]. This trial prescribed a radiation dose of 59.4 Gy in 33 fractions over 60 days. There were two cohorts. Cohort 1 ($n = 19$) had a planned 2 week break in the radiation after 36 Gy was given and cohort 2 ($n = 13$) had no planned break. The 5-year overall survival for cohorts 1 and 2 was 58% and 84%, respectively. A comparison of outcomes of patients treated on RTOG 8704 (50.4 Gy) versus RTOG 9208 (59.4 Gy split course) revealed that overall, disease-free, and colostomy-free survival were inferior in patients treated with split course radiation [94]. In a recent analysis of pooled data from RTOG 9811 and RTOG 8704, it was shown that total treatment time but not total RT duration was significantly associated with colostomy failure and local failure on univariate analysis [95]. It was suggested that induction chemotherapy may contribute to local failure by increasing total treatment time. Finally, the results of the ACT II randomized trial showed a high complete response and 3-year relapse-free survival of 74% with 50.4 Gy chemoradiation [37]. The good results were attributed to the lack of a treatment break. Treatment breaks in general should be avoided whenever possible. However, this may be unavoidable due to treatment-related toxicity like skin desquamation and diarrhea [96]. IMRT has been shown to reduce toxicity and RT duration compared with 3DCRT. However, no differences in locoregional control, overall, and colostomy-free survival were noted (Tables 10.3 and 10.4).

Quality of Life for Patients Treated for Anal Cancer

The majority of patients with anal SCCA who are treated with chemotherapy and radiation have excellent outcomes [34]. However, immediate side effects and toxicity may adversely affect the quality of life (QoL). The immediate and late effects include sexual dysfunction, urological/GI complaints, financial difficulties, fatigue, and a reduction in emotional and social well-being [97].

Acute effects of chemoradiation for anal carcinomas include diarrhea, mucositis, skin erythema, and myelosupression. Late complications include anal ulcers, stricture, stenosis, fistulae, and necrosis.

Allal *et al.* evaluated the QoL of 41 patients with anal SCCA (35 female and six male), after radiation alone or combined chemoradiation. Patients treated with radiation with or without chemotherapy rated their QoL to be similar to that of the general population with the exception of noting more frequent diarrhea [98]. Although 50% of these patients reported suboptimal anal function, 71% reported that they were satisfied with their current function. Of note, however, the sexual functioning score in this study was very low, with only 35% of patients reporting some sexual activity. Moreover, the extent of this activity varied greatly among patients and never reached the maximum level of functioning in any patient. Because genital organs are in close proximity to the high-dose treatment volume, this high degree of sexual dysfunction is consistent with the studies of women with gynecological cancers [99] and men with prostate cancers [100], in whom loss of sexual desire and/or orgasm, dyspareunia, and loss of potency are frequent.

Das *et al.* also evaluated long-term QoL of 32 patients with anal SCCA who were treated with radiotherapy or chemoradiation. These patients had acceptable overall QoL scores, but poor sexual functioning scores. Of note, younger patients were found to have lower QoL and sexual functioning scores [101].

Proactive Approaches to Management of Side Effects

Sexual Side Effects

Proactive care and prompt responses to onset of side effects can help minimize immediate and long-term effects. For women receiving pelvic radiation, the early and ongoing use of dilators, moisturizers, and lubricants should be encouraged, with clear information given about its importance. Vaginal foreshortening due to fibrosis is a significant subacute and late side effect of pelvic irradiation. Cullen *et al.* suggest eight care recommendations that address the concerns of women treated with pelvic radiation: (i) introducing the dilator in a light and straightforward manner; (ii) enhance dilator accessibility; (iii) introduce the dilator early in treatment; (iv) emphasize health maintenance over intercourse as a benefit of dilator use; (v) explore and acknowledge women's values and views on sexuality; (vi) increased awareness and sensitivity to emotional reactions; (vii) enhance psychoeducational resources for supporting vaginal dilator use; (viii) ensure consistent institutional practice when introducing the dilator. Early involvement of support services, including physical therapists, pelvic rehab specialists, dieticians, and psychosocial support can be very helpful. Also, topical estrogen, vaginal moisturizers, lubricants, and vaginal dilators can help improve sexual function in women. Minimizing radiotherapy dose to a portion of the anterior wall of the vaginal vault may also be helpful. Phosphodiesterase inhibitors, such as sildenafil, can help improve sexual function in men after anal cancer treatment.

Mirabeau-Beale *et al.* evaluated 95 consecutive women who were treated for locally advanced anal cancer between 2003 and 2012 [102]. Sixty-four percent of patients developed grade 2 and 3 vaginal stenosis. The development of vaginal stenosis was more common in younger patients, with a higher dose of radiation, and associated with years of radiation therapy provided.

Fertility Preservation

It is essential that all disciplines discuss fertility preservation and refer patients of child-bearing age to a reproductive endocrinologist [103,104].

GI Side Effects

Articles have reviewed the appropriate management of GI and sexual dysfunction after pelvic radiotherapy [105–107]. Opiate agonists such as loperamide, bulking agents, and a low-fiber diet can help decrease GI symptoms, like diarrhea. Sacral nerve stimulation may be a possible treatment for fecal and urinary incontinence [108].

Conclusion

Concurrent chemoradiation for curative intent remains the standard of care for locally advanced anal cancer. Although the role of chemotherapy as a radiation sensitization has largely remained unchanged, the multidisciplinary management is now focused on prolonging the duration of surveillance before making a critical decision regarding salvage surgery as well as acute and chronic toxicities. Novel approaches will likely include the role immunotherapy as a potential treatment option for both early and late stage disease.

References

1 Siegel R, Miller KD, Jemal A. Cancer statistics, 2017. *CA Cancer J Clin* 2017;67(1):7–30.
2 NCCN. NCCN Guidelines for Anal Carcinoma, 2016. Version 2.2016.
3 Ahmed S, Eng C. Optimal treatment strategies for anal cancer. *Curr Treat Options Oncol* 2014;15(3):443–55.
4 Eng C, Ahmed S. Optimal management of squamous cell carcinoma of the anal canal: where are we now? *Expert Rev Anticancer Ther* 2014;14(8):877–86.
5 Nelson VM, Benson AB. Epidemiology of anal cancer. *Surg Oncol Clin N Am* 2017;26(1):9–15.
6 Palefsky JM. Screening to prevent anal cancer: current thinking and future directions. *Cancer Cytopathol* 2015;123(9):509–10.
7 Wang CJ, Sparano J, Palefsky JM. Human immunodeficiency virus/AIDS, human papilloma virus, and anal cancer. *Surg Oncol Clin* 2017;26(1):17–31
8 Uronis HE, Bendell JC. Anal cancer: an overview. *Oncologist* 2007;12(5):524–34.
9 Joura EA, Guiliano AR, Iverson OE, *et al.* A 9-valent HPV vaccine against infection and intraepithelial neoplasia in women N Engl J Med 2015;372(8):711–23.
10 Bilimoria KY, Bentrem DJ, Rock CE, *et al.* Outcomes and prognostic factors for squamous-cell carcinoma of the anal canal: analysis of patients from the National Cancer Data Base. *Dis Colon Rectum* 2009;52:624–31.
11 Moore HG, Guillem JG. Anal neoplasms. *Surg Clin North Am* 2002;82(6):1233–51.
12 Klas JV, Rothenberger DA, Wong WD, *et al.* Malignant tumors of the anal canal: the spectrum of disease, treatment, and outcomes. *Cancer* 1999;85(8):1686–93.
13 Welton ML, Steele SR, Goodman KA, *et al.* Anus. In: M Amin, S Edge, R Greene, *et al.* (eds) *AJCC Cancer Staging Manual 8th Edition*. New York: Springer, 2017.
14 Wade DS, Herrera L, Castillo NB, *et al.* Metastases to the lymph nodes in epidermoid carcinoma of the anal canal studied by a clearing technique. *Surg Gynecol Obstet* 1989;169(3):238–42.
15 Davey P, Saibil EA, Wong R. Bipedal lymphography in the management of carcinoma of the anal canal. *Br J Radiol* 1996;69(823):632–5.
16 Ajani JA, Winter KA, Gunderson LL, *et al.* Prognostic factors derived from a prospective database dictate clinical biology of anal cancer: the intergroup trial (RTOG 98–11). *Cancer* 2010;116(17):4007–13.
17 Bartelink, H, Roelofsen F, Eschwege F, *et al.* Concomitant radiotherapy and chemotherapy is superior to radiotherapy alone in the treatment of locally advanced anal cancer: results of a phase III randomized trial of the European Organization for Research and Treatment of Cancer Radiotherapy and Gastrointestinal Cooperative Groups. *J Clin Oncol* 1997;15(5):2040–9.
18 Boman BM, Moertel CG, O'Connell MJ, *et al.* Carcinoma of the anal canal. A clinical and pathologic study of 188 cases. *Cancer* 1984;54(1):114–25.
19 Frost DB, Richards PC, Montague ED, *et al.* Epidermoid cancer of the anorectum. *Cancer* 1984;53(6):1285–93.
20 Wexler A, Berson AM, Goldstone SE, *et al.* Invasive anal squamous-cell carcinoma in the HIV-positive patient: outcome in the era of highly active antiretroviral therapy. *Dis Colon Rectum* 2008;51(1):73–81.
21 Nigro ND, Vaitkevicius VK, Considine B, Jr, Combined therapy for cancer of the anal canal: a preliminary report. *Dis Colon Rectum* 1974;17(3):354–6.
22 Leichman L, Nigro N, Vaitkevicius VK, *et al.* Cancer of the anal canal. Model for preoperative adjuvant combined modality therapy. *Am J Med* 1985;78(2):211–5.
23 UKCCCR Anal Cancer Trial Working Party. Epidermoid anal cancer: results from the UKCCCR randomised trial of radiotherapy alone versus radiotherapy, 5-fluorouracil, and mitomycin. UKCCCR Anal Cancer Trial Working Party. UK Co-ordinating Committee on Cancer Research. Lancet 1996;348(9034):1049–54.
24 Northover J, Glynne-Jones R, Sebag-Montefiore D, *et al.* Chemoradiation for the treatment of epidermoid anal cancer: 13-year follow-up of the first randomised UKCCCR Anal Cancer Trial (ACT I). *Br J Cancer* 2010;102(7):1123–8.
25 Bartelink H, Roelofsen F, Eschwege F, *et al.* Concomitant radiotherapy and chemotherapy is superior to radiotherapy alone in the treatment of locally advanced anal cancer: results of a phase III randomized trial of the European Organization for Research and Treatment of Cancer Radiotherapy and Gastrointestinal Cooperative Groups. *J Clin Oncol* 1997;15(5):2040.
26 Shiraha Y, Sakai K, Teranaka T. Clinical trials of mitomycin C, a new antitumor antibiotic; preliminary report of results obtained in 82 consecutive cases in the field of general surgery. *Antibiot Annu* 1958;6:533–40.

27 Cantrell JE, Jr., Phillips TM, Schein PS. Carcinoma-associated hemolytic-uremic syndrome: a complication of mitomycin C chemotherapy. *J Clin Oncol* 1985;3(5):723–34.
28 Thomas CR, Jr., Stelzer KJ, Douglas JG *et al.* Common emergencies in cancer medicine: infectious and treatment-related syndromes, *Part II. J Natl Med Assoc* 1994;86(11):839–52.
29 Zakarija, A, Bennett C. Drug-induced thrombotic microangiopathy. *Semin Thromb Hemost* 2005;31(6):681–90.
30 Rosenberg B, Vancamp L, Krigas T. Inhibition of cell division in Escherichia Coli by electrolysis products from a platinum electrode. *Nature* 1965;205:698–9.
31 Flam M, John M, Pajak TF, *et al.* Role of mitomycin in combination with fluorouracil and radiotherapy, and of salvage chemoradiation in the definitive nonsurgical treatment of epidermoid carcinoma of the anal canal: results of a phase III randomized intergroup study. *J Clin Oncol* 1996;14(9):2527–39.
32 Chakravarthy AB, Catalano PJ, Martenson JA, *et al.* Long-term follow-up of a Phase II trial of high-dose radiation with concurrent 5-fluorouracil and cisplatin in patients with anal cancer (ECOG E4292). *Int J Radiat Oncol Biol Phys* 2011;81(4):e607–13.
33 Doci R, Zucali R, La Monica G, *et al.* Primary chemoradiation therapy with fluorouracil and cisplatin for cancer of the anus: results in 35 consecutive patients. *J Clin Oncol* 1996;14(12):3121–5.
34 Ajani JA, Winter KA, Gunderson LL, *et al.* Fluorouracil, mitomycin, and radiotherapy vs fluorouracil, cisplatin, and radiotherapy for carcinoma of the anal canal: a randomized controlled trial. *JAMA* 2008;299(16):1914–21.
35 Gunderson LL, Winter KA, Ajani JA, *et al.* Long-term update of US GI intergroup RTOG 98-11 phase III trial for anal carcinoma: survival, relapse, and colostomy failure with concurrent chemoradiation involving fluorouracil/mitomycin versus fluorouracil/cisplatin. *J Clin Oncol* 2012;30(35):4344–51.
36 Peiffert D, Tournier-Rangeard L, Gerard JP, *et al.* Induction chemotherapy and dose intensification of the radiation boost in locally advanced anal canal carcinoma: final analysis of the randomized UNICANCER ACCORD 03 trial. *J Clin Oncol* 2012; 30(16):1941–8.
37 James RD, Glynne-Jones R, Meadows HM, *et al.* Mitomycin or cisplatin chemoradiation with or without maintenance chemotherapy for treatment of squamous-cell carcinoma of the anus (ACT II): a randomised, phase 3, open-label, 2 x 2 factorial trial. *Lancet Oncol* 2013;14(6):516–24.
38 Cummings BJ, Keane TJ, O'Sullivan B, *et al.* Epidermoid anal cancer: treatment by radiation alone or by radiation and 5-fluorouracil with and without mitomycin C. *Int J Radiat Oncol Biol Phys* 1991;21(5):1115–25.
39 Brooks CJ, Lee YK, Aitken K, *et al.* Organ-sparing intensity-modulated radiotherapy for anal cancer using the ACTII schedule: a comparison of conventional and intensity-modulated radiotherapy plans. *Clin Oncol (R Coll Radiol)* 2013;25(3):155–61.
40 Chen YJ, Liu A, Tsai PT, *et al.* Organ sparing by conformal avoidance intensity-modulated radiation therapy for anal cancer: dosimetric evaluation of coverage of pelvis and inguinal/femoral nodes. *Int J Radiat Oncol Biol Phys* 2005;63(1):274–81.
41 Clivio A, Fogliata A, Franzetti-Pellanda A, *et al.* Volumetric-modulated arc radiotherapy for carcinomas of the anal canal: a treatment planning comparison with fixed field IMRT. *Radiother Oncol* 2009;92(1):118–24.
42 Joseph KJ, Syme A, Small C, *et al.* A treatment planning study comparing helical tomotherapy with intensity-modulated radiotherapy for the treatment of anal cancer. *Radiother Oncol* 2010;94(1):60–6.
43 Lin, A, Ben-Josef E. Intensity-modulated radiation therapy for the treatment of anal cancer. *Clin Colorectal Cancer* 2007;6(10):716–9.
44 Menkarios C, Azria D, Laliberte B, *et al.* Optimal organ-sparing intensity-modulated radiation therapy (IMRT) regimen for the treatment of locally advanced anal canal carcinoma: a comparison of conventional and IMRT plans. *Radiat Oncol* 2007;2:41.
45 Stieler F, Wolff D, Lohr F, *et al.* A fast radiotherapy paradigm for anal cancer with volumetric modulated arc therapy (VMAT). *Radiat Oncol* 2009;4:48.
46 Vieillot S, Azria D, Lemanski C, *et al.* Plan comparison of volumetric-modulated arc therapy (RapidArc) and conventional intensity-modulated radiation therapy (IMRT) in anal canal cancer. *Radiat Oncol* 2010;5:92.
47 Chuong M, Freilich J, Hoffe S, *et al.* Intensity-modulated radiation therapy versus conventional radiation therapy for squamous cell carcinoma of the anal canal. *Gatrointest Cancer Res* 2013;6(2):39–45.
48 Kachnic LA, Winter K, Myerson RJ, *et al.* RTOG 0529: a Phase 2 evaluation of dose-painted intensity modulated radiation therapy in combination with 5-Fluorouracil and mitomycin-C for the reduction of acute morbidity in carcinoma of the anal canal. *Int J Radiat Oncol Biol Phys* 2013;86(1)27–33.
49 Bazan JG, Hara W, Hsu A, *et al.* Intensity-modulated radiation therapy versus conventional radiation therapy for squamous cell carcinoma of the anal canal. *Cancer* 2011;117(15):3342–51.
50 Dewas CV, Maingon P, Dalban C, *et al.* Does gap-free intensity modulated chemoradiation therapy provide a greater clinical benefit than 3D conformal chemoradiation in patients with anal cancer? *Radiat Oncol* 2012;7:201.
51 Call JA, Haddock MG, Quevedo JF, *et al.* Intensity-modulated radiotherapy for squamous cell carcinoma of the anal canal: efficacy of a low daily dose to clinically negative regions. *Radiat Oncol* 2011;6:134.
52 Chuong MD, Hoffe SE, Weber J, *et al.* Outcomes of anal cancer treated with definitive IMRT-based chemoradiation. *J Radiat Oncol* 2012;1:165–72.
53 DeFoe SG, Beriwal S, Jones H, *et al.* Concurrent chemotherapy and intensity-modulated radiation therapy for anal carcinoma–clinical outcomes in a large National Cancer Institute-designated integrated cancer centre network. *Clin Oncol (R Coll Radiol)* 2012;24(6):424–31.
54 Kachnic LA, Tsai HK, Coen JJ, *et al.* Dose-painted intensity-modulated radiation therapy for anal cancer: a multi-institutional report of acute toxicity and response to therapy. *Int J Radiat Oncol Biol Phys* 2012;82(1):153–8.

55 Kachnic LA, Winter K, Myerson RJ, *et al.* RTOG 0529: A Phase 2 Evaluation of Dose-Painted Intensity Modulated Radiation Therapy in Combination With 5-Fluorouracil and Mitomycin-C for the Reduction of Acute Morbidity in Carcinoma of the Anal Canal. *Int J Radiat Oncol Biol Phys* 2013;86(1):27–33.

56 Milano MT, Jani AB, Farrey KJ, *et al.* Intensity-modulated radiation therapy (IMRT) in the treatment of anal cancer: toxicity and clinical outcome. *Int J Radiat Oncol Biol Phys* 2005;63(2):354–61.

57 Mitchell MP, Abboud M, Eng C, *et al.* Intensity-modulated radiation therapy with concurrent chemotherapy for anal cancer: outcomes and toxicity. *Am J Clin Oncol* 2014;37(5):461–6.

58 Pepek JM, Willett CG, Wu QJ, *et al.* Intensity-modulated radiation therapy for anal malignancies: a preliminary toxicity and disease outcomes analysis. *Int J Radiat Oncol Biol Phys* 2010;78(5):1413–9.

59 Salama JK, Mell LK, Schomas DA, *et al.* Concurrent chemotherapy and intensity-modulated radiation therapy for anal canal cancer patients: a multicenter experience. *J Clin Oncol* 2007;25(29):4581–6.

60 Vieillot S, Fenoglietto P, Lemanski C, *et al.* IMRT for locally advanced anal cancer: clinical experience of the Montpellier Cancer Center. *Radiat Oncol* 2012;7:45.

61 Herman JM, Thomas CR, Jr. RTOG 0529: Intensity modulated radiation therapy and anal cancer a step in the right direction? *Int J Radiat Oncol Biol Phys* 2013;86(1):8–10.

62 Dasgupta T, Rothenstein D, Chou JF, *et al.* Intensity-modulated radiotherapy vs conventional radiotherapy in the treatment of anal squamous cell carcinoma: a propensity score analysis. *Radiother Oncol* 2013;107(2):189–94.

63 Saarilahti K, Arponen P, Vaalavirta L, *et al.* The effect of intensity-modulated radiotherapy and high dose rate brachytherapy on acute and late radiotherapy-related adverse events following chemoradiotherapy of anal cancer. *Radiother Oncol* 2008; 87(3):383–90.

64 Mistrangelo DM, Bello M, Cassoni P, *et al.* Value of staging squamous cell carcinoma of the anal margin and canal using the sentinel lymph node procedure: an update of the series and a review of the literature. *Br J Cancer* 2013;108(3):527–32.

65 Cummings BJ, Thomas GM, Keane TJ, *et al.* Primary radiation therapy in the treatment of anal canal carcinoma. *Dis Colon Rectum* 1982;25(8):778–82.

66 Salmon RJ, Fenton J, Asselain B, *et al.* Treatment of epidermoid anal canal cancer. *Am J Surg* 1984;147(1):43–8.

67 Stewart D, Yan Y, Kodner IJ, *et al.* Salvage surgery after failed chemoradiation for anal canal cancer: should the paradigm be changed for high-risk tumors? *J Gastrointest Surg* 2007;11(12):1744–51.

68 Mitchell SE, Mendenhall WM, Zlotecki RA, *et al.* Squamous cell carcinoma of the anal canal. *Int J Radiat Oncol Biol Phys* 2001;49(4):1007–13.

69 Myerson RJ, Kong F, Birnbaum EH, *et al.* Radiation therapy for epidermoid carcinoma of the anal canal, clinical and treatment factors associated with outcome. *Radiother Oncol* 2001;61(1):15–22.

70 Ortholan C, Resbeut M, Hannoun-Levi JM, *et al.* Anal canal cancer: management of inguinal nodes and benefit of prophylactic inguinal irradiation (CORS-03 Study). *Int J Radiat Oncol Biol Phys* 2012;82(5):1988–95.

71 Gerard JP, Chapet O, Samiei F, *et al.* Management of inguinal lymph node metastases in patients with carcinoma of the anal canal: experience in a series of 270 patients treated in Lyon and review of the literature. *Cancer* 2001;92(1):77–84.

72 Matthews JH, Burmeister BH, Borg M, *et al.* T1-2 anal carcinoma requires elective inguinal radiation treatment–the results of Trans Tasman Radiation Oncology Group study TROG 99.02. *Radiother Oncol* 2011;98(1):93–8.

73 Zilli T, Betz M, Bieri S, *et al.* Elective inguinal node irradiation in early-stage T2N0 anal cancer: prognostic impact on locoregional control. *Int J Radiat Oncol Biol Phys* 2013;87(1):60–6.

74 Chiao EY, Giordano TP, Richardson P, *et al.* Human immunodeficiency virus-associated squamous cell cancer of the anus: epidemiology and outcomes in the highly active antiretroviral therapy era. *J Clin Oncol* 2008;26(3):474–9.

75 Seo Y, Kinsella MT, Reynolds HL, *et al.* Outcomes of chemoradiotherapy with 5-Fluorouracil and mitomycin C for anal cancer in immunocompetent versus immunodeficient patients. *Int J Radiat Oncol Biol Phys* 2009;75(1):143–9.

76 Oehler-Janne C, Huguet F, Provencher S, *et al.* HIV-specific differences in outcome of squamous cell carcinoma of the anal canal: a multicentric cohort study of HIV-positive patients receiving highly active antiretroviral therapy. *J Clin Oncol* 2008;26(15):2550–7.

77 Klencke BJ, JPalefsky M. Anal cancer: an HIV-associated cancer. *Hematol Oncol Clin North Am* 2003;17(3):859–72.

78 Deniaud-Alexandre E, Touboul E, Tiret E, *et al.* Results of definitive irradiation in a series of 305 epidermoid carcinomas of the anal canal. *Int J Radiat Oncol Biol Phys* 2003;56(5):1259–73.

79 Eng C, Pathak P. Treatment options in metastatic squamous cell carcinoma of the anal canal. *Curr Treat Options Oncol* 2008;9(4–6):400–7.

80 James R, Wan S, Glynne-Jones R, *et al.* 2009 ASCO Annual Meeting. J Clin Oncol 2009;27:18 s.

81 Jemal A, Bray F, Center MM, *et al.* Global cancer statistics. *CA Cancer J Clin* 2011;61(2):69–90.

82 Lynch TJ, Patel T, Dreisbach L, *et al.* Cetuximab and first-line taxane/carboplatin chemotherapy in advanced non-small-cell lung cancer: results of the randomized multicenter phase III trial BMS099. *J Clin Oncol* 2010;28(6):911–7.

83 Hainsworth JD, Burris Iii HA, Meluch AA, *et al.* Paclitaxel, carboplatin, and long-term continuous infusion of 5-fluorouracil in the treatment of advanced squamous and other selected carcinomas. *Cancer* 2001;92(3):642–9.

84 Bendell, JC, *et al.* Checkpoint kinase (CHK) 1/2 inhibitor LY2606368 in a phase I, dose-expansion study in patients (pts) with metastatic squamous cell carcinoma (mSCC) of the anus, in 2015 ASCO Annual Meeting, 2015. J Clin Oncol, Chicago, USA.

85 Morris V, Eng C. Metastatic anal cancer and novel agents. *Surg Oncol Clin N Am* 2017;26(1):133–42.

86 Morris V, Eng C. Summary of emerging targets in anal cancer: the case for an immunotherapy based-approach. *J Gastrointest Oncol* 2016;7(5):721–6.

87 Morris V, *et al.* ASCO 2016. J Clin Oncol 2016;34(suppl; abstr 3503).
88 http://ir.advaxis.com/press-releases/detail/1094/advaxis-presents-preliminary-data-from-a-phase-12-trial-of (accessed 28 September 2017).
89 Mullen JT, Rodriguez-Bigas MA, Chang GJ, *et al.* Results of surgical salvage after failed chemoradiation therapy for epidermoid carcinoma of the anal canal. *Ann Surg Oncol* 2007;14(2):478–83.
90 Schiller DE, Cummings BJ, Rai S, *et al.* Outcomes of salvage surgery for squamous cell carcinoma of the anal canal. *Ann Surg Oncol* 2007;14(10):2780–9.
91 Renehan AG, Saunders MP, Schofield PF, *et al.* Patterns of local disease failure and outcome after salvage surgery in patients with anal cancer. *Br J Surg* 2005;92(5):605–14.
92 Eeson G, Foo M, Harrow S, *et al.* Outcomes of salvage surgery for epidermoid carcinoma of the anus following failed combined modality treatment. *Am J Surg* 2011;201(5):628–33.
93 Ng M, Leong T, Chander S, *et al.* Australasian Gastrointestinal Trials Group (AGITG) contouring atlas and planning guidelines for intensity-modulated radiotherapy in anal cancer. *Int J Radiat Oncol Biol Phys* 2012;83(5):1455–62.
94 Konski A, Garcia M, Jr., John M, *et al.* Evaluation of planned treatment breaks during radiation therapy for anal cancer: update of RTOG 92-08. *Int J Radiat Oncol Biol Phys* 2008;72(1):114–8.
95 Ben-Josef E, Moughan J, Ajani JA, *et al.* Impact of overall treatment time on survival and local control in patients with anal cancer: a pooled data analysis of Radiation Therapy Oncology Group trials 87-04 and 98-11. *J Clin Oncol* 2010;28(34):5061–6.
96 Roohipour R, Patil S, Goodman KA, *et al.* Squamous-cell carcinoma of the anal canal: predictors of treatment outcome. *Dis Colon Rectum* 2008;51(2):147–53.
97 Welzel G, Hagele V, Wenz F, *et al.* Quality of life outcomes in patients with anal cancer after combined radiochemotherapy. *Strahlenther Onkol* 2011;187(3):175–82.
98 Allal AS, Sprangers MA, Laurencet F, Reymond MA, Kurtz JM. Assessment of long-term quality of life in patients with anal carcinomas treated by radiotherapy with or without chemotherapy. *Br J Cancer* 1999;80:1588–94.
99 Andersen BL, Anderson B, deProsse C. Controlled prospective longitudinal study of women with cancer: I. Sexual functioning outcomes. *J Consult Clin Psychol* 1989;57(6):683–91.
100 Crook J, Esche B, Futter N. Effect of pelvic radiotherapy for prostate cancer on bowel, bladder, and sexual function: the patient's perspective. *Urology* 1996;47(3):387–94.
101 Das P, Cantor SB, Parker CL, *et al.* Long-term quality of life after radiotherapy for the treatment of anal cancer. *Cancer* 2010;116(4):822–9.
102 Mirabeau-Beale K, Hong TS, Niemierko A, *et al.* Clinical and treatment factors associated with vaginal stenosis after definitive chemoradiation for anal canal cancer. *Pract Radiat Oncol* 2015;5(3):e113–8.
103 Robinson RD, Knudtson JF. Fertility preservation in patients receiving chemotherapy or radiotherapy. *Mo Med* 2014;111(5):434–8.
104 Gwede C, Vadaparampil S, Hoffe S, *et al.* The role of radiation oncologists and discussion of fertility preservation in young cancer patients. *Pract Radiat Oncol* 2013; 2:242–7.
105 Andreyev HJ. Gastrointestinal problems after pelvic radiotherapy: the past, the present and the future. *Clin Oncol (R Coll Radiol)* 2007;19(10):790–9.
106 Krychman ML, Pereira L, Carter J, *et al.* Sexual oncology: sexual health issues in women with cancer. *Oncology* 2006;71(1–2):18–25.
107 Peltier A, van Velthoven R, Roumeguere T. Current management of erectile dysfunction after cancer treatment. *Curr Opin Oncol* 2009;21(4):303–9.
108 Norderval S, Rydningen M, Lindsetmo RO, *et al.* Sacral nerve stimulation. *Tidsskr Nor Laegeforen* 2011;131(12):1190–3.

11

Gastrointestinal Stromal Tumors

Rian M. Hasson Charles[1], Stanley W. Ashley[2], and Chandrajit P. Raut[2,3]

[1] Mayo Clinic, Rochester, Minnesota, USA
[2] Brigham and Women's Hospital; Harvard Medical School, Boston, Massachusetts, USA
[3] Dana-Farber Cancer Institute, Boston, Massachusetts, USA

Introduction

Gastrointestinal stromal tumors (GISTs) are the most common sarcoma and account for 80% of gastrointestinal mesenchymal neoplasms, but are still considered rare neoplasms, representing only 0.1–3% of all gastrointestinal malignancies. They are thought to arise from the interstitial cells of Cajal, which are components of the intestinal autonomic nervous system and serve as intestinal pacemakers [1]. Due to ambiguity in previous methods of diagnosis, GISTs were often misdiagnosed as intestinal leiomyomas, leiomyosarcomas, leiomyoblastomas, Schwannomas, gastrointestinal autonomic nerve tumors, or other similar soft tissue histologies [2]. However, two key developments in the last 15 years have enhanced the understanding and treatment of GISTs: (i) the identification of constitutively active signals (oncogenic mutation of the *c-KIT* and *platelet-derived growth factor alpha* (*PDGFRA*) genes encoding receptor tyrosine kinases) [3], and (ii) the development of tyrosine kinase inhibitors (TKIs) that suppress tumor growth by specifically targeting and inhibiting this signal [4]. This advent of effective therapy has dramatically improved outcomes for patients with GIST, thus redefining the role for surgical intervention. Moreover, developments in the management of GIST have come to represent a proof of principle in regard to translational therapeutics in oncology, confirming that specific inhibition of tumor-associated receptor tyrosine kinase activity may be an effective cancer treatment. This chapter reviews the biology, diagnosis, treatment, and persistent clinical challenges that describe these mesenchymal neoplasms.

Incidence

The most recent data from the National Cancer Institute's Surveillance, Epidemiology, and End Results (SEER) program showed a near doubling of the incidence of all GI mesenchymal tumors reported (over 80% were GIST), which is likely due to increased identification and recognition [5]. Currently, the incidence in the United States is estimated to be approximately 5,000 new cases per year [6]. International population-based studies have estimated an annual incidence rate ranging from 10 to 15 cases per million population, and a prevalence of approximately 129 persons per million [7,8].

Etiology and Risk Factors

There are no racial, ethnic, or gender predilections for GIST. The median age at diagnosis is 60 years. GISTs rarely occur in children, except as part of a familial syndrome or Carney triad [9]. Unlike adults children (i) tend to present with multifocal gastric GISTs, (ii) their neoplasms are wild-type for *KIT* and *PDGFRA*, and (iii) their tumors have a higher incidence of lymph node metastases [10].

Hereditary GIST

Though familial cohorts with germline *KIT* or *PDFGRA* mutations have been reported, the overwhelming majority of GISTs are sporadic. Key differences between individuals with GISTs secondary to germline *KIT* mutations versus sporadic GISTs include younger presentation, multifocal disease manifested at presentation, and rare metastatic disease dissemination [11]. The phenotype of kindred GIST populations with germline *KIT* mutations includes skin hyperpigmentation and diffuse hyperplasia of the intestinal myenteric plexus. Cases of associated melanoma, breast, and esophageal cancers have also been reported [12].

Gastric GISTs can be a component of Carney triad and Carney–Stratakis syndrome, and often exhibit a chronic, yet indolent, course. Carney triad consists of gastric GIST (previously thought to be leiomyosarcoma), functional extra-adrenal paragangliomas, and pulmonary chondromas [13]. Esophageal leiomyomas and adrenal cortical adenomas have more recently been added as components of the syndrome. Approximately

The American Cancer Society's Oncology in Practice: Clinical Management, First Edition. Edited by The American Cancer Society.

80% are diagnosed before the age of 30 and approximately 85% occur in women. GISTs found in patients with Carney triad do not have somatic *KIT* or *PDGFRA* mutations. Carney–Stratakis syndrome describes familial cases expressing GISTs and paragangliomas [14]. Mutations in genes encoding several succinate dehydrogenase subunits have been reported in Carney–Stratakis syndrome kindreds [15].

Approximately 7% of individuals with the autosomal dominant disorder von Recklinghausen's neurofibromatosis (NF1) have GIST. Contrary to the equal sex distribution noted for type 1 and/or atypical NF1 deletions, these NF1-associated GISTs have a higher incidence in women (1.4:1), and are most commonly manifested by a multifocal presence in the small intestine [16]. While these individuals express *KIT* and *PDGFRA* point mutations in 8% and 6% of their GISTs respectively, *NF1* mutations have not been identified in non-NF1 individuals with sporadic GISTs [17–19].

Clinical Presentation

Primary Tumors

In one early study, 69% of GISTs were symptomatic, 21% were discovered incidentally at surgery, and 10% were discovered at autopsy [20]. GISTs commonly arise in the stomach (50–70%), small intestine (25–35%), colon and rectum (5–10%), mesentery or omentum (7%), and esophagus (<5%), but may occasionally arise in the duodenal ampulla, appendix, gallbladder, and urinary bladder. GISTs are often friable and highly vascular, and commonly present with bleeding. They may cause life-threatening hemorrhage by erosion into the bowel lumen [21]. Alternatively, intestinal obstruction may lead to frank perforation or tumor rupture resulting in potentially catastrophic intraperitoneal bleeding and/or dissemination by peritoneal seeding. Smaller tumors often remain asymptomatic, only incidentally detected on radiographic studies, during endoscopy or at laparotomy.

Metastatic Disease

Presentation with metastatic disease occurs in approximately 15–50% of patients with GIST. Common sites include the liver, peritoneum, and omentum, while metastases to lymph nodes and extra-abdominal structures (brain, bone, lung, and subcutaneous tissues) occurs in <5% of patients. Extra-abdominal metastases are usually only noted later in the course of the disease [22].

Diagnosis

Radiographic Studies

Contrast-enhanced computed tomography (CT) of the abdomen and pelvis is the initial imaging study of choice for a suspected or confirmed GIST. Primary GISTs typically appear as well-circumscribed masses within the walls of hollow viscera on CT (Figure 11.1(a)), while magnetic resonance imaging (MRI) may help characterize metastatic liver or primary perirectal disease (Figure 11.1(b)) [23]. Although [^{18}F]fluoro-2-deoxy-D-glucose positron emission tomography (FDG-PET) may help characterize masses ambiguous on CT, monitor response to therapy, and detect emergence of drug-resistant clones for most patients with suspected neoplasms, it is not *de rigueur* for the routine management of patients with primary advanced disease. Recommendations concerning the utility of PET in patients with metastatic GIST have been equivocal. Consequently, they may be used sparingly.

Endoscopy, Fine-Needle Aspiration, and Biopsy

The endoscopic appearance of a primary GIST is typically a submucosal lesion often indistinguishable from GI leiomyomas. GIST may be located in either the upper or lower GI tract [24] and ulceration may or may not be present. Upper endoscopy with endoscopic biopsy has a low diagnostic yield (17–42%), and endoscopic ultrasound alone has not been found necessary to evaluate a confirmed GIST. Conversely, endoscopic ultrasound-guided fine-needle aspiration (FNA) has a diagnostic yield and sensitivity nearing 80%. Immunohistochemistry [25] or reverse-transcriptase polymerase chain reaction analysis of FNA specimens for *KIT* mutations may be required to confirm a diagnosis definitively.

Preoperative biopsy is not routinely necessary for a primary, resectable mass suspicious for GIST. In theory, biopsy may rupture a suspected GIST, increasing the risk of dissemination. However, biopsy may be appropriate if neoadjuvant therapy is a consideration, if the differential diagnosis includes entities such as lymphoma that would dictate a different treatment, or if there is metastatic disease.

Histopathology and Molecular Pathology

In 1983, Mazur and Clark proposed the term "GIST" to describe "intraabdominal nonepithelial neoplasms that lacked the ultrastructural features of smooth muscle cells and the immunohistochemical characteristics of Schwann cells" [26]. GISTs are classified histologically into one of three categories: epithelioid type, spindle cell type, or mixed type. While most gastric GISTs feature an *epithelioid* phenotype, esophageal, small intestinal, colonic, and anorectal tumors more often feature *spindle cell* morphology.

Hirota *et al.* reported two critical findings in 1998 [3]: (i) near-universal expression of the transmembrane receptor tyrosine kinase KIT in GIST, and (ii) gain-of-function mutations in the corresponding c-*KIT* proto-oncogene. Normally activated by binding Kit ligand, also known as "steel factor" or "stem cell factor", the KIT receptor plays a critical role in hematopoiesis, and gametogenesis, and the maintenance of intestinal pacemaker cells.

More than 85% of GISTs have activating *KIT* mutations, and mutated Kit remains constitutively active even in the absence of ligand binding resulting in both unregulated cell growth and malignant transformation [27]. These mutations commonly occur in exon 11 (57– 95% of cases), exon 9 (10–18%), and exons 13 and 17 (both 1–4% respectively) [28–30]. GISTs with *KIT* exon 9 mutations predominantly arise in the small intestine,

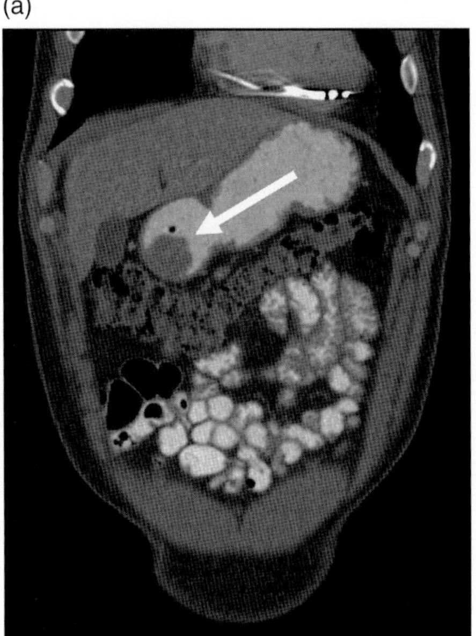

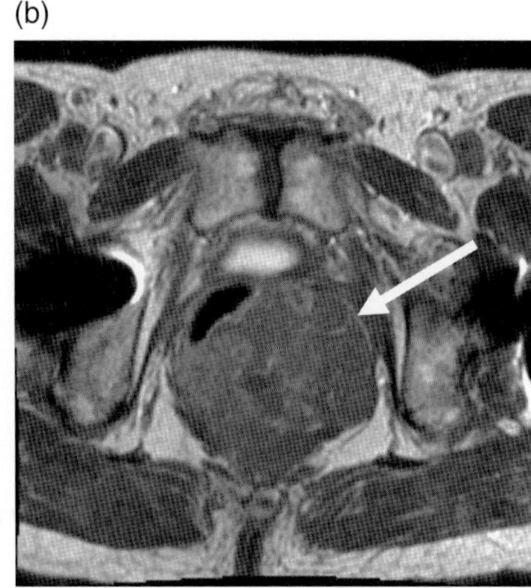

Figure 11.1 Cross-sectional imaging depicting (a) a computed tomography image of a distal gastric GIST (arrow) and (b) a magnetic resonance image of a nearly obstructing rectal GIST (arrow).

and homozygous mutant GISTs are often associated with metastatic disease. Mast/stem cell growth factor receptor (SCFR), also known as tyrosine-protein kinase Kit, proto-oncogene c-Kit, or CD117, is a protein that is encoded by the *KIT* gene in humans [31]. The presence of CD117 immunoreactivity does not necessarily correlate with a *KIT* gene mutation, and conversely a *KIT* mutation can exist in the absence of CD117 immunoreactivity. Nevertheless, because CD117 expression (KIT-positivity) is characteristic of most GISTs, and is not characteristic of other gastrointestinal smooth muscle tumors such as leiomyosarcoma, GISTs are now identified by immunohistochemical staining for this antigen, a practice that has enhanced the understanding of the prevalence of this disease [32].

Activating mutations in a gene encoding a related receptor tyrosine kinase, platelet-derived growth factor receptor alpha (*PDGFRA*), have been identified in approximately 35% of GISTs lacking *KIT* mutations [9]. *PDGFRA* mutations in GISTs have been identified in exon 18 (2–6%), exon 12 (1–2%), and in exon 14 (<1% of the time) [9,10,33]. No differences in the activation of downstream signaling intermediates have been observed between *PDGFRA*-mutant and *KIT*-mutant tumors, suggesting that mutant *PDGFRA* provides oncogenic signals that parallel those of mutant *KIT*.

Wild-type GISTs exhibit no detectable *KIT* or *PDGFRA* mutations and utilize other pathways for pathogenesis [34]. Overexpression of insulin-like growth factor-1 receptor in addition to several reported mutations of succinate dehydrogenase subunits and *BRAF* have also been identified in a small percentage of wild-type tumors [35–37].

Prognostic Factors

While tumors under 1 cm are likely have a low risk of recurrence, no tumors can be definitively called benign. The three established, independently prognostic factors are tumor site of origin, tumor size (single largest dimension), and mitotic index (the most important and strongest predictor of recurrence) (Figure 11.1) [38]. Small bowel GISTs have a higher risk of progression than gastric GISTs of comparable size and mitotic count with jejunal and ileal tumors having the highest rate of metastasis followed by duodenal and rectal tumors respectively (Table 11.1).

A validated nomogram [39] assigns points for each of these three prognostic factors. The probability of remaining recurrence-free at 2 and 5 years can then be predicted by using the point totals in a summative manner (Figure **11.2**). It is important to note that the nomogram bases the probability of recurrence on a cohort of patients diagnosed in the pretyrosine kinase inhibitor (TKI) therapy era.

Point mutations can also affect prognosis, and location is important. Insertions of *KIT* exon 11 appear to have a favorable prognosis, while deletions involving amino acid W557 and/or K558 have a poor prognosis [40]. Patients with *PDGFRα* exon 18 D842V mutations are resistant to imatinib therapy, whereas those with mutations in exon 12 are responsive to imatinib [12]. Additional adverse prognostic factors observed in some but not all studies included *KIT* exon 9 mutations, aneuploidy, high cellular proliferation index, and telomerase expression.

Staging

The most common system used for the staging of GISTs is the TNM system of the American Joint Committee on Cancer (AJCC) [41]. Once the T, N, and M categories have been assigned, the mitotic rate in combination with TNM classification is combined with the starting tumor location to predict prognosis. Hence, GISTs that start in the stomach or omentum are classified in one group, while GISTs of the esophagus, small intestine, colon, rectum, and/or peritoneum are separately defined. Tumors are finally described as *resectable* or *unresectable* depending on size, location, spread, and the

Table 11.1 Risk assessment for primary gastrointestinal stromal tumors. Source: Miettinen and Lasota [38]. Reproduced with permission of Elsevier. Risk of recurrence is based on data from the preimatinib era.

		Patients with progressive disease/risk classification, based on site of origin (%)			
Mitotic rate	**Tumor size (cm)**	**Stomach**	**Duodenum**	**Jejunum/ileum**	**Rectum**
≤5 per 50 HPF	≤2	0	0	0	0
	>2, ≤5	1.9/very low	8.3/low	4.3/ ow	8.5/low
	>5, ≤10	3.6/low	–*	24/moderate	–*
	>10	12/moderate	34/high	52/high	57/high
>5 per 50 HPF	≤2	–*	–*	–*	54/high
	>2, ≤5	16/moderate	50/high	73/high	52/high
	>5, ≤10	55/high	–*	85/high	–*
	>10	86/high	86/high	90/high	71/high

HPF, high-power field; *,insufficient data.

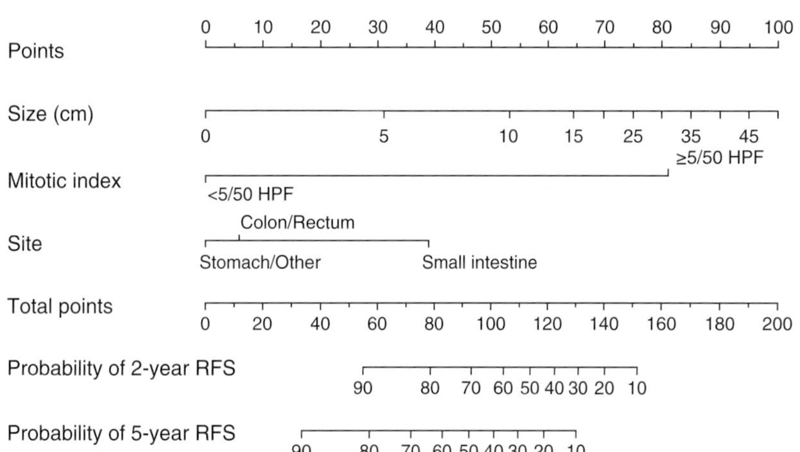

Figure 11.2 Normogram to predict the probabilities of 2-year and 5-year recurrence-free survival. Points are assigned for size, mitotic index, and site of origin by drawing a line upward from the corresponding values to the "points" line. The sum of these three points, plotted on the "total points" line, corresponds to predictions of 2-year and 5-year recurrence-free survival (RFS). HPF, high-power field. Source: Gold *et al.* [39]. Reproduced with permission of Elsevier.

ability of the patient to sustain an operative resection. Tumors may be defined as *marginally resectable* if complete removal is uncertain.

Therapy for Primary Disease

Pre-Operative Therapy for Primary Disease

The identification of effective, relatively well-tolerated, orally available TKIs including imatinib mesylate, sunitinib malate, and regorafenib have dramatically changed treatment practices. Imatinib selectively inhibits several tyrosine kinases, including KIT, PDGFRA, and BCR-ABL. Up to 80% of patients with metastatic GIST show a radiographic partial or complete response on imatinib or demonstrate stable disease. This success prompted investigation of its use in the perioperative period given the high incidence of recurrence often seen following resection of primary, nonmetastatic GIST [42–46].

In the Radiation Therapy Oncology Group (RTOG) 0312 phase II trial [43,47] patients with primary GIST measuring ≥5 cm (group A) or resectable recurrent/metastatic GIST measuring ≥2 cm (group B) received neoadjuvant imatinib (600 mg/day) for 8–12 weeks prior to surgical intervention, followed by maintenance postoperative imatinib for a duration of 2 years. Estimated 5-year progression-free survival (PFS) was 57% in group A and 30% in group B while 5-year overall survival (OS) was 77% in group A and 68% in group B, respectively. With regards to disease-specific survival, in group A, seven of 11 patients experienced disease progression >2 years from registration, and six of seven of the patients with progression had stopped imatinib before progression. In group B, disease progressed in 10 of 13 patients >2 years from registration, and six of 10 patients with progression had stopped imatinib before progression. This first multi-institutional neoadjuvant study confirmed the use of neoadjuvant imatinib as a safe practice. The authors also suggested considering longer treatment durations in intermediate-to-high-risk GIST patients receiving adjuvant therapy especially given that a high percentage of patients experienced disease progression after discontinuation of maintenance imatinib following surgery.

In a single-institution study of neoadjuvant imatinib administered for 3, 5, or 7 days prior to surgery (followed by 2 years of postoperative imatinib), tumors resected from individuals treated with preoperative imatinib demonstrated increased tumor apoptosis compared to treatment-naïve patients [47].

The German APOLLON study [48] was a prospective, open label, phase II study evaluating the effects of neoadjuvant treatment on patients with locally advanced KIT- or PDGFRA-positive GISTs. Enrolled patients received imatinib daily for 6 months, in the absence of disease progression or unacceptable toxicity. At 8 weeks, patients underwent FDG-PET examination to assess response in parallel to CT imaging. Unlike other trials, patients did not receive adjuvant treatment postoperatively as this was a purely neoadjuvant study. R0 resections were performed in 30/34 patients, and two patients showed M1 disease at resection. This study concluded that neoadjuvant treatment with imatinib for 6 months was not only a safe treatment in patients with locally advanced disease, but also that the extent of the operation could be significantly downstaged following pretreatment.

Although many studies have documented that imatinib significantly improves the outcomes of most patients with advanced GIST (as discussed later), demonstrating its utility in the neoadjuvant setting is challenging, and there are still unanswered questions. Defining a duration of treatment for those that are responsive would be helpful. Furthermore, it is unclear what long-term survival benefits there are to neoadjuvant imatinib therapy.

Though it is still unclear when precisely to use neoadjuvant imatinib in practice, situations where tumor shrinkage potentially allows the scope of an operation to be downstaged or simplified offer good indications for its use, as evidenced by the APOLLON study, and illustrated in Figure 11.3. In the case study demonstrated in Figure 11.3, pretreatment and post-treatment/preoperative axial MRI images of a patient with a rectal GIST treated with neoadjuvant imatinib showing dramatic shrinkage of tumor. The patient initially presented with partially obstructive symptoms, but due to rapid improvement of symptoms on imatinib, he was able to avoid a diverting colostomy. After completion of 7 months of neoadjuvant imatinib, he underwent a transanal full thickness rectal wall resection of his GIST with excellent preservation of sphincter function. Alternatively, shrinking a tumor to permit laparoscopic as opposed to open resection, even if the extent of resection is unlikely to change, may be another indication for neoadjuvant imatinib.

Surgery

Technique

Regardless of whether neoadjuvant therapy is used, the standard of care and only potentially curative therapy for patients with primary, localized, and resectable GISTs is surgical intervention [49,50]. The abdomen should be thoroughly explored at laparotomy to identify and remove any previously undetected metastatic peritoneal deposits (although if metastatic disease is known preoperatively, systemic therapy with imatinib should be first-line therapy, not surgery). GISTs generally do not invade other organs beyond the site of origin despite CT appearance, although primary tumors may demonstrate inflammatory adhesions to surrounding organs. In a series of 140 patients with primary gastric GISTs, wedge resections were performed in 68%, partial gastrectomies in 28%, and total gastrectomies in only 4% [51]. In cases where the tumor size is quite large and invasive into surrounding critical organs, a more extensive resection (total gastrectomy for a large proximal gastric GIST, pancreaticoduodenectomy for a periampullary GIST, or abdominoperineal resection for a low rectal GIST) may be necessary. However, several recent multi-institutional retrospective series have questioned the need for these resections given that neoadjuvant imatinib may

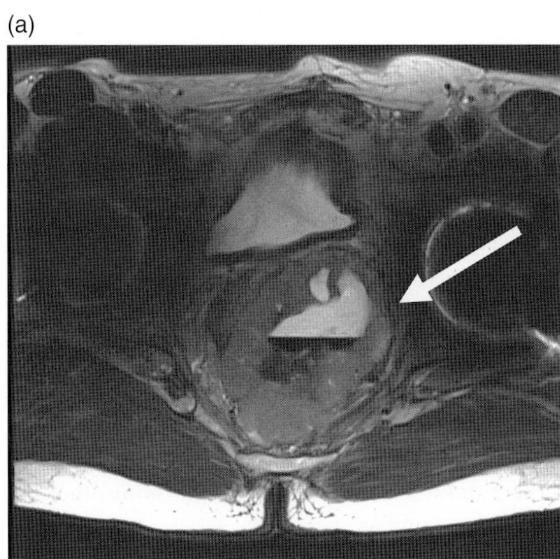
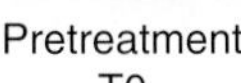

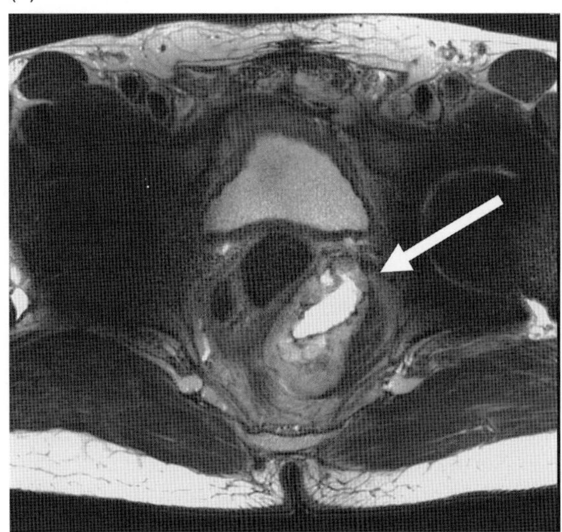

Figure 11.3 Pretreatment (a) and post-treatment (b) axial magnetic resonance images of a patient with a rectal GIST treated with neoadjuvant imatinib. Patient initially presented with partial obstructive symptoms, but due to rapid improvement of symptoms on imatinib, he did not require a diverting colostomy. After 8 months of neoadjuvant imatinib, he underwent a transanal full thickness rectal wall resection of his GIST with excellent preservation of sphincter function.

downstage the scope of the operation. In adult patients, lymphadenectomy is not required since lymph nodes are rarely involved, while lymphadenectomy in pediatric patients is generally considered on a case by case basis given their higher frequency of nodal involvement [52,53].

The goal of the operation should be an R0 (no residual gross or microscopic disease) resection. Multiple studies have shown that a macroscopically complete resection with negative or positive microscopic margins (R0 or R1 resection, respectively) is associated with better prognosis than a macroscopically incomplete resection (R2 resection). Violation of the tumor capsule or tumor rupture during surgery is associated with an increased risk of recurrence (virtually that of metastatic disease), and should therefore be avoided. Although the optimal margin of resection is still unclear, post hoc analysis of a randomized trial evaluating the utility of adjuvant imatinib mesylate therapy for 1 year after resection of primary GISTs at least 3 cm in size demonstrated that regardless of the use of adjuvant imatinib, there was no significant difference in recurrence-free survival (RFS) for patients undergoing an R0 versus R1 resection [54]. There are no data indicating that patients who have an R1 resection require re-excision, and lack of difference in RFS between patients undergoing R0 versus R1 resection suggests that re-excision may be avoided. However, given the fact that margins may retract after resection, or the pathologist may trim the staple line (converting a technically negative microscopic margin into a positive one), all cases of positive microscopic margins should be carefully reviewed by a multidisciplinary team of pathologists and surgical and medical oncologists to assess the need for re-excision. The impact of this intervention on OS still remains unknown.

All GISTs 2 cm in size or greater should be resected when possible, as none of these can be considered benign; however, the natural history of GISTs under 2 cm in size is unclear, and their management is more debatable. While the low risk of progression of GISTs under 2 cm may support a more conservative approach, an accurate mitotic index cannot be determined by biopsy or FNA and therefore observation for these tumors is difficult to recommend. As such, resection of GIST measuring 1–2 cm should be considered, and the risks and benefits of surgery versus observation should be reviewed with the patient. Given the higher risk of aggressive behavior of small bowel and colon GISTs, any tumor in these locations should be resected irrespective of size. Conversely, multiple studies have established that subcentimeter gastric GISTs are relatively common, were detected in 10–35% of patients undergoing resection for other gastrointestinal malignancies [55–57] and were detected in approximately 23% of autopsies in adults over the age of 50 [58]. Despite their relative frequency, few of these neoplasms appear to become clinically relevant and most gastric GISTs under 1 cm in size may be followed. Until further data are available, the most appropriate management of such small tumors remains uncertain.

Although endoscopic resection of small gastric GISTs has been reported, this cannot be recommended. Because GISTs involve the muscularis propria, attempts at endoscopic resection risk leaving gross tumor behind and could result in perforation due to the depth of the lesion. All small GISTs that are symptomatic (e.g., hemorrhage from erosion through the mucosa) or increase in size on serial follow-up should be resected, regardless of their size.

Two early studies confirmed both the safety and feasibility of a laparoscopic approach when resecting GISTs, and laparoscopic or laparoscopy-assisted resection of primary GISTs may be performed using standard oncologic principles [59,60]. More recent studies [61,62]. demonstrated that compared with open resection, laparoscopic resection of gastric GISTs offers the advantages of less trauma, faster recovery, less blood loss, and shorter hospital stay. Furthermore, laparoscopic resection of gastric GIST can be performed more safely, more effectively, and with faster postoperative recovery using a gasless technique when compared to a standard open technique [63].

Postoperative Therapy for Primary Disease

Several prospective trials have explored the role of adjuvant therapy with imatinib combined with resection of primary disease (Table 11.2) [49,64–69]. In the phase III ACOSOG Z9001 trial [66], patients were randomized to receive either placebo or imatinib postoperatively for 12 months following complete resection of primary GISTs at least 3 cm in size. Interim analysis confirmed that the 1-year RFS was significantly better in the imatinib arm (97% vs 83%, $P = 0.0000014$), and the trial was halted early. Interestingly, once recurrences were observed, the slopes of the Kaplan–Meier curves representing the two treatment arms were similar. This suggested that 1 year of adjuvant imatinib may delay recurrence of primary GIST, but may not necessarily cure patients during this short follow-up interval. Furthermore, there was no difference observed in OS between the two treatment arms.

In the phase III SSG XVIII trial [44], patients with high risk or more clinically advanced GISTs were randomized to receive imatinib postoperatively for 12 months versus 36 months following complete resection. This trial confirmed that patients treated with 36 months of adjuvant imatinib had longer 5-year RFS than those treated with 12 months of adjuvant imatinib (66% vs 48%, $P < 0.01$). More importantly, it demonstrated that patients treated with a longer duration of imatinib had an improved 5-year OS (92% vs 82%, $P = 0.02$).

Casali *et al.* conducted an open-label randomized trial evaluating adjuvant imatinib for 2 years in localized, surgically resected, high/intermediate risk GIST [45]. Specifically, patients were randomized between 2 years of postoperative imatinib (400 mg daily) and no postoperative treatment. With a median follow-up of 4.7 years, there was no statistically significant difference in imatinib-free survival though there was a trend in favor of imatinib when the analysis was limited to patients at high risk of recurrence. Imatinib did confer improved RFS at 3 years and at 5 years ($P < 0.001$), confirming other studies. Five-year OS was similar.

The PERSIST-5 trial (5 years of adjuvant imatinib) [69] has completed accrual. Based on the available data, the current standard of care is that patients with intermediate- to high-risk GIST should be treated with a minimum of 36 months of adjuvant imatinib. Any adjuvant therapy of 1 year's duration or longer improves RFS, but improvement in OS is not seen until completion of 3 years of therapy.

Table 11.2 Multi-institutional trials of the use of neoadjuvant or adjuvant imatinib in the perioperative management of resected primary gastrointestinal stromal tumors.

Trial	Imatinib therapy	Design	Eligibility	Dose	Primary endpoint	Status
RTOG S0132 [42]	Neoadjuvant	Phase II	Any of the following: 1) Primary tumor ≥5 cm 2) Recurrent tumor ≥2 cm Potentially resectable	600 mg daily × 8–10 weeks preoperatively + 600 mg daily × 24 months postoperatively	RFS	Published
ACOSOG Z9000 [64]	Adjuvant	Phase II	Any of the following: 1) Tumor ≥10 cm 2) Rupture/hemorrhage 3) Multiple tumors (<5) Complete resection	400 mg daily × 12 months	RFS	Published
ACOSOG Z9001 [65]	Adjuvant	Phase III	Tumor ≥3 cm Complete resection	400 mg daily vs placebo × 12 months	RFS	Published
China Gastrointestinal Cooperative Group [66]	Adjuvant	Phase II	Any of the following: 1) Tumor >5 cm 2) Mitotic rate >5/50 HPF	400 mg daily × 12 months	RFS	Published
SSG XVIII [65]	Adjuvant	Phase III	Any of the following: 1) Tumor ≥10 cm 2) Rupture 3) Mitotic rate >10 4) Tumor >5 cm + mitotic rate >5 5) Primary tumor + liver/peritoneal metastases Complete resection	400 mg daily × 12 months or 36 months	RFS	Published
EORTC 62024 [45]	Adjuvant	Phase III	Any of the following: 1) Tumor >5 cm 2) Mitotic rate >10 3) Tumor <5 cm + mitotic count 6–10/50 HPF Complete resection	400 mg daily vs no treatment × 24 months	Imatinib failure-free survival	Published
Korea [67]	Adjuvant	Phase II	Any of the following: 1) Tumor >5 cm + mitotic count > 5/50 HPF 2) Tumor >10 cm 3) Mitotic count >10/50 HPF Complete resection	400 mg daily × 24 months	RFS	Published
CSTI571BUS282 [69]	Adjuvant	Phase II	Any of the following: 1) Tumor ≥2 cm + mitotic count ≥5/50 HPF 2) Any nongastric tumor ≥5 cm Complete resection	400 mg daily × 5 years	RFS	Reported

ACOSOG, American College of Surgeons Oncology Group; EORTC, European Organisation for Research and Treatment of Cancer; HPF, high power fields; RTOG, Radiation Therapy Oncology Group; RFS, recurrence-free survival.

Therapy for Advanced Disease

Targeted Therapy

Unfortunately, despite a macroscopically complete resection, up to 50% of patients with primary GIST will recur at a median of 24 months [71]. An R0 or R1 resection is associated with 5-year OS rates of 34–63% whereas R2 resection is associated with 5-year OS as low as 8%. Most recurrences occur along the peritoneal and serosal surfaces or within the liver. Lung and other soft tissue metastases only develop late in the course of progressive disease. True local recurrences are rare in the absence of a macroscopically incomplete resection, and most recurrences present as disseminated disease. The three risk factors most predictive of recurrence are tumor site of origin, primary tumor size, and mitotic count [72].

Imatinib mesylate, sunitinib malate, and regorafenib are approved for the treatment of metastatic GIST. Imatinib is the first-line therapy for advanced (unresectable primary or metastatic) GIST [73,74]. The starting dose is generally 400 mg once daily. In patients who develop progressive disease on 400 mg, dose escalation up to 400 mg twice daily may be effective; however, greater toxicity and more dose reductions are generally required at doses above 400 mg per day. Toxicities may include headache, fatigue, nausea, diarrhea, edema, muscle cramps, dermatitis, anemia, and neutropenia. Fortunately, >70% of side effects are mild to moderate in severity and often resolve with continuing therapy. Following imatinib treatment, partial responses or stable disease were observed in nearly 85% of patients. Median time to PFS and OS was 18–20 months and 51–55 months, respectively.

KIT mutation location correlates with response to imatinib therapy. Patients whose GIST harbored an exon 11 mutation had a much higher response rate of 72%, while only 32% of patients with exon 9 *KIT* mutants and 12% of wild-type *KIT* patients responded to imatinib [75]. Furthermore, the median event-free survival for patients whose tumors had mutations of exon 11 and were treated with imatinib was 22.5 months, compared to 6.6 months for patients with mutations in exon 9 [76]. In a meta-analysis of the two large phase III studies, a slight advantage in PFS was noted in patients initially treated with higher dose imatinib, but that advantage was essentially limited to patients with *KIT* exon 9 mutations, and there was no overall survival advantage [77].

Sunitinib is a multitargeted TKI whose targets include KIT, PDGFR, the ret proto-oncogene receptor (RET), Fms-like tyrosine kinase-3 receptor (Flt3), and vascular endothelial growth factor receptor (VEGFR1, VEGFR2, VEGFR3). If patients continue to progress on escalating doses of imatinib or do not tolerate imatinib, then second-line sunitinib is started. Initially dosed as 50 mg daily in a 4-week-on-2-week-off cycle, many oncologists now favor a continuous dosing regimen of 37.5 mg daily. A placebo-controlled phase III trial [70] demonstrated significant improvement in time to progression in patients treated with sunitinib compared to those treated with placebo (27.3 weeks vs 6.4 weeks, respectively), as well as PFS and OS.

Regorafenib recently demonstrated benefit as a third-line agent providing significant improvement in progression-free survival compared with placebo in a randomized, placebo-controlled, phase 3 trial [78].

Other TKIs evaluated or currently under investigation include pazopanib, dasatinib, masitinib, nilotinib, sorafenib, and vatalanib among others. Crenolanib is a novel PDGFRA kinase inhibitor undergoing evaluation in GIST patients whose tumors carry a *PDGFRA* D842V mutation resistant to most other kinases available [79]. Pazopanib is a multitargeted receptor TKI and was recently shown in a randomized, open-label phase II study to improve progression-free survival of patients with advanced GIST resistant to imatinib and sunitinib [80]. Other potential non-TKI molecules for targeted therapy include heat shock protein-90 [81], mammalian target of rapamycin (mTOR) [82], histone deacetylase [83], and insulin-like growth factor type I receptor [84].

The French randomized imatinib discontinuation study BFR14 demonstrated that patients with GIST on imatinib who stop imatinib therapy after 1 year, 3 and 5 years had a much higher rate of disease progression than those who continued on therapy [85–87]. Therefore, once metastatic disease develops, patients should remain on some therapy indefinitely.

Surgery

Investigators have pursued a strategy of aggressive cytoreductive surgery in patients with advanced, metastatic GIST on TKI therapy, given the fact that pathologic complete responses are rare (<5% of patients), the majority of patients experience durable periods of partial response or stable disease on imatinib, and response to imatinib is not maintained indefinitely (median time to progression, 18–24 months). Once drug resistance develops, disease progression may present in either a limited (progression at one site of tumor, with other tumor deposits showing ongoing response to TKI) or generalized (progression at more than one site) fashion.

Many single-institution retrospective studies have documented the PFS and OS rates following extensive cytoreductive surgery in patients with advanced GIST treated with TKI therapy. The goal for advanced or metastatic GISTs is to perform a macroscopically complete (R0 or R1) resection when safely possible. However, the disease frequently may be too extensive to be completely resected, in which case progressing lesions are preferentially removed. The best results are generally observed in patients whose disease is still responsive to TKI therapy at the time of surgery (78% in patients with responsive disease compared to 7% of patients with generalized progression, $P < 0.0001$) [88]. Furthermore, the ability to remove all macroscopic disease is greatest in patients demonstrating ongoing response to TKI therapy (bulky residual disease remained postoperatively in only 4% of patients with responsive disease compared to 43% of patients with generalized progression). This seems more applicable to patients undergoing surgery while still on imatinib, and less relevant for patients undergoing surgery on sunitinib, where selection bias may cloud the impact of response to therapy on eventual outcomes [89].

Even though cytoreductive surgery is feasible, there is still no evidence that outcomes are superior or even equal to those for patients who continue on TKI therapy without surgery. Conversely, patients with generalized progression have not been shown to derive any benefit from cytoreductive surgery and are best treated nonoperatively. Nevertheless, these patients may need urgent surgery for palliative or emergency purposes if obstruction or hemorrhage occurs.

Surveillance

Patients who have had resection of a primary GIST should undergo a history, physical examination, and abdomen/pelvis CT scan with intravenous contrast every 3–6 months during the first 3–5 years, and then annually thereafter according to the NCCN consensus panel recommendations [90,91]. CT scans of the head, chest, or other extra-abdominal areas are unnecessary given the rarity of pulmonary or extra-abdominal metastases. Screening using routine PET scans is also unnecessary. Imaging intervals of 3–6 months are standard for patients in the first 5 years of post-treatment follow-up, with less frequent annual evaluation thereafter given that most recurrences occur within the first 5 years after surgery. At present there are no specific serum-based markers in routine use to detect recurrent GIST, though this is an active area of development [92,93].

References

1 Heinrich MC, Rubin BP, Longley BJ, Fletcher JA. Biology and genetic aspects of gastrointestinal stromal tumors: KIT activation and cytogenetic alterations. *Hum Pathol* 2002;33(5):484–95.

2 Fletcher CD, Berman JJ, Corless C, *et al.* Diagnosis of gastrointestinal stromal tumors: a consensus approach. *Hum Pathol* 2002;33(5):459–65.

3 Hirota S, Isozaki K, Moriyama Y, *et al.* Gain-of-function mutations of c-kit in human gastrointestinal stromal tumors. *Science* 1998;23;279(5350):577–80.

4 FDA.gov (Internet) Food and Drug Administration 2008 (updated December 7, 2010, cited December 23, 2008). Available from: http://www.fda.gov/Safety/MedWatch/SafetyInformation/ucm2553333.htm

5 Perez EA, Livingstone AS, Franceschi D, *et al.* Current incidence and outcomes of gastrointestinal mesenchymal tumors including gastrointestinal stromal tumors. *J Am Coll Surg* 2006;202(4):623–9.

6 Bamboat AM, DeMatteo RP. Updates on the management of gastrointestinal stromal tumors. *Surg Oncol Clin N Am* 2012; 21:301–16.

7 Rubin JL, Sanon M, Taylor DC, *et al.* Epidemiology, survival, and costs of localized gastrointestinal stromal tumors. *Int J Gen Med* 2011;4:121–30.

8 Søreide K, Sandvik OM, Søreide JA, *et al.* Global epidemiology of gastrointestinal stromal tumours (GIST): a systematic review of population-based cohort studies. *Cancer Epidemiol* 2016;40:39–46.

9 Benesch M, Wardelmann E, Ferrari A, Brennan B, Verschuur A. Gastrointestinal stromal tumors (GIST) in children and adolescents: a comprehensive review of the current literature. *Pediatr Blood Cancer* 2009;53(7):117–9.

10 Pappo AS, Janeway KA. Pediatric gastrointestinal stromal tumors. *Hematol Oncol Clin North Am* 2009;23(1):15–34.

11 Antonescu CR. Gastrointestinal stromal tumor (GIST) pathogenesis, familial GIST, and animal models. *Semin Diagn Pathol* 2006;23(2):63–9.

12 Li FP, Fletcher JA, Heinrich MC, *et al.* Familial gastrointestinal stromal tumor syndrome: phenotypic and molecular features in kindred. *J Clin Oncol* 2005;23(12):2735–43.

13 Carney JA, Sheps SG, Go VL, Gordon H. The triad of gastric leiyomyosarcoma, functioning extra-adrenal paraganglioma and pulmonary chondroma. *N Engl J Med* 1977;296(26):1517–8.

14 Stratakis CA, Carney JA. The triad of paragangliomas, gastric stromal tumours and pulmonary chondromas (Carney triad), and the dyad of paragangliomas and gastric stromal sarcomas (Carney-Stratakis syndrome): molecular genetics and clinical implications. *J Intern Med* 2009;266(1):43–52.

15 Gaal J, Stratakis CA, Carney JA, *et al.* SDHB immunohistochemistry: a useful tool in the diagnosis of Carney-Stratakis and Carney triad gastrointestinal stromal tumors. *Mod Pathol* 2011;24(1):147–51.

16 Andersson J, Sihto H, Meis-Kindblom JM, *et al.* NF1-associated gastrointestinal stromal tumors have unique clinical, phenotypic, and genotypic characteristics. *Am J Surg Pathol* 2005;29(9):1170–6.

17 Yantiss RK, Rosenberg AE, Sarran L, Besmer P, Antonescu CR. Multiple gastrointestinal stromal tumors in type I neurofibromatosis: a pathologic and molecular study. *Mod Pathol* 2005;18:475–84.

18 Miettinen M, Fetsch JF, Sobin LH, Lasota J. Gastrointestinal stromal tumors in patients with neurofibromatosis 1: a clinicopathologic and molecular genetics study of 45 cases. *Am J Surg Pathol* 2006;30:90–6.

19 Mussi C, Schildhaus HU, Gronchi A, Wardelmann E, Hohenberger P. Therapeutic consequences from molecular biology for gastrointestinal stromal tumor patients affected by neurofibromatosis type 1. *Clin Cancer Res* 2008;14:4550–5.

20 Katz SC, DeMatteo RP. Gastrointestinal stromal tumors and leiomyosarcomas. *J Surg Oncol* 2008;97(4):350–9.

21 Chaudhry UI, DeMatteo RP. Management of resectable gastrointestinal stromal tumor. *Hematol Oncol Clin Noth Am* 2009;23(1):79–96.

22 Patnaik S, Jyotsnarani Y, Rammurti S. Radiological features of metastatic gastrointestinal stromal tumors. *J Clin Imaging Sci* 2012;2:43.

23 Bley TA, Tittelbach-Helmrich D, Baumann T, *et al.* Sliding multislice MRI for abdominal staging of rectal gastrointestinal stromal tumours. *In Vivo* 2007;21(5):891–4.

24 Voiosu T, Voiosu A, Rimbas M, Voiosu R. Endoscopy: possibilities and limitations in the management of GIST of the upper GI tract. *Rom J Intern Med* 2012;50(1):7–11.

25 Watson RR, Binmoeller KF, Hamerski CM, *et al.* Yield and performance characteristics of endoscopic ultrasound-guided fine needle aspiration for diagnosing upper GI tract stromal tumors. *Dig Dis Sci.* 2011;56(6):1757–62.

26 Mazur MT, Clark HB. Gastric stromal tumors. Reappraisal of histogenesis. *Am J Surg Pathol* 1983;7(6):507–19.

27 Hornick JL, Fletcher CD. The role of KIT in the management of patients with gastrointestinal stromal tumors. *Hum Pathol* 2007;38(5):679–87.

28 Tarn C, Merkel E, Canutescu AA, Shen W, Skorobogatko Y, Heslin MJ, *et al.* Analysis of KIT mutations in sporadic and familial gastrointestinal stromal tumors: therapeutic implications through protein modeling. *Clin Cancer Res* 2005;11(10):3668–77.

29 Lasota J, Miettinen M. KIT and PDGFRA mutations in gastrointestinal stromal tumors (GISTs). *Semin Diagn Pathol* 2006;23(2):91–102.

30 Lasota J, Miettinen M. Clinical significance of oncogenic KIT and PDGFRA mutations in gastrointestinal stromal tumours. *Histopathology* 2008;53(3):245–66.

31 Andre C, Hampe A, Lachaume P, *et al.* Sequence analysis of two genomic regions containing the KIT and the FMS receptor tyrosine kinase genes. *Genomics* 1997;39(2): 216–26.

32 Liu FY, Qi JP, Xu FL, Wu AP. Clinicopathological and immunohistochemical analysis of gastrointestinal stromal tumor. *World J Gastroenterol* 2006;12(26):4161–5.

33 Corless CL, Schroeder A, Griffith D, *et al.* PDGFRA mutations in gastrointestinal stromal tumors: frequency, spectrum and in vitro sensitivity to imatinib. *J Clin Oncol* 2005;23(23):5357–64.

34 Panteleo MA, Astolfi A, Nannini M, *et al.* Differential expression of neural markers in KIT and PDGFRA wild-type gastrointestinal stromal tumours. *Histopathology* 2011;59(6):1071–80.

35 Gill AJ. Succinate dehydrogenase (SDH) and mitochondrial driven neoplasia. *Pathology* 2012;44(4):285–92.

36 Patil DT, Rubin BP. Genetics of gastrointestinal stromal tumors: a heterogeneous family of tumors? *Surg Pathol Clin* 2015;8(3):515–24.

37 Hostein I, Faur N, Primois C, Boury F, Denard J, Emile JF, *et al.* BRAF mutation status in gastrointestinal stromal tumors. *Am J Clin Pathol* 2010;133(1):141–8.

38 Miettinen M, Lasota J. Gastrointestinal stromal tumors: pathology and prognosis at different sites. *Semin Diagn Pathol* 2006;23(2):70–83.

39 Gold JS, Gönen M, Gutiérrez A, *et al.* Development and validation of a prognostic nomogram for recurrence-free survival after complete surgical resection of localized primary gastrointestinal stromal tumour: a retrospective analysis. *Lancet Oncol* 2009;10(11):1045–52.

40 Andersson J, Bümming P, Meis-Kindblom JM, *et al.* Gastrointestinal stromal tumors with KIT exon 11 deletions are associated with poor prognosis. *Gastroenterology* 2006;130(6):1573–81.

41 DeMatteo RP, Maki RG, Agulnik M, *et al.* Gastrointestinal stromal tumor. In: MB Amin (ed) *AJCC Cancer Staging Manual*, Eighth Edition. New York: Springer, 2017.

42 Eisenberg BL, Harris J, Blanke CD, *et al.* Phase II trial of neoadjuvant /adjuvant imatinib mesylate (IM) for advanced primary and metastatic/recurrent operable gastrointestinal stromal tumor (GIST): early results of RTOG 0123/ACRIN 6665. *J Surg Oncol* 2009;99(1):42–7.

43 DeMatteo RP, Ballman KV, Antonescu CR, *et al.* Adjuvant imatinib mesylate after resection of localised, primary gastrointestinal stromal tumour: a randomised, double blind, placebo-controlled trial. Lancet 2009;373 (9669).

44 Joensuu H, Eriksson M, Sundby Hall K, *et al.* One vs three years of adjuvant imatinib for operable gastrointestinal stromal tumor: a randomized trial. *JAMA* 2012;307(12):1265–72.

45 Casali PG, Cesne AL, Velasco AP, *et al.* Time to definitive failure to the first tyrosine kinase inhibitor in localized GI stromal tumors treated with imatinib as an adjuvant: a European Organisation for Research and Treatment of Cancer Soft Tissue and Bone Sarcoma Group Intergroup Randomized Trial in Collaboration With the Australasian Gastro-Intestinal Trials Group, UNICANCER, French Sarcoma Group, Italian Sarcoma Group, and Spanish Group for Research on Sarcomas. *J Clin Oncol* 2015;33(36):4276–83.

46 Wang D, Zhang Q, Blanke CD, *et al.* Phase II trial of neoadjuvant/recurrent operable gastrointestinal stromal tumors: long-term follow – up results of Radiation Therapy Oncology Group 0132. *Ann Surg Oncol* 2012;19(4):1074–80.

47 McAuliffe JC, Hunt KK, Lazar AJ, *et al.* A randomized, phase II study of preoperative plus postoperative imatinib in GIST: evidence of rapid radiographic response and temporal induction of tumor cell apoptosis. *Ann Surg Oncol* 2009;16(4):910–9.

48 Hohenberger P, Langer C, Wendtner CM, *et al.* Neoadjuvant treatment of locally advanced GIST: results of APOLLON, a prospective, open label phase II study in KIT- or PDGFRA-positive tumors. J Clin Oncol 2012;30(suppl; abstr 10031).

49 Raut CP, Ashley SW. How I do it: surgical management of gastrointestinal stromal tumors. *J Gastrointest Surg* 2008;12(9):1592–9.

50 Fairweather M, Raut CP. Surgical management of GIST and intra-abdominal visceral leiomyosarcomas. *J Surg Oncol* 2015;111(5):562–9.

51 Fujimoto Y, Nakanishi Y, Yochimura K, Shimoda T. Clinicopathologic study of primary malignant gastrointestinal stromal tumor of the stomach, with special reference to prognostic factors: analysis of results in 140 surgically resected patients. *Gastric Cancer* 2003;6(1):39–48.

52 Prakash S, Sarran L, Socci N, *et al.* Gastrointestinal stromal tumors in children and young adults: a clinicopathologic, molecular, and genomic study of 15 cases and review of the literature. *J Pediatr Hematol Oncol* 2005;27(4):179–87.

53 Rege TA, Wagner AJ, Corless CL, Heinrich MC, Hornick JL. Pediatric-type gastrointestinal stromal tumors in adults: distinctive histology predicts genotype and clinical behavior. *Am J Surg Pathol* 2011;35(4):495–504.

54 DeMatteo RP, Ballman KV, Antonescu CR, *et al.* Adjuvant imatinib mesylate after resection of localized, primary gastrointestinal stromal tumour: a randomized, double-blind, placebo-controlled trial. *Lancet* 2009;373(9669):1097–104.

55 Kawanowa K, Sakuma Y, Sakurai S, *et al.* High incidence of microscopic gastrointestinal stromal tumors in the stomach. *Human Pathol* 2006;37(12):1527–35.

56 Cai R, Ren G, Wang DB. Synchronous adenocarcinoma and gastrointestinal stromal tumors in the stomach. *World J Gastroenterol* 2013;19(20):3117–23.

57 Yan Y, Li Z, Liu Y, *et al.* Coexistence of gastrointestinal stromal tumors and gastric adenocarcinomas. *Tumour Biol* 2013;34(2):919–27.

58 Agaimy A, Wünsch PH, Hofstaedter F, *et al.* Minute gastric sclerosing stromal tumors (GIST tumorlets) are common in adults and frequently show c-KIT mutations. *Am J Surg Pathol* 2007;31(10):113–20.

59 Novitsky YW, Kercher KW, Sing RF, Heniford BT. Long-term outcomes of laparoscopic resection of gastric gastrointestinal stromal tumors. *Ann Surg* 2006;243(6):738–45; discussion 745–7.

60 Otani Y, Furukawa T, Yoshida M, *et al.* Operative indications for relatively small (2–5 cm) gastrointestinal stromal tumor of the stomach based on analysis of 60 operated cases. *Surgery* 2006;139(4):484–92.

61 Shu ZB, Sun LB, Li JP, Li YC, Ding DY. Laparoscopic versus open resection of gastric gastrointestinal stromal tumors. *Chin J Cancer Res* 2013;25(2):175–82.

62 De Vogelaere K, Hoorens A, Haentijens P, Delvaux G. Laparoscopic versus open resection of gastrointestinal stromal tumors or the stomach. *Surg Endosc* 2013;27(5): 1546–54.

63 Lee PC, Lai PS, Yang CY, *et al.* A gasless laparoscopic technique of wide excision for gastric gastrointestinal stromal tumor vs open method. *World J Surg Oncol* 2013;11:44.

64 Dematteo RP, Ballman KV, Antonescu CR, *et al.* Long-term results of adjuvant imatinib mesylate in localized, high-risk, primary gastrointestinal stromal tumor: ACOSOG Z9000 (Alliance) Intergroup Phase 2 Trial. *Ann Surg* 2013;258(3):422–9.

65 Reichardt P, Joensuu H, Blay JY. New fronts in the adjuvant treatment of GIST. *Cancer Chemother Pharmacol* 2013;72(4):715–23

66 Zhan WH, Wang PZ, Shao YF, *et al.* Efficacy and safety of adjuvant post-surgical therapy with imatinib in gastrointestinal stromal tumor patients with high risk of recurrence: interim analysis from a multicenter prospective clinical trial. (Article in Chinese.) *Zhonghua Wei Chang Wai Ke Za Zhi* 2006;9(5):383–7.

67 Kang YK, Kang BW, Im SA, *et al.* Two-year adjuvant imatinib mesylate after complete resection of localized, high-risk GIST with KIT exon 11 mutation. *Cancer Chemother Pharmacol* 2013;71(1):43–51.

68 DeMatteo RP, Ballman KV, Antonescu CR, *et al.* Adjuvant imatinib mesylate after resection of localized, primary gastrointestinal stromal tumour: arandomised, double-blind, placebo-controlled trial. *Lancet* 2009;373:1097–104.

69 Raut CP, Espat J, Maki RG, *et al.* PERSIST-5: five year extended treatment with adjuvant imatinib for patients with intermediate/high risk primary gastrointestinal stromal tumor (GIST). 2017 ASCO Annual Meeting. *J Clin Oncol* 2017;35:(suppl; abstr 11009).

70 Demetri, GD, van Oosterom AT, Garrett CR, *et al.* Efficacy and safety of sunitinib in patients with advanced gastrointestinal stromal tumour after failure of imatinib: a randomized controlled trial. *Lancet* 2006;368(9544): 1329–38.

71 DeMatteo RP, Lewis JJ, Leung D, *et al.* Two hundred gastrointestinal stromal tumors: recurrence patterns and prognostic factors for survival. *Ann Surg* 2000;231(1):51–8.

72 DeMatteo RP, Gold JS, Saran L, *et al.* Tumor mitotic rate, size, and location independently predict recurrence after resection of primary gastrointestinal stromal tumor (GIST). *Cancer* 2008;112(3):608–15.

73 Blanke CD, Rankin C, Demetri GD, *et al.* Phase III randomized, intergroup trial assessing imatinib mesylate at two dose levels in patients with unresectable or metastatic gastrointestinal stromal tumors expressing the kit receptor tyrosine kinase: S0033. *J Clin Oncol* 2008;26(4):626–32.

74 Verweij, J, Casali PG, Zalcberg J, *et al.* Progression-free survival in gastrointestinal stromal tumours with high-dose imatinib: randomised trial. *Lancet* 2004;364(9440):1127–34.

75 Heinrich MC, Corless CL, Demetri GD, *et al.* Kinase mutations and imatinib response in patients with metastatic gastrointestinal stromal tumor. *J Clin Oncol* 2003;21(23):4342–9.

76 Debiec-Rychter M, Sciot R, Le Cesne A, *et al.* KIT mutations and dose selection for imatinib in patients with advanced gastrointestinal stromal tumours. *Eur J Cancer* 2006;42(8):1093–103.

77 Gastrointestinal Stromal Tumor Meta-Analysis Group (MetaGIST). Comparison of two doses of imatinib for the treatment of unresectable or metastatic gastrointestinal stromal tumors: a meta analysis of 1,640 patients. *J Clin Oncol* 2010;28(7):1247–53.

78 Demetri GD, Reichardt P, Kang YK, *et al.* Efficacy and safety of regorafenib for advanced gastrointestinal stromal tumours after failure of imatinib and sunitinib (GRID): an international, multicentre, randomized, placebo-controlled, phase 3 trial. *Lancet* 2013;381(9863):295–302.

79 Heinrich MC, Griffith D, McKinely A, *et al.* Crenolanib inhibits the drug resistant PDGFRA D842V mutation associated with imatinib-resistant gastrointestinal stromal tumors. *Clin Cancer Res* 2012;18(16):4375–84.

80 Mir O, Cropet C, Toulmonde M, Le Cesne A, Molimard M, Bompas E, Cassier P, Ray-Coquard I, Rios M, Adenis A, Italiano A. Pazopanib plus best supportive care versus best supportive care alone in advanced gastrointestinal stromal tumours resistant to imatinib and sunitinib (PAZOGIST): a randomised, multicentre, open-label phase 2 trial. *The Lancet Oncology.* 2016 May 31;17(5):632–41.

81 Bauer S, Yu LK, Demetri GD, Fletcher JA. Heat shock protein 90 inhibition in imatinib-resistant gastrointestinal stromal tumor. *Cancer Res* 2006;66(18):9153–61.

82 Schöffski P, Reichardt P, Blay JY, Dumez H, Morgan JA, Ray-Coguard I, *et al.* A phase I-II study of everolimus (RAD001) in combination with imatinib in patients with imatinib-resistant gastrointestinal stromal tumors. *Ann Oncol* 2010;21(10):1990–8.

83 Floris G, Debiec-Rychter M, Sciot R, Stefan C, Fieuws S, Machiels K, *et al.* High efficacy of panobinostat towards human gastrointestinal stromal tumors in a xenograft mouse model. *Clin Cancer Res* 2009 Jun 15;15(12):4066–76.

84 Tarn C, Rink L, Merkel E, Flieder D, Pathak H, Koumbi D, *et al.* Insulin-like growth factor 1 receptor is a potential therapeutic target for gastrointestinal stromal tumors. *Proc Natl Acad Sci U.S.A.* 2008;105(24):8387–92.

85 Blay JY, Le Cesne A, Ray-Coquard I, Bui B, Duffaud F, Delbaldo C, *et al.* Prospective multicentric randomized phase III study of imatinib in patients with advanced gastrointestinal

stromal tumors comparing interruption versus continuation of treatment beyond 1 year: the French Sarcoma Group. *J Clin Oncol* 2007;25(9):1107–13.

86 Le Cesne A, Ray-Coquard I, Bui BN, Adenis A, Rios M, Bertucci F, *et al.* Discontinuation of imatinib in patients with advanced gastrointestinal stromal tumours after 3 years of treatment: an open-label multicentre randomized phase 3 trial. *Lancet Oncol* 2010;11:942–9.

87 Blay JY, Adenis A, Ray-Coquard I, Cassier PA, Le Cesne A. Is there a role for discontinuing imatinib in patients with advanced gastrointestinal stromal tumour? *Current Opn Oncol* 2009;21(4):360–6.

88 Raut CP, Posner M, Desai J, Morgan JA, George S, Zahrieh D, *et al.* Surgical management of advanced gastrointestinal stromal tumors after treatment with targeted systemic therapy using kinase inhibitors. *J Clin Oncol* 2006;24(15): p. 2325–31.

89 Raut CP, Wang Q, Manola J, Morgan JA, George S, Wagner AJ, *et al.*, Cytoreductive surgery in patients with metastatic gastrointestinal stromal tumor treated with sunitinib maleate. *Ann Surg Oncol* 2010 Feb;17(2): 407–15.

90 Demetri GD, von Mehren M, Antonescu CR, DeMatteo RP, Ganjoo KN, Maki RG, *et al.* NCCN Task Force report: update on the management of patients with gastrointestinal stromal tumors. *J Natl Compr Canc Netw.* 2010 Apr;8 Suppl 2:S1–41.

91 Von Mehren M, Randall RL, Benjamin RS, Boles S, Bui MM, *et al.* Clinical practice guidelines in oncology. Soft tissue sarcoma V 1.2017. December 21, 2016. Nccn.org. accessed January 12, 2017.

92 Demetri, GD, Jeffers M, Reichardt P, Yoon-Koo K, Jean-Yves B, Rutkowski P, *et al.* Mutational analysis of plasma DNA from patients (pts) in the phase III GRID study of regorafinib (REG) versus placebo (PL) in tyrosine kinase inhibitor (TKI)-refractory GIST: Correlating genotype with clinical outcomes. *J Clin Oncol* 31, 2013 (suppl:abstr 10503).

93 Duffy MJ, Lamerz R, Haglund C, Nicolini A, Kalousová M, Holubel L. Tumor markers in colorectal cacer, gastric cancer and gastrointestinal stromal cancers: European group on tumor markers (EGTM) 2014 guidelines update. *Int J Cancer.* 2014;134(11):2513–22.

Section 3

Head and Neck

12

Oral Cavity and Oropharyngeal Cancer

Avinash V. Mantravadi[1] *and Michael G. Moore*[2]

[1] *Indiana University School of Medicine, Indianapolis, Indiana, USA*
[2] *The University of California at Davis Medical Center, Sacramento, California, USA*

Introduction

The oral cavity and oropharynx are complex subsites of the upper aerodigestive tract that play a significant role in functions such as mastication, articulation, swallowing, and breathing. Consequently, when managing malignancies in these areas, decisions must be made to optimize cancer cure while minimizing functional morbidity. Moreover, due to the prominent role the lips and upper and lower jaws play in the structure of the face, cosmetic outcomes must also be considered. This chapter will address the epidemiology and risk factors of oral and oropharyngeal cancer and will outline the basic anatomy of each region. Typical clinical presentations and appropriate workup for cancers in these locations will be discussed, along with a summary of the contemporary staging systems as well as fundamentals of treatment.

Incidence and Mortality

The American Cancer Society estimates that approximately 49,760 persons are diagnosed with oral or oropharyngeal cancer, and nearly 9,700 individuals die from this disease each year in the United States (US)[1]. Squamous cell carcinomas comprise approximately 85% of the cancers in this region, with the remaining tumors arising from minor salivary glands (salivary cancers), lymphoid tissue (lymphoma), teeth and related structures (odontogenic cancers), or surrounding tissue (sarcomas). Incidence rates for oral cavity and pharynx cancer increased by an average of 0.8% per year from 2004 to 2013 and death rates declined by an average of 0.6% per year during that period [2].

Etiology and Risk Factors

Men are affected by oral and pharyngeal cancer more than twice as frequently as women (incidence rates 16.7 and 6.2 cases per 100,000 individuals per year). Incidence rates in the US are highest among Whites, lowest among Hispanics, and intermediate for other racial and ethnic groups. The average ages at the times of diagnosis and death are 62 years and 67 years, respectively [2].

The primary risk factors for the development of oral and oropharyngeal squamous cell cancer are tobacco and alcohol use, with up to 75% of cases resulting from exposure to these substances. Although each factor is known to increase the risk of malignancy, studies have shown that the effects of chronic exposure to both tobacco and alcohol together is synergistic and increases risk exponentially. Sun exposure increases the risk of forming cancer of the lower lip while the use of smokeless tobacco and betel quid can result in carcinogenesis to the areas in regular contact with the substance such as the associated gums, cheek mucosa, and/or lip. Although the incidence of tobacco-related cancers has declined in North America and Western Europe due to increased awareness of harmful effects and decreased tobacco use, the cultural and dietary use of carcinogenic substances such as betel quid contributes significantly to the increasing incidence in regions such as the Indian subcontinent. Genetic predisposition also plays a role in the development of oral and oropharyngeal cancers, as a family history of a first degree relative with head and neck cancer results in a 1.7-fold increase in the risk of disease development [3, 4].

In recent years, human papillomavirus (HPV) has been shown to play a role in the development of head and neck squamous cell carcinoma, particularly in the oropharynx originating in the mucosa overlying the tonsils and base of tongue. These tumors, usually associated with prior infection with HPV subtype 16, are the primary reason why the incidence of oropharyngeal cancer has been increasing in recent years while tobacco-related cancers are becoming less common [5]. HPV infects only within the stratified epithelial layer of the skin, oral cavity/oropharynx, and anogenital tract. A complex interaction between the immune system and expression of viral oncogenes *E6* and *E7* subsequently takes place, ultimately leading to inactivation

The American Cancer Society's Oncology in Practice: Clinical Management, First Edition. Edited by The American Cancer Society.

of tumor suppressor proteins and the promotion of neoplastic cell growth. The sexually transmitted nature of this disease is highlighted by studies that have shown an increased risk of oropharyngeal carcinoma in patients with an increased number of sexual and oral-sexual partners. A history of HIV positivity also greatly increases the risk of HPV-related oropharyngeal carcinoma, resulting in increased rates of head and neck cancers in geographic regions affected by high rates of HIV infection such as Africa [3, 4]. An improved understanding of the role of HPV in the development of oropharyngeal carcinoma is significant in that HPV-related tumors often have a different clinical presentation and a significantly better response to treatment and survival rate than non-HPV-related tumors [6–9].

Prevention

For oral cavity cancer, avoidance of exposure to common risk factors such as tobacco and alcohol is the most appropriate means for prevention. Maintaining good oral hygiene and dental care may also reduce the risk of cancer development along with regular screenings by dental professionals.

With regard to oropharyngeal cancer, in 2006, HPV-vaccination was first approved in the US [10] and vaccines against additional HPV types were subsequently approved. Current recommendations by the Centers for Disease Control are for boys and girls to receive three doses of a quadravalent or nonavalent vaccine starting at ages 11–12. Doses are given as an intramuscular injection at 0, 1 and 6 months. For those who can complete a two-dose regimen before age 15 with doses 6–12 months apart, a third dose is not required [11]. These vaccines are safe and have proven effective in preventing oral HPV infections, when compared to placebo [12]. However, due to the long time interval between exposure to carcinogenesis, as well as the lack of observable precursor lesions, a trial proving prevention of oropharyngeal cancer with the vaccine is unlikely.

Anatomy

The oral cavity includes the territory from the lips to the junction between the hard and soft palate above and the circumvallate papillae on the tongue below, which delineates the border between the oral tongue (anterior two-thirds) and tongue base (posterior one-third). The major subsites include the lips, buccal mucosa, maxillary and mandibular alveolar ridges, floor of mouth (FOM), oral tongue, retromolar trigone, and hard palate.

The lip has both cutaneous and mucosal portions, and for the purposes of this discussion the "oral cavity" portion of the lip can be considered that which comes in contact with the opposing lip. This comprises the anterior-most portion of the oral vestibule and is essential to oral sphincter functions required for adequate oral intake and speech articulation. The remainder of the vestibule is formed by the buccal mucosa, which lines the inner lips and cheek (Figure 12.1(a) and (b)). Loss of this tissue due to cancer may result in poor oral competence and drooling. The alveolar ridges include the mucosa of the gums on both the buccal (towards the cheek and lips) and lingual surface (towards the FOM) of the mandible. The retromolar trigone is a triangular-shaped region overlying the mandible behind the last molar tooth (Figure 12.1(b)). Cancers in this region frequently involve the underlying mandible early in their course. The mucosa of the maxillary gums are also included in this region. The mucosa of the hard palate is firmly adherent to the maxilla and as a result, cancers in this region often demonstrate early bony involvement.

The FOM mucosa extends from the alveolar ridge of the mandible to the undersurface of the tongue (ventral tongue) and along each side under the tongue to the anterior tonsillar pillar. Loss of FOM mucosa may result in tethering of the tongue with subsequent impact on swallowing and speech articulation (Figure 12.1(c)).

The oral tongue (anterior to the circumvallate papillae; the anterior two-thirds of the tongue) is considered part of the oral cavity, while the base of tongue (posterior to the circumvallate papillae; the posterior third of the tongue) is considered a part of the oropharynx and will be discussed in greater detail later in this chapter. The oral tongue consists of four anatomic areas – the tip, the lateral borders (sides), the dorsal tongue (top surface), and ventral tongue (undersurface) – see Figure 1(d). The functional consequence of surgical removal of these areas depends on which of these subsites are involved, with speech, swallowing, and oral competence frequently being affected.

Anatomy of the Oropharynx

The oropharynx is the area of the throat that lies behind the oral cavity, and is bordered by the nasopharynx above, and the hypopharynx and larynx below (Figure 12.2). Anatomically, this region starts at the junction of the hard and soft palate superiorly, and extends inferiorly with its anterior extent being the anterior tonsillar pillars and the circumvallate papillae that separate the oral tongue from the tongue base. The junction of the tongue base and the epiglottis is termed the vallecula, and represents the boundary between the oropharynx and the larynx.

The different subsites of the oropharynx include the tonsillar fossae (which contain the palatine tonsils), soft palate, tongue base (which contain lingual tonsil tissue), and posterior pharyngeal wall (Figure 12.3). The tonsils and tongue base make up part of Waldeyer's ring, are composed mainly of lymphoid tissue lined by epithelial crypts assisting in immune surveillance, and are the areas that are primarily involved with oropharyngeal cancer related to the human papillomavirus.

The oropharynx plays a critical role in swallowing and speech. During a normal swallow, the oral tongue propels the bolus to the oropharynx where the tongue and tongue base elevate and oppose the palate. The soft palate along with the pharyngeal constrictor muscles serve to close off the entry to the nasopharynx to ultimately guide the bolus inferiorly during the pharyngeal phase. Insufficiency of palatal function results in leakage of food or drink into the nasopharynx

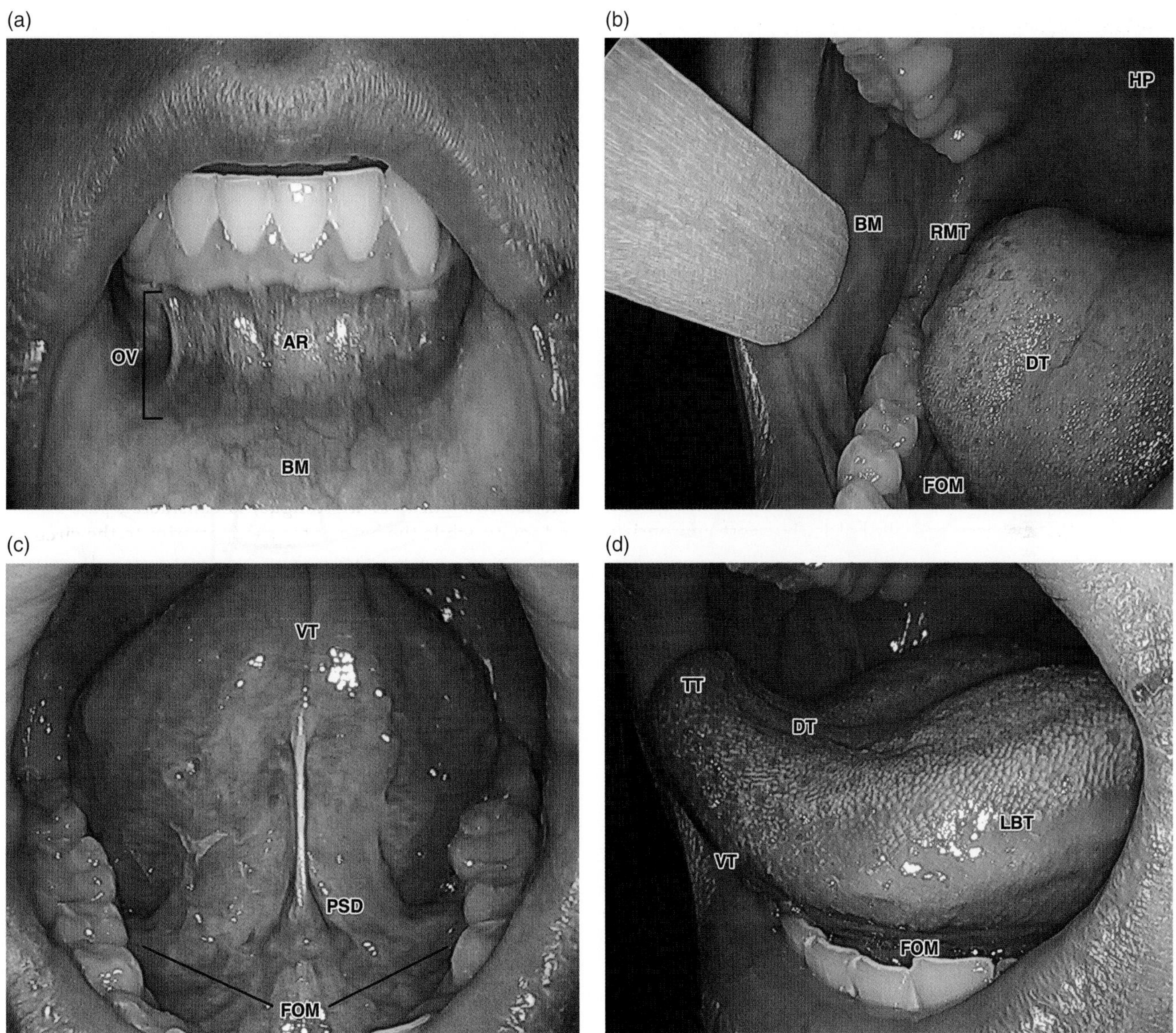

Figure 12.1 (a) This view of the oral cavity demonstrates the oral vestibule (OV), anterior buccal mucosa (BM), and the buccal surface of the mandibular alveolar ridge (AR). (b) This view of the lateral oral cavity with cheek retracted with tongue blade demonstrates lateral buccal mucosa (BM), retromolar trigone (RMT), hard palate (HP), dorsal surface of tongue (DT), and floor of mouth mucosa (FOM). (c) Transoral view with the tongue elevated, showing the ventral surface of the tongue (VT), paired papillae of the submandibular (Wharton's) duct (PSD), and floor of mouth mucosa (FOM). (d) The four anatomic regions of the oral tongue: the tongue tip (TT), lateral border (LBT), dorsal (DT) and ventral (VT) surfaces. The floor of mouth (FOM) is also visible.

during swallowing, and during speech, large amounts of air can escape through the nose causing speech to sound hollow and hypernasal.

Lymphatic Drainage

Oral cavity cancers that metastasize to lymph nodes in the neck can be expected to spread to the submandibular and submental (level I) nodes, as well as the superior deep jugular basin (level II and III) (Figure 12.4) [13]. Lateral oral tongue cancers may also involve level IV nodes in some instances [14, 15]. This knowledge has allowed for more targeted and limited surgery to address these cancers, thereby decreasing potential complications associated with more traditional techniques. Cancers located near the midline of the lip, FOM, and tongue are at increased risk for metastasizing to lymph nodes in the contralateral neck, such that both necks require treatment.

For oropharyngeal cancers, the first echelon of lymphatic drainage is to level II on the side of the primary cancer. However, levels III and IV are often involved. Lymph node metastases of tonsil and tongue base tumors are classically large and contain cystic central compartments representing tissue necrosis. Consequently, these neck masses may often be mistaken for congenital neck masses such as branchial cleft cysts or suppurative lymphadenitis. In adult patients, it is imperative that the clinician keep a high index of suspicion for malignancy in order to avoid delay in diagnosis. While tonsil cancer metastases are typically on the same side as the primary tumor, tongue base cancers and those of the soft palate and posterior pharyngeal wall often spread to either side of the neck.

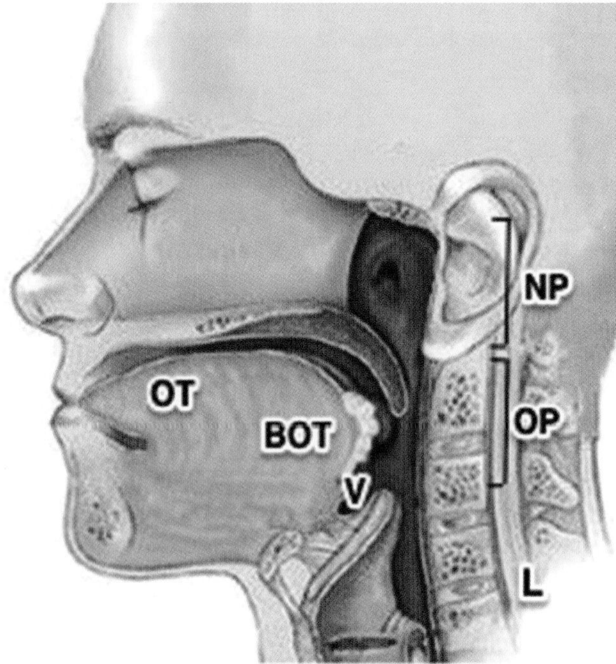

Figure 12.2 Sagittal view of the head and neck, showing the delineation between the oral tongue (OT) and the base of tongue (BOT). The relationship between the oropharynx (OP) with the nasopharynx (NP – superior) and larynx (L – below) is demonstrated. The vallecula (V) marks the junction between the oropharynx and the larynx.

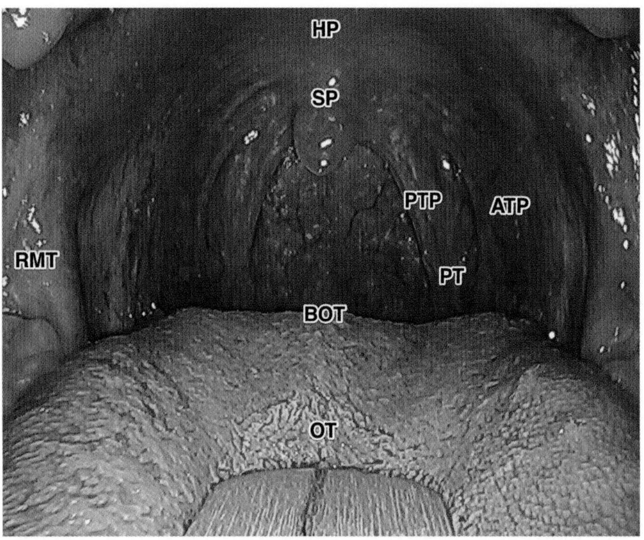

Figure 12.3 The oral tongue (OT) or anterior two-thirds of the tongue is considered part of the oral cavity, while the base of tongue (BOT) is a component of the oropharynx. The retromolar trigone (RMT) is the posterolateral extent of the oral cavity. The oropharynx begins at the junction between the hard palate (HP) and soft palate (SP). The palatine tonsil (PT) lies between the anterior (ATP) and posterior (PTP) tonsillar pillars.

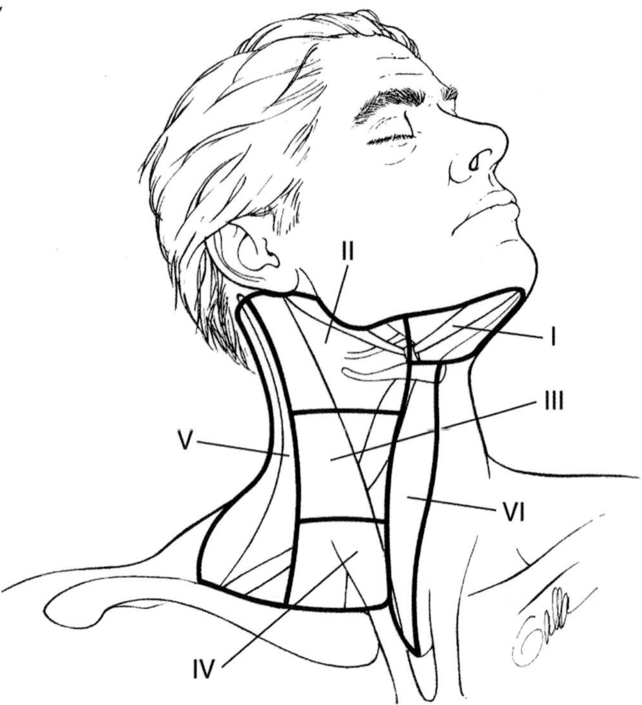

Figure 12.4 Location of the six major lymph node basins within the head and neck. Source: Janfaza *et al.* [10]. Reproduced with permission of Wolters Kluwer.

Pathology

Common precancerous lesions in the oral cavity and oropharynx include leukoplakia, a white keratotic patch in the oral mucosa that cannot be rubbed off. Leukoplakia sometimes results from chronic irritation of the oral mucosa, and has been shown to convert to invasive carcinoma up to 18% of the time [16]. Erythroplakia, a red mucosal plaque, is not associated with chronic irritation or oral trauma but has a higher likelihood of malignant transformation than leukoplakia. Lichen planus, characterized by lacy or velvety white lines at the buccal mucosa, has also shown premalignant potential.

Squamous cell carcinoma, arising from the oral and oropharyngeal epithelium, comprises more than 90% of all malignant lesions in this region, and as a result the remainder of this section will focus on this disease process. Nonmucosal malignancies make up the remaining <10% of cancers in these regions. These include minor salivary gland carcinomas (adenoid cystic carcinoma, mucoepidermoid carcinoma, and polymorphous low grade adenocarcinoma), Kaposi sarcoma associated with AIDS, primary mucosal melanoma, lymphomas arising in the lymphoid tissue of the tonsils or tongue base, and sarcomas.

Pathogenesis

Slaughter *et al.* first described the concept of "field cancerization" in 1953 [17], which demonstrated histologically abnormal epithelium adjacent to and distant from primary cancers in the oral cavity. This concept has been further expanded to demonstrate that all mucosal surfaces exposed to a known carcinogen are at risk for malignant growth, and has been used to explain the presence of multiple synchronous cancers throughout the head, neck, lung, and esophagus. Lesions can be observed to demonstrate a progression from normal mucosa to premalignant lesions to invasive cancer.

Clinical Presentation

Presenting symptoms of oral cavity and oropharyngeal cancers depend on the location and extent of the tumor. The most common presenting symptom for patients with cancer of the oral cavity is a painful lesion in the mouth. Patients may also present with bleeding from the oral cavity, loose teeth, or ill-fitting dentures. Asymptomatic lesions are often discovered on routine dental or medical examinations or present as a nonhealing ulcer or wound after minor dental trauma. Cancer of the FOM may involve the papilla of the submandibular duct and obstruct salivary outflow, leading to tenderness and enlargement of the submandibular gland. Bacterial colonization of an ulcerated cancer can produce a foul odor.

Unlike oral cavity lesions, oropharyngeal cancers, due to the large potential space of the pharynx, are often not identified in their early stages. Symptoms tend to be vague and mimic common, benign conditions such as pharyngitis and cervical lymphadenitis. As a result, additional workup is often not performed until initial treatment regimens have failed.

As disease progresses, patients may notice a change in their voice (classically a muffled voice) and may develop more difficulty breathing when lying on their back or on the side opposite the tumor. Deep infiltration of the cancer may extend into the nearby muscular sling around the jaw, or pterygoid muscles. This often generates considerably more discomfort and can result in referral of pain to the ear on the same side (otalgia). Additionally, when there is significant pterygoid muscle extension, patients may have difficulty with mouth opening (trismus) and even numbness of the tongue on the affected side (due to extension around the lingual nerve). Invasion into the mandible often elicits deep aching pain and can generate numbness of the ipsilateral lip once the inferior alveolar nerve is involved.

Because of the relatively early onset of symptoms and ease with which a patient or healthcare provider can access the oral cavity for examination, it is rare for a patient with cancer of the oral cavity to present with a neck mass in the absence of oral cavity symptoms or a known primary lesion. In contrast, the most common presenting symptom for an HPV-related oropharyngeal cancer is an enlarged neck mass, whereas the most common symptom for an HPV-negative oropharyngeal cancer is throat pain [7].

Evaluation and Workup

Initial evaluation of a patient with suspected cancer of the oral cavity or oropharynx requires a detailed history and physical examination, imaging studies to include metastatic workup, tissue biopsy, and often an examination under anesthesia.

History and Physical Examination

Initial evaluation should start with a detailed timeline of symptoms including information on onset, duration, consistency, and periods of resolution. The presence of pain is an important factor in delineating suspicion for benign or malignant disease. Dental issues including the presence of loose teeth or alteration of the patient's normal dental occlusion should be noted.

An assessment of tobacco and alcohol abuse is particularly relevant since they are the primary risk factors for squamous cell carcinoma of the head and neck. However, risk factors for exposure to high risk human papillomavirus should also be evaluated with a thorough sexual history, including the number of sexual partners, age of first sexual encounter, and participation in oral sex [18, 19]. A history of occupational or recreational sun exposure and frequent sunburns should be noted, as this places patients at increased risk for carcinoma of the lower lip. Prior treatment of head and neck cancers including previous head and neck irradiation should be recorded. The patient's past medical and surgical history, family history, social history, and occupational history are also important.

A review of systems may provide a better understanding of the patient's overall health. For cancer of the oropharynx, dysphagia and difficulty lying supine are important to note. Weight loss should also be documented as it may represent malnutrition and/or a manifestation of distant metastases.

The physical examination should start with a thorough head and neck evaluation. Meticulous inspection of the entire oral cavity and oropharynx should be performed with a headlight to allow freedom of both hands to expose the mucosal surfaces with tongue blades (Figure 12.5). The appearance and size of the lesion, as well as its location and all involved structures should be noted. Determination of whether the lesion crosses the midline provides valuable information for treatment planning. Bimanual palpation is critical to assess the depth, and whether deeper muscles and/or bone appear involved. Indirect (mirror) laryngoscopy is performed to assess the oropharynx and laryngeal structures. However, due to the elevated risk of second primary malignancies, the improved, magnified visualization afforded by flexible fiberoptic pharyngolaryngoscopy is

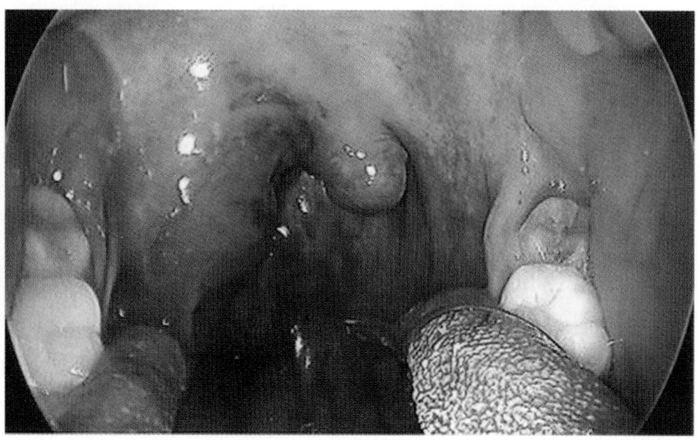

Figure 12.5 Transoral view showing an exophytic cancer of the right tonsil.

optimal to determine the extent of tumor involvement and to rule out an additional cancer. Ensuring a patent and safe airway is of paramount importance in advanced lesions, and may require awake tracheotomy in the operating room prior to the completion of the initial workup. The presence of enlarged cervical lymph nodes in the setting of primary oral and oropharyngeal malignancies has important prognostic and therapeutic implications, and therefore detailed palpation of all levels of the neck is critical to the initial evaluation. Any neck masses should be assessed for size, location, tenderness, consistency, pulsation, and mobility from the overlying skin and deep neck structures.

Imaging

Initial imaging should be selected to evaluate both the primary tumor as well as the cervical lymph node basins. Contrasted computed tomography (CT) (Figure 12.6(a)) and magnetic resonance imaging (MRI) (Figure 12.6(b)) are available modalities, each with its own unique advantages. CT is most commonly used due to its decreased cost and time required for testing, but these images do require exposure to ionizing radiation and may be limited in patients with a history of dental work which creates significant imaging artifact. MRI is often preferred in these situations. CT is effective for assessment of depth of invasion and involvement of adjacent structures, and is superior for detecting cortical bone erosion. MR is superior to CT in the assessment of tongue-base involvement, as well as to determine invasion of the mandibular bone marrow space or perineural spread of tumor [20].

Routine metastatic workup includes imaging of the chest, via chest X-ray or noncontrasted CT. Positron emission tomography/CT may also be utilized to rule out metastatic disease. However, its routine use for this purpose is recommended only for those patients with clinical stage III and IV disease [21].

Tissue Biopsy/Examination under Anesthesia

A biopsy specimen should be obtained at the time of the patient's initial presentation. The majority of oral cavity lesions are accessible for biopsy in the clinic setting using local anesthesia. For most oropharyngeal lesions and those oral cavity tumors inaccessible to office biopsy, a specimen may be obtained with the patient under general anesthesia. All biopsies from the oropharynx, when possible, should be sent for p16 immunohistochemistry and high-risk HPV *in situ* hybridization [22]. New techniques such as *in situ* hybridization looking at high-risk HPV E6/E7 mRNA are also being advocated [23]. If the extent of disease is poorly visualized in the clinic setting, particularly in patients with a history of previous chemoradiation, an examination under general anesthesia including direct laryngoscopy and esophagoscopy is required. This is often performed in patients with oral cavity or oropharyngeal cancer either as a part of their initial workup or at the time of surgical management, due to the high prevalence of second malignancies as discussed earlier.

Staging

Staging of oral cavity and oropharyngeal squamous cell carcinoma follow the tumor, node, metastasis (TNM) staging system from the American Joint Committee for Cancer (AJCC) Cancer Staging Manual (8th Edition, 2017) [24–26] and the Union for International Cancer Control (UICC), which includes information garnered from clinical examinations and imaging studies (Table 12.1). The size of the tumor (T), presence or absence of metastasis to the cervical lymph nodes (N), and presence or absence of distant metastasis (M) are combined in this system.

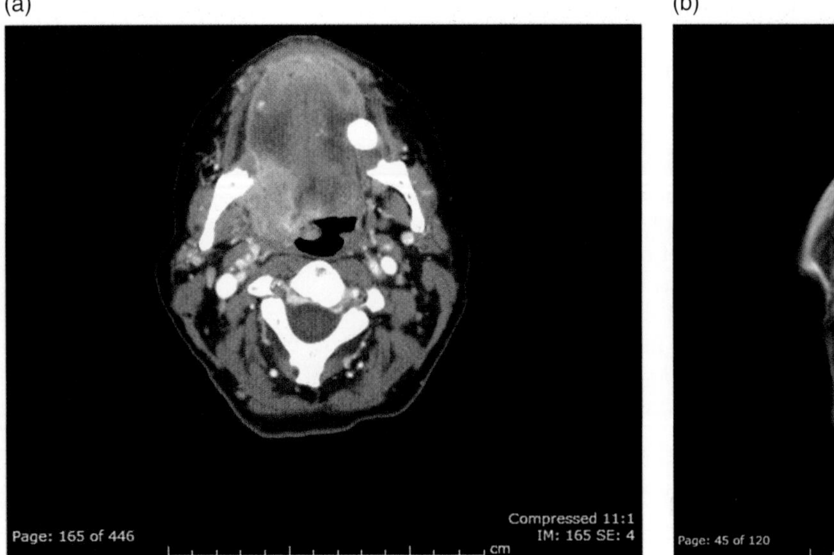

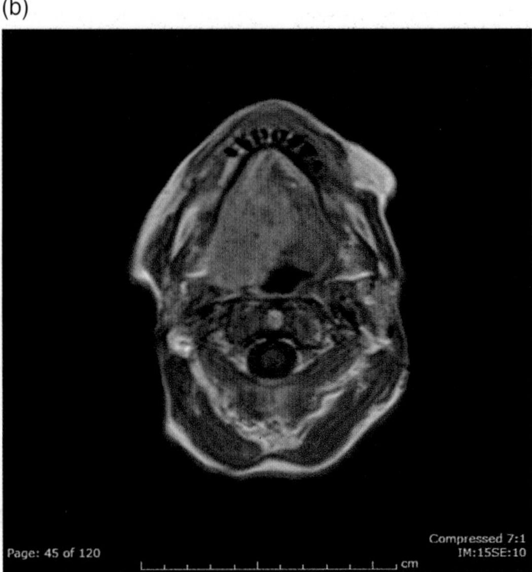

Figure 12.6 (a) Axial computed tomography image with intravenous contrast showing an endophytic right tongue base cancer with adherence to the adjacent mandible. (b) Magnetic resonance image demonstrating the significant submucosal extension of a right sided oral tongue cancer. Notice the loss of the normal muscle architecture of the patient's right tongue.

Table 12.1 Staging of oral cavity and oropharyngeal squamous cell carcinoma.

Oral cavity tumor categories [21]

T category	T criteria
TX	Primary tumor cannot be assessed
Tis	Carcinoma *in situ*
T1	Tumor ≤2 cm, ≤5 mm depth of invasion (DOI) DOI is depth of invasion and not tumor thickness.
T2	Tumor ≤2 cm, DOI >5 mm and ≤10 mm *or* tumor >2 cm but ≤4 cm, and ≤10 mm DOI
T3	Tumor >4 cm *or* any tumor >10 mm DOI
T4	Moderately advanced or very advanced local disease
T4a	Moderately advanced local disease (Lip) Tumor invades through cortical bone or involves the inferior alveolar nerve, floor of mouth, or skin of face (i.e., chin or nose) (Oral cavity) Tumor invades adjacent structures only (e.g., through cortical bone of the mandible or maxilla, or involves the maxillary sinus or skin of the face) Note: Superficial erosion of bone/tooth socket (alone) by a gingival primary is not sufficient to classify a tumor as T4.
T4b	Very advanced local disease Tumor invades masticator space, pterygoid plates, or skull base and/or encases the internal carotid artery

Oropharyngeal tumor categories [22]

Oropharynx (p16-)

T category	T criteria
TX	Primary tumor cannot be assessed
Tis	Carcinoma *in situ*
T1	Tumor 2 cm or smaller in greatest dimension
T2	Tumor larger than 2 cm but not larger than 4 cm in greatest dimension
T3	Tumor larger than 4 cm in greatest dimension or extension to lingual surface of epiglottis
T4	Moderately advanced or very advanced local disease
T4a	Moderately advanced local disease Tumor invades the larynx, extrinsic muscle of tongue, medial pterygoid, hard palate, or mandible[1]
T4b	Very advanced local disease Tumor invades lateral pterygoid muscle, pterygoid plates, lateral nasopharynx, or skull base or encases carotid artery

[1] Note: Mucosal extension to lingual surface of epiglottis from primary tumors of the base of the tongue and vallecula does not constitute invasion of the larynx.

Oropharynx (HPV+) [23]

T category	T criteria
T0	No primary identified
T1	Tumor 2 cm or smaller in greatest dimension
T2	Tumor larger than 2 cm but not larger than 4 cm in greatest dimension
T3	Tumor larger than 4 cm in greatest dimension or extension to lingual surface of epiglottis
T4	Moderately advanced local disease Tumor invades the larynx, extrinsic muscle of tongue, medial pterygoid, hard palate, or mandible or beyond[1]

[1]Mucosal extension to lingual surface of epiglottis from primary tumors of the base of the tongue and vallecula does not constitute invasion of the larynx.

(*Continued*)

Table 12.1 (Continued)

Nodal clinical categories for oral cavity cancer and HPV – oropharyngeal cancer

N category	N criteria
NX	Regional lymph nodes cannot be assessed
N0	No regional lymph node metastasis
N1	Metastasis in a single ipsilateral lymph node, 3 cm or smaller in greatest dimension ENE(−)
N2	Metastasis in a single ipsilateral node larger than 3 cm but not larger than 6 cm in greatest dimension and ENE(−); *or* metastases in multiple ipsilateral lymph nodes, none larger than 6 cm in greatest dimension and ENE(−); *or* in bilateral or contralateral lymph nodes, none larger than 6 cm in greatest dimension, and ENE(−)
N2a	Metastasis in a single ipsilateral node larger than 3 cm but not larger than 6 cm in greatest dimension, and ENE(−)
N2b	Metastasis in multiple ipsilateral nodes, none larger than 6 cm in greatest dimension, and ENE(−)
N2c	Metastasis in bilateral or contralateral lymph nodes, none larger than 6 cm in greatest dimension, and ENE(−)
N3	Metastasis in a lymph node larger than 6 cm in greatest dimension and ENE(−); *or* metastasis in any node(s) and clinically overt ENE(+)
N3a	Metastasis in a lymph node larger than 6 cm in greatest dimension and ENE(−)
N3b	Metastasis in any node(s) and clinically overt ENE(+)

Note: a designation of “U” or “L” may be used for any N category to indicate metastasis above the lower border of the cricoid (U) or below the lower border of the cricoid (L).
Similarly, clinical and pathological extranodal extension (ENE) should be recorded as ENE(−) or ENE(+).

Nodal clinical categories for HPV+ oropharyngeal cancer

N category	N criteria
NX	Regional lymph nodes cannot be assessed
N0	No regional lymph node metastasis
N1	One or more ipsilateral lymph nodes, none larger than 6 cm
N2	Contralateral or bilateral lymph nodes, none larger than 6 cm
N3	Lymph node(s) larger than 6 cm

Nodal pathologic categories for oral cavity cancer and HPV- oropharyngeal cancer

N category	N criteria
NX	Regional lymph nodes cannot be assessed
N0	No regional lymph node metastasis
N1	Metastasis in a single ipsilateral lymph node, 3 cm or smaller in greatest dimension and ENE(−)
N2	Metastasis in a single ipsilateral lymph node, 3 cm or smaller in greatest dimension and ENE(+); *or* larger than 3 cm but not larger than 6 cm in greatest dimension and ENE(−); *or* metastases in multiple ipsilateral lymph nodes, none larger than 6 cm in greatest dimension and ENE(−); *or* in bilateral or contralateral lymph nodes, none larger than 6 cm in greatest dimension, ENE(−)
N2a	Metastasis in single ipsilateral or contralateral node 3 cm or smaller in greatest dimension and ENE(+); *or* a single ipsilateral node larger than 3 cm but not larger than 6 cm in greatest dimension and ENE(−)
N2b	Metastasis in multiple ipsilateral nodes, none larger than 6 cm in greatest dimension and ENE(−)
N2c	Metastasis in bilateral or contralateral lymph nodes, none larger than 6 cm in greatest dimension and ENE(−)
N3	Metastasis in a lymph node larger than 6 cm in greatest dimension and ENE(−); *or* in a single ipsilateral node larger than 3 cm in greatest dimension and ENE(+); *or* multiple ipsilateral, contralateral or bilateral nodes any with ENE(+)
N3a	Metastasis in a lymph node larger than 6 cm in greatest dimension and ENE(−)
N3b	Metastasis in a single ipsilateral node larger than 3 cm in greatest dimension and ENE(+); *or* multiple ipsilateral, contralateral or bilateral nodes any with ENE(+)

Note: a designation of “U” or “L” may be used for any N category to indicate metastasis above the lower border of the cricoid (U) or below the lower border of the cricoid (L).
Similarly, clinical and pathological ENE should be recorded as ENE(−) or ENE(+).

Table 12.1 (Continued)

Nodal pathologic categories for HPV+ oropharyngeal cancer	
N category	**N criteria**
NX	Regional lymph nodes cannot be assessed
pN0	No regional lymph node metastasis
pN1	Metastasis in 4 or fewer lymph nodes
pN2	Metastasis in more than 4 lymph nodes
Distant metastasis categories for oral cavity, HPV- oropharyngeal cancer, and HPV+ oropharyngeal cancer	
M category	**M criteria**
M0	No distant metastasis
M1	Distant metastasis

Source: Ridge *et al.* [21]. Used with permission of the American College of Surgeons, Chicago, Illinois. The original source for this information is the AJCC Cancer Staging Manual, 8th edn (2017), which is published by Springer Science + Business Media.

Of note, this newly published staging system now takes into account differences in the clinical behavior of HPV+ and HPV- oropharyngeal cancer. In addition, the negative impact of depth of invasion for oral cavity cancers is also incorporated into the staging of the primary site (Table 12.2).

Management

Successful management of oral and oropharyngeal cancers requires participation from many members of a multidisciplinary team including head and neck oncologic and reconstructive surgery, radiation and medical oncology, dedicated head and neck pathology and radiology, dentistry, maxillofacial prosthodontics, and speech and swallowing pathology. The main treatment options include surgery, radiation, and chemotherapy, or some combination thereof. Chemotherapy is not used as a primary treatment modality alone, but rather as an adjunct to radiation therapy to increase its effectiveness (radiosensitizer). It may on occasion be given alone for palliation in patients with unresectable disease or distant metastases.

Early-stage tumors (stage I and II) can be treated with either surgery or radiation alone with equal effectiveness, each of which has unique advantages and disadvantages. The choice of treatment should depend on several patient-related factors:

1) Comorbidities and ability to undergo general anesthesia
2) Social support (patient's capacity to attend daily radiation treatments for up to 7 weeks, or the availability of support to help with postoperative care)
3) The degree of anticipated loss of function after surgical removal of tumor or radiation therapy to the oral cavity
4) Patient preference after full informed discussion of available treatment options.

Advanced-stage tumors (stage III and IV) generally mandate multimodality treatment, either with surgery followed by radiation with or without chemotherapy or upfront chemoradiation, reserving surgery for salvage [27].

Table 12.2 AJCC prognostic stage groups for oral cavity cancer, HPV- oropharyngeal cancer and HPV+ oropharyngeal cancer.

AJCC prognostic stage groups for oral cavity cancer [21]			
When T is...	**And N is...**	**And M is...**	**Then the stage group is...**
T1	N0	M0	I
T2	N0	M0	II
T3	N0	M0	III
T1, 2, 3	N1	M0	III
T4a	N0,1	M0	IVA
T1, 2, 3, 4a	N2	M0	IVA
Any T	N3	M0	IVB
T4b	Any N	M0	IVB
Any T	Any N	M1	IVC
AJCC prognostic stage groups for HPV- oropharyngeal cancer [22]			
When T is...	**And N is...**	**And M is...**	**Then the stage group is...**
Tis	N0	M0	0
T1	N0	M0	I
T2	N0	M0	II
T3	N0	M0	III
T1, T2, T3	N1	M0	III
T4a	N0,N1	M0	IVA
T1, T2, T3, T4a	N2	M0	IVA
Any T	N3	M0	IVB
T4b	Any N	M0	IVB
Any T	Any N	M1	IVC

(Continued)

Table 12.2 (Continued)

AJCC prognostic stage groups for HPV+ oropharyngeal cancer [23]

Clinical

When T is...	And N is...	And M is...	Then the stage group is...
T0, T1 or T2	N0 or N1	M0	I
T0, T1 or T2	N2	M0	II
T3	N0, N1 or N2	M0	II
T0, T1, T2, T3 or T4	N3	M0	III
T4	N0, N1, N2 or N3	M0	III
Any T	Any N	M1	IV

Pathological

When T is...	And N is...	And M is...	Then the stage group is...
T0, T1 or T2	N0, N1	M0	I
T0, T1 or T2	N2	M0	II
T3 or T4	N0, N1	M0	II
T3 or T4	N2	M0	III
Any T	Any N	M1	IV

Source: Amin *et al.* [53]. Used with permission of the American College of Surgeons, Chicago, Illinois. The original source for this information is the AJCC Cancer Staging Manual, 8th edn (2017), which is published by Springer Science + Business Media.

Surgery

Oral Cavity

In the mid 1900s, surgery for oral cavity cancer resulted in significant functional loss, and the lack of viable reconstructive options left many patients with cosmetic and functional deformities. However, modern advances in reconstructive, prosthetic, and rehabilitation strategies have revolutionized surgical treatment for these cancers and has made it the first line therapy for cancers in this region.

Surgery for early-stage disease allows for one-stage treatment without the need for daily radiation treatments spread out over 6–7 weeks. Most early-stage cancers of the oral cavity can be approached transorally and should be removed with at least a 1 cm margin of normal-appearing tissue around the tumor. The defect may be closed primarily, left open to heal by secondary intention, or skin grafted. Because of the relatively small amount of tissue lost, functions such as speech articulation and swallowing are often preserved. Salivary flow is usually unaffected after surgery alone. However, the amount of functional disability after surgery is ultimately dependent on the extent of the surgical resection.

Advanced-stage lesions often involve multiple subsites within the oral cavity and leave a larger defect after tumor removal, which may result in a communication between the nonsterile saliva-containing oral cavity and the soft tissues of the neck. Such a communication must be addressed surgically at the time of tumor removal to prevent salivary drainage over the neck vessels and potential life-threatening complications such as carotid artery rupture. In these instances, complex reconstruction using a locoregional flap or free tissue transfer (free flaps) is effective in preserving residual function and creating a barrier between the nonsterile oral cavity and the neck, thereby restoring continuity to the aerodigestive tract.

Surgery may not be considered primarily if the extent of the resection results in a prohibitive functional morbidity for the patient, or in patients incapable of undergoing general anesthesia. General contraindications to upfront surgery for advanced oral cancer include encasement of the internal carotid artery, the presence of dermal or distant metastases, and involvement of the masticator space and/or prevertebral fascia. A number of factors must be considered when planning surgery for oral cavity cancer.

Status of the Mandible

If there is clinical or radiologic evidence of mandibular invasion, the degree of involvement must be determined. The segment of involved mandible will require removal at the time of tumor resection, and most often requires free flap reconstruction to preserve mandibular function and prevent significant cosmetic deformity (Figure 12.7).

Degree of Tongue Involvement

Early tongue cancers can be removed and closed primarily or left to heal by secondary intention with excellent functional results. In more advanced tumors, nearly the entire oral tongue (anterior to the circumvallate papillae) can be removed and appropriately reconstructed with vascularized tissue while preserving the capacity to swallow without aspiration, due to the preserved tongue base that retains its capacity to propel a food bolus to the esophagus and elevate the larynx during a normal swallow (Figure 12.8).

Composite Nature of Anticipated Defect

Oral cancers that involve more than one subsite (e.g. FOM tumor involving tongue, buccal mucosa involving mandible) require reconstruction of each subsite for optimal functional preservation postoperatively to prevent issues such as tongue tethering and poor cosmetic outcome. A sound understanding of the relevant functional anatomy allows the appropriate choice of reconstruction.

Treatment of the Neck

Neck dissection has evolved considerably since first described by Crile in the early 1900s [28], from the traditional radical neck dissection that removed both lymphatic and nonlymphatic structures resulting in significant shoulder and cosmetic morbidity, to the modified radical neck dissection, which removes the lymphatics in the neck while sparing the internal jugular vein, spinal accessory nerve, and/or sternocleidomastoid muscle. If clinically evident cervical metastases are present, the patient should undergo modified radical neck dissection at the time of surgery to remove the primary tumor. Patients with tumors close to the midline or crossing

(a)

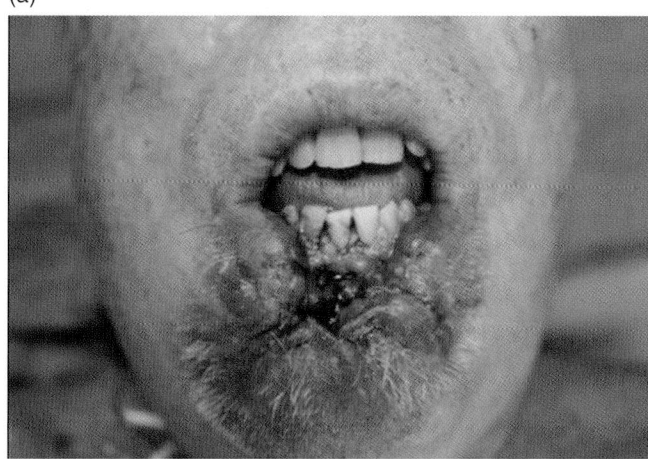

(b)

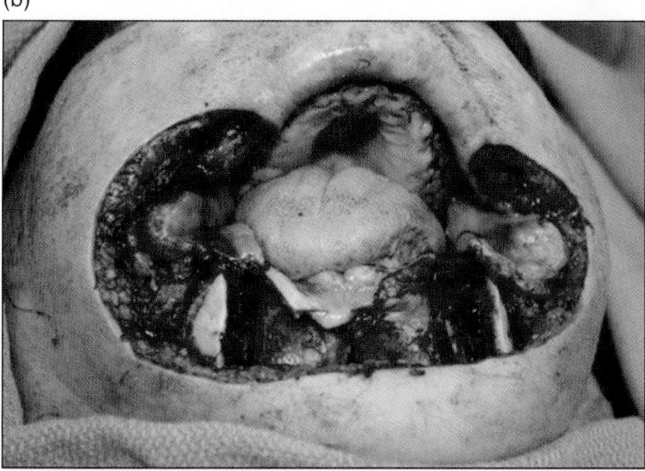

(c)

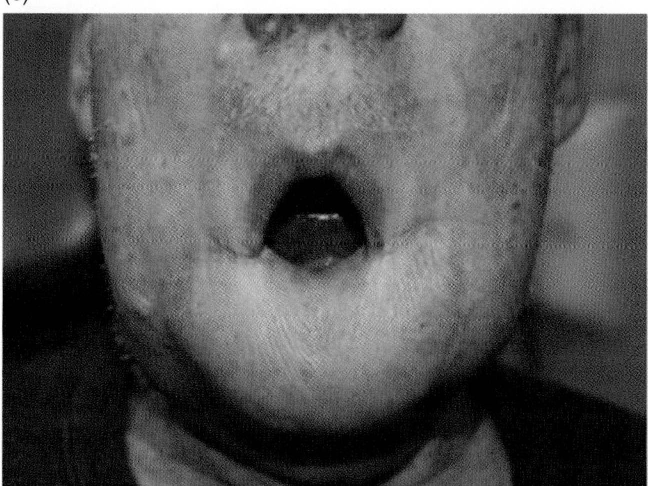

Figure 12.7 This patient with an endophytic cancer of the lower lip required resection of the lip, chin skin, and underlying mandible with subsequent reconstruction using a fibula free flap.

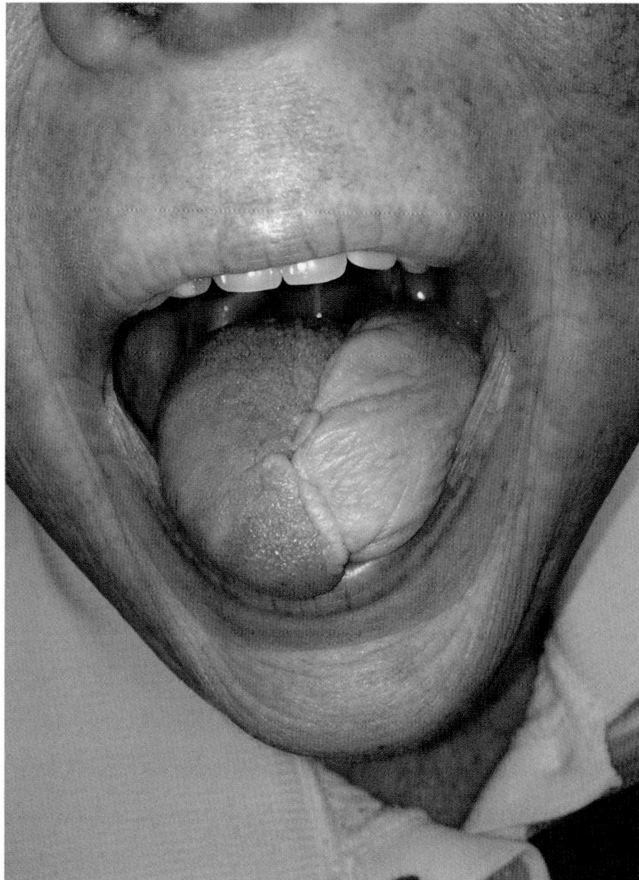

Figure 12.8 This patient underwent repair of a hemiglossectomy defect with a radial forearm free flap. Notice the excellent contour of the neotongue.

the midline should undergo bilateral neck dissections due to the rich lymphatic drainage of the oral cavity. While radical or modified radical neck dissection is still performed for advanced disease (N2 and N3) due to tumor adherence to these structures, selective neck dissection (including levels I, II, and III) is often performed for early-stage disease even in absence of clinically evident metastasis. Up to 30–35% of patients with no palpable cervical lymph nodes are found to have pathologic evidence of metastases at the time of surgery. Therefore, an elective rather than observation and a therapeutic neck dissection is recommended as it has been shown to improve overall survival [29].

Importance of Pre- and Postoperative Speech and Swallow Therapy

Speech and swallowing rehabilitation play a critical role in restoration of function postoperatively. This aspect of care cannot be overemphasized as it can greatly impact patients' quality of life after surgery [30, 31].

Role for Oral and Maxillofacial Prosthodontics

Cancers of the alveolar ridge or hard palate treated with surgery resulting in a communication between the oral and sinonasal cavities can often be rehabilitated with the use of an oral obturator to separate the two spaces and preserve oral intake. In these cases, reconstruction is accomplished by the prosthetic and does not require any additional surgery.

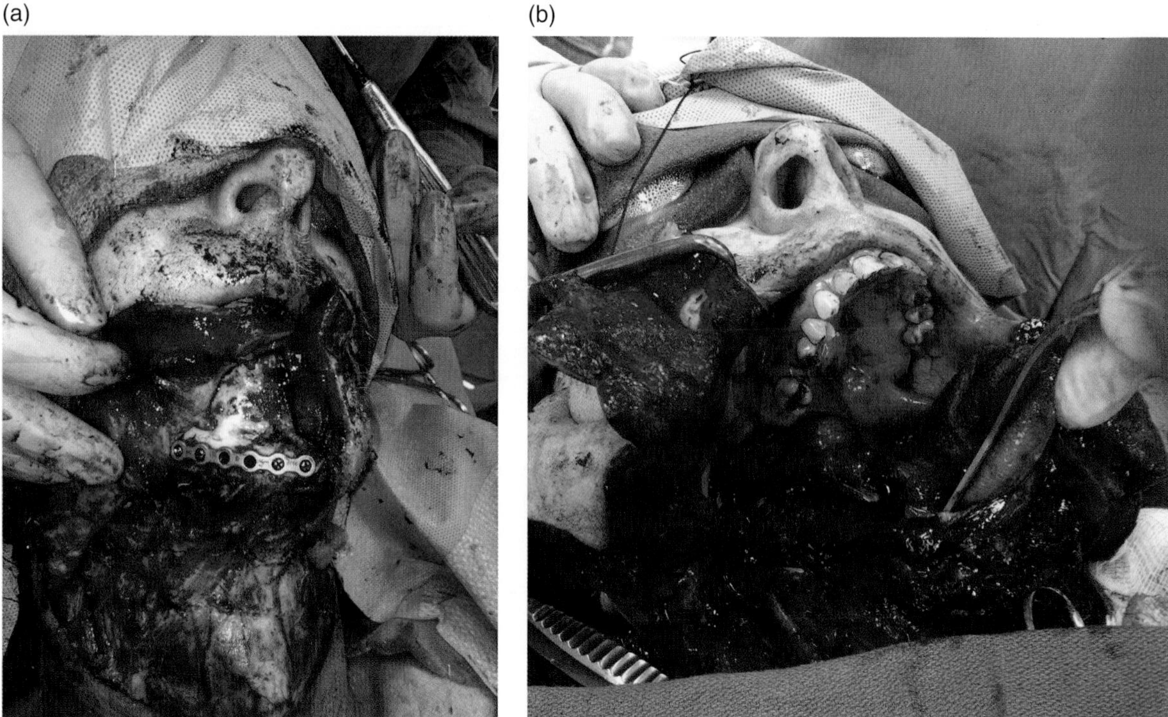

Figure 12.9 (a) In the transmandibular approach to the oropharynx, a soft tissue incision is made and the approach allows for the underlying mandible to be isolated and preplated. At the end of the procedure, the plate will be replaced onto the mandible to allow for appropriate realignment of the bone. (b) A sagittal osteotomy is then performed and the floor of mouth soft tissue attachments are liberated. At this point, the mandible is "swung" to the side to allow for direct access to the oropharynx. This allows for controlled tumor removal while maintaining access to the adjacent neurovascular structures.

Oropharyngeal Cancer

Transoral Surgery for the Oropharynx

When managing tumors of the oropharynx, priorities in order of importance include successful eradication of disease, followed by maintenance of speech and swallowing function. The traditional approach to treatment in the 1980s and 1990s involved open surgical resection with postoperative radiation therapy [32, 33]. Although this provided excellent local and regional control, the functional consequence included a 29% rate of requiring either a long-term gastrostomy or tracheostomy tube. Due to this morbidity and the significant rate of distant metastases in these patients, treatment regimens began to shift to chemoradiation therapy [34].

The application of transoral laser microsurgery by Steiner *et al.* reintroduced upfront surgery as a viable treatment option for tumors of the oropharynx, with excellent rates of feeding tube independence [35]. With this approach, the tumor is typically intentionally transected allowing for careful delineation of the margin of the tumor and adjacent normal tissue.

Over the past decade, robotic surgical systems have been utilized for resection of tumors of the tonsil [36] and tongue base [37]. Using this approach, angled scopes and small robotic arms with capabilities of wristed instrumentation allow for *en bloc* tumor removal in locations such as the tongue base where a direct line of sight is challenging to obtain. In this technique, a mouth gag is used to achieve access for the instruments, which are docked to robotic "arms". The movement of these instruments and the endoscope are controlled by the surgeon who sits at a remote console.

Open Surgical Approaches to the Oropharynx

In situations where persistent or recurrent disease is present after chemoradiation therapy, or when patients are not a candidate for a transoral resection of the tumor (i.e. there is significant extension to the parapharyngeal space and/or pterygoid musculature), an open approach to the oropharynx can be employed. One example is the transmandibular approach (Figure 12.9).

Through this approach, excellent exposure is provided to the entire oropharynx as well as its relationship to the adjacent carotid arterial system. The consequences of the surgery are related to the functional impairment through the release of the FOM muscular attachments and the resulting impact on swallowing, speech and breathing physiology, as well as the cosmetic deformity that accompanies an incision through the lower lip. Similar to what is seen following removal of advanced oral cavity tumors, a large communication is created from the pharynx to the neck. Consequently, to allow for appropriate healing and to avoid fistula formation, regional or free flap reconstruction is often required.

Radiation Therapy

Traditional external beam radiation therapy (EBRT) results in significant side effects when used for treatment of head and neck cancers due to radiation effects on normal tissue close to the primary tumor. Skin fibrosis of the neck, altered taste, mucositis, osteoradionecrosis of the mandible, and chronic dry mouth due to altered salivary outflow are common. Modern advances in radiation techniques, including hyperfractionation and intensity modulated radiation therapy, have greatly improved the capacity to deliver maximal radiation to the tumor bed while minimizing the dose and side effects to the surrounding tissues, including the salivary glands, mandible, spinal cord, and brachial plexus.

Treatments are generally administered daily over a 6–7 week course to a total dose of 65–75 Gy if used as a primary treatment for oral cavity cancer, but this dose may be reduced if administered in the postoperative (adjuvant) setting. For early-stage lesions, radiation may be used as a primary treatment alone with the primary advantages being that it is useful in patients unsuitable for general anesthesia or in those who wish to avoid surgery. However, the side effects of dry mouth, mucositis, and altered taste remain significant, and the duration of treatment is extended when compared to surgery. In addition, full dose radiation can only be given once due to the potential for significant side effects with a second dose, such as a weakening of the carotid artery which can result in aneurysm formation and life-threatening complications [38].

Interstitial radiation implants (brachytherapy) can deliver radiotherapy to the primary tumor site as an adjunct to traditional EBRT. This form of treatment involves placement of catheters within the tumor and application of radioisotopes to the primary site directly, thereby concentrating the dose to the primary and potentially sparing surrounding structures and decreasing the required dose of EBRT. Doses may range from 40 to 60 Gy given over 5–10 days. Brachytherapy also may play a potential role in the setting of recurrent disease in a patient who has previously received EBRT [39]. Disadvantages include a potentially increased risk of osteoradionecrosis of the mandible due to dose concentration and the need for general anesthesia for placement and removal of catheters.

Chemotherapy

As noted earlier, the role of chemotherapy in head and neck cancer is primarily as a radiosensitizer. Advanced-stage tumors found to be unsuitable for surgery due to patient comorbidities and/or unresectable disease may be treated primarily with concurrent chemoradiotherapy, and studies have established significant improvement in survival and locoregional control over radiation alone [40–42]. In the postoperative setting, chemotherapy is given in addition to radiation therapy in patients with noted extracapsular lymph node spread or positive surgical margins on pathologic assessment of neck dissection and primary tumor specimens, respectively. The addition of chemotherapy to postoperative RT has been shown to improve disease-free survival in these instances [43–45]. However, in patients with HPV+ oropharyngeal cancer, due to their favorable prognosis, there is ongoing study looking at the safety and efficacy of select "de-escalation" protocols, with a goal being to maintain oncologic control while minimizing the side effects of therapy [46, 47].

The most commonly used agents for primary chemoradiotherapy include cisplatin or carboplatin alone or in combination with paclitaxel or 5-fluorouracil (5-FU). These agents have been used in various combinations and treatment schedules, but no studies have shown a significant difference in the impact of these variations. In the postoperative setting, cisplatin is most often administered alone during radiation therapy intravenously at a dose of 100 mg/m^2 on days 1, 22, and 43 or 40–50 mg/m^2 weekly for 6–7 weeks [48]. Side effects of these agents includes renal and ototoxicity [49]. Recent studies have focused on the addition of cetuximab, a monocolonal antibody that blocks the epidermal growth factor receptor that may be overexpressed in squamous cell carcinoma of the head and neck [50]. This agent has shown particular benefit when administered during radiation in patients unable to tolerate traditional chemotherapy [51].

Follow-Up and Survivorship

Long-term clinical follow-up in a surveillance setting is of critical importance in the management of cancers of the oral cavity and oropharynx. Patients remain at risk not only for disease recurrence after treatment but for the development of second primary head and neck malignancies due to the effects of field cancerization. Complete head and neck clinical examination, including fiberoptic pharyngolaryngoscopy, should be performed every 1–3 months during the first year, every 2–6 months during the second year, and every 4–8 months in the third, fourth and fifth years after the completion of treatment. Baseline post-treatment imaging (positron emission tomography/CT, CT, MRI) is obtained at least 3 months after the completion of treatment, but only as clinically indicated thereafter. Chest imaging should be obtained on an annual basis in patients with a history of smoking.

Disciplines involved in surveillance should include otolaryngology, radiation oncology, medical oncology, primary care, dental, and speech/swallow therapy. Common long-term side effects of radiation therapy to the head and neck include altered taste, lymphedema and neck skin fibrosis, dry mouth, dysphagia, and hypothyroidism. Swallow function should be assessed prior to, during, and after completion of treatment and may require long-term therapy. Thyroid-stimulating hormone should be monitored every 6–12 months and thyroid hormone replacement should be initiated and adjusted as indicated. Dry mouth resulting from alteration of mucosal minor salivary gland function is managed with salivary replacements and frequent hydration. Smoking cessation counseling and interventions should be continued if not previously successful [27, 52].

Conclusion

The oral cavity and oropharynx are complex subsites of the upper aerodigestive tract. While prevention is optimal, once these areas are affected by cancer, initial workup should allow for accurate staging of the tumors and should assess for additional primary lesions. After the extent of disease has been determined, a multidisciplinary approach to care should be provided to optimize cancer cure while minimizing functional impairment and cosmetic deformity.

References

1 Siegel RL, Miller KD, Jemal A. Cancer statistics, 2017. *CA Cancer J Clin* 2017;67(1):7–30.

2 Howlader N, Noone AM, Krapcho M, *et al.* (eds). SEER Cancer Statistics Review, 1975–2013, National Cancer Institute. Bethesda, MD. http://seer.cancer.gov/csr/1975_2013/, based on November 2015 SEER data submission, posted to the SEER web site, April 2016.

3 Mehanna H, Paleri V, West C, Nutting C. Head and neck cancer – Part 1: epidemiology, presentation, and prevention. *BMJ* 2010;341(7774):663–6.

4 Zandberg DP, Bhargava R, Badin S, Cullen KJ. The role of human papillomavirus in nongenital cancers. *CA Cancer J Clin* 2013;63(1):57–81.

5 Shiboski CH, Schmidt BL, Jordan RC. Tongue and tonsil carcinoma: increasing trends in the US population ages 20–44 years. *Cancer* 2005;103:1843–9.

6 Chaturvedi AK, Engels EA, Pfeiffer RM, *et al.* Human papillomavirus and rising oropharyngeal cancer incidence in the United States. *J Clin Oncol* 2011;29(32):4294–301.

7 McIlwain WR, Sood AJ, Nguyen SA, Day TA. Initial symptoms in patients with HPV-positive and HPV-negative oropharyngeal cancer. *JAMA Otolaryngol Head Neck Surg* 2014;140(5):441–7.

8 Ang KK, Harris J, Wheeler R, *et al.* Human papillomavirus and survival of patients with oropharyngeal cancer. *N Engl J Med* 2010;363:24–35.

9 Fakhry C, Westra WH, Li S, Cmelak A, *et al.* Improved survival with human papillomavirus-positive head and neck squamous cell carcinoma in a prospective clinical trial. *J Natl Cancer Inst* 2008;100(4):261–9.

10 Janfaza P, Nadol Jr JB, Galla RJ, Fabian RL, Montgomery WW. *Surgical Anatomy of the Head and Neck.* Philadelphia: Lippincott, Williams and Wilkins, 2001.

11 Gardasil (human papillomavirus quadrivalent [types 6, 11, 16, 18] vaccine, recombinant): product information and supporting documents. Food and Drug Administration. http://www.fda.gov/BiologicsBloodVaccines/Vaccines/ApprovedProducts/ucm094042.htm (accessed 2 October 2017).

12 CDC recommends only two HPV shots for younger adolescents. www.cdc.gov/media/releases/2016/p1020-hpv-shots.html (accessed 2 October 2017).

13 Herrero R, Hildesheim A, Gonzalez P, *et al.* Reduced prevalence of oral human papillomavirus (HPV) 4 years after bivalent HPV vaccination in a randomized clinical trial in Costa Rica. *PLoS One* 2013;8(7).

14 Rouviere H. *Anatomy of the Human Lymphatic System.* Ann Arbor: Edward Brothers, 1938.

15 Lindberg R. Distribution of cervical lymph node metastasis from squamous cell carcinoma of the upper respiratory and digestive tracts. *Cancer* 1972;29:1446–9.

16 Kannan S, Balaram P, Pillai MR, *et al.* Ultrastructural variations and assessment of malignant transformation risk in oral leukoplakia. *Pathol Res Pract* 1993;189:1169–80.

17 Slaughter DP, Southwick HW, Smejkal W. "Field cancerization" in oral stratified squamous epithelium: clinical implications of multicentric origin. *Cancer* 1953;6:963–8.

18 D'Souza G, Agrawal Y, Halpern J, Bodison S, Gillison ML. Oral sexual behaviors associated with prevalent oral human papillomavirus infection. *J Infect Dis* 2009;199:1263–9.

19 Gillison ML. Human papillomavirus-associated head and neck cancer is a distinct epidemiologic, clinical, and molecular entity. *Semin Oncol* 2004;31:744–54.

20 Caldemeyer KS, Matthews VP, Righi PD, *et al.* Imaging features and clinical significance of perineural spread or extension of head and neck tumors. *Radiographics* 1998;18:97–110.

21 Fogh SE, Champ C, Kubicek GJ, *et al.* Value of FDG-PET for detecting metastatic lesions in head and neck cancer. *J Clin Oncol* 2008;26(15S):6047.

22 Robinson M, Sloan P, Shaw R. Refining the diagnosis of oropharyngeal squamous cell carcinoma using human papillomavirus testing. *Oral Oncol* 2010;46(7):492–6.

23 Mirghani H, Casiraghi O, Guerlain, *et al.* Diagnosis of HPV driven oropharyngeal cancers: Comparing p16 based algorithms with the RNAscope HPV-test. *Oral Oncol* 2016;62:101–8.

24 Ridge JA, Lydiatt WM, Patel SG, *et al.* (eds) *AJCC Cancer Staging Manual*, 8th edn. New York: Springer Nature, 2017.

25 Lydiatt WM, Ridge JA, Patel SG, *et al.* Oropharynx (p16-) and hypopharynx. In M Amin, S Edge, FL Greene, *et al.* (eds) *AJCC Cancer Staging Manual*, 8th edn. New York: Springer Nature, 2017.

26 O'Sullivan B, Lydiatt WM, Haughey BH, *et al.* HPV-Mediated (p16+) oropharyngeal cancer. In M Amin, S Edge, FL Greene, *et al.* (eds) *AJCC Cancer Staging Manual*, 8th edn. New York: Springer Nature, 2017.

27 Pfister FG, Spencer S, Adelstein D, *et al.* NCCN Clinical Practice Guidelines in Oncology, Head and Neck Cancer Version 2.2016. nccn.org (accessed 2 October 2017).

28 Crile G. Excision of cancer of the head and neck: with special reference to the plan of dissection based on 132 operations. *JAMA* 1906;47:1780–85.

29 D'Cruz AK, Vaish R, Kapre N, *et al.* Elective versus therapeutic neck dissection in node-negative oral cancer. *N Engl J Med* 2015;373(6):521–9.

30 Logemann JA, Pauloski BR, Rademaker AW, Colangelo LA. Speech and swallowing rehabilitation for head and neck cancer patients. *Oncology* 1997;11(5):651–6.

31 Mittal BB, Pauloski BR, Haraf DJ, *et al.* Swallowing dysfunction – preventative and rehabilitation strategies in patients with head-and-neck cancers treated with surgery, radiotherapy, and chemotherapy: a critical review. *Int J Radiat Oncol Biol Phys* 2003;57:1219–30.

32 Machtay M, Perch S, Markiewicz D, *et al.* Combined surgery and postoperative radiotherapy for carcinoma of the base of tongue: analysis of treatment outcome and prognostic value of margin status. *Head Neck* 1997;19:494–9.

33 Zhen W, Karnell LH, Hoffman HT, *et al.* The National Cancer Data Base report on squamous cell carcinoma of the base of tongue. *Head Neck* 2004;26:660–74.

34 Koch WM. Head and neck surgery in the era of organ preservation therapy. *Semin Oncol* 2000;27(4 Suppl 8):5–12.

35 Steiner W, Fierek O, Ambrosch P, *et al.* Transoral laser microsurgery for squamous cell carcinoma of the base of the tongue. *Arch Otolaryngol Head Neck Surg* 2003;129:36–43.
36 Weinstein GS, O'Malley BW Jr, Snyder W, Sherman E, Quon H. Transoral robotic surgery: radical tonsillectomy. *Arch Otolaryngol Head Neck Surg* 2007;133(12):1220–6.
37 O'Malley BW Jr, Weinstein GS, Hockstein NG. Transoral robotic surgery (TORS) for base of tongue neoplasms. *Laryngoscope* 2006;116(8):1465–72.
38 McDonald MW, Moore MG, Johnstone PA. Risk of carotid artery blowout after reirradiation of the head and neck: a systematic review. *Int J Radiat Oncol Biol Phys* 2012;82(3):1083–9.
39 Stannard C, Maree G, Tovey S, Hunter A, Wetter J. Iodine-125 brachytherapy in the management of squamous cell carcinoma of the oral cavity and oropharynx. *Brachytherapy* 2014;13(4):405–12.
40 Kohno N, Kitahara S, Tamura E, *et al.* Concurrent chemoradiotherapy with low-dose cisplatin plus 5-fluorouracil for the treatment of patients with unresectable head and neck cancer. *Oncology* 2002;63:226–31.
41 Adelstein DJ, Li Y, Adams GL, *et al.* An intergroup phase III comparison of standard radiation therapy and two schedules of concurrent chemoradiotherapy in patients with unresectable squamous cell head and neck cancer. *J Clin Oncol* 2003;21:92–8.
42 Brizel DM, Albers ME, Fisher SR *et al.* Hyperfractionated irradiation with or without concurrent chemotherapy for locally advanced head and neck cancer. *N Engl J Med* 1998;338:1798–804.
43 Johnson JT, Wagner RL, Myers EN. A long term assessment of adjuvant chemotherapy on outcome of patients with extracapsular spread of cervical metastases from squamous cell carcinoma of the head and neck. *Cancer* 1996;77:1181–5.
44 Bernier J, Ozsahin M, Lefebvre JL, *et al.* Postoperative irradiation with or without concomitant chemotherapy for locally advanced head and neck cancer. *New Engl J Med* 2004;350(19):1945–52.
45 Cooper JS, Pajak TF, Forastiere AA, *et al.* Postoperative concurrent radiotherapy and chemotherapy for high risk squamous cell carcinoma of the head and neck. *New Engl J Med* 2004;350(19):1937.
46 Kelly JR, Husain ZA, Burtness B. Treatment de-intensification strategies for head and neck cancer. *Eur J Cancer* 2016;68:125–33.
47 Bhatia A, Burtness B. Human papillomavirus-associated oropharyngeal cancer: defining risk groups and clinical trials. *J Clin Oncol* 2015;33(29):3243–50.
48 Bachaud JM, Cohen-Jonathan E, Alzieu C, *et al.* Combined postoperative radiotherapy and weekly cisplatin infusion for locally advanced head and neck carcinoma: final report of a randomized trial. *Int J Radiat Oncol Biol Phys* 1996;36(5):999–1004.
49 Rades D, Ulbricht T, Hakim SG, Schild SE. Cisplatin superior to carboplatin in adjuvant radiochemotherapy for locally advanced cancers of the oropharynx and oral cavity. *Strahlenther Onkol* 2012;188(1):42–8.
50 Harari PM, Harris J, Kies MS, *et al.* Postoperative chemoradiotherapy and cetuximab for high-risk squamous cell carcinoma of the head and neck: Radiation Therapy Oncology Group RTOG-0234. *J Clin Oncol* 2014;10;32(23): 2486–95.
51 Bonner JA, Harari PM, Giralt J, *et al.* Radiotherapy plus Cetuximab for squamous cell carcinoma of the head and neck. *N Engl J Med* 2006;354:567–78.
52 Cohen EE, LaMonte SJ, Erb NL, *et al.* American Cancer Society head and neck cancer survivorship care guideline. *CA Cancer J Clin* 2016;66(3):203–39.
53 Amin M, Edge S, Greene FL, *et al.* (eds) *AJCC Cancer Staging Manual*, 8th edn. New York: Springer Nature, 2017.

13

Salivary Gland Cancer

Daniel Brickman[1] *and Neil D. Gross*[2]

[1] *Levine Cancer Institute, Carolinas HealthCare System, Charlotte, North Carolina, USA*
[2] *The University of Texas MD Anderson Cancer Center, Houston, Texas, USA*

Incidence and Mortality Statistics

Major and minor salivary gland cancers are rare, comprising approximately 3% of all head and neck cancers [1]. The estimated incidence rate is 1.3 per 100,000 persons per year in the United States, and is higher for males than females (1.7 vs 1.0, respectively) [2]. The incidence of presentation increases with age, peaking at ages 65–74 years. Fewer than 5% of all salivary gland neoplasms occur in children, but when diagnosed in children they are much more likely to be malignant than those in adults [3]. Approximately 2.2% of salivary gland cancers are diagnosed in individuals younger than 20 years [2]. The mortality rate for salivary gland cancer is 0.2 per 100,000 persons per year in the United States [2].

Of all salivary neoplasms, the majority occurs in the parotid gland and the fewest in the sublingual gland. Importantly, there is an inverse relationship between the overall incidence of major salivary gland neoplasms by site and the likelihood of malignancy (Table 13.1). For example, the parotid gland is the most common site for a salivary gland neoplasm and the majority of parotid gland neoplasms are benign.

The frequency of the different histologic types of salivary gland cancer varies depending on the gland and site. The most common salivary gland cancer is mucoepidermoid carcinoma. The next most common salivary gland cancer is adenoid cystic carcinoma, followed by adenocarcinoma, malignant mixed tumor, acinic cell carcinoma, and squamous cell carcinoma (Table 13.2). When considering the histologic types by anatomic site, mucoepidermoid carcinoma is the most frequent malignancy of the parotid, while adenoid cystic carcinoma is the most frequent malignancy of the submandibular and minor salivary glands except in the nasal cavity and paranasal sinuses. Adenocarcinoma is the most common salivary gland cancer identified in the nasal cavity and paranasal sinuses [1, 4, 5].

Risk Factors

The rarity of salivary gland cancers limits knowledge about the pathogenesis and possible strategies for prevention. Radiation exposure has been documented as a risk factor for the development of salivary gland cancer among atomic bomb survivors and among childhood cancer survivors treated with head and neck irradiation [6]. Increased risk of sinonasal salivary gland cancer has additionally been linked to occupational exposure to nickel compounds, chronic exposure to wood dust (especially soft wood) and chemicals used in the leather tanning industry, as well as employment in the rubber industry [7]. Unlike other cancers of the upper aerodigestive tract, the role of tobacco and alcohol in the development of salivary gland cancer has not been fully established [8]. There is no known genetic predisposition to salivary gland cancer. It is important to note that squamous cell carcinoma of the skin can metastasize to lymph nodes within the parotid gland and be confused with a primary salivary gland cancer. Increased rates of salivary gland cancers have been seen after radiation exposures such as radioactive iodine treatment for thyroid cancer and environmental exposures [9, 10].

Pathology

Due to the heterogeneity of salivary gland cancers, their behavior and resulting clinical management are highly dependent on their histologic type and grade. Thus, knowledge of the types of cancer and the pathologic classification is critical. First, it is important to consider the normal histology of the salivary gland because cancer arises from the same cell types that are present in the normal gland. Salivary glands contain acini composed of either serous or mucous cells or a mixture of both. The fluid secreted by the parotid gland is almost exclusively serous, while that from the sublingual gland is almost exclusively mucous.

The American Cancer Society's Oncology in Practice: Clinical Management, First Edition. Edited by The American Cancer Society.

Table 13.1 Rates of salivary gland malignancy by size.

Gland	Salivary tumors (%)	Malignant salivary tumors (5)
Parotid	73	15
Submandibular	11	37
Sublingual	0.3	86
Minor	14	46

Source: adapted from Eveson and Cawson [11].

Table 13.2 Relative incidence of malignant salivary gland neoplasms.

Histologic type	%
Mucoepidermoid	34
Adenoid cystic carcinoma	22
Adenocarcinoma	18
Malignant mixed tumor	13
Acinic cell carcinoma	7
Squamous cell carcinoma	4
Others	3

Source: adapted from Spiro [1].

The fluid secreted from the submandibular gland is a mixture of serous and mucous. The ducts form tubular structures within the glands. Both the acini and ducts have supportive cells called myoepithelial cells along their periphery. Therefore, all salivary gland neoplasms can be roughly classified on the basis of the type of normal salivary gland cell from which they arise: acinar, ductal, or myoepithelial. It is likely that salivary cancers will be better classified according to molecular characteristics in the future. Of note, salivary gland cancers can arise *de novo* or via malignant conversion from a benign neoplasm (pleomorphic adenoma to carcinoma ex pleomorphic adenoma, basal cell adenoma to basal cell adenocarcinoma, myoepithelioma to myoepithelial carcinoma).

Mucoepidermoid Carcinoma

Mucoepidermoid carcinoma (MEC) is the most common salivary gland cancer [1]. Most cases occur in the major salivary glands, but MEC can also arise from minor salivary glands in the oral cavity. Clinically, MEC is slightly more common in women with a mean age of approximately 45 years. MEC is also the most common pediatric salivary gland cancer. The usual presentation is a painless, slow-growing mass. Intraoral MEC may mimic a mucocele or vascular lesion [11]. Microscopically, a hallmark feature of MEC is the presence of three cell types: mucous, squamoid, and intermediate. Histologic grading correlates strongly with clinical behavior [12, 13]. In general, low-grade MEC has a prominent cystic component and abundant well-differentiated mucous cells with little cytologic atypia and low mitotic activity. High grade MEC are more solid with squamoid and intermediate cells predominating with cytologic atypia, mitotic activity, necrosis, and infiltrative growth. Low-grade MEC rarely metastasizes or results in death. MEC of the submandibular gland is more likely to recur and metastasize than MEC of other sites.

Adenoid Cystic Carcinoma

Adenoid cystic carcinoma (ACC) is also a common salivary gland cancer, being notorious for its infiltrative growth with a predilection for perineural spread and slowly progressive behavior with recurrences and spread over many years [14]. ACC occurs with an even distribution among all salivary gland sites, both genders, and with a peak incidence between 50 and 60 years of age [15–17]. Grossly, ACC appears well circumscribed but unencapsulated, while microscopically, there are three growth architectures: tubular, cribriform, and solid. A frequent histologic feature of ACC is perineural invasion, which is identified in approximately 70–75% of cases and correlates with a worse prognosis [18, 19].

Polymorphous Adenocarcinoma

Polymorphous adenocarcinoma is a typically a low grade salivary gland cancer first recognized as a distinct entity in the mid-1980s [20]. Polymorphous adenocarcinoma arises almost exclusively from the minor salivary glands, especially at the junction of the hard and soft palate [20]. Polymorphous adenocarcinoma is twice as common in women as men and tends to present in the fourth to sixth decades as an asymptomatic slow-growing mass [21]. Microscopically, the architectural features of this polymorphous adenocarcinoma are variable but a common appearance within the tumor is concentric whorling of the nests around each other in a single-file arrangement. Most cases of polymorphous adenocarcinoma show perineural invasion [21, 22]. Lymph node metastases are uncommon with large series not having any patients with nodal disease at presentation and local recurrence occurs in 10–15% of patients. Distant metastases are equally as uncommon and patients with polymorphous adenocarcinoma have an excellent long-term prognosis with greater than 95% disease-free survival at 10 years, though few patients have been shown to die from distant disease at up to 14 years from initial treatment. [21, 22].

Acinic Cell Carcinoma

Acinic cell carcinoma is a salivary gland cancer with cells showing differentiation toward cells of the normal salivary gland acini. However, acinic cell carcinoma may also show focal ductal and/or myoepithelial differentiation. Acinic cell carcinoma account for approximately 10% of all salivary gland cancers [11, 15, 23]. More than 90% occur in the parotid, over a wide age spectrum from children to the elderly [24, 25]. Acinic cell carcinoma typically presents as a slowly growing mass, which is only occasionally painful and rarely associated with a facial palsy [24, 25]. The microscopic presentation is variable, with four principal histologic patterns: solid/lobular, microcystic, papillary–cystic, and follicular. Acinic cell carcinoma can recur in up to one-third of cases, underscoring the importance of complete resection [24, 25]. Although classically regarded as low-grade malignancies, 10–15% of acinic cell carcinoma will metastasize locally to regional lymph nodes or distantly to the lung and bones. Acinic cell carcinoma is also notorious for having a protracted clinical course with late recurrences [26]. Survival is approximately 80% at 5 years and 70% at 10 years [24, 26].

Carcinoma Ex Pleomorphic Adenoma

Carcinoma ex pleomorphic adenoma is defined as cancer arising from a benign mixed tumor (pleomorphic adenoma). Carcinoma ex pleomorphic adenoma is most common in the parotid gland, followed by the submandibular gland, the minor salivary glands, and the sublingual gland. [27]. Most patients are in their sixth and seventh decades and the classic history is a patient with a longstanding slow-growing mass that suddenly undergoes rapid, painful growth [27, 28]. Microscopically, these cancers show a cytologically malignant epithelial component that invades beyond the borders of a residual pleomorphic adenoma. The prognosis is dependent on the extent of invasion. These cancers are notorious for aggressive clinical behavior and have a survival ranging from 26 to 65% at 5 years and 0 to 38% at 20 years [28].

Metastasizing Mixed Tumors

Metastasizing mixed tumors are exceedingly rare salivary gland cancers that have the bland morphology of a benign mixed tumor without significant cytologic atypia or mitotic activity, but inexplicably metastasize either to local lymph nodes or to distant sites including bone and lung. [29]. Often, there is a prior protracted clinical course with multiple recurrences at the primary site before metastasis occurs [30]. The mean time between presentation of the primary tumor and detection of metastatic disease is 12 years [30].

Salivary Duct Carcinoma

Salivary duct carcinoma is a relatively recently described distinct salivary gland cancer that was previously categorized generically as a salivary adenocarcinoma [31]. This cancer accounts for fewer than 10% of salivary gland cancers. Males are more commonly affected and patients generally present in the sixth decade with a rapidly growing parotid mass. A minority have facial nerve involvement and occasional facial skin ulceration [32]. Between 70% and 90% of cases arise in the parotid. [33, 34]. Histologically, salivary duct carcinoma has a similar appearance to high-grade ductal carcinoma of the breast with large and prominent ductal carcinoma in-situ component and a cribriform pattern. [31]. Salivary duct carcinomas can be positive for Her2/neu which can be important for adjuvant treatment options. [35, 36]. Salivary duct carcinoma is aggressive with 30–40% of patients developing local recurrence and between 50 and 75% developing distant metastases and dying of their disease. [33, 34].

Squamous Cell Carcinoma

Squamous cell carcinoma (SCC) frequently metastasizes from cutaneous or oral cancers to lymph nodes within the parotid gland. However, primary salivary gland SCC is rare and represents fewer than 1% of all salivary gland cancers [37]. Most patients with SCC are in their sixth to eighth decades, and sometimes there is a history of prior radiation therapy. Of these, 80–90% arise in the parotid gland, and 10–20% in the submandibular gland [37]. SCC frequently metastasizes to regional lymph nodes, so they are often advanced stage at the time of diagnosis. Microscopically, salivary gland SCC appears identical to SCC of the upper aerodigestive tract with prominent desmoplasia and perineural invasion and early extension into periglandular soft tissue [37, 38]. Primary SCC is aggressive, with a 5-year survival of approximately 20–50%. [38].

Small Cell Carcinoma

Small cell carcinoma represents approximately 2% of all salivary gland cancers [39, 40]. This cancer typically presents as a painless mass usually in patients in their sixth and seventh decades. Many patients present with associated cervical lymphadenopathy and/or facial nerve palsy. Microscopically, small cell carcinoma consists of sheets of small cells with dark nuclei, brisk mitotic activity, and scant cytoplasm; immunohistochemistry shows one or more neuroendocrine markers [40]. It is critical for these cancers to be differentiated from primary lung small cell carcinoma which is far more common and carries a worse prognosis, with an estimated 2- and 5-year survival of 70 and 46% respectively [39, 40]. Lymph node metastases are frequent, as are distant metastases to the liver, lung, brain, and bones.

Epithelial–Myoepithelial Carcinoma

Epithelial–myoepithelial carcinomas account for approximately 0.5–1% of salivary gland cancers. They occur in older patients and predominantly in the parotid gland. Microscopically, the classic appearance of epithelial–myoepithelial carcinoma is of duct structures with eosinophilic lining cells (the "epithelial" component), overlying and surrounded by prominent clear cells (the "myoepithelial" component). In these lesions, the recurrence rate was 36.3%, but death was rare with 5-year and 10-year disease-specific survivals of 93.5% and 81.8% respectively [41].

Basal Cell Adenocarcinoma

Basal cell adenocarcinoma is the rare, malignant counterpart to basal cell adenoma. The majority arise in the parotid gland and consists of basaloid cells in tubular, trabecular, solid, or membranous patterns [42]. Local recurrence occurs in a minority of patients, and metastases to regional lymph nodes in fewer than 10%. Overall, the prognosis is excellent.

Myoepithelial Carcinoma

Myoepithelial carcinoma is the uncommon malignant counterpart to myoepithelioma. About 60% occur in the parotid gland [43]. Myoepithelial carcinoma can have diverse cell types including epithelioid, spindled, plasmacytoid or hyaline, or clear cell. These cancers have infiltrative peripheral borders. The prognosis of patients with myoepithelial carcinoma is highly variable with roughly one-third of patients developing multiple local recurrences and one-third of patients dying of metastatic disease.

Adenocarcinoma

Adenocarcinoma is a salivary gland cancer that exhibits ductal differentiation but otherwise lacks the histologic features that define other types of salivary gland cancer. There is an equal distribution between major and minor salivary glands [44, 45].

Adenocarcinoma can range in presentation from low- to high-grade cancers. In general, the prognosis for adenocarcinoma is worse than for most other salivary gland carcinoma with reported 10-year survival rates of 55% and 15-year survival rates of 41%, 34%, and 28% for low, intermediate, and high grade tumors, respectively [44, 45].

Lymphoma

Primary lymphoma of the major salivary glands comprises approximately 2% of all primary salivary gland cancers. Most patients with lymphoma of the salivary gland are between 50 and 70 years of age and present with a solitary, painless mass. The microscopic appearance, treatment, and survival depend on the specific type of lymphoma, which are most likely to be MALT followed by follicular and diffuse large B cell [46]. These can be related to either with Sjogren's syndrome or hepatitis C virus infection [47].

Metastasis to the salivary glands or parotid lymph nodes is a frequent occurrence. The parotid lymph nodes drain skin from the scalp, face, and ear, so skin tumors such as SCC and melanoma account for approximately 80–90% of metastases. The opposite distribution is seen for the submandibular gland, with 85% of metastases coming from infraclavicular primary tumors (breast, kidney, and lung) [48].

Diagnosis

Examination

The clinical presentation of salivary gland cancer can range from indolent asymptomatic masses to rapidly growing painful masses with progressive nerve palsies. In general, episodic swelling and pain are a sign of salivary gland duct obstruction, whereas constant pain is more worrisome for malignancy. Inflammation of a salivary gland, sialadenitis, is more common than salivary gland cancer. However, the latter must be considered in the evaluation of any salivary gland swelling with pain. Approximately 10% of parotid gland cancers present with associated facial paralysis, and this portends a poor prognosis [49, 50]. Facial nerve weakness in the setting of a parotid mass should be considered a sign of salivary gland cancer until proven otherwise.

The parotid glands are the largest of the major salivary glands and are unique in that they contain intraglandular lymph nodes. The parotid gland can be divided into a superficial and a deep lobe by the plane in which the facial nerve branches course. These lobes are primarily defined for surgical treatment purposes, but anatomically most of the 10–20 intraglandular lymph nodes are in the superficial lobe. A thorough examination of the parotid gland includes palpation of the gland and neck, assessment of the overlying skin, bimanual palpation of the buccal space, which includes Stensen duct, examination of the oropharynx and nasopharynx, and a thorough evaluation of facial nerve function and symmetry. Deep lobe parotid gland cancers can involve the parapharyngeal space and present as a submucosal bulging mass in the oropharynx and/or nasopharynx, distorting the soft palate or obstructing the Eustachian tube. Deep lobe parotid gland cancers may also be associated with cranial neuropathies, manifesting as a decreased gag reflex, aspiration, asymmetric palate elevation, hoarseness, dysphagia, shoulder weakness, or paresis of the tongue. These cancers can also cause trismus via infiltration into the masticator space.

The submandibular glands are located in the submandibular triangle of the neck and extend to the medial aspect of the mandible. These glands are closely associated with the lingual nerve, hypoglossal nerve, facial artery and vein, and overlying marginal mandibular branch of the facial nerve. They drain into the floor of the mouth via Wharton's duct. Bimanual palpation of any submandibular gland tumor should be performed to assess the extent of the tumor and to determine if there is fixation to adjacent structures such as the mandible or skin. A careful neurologic examination should also be performed to assess nerve involvement including numbness of the tongue, weakness of the tongue, or weakness of the lower lip. Careful examination of the neck is also important because 25–28% of submandibular gland cancers will metastasize to regional lymph nodes [1].

The paired sublingual glands are located in the floor of the mouth, lateral to Wharton's duct in the submucosal compartment. The drainage of these glands is via Bartholin's ducts. As with submandibular gland tumors, bimanual palpation of the floor of the mouth is important to assess the extent and possible fixation of sublingual gland tumors to the mandible. Because the sublingual gland is also associated with the lingual and hypoglossal nerves, a careful neurologic examination is important. Any mass of the sublingual gland should warrant high clinical suspicion because the likelihood of malignancy is high [11].

Minor salivary gland tissue is found throughout the upper aerodigestive tract, with the majority located in the oral cavity, especially in the submucosa of the hard palate. Minor salivary glands have minimal capsular tissue, making local invasion of tumors into surrounding tissue common. Patients with minor salivary gland cancer most often present with a painless submucosal lump, but there is frequently fixation of the overlying mucosa. Approximately one-quarter of patients with minor salivary gland cancer will complain of local pain or paresthesia/anesthesia concerning for nerve invasion [51]. Other presenting symptoms may include nasal airway obstruction, sinusitis, eustachian tube dysfunction, or hoarseness.

Imaging

Magnetic resonance imaging (MRI) is a common imaging modality used to assess salivary gland pathology. It has a high level of soft tissue clarity and therefore provides useful information about the extent of the disease. Benign and malignant salivary gland neoplasms are well visualized on T1-weighted images because they are easily distinguished from the fatty parenchyma of the gland, which appears hyperintense [7]. In general, low-grade salivary gland cancers have high T2-weighted signal intensities whereas high-grade cancers tend to have low-to-intermediate signal intensities on T2-weighted imaging. MRI may be able to differentiate specific characteristics of malignant lesions [52]. Contrast material such as gadolinium can be helpful to assess bone involvement and perineural spread. Computed tomography (CT) with intravenous contrast

Table 13.3 Staging for major salivary gland cancer.

Primary tumor (T)	
Tx	Primary tumor cannot be assessed
T0	No evidence of primary tumor
T1	Tumor 2 cm or smaller in greatest dimension without extraparenchymal extension
T2	Tumor larger than 2 cm but not larger than 4 cm in greatest dimension without extraparenchymal extension
T3	Tumor larger than 4 cm and/or tumor having extraparenchymal extension
T4a	Moderately advanced disease. Tumor invades skin, mandible, ear canal, and/or facial nerve
T4b	Very advanced disease. Tumor invades skull base and/or pterygoid plates and/ or encases carotid artery

Extraparenchymal extension is clinical or macroscopic evidence of invasion of soft tissues. Microscopic evidence alone does not constitute extraparenchymal extension for classification purposes.

Regional lymph nodes (N), clinical N (cN)	
Nx	Regional lymph nodes cannot be assessed
N0	No regional lymph node metastasis
N1	Metastasis in a single ipsilateral lymph node, 3 cm or smaller in greatest dimension and extranodal extension (ENE) (−)
N2a	Metastasis in a single ipsilateral node larger than 3 cm but not larger than 6 cm in greatest dimension and ENE(−)
N2b	Metastasis in multiple ipsilateral nodes, none larger than 6 cm in greatest dimension and ENE(−)
N2c	Metastasis in bilateral or contralateral lymph nodes, none larger than 6 cm in greatest dimension and ENE(−)
N3a	Metastasis in a lymph node larger than 6 cm in greatest dimension and ENE(−)
N3b	Metastasis in any node(s) with clinically overt ENE(+)

Note: a designation of "U" or "L" may be used for any N category to indicate metastasis above the lower border of the cricoid (U) or below the lower border of the cricoid (L).
Similarly, clinical and pathological ENE should be recorded as ENE(−) or ENE(+).

Regional lymph nodes (N), pathological N (pN)	
Nx	Regional lymph nodes cannot be assessed
N0	No regional lymph node metastasis
N1	Metastasis in a single ipsilateral lymph node, 3 cm or smaller in greatest dimension and ENE(−)
N2a	Metastasis in single ipsilateral or contralateral node 3 cm or smaller in greatest dimension and ENE(+) *or* a single ipsilateral node larger than 3 cm but not larger than 6 cm in greatest dimension and ENE(−)
N2b	Metastasis in multiple ipsilateral nodes, none larger than 6 cm in greatest dimension and ENE(−)
N2c	Metastasis in bilateral or contralateral lymph nodes, none larger than 6 cm in greatest dimension and ENE(−)
N3a	Metastasis in a lymph node larger than 6 cm in greatest dimension and ENE(−)
N3b	Metastasis in a single ipsilateral node larger than 3 cm in greatest dimension and ENE(+); *or* multiple ipsilateral, contralateral, or bilateral nodes any with ENE(+)

Distant metastasis (M)	
Mx	Distant metastasis cannot be assessed
M0	No distant metastasis
M1	Distant metastasis

Stage grouping			
0	Tis	N0	M0
I	T1	N0	M0
II	T2	N0	M0
III	T3	N0	M0
III	T0, T1, T2, T3	N1	M0
IVA	T4a	N0, N1	M0
IVA	T0, T1, T2, T3, T4a	N2	M0
IVB	Any T	N3	M0
IVB	T4b	Any N	M0
IVC	Any T	Any N	M1

Source: Lydiatt, *et al.* 2017 [55]. Used with permission of the American College of Surgeons, Chicago, Illinois. The original source for this information is the AJCC Cancer Staging Manual, 8th edn (2017), which is published by Springer Science + Business Media.

is also widely used in evaluating salivary gland pathology primarily because of the speed of acquisition. CT is particularly useful for evaluating cortical bone erosion from adjacent tumors. CT is much better than MRI in visualizing small salivary duct stones and can be helpful differentiating masses from sialolithiasis.

Biopsy

A biopsy is required to make the diagnosis of salivary gland cancer. Minimally-invasive pretreatment diagnosis has been made possible by fine-needle aspiration (FNA) biopsies. FNA is well tolerated and safe, with a much lower risk of tumor seeding than open or large needle biopsy [53]. The variety of different salivary gland cancers and their widely overlapping histologies may preclude definitive classification on FNA alone, but this may be improved with the use of immunohistochemistry. Sensitivity and specificity estimates for determining malignant versus benign disease using FNA are 0.80 and 0.97 respectively [53]. With this in mind, FNA has the major benefit of stratification of parotid masses into benign versus malignant groupings which can dictate the need for surgical intervention. Intraoperative frozen section has utility in assessing the extent of tumor spread to local/regional tissues, assessing surgical margins, and establishing the diagnosis in cases where the preoperative FNA biopsy was not diagnostic [54].

Staging

Clinical staging of salivary gland cancers is important for prognosis and treatment decisions. The TNM staging classification for major salivary gland cancers published in the American Joint Committee on Cancer (AJCC) Cancer Staging Manual Eighth Edition is the classification most commonly used (Table 13.3). Minor salivary gland carcinomas are staged according to the anatomic site of origin (e.g., oral cavity, sinus, and larynx). It is important to note that the current AJCC iteration of nodal (N) categorization includes extranodal extension (ENE). Nodal metastases with gross ENE are effectively upstaged to a higher N category.

Treatment

General

Salivary gland cancers are primarily treated surgically when resectable. Unresectable salivary gland cancers can be treated with radiation and or chemotherapy as palliation. Surgery alone is often adequate for early stage, low-grade salivary gland cancers. However, adjuvant radiation therapy is advised for all advanced stage and high grade cancers. [56]. Early stage cancers can be thought of as T1–2 lesions without nodal involvement. Advanced stage cancers are T3–4, or those with nodal disease. Patients high-grade salivary gland cancers including high-grade MEC, undifferentiated carcinoma, SCC, adenocarcinoma, carcinoma ex pleomorphic adenoma, and salivary duct carcinoma tend to have a high incidence of nodal metastases and a poorer prognosis. Low-grade salivary gland cancers include acinic cell carcinoma, low-grade mucoepidermoid carcinoma, low-grade adenocarcinoma (including basal cell and mucinous adenocarcinoma), and papillary cystadenocarcinoma. Intermediate-grade salivary gland cancers include adenoid cystic carcinoma and epithelial–myoepithelial carcinoma.

Radiation is not typically used as primary therapy in salivary malignancies, but can be considered for patients with advanced-stage, incompletely resectable tumors. Only 20% of patients with stage IV disease will be cured with RT alone [56]. The use of postoperative radiation therapy appears to improve locoregional control rates following resection of advanced stage or high grade salivary gland cancers. Five-year local control rates for patients in this study with stage III–IV disease after surgery and RT compared with surgery alone were 51% versus 17% [57]. There may be advantages to special methods of radiation therapy, including neutron beam and proton therapy, but definitive studies are still needed to define the optimum approach. [58]. Brachytherapy may play a role in the future for treatment of these lesions in the postoperative setting [59].

The use of systemic chemotherapy in the treatment of salivary gland cancer is currently limited to clinical trials and the palliative treatment of unresectable, recurrent, and metastatic disease. Response rates to chemotherapy alone tend to be partial and in about 40% of patients [60]. A variety of agents have been explored but measuring their effectiveness has been limited by small retrospective studies. Platinum-based chemotherapy has the strongest evidence for potential benefit in salivary gland cancer and remains under investigation. Currently, NRG (formerly RTOG) 1008 is studying the effect of the addition of adjuvant platinum therapy to radiation alone for resected high-risk salivary gland cancers. Attention has also been directed to the role for directed therapy against biologic targets expressed in these cancers including receptor tyrosine kinases such as c-KIT and members of the ErbB family. Her2/neu is frequently expressed in a subset of salivary gland cancers, namely salivary duct carcinoma, and has been used in targeted therapy [37, 61]. There are promising data indicating that targeted therapy in combination with conventional chemotherapy may have a synergistic effect.

Surgical Management

Parotidectomy is the indicated operation for a salivary gland cancer of the parotid gland [62]. The parotid gland can be divided into a superficial and a deep lobe by a sagittal plane defined by branches of the facial nerve. A superficial parotidectomy is generally adequate treatment for salivary gland cancers confined to the lateral lobe of the parotid. Dissection deep to the facial nerve may be required for salivary gland cancers that invade the deep lobe. A total parotidectomy is indicated for parotid gland cancers that involve the facial nerve and often for any salivary gland cancer originating within the deep lobe. If the facial nerve is involved by cancer, it should be resected to negative margins using frozen section analysis. In general, if the preoperative facial nerve function is intact, then the nerve is most likely not invaded, and all attempts should be made to preserve it. Conversely, preoperative paresis heralds invasion of the nerve. Advanced parotid gland cancers may extend to adjacent structures including muscle, bone, pharyngeal mucosa, and the overlying skin. This may require a partial mandibulectomy, a lateral or partial temporal bone resection, an extended resection of pharyngeal mucosa, or a resection of facial skin.

For cancers of the submandibular gland, oncologic resection of the gland often requires removal of the surrounding nodal groups. Structures at risk during this operation include the marginal mandibular branch of the facial nerve which is necessary for a symmetric smile, the lingual nerve which carries taste information from the ipsilateral tongue, and the hypoglossal nerve which moves the tongue on the same side. Submandibular gland cancer surgery is usually performed through a neck incision but can be accomplished via a transoral or combined approach. More advanced submandibular gland cancers require a more aggressive approach including possible mandibulectomy, floor of mouth resection, and/or partial glossectomy. The surgical management of minor salivary gland cancers is dictated by the specific site of the cancer. For example, a minor salivary gland cancer of the larynx may be amenable to transoral laser resection, while a cancer of the base of the tongue may be well suited for transoral robotic surgery. The most frequent location of a minor salivary gland cancer is the palate, and in these situations, transoral approaches are adequate and can be used in conjunction with partial or total maxillectomy for extensive lesions [63].

Neck dissection is a critical component of the surgical management of many salivary gland cancers. An ipsilateral neck dissection should be performed in patients with palpable or radiographically enlarged cervical lymph nodes and in patients with high grade histology. When a neck dissection is performed, a selective neck dissection (levels I–IV) is generally adequate. The decision on whether to perform an elective neck dissection can be controversial depending on the site, stage, and grade of the salivary gland cancer. The site of the primary cancer is associated with the frequency of occult nodal involvement. Tumors of the submandibular and sublingual gland have a higher incidence of occult metastasis to the cervical lymph nodes than those of the parotid gland. The size of the primary cancer and the presence of extraglandular extension have also been correlated with risk of metastases. Other features that have been associated with a higher risk of occult metastases are the histologic type and grade of the primary cancer.

Prognosis

The overall 10-year, disease-free survival rate of patients with salivary gland cancers ranges from 47 to 74% [15]. A predictive nomogram has been developed to help estimate survival [64]. Salivary gland cancers are heterogeneous and specific information regarding survival after treatment can vary significantly by histology. In general, several clinical characteristics of the primary cancer are recognized to be predictive of outcome. Primary cancer staging, which accounts for both size and the presence of extraglandular involvement, has a significant impact on prognosis. For example, salivary gland cancers with facial nerve involvement are more likely to recur and or metastasize than cancers without facial nerve involvement. The site of the primary cancer is also associated with prognosis. In particular, patients with submandibular and sublingual gland cancers tend to have more frequent metastases and a worse outcome than patients with parotid gland cancer. Advanced age, male gender, and local tissue invasion appear to portend a worse clinical outcome. Perineural invasion and spread as well as local bone invasion have also been shown to be independently associated with an increased risk of local recurrence and shorter overall survival. Last, the presence of positive surgical margins has been shown to be associated with a worse clinical outcome. Recently, lymph node density has been described as a prognostic feature [65].

Follow-Up and Survivorship

Surgery and postoperative radiotherapy result in good outcomes with minimal side effects and preservation in quality of life over time in patients with salivary gland cancers [66]. One of the major long-term side effects after treatment for salivary gland cancer is the xerostomia that is induced by radiotherapy in the head and neck region. Treatment consists of supportive care, artificial saliva substitutes, and aggressive dental hygiene [67, 68]. Other considerations include relevant anatomy that is sacrificed in the treatment of the tumor, mainly the facial nerve. Reanimation techniques are varied depending on the extent of damage to the nerve and can be performed at the time of the primary surgery or in secondary operations.

Long-term monitoring of patients after treatment consists of routine physical examination and imaging. Most practitioners follow patients with head and neck cancers for about 5 years, with more frequent examinations in the first 2 years. The use of imaging for follow-up remains controversial, but consists mostly of cross-sectional imaging to evaluation of the primary site and positron emission tomography scans for distant metastatic workup. Imaging studies can be obtained on a predetermined schedule or to assess new symptomatology.

References

1 Spiro RH. Salivary neoplasms: overview of a 35-year experience with 2,807 patients. *Head Neck Surg* 1986;8(3):177–84.

2 Howlader N, Noone AM, Krapcho M, *et al.* (eds). SEER Cancer Statistics Review, 1975–2013, National Cancer Institute, Bethesda, MD. http://seer.cancer.gov/csr/1975_2013/, based on November 2015 SEER data submission, posted to the SEER web site, April 2016.

3 Shapiro NL, Bhattacharyya N. Clinical characteristics and survival for major salivary gland malignancies in children. *Otolaryngol Head Neck Surg* 2006;134(4): 631–4.

4 Hunter RM, Davis BW, Gray GF, Jr, Rosenfeld L. Primary malignant tumors of salivary gland origin. A 52-year review. *Am Surg* 1983;49(2):82–9.

5 Pinkston JA, Cole P. Incidence rates of salivary gland tumors: results from a population-based study. *Otolaryngol Head Neck Surg* 1999;120(6):834–40.
6 Boukheris H, Stovall M, Gilbert ES, *et al.* Risk of salivary gland cancer after childhood cancer: a report from the Childhood Cancer Survivor Study. *Int J Radiat Oncol Biol Phys* 2013;85(3):776–83.
7 Flint PW, Cummings CW. *Cummings Otolaryngology: Head and Neck Surgery*, 5th edn. Philadelphia: Mosby/Elsevier, 2010:2963, cxciv.
8 Horn-Ross PL, Ljung BM, Morrow M. Environmental factors and the risk of salivary gland cancer. *Epidemiology* 1997;8(4):414–19.
9 Iyer NG, Morris LG, Tuttle RM, Shaha AR, Ganly I. Rising incidence of second cancers in patients with low-risk (T1N0) thyroid cancer who receive radioactive iodine therapy. *Cancer* 2011;117(19):4439–46.
10 Land CE, Saku T, Hayashi Y, *et al.* Incidence of salivary gland tumors among atomic bomb survivors, 1950–1987. Evaluation of radiation-related risk. *Radiat Res* 1996;146(1):28–36.
11 Eveson JW, Cawson RA. Salivary gland tumours. A review of 2410 cases with particular reference to histological types, site, age and sex distribution. *J Pathol* 1985;146(1):51–8.
12 Spiro RH, Huvos AG, Berk R, Strong EW. Mucoepidermoid carcinoma of salivary gland origin. A clinicopathologic study of 367 cases. *Am J Surg* 1978;136(4):461–8.
13 Auclair PL, Goode RK, Ellis GL. Mucoepidermoid carcinoma of intraoral salivary glands. Evaluation and application of grading criteria in 143 cases. *Cancer* 1992;69(8):2021–30.
14 Beckhardt RN, Weber RS, Zane R, *et al.* Minor salivary gland tumors of the palate: clinical and pathologic correlates of outcome. *Laryngoscope* 1995;105(11):1155–60.
15 Renehan A, Gleave EN, Hancock BD, Smith P, McGurk M. Long-term follow-up of over 1000 patients with salivary gland tumours treated in a single centre. *Br J Surg* 1996;83(12):1750–4.
16 Spiro RH, Huvos AG, Strong EW. Adenoid cystic carcinoma of salivary origin. A clinicopathologic study of 242 cases. *Am J Surg* 1974;128(4):512–20.
17 Spiro RH, Huvos AG. Stage means more than grade in adenoid cystic carcinoma. *Am J Surg* 1992;164(6):623–8.
18 Fordice J, Kershaw C, El-Naggar A, Goepfert H. Adenoid cystic carcinoma of the head and neck: predictors of morbidity and mortality. *Arch Otolaryngol Head Neck Surg* 1999;125(2):149–52.
19 Szanto PA, Luna MA, Tortoledo ME, White RA. Histologic grading of adenoid cystic carcinoma of the salivary glands. *Cancer* 1984;54(6):1062–9.
20 Evans HL, Batsakis JG. Polymorphous low-grade adenocarcinoma of minor salivary glands. A study of 14 cases of a distinctive neoplasm. *Cancer* 1984;53(4):935–42.
21 Evans HL, Luna MA. Polymorphous low-grade adenocarcinoma: a study of 40 cases with long-term follow up and an evaluation of the importance of papillary areas. *Am J Surg Pathol* 2000;24(10):1319–1328.
22 Castle JT, Thompson LD, Frommelt RA, Wenig BM, Kessler HP. Polymorphous low grade adenocarcinoma: A clinicopathologic study of 164 cases. *Cancer.* 1999;86(2):207–219.
23 Spitz MR, Tilley BC, Batsakis JG, Gibeau JM, Newell GR. Risk factors for major salivary gland carcinoma. A case-comparison study. *Cancer.* 1984;54(9):1854–1859.
24 Spiro RH, Huvos AG, Strong EW. Acinic cell carcinoma of salivary origin. A clinicopathologic study of 67 cases. *Cancer.* 1978;41(3):924–935.
25 Ellis GL, Corio RL. Acinic cell adenocarcinoma. A clinicopathologic analysis of 294 cases. *Cancer.* 1983;52(3):542–549.
26 Lewis JE, Olsen KD, Weiland LH. Acinic cell carcinoma. clinicopathologic review. *Cancer.* 1991;67(1):172–179.
27 Spiro RH, Huvos AG, Strong EW. Malignant mixed tumor of salivary origin: A clinicopathologic study of 146 cases. *Cancer.* 1977;39(2):388–396.
28 Olsen KD, Lewis JE. Carcinoma ex pleomorphic adenoma: A clinicopathologic review. *Head Neck.* 2001;23(9):705–712.
29 Qureshi AA, Gitelis S, Templeton AA, Piasecki PA. "Benign" metastasizing pleomorphic adenoma. A case report and review of literature. *Clin Orthop Relat Res.* 1994;(308)(308):192–198.
30 Nouraei SA, Ferguson MS, Clarke PM, *et al.* Metastasizing pleomorphic salivary adenoma. *Arch Otolaryngol Head Neck Surg* 2006;132(7):788–793.
31 Chen KT, Hafez GR. Infiltrating salivary duct carcinoma. A clinicopathologic study of five cases. *Arch Otolaryngol.* 1981;107(1):37–39.
32 Lewis JE, McKinney BC, Weiland LH, Ferreiro JA, Olsen KD. Salivary duct carcinoma. clinicopathologic and immunohistochemical review of 26 cases. *Cancer.* 1996;77(2):223–230.
33 Brandwein MS, Jagirdar J, Patil J, Biller H, Kaneko M. Salivary duct carcinoma (cribriform salivary carcinoma of excretory ducts). A clinicopathologic and immunohistochemical study of 12 cases. *Cancer.* 1990;65(10):2307–2314.
34 Jaehne M, Roeser K, Jaekel T, *et al.* Clinical and immunohistologic typing of salivary duct carcinoma: A report of 50 cases. *Cancer.* 2005;103(12):2526–2533.
35 Barnes L, Rao U, Contis L, *et al.* Salivary duct carcinoma. part II. immunohistochemical evaluation of 13 cases for estrogen and progesterone receptors, cathepsin D, and c-erbB-2 protein. *Oral Surg Oral Med Oral Pathol* 1994;78(1):74–80.
36 Johnson CJ, Barry MB, Vasef MA, Deyoung BR. Her-2/neu expression in salivary duct carcinoma: an immunohistochemical and chromogenic in situ hybridization study. *Appl Immunohistochem Mol Morphol* 2008;16(1):54–8.
37 Batsakis JG. Primary squamous cell carcinomas of major salivary glands. *Ann Otol Rhinol Laryngol* 1983;92(1 Pt 1):97–8.
38 Gaughan RK, Olsen KD, Lewis JE. Primary squamous cell carcinoma of the parotid gland. *Arch Otolaryngol Head Neck Surg* 1992;118(8):798–801.
39 Gnepp DR, Corio RL, Brannon RB. Small cell carcinoma of the major salivary glands. *Cancer* 1986;58(3):705–14.
40 Nagao T, Gaffey TA, Olsen KD, Serizawa H, Lewis JE. Small cell carcinoma of the major salivary glands: clinicopathologic study with emphasis on cytokeratin 20 immunoreactivity and clinical outcome. *Am J Surg Pathol* 2004;28(6):762–70.
41 Seethala RR, Barnes EL, Hunt JL. Epithelial-myoepithelial carcinoma: a review of the clinicopathologic spectrum and

immunophenotypic characteristics in 61 tumors of the salivary glands and upper aerodigestive tract. *Am J Surg Pathol* 2007;31(1):44–57.

42 Muller S, Barnes L. Basal cell adenocarcinoma of the salivary glands. report of seven cases and review of the literature. *Cancer* 1996;78(12):2471–7.

43 Savera AT, Sloman A, Huvos AG, Klimstra DS. Myoepithelial carcinoma of the salivary glands: a clinicopathologic study of 25 patients. *Am J Surg Pathol* 2000;24(6):761–74.

44 Wahlberg P, Anderson H, Biorklund A, Moller T, Perfekt R. Carcinoma of the parotid and submandibular glands – a study of survival in 2465 patients. *Oral Oncol* 2002;38(7):706–13.

45 Spiro RH, Huvos AG, Strong EW. Adenocarcinoma of salivary origin. clinicopathologic study of 204 patients. *Am J Surg* 1982;144(4):423–31.

46 Dunn P, Kuo TT, Shih LY, *et al.* Primary salivary gland lymphoma: a clinicopathologic study of 23 cases in Taiwan. *Acta Haematol* 2004;112(4):203–8.

47 Ambrosetti A, Zanotti R, Pattaro C, *et al.* Most cases of primary salivary mucosa-associated lymphoid tissue lymphoma are associated either with sjoegren syndrome or hepatitis C virus infection. *Br J Haematol* 2004;126(1):43–9.

48 Seifert G, Hennings K, Caselitz J. Metastatic tumors to the parotid and submandibular glands–analysis and differential diagnosis of 108 cases. *Pathol Res Pract* 1986;181(6):684–92.

49 Eneroth CM. Facial nerve paralysis. A criterion of malignancy in parotid tumors. *Arch Otolaryngol* 1972;95(4):300–4.

50 Witt RL. Major salivary gland cancer. *Surg Oncol Clin N Am* 2004;13(1):113–27.

51 Vander Poorten VL, Balm AJ, Hilgers FJ, *et al.* Stage as major long term outcome predictor in minor salivary gland carcinoma. *Cancer* 2000;89(6):1195–204.

52 Kashiwagi N, Takashima S, Tomita Y, *et al.* Salivary duct carcinoma of the parotid gland: clinical and MR features in six patients. *Br J Radiol* 2009;82(982):800–4.

53 Schmidt RL, Hall BJ, Wilson AR, Layfield LJ. A systematic review and meta-analysis of the diagnostic accuracy of fine-needle aspiration cytology for parotid gland lesions. *Am J Clin Pathol* 2011;136(1):45–59.

54 Seethala RR, LiVolsi VA, Baloch ZW. Relative accuracy of fine-needle aspiration and frozen section in the diagnosis of lesions of the parotid gland. *Head Neck* 2005;27(3):217–23.

55 Lydiatt WM, Mukherji SK, O'Sullivan B, Patel SG, Shah JP. Major Salivary glands. In M Amin, S Edge, FL Greene, D Byrd, R Brookland (eds) AJCC Cancer Staging Manual, 8th edn.New York: Springer Nature, 2017.

56 Mendenhall WM, Morris CG, Amdur RJ, Werning JW, Villaret DB. Radiotherapy alone or combined with surgery for salivary gland carcinoma. *Cancer* 2005;103(12):2544–50.

57 Armstrong JG, Harrison LB, Spiro RH, *et al.* Malignant tumors of major salivary gland origin. A matched-pair analysis of the role of combined surgery and postoperative radiotherapy. *Arch Otolaryngol Head Neck Surg* 1990;116(3):290–3.

58 Laramore GE, Krall JM, Griffin TW, *et al.* Neutron versus photon irradiation for unresectable salivary gland tumors: final report of an RTOG-MRC randomized clinical trial. radiation therapy oncology group. medical research council. *Int J Radiat Oncol Biol Phys* 1993;27(2):235–40.

59 Mao MH, Zhang JG, Zhang J, *et al.* Postoperative [(1)(2)(5)I] seed brachytherapy in the treatment of acinic cell carcinoma of the parotid gland: with associated risk factors. *Strahlenther Onkol* 2014;190(11):1008–14.

60 Suen JY, Johns ME. Chemotherapy for salivary gland cancer. *Laryngoscope* 1982;92(3):235–9.

61 Haddad R, Colevas AD, Krane JF, *et al.* Herceptin in patients with advanced or metastatic salivary gland carcinomas. A phase II study. *Oral Oncol* 2003;39(7):724–7.

62 Woods JE, Chong GC, Beahrs OH. Experience with 1,360 primary parotid tumors. *Am J Surg* 1975;130(4):460–2.

63 Vander Poorten V, Hunt J, Bradley PJ, *et al.* Recent trends in the management of minor salivary gland carcinoma. *Head Neck* 2014;36(3):444–55.

64 Ali S, Palmer FL, Yu C, *et al.* Postoperative nomograms predictive of survival after surgical management of malignant tumors of the major salivary glands. *Ann Surg Oncol* 2014;21(2):637–42.

65 Hong HR, Roh JL, Cho KJ, *et al.* Prognostic value of lymph node density in high-grade salivary gland cancers. *J Surg Oncol* 2015;111(6):784–9.

66 Al-Mamgani A, van Rooij P, Verduijn GM, Meeuwis CA, Levendag PC. Long-term outcomes and quality of life of 186 patients with primary parotid carcinoma treated with surgery and radiotherapy at the Daniel Den Hoed Cancer Center. *Int J Radiat Oncol Biol Phys* 2012;84(1):189–95.

67 Jensen SB, Pedersen AM, Vissink A, *et al.* A systematic review of salivary gland hypofunction and xerostomia induced by cancer therapies: prevalence, severity and impact on quality of life. *Support Care Cancer* 2010;18(8):1039–60.

68 Cohen EE, LaMonte SJ, Erb NL, *et al.* American Cancer Society Head and Neck Cancer Survivorship Care Guideline. *CA Cancer J Clin* 2016;66(3):203–39.

14

Larynx Cancer

Emma B. Holliday[1], Blaine D. Smith[2], Neil D. Gross[1], Clifton D. Fuller[1], and David I. Rosenthal[1]

[1] The University of Texas MD Anderson Cancer Center, Houston, Texas, USA
[2] Duke University Medical Center, Durham, North Carolina, USA

Incidence and Mortality

Larynx cancer accounts for nearly 25% of all head and neck cancers in the United States (US), although it only makes up 1% of all new cancer diagnoses overall; in 2017, there are estimated to be 13,360 new cases (10,570 men and 2,790 women) of larynx cancer and 3,660 deaths (2,940 men and 720 women) from the disease [1]. In the US, glottic larynx cancer comprises approximately 75% of all laryngeal cancers, with supraglottic and subglottic larynx cancers only accounting for 24% and 1–2% of all laryngeal tumors, respectively. However, in Mediterranean and Scandinavian countries, proportions of supraglottic tumors have been reported to be higher [2, 3]. In the US, incidence and mortality rates are highest among African Americans and lowest among Asian Americans and Pacific Islanders. Incidence and mortality rates for men have been declining since the late 1970s/early 1980s; these rates peaked for women during the late 1980s/early 1990s but have been declining since then [4]. The median age at diagnosis is 65 years [4].

Additionally, while the incidence of nontobacco-related head and neck cancers (e.g., human papillomavirus (HPV)-associated oropharyngeal squamous cell carcinoma) have increased, the incidence of tobacco-related head and neck cancers (e.g., laryngeal squamous cell cancer) has decreased. Interestingly, the survival of laryngeal cancer declined over the same time period even as the survival rates have steadily improved for cancers in other head and neck subsites [4–8]. This may reflect the widespread adoption of organ preservation strategies for the treatment of advanced-stage larynx cancer in lieu of primary surgery [7].

Etiology and Risk Factors

The strongest risk factors for the development of larynx cancer are cigarette smoking and alcohol consumption. It is often difficult to separate out the effects of tobacco and alcohol in epidemiologic studies because smokers are more likely to be drinkers and vice versa. Even so, cigarette smoking appears to contribute more to larynx cancer risk than excessive alcohol consumption [9]. It has been estimated that greater than 50% of larynx cancer cases are attributable to smoking [10]. Other risk factors have been postulated including laryngopharyngeal reflux, which can cause chronic irritation of the laryngeal mucosa [11]. Additionally, exposures to asbestos, diesel fumes, rubber fumes, or wood dust have been identified as risk factors [12]. Most occupational exposures have been shown to confer little excess risk, and even suspected exposure-related larynx cancers are thought to be confounded by coexisting tobacco use [12]. Frequent or extreme vocal use, such as in the case of professional singers or lecturers, has also been cited as a risk factor [13]. Finally, although human papillomavirus (HPV) has been cited as a causative agent for oropharyngeal carcinoma, and laryngeal papillomatosis is caused by low-risk HPV types 6 and 11, there are relatively scant data supporting an association of HPV infection with laryngeal carcinoma [14]. A recent meta-analysis suggests the prevalence of HPV in larynx cancer is between 20 and 30% [15], but the role of HPV infection in the pathogenesis of larynx cancer remains uncertain, as studies have reported that normal laryngeal specimens and larynx cancers harbor high-risk HPV DNA at similar frequencies (up to 19%) [16].

Prevention

Prevention of larynx cancer is best achieved by lifestyle modifications aimed at reducing the risk factors outlined above, namely smoking cessation and, to a lesser extent, moderating alcohol consumption. Current smokers should be encouraged to quit, as the excess cancer risk does decline after cessation and returns to baseline risk after 20 years, and other medical benefits are more immediate [17]. Although no practical or cost-effective screening regimens exist for asymptomatic patients, occasionally patients with premalignant lesions of the larynx will come to medical attention. Hoarseness is the only early

The American Cancer Society's Oncology in Practice: Clinical Management, First Edition. Edited by The American Cancer Society.

symptom for glottis cancer often leading to earlier diagnosis, while supraglottic cancer remains asymptomatic longer for most patients leading to diagnosis in later stages [18]. Often this prompts fiberoptic examination and biopsy of any visible abnormalities. Patients with confirmed premalignant laryngeal lesions including severe dysplasia or carcinoma *in situ* have a risk of malignant transformation as high as 30% [19]. As the transition between precarcinoma to carcinoma can often take years, surveillance with early intervention can prevent or catch early any progression to invasive cancer. The preferred treatment approach for premalignant epithelial laryngeal lesions varies by institution and practitioner, but options include surgical excision, carbon dioxide laser excision, photodynamic therapy and radiation therapy.

Pathology

Over 95% of malignant tumors of the larynx are squamous cell carcinomas. Verrucous carcinoma is a subtype of squamous cell carcinoma that accounts for fewer than 5% of all larynx cancers [20]. It is exophytic and bulky with papillomatous projections that have a broad base [21]. In comparison with usual squamous cell carcinomas, verrucous carcinomas are thought to be lower grade, and perhaps not as responsive to irradiation. Poorly differentiated sarcomatoid squamous variants may also not be as responsive to irradiation. Other less common histologies include lymphoma, plasmacytoma, soft tissue sarcoma, chondrosarcoma, melanoma, small cell carcinoma, adenocarcinoma, adenoid cystic carcinoma, and metastatic disease [13].

Diagnosis

Typical presenting symptoms depend on subsite and extent of disease. Small cancers of the true vocal cords cause hoarseness or a change in vocal quality, whereas sore throat (odynophagia) and ear pain (otalgia) are more likely with supraglottic cancers. Unilateral otalgia is, in fact, a common presenting complaint, caused by referred pain mediated by involvement of the auricular nerve of Arnold, which innervates the supraglottic larynx. Tumors of the subglottic larynx are rare, but when they occur, typically present with symptoms of advanced disease including hemoptysis and upper airway obstruction with stridor, hoarseness, and odynophagia. The incidence of lymph node metastases also varies widely by subsite and tumor size. The true vocal cords have practically no lymphatic drainage, so cancers that are truly localized to the glottis have a negligible chance of nodal metastases. The risk increases when there is supra- or subglottic extension. The supraglottis, conversely, has rich lymphatic drainage, and approximately half of all patients with supraglottic cancer will have palpable or radiographically apparent lymph nodes at presentation [22]. The rate of nodal metastases is 20–30% for even T1 supraglottic larynx cancers. The subglottis also has a draining lymphatic network, and approximately 20% of patients with subglottic cancer will present with clinically apparent lymph nodes at presentation [23].

The diagnostic work up for a patient with suspected larynx cancer should begin with a thorough history and physical examination. The neck and supraclavicular region should be palpated for any clinically apparent lymph nodes and the thyroid cartilage palpated for tenderness. The examination should also include inspection of the larynx through mirror or fiberoptic examination to observe any mucosal abnormalities, assess the airway, and assess vocal cord mobility. Imaging should be considered for any suspected malignancy, usually either fine-cut computed tomography (CT) with contrast or a gadolinium-enhanced magnetic resonance imaging (MRI). Figure 14.1 shows representative images from a fiberoptic endoscope and CT from a patient with T2 glottic larynx cancer. Positron emission tomography imaging can be considered for stage III–IV disease, although its routine use in upfront staging of larynx cancer remains controversial [24]. Chest imaging is recommended by the National Comprehensive Cancer Network (NCCN) only as clinically indicated by new respiratory symptoms [25]. A biopsy is ultimately required to establish the diagnosis of cancer, and is usually performed in the operating room under anesthesia with rigid endoscopy. Videostroboscopy can be considered for functional evaluation and provides durable documentation of baseline tumor characteristics and vocal cord function. Multidisciplinary evaluation is also a recommended part of the workup with consultations made to surgical, radiation, and medical oncology specialists. Evaluation by dental, nutrition, speech and swallowing, and audiology experts can also be considered for baseline evaluation as clinically indicated [25].

Staging

The most widely used staging system for larynx cancer is the tumor-node-metastasis (TNM) system of the American Joint Committee on Cancer (AJCC) and the Union for International Cancer Control (UICC). There are slightly different staging classification systems for the three distinct subsites of the larynx [26]. The glottis is comprised of the true vocal cords, anterior, and posterior commissures as well as the area 5 mm inferior to the free margin of the true vocal cords. The supraglottis includes the false vocal cords, arytenoids, suprahyoid epiglottis, infrahyoid epiglottis, and aryepiglottic folds. The subglottis includes the region extending from 5 mm below the free margin of the true vocal cords to the inferior margin of the cricoid cartilage. It is important to note that the current AJCC iteration of nodal (N) categorization includes extranodal extension (ENE). Nodal metastases with gross ENE are effectively upstaged to a higher N category. The classification from the most recent version, 8th edition (2017), is shown in Table 14.1 [26].

Treatment

The treatment options for larynx cancer vary based on site and stage, roughly divided into early (stage I–II) and advanced (stage III–IV). Early stage larynx cancers have small primary mucosal lesions with no lymph node involvement and can often be treated with a single modality approach. Advanced larynx cancers have

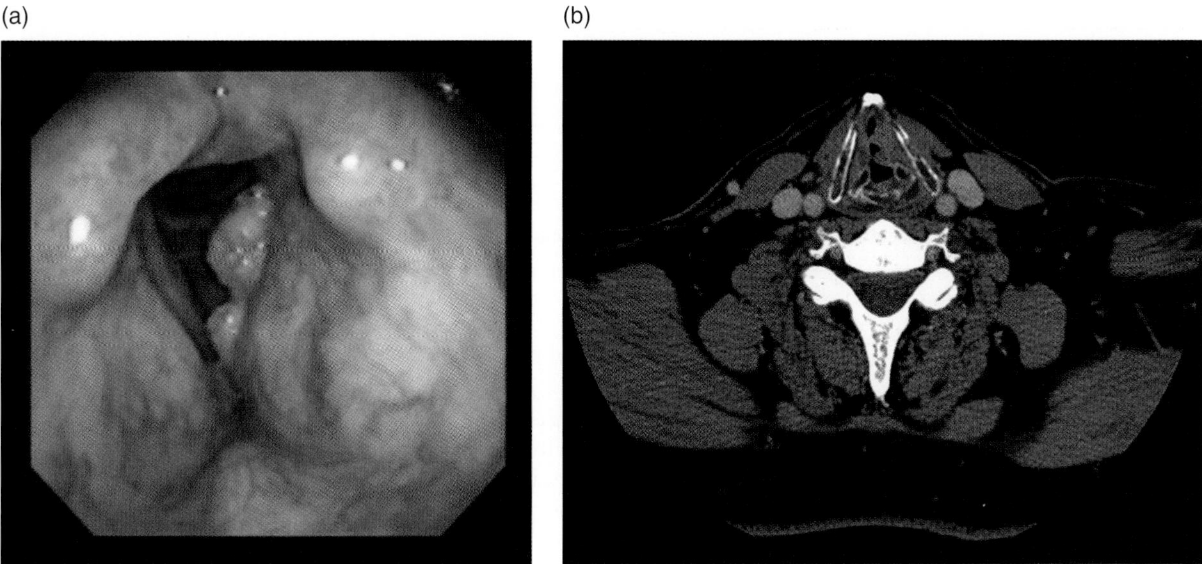

Figure 14.1 (a) Squamous cell carcinoma of the left true vocal cord involving the anterior commissure. On phonation, the patient's left true vocal cord showed decreased mobility. (b) Computed tomography of the neck with contrast from a patient with squamous cell carcinoma of the left true vocal cord involving the anterior commissure.

larger primary mucosal lesions and/or positive lymph nodes and require multimodality treatment. Nonsurgical organ-preservation radiation and chemotherapy is generally favored for advanced larynx cancers that would otherwise require total laryngectomy. Partial laryngectomy, done either open or endoscopically, may be an option for well-selected patients.

Early Stage Glottic Cancer

As vocal symptoms appear even when these cancers are very small, most patients with glottic cancer present with early-stage disease. Fortunately, outcomes with definitive local therapy are excellent, with 5-year overall survival (OS) often in excess of 85% [27]. Voice-preserving therapy is preferred for patients with T1 or T2 larynx cancer and no lymph node involvement, either with radiation therapy (RT) or a voice-preserving surgery such as transoral endoscopic excision (either with or without robotic assistance) or transoral laser microsurgical resection [25]. There have been no randomized trials comparing surgical versus RT-based treatment, so the decision often varies widely by institution, clinician, and patient. Factors to consider include tumor size, location, vocal cord mobility, expected post-treatment voice, endoscopic access, patient preference and occupation, availability, and cost [28]. In the US, RT is common due to higher rates of voice preservation [29, 30], although this is still controversial [31]. Newer studies suggest that after an initial decrease in vocal quality after endoscopic resection, most patients return to their presurgical vocal quality [32]. The Cochrane Collaboration attempted to compare the efficacy of open partial laryngectomy, endolaryngeal excision (with or without laser), and RT for early glottic laryngeal cancer. On combined analysis, they reported 5-year disease-free survival to be 71.1% following RT and 100% following surgery for T1 glottic cancers ($P > 0.05$) and 60.1% following RT and 78.1% following surgery for T2 cancers ($P = 0.036$). However, there were no data analyzed for treatment toxicity, quality of life, voice outcomes, or cost and the authors found insufficient evidence to guide management decisions on the most effective treatment [33].

Patients with superficial, well-circumscribed T1a cancers may be amenable to surgery with excellent voice quality. The likelihood of a good voice outcome after surgery diminishes with the extent and bulk of the cancer. Further, local control (LC) after endoscopic resection has been reported to be lower than after RT [34]. For these reasons, RT is often preferred over surgery in the US for early stage larynx cancer. For patients with a cancer that involves both vocal cords or the anterior commissure, RT is preferred, to decrease the risk for glottic webbing and permanent hoarseness. However, as surgeons become more comfortable with the modality, some centers now favor transoral laser microsurgical resection even for lesions in which both vocal cords [35] or the anterior commissure is involved [36]. RT is typically delivered via two opposed lateral photon fields to cover the entire larynx. At least 2 Gy per day has been shown to improve LC. One common regimen is 63 Gy in 2.25 Gy daily fractions for T1 tumors [37]. For T2 tumors, RT can result in larynx preservation rates of up to 88% [38]. Similar to the treatment of T1 tumors, increased daily radiation dose increases LC, whether in the form of daily radiation fractions greater than 2 Gy (called hypofractionation) or twice daily radiation fractions of 1.2 Gy (called hyperfractionation) [39, 40]. For patients with vertical extension but preserved vocal cord mobility, the once daily hypofractionation approach is common, with 65.25 Gy in 2.25 Gy daily fractions [39]. Patients with impaired vocal cord mobility have poorer outcomes with once daily RT alone and require either 70 Gy/6–7 weeks or concurrent chemoradiotherapy (CRT), similar to those with T3 tumors. According to the NCCN, 66 Gy in 2 Gy daily fractions and 70 Gy in 2 Gy daily fractions

Table 14.1 Classification of larynx cancer according to the AJCC 8th edn (2017).

Primary tumor (T-category)		
Glottis	TX	Primary tumor cannot be assessed
	Tis	Carcinoma *in situ*
	T1	Tumor limited to the vocal cord(s) (may involve anterior or posterior commissure) with normal mobility
	T1a	Tumor limited to one vocal cord
	T1b	Tumor involves both vocal cords
	T2	Tumor extends to supraglottis and/or subglottis, and/or with impaired cord mobility
	T3	Tumor limited to the larynx with vocal cord fixation and/or invasion of paraglottic space and/or inner cortex of the thyroid cartilage
	T4	Moderately advanced or very advanced
	T4a	Moderately advanced local disease Tumor invades through the outer cortex of the thyroid cartilage and/or invades tissues beyond the larynx (e.g., trachea, cricoid cartilage, soft tissues of neck including deep extrinsic muscle of the tongue, strap muscles, thyroid or esophagus)
	T4b	Very advanced local disease Tumor invades prevertebral space, encases carotid artery, or invades mediastinal structures
Supraglottis	TX	Primary tumor cannot be assessed
	Tis	Carcinoma *in situ*
	T1	Tumor limited to one subsite of supraglottis with normal vocal cord mobility
	T2	Tumor invades mucosa of more than one adjacent subsite of supraglottis or glottis or region outside the supraglottis (e.g., mucosa of base of tongue, vallecula, medial wall of pyriform sinus) without fixation of the larynx
	T3	Tumor limited to larynx with vocal cord fixation and/or invades any of the following: postcricoid area, preepiglottic space, paraglottic space, and/or inner cortex of thyroid cartilage
	T4	Moderately advanced or very advanced
	T4a	Moderately advanced local disease Tumor invades through the outer cortex of the thyroid cartilage and/or invades tissues beyond the larynx (e.g., trachea, soft tissues of neck including deep extrinsic muscle of the tongue, strap muscles, thyroid or esophagus)
	T4b	Very advanced local disease Tumor invades prevertebral space, encases carotid artery, or invades mediastinal structures
Subglottis	TX	Primary tumor cannot be assessed
	Tis	Carcinoma *in situ*
	T1	Tumor limited to the subglottis
	T2	Tumor extends to the vocal cord(s) with normal or impaired mobility
	T3	Tumor limited to larynx with vocal cord fixation and/or invasion of paraglottic space and/or inner cortex of the thyroid cartilage
	T4	Moderately advanced or very advanced
	T4a	Moderately advanced local disease Tumor invades cricoid or thyroid cartilage and/or invades tissues beyond the larynx (e.g., trachea, soft tissues of neck including deep extrinsic muscle of the tongue, strap muscles, thyroid or esophagus)
	T4b	Very advanced local disease Tumor invades prevertebral space, encases carotid artery, or invades mediastinal structures
Regional lymph nodes (N-category)		
Clinical N (cN)	NX	Regional lymph nodes cannot be assessed
	N0	No regional lymph node metastasis
	N1	Metastasis in a single ipsilateral lymph node, 3 cm or smaller in greatest dimension and ENE(−)
	N2	Metastasis in a single ipsilateral node, larger than 3 cm but not larger than 6 cm in greatest dimension and ENE(−); *or* metastases in multiple ipsilateral lymph nodes, none larger than 6 cm in greatest dimension and ENE(−); *or* metastasis in bilateral or contralateral lymph nodes, none larger than 6 cm in greatest dimension and ENE(−)
	N2a	Metastasis in a single ipsilateral node, larger than 3 cm but not larger than 6 cm in greatest dimension and ENE(−)
	N2b	Metastases in multiple ipsilateral nodes, none larger than 6 cm in greatest dimension and ENE(−)
	N2c	Metastasis in bilateral or contralateral nodes, none larger than 6 cm in greatest dimension and ENE(−)
	N3	Metastasis in a lymph node, larger than 6 cm in greatest dimension and ENE(−); *or* metastasis in any lymph node(s) with clinically overt ENE(+)
	N3a	Metastasis in a lymph node, larger than 6 cm in greatest dimension and ENE(−)
	N3b	Metastasis in any lymph node(s) with clinically overt ENE(+)

Table 14.1 (Continued)

Pathological N (pN)	NX	Regional lymph nodes cannot be assessed
	N0	No regional lymph node metastasis
	N1	Metastasis in a single ipsilateral lymph node, 3 cm or smaller in greatest dimension and ENE(−)
	N2	Metastasis in a single ipsilateral lymph node, 3 cm or smaller in greatest dimension and ENE(+); *or* metastasis in a single ipsilateral lymph node, larger than 3 cm but not larger than 6 cm in greatest dimension and ENE(−); *or* metastases in multiple ipsilateral lymph nodes, none larger than 6 cm in greatest dimension and ENE(−); *or* metastasis in bilateral or contralateral lymph nodes, none larger than 6 cm in greatest dimension and ENE(−)
	N2a	Metastasis in a single ipsilateral or contralateral node, 3 cm or smaller in greatest dimension and ENE(+); *or* metastasis in a single ipsilateral node, larger than 3 cm but not larger than 6 cm in greatest dimension and ENE(−)
	N2b	Metastases in multiple ipsilateral nodes, none larger than 6 cm in greatest dimension and ENE(−)
	N2c	Metastasis in bilateral or contralateral lymph nodes, none larger than 6 cm in greatest dimension and ENE(−)
	N3	Metastasis in a lymph node, larger than 6 cm in greatest dimension and ENE(−); *or* metastasis in a single ipsilateral node, larger than 3 cm in greatest dimension and ENE(+); *or* metastases in multiple ipsilateral, contralateral, or bilateral lymph nodes and any with ENE(+)
	N3a	Metastasis in a lymph node, larger than 6 cm in greatest dimension and ENE(−)
	N3b	Metastasis in a single ipsilateral node, larger than 3 cm in greatest dimension and ENE(+); *or* metastases in multiple ipsilateral, contralateral, or bilateral lymph nodes and any with ENE(+)
Note: a designation of "U" or "L" may be used for any N category to indicate metastasis above the lower border of the cricoid (U) or below the lower border of the cricoid (L).		
Distant metastatic disease (M-category)		
	M0	No distant metastasis
	M1	Distant metastasis

Stage grouping[1]

0	Tis	N0	M0
I	T1	N0	M0
II	T2	N0	M0
III	T3	N0	M0
	T1–T3	N1	M0
IVA	T4a	N0–N1	M0
	T1–T4a	N2	M0
IVB	T4b	Any N	M0
	Any T	N3	M0
IVC	Any T	Any N	M1

Source: Amin *et al.* [26]. Used with permission of the American College of Surgeons, Chicago, Illinois. The original source for this information is the AJCC Cancer Staging Manual, 8th edn (2017), which is published by Springer Science + Business Media.

[1] Definitions apply to all subsites.

are also suitable definitive radiation regimens [25]. A recent randomized trial showed no survival benefit of twice daily radiation when compared with daily treatment but did show a trend towards increased local control [41]. Upfront open partial laryngoectomy is performed through a midline neck incision, and it is typically reserved for patients who cannot receive either transoral laser excision or RT. A temporary tracheostomy is required in the postoperative period, though permanent tracheostomy is rarely needed. Although one vocal cord is spared and speech is preserved, the voice is typically permanently raspy after this procedure. Chemotherapy is not a standard part of the treatment plan for most patients with early stage glottic cancer. Additionally, the low risk of lymph node metastasis means that the neck is not typically addressed either when surgery or RT is used as the primary treatment modality except for patients with impaired vocal cord mobility or significant supraglottic involvement.

The lymph nodes of the neck are divided into five levels. Level I nodes are located in the submental and submandibular regions. Level II nodes are located between the sternocleidomastoid muscle to the submandibular gland and extend from the base of skull down to the hyoid bone. Level III nodes are located between the common carotid artery and the sternocleidomastoid muscle and extend from the hyoid bone down to the cricoid cartilage. Level IV nodes extend below level III from the cricoid cartilage down to the clavicle. Level V nodes are located in the posterior triangle, posterior to levels II–IV. The larynx drains to lymph nodes in levels II and III. Therefore, it is primarily these levels that are addressed with surgery or radiation in cases of more advanced disease.

Early Stage Supraglottic Cancer

Similar to patients with early stage glottic cancer, the primary intent for patients with early stage supraglottic cancer is to achieve cure with local therapy while maintaining organ and voice preservation. Also similar to glottic cancer, endoscopic laser or robotic-assisted resection is an option for patients with superficial, well-demarcated tumors, as studies have shown equal outcome and less morbidity when compared to open procedures. Patients undergoing endoscopic laser resection have shorter hospital stays, lower tracheostomy rates, and less time to restoration of swallowing compared to open approaches [42, 43]. When either surgery is performed, an ipsilateral lymph node dissection is considered, due to the higher chance of occult lymph node metastasis [25]. There have been no randomized controlled trials comparing surgery with RT for early stage supraglottic cancer. The retrospective data that do exist are sometimes difficult to interpret because of inherent differences between the groups and oncologic outcomes are likely similar. Based on limited poor quality data, a primary surgical approach may afford patients better LC than with upfront RT [44]. Patients must be carefully selected, however, because comorbid medical conditions and extent of tumor often preclude patients from being good surgical candidates. Surgical staging may lead to upstaging, and patients may require postoperative radiation (PORT) if upstaged to T3 or T4 tumors, if positive lymph nodes are found, or if negative margins cannot be achieved. Because PORT can magnify the toxicities of surgery, giving primary RT may be preferred when upstaging is likely. LC has been reported to be 84% with supraglottic surgery versus 79% with initial RT. However, local failure after primary RT are more easily salvaged than local failure after surgery and such salvage procedures carry less morbidity. LC after primary radiation and surgical salvage has been reported to be as high as 90%, with a larynx preservation rate of 83% [44]. When RT is used as the primary modality, the dose, targets, and fractionation depend on the size of the tumor. Because of the rich lymphatic drainage of the supraglottis, bilateral cervical lymph nodes are treated with RT even for clinically N0 patients. RT is delivered to the larynx and cervical lymph nodes from levels II–IV. The lymph nodes receive 50 Gy in 2 Gy fractions and the primary tumor plus margin receive an additional 16 Gy in eight fractions for a total of 66 Gy [45]. Patients with T1 and T2 cancers are typically treated with RT alone, whereas patients with bulky or deep infiltrative T2 cancers may benefit from escalated therapy either in the form of concurrent CRT with cisplatin [46] or with a hyperfractionated or hypofractionated RT regimen. Also in contrast to glottic cancers, a more conformal intensity-modulated radiation therapy technique is often used for supraglottic cancers in order to spare dose to normal structures such as salivary tissue [45].

Early Stage Subglottic Cancer

Cancers seldom arise from the subglottic area, but when they do, they are often very advanced at presentation. This is because cancers in the subglottic region do not cause the noticeable symptoms of vocal change that prompt early presentation and diagnosis for patients with glottic cancer. The most oncologically effective treatment strategy in these cases is a wide-field laryngectomy with bilateral paratracheal lymph node dissection. LC is reported to be 50–70% and OS is reported to be 40–70% [47, 48] with this aggressive primary surgical approach. The addition of PORT to laryngectomy can increase 5-year LC upwards of 80% [49]. LC and OS are much lower for nonoperative patients with subglottic cancer, reported as low as 50–70% and 25–50%, respectively, in retrospective reviews of patients treated with primary RT [50, 51]. CRT may increase LC and has been studied for organ preservation in subglottic cancer with promising results [52].

Advanced Larynx Cancer

No matter the laryngeal subsite of origin, stage III–IV cancers of the larynx are largely treated in the same manner. Patients with locally advanced laryngeal cancer fare much worse than their early stage counterparts, with 5-year survival rates ranging from 30 to 60% [53].

Historically, patients with locally advanced larynx cancer received a total laryngectomy, ipsilateral thyroidectomy, and ipsilateral or bilateral neck lymph node dissection. A select number of patients may be candidates for partial laryngeal surgery. However, now patients with node-positive laryngeal cancer and/or large T3 cancers who have adequate performance status and desire larynx preservation can receive organ preservation cisplatin-based CRT [25]. The VA Laryngeal Cancer Study first established CRT as a means of achieving both cure and larynx preservation by comparing surgical and nonsurgical approaches for patients with stage III and IV laryngeal cancer. The two arms of the trial were: (i) total laryngectomy followed by PORT and (ii) two cycles of induction cisplatin 100 mg/m^2 and 1000 mg/m^2 continuous infusion 5-fluorouracil (5-FU) followed by restaging. Those who responded received a third cycle and then definitive RT to 70 Gy in 2 Gy daily fractions. Nonresponders underwent total laryngectomy and PORT. Local failure was higher in the nonsurgical arm (12 vs 2%), but OS was 68% in both groups, and the nonsurgical arm achieved a 64% larynx preservation rate [54].

The current preferred nonsurgical treatment is to administer CRT with an RT dose of 70 Gy in 2 Gy daily fractions and concurrent cisplatin is 100 mg/m^2 given on days 1, 22, and 43. This regimen is derived from a randomized controlled trial, RTOG 91-11, that enrolled patients with stage III and IV tumors. The arms of the trial were: (i) 5-FU/cisplatin induction chemotherapy followed by RT (the VA regimen) that was the reference and the two experimental arms were (ii) concurrent CRT with cisplatin 100 mg/m^2 on days 1, 22, and 42 and (iii) the same RT alone. The initial results of this study showed higher 2-year larynx preservation rates for CRT when compared with induction chemotherapy and RT alone (88% compared to 74% and 69%, respectively) and no difference in OS between the arms [55]. A 10-year update of these results showed persistence of the LC benefit of CRT, but showed a trend toward improved OS in the induction arm. Although not statistically significant, the survival appears to be better for patients receiving induction chemotherapy, as there was a higher noncancer-related mortality among patients treated with CRT [56]. This suggests that CRT may worsen function, lead to aspiration, and lead to other later systemic causes of mortality. Figure 14.2 shows representative images from a radiation treatment plan for a patient treated

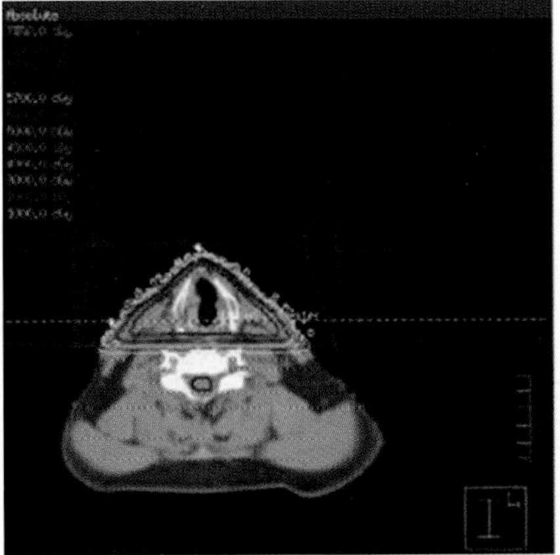
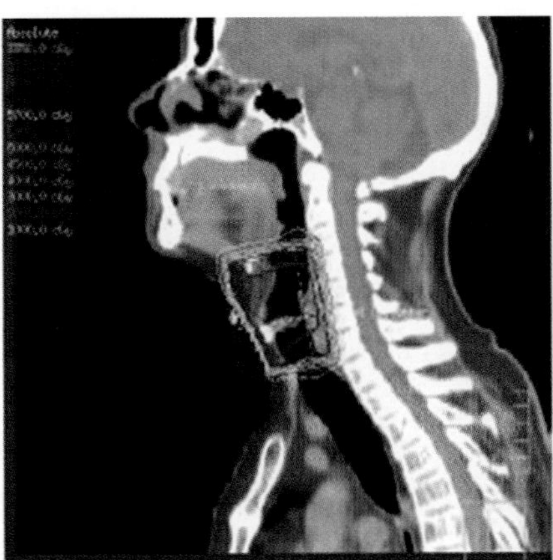
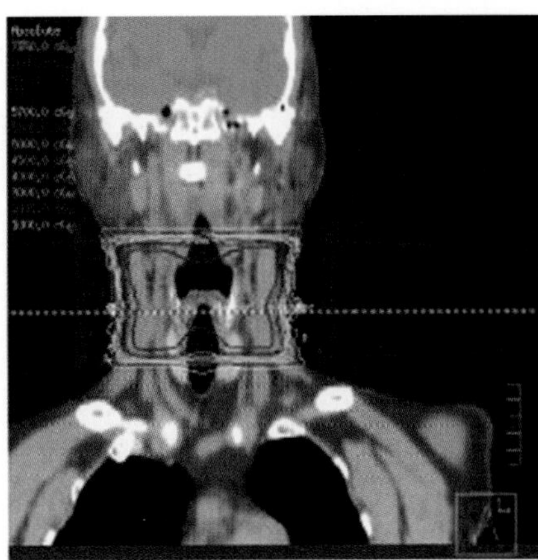

Figure 14.2 Radiation treatment planning images for a patient with advanced stage squamous cell carcinoma of the right vocal cord treated with radiation and chemotherapy.

with CRT for T3N0 glottic cancer. The use of cetuximab as the concurrent agent during radiation therapy has garnered interest for reducing toxicity. Retrospective data suggests cetuximab with RT improves larynx preservation for laryngeal cancers compared with radiation alone [57, 58], but the efficacy of cetuximab for laryngeal tumors should be validated in a prospective setting prior to becoming the standard of care [59].

A refinement in induction strategy or patients with locally advanced larynx cancer is to give induction chemotherapy with docetaxel, cisplatin, and 5-FU (TPF) [25, 60, 61]. The response to therapy can then be used to tailor further treatment. If there is a complete response in the primary tumor, definitive RT alone can be given. A recent phase II study suggests patients who respond well to induction TPF may also benefit by adding cetuximab to radiation, although further study in the phase III setting is certainly warranted [62]. If there is a partial response, RT alone or CRT can be given. A neck dissection is recommended after completion of RT for any residual neck nodes that do not resolve on clinical examination and imaging studies on followup. If there is no response or progression while on chemotherapy, laryngectomy can be considered, as this was the treatment for patients on the VA Laryngeal Cancer Study who progressed on induction chemotherapy [54]. However, the use of induction chemotherapy was a source of disagreement for NCCN panel members, leading to its receipt of a category 2B ("based on lower-level evidence, there is NCCN consensus that the intervention is appropriate") or 3 ("based on any level of evidence, there is major NCCN disagreement that the intervention is appropriate") recommendation, depending on the setting [25].

Patients with T4 laryngeal squamous cell cancer are usually advised total laryngectomy and lymph node dissection with or without PORT [63, 64]. Approximately 25% of the patients included in the VA Laryngeal Cancer Study had T4 cancers, and these patients were found to have unacceptably high rates of failure. Of the T4 patients randomized to the nonsurgical arm and treated with induction chemotherapy, 56% required salvage laryngectomy [54]. Based on these results, patients with bulky cancers involving >1 cm of the base of tongue or extending completely through the thyroid cartilage were excluded from RTOG 91-11 [55]. Several retrospective series and recent SEER analyses have confirmed the benefit of PORT for patients with T4 disease, especially in node-positive patients, so PORT is now standard for larynx cancer patients with intermediate to high-risk clinical, surgical, or pathologic factors [65, 66]. PORT is given to a dose of 60 Gy in 2 Gy daily fractions and is delivered to the entire postoperative bed as well as the bilateral neck lymph nodes. Positive surgical margins and lymph nodes with extracapsular extension are indications to give postoperative CRT [67, 68]. Figure 14.3 shows the radiation treatment plan for a patient who was treated with postoperative CRT after total laryngectomy.

There is emerging interest in considering definitive CRT for patients with T4 tumors who either are not medically fit for, or who decline surgery. LC for these nonsurgical patients has been reported from 56 to 82% with CRT [69–72]. Although LC is certainly lower than in surgical series, some patients and practitioners are willing to take this risk in favor of the possibility of organ preservation. Induction chemotherapy is often utilized in this setting as well [25]. However, patients must be chosen appropriately, as it is recognized that patients with T4 laryngeal cancers may initially present with an impaired airway or impaired airway protection, loss of laryngeal sensation or impaired swallowing function [73, 74]. Function will generally worsen after RT so this strategy is ill-advised in patients with any evidence of impaired laryngeal operation on presentation as radical efforts taken to preserve an "ornamental" larynx that does not protect the airway are foolhardy [75, 76]. Furthermore, salvage rates for T4 RT failures are poor, as opposed to T3, so many patients are at increased risk for demise with uncontrolled cancer in the neck.

Follow-Up and Survivorship

After completion of therapy, patients are monitored for disease recurrence and functionality as well as for treatment-related toxicities and second primaries [77]. One common follow-up schedule includes history, physical examination, and fiberoptic examination every 3–4 months for the first 2 years, every 6 months for the third to fifth years and annually after 5 years. Thyroid-stimulating hormone levels should be obtained every 6 months in patients who received radiation and thyroid supplementation

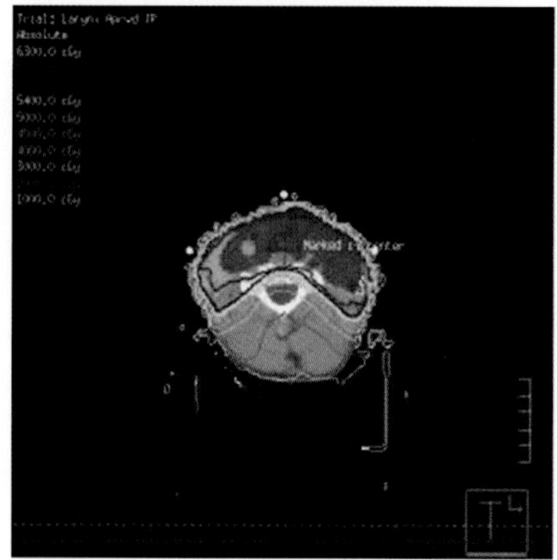
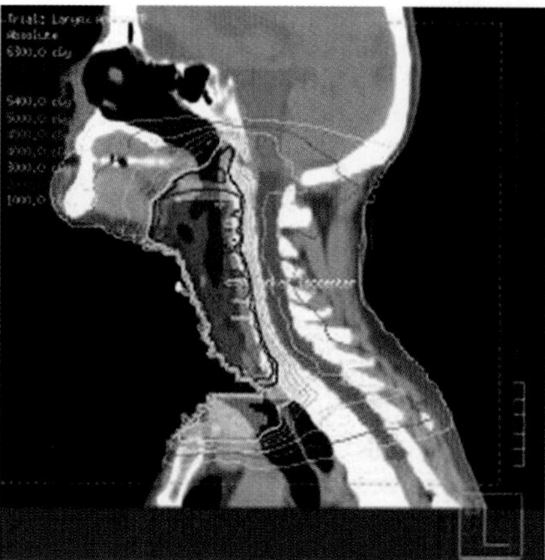
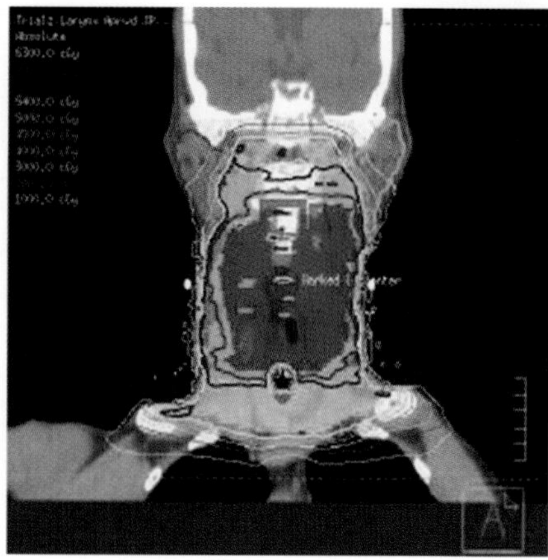

Figure 14.3 Radiation treatment planning images for a patient with advanced stage squamous cell carcinoma of the larynx after surgery (total laryngectomy) treated with postoperative radiation to a total dose of 60 Gy in 30 fractions and concurrent cisplatin chemotherapy.

given for clinically hypothyroid patients. Chest imaging can be considered for patients who develop new symptoms, or for patients with a significant smoking history who meet criteria for CT screening for lung cancer (see Chapter 11 in *The American Cancer Society's Principles of Oncology: Prevention to Survivorship*). Speech and swallowing therapy should be continued during the follow-up period, including assessment of functional oropharyngeal swallow and sensate airway protection. Post-treatment imaging may be obtained at the first follow-up, depending on the initial stage of the cancer. The NCCN recommends no further imaging after initial restaging for patients without worrisome signs or symptoms [25]. However, surveillance imaging should customized to the individual. For example, laryngeal cancer patients treated for node-positive disease may benefit from more intensive imaging follow-up. Most local recurrences occur within the first 2 years. However, patients with laryngeal cancer also have a high risk of developing a second primary cancer of the upper aerodigestive tract, particularly those patients with a history of heavy tobacco use. One large, pooled cancer registry study showed laryngeal cancer patients developed a second primary cancer at a rate of approximately 1–3% per year [78].

References

1 Seigel RL, Miller KD, Jemal A. Cancer Statistics, 2017. *CA Cancer J Clin* 2017;67(1):7–30.

2 Tamarit Conejeros JM, Carrasco Llatas M, Estelles Ferriol E, *et al.* Supraglottic and glottis carcinomas. Study of the incidence in the last 31 years. *Acta Otorrinolaringol Esp* 2007;58:449–53.

3 Virtaniemi JA, Hirvikoski PP, Kumpulainen EJ, *et al.* Is the subsite distribution of laryngeal cancer related to smoking habits? *Acta Oncol* 2000;39:77–9.

4 Howlader N, Noone AM, Krapcho M, *et al.* (eds) SEER Cancer Statistics Review, 1975–2011, National Cancer Institute, Bethesda, MD. http://seer.cancer.gov/csr/1975_2011/, based on November 2013 SEER data submission, posted to the SEER web site, April 2014. http://seer.cancer.gov/csr/1975_2011/results_merged/sect_12_larynx.pdf

5 Simard EP, Torre LA, Jemal A. International trends in head and neck cancer incidence rates: differences by country, sex and anatomic site. *Oral Oncol* 2014;50:387–403.

6 Johnson-Obaseki S, McDonald JT, Corsten M, *et al.* Head and neck cancer in Canada: trends 1992–2007. *Otolaryngol Head Neck Surg* 2012;147:74–8.

7 Hofman HT, Porter K, Karnell LH, *et al.* Laryngeal cancer in the United States: changes in demographics, patterns of care and survival. *Laryngoscope* 2006;116(9 Pt 2 Suppl 111):1–13.

8 van Dijk BA, Karim-Kos HE, Coebergh JW, *et al.* Progress against laryngeal cancer in The Netherlands between 1989 and 2010. *Int J Cancer* 2014;134:674–81.

9 Islami F, Tramacere I, Rota M, *et al.* Alcohol drinking and laryngeal cancer: overall and dose-risk relation – a systematic review and meta-analysis. *Oral Oncol* 2010;46(11):802–10.

10 Moura MA, Bergmann A, Aguiar SS, *et al.* The magnitude of the association between smoking and the risk of developing cancer in Brazil: a multicenter study. *BMJ Open* 2014;4(2):e003736.

11 Coca-Pelaz A, Rodrigo JP, Takes RP, *et al.* Relationship between reflux and laryngeal cancer. *Head Neck* 2013;35:1814–18.

12 Brown T, Darnton A, Fortunato L, *et al.* Occupational cancer in Britain. *Br J Cancer* 2012;107 Suppl 1:S56–70.

13 Cahlon O, Lee N, Le QT, *et al.* Cancer of the larynx. In: RT Hoppe, TL Phillips, M Roach III (eds) *Leibel and Phillips Textbook of Radiation Oncology*, 3rd edn. Philadelphia: Elsevier Saunders, 2010:642.

14 Anantharaman D, Gheit T, Waterboer T, *et al.* Human papillomavirus infections and upper aero-digestive tract cancers: the ARCAGE study. *J Natl Cancer Inst* 2013;105(8):536–45.

15 Gama RR, Carvalho AL, Filho AL, *et al.* Detection of human papillomavirus in laryngeal squamous cell carcinoma: systematic review and meta-analysis. *Laryngoscope* 2016;126:885–93.

16 Kreimer AR, Clifford GM, Boyle P, *et al.* Human papillomavirus types in head and neck squamous cell

carcinomas worldwide: a systematic review. *Cancer Epidemiol Biomarkers Prev* 2005;14:467–75.

17 Lewin F, Novell SE, Johansson H, *et al.* Smoking tobacco, oral snuff, and alcohol in the etiology of squamous cell carcinoma of the head and neck: a population based case-referent study in Sweden. *Cancer* 1998;82:1367–75.

18 Bouquot JE, Gnepp DR. Laryngeal precancer: a review of the literature, commentary, and comparison with oral leukoplakia. *Head Neck* 1991;13:488–97.

19 Mehanna H, Paleri V, Robson A, *et al.* Consensus statement by otorhinolaryngologists and pathologists on the diagnosis and management of laryngeal dysplasia. *Clin Otolaryngol* 2010;35:170–6.

20 Kraus FT, Perez-Mesa C. Verrucous carcinoma: clinical and pathologic study of 105 cases involving oral cavity, larynx, and genitalia. *Cancer* 1966;19:26–38.

21 Ryan RE Jr., DeSanto LW, Devine KD, *et al.* Verrucous carcinoma of the larynx. *Laryngoscope* 1977;87:1989–94.

22 Lindberg R. Distribution of cervical lymph node metastases from squamous cell carcinoma of the upper respiratory and digestive tracts. *Cancer* 1972;29:1446–9.

23 McGavran M, Bauer W, Ogura J. The incidence of cervical lymph node metastasis from epidermoid carcinoma of the larynx and their relationship to certain characteristics of the primary tumor. A study based on the clinical and pathological findings for 96 patients treated by primary en bloc laryngectomy and radical neck dissection. *Cancer* 1961;14:66.

24 Lv Y, Zheng H, Wang Q, *et al.* Value of (18)F-FDG PET/CT in the diagnosis of laryngeal carcinoma. *Nan Fang Yi Ke Da Xue Xue Bao* 2012;32:1486–90.

25 NCCN Clinical Practice Guidelines in Oncology: Cancer of the Glottic Larynx. Version 2.2016. October 11, 2016. Nccn.org. Accessed January 11, 2016.

26 Amin MB, Edge SB, Greene FL, *et al.* (eds) *AJCC Cancer Staging Manual*, 8th edn. New York: Springer Nature, 2017.

27 Shah JP, Karnell LH, Hoffman HT, *et al.* Patterns of care for cancer of the larynx in the United States. *Arch Otolaryngol Head Neck Surg* 1997;123:475–83.

28 Groome PA, O'Sullivan B, Irish JC, *et al.* Canada and the SEER areas of the United States: do different management philosophies produce different outcome profiles? *J Clin Epidemiol* 2001;54:301–15.

29 Mendenhall WM, Werning JW, Hinerman RW, *et al.* Management of T1-T2 glottic carcinomas. *Cancer* 2004;100:1786–92.

30 Smee R, Bridger GP, Williams J, *et al.* Early glottic carcinoma: results of treatment by radiotherapy. *Austr Radiol* 2000;44:53–9.

31 Loughran S, Calder N, MacGregor FB, *et al.* Quality of life and voice following endoscopic resection or radiotherapy for early glottic cancer. *Clin Otolaryngol* 2005;30:42–7.

32 Mendelsohn AH, Matar N, Bachy V, Lawson G, Remacle M. Longitudinal voice outcomes following advanced CO2 laser cordectomy for glottic cancer. *J Voice* 2015;29:772–5.

33 Dey P, Arnold D, Wight R, *et al.* Radiotherapy versus open surgery versus endolaryngeal surgery (with or without laser) for early laryngeal squamous cell carcinoma. *Cochrane Database Syst Rev 2002*;2:CD002027, updated 2010.

34 Spector JG, Sessions DG, Chao KS, *et al.* Stage I (T1 N0 M0) squamous cell carcinoma of the laryngeal glottis: therapeutic results and voice preservation. *Head Neck* 1999;21:707–17.

35 Weiss BG, Ihler F, Pilavakis Y, *et al.* Transoral laser microsurgery for T1b glottic cancer: review of 51 cases. *Eur Arch Otorhinolaryngol* 2016;27(4):1997–2004.

36 Stephenson KA, Fagan JJ. Transoral laser resection of glottic carcinoma: what is the significance of anterior commissure involvement? *J Laryngol Otol* 2017;131(2):168–72.

37 Yamazaki H, Nishiyama K, Tanaka E, *et al.* Radiotherapy for early glottis carcinoma (T1N0M0): results of prospective randomized study of radiation fraction size and overall treatment time. *Int J Radiat Oncol Biol Phys* 2006;64:77–82.

38 Frata P, Cellai E, Magrini SM, *et al.* Radical radiotherapy for early glottis cancer: results in a series of 1087 patients from two Italian radiation oncology centers. II. The case of T2N0 disease. *Int J Radiat Oncol Biol Phys* 2005;63:1387–94.

39 Garden AS, Forster K, Wong PF, *et al.* Results of radiotherapy for T2N0 glottic carcinoma: does the "2" stand for twice-daily treatment? *Int J Radiat Oncol Biol Phys* 2003;55:322–8.

40 Trotti A, Pajak T, Emami B, *et al.* A randomized trial of hyperfractionation versus standard fractionation in T2 squamous cell carcinoma of the vocal cord. *Int J Radiat Oncol Biol Phys* 2006;66:S15.

41 Trotti A 3rd, Zhang Q, Bentzen SM, *et al.* Randomized trial of hyperfractionation versus conventional fractionation in T2 squamous cell carcinoma of the vocal cord (RTOG 9512). *Int J Radiat Oncol Biol Phys* 2014;89:958–63.

42 Preuss SF, Cramer K, Klussmann JP, *et al.* Transoral laser surgery for laryngeal cancer: outcome, complications, and prognostic factors in 275 patients. *Eur J Surg Oncol* 2008;35:235–40

43 Cabanillas R, *et al.* Oncologic outcomes of transoral laser surgery of supraglottic carcinoma compared with a transcervical approach. *Head Neck* 2008;30:750–5.

44 Orus C, Leon X, Vega M, *et al.* Initial treatment of early stages (I,II) of supraglottic squamous cell carcinoma: partial laryngectomy versus radiotherapy. *Eur Arch Otorhinolaryngol* 2000;257:512–16.

45 Ang KK, Garden AS. Larynx. In: KK Ang, AS Garden (eds) *Radiotherapy for Head and Neck Cancers: Indications and Techniques*, 4th edn. Philadelphia: Wolters Kluwer/Lippincott Williams & Wilkins, 2012:151–3.

46 Suzuki G, Yamazaki H, Ogo E, *et al.* Multimodal treatment for t1-2 supraglottic cancer: the impact of tumor location. *Anticancer Res* 2014;34:203–7.

47 Dahm JD, Sessions DG, Paniello RC, *et al.* Primary subglottic cancer. *Laryngoscope* 1998;108:741–6.

48 Santoro R, Turelli M, Polli G. Primary carcinoma of the subglottic larynx. *Eur Arch Otorhinolaryngol* 2000;257:548–51.

49 Smee RI, Williams JR, Bridger GP. The management dilemmas of invasive subglottic carcinoma. *Clin Oncol (R Coll Radiol)* 2008;20:751–6.

50 Paisley S, *et al.* Results of radiotherapy for primary subglottic squamous cell carcinoma. *Int J Radiat Oncol Biol Phys* 2002;52:1245–50.

51 Warde P, Harwood A, Keane T. Carcinoma of the subglottis: results of initial radical radiation. *Arch Otolaryngol Head Neck* 1987;44:755–65.

52 Hata M, Taguchi T, Koike I, *et al.* Efficacy and toxicity of (chemo)radiotherapy for primary subglottic cancer. *Strahlenther Onkol* 2013;189:26–32.

53 Spector GJ, *et al.* Management of stage IV glottic carcinoma: therapeutic outcomes. *Laryngoscope* 2004;114:1438–46.

54 The Department of Veterans Affairs Laryngeal Study Group. Induction chemotherapy plus radiation compared with surgery plus radiation in patients with advanced laryngeal cancer. *N Engl J Med* 1991;324:1685–90.

55 Forastiere AA, Goepfert H, Maor M, *et al.* Concurrent chemotherapy and radiotherapy for organ preservation in advanced laryngeal cancer. *N Engl J Med* 2003;349:2091–8.

56 Forastiere AA, Zhang Q, Weber RS, *et al.* Long-term results of RTOG 91-11: a comparison of three nonsurgical treatment strategies to preserve the larynx in patients with locally advanced larynx cancer. *J Clin Oncol* 2013;31:845–52.

57 Bonner J, Giralt J, Harari P, *et al.* Cetuximab and radiotherapy in laryngeal preservation for cancers of the larynx and hypopharynx: a secondary analysis of a randomized clinical trial. *JAMA Otolaryngol Head Neck Surg* 2016;142:842–9.

58 Saba NF, Shin DM. The challenges of laryngeal preservation – is it the systemic agent or the proper sequence of therapy? *JAMA Otolaryngol Head Neck Surg* 2016;142:849–50.

59 Magrini SM, Buglione M, Corvo R, *et al.* Cetuximab and radiotherapy versus cisplatin and radiotherapy for locally advanced head and neck cancer: a randomized phase II trial. *J Clin Oncol* 2016;34:427–35.

60 Posner MR, Hershock DM, Blajman CR, *et al.* Cisplatin and fluorouracil alone or with docetaxel in head and neck cancer. *N Engl J Med* 2007;357:1705–15.

61 Pointreau Y, Garaud P, Chapet S, *et al.* Randomized trial of induction chemotherapy with cisplatin and 5-fluorouracil with or without docetaxel for larynx preservation. *J Natl Cancer Inst* 2009;101:489–506.

62 Mesia R, Garcia-Saenz JA, Lozano A, *et al.* Could the addition of cetuximab to conventional radiation therapy improve organ preservation in those patients with locally advanced larynx cancer who respond to induction chemotherapy? An Organ Preservation Spanish Head and Neck Cancer Cooperative Group Phase 2 Study. *Int J Radiat Oncol Biol Phys* 2016;97(3):473–80.

63 Jesse RH. The evaluation of treatment of patients with extensive squamous cancer of the vocal cords. *Laryngoscope* 1975;85:1424–9.

64 Grover S, Swisher-McClure S, Mitra N, *et al.* Total laryngectomy versus larynx preservation for T4a larynx cancer: patterns of care and survival outcomes. *Int J Radiat Oncol Biol Phys* 2015;92:594–601.

65 Kao J, Lavaf A, Teng MS, *et al.* Adjuvant radiotherapy and survival for patients with node-positive head and neck cancer: an analysis by primary site and nodal stage. *Int J Radiat Oncol Biol Phys* 2008;71:362–70.

66 Groome PA, O'Sullivan B, Irish JC, *et al.* Management and outcome differences in supraglottic cancer between Ontario, Canada, and the Surveillance, Epidemiology, and End Results areas of the United States. *J Clin Oncol* 2003;21:496–505.

67 Bernier J, Domenge C, Ozshin M, *et al.* Postoperative irradiation with or without concomitant chemotherapy for locally advanced head and neck cancer. *N Engl J Med* 2004;350:1945–52.

68 Cooper JS, Pajak TF, Forastiere AA, *et al.* Postoperative concurrent radiotherapy and Chemotherapy for high-risk squamous-cell carcinoma of the head and neck. *N Engl Med.* 2004;350:1937–44.

69 Harwood AR, Rawlinson E. The quality of life of patients following treatment for laryngeal cancer. *Int J Radiat Oncol Biol Phys* 1983;9:335–8.

70 Hinerman RW, Mendenhall WM, Morris CG, *et al.* T3 and T4 true vocal cord squamous carcinomas treated with external beam irradiation: a single institution's 35 year experience. *Am J Clin Oncol* 2007;30:181–5.

71 Knab BR, Salama JK, Solanki A, *et al.* Functional organ preservation with definitive chemoradiotherapy for T4 laryngeal squamous cell carcinoma. *Ann Oncol* 2008;19:1650–4.

72 Worden FP, Moyer J, Lee JS, *et al.* Chemoselection as a strategy for organ preservation in patients with T4 laryngeal squamous cell carcinoma with cartilage invasion. *Laryngoscope* 2009;119:1510–17.

73 Aviv JE, Liu H, Parides M, *et al.* Laryngopharyngeal sensory deficits in patients with laryngopharyngeal reflux and dysphagia. *Ann Otol Rhinol Laryngol* 2000;109:1000–6.

74 Aviv JE, Spitzer J, Cohen M, *et al.* Laryngeal adductor reflex and pharyngeal squeeze as predictors of laryngeal penetration and aspiration. *Laryngoscope* 2002;112:338–41.

75 Agarwal J, Dutta D, Palwe V, *et al.* Prospective subjective evaluation of swallowing function and dietary pattern in head and neck cancers treated with concomitant chemo-radiation. *J Cancer Res Ther* 2010;6(1):15–21.

76 Pauloski BR, Rademaker AW, Logemann JA, *et al.* Speech and swallowing in irradiated and nonirradiated postsurgical oral cancer patients. *Otolaryngol Head Neck Surg* 1998;118:616–24.

77 Cohen EE, LaMonte SJ, Erb NL, *et al.* American Cancer Society Head and Neck Cancer Survivorship Care Guideline. *CA Cancer J Clin* 2016;66(3):203–39.

78 Chuang SC, Scelo G, Tonita JM, *et al.* Risk of second primary cancer among patients with head and neck cancers: a pooled analysis of 13 cancer registries. *Int J Cancer* 2008;123:2390–6.

15

Nasal and Paranasal Sinus Cancer

Emma B. Holliday, Michael E. Kupferman, Clifton D. Fuller, and Ehab Hanna

The University of Texas MD Anderson Cancer Center, Houston, Texas, USA

Incidence and Mortality

Cancers of the paranasal sinuses and nasal cavity account for approximately 3% of all head and neck malignancies, and fewer than 0.5% of all human malignancies. Their estimated incidence rate in the United States is 0.556 cases per 100,000 population per year [1]. Sinonasal cancers are comprised of several different histologies and specific anatomic sites. Over 50% of sinonasal cancers are squamous cell carcinomas (SCC), with adenocarcinoma as the second most common histology, and adenoid cystic carcinoma (ACC), esthesioneuroblastoma (ENB), mucosal melanoma (MM) and lymphoma more rarely seen. The most common sites of disease are the nasal cavity and the maxillary sinus. A recent population-based study spanning the 1970s to the 2000s showed that the incidence of sinonasal cancer has remained relatively stable [1].

Unfortunately, most patients with sinonasal cancers present with late stage disease due to the ability of these tumors to grow silently for many years in sinus cavities without causing symptoms. The mortality from sinonasal cancers is roughly half the incidence [2]. The prognosis of patients with sinonasal tumors is relatively poor, with published 5-year survival ranging from 22 to 67% in single institution series, though the wide range of survival is likely a reflection of the varied natural histories of the different histologies [3–6].

Etiology and Risk Factors

Sinonasal cancers are second only to mesothelioma in the proportion of cases associated with occupational exposure [7]. The World Health Organization's International Agency for Research on Cancer classifies seven environmental and/or occupational agents, mixtures, and exposure circumstances as having sufficient evidence of nasal and paranasal sinus carcinogenicity (isopropyl alcohol production, leather dust, nickel compounds, radium-226 and its decay products, radium-228 and its decay products, tobacco smoking, and wood dust) and also classifies four as having limited evidence (carpentry and joinery, chromium (VI) compounds, formaldehyde, and textile manufacturing) [8]. There is interest in the possible etiologic role of the human papillomavirus (HPV) in cancers of the nasal cavity and paranasal sinuses, and a meta-analysis of studies published reported that 27% of cases tested positive for a marker of HPV infection [9]. Recent reviews note that HPV-positive sinonasal carcinomas tend to have a nonkeratinizing morphology and that the presence of transcriptionally-active HPV suggests biological relevance [10, 11].

Pathology

Several distinct histologic entities can arise in the nasal cavity and paranasal sinuses. SCC is the most common malignancy in this location, accounting for over 50% of all tumors. Adenocarcinoma is the second most common sinonasal histology overall [1]. Other subtypes include lymphoepithelial carcinoma, sinonasal undifferentiated carcinoma (SNUC), neuroendocrine tumors, including carcinoid and small cell carcinoma, and salivary gland-type carcinomas [12, 13]. Included in salivary gland-type carcinomas are ACC, acinic cell carcinoma, mucoepidermoid carcinoma, epithelial–myoepithelial cell carcinoma, clear cell carcinoma, carcinoma ex pleomorphic adenoma, and polymorphous low-grade adenocarcinoma [13].

ACC accounts for 15% of sinonasal cancers [1]. The three histological subtypes described, ranging from least to most aggressive, are: tubular, cribriform, and solid, although many tumors are comprised of a combination of each of these. These tumors are notorious for exhibiting perineural invasion along both named and unnamed nerves, and intracranial spread via branches of V_2 and V_3 is not uncommon. While ACC has a slow-growth pattern and is often amenable to surgical resection when perineural invasion is absent, distant metastasis may develop in as many as 40% of patients, and recurrences 10 years

The American Cancer Society's Oncology in Practice: Clinical Management, First Edition. Edited by The American Cancer Society.

after initial therapy are not uncommon. Lymphatic spread occurs in 10–25% of patients. However, 5-year overall survival can be as high as 40–60% [14]. ENB arise from the olfactory neuroepithelium and have unique biological and clinical behavior. These lesions are locally aggressive with a propensity for skull base invasion. MM accounts for 6% of head and neck melanomas and occurs primarily in the oral cavity and nasal cavity. Intranasally, the lesions appear pigmented and polypoid and are friable. The biological behavior of MM is characterized by locoregional recurrence and distant metastasis. Even though surgery, in combination with postoperative radiation, can give local control as high as 85%, most patients ultimately fail distantly and long-term survival is rare [15, 16].

One of the most aggressive neoplasms of the paranasal sinuses is SNUC. Extension beyond the confines of the paranasal sinuses is common, with intracranial, cranial nerve, and orbital involvement frequently evident on presentation. Local failure and distant metastasis occurs in approximately 23% and 25% of patients, respectively, and overall survival at 5 years was 65% in a series of 16 cases from a single academic center [17]. However, the 5-year survival rate was 42.2% among 460 patient records entered into the National Cancer Database from 2005 to 2013 [18]. It is imperative that these tumors be distinguished histologically from other "small round blue-cell tumors" of the sinuses that are treated differently, such as small cell neuroendocrine carcinoma, rhabdomyosarcoma, T-cell lymphoma and MM.

Diagnosis

Upon suspicion of a sinonasal cancer, the patient should undergo a thorough history and physical examination [19]. Common presenting symptoms often include sinus pressure or nasal obstruction, epistaxis or nasal discharge, headaches, facial swelling, or facial pain. Complaints of blurred vision, diplopia, parasthesias or hypesthesias along the branches of the trigeminal nerve should prompt further investigation into possible base of skull involvement. Although a full physical examination is prudent, a careful rigid or flexible nasal endoscopy can be particularly helpful in assessing the extent of disease as well as obtaining biopsy when the histological diagnosis is in doubt. In-office biopsy should be avoided prior to formal axial and coronal imaging and should also be avoided when the superior margin of the tumor cannot be visualized as it risks a cerebrospinal leak or uncontrolled epistaxis that can be difficult to control in the clinic setting.

Complete imaging of the head and neck, either with a contrast computed tomography (CT) or magnetic resonance imaging (MRI), is necessary to adequately stage all sinonasal malignancies [19]. Often both are obtained for pretreatment planning as CT better identifies bony invasion, neural foramina widening, and involved lymph nodes, while MRI better identifies soft tissue, dural, and perineural invasion [20]. An example of MRI images from a patient with T4N0 ENB can be seen in Figure 15.1. Chest imaging can be obtained if clinically indicated, such as in cases of respiratory symptoms, high burden of nodal disease, or ACC histology, which has a higher propensity for metastatic disease. Positron emission tomography-CT scan is often ordered for patients with advanced disease. If a biopsy cannot be safely obtained in the office setting, a biopsy under the appropriate image-guidance should be scheduled. The transnasal route is preferred, and canine fossa puncture or Caldwell–Luc approach should be avoided. Finally, as head and neck cancers are best managed in the multidisciplinary setting, referrals should be made to surgical oncology, radiation oncology, medical oncology, as well as dental, nutrition, and ophthalmologic specialists, depending on the location, histology, and extent of disease.

Staging

The most widely used staging system for sinonasal cancers is the tumor-node-metastasis (TNM) system of the American Joint Committee on Cancer and Union of International Cancer Control [21]. There is a different staging system for tumors of the maxillary sinus from that used for ethmoid sinus and nasal cavity tumors. The nodal staging system for maxillary, ethmoid, and nasal cavity tumors is the same as for other sites in the head

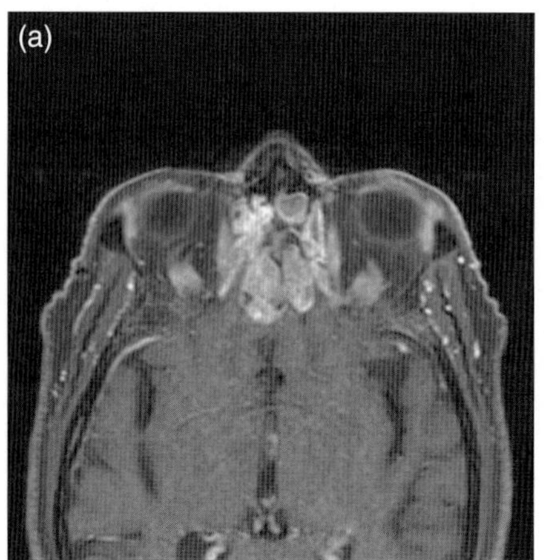

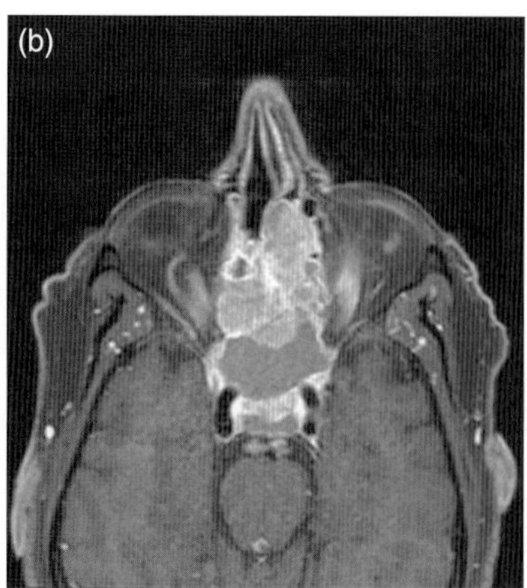

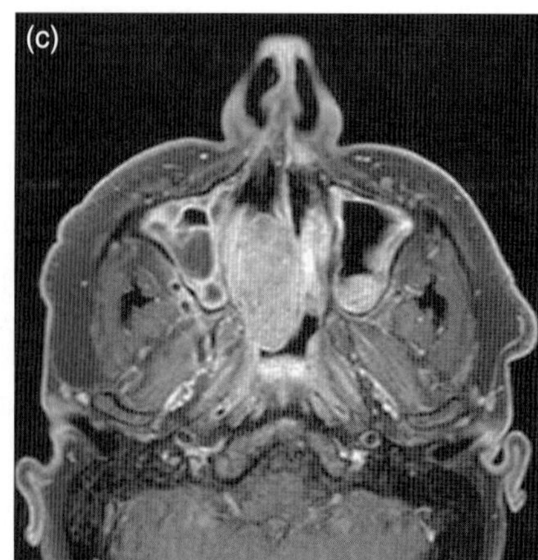

Figure 15.1 (a–c) Representative axial images from a T1-weighted MRI with contrast from a patient with a T4N0 esthesioneuroblastoma measuring 6.5 cm filling the posterior right nasal cavity from the palate to the cribiform plate extending through the sphenopalatine foramen into the medial aspect of the right pterygopapatine fossa, encroaching the right posterior medial orbit, extending to the left sphenoid sinus, and including an intracranial component. There was no lateral retropharyngeal or cervical lymphadnopathy.

and neck, and depends on the number, size, and laterality of involved lymph nodes. ENB have their own staging system called the Kadish–Morita Staging System [22]. The classification from the most recent American Joint Committee on Cancer version, 8th edition [21], is shown in Table 15.1.

Treatment

Surgical resection remains the cornerstone of curative treatment for squamous cell carcinomas and minor salivary gland malignancies of the nasal cavity and paranasal sinuses. Early stage tumors are sometimes diagnosed incidentally upon pathologic evaluation of a polypectomy or other procedure for a presumed benign process. If a nononcologic procedure is performed prior to pathologic diagnosis, a re-excision should be attempted, because confirmation of T1 category can obviate the need for postoperative radiation. However, adjuvant radiation is indicated for T2–T4a tumors for the purpose of improving local control [23–27]. Systemic therapy should be included for patients with ENB, MM, and SNUC [28–39]. The role of chemotherapy for SCC is an emerging question [40, 41]. Definitive chemoradiation or radiation alone is recommended for T4b, nonmetastatic patients, and also for patients who are medically or otherwise inoperable [19, 42]. Surgical salvage may be necessary for residual or recurrent disease, if feasible, and 5-year overall survival rates after salvage surgery in this setting have been reported to be approximately 30% [43]. However, as the rarity and heterogeneity of sinonasal malignancies preclude large, randomized controlled trials, most of the published data that inform our current standards of care come from retrospective reviews that include patients treated over long periods of time during which imaging, surgery, radiotherapy, and chemotherapy techniques have changed.

Surgical Management of the Primary Tumor

The preferred surgical approach typically depends on the location of the tumor. Centrally located tumors are most easily accessed by a lateral rhinotomy incision, which can be extended onto the infraorbital rim (Weber–Ferguson incision) or the supraorbital rim (Lynch incision) for extended access to the maxillary sinus, frontal sinus, orbit, and central skull base [44, 45]. Laterally located tumors are best resected with a medial maxillectomy, while tumors of the inferior maxillary sinus are best resected with an infrastructure maxillectomy. Craniofacial resection is necessary for tumors that involve the cribriform plate, and an orbital exenteration is included when there is frank invasion of the orbital periosteum and fat, extraocular musculature, or the globe itself [44, 45].

Endoscopic resections can allow for magnified visualization of the anatomy which has led to increasing interest in this approach. The efficacy and safety of endoscopic resections are currently under investigation by various groups, as it has been shown to have better quality of life [46] and faster recovery time [47]. Transnasal endoscopic resection has been suggested to be a reasonable alternative to craniofacial resection for T1–T2 sinonasal malignancies in a recent meta-analysis with similar 5-year locoregional control, disease-specific survival, and overall

Table 15.1 Classification of sinonasal cancer.

Primary tumor (T-category)		
Maxillary sinus	T1	Limited to the maxillary sinus mucosa with no erosion or bone destruction
	T2	Bone erosion/destruction including hard palate, middle nasal meatus, except for posterior wall of maxillary sinus and pterygoid plates
	T3	Invasion of bone of posterior wall of maxillary sinus, subcutaneous tissues, floor or medial wall or orbit, pterygoid fossa, ethmoid sinuses
	T4a	Invasion of anterior orbital contents, skin of cheek, pterygoid plates, infratemporal fossa, cribiform plate, sphenoid or frontal sinuses
	T4b	Invasion of orbital apex, dura, brain, middle cranial fossa, nasopharynx, clivus, or cranial nerves except for V2.
Nasal cavity and ethmoid sinus	T1	Limited to any one subsite, with or without bony invasion
	T2	Invasion into two subsites in a single region or extending to adjacent region in the nasoethmoidal complex, with or without bony invasion
	T3	Invasion of medial wall or floor of orbit, maxillary sinus, palate or cribiform plate
	T4a	Invasion into anterior orbital contents, skin of nose or cheek, minimal extension into anterior cranial fossa, pterygoid plates, sphenoid or frontal sinuses
	T4b	Invasion into orbital apex, dura, brain, middle cranial fossa, nasopharynx, clivus, or cranial nerves other than V2.
Olfactory esthesio-neuroblastoma	T1	Tumor isolated to nasal cavity and ethmoid sinuses
	T2	Tumor extends to sphenoid sinus or cribiform plate
	T3	Tumor extends to anterior cranial fossa or orbit, no dural invasion
	T4	Tumor invades dura or brain parenchyma
Regional lymph nodes (N-category)[1]		
	N0	No regional lymph node metastasis
	N1	Metastasis in a single ipsilateral lymph node, ≤3cm in greatest dimension
	N2a	Metastasis in a single ipsilateral lymph node, >3cm and ≤6cm
	N2b	Metastasis in multiple ipsilateral lymph nodes, none >6cm
	N2c	Metastasis in bilateral or contralateral lymph nodes, none >6cm
	N3	Metastasis in a lymph node >6cm
Distant metastatic disease (M-category)[2]		
	M0	No distant metastasis
	M1	Distant metastasis present

Source: AJCC 8th edn (2017). Used with permission of the American College of Surgeons, Chicago, Illinois. The original source for this information is the AJCC Cancer Staging Manual, 8th edn (2017), which is published by Springer Science+Business Media.

[1] Definitions apply to all subsites except for olfactory esthesioneuroblastoma which uses a N0 versus N1 system for positive and negative nodal metastases, respectively.

[2] Definitions apply to all subsites.

survival [48]. Figure 15.2 depicts clinical endoscopic and CT imaging pre- and postoperatively for a patient with T4N0 esthesioneuroblastoma who underwent endoscopic resection.

Although patients with certain histologies such as ACC or MM are at increased risk for distant failure, the overall predominant pattern of failure for patients with sinonasal malignancies is local failure [3, 15, 17]. The best established risk factors for recurrence after surgical resection are advanced T-category, involved lymph nodes, aggressive histologic type, suprastructural location, and positive surgical margins [3, 6, 43, 49]. Published series that included all histologies and stages of disease report 5-year local control, disease-free, and overall survival rates to all be approximately 50% [3].

Management of the Neck

The lymphatic drainage of the paranasal sinuses and nasal cavity includes levels I–III as well as the retropharyngeal nodes. Patients with tumors in the sinonasal region are at risk for lymphatic spread due to the rich vascular network in this area. Approximately 10–20% of patients present with clinically involved lymph nodes [42], although this percentage varies by histology [50, 51].

Thus, elective regional lymph node dissections remain controversial due to the risk of overtreatment of the many patients without lymph node metastases. Currently, elective neck dissection is generally not advocated for early-stage lesions. However, patients with T3 or T4 lesions have a greater risk for the development of cervical metastasis during the course of disease, and thus elective neck dissection should be considered [19]. There is some interest in adopting a strategy employing a sentinel lymph node biopsy for patients with sinonasal malignancies, but this is still considered investigational [52, 53].

Radiation Therapy

The main role of radiation therapy in the treatment of sinonasal malignancies is in the postoperative setting in the case of T1–T4a disease [19]. However, there has been some recent interest in treatment strategies either involving a function-preserving/debulking surgery followed by either external beam radiation therapy [23] or brachytherapy [54] in order to avoid a particularly morbid or disfiguring operation. Additionally, radiation can be used as definitive local therapy for cases of T4b disease or less advanced disease in medically inoperable patients.

Early retrospective studies showed that the addition of postoperative radiation therapy improved local control [25, 27, 55, 56]. Doses of 60 Gy are commonly considered adequate for postoperative cases with gross total resection. Total doses of 63–70 Gy are more commonly given in cases of positive margins or gross residual disease. Earlier techniques used to deliver radiation therapy resulted in the exposure of surrounding tissues, such as the brainstem, pituitary gland, and optic structures, to high doses of radiation. The brainstem and the majority of the optic structures are typically thought to be able to tolerate only 54 Gy at standard fractionation [57], which makes safe delivery of meaningful doses challenging. Complications of radiotherapy to the paranasal sinuses and orbit include: optic neuritis, cataracts, blindness, skull base osteoradionecrosis, temporal and frontal lobe necrosis, pan-hypopituitarism, carotid artery stenosis, and spinal cord necrosis. Although protecting adjacent normal tissues from radiation is an important goal, it is one that must be balanced with adequate tumor coverage [58].

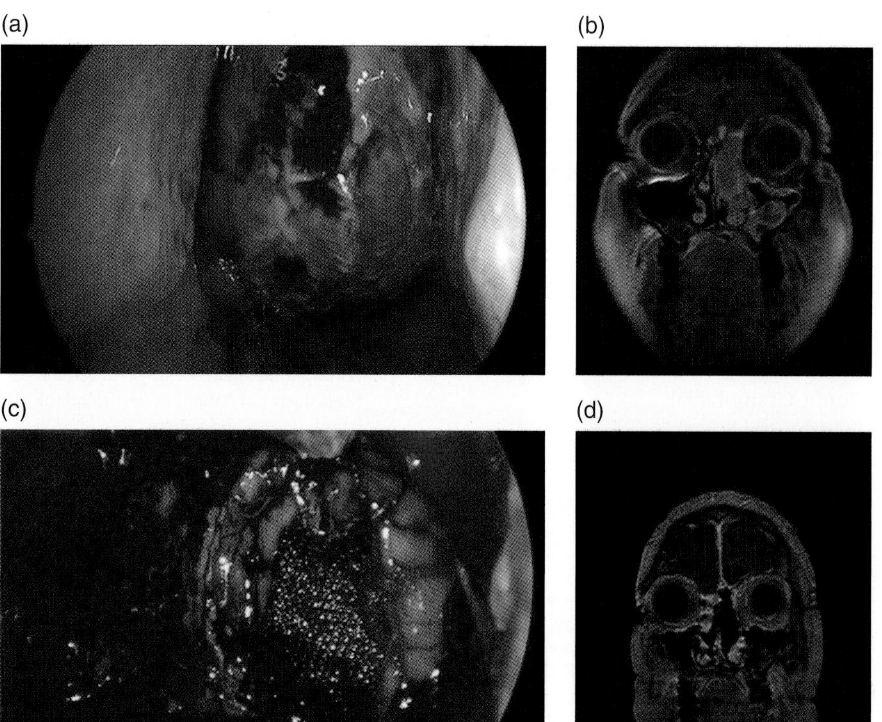

Figure 15.2 These are preoperative (a) and (b) and postoperative (c) and (d) gross intraoperative (a) and (c) and coronal CT images (b) and (d) for a patient with a T4N0 esthesioneuroblastoma. He received endoscopic resection followed by postoperative radiation therapy. He was found to be disease-free at 3 years after completion of therapy.

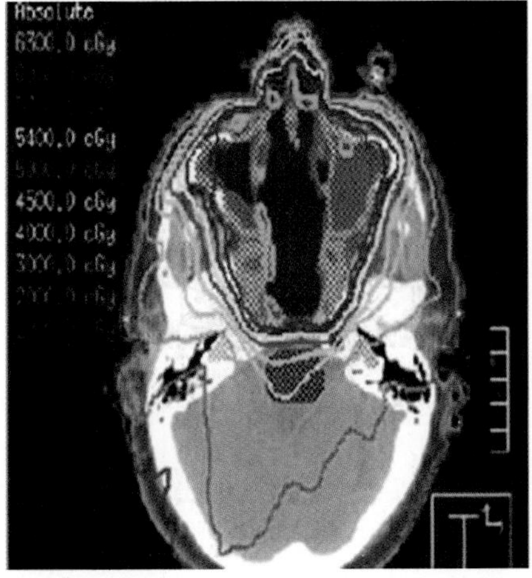

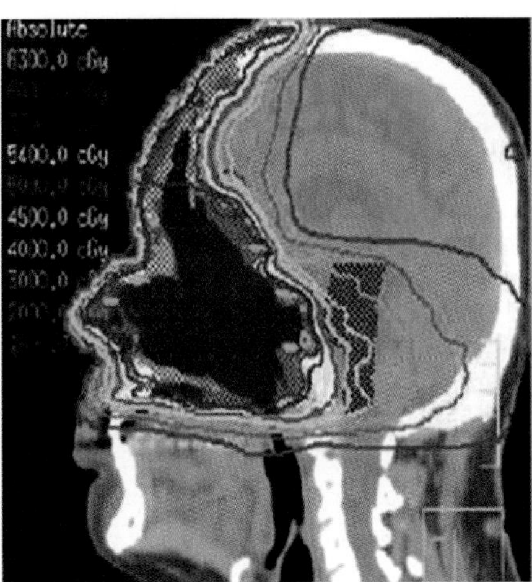

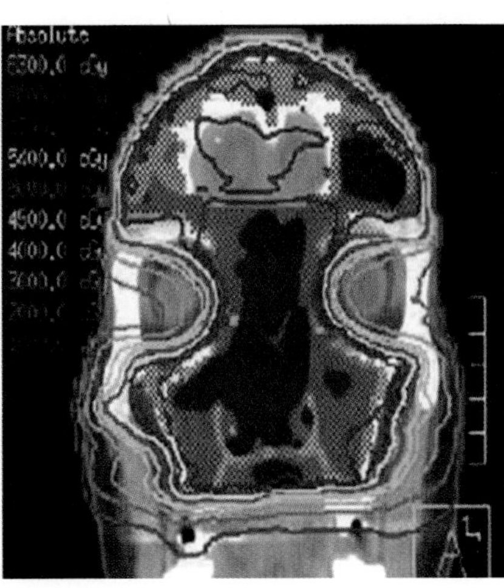

Figure 15.3 Representative axial, sagittal, and coronal images from a radiation treatment plan for a patient with T4N0 esthesioneuroblastoma (whose preoperative MRI images are shown in Figure 15.1). This patient underwent a endoscopic approach to the extradural component of tumor, posterior septectomy, bilateral maxillary antrostomies, bilateral ethmoidectomies and bilateral sphenoidectomies with tissue removal. Neurosurgery then performed a bifrontal craniotomy approach to the anterior skull base and resected the intradural tumor component.The patient had a gross total resection. This patient went on to receive postoperative radiation therapy to a total dose of 60 Gy in 30 daily fractions of 2 Gy each using intensity-modulated radiation therapy to the postoperative bed plus margin.

The advent of intensity-modulated radiation therapy (IMRT) allows for the more conformal delivery of radiation therapy. Although comparative retrospective studies showed tumor control and survival were not improved with the adoption of IMRT, the decreased rates of optic and other toxicities were encouraging with this new technology [23, 24, 26]. Figure 15.3 depicts a radiation treatment plan using IMRT. More recently, there has been interest in the use of proton beam radiation for tumors in the sinonasal region. Protons are well-suited for treatment of tumors in this area because of their favorable physical properties [59, 60]. Proton beam radiation has the potential to limit radiation toxicity [61]. Single-institution studies have shown the safety of proton beam radiation in the treatment of patients with T4b or recurrent tumors both with and without the use of concurrent chemotherapy [62–66].

Systemic Therapy

The role of chemotherapy in sinonasal malignancies continues to evolve. For SNUC, ENB, rhabdomyosarcoma, and T-cell lymphomas, systemic chemotherapy in combination with external beam radiation has been shown to be beneficial in terms of control and survival [28–37]. Patients with ACC are often given single agent cisplatin concurrently with postoperative radiation, but this varies by institutional practice [67]. The role of chemotherapy in SCC and adenocarcinomas is even less clearly defined. Most regimens are platin-based in combination with 5-fluorouracil or a taxane. Some patients have enjoyed significant reduction in tumor burden when treated with concomitant chemotherapy and radiation therapy, although this approach awaits further validation in larger studies [51]. In the recurrent or metastatic setting, salvage chemotherapy can be offered for palliation [19]. Preliminary studies have shown that patients with sinonasal SCC whose tumors have epidermal growth factor receptor expression have shorter disease-free survival, suggesting there may be a role for epidermal growth factor receptor-directed therapy in the future [68].

Follow-Up and Survivorship

Recommended follow-up for patients treated for sinonasal malignancies is similar to what is recommended for other head and neck cancer patients. For the first year after treatment is complete, physical examinations, including fiberoptic examinations, should be performed every 3 months. In the second year after treatment is complete, examinations can be spaced out to every 4 months, and in years 3–5, examinations can be spaced out to every 6–12 months. After 5 years, patients should continue to be followed annually [19]. Patients with ACC are at particularly high risk for late relapse, with documented relapses as late as 15–20 years after the primary diagnosis [69]. Imaging with either a CT with contrast or an MRI should be performed 4–6 months after treatment and then as clinically indicated based on symptoms [19]. Patients with MM may benefit from systemic restaging depending on their presenting stage. Chest imaging can be considered also, particularly for those with positive lymph nodes or with ACC, which has a propensity for spread to the lungs [19]. Patients treated with radiation have the potential to develop late toxicities related to treatment. Single-institution series with long-term follow-up have reported blindness in one patient that occurred 7 years after completion of treatment and two patients who developed symptomatic temporal lobe radionecrosis more than 1 year after completion of treatment [70]. This reinforces the importance of long-term follow-up for these patients not only to screen for recurrence but also to monitor for and document late treatment-related complications.

References

1 Turner JH, Reh DD. Incidence and survival in patients with sinonasal cancer: a historical analysis of population-based data. *Head Neck* 2012;34;877–85.

2 Youlden DR, Cramb SM, Peters S, *et al.* International comparisons of the incidence and mortality of sinonasal cancer. *Cancer Epidemiol* 2013;37;770–9.

3 Khademi B, Moradi A, Hoseini S, Mohammadianpanah M. Malignant neoplasms of the sinonasal tract: report of 71 patients and literature review and analysis. *Oral Maxillofac Surg* 2009;13;191–9.

4 Jakobsen MH, Larsen SK, Kirkegaard J, Hansen HS. Cancer of the nasal cavity and paranasal sinuses. Prognosis and outcome of treatment. *Acta Oncol* 1997;36;27–31.

5 D'Aguillo CM, Kanumuri VV, Khan MN, *et al.* Demographics and survival trends of sinonasal adenocarcinoma from 1973 to 2009. *Int Forum Allergy Rhinol* 2014;4:771–6.

6 Bugra Cengiz A, Uyar M, Comert E, *et al.* Sinonasal tract malignancies: prognostic factors and surgery outcomes. *Iran Red Crescent Med J* 2013;15;e14118.

7 Rushton L, Hutchings SJ, Fortunato L, *et al.* Occupational cancer burden in Great Britain. *Br J Cancer* 2012;107 Suppl 1;S3–7.

8 International Agency for Research on Cancer Monographs on the Evaluation of Carcinogenic Risks to Humans, updated 24 October 2016. http://monographs.iarc.fr/ENG/Classification/Table4.pdf. (accessed 4 October 2017).

9 Syrjanen K, Syrjanen S. Detection of human papillomavirus in sinonasal carcinoma: systematic review and meta-analysis. *Hum Pathol* 2013;44;983–91.

10 Lewis Jr JS, Westra WH, Thompson LD, *et al.* The sinonasal tract: another potential "hot spot" for carcinomas with transcriptionally-active human papillomavirus. *Head Neck Pathol* 2014;8(3):241–9.

11 Lewis JS Jr. Sinonasal squamous cell carcinoma: a review with emphasis on emerging histologic subtypes and the role of human papillomavirus. *Head Neck Pathol* 2016;10(1):60–7.

12 Barnes L, Eveson JW, Reichart P, *et al.* WHO histological classification of tumours of the nasal cavity and paranasal sinuses. In: L Barnes, JW Eveson, P Reichart, D Sidransky (eds) *Pathology and Genetics of Head and Neck Tumours.* Lyon, France: IARC Press, 2005:10–11.

13 World Health Organization Classification of Tumours. http://www.iarc.fr/en/publications/pdfs-online/pat-gen/bb9/bb9-chap1.pdf (accessed 4 October 2017).

14 Amit M, Binenbaum Y, Sharma K, *et al.* Adenoid cystic carcinoma of the nasal cavity and paranasal sinuses: a meta-analysis. *J Neurol Surg B Skull Base* 2013;74;118–25.

15 Tajudeen BA, Vorasubin N, Sanaiha Y, *et al.* Sinonasal mucosal melanoma: 20-year experience at a tertiary referral center. *Int Forum Allergy Rhinol* 2014;4;592–7.

16 Lombardi D, Bottazzoli M, Turri–Zanoni M, *et al.* Sinonasal mucosal melanoma: a 12-year experience of 58 cases. *Head Neck.* 2016;38(Suppl 1):E1737–45.

17 Yoshida E, Aouad R, Fragoso R, *et al.* Improved clinical outcomes with multi-modality therapy for sinonasal undifferentiated carcinoma of the head and neck. *Am J Otolaryngol* 2013;34;658–63.

18 Khan MN, Konuthula N, Parasher A, *et al.* Treatment modalities in sinonasal undifferentiated carcinoma: an analysis from the national cancer database. *Int Forum Allergy Rhinol* 2017;7(2):205–10.

19 Pfister FG, Spencer S, Adelstein D, *et al.* NCCN Clinical Practice Guidelines in Oncology, Head and Neck Cancer. Version 2.2016.nccn.org. Accessed 19 January 2017.

20 Gomaa MA, Hammad MS, Abdelmoghny A, *et al.* Magnetic resonance imaging versus computed tomography and different imaging modalities in evaluation of sinonasal neoplasms diagnosed by histopathology. *Clin Med Insights Ear Nose Throat* 2013;6;9–15.

21 Kraus DH, Lydiatt WM, Patel SG, *et al.* Nasal cavity and paranasal sinuses. In: Amin MB, Edge SB, Greene FL, *et al.* (eds) *AJCC Cancer Staging Manual*, 8th edn. New York: Springer Nature, 2017.

22 Kadish S, Goodman M, Wang CC. Olfactory neuroblastoma. A clinical analysis of 17 cases. *Cancer* 1976;37;1571–6.

23 Jansen EP, Keus RB, Hilgers FJ, *et al.* Does the combination of radiotherapy and debulking surgery favor survival in paranasal sinus carcinoma? *Int J Radiat Oncol Biol Phys* 2000;48;27–35.

24 Duthoy W, Boterberg T, Claus F, *et al.* Postoperative intensity-modulated radiotherapy in sinonasal carcinoma: clinical results in 39 patients. *Cancer* 2005;104;71–82.

25 Padovani L, Pommier P, Clippe SS, *et al.* Three-dimensional conformal radiotherapy for paranasal sinus carcinoma: clinical results for 25 patients. *Int J Radiat Oncol Biol Phys* 2003;56;169–76.

26 Hoppe BS, Stegman LD, Zelefsky MJ, *et al.* Treatment of nasal cavity and paranasal sinus cancer with modern radiotherapy techniques in the postoperative setting – the MSKCC experience. *Int J Radiat Oncol Biol Phys* 2007;67;691–702.

27 Gabriele AM, Airoldi M, Garzaro M, *et al.* Stage III–IV sinonasal and nasal cavity carcinoma treated with three-dimensional conformal radiotherapy. *Tumori* 2008;94;320–6.

28 Al-Mamgani A, van Rooij P, Mehilal R, *et al.* Combined-modality treatment improved outcome in sinonasal undifferentiated carcinoma: single-institutional experience of 21 patients and review of the literature. *Eur Arch Otorhinolaryngol* 2013;270;293–9.

29 Mourad WF, Hauerstock D, Shourbaji RA, *et al.* Trimodality management of sinonasal undifferentiated carcinoma and review of the literature. *Am J Clin Oncol* 2013;36;584–8.

30 Lin EM, Sparano A, Spalding A, *et al.* Sinonasal undifferentiated carcinoma: a 13-year experience at a single institution. *Skull Base* 2010;20;61–7.

31 Babin E, Rouleau V, Vedrine PO, *et al.* Small cell neuroendocrine carcinoma of the nasal cavity and paranasal sinuses. *J Laryngol Otol* 2006;120;289–97.

32 Chen AM, Daly ME, El-Sayed I, *et al.* Patterns of failure after combined-modality approaches incorporating radiotherapy for sinonasal undifferentiated carcinoma of the head and neck. *Int J Radiat Oncol Biol Phys* 2008;70;338–43.

33 Mendenhall WM, Mendenhall CM, Riggs CE, Jr., *et al.* Sinonasal undifferentiated carcinoma. *Am J Clin Oncol* 2006;29;27–31.

34 Kim BS, Vongtama R, Juillard G. Sinonasal undifferentiated carcinoma: case series and literature review. *Am J Otolaryngol* 2004;25;162–6.

35 Diaz EM, Jr., Johnigan RH, 3rd, Pero C, *et al.* Olfactory neuroblastoma: the 22-year experience at one comprehensive cancer center. *Head Neck* 2005;27;138–49.

36 Smith SR, Som P, Fahmy A, *et al.* A clinicopathological study of sinonasal neuroendocrine carcinoma and sinonasal undifferentiated carcinoma. *Laryngoscope* 2000;110;1617–22.

37 McLean JN, Nunley SR, Klass C, *et al.* Combined modality therapy of esthesioneuroblastoma. *Otolaryngol Head Neck Surg* 2007;136;998–1002.

38 Ozsahin M, Gruber G, Olszyk O, *et al.* Outcome and prognostic factors in olfactory neuroblastoma: a rare cancer network study. *Int J Radiat Oncol Biol Phys* 2010;78;992–7.

39 Kondo N, Takahashi H, Nii Y, Nagao J. Olfactory neuroblastoma: 15 years of experience. *Anticancer Res* 2012;32;1697–703.

40 Noronha V, Patil VM, Joshi A, *et al.* Induction chemotherapy in technically unresectable locally advanced carcinoma of maxillary sinus. *Chemother Res Pract* 2014;2014;487872.

41 Sohrabi S, Drabick JJ, Crist H, *et al.* Neoadjuvant concurrent chemoradiation for advanced esthesioneuroblastoma: a case series and review of the literature. *J Clin Oncol* 2011;29;e358–61.

42 Le QT, Fu KK, Kaplan MJ, *et al.* Lymph node metastasis in maxillary sinus carcinoma. *Int J Radiat Oncol Biol Phys* 2000;46;541–9.

43 Li XM, Li J, Di B, *et al.* [Recurrence and surgical salvage of sinonasal squamous cell carcinoma]. *Zhonghua Er Bi Yan Hou Tou Jing Wai Ke Za Zhi* 2013;48;186–90.

44 McCutcheon IE, Blacklock JB, Weber RS, *et al.* Anterior transcranial (craniofacial) resection of tumors of the paranasal sinuses: surgical technique and results. *Neurosurgery* 1996;38;471–9;discussion 479–80.

45 Lund VJ, Howard DJ, Wei WI, Cheesman AD. Craniofacial resection for tumors of the nasal cavity and paranasal sinuses – a 17-year experience. *Head Neck* 1998;20;97–105.

46 Castelnuovo P, Lepera D, Turri-Zanoni M, *et al.* Quality of life following endoscopic endonasal resection of anterior skull base cancers. *J Neurosurg* 2013;119;1401–9.

47 Vergez S, Martin-Dupont N, Lepage B, *et al.* Endoscopic vs transfacial resection of sinonasal adenocarcinomas. *Otolaryngol Head Neck Surg* 2012;146;848–53.

48. Higgins TS, Thorp B, Rawlings BA, Han JK. Outcome results of endoscopic vs craniofacial resection of sinonasal malignancies: a systematic review and pooled-data analysis. *Int Forum Allergy Rhinol* 2011;1;255–61.

49 Michel J, Fakhry N, Mancini J, *et al.* Sinonasal squamous cell carcinomas: clinical outcomes and predictive factors. *Int J Oral Maxillofac Surg* 2014;43;1–6.

50 Wiseman SM, Popat SR, Rigual NR, *et al.* Adenoid cystic carcinoma of the paranasal sinuses or nasal cavity: a 40-year review of 35 cases. *Ear Nose Throat J* 2002;81;510–14, 516–17.

51 Patel SG, Prasad ML, Escrig M, *et al.* Primary mucosal malignant melanoma of the head and neck. *Head Neck* 2002;24;247–57.

52 Ene P, Popescu RC, Voiculescu S, *et al.* Sentinel lymph node – work hypothesis in sinonasal carcinoma treatment. *Maedica (Buchar)* 2011;6;308–12.

53 Fernandez JM, Santaolalla F, Del Rey AS, *et al.* Preliminary study of the lymphatic drainage system of the nose and paranasal sinuses and its role in detection of sentinel metastatic nodes. *Acta Otolaryngol* 2005;125;566–70.

54 Teudt IU, Meyer JE, Ritter M, *et al.* Perioperative image-adapted brachytherapy for the treatment of paranasal sinus and nasal cavity malignancies. *Brachytherapy* 2014;13;178–86.

55 Tran L, Sidrys J, Horton D, *et al.* Malignant salivary gland tumors of the paranasal sinuses and nasal cavity. The UCLA experience. *Am J Clin Oncol* 1989;12;387–92.

56 Goepfert H, Luna MA, Lindberg RD, White AK. Malignant salivary gland tumors of the paranasal sinuses and nasal cavity. *Arch Otolaryngol* 1983;109;662–8.

57 Debus J, Hug EB, Liebsch NJ, *et al.* Brainstem tolerance to conformal radiotherapy of skull base tumors. *Int J Radiat Oncol Biol Phys* 1997;39;967–75.

58 Fried DV, Zanation AM, Huang B, *et al.* Patterns of local failure for sinonasal malignancies. *Pract Radiat Oncol* 2013;3;e113–20.

59 Mock U, Georg D, Bogner J, *et al.* Treatment planning comparison of conventional, 3D conformal, and intensity-modulated photon (IMRT) and proton therapy for paranasal sinus carcinoma. *Int J Radiat Oncol Biol Phys* 2004;58;147–54.

60 Lomax AJ, Goitein M, Adams J. Intensity modulation in radiotherapy: photons versus protons in the paranasal sinus. *Radiother Oncol* 2003;66;11–18.

61 van de Water TA, Bijl HP, Schilstra C, *et al.* The potential benefit of radiotherapy with protons in head and neck cancer with respect to normal tissue sparing: a systematic review of literature. *Oncologist* 2011;16;366–77.

62 Weber DC, Chan AW, Lessell S, *et al.* Visual outcome of accelerated fractionated radiation for advanced sinonasal malignancies employing photons/protons. *Radiother Oncol* 2006;81;243–9.

63 Okano S, Tahara M, Zenda S, *et al.* Induction chemotherapy with docetaxel, cisplatin and S-1 followed by proton beam therapy concurrent with cisplatin in patients with T4b nasal and sinonasal malignancies. *Jpn J Clin Oncol* 2012;42;691–6.

64 Fukumitsu N, Okumura T, Mizumoto M, *et al.* Outcome of T4 (International Union Against Cancer Staging System, 7th edition) or recurrent nasal cavity and paranasal sinus carcinoma treated with proton beam. *Int J Radiat Oncol Biol Phys* 2012;83;704–11.

65 Zenda S, Kohno R, Kawashima M, *et al.* Proton beam therapy for unresectable malignancies of the nasal cavity and paranasal sinuses. *Int J Radiat Oncol Biol Phys* 2011;81;1473–8.

66 Chera BS, Malyapa R, Louis D, *et al.* Proton therapy for maxillary sinus carcinoma. *Am J Clin Oncol* 2009;32;296–303.

67 Samant S, van den Brekel MW, Kies MS, *et al.* Concurrent chemoradiation for adenoid cystic carcinoma of the head and neck. *Head Neck* 2012;34;1263–8.

68 Takahashi Y, Bell D, Agarwal G, *et al.* Comprehensive assessment of prognostic markers for sinonasal squamous cell carcinoma. *Head Neck* 2013;36;1094–102.

69 van Weert S, Bloemena E, van der Waal I, *et al.* Adenoid cystic carcinoma of the head and neck: a single-center analysis of 105 consecutive cases over a 30-year period. *Oral Oncol* 2013;49;824–9.

70 Hoppe BS, Nelson CJ, Gomez DR, *et al.* Unresectable carcinoma of the paranasal sinuses: outcomes and toxicities. *Int J Radiat Oncol Biol Phys* 2008;72;763–9.

16

Nasopharyngeal Cancer

Jamie M. Pawlowski[1], Emma B. Holliday[2], and Clifton D. Fuller[2]

[1] The University of Texas Health Science Center at San Antonio, San Antonio, Texas, USA
[2] The University of Texas MD Anderson Cancer Center, Houston, Texas, USA

Incidence and Mortality

Nasopharyngeal cancer (NPC) is a rare malignancy. In 2012, there were estimated to be 87,000 new cases (61,000 men and 26,000 women) of NPC worldwide and 51,000 deaths (36,000 men and 15,000 women) from the disease, or 0.6% of all cancer deaths. NPC demonstrates marked racial and geographical variations with the highest incidence observed in Southeast Asia, East Asia, Polynesia, North Africa, and in native peoples of the Arctic region [1, 2]. In the United States (US), there were estimated to be 2,300 new cases (1,600 men and 700 women) of NPC and 900 deaths (600 men and 300 women) from the disease in 2012 [2].

The incidence rate is much higher among Asian Americans (3.03 cases per 100,000 persons per year) than in the US population (0.74 cases per 100,000 persons per year). Fortunately, the incidence of NPC has been declining in East Asian countries since the 1970s [3, 4]. The risk of developing NPC increases with age, with a median age at diagnosis of 55 years in the US [5]. However, NPC can also occur in children, and when it does, it typically presents with a more advanced stage at diagnosis [6].

Etiology and Risk Factors

Risks factors for NPC vary based on histologic type (see Pathology section). The strongest risk factor associated with the development of the nonkeratinizing, undifferentiated form of NPC is the Epstein–Barr virus (EBV) [7–10]. When EBV infects nasopharyngeal epithelium, the cells are stimulated to divide primarily by viral expression of latent membrane protein 1 (LMP1) and Epstein–Barr nuclear antigen 1 (EBNA-1). This makes the cell's DNA more susceptible to genetic mutations thereby increasing susceptibility to NPC [9, 10]. In fact, recent studies suggest that a high EBV DNA level is correlated with a worse overall prognosis [11]. The keratinizing form of NPC is associated with tobacco use [1]. Additional risk factors include genetic predisposition and dietary practices such as heavy consumption of salted fish or preserved foods [3, 12–14].

Prevention

Prevention of NPC is best achieved by lifestyle modification aimed at reducing the environmental risk factors outlined above, that is, cessation of tobacco use and diet modifications. Although routine screening regimens do not yet exist, promising strategies are being evaluated due to the high cure rate of early-stage NPC [15]. Additionally, EBV DNA levels have prognostic significance and may one day be useful in monitoring for treatment response and to detect recurrence [16, 17].

Pathology

NPC is classified by multiple histologic variants; over 75% of NPC is nonkeratinizing squamous cell carcinoma (SCC) that can be further subdivided into differentiated and undifferentiated forms. Undifferentiated NPC, historically known as lymphoepithelioma, represents over 99% of cases in endemic areas and comprises 60–95% of all NPC cases. It has the most favorable prognosis and is associated with the presence of EBV DNA. The remaining 25% of NPC is classified as keratinizing SCC, a sporadic form with more variable prognoses [1]. Recently, another histologic subtype was added to the NPC classification, called basaloid SCC. This is a very rare histology that displays aggressive behavior and a poor prognosis [18]. Other tumor types that can arise in the nasopharynx include lymphoma, minor salivary gland tumors, melanomas, and sarcomas, but these are outside the scope of this chapter [19, 20].

The American Cancer Society's Oncology in Practice: Clinical Management, First Edition. Edited by The American Cancer Society.

Diagnosis

NPC most commonly arises from the pharyngeal recess, also called the Fossa of Rosenmuller. Due to this location, many patients may remain asymptomatic for a prolonged period [21]. The most common presenting symptom is a neck mass due to cervical nodal metastases [22]. Additional complaints result from tumor invasion into local structures. These symptoms may include headache, epistaxis, nasal obstruction, otalgia, or tinnitus [21, 22]. NPC may also cause cranial nerve deficits from local extension. If cranial nerves II, III, IV, and V1-2 are affected, it can lead to unilateral ptosis, ophthalmoplegia, diplopia, and amaurosis. These cranial nerve deficits can be caused by direct tumor extension through the foramen lacerum into the cavernous sinus, also known as petrosphenoidal syndrome of Jacod. The cervical sympathetic trunk and cranial nerves IX–XII can also be affected, leading to changes in taste, dysphagia, numbness of the soft palate, paresis of the soft palate, vagal dysfunction, and Horner's syndrome, also known as the retroparotid syndrome of Villaret. This syndrome is caused by lateral tumor extension into the pharyngeal space [23]. If Horner's syndrome is not present, this constellation of symptoms characterized by unilateral palsy of cranial nerves IX–XII is also known as Collet–Sicard syndrome [24].

The diagnostic workup for a patient with suspected NPC should begin with a thorough history and physical, including a complete head and neck examination. A mirror or fiberoptic examination is indicated to observe the postnasal space. Imaging of the head and neck should be considered for any suspected malignancy, either with a computed tomography (CT) with contrast or a magnetic resonance image (MRI) with gadolinium [25]. MRI is preferred over CT due to its superior ability to demonstrate soft tissue and bony involvement, which can dramatically change the tumor staging [26]. If the patient is at high risk for distant metastases as suggested by the presence of positive lymph nodes or advanced primary tumor (T3–T4), then further imaging should be performed, preferably with positron emission tomography (PET) CT and/or bone scan [25, 27, 28]. These imaging studies are needed to assign an appropriate stage to the tumor and to assist with treatment planning, particularly for radiation therapy (RT). A biopsy is ultimately required to establish the diagnosis of cancer, and it is usually obtained with rigid endoscopy in the operating room. Multidisciplinary evaluation is recommended with referral to surgical, radiation, and medical oncology specialists. Additionally, evaluation by dental, nutrition, speech pathology, and audiology experts may be clinically indicated to establish baseline function prior to treatment and to educate patients on the prevention and monitoring of treatment-related side effects [25].

Staging

The most widely used staging system for NPC is the tumor-node-metastasis (TNM) staging system from the International Union Against Cancer and the American Joint Committee on Cancer (AJCC) [28]. The most recent version of the TNM classification, from the 8th edition of the AJCC (2017), is shown in Table 16.1. The TNM staging system is used as the basis for treatment recommendations, and it carries prognostic significance. Since most NPC present with lymphadenopathy, it should be known that the most probable primary lymph node drainage sites of the nasopharynx are the lateral retropharyngeal nodes and the level II lymph nodes [29]. The most common site of distant metastases is bone, followed by liver, lung, and brain [30]. Staging of NPC is notably different from other head and neck tumors in that T-category is determined by degree of tumor extension and not by size alone. Additionally, extensive changes were made from the 7th edition of AJCC staging system. The category T0 was added for an unidentified primary

Table 16.1 Classification of nasopharyngeal cancer.

Primary tumor (T-category)			
TX	Primary tumor cannot be assessed		
T0	No tumor identified, but EBV-positive cervical node(s) are present		
T1	Tumor limited to nasopharynx, or tumor extends to oropharynx and/or nasal cavity without parapharyngeal extension		
T2	Tumor extends to parapharyngeal space, and/or adjacent soft tissue involvement (medial pterygoid, lateral pterygoid, prevertebral muscles)		
T3	Tumor involves bony structures of skull base, cervical vertebra, pterygoid structures, and/or paranasal sinuses		
T4	Tumor with intracranial extension, involvement of cranial nerves, hypopharynx, orbit, parotid gland, and/or extensive soft tissue infiltration beyond the lateral surface of the lateral pterygoid muscle		
Regional lymph nodes (N-category)			
NX	Regional lymph nodes cannot be assessed		
N0	No regional lymph node metastasis		
N1	Unilateral metastasis in cervical lymph node(s), and/or unilateral or bilateral metastasis in retropharyngeal lymph node(s), 6 cm or less in greatest dimension, above the caudal border of cricoid cartilage		
N2	Bilateral metastasis in cervical lymph node(s), 6 cm or less in greatest dimension, above the caudal border of cricoid cartilage		
N3	Unilateral or bilateral metastasis in cervical lymph node(s), larger than 6 cm in greatest dimension, and/or extension below the caudal border of cricoid cartilage		
Distant metastatic disease (M-category)			
M0	No distant metastasis		
M1	Distant metastasis		
Stage grouping			
0	Tis	N0	M0
I	T1	N0	M0
II	T0–T1 T2	N1 N0–N1	M0 M0
III	T0–T2 T3	N2 N0–N2	M0 M0
IVA	T4 Any T	N0–N2 N3	M0 M0
IVB	Any T	Any N	M1

Source: AJCC 8th edn (2017). Used with permission of the American College of Surgeons, Chicago, Illinois. The original source for this information is the AJCC Cancer Staging Manual, 8th edn (2017), which is published by Springer Science+Business Media.

tumor with EBV-positive cervical lymph nodes. T2 now encompasses not only posterolateral involvement, but also adjacent muscle involvement. T3 and T4 criteria now have specific tissue descriptions to avoid ambiguity. N3a and N3b were merged into a single N3 category with a new definition. Finally, the previous Stage IVB was merged with IVA, and the previous Stage IVC was changed to IVB [28].

Treatment

The treatment options for NPC vary based on stage, divided approximately into early (T1–T2 without nodal involvement) and advanced. Very early-stage tumors can be treated with RT alone. More advanced NPC have either a larger primary tumor size and/or positive lymph nodes, and these require multimodality management to include both radiation and systemic therapy [25].

Early-Stage Nasopharyngeal Carcinoma

Patients with stage I NPC (T1, N0, M0) can be treated definitively with RT alone. The role of surgery is limited to the initial biopsy for histologic confirmation or for persistent disease. The deep anatomical location of NPC and its close proximity to crucial neurovascular structures make for a difficult surgical approach with significant associated morbidity. The local control rate for definitive RT of early-stage nasopharyngeal tumors ranges from 75 to 90%, but larger primary tumors have a much lower local control rate with RT alone [31, 32]. The conventional RT approach uses two opposed lateral photon fields to cover the entire primary tumor and the upper neck lymphatics with careful attention to minimize the radiation dose to nearby critical organs, including the spinal cord, eyes, middle and inner ears, temporal lobes, and parotid glands. However, several reports have demonstrated good outcomes with a newer form of RT called intensity-modulated radiation therapy (IMRT) [33, 34]. IMRT is preferred over conventional RT to minimize the dose to critical structures and to improve the side effect profile, including a significant reduction in xerostomia, hearing deficits, and other late effects [35, 36]. Dose determination for definitive RT with IMRT was evaluated with a phase II study that included all stages of NPC. This study used doses of 70 Gy to the primary tumor with a 5 mm margin, and 59.9 Gy to an intermediate risk volume that included the entire nasopharynx, retropharyngeal nodes, skull base and clivus, pterygoid fossae, parapharyngeal space, sphenoid sinus, posterior third of the nasal cavity, maxillary sinuses, and lymph node levels I–V bilaterally. A simultaneous integrated boost technique was used to deliver both dose levels in 33 fractions [37]. Common regimens for definitive RT for early-stage NPC use 66–70.2 Gy in 1.8–2.12 Gy/fraction to the primary tumor and 44–63 Gy in 1.6–2 Gy/fraction as prophylactic treatment to the node-negative upper neck due to the high likelihood of subclinical spread [25, 38, 39].

Advanced Nasopharyngeal Carcinoma

Advanced NPC requires multimodality treatment because of the significant risk of isolated local recurrence or distant metastases after definitive RT alone [40, 41]. Concurrent RT and chemotherapy with a platinum-based agent (used to sensitize the tumor to radiation) is the most effective method to improve overall survival (OS) in locally advanced NPC [42, 43]. The RT dose used for concurrent chemoradiation (CRT) is typically 70–70.2 Gy in 1.8–2 Gy/fraction targeting the primary tumor and involved lymph nodes. Sites of suspected clinical spread receive lower doses of 44–63 Gy in 1.6–2 Gy/fraction. Similar to early-stage disease, the use of IMRT is preferred [25]. The first trial to demonstrate a benefit of CRT over RT alone for locally advanced NPC was the Intergroup 0099 trial [44]. This trial enrolled patients with stage III–IV NPC, although the 4th edition of the AJCC staging system was used. At that time, patients with any extension into the oropharynx or nasal cavity were considered T3, whereas now they would be considered T1. The CRT arm of the study used RT to 70 Gy with cisplatin 100 mg/m^2 on days 1, 22, and 43. The first two cycles of chemotherapy were given concurrent with radiation and the third cycle was given adjuvantly. The study closed early due to the significant survival benefit of the CRT compared to RT alone (3 year OS 46% vs 76%) as well as decreased local, regional, and distant recurrence rates with CRT. Similar studies were modeled after the Intergroup regimen, and they confirmed an advantage of CRT compared to RT alone for locoregionally advanced NPC [45, 46]. A meta-analysis of eight trials that included 1,753 patients also demonstrated that for locally advanced NPC, the addition of chemotherapy led to a small but significant improvement in 5-year OS (56% vs 62%) and 5-year event-free survival (42% vs 52%), a benefit observed primarily with concurrent CRT [47].

The use of adjuvant chemotherapy after CRT is also recommended as part of the multimodality treatment strategy for advanced NPC. However, the National Comprehensive Cancer Network (NCCN) recently downgraded the adjuvant chemotherapy recommendation from category 1 ("Based upon high-level evidence, there is uniform NCCN consensus that the intervention is appropriate") to category 2B ("Based upon lower-level evidence, there is uniform NCCN consensus that the intervention is appropriate") [25]. This recommendation changed in part because of a phase III randomized trial that compared CRT (cisplatin) with or without adjuvant chemotherapy (cisplatin and 5-fluorouracil) [48]. There was no statistically significant improvement in the 2-year failure-free survival (86% vs 84%), although long-term follow up in this study is required to help clarify the role of adjuvant chemotherapy. A recent meta-analysis evaluating 19 trials that included 4,806 patients confirmed that concurrent CRT significantly improves OS and is favored over adjuvant or induction chemotherapy alone. This meta-analysis did not determine whether there was an oncologic benefit with concurrent plus adjuvant chemotherapy versus concurrent CRT alone, but it did demonstrate that concurrent plus adjuvant chemotherapy had the highest frequency of acute toxicities including neutropenia, mucositis, nausea, and vomiting [43].

Induction chemotherapy prior to CRT is a bit more controversial. It currently has a category 3 recommendation from the NCCN ("Based on any level of evidence, there is major NCCN disagreement that the intervention is appropriate") [25]. Two phase II studies have demonstrated a potential role for induction chemotherapy, with a 3-year OS that ranges from 85 to

95% [49, 50]. Two recent phase III trials have confirmed that induction chemotherapy plus concurrent CRT offers improved tumor control, particularly at distant sites, when compared to concurrent CRT alone [51, 52]. Only the induction chemotherapy regimen of docetaxel, cisplatin, and 5-fluorouracil (TPF) demonstrated an improved OS [52]. Additionally, the tumor's response to induction chemotherapy may be a powerful prognostic factor for survival [53].

In summary, concurrent CRT offers the most pronounced benefit for the management of locally advanced nasopharyngeal cancer, and it can be used in conjunction with adjuvant or induction chemotherapy, although further studies are required to clarify the role of adjuvant and induction chemotherapy in the concomitant setting [25].

The management of patients with metastatic NPC uses a systemic combination regimen. Wide ranges of chemotherapy options demonstrate antitumor activity, but no randomized clinical trial has been conducted to define the optimal regimen. However, platinum-based agents have consistently shown the highest reported response rates for metastatic NPC, ranging from 65 to 75% complete or partial response [54].

Follow-up and Survivorship

After NPC patients have completed therapy, they are monitored for disease recurrence, treatment-related toxicities, and secondary malignancies. Follow-up examinations typically include a thorough history, physical examination, and fiberoptic examination every 3 months for the first 2 years, every 4–6 months for years 3–5, and annually thereafter. Post-treatment imaging of primary tumor site and neck is recommended for T3–T4 or N2–N3 disease if clinically indicated based on signs and symptoms. Chest imaging may be considered if patients develop new symptoms or if they have a significant smoking history and meet criteria for CT screening for lung cancer. Thyroid-stimulating hormone levels should be obtained every 6–12 months if the neck was irradiated, and thyroid hormone supplementation should be given if the patient is clinically hypothyroid. Speech, swallowing, hearing, and dental assessment should be continued during the follow up period [25]. Patients with NPC have a propensity to recur later compared to other head and neck cancers, most frequently due to local or regional failure [40, 55]. Therefore, it is important to maintain a regimented follow-up schedule.

References

1 Barnes L, Eveson JW, Reichart P, Sidransky D. *Pathology and Genetics of Head and Neck Tumors. World Health Organization Classification of Tumours.* IARC Press: Lyon, 2005.

2 Ferlay J, Soerjomataram I, Dikshit R, *et al.* Cancer incidence and mortality worldwide: sources, methods and major patterns in GLOBOCAN 2012. *Int J Cancer* 2015; 136(5):E359–86.

3 Tsao SW, Yip YL, Tsang CM, *et al.* Etiological factors of nasopharyngeal carcinoma. *Oral Oncol* 2014; 50(5):330–8.

4 Huang TR, Zhang SW, Chen WQ, *et al.* Trends in nasopharyngeal carcinoma mortality in China, 1973–2005. *Asian Pac J Cancer Prev* 2012;13(6):2495–502.

5 Wang Y, Zhang Y, Ma S. Racial differences in nasopharyngeal carcinoma in the United States. *Cancer Epidemiol* 2013; 37(6):793–802.

6 Sultan I, Casanova M, Ferrari A, *et al.* Differential features of nasopharyngeal carcinoma in children and adults: a SEER study. *Pediatr Blood Cancer* 2010;55(2):279–84.

7 Gullo C, Low WK, Teoh G. Association of Epstein-Barr virus with nasopharyngeal carcinoma and current status of development of cancer-derived cell lines. *Ann Acad Med Singapore* 2008;37(9):769–77.

8 Kijima T, Kinukawa N, Gooding WE, *et al.* Association of Epstein-Barr virus with tumor cell proliferation: clinical implication in nasopharyngeal carcinoma. *Int J Oncol* 2001; 18(3):479–85.

9 Liebowitz D. Nasopharyngeal carcinoma: the Epstein–Barr virus association. *Semin Oncol* 1994;21(3):376–81.

10 Shen JJ, Niu WN, Zhou M, *et al.* Association of Epstein Barr virus A73 gene polymorphism with nasopharyngeal carcinoma. *Genet Test Mol Biomarkers* 2015; 19(4):187–90.

11 Lu L, Li J, Zhao C, *et al.* Prognostic efficacy of combining tumor volume with Epstein–Barr virus DNA in patients treated with intensity-modulated radiotherapy for nasopharyngeal carcinoma. *Oral Oncol* 2016;60:18–24.

12 Farrow DC, Vaughan TL, Berwick M, *et al.* Diet and nasopharyngeal cancer in a low-risk population. *Int J Cancer* 1998;78(6):675–9.

13 Yuan JM, Wang XL, Xiang YB, *et al.* Preserved foods in relation to risk of nasopharyngeal carcinoma in Shanghai, *China. Int J Cancer* 2000; 85(3):358–63.

14 Ung A, Chen CJ, Levine PH, *et al.* Familial and sporadic cases of nasopharyngeal carcinoma in Taiwan. *Anticancer Res* 1999; 19(1B):661–5.

15 Ng WT, Yau TK, Yung RW, *et al.* Screening for family members of patients with nasopharyngeal carcinoma. *Int J Cancer* 2005;113(6):998–1001.

16 Haws L Jr, Haws BT. Aerodigestive cancers: pharyngeal cancer. *FP Essent* 2014; 424:18–25.

17 Lin JC, Wang WY, Chen KY, *et al.* Quantification of plasma Epstein–Barr virus DNA in patients with advanced nasopharyngeal carcinoma. *N Engl J Med* 2004;350(24):2461–70.

18 Muller E, Beleites E. The basaloid squamous cell carcinoma of the nasopharynx. *Rhinology* 2000; 38(4):208–11.

19 El-Banhawy OA, El-Desoky I. Low-grade primary mucosa-associated lymphoid tissue lymphoma of the nasopharynx: clinicopathological study. *Am J Rhinol* 2005;19(4):411–16.

20 Barton RT. Mucosal melanomas of the head and neck. *Laryngoscope* 1975;85(1):93–9.

21 Neel HB, 3rd. Nasopharyngeal carcinoma: diagnosis, staging, and management. *Oncology (Williston Park)* 1992;6(2):87–95; discussion 99–102.

22 Hsu MM, Tu SM. Nasopharyngeal carcinoma in Taiwan. Clinical manifestations and results of therapy. *Cancer* 1983; 52(2):362–8.

23 Handley TP, Miah MS, Majumdar S, *et al.* Collet-Sicard syndrome from thrombosis of the sigmoid-jugular complex: a

case report and review of the literature. Int *J Otolaryngol* 2010; 2010:10.1155/2010/203587. Epub 2010 Jul 25.

24 Li JX, Lu TX, Huang Y, *et al.* Clinical features of 337 patients with recurrent nasopharyngeal carcinoma. *China J Cancer* 2010; 29(1):82–6.

25 National Comprehensive Cancer Network: Cancer of the Nasopharynx. Version 2.2014; Available at: www.nccn.org (accessed 5 October 2017).

26 Liao XB, Mao YP, Liu LZ, *et al.* How does magnetic resonance imaging influence staging according to AJCC staging system for nasopharyngeal carcinoma compared with computed tomography? *Int J Radiat Oncol Biol Phys* 2008;72(5):1368–77.

27 Caglar M, Ceylan E, Ozyar E. Frequency of skeletal metastases in nasopharyngeal carcinoma after initiation of therapy: should bone scans be used for follow-up? *Nucl Med Commun* 2003;24(12):1231–6.

28 Amin MB, Edge SB, Greene FL, *et al.* (eds) *AJCC Cancer Staging Manual*, 8th edn. New York: Springer, 2017.

29 Ho FC, Tham IW, Earnest A, *et al.* Patterns of regional lymph node metastasis of nasopharyngeal carcinoma: a meta-analysis of clinical evidence. *BMC Cancer* 2012; 12:98–2407–12–98.

30 Hui EP, Leung SF, Au JS, *et al.* Lung metastasis alone in nasopharyngeal carcinoma: a relatively favorable prognostic group. A study by the Hong Kong Nasopharyngeal Carcinoma Study Group. *Cancer* 2004;101(2):300–6.

31 Lee AW, Poon YF, Foo W, *et al.* Retrospective analysis of 5037 patients with nasopharyngeal carcinoma treated during 1976–1985: overall survival and patterns of failure. *Int J Radiat Oncol Biol Phys* 1992;23(2):261–70.

32 Mesic JB, Fletcher GH, Goepfert H. Megavoltage irradiation of epithelial tumors of the nasopharynx. *Int J Radiat Oncol Biol Phys* 1981;7(4):447–53.

33 Kam MK, Leung SF, Zee B, *et al.* Prospective randomized study of intensity-modulated radiotherapy on salivary gland function in early-stage nasopharyngeal carcinoma patients. *J Clin Oncol* 2007; 25(31):4873–9.

34 Wang W, Feng M, Fan Z, *et al.* Clinical outcomes and prognostic factors of 695 nasopharyngeal carcinoma patients treated with intensity-modulated radiotherapy. *Biomed Res Int* 2014;2014:814948.

35 Nutting CM, Morden JP, Harrington KJ, *et al.* Parotid-sparing intensity modulated versus conventional radiotherapy in head and neck cancer (PARSPORT): a phase 3 multicentre randomised controlled trial. *Lancet Oncol* 2011;12(2):127–36.

36 Zheng Y, Han F, Xiao W, *et al.* Analysis of late toxicity in nasopharyngeal carcinoma patients treated with intensity modulated radiation therapy. *Radiat Oncol* 2015; 10:17–014–0326–z.

37 Chen A, Lee N, Yang C, *et al.* Comparison of intensity-modulated radiotherapy using helical tomotherapy and segmental multileaf collimator-based techniques for nasopharyngeal carcinoma: dosimetric analysis incorporating quality assurance guidelines from RTOG 0225. *Technol Cancer Res Treat* 2010;9(3):291–8.

38 Wei WI, Sham JS. Nasopharyngeal carcinoma. *Lancet* 2005; 365(9476):2041–54.

39 Li JG, Yuan X, Zhang LL, *et al.* A randomized clinical trial comparing prophylactic upper versus whole-neck irradiation in the treatment of patients with node-negative nasopharyngeal carcinoma. *Cancer* 2013;119(17):3170–6.

40 Sanguineti G, Geara FB, Garden AS, *et al.* Carcinoma of the nasopharynx treated by radiotherapy alone: determinants of local and regional control. *Int J Radiat Oncol Biol Phys* 1997;37(5):985–96.

41 Johansen LV, Mestre M, Overgaard J. Carcinoma of the nasopharynx: analysis of treatment results in 167 consecutively admitted patients. *Head Neck* 1992;14(3):200–7.

42 Langendijk JA, Leemans CR, Buter J, *et al.* The additional value of chemotherapy to radiotherapy in locally advanced nasopharyngeal carcinoma: a meta-analysis of the published literature. *J Clin Oncol* 2004;22(22):4604–12.

43 Blanchard P, Lee A, Marguet S, *et al.* Chemotherapy and radiotherapy in nasopharyngeal carcinoma: an update of the MAC-NPC meta-analysis. *Lancet Oncol* 2015;16(6):645–55.

44 Al-Sarraf M, LeBlanc M, Giri PG, *et al.* Chemoradiotherapy versus radiotherapy in patients with advanced nasopharyngeal cancer: phase III randomized Intergroup study 0099. *J Clin Oncol* 1998;16(4):1310–17.

45 Wee J, Tan EH, Tai BC, *et al.* Randomized trial of radiotherapy versus concurrent chemoradiotherapy followed by adjuvant chemotherapy in patients with American Joint Committee on Cancer/International Union against cancer stage III and IV nasopharyngeal cancer of the endemic variety. *J Clin Oncol* 2005; 23(27):6730–38.

46 Chan AT, Leung SF, Ngan RK, *et al.* Overall survival after concurrent cisplatin-radiotherapy compared with radiotherapy alone in locoregionally advanced nasopharyngeal carcinoma. *J Natl Cancer Inst* 2005; 97(7):536–9.

47 Baujat B, Audry H, Bourhis J, *et al.* Chemotherapy in locally advanced nasopharyngeal carcinoma: an individual patient data meta-analysis of eight randomized trials and 1753 patients. *Int J Radiat Oncol Biol Phys* 2006;64(1):47–56.

48 Chen L, Hu CS, Chen XZ, *et al.* Concurrent chemoradiotherapy plus adjuvant chemotherapy versus concurrent chemoradiotherapy alone in patients with locoregionally advanced nasopharyngeal carcinoma: a phase 3 multicentre randomised controlled trial. *Lancet Oncol* 2012;13(2):163–71.

49 Hui EP, Ma BB, Leung SF, *et al.* Randomized phase II trial of concurrent cisplatin-radiotherapy with or without neoadjuvant docetaxel and cisplatin in advanced nasopharyngeal carcinoma. *J Clin Oncol* 2009;27(2):242–9.

50 Bae WK, Hwang JE, Shim HJ, *et al.* Phase II study of docetaxel, cisplatin, and 5-FU induction chemotherapy followed by chemoradiotherapy in locoregionally advanced nasopharyngeal cancer. *Cancer Chemother Pharmacol* 2010; 65(3):589–95.

51 Cao SM, Yang Q, Guo L, *et al.* Neoadjuvant chemotherapy followed by concurrent chemoradiotherapy versus concurrent chemoradiotherapy alone in locally advanced nasopharyngeal carcinoma: A phase III multicentre randomised controlled trial. *Eur J Cancer* 2017;75:14–23.

52 Sun Y, Li WF, Chen NY, *et al.* Induction chemotherapy plus concurrent chemoradiotherapy versus concurrent chemoradiotherapy alone in locoregionally advanced nasopharyngeal carcinoma: a phase 3, multicentre, randomised controlled trial. *Lancet* 2016;17(11):1509–20.

53 Peng H, Chen L, Li WF, *et al.* Tumor response to neoadjuvant chemotherapy predicts long-term survival outcomes in patients with locoregionally advanced nasopharyngeal carcinoma: A secondary analysis of a randomized phase 3 clinical trial. *Cancer* 2017;123(9):1643–52.

54 Jin Y, Shi YX, Cai XY, *et al.* Comparison of five cisplatin-based regimens frequently used as the first-line protocols in metastatic nasopharyngeal carcinoma. *J Cancer Res Clin Oncol* 2012; 138(10):1717–25.

55 Bailet JW, Mark RJ, Abemayor E, *et al.* Nasopharyngeal carcinoma: treatment results with primary radiation therapy. *Laryngoscope* 1992;102(9):965–72.

Section 4

Urinary System

17

Renal Cell Carcinoma

Jonathan Mathias[1] *and Brian Rini*[2]

[1] *Cleveland Clinic, Cleveland, Ohio, USA*
[2] *Taussig Cancer Institute, Cleveland, Ohio, USA*

Incidence and Mortality

Statistical data are compiled by the National Cancer Institute's Surveillance, Epidemiology, and End Results (SEER) Program for the category of "cancer of the kidney and renal pelvis" [1].

The incidence rate of cancers of the kidney and renal pelvis, overall, based on cases diagnosed from 2009 to 2013, was approximately 15.6 per 100,000 men and women per year. During the same time period, the age-adjusted death rate was 3.9 per 100,000 per year. From 1997 to 2008, the incidence rate increased by an average of 3.2% per year (largely due to increased detection of asymptomatic tumors by diagnostic imaging during this period), and has remained stable from 2008 to 2013 (the most recent year with incidence data available). The death rate for cancers of the kidney and renal pelvis declined by an average of 0.7% per year from 1995 to 2013.

The lifetime risk of developing cancer of the kidney and renal pelvis is approximately 1.6%.

According to the American Cancer Society, approximately 63,990 new cancers of the kidney and renal pelvis are diagnosed (3.8% of cancer diagnoses) and approximately 14,400 deaths from cancers from these cancers occur (2.4% of cancer deaths) annually in the United States. It is the sixth most common cancer in men and tenth in women [2].

These overall statistics largely reflect those of RCC, which is the most common cancer of the kidney and renal pelvis. The remainder of this chapter focuses on RCC. Wilms tumor is discussed in Chapter 47.

Risk Factors

Cigarette Smoking

Cigarette smoking has been shown to be strongly linked with RCC. It is estimated to account for about 20–30% of renal cell cancers [3, 4]. There is also a clear dose-dependent risk (twofold in men and 1.6-fold in women) in heavy smokers (more than 21 cigarettes a day) [5]. Smoking cessation has shown to lower risk with a 15–30% decrease in risk 10–15 years after quitting [4]. Secondhand or environmental tobacco smoke has also been shown to be associated with an increased risk of RCC [6, 7].

Obesity

Obesity has been strongly linked to RCC in multiple case control and cohort studies [8–11]. Increasing BMI and weight gain in early and middle adulthood are also strongly correlated with RCC [2, 11]. Close to 30% of RCC can be attributed to obesity [4, 10].

Hypertension

Hypertension is a well-established risk factor for RCC. Poorly controlled hypertension increases risk and better controlled hypertension shows a decrease in risk [12, 13]. Epidemiologic data points to hypertension rather than antihypertensive medications as associated with RCC risk [13].

End-Stage Renal Disease/Acquired Cystic Kidney Disease

Individuals with end-stage renal disease (ESRD) have an increased incidence of RCC and the risk appears to increase with increasing length of dialysis [14]. Chronic kidney disease stages 3 and 4 might also be associated with RCC [15, 16]. Acquired cystic kidney disease is associated with chronic kidney disease and ESRD and carries an increased risk for developing RCC [17]. Acquired cystic kidney disease in native kidneys in transplant patients also carries a substantial risk [18].

Other Factors

There is an increased incidence of RCC in African Americans, but not a corresponding increase in mortality, suggesting a less aggressive disease course [19]. Eating a diet rich in fruits, vegetables, and fiber has been shown in some studies to be protective, but the data are not definitive [20, 21]; in addition a

The American Cancer Society's Oncology in Practice: Clinical Management, First Edition. Edited by The American Cancer Society.

protein-rich diet has not been shown to increase risk [22]. Alcohol use is not a risk factor and moderate consumption might be protective [23].

Renal Cysts

Renal cysts are acquired lesions of the kidney and their incidence increases with age [24]. Up to a third of individuals over the age of 50 will have cysts on imaging [19, 24, 25]. Cysts are classified using CT imagery and based on the Bosniak classification scheme which looks at cyst wall thickness, presence of septae, calcifications, and enhancement on CT imaging. Category I cysts are simple cysts without septae, wall thickness, or calcifications. Category II cysts have few hairline septae, and fine calcifications in the wall or septa. Category I and II cysts are benign and no follow-up is necessary. Category IIF (F for follow-up) cysts have multiple septae and thick calcifications, but do not enhance on CT scan. These need follow-up with CT scans at 3, 6, 12 months and then annually [26]. Category III cysts have multiple septae, thick calcifications, and they enhance on CT. They have a high malignant potential and need to be surgically treated even though some may be benign. Category IV cysts are malignant lesions and have a soft tissue component, in addition to having properties of category III cysts [27].

Polycystic kidney disease (austosomal dominant/autosomal recessive) are inherited cystic kidney diseases. There is no increased incidence of RCC in these patients as compared to that of the general population [28].

Genetic Predispositions

About 2–3% of cases are familial, mostly related to autosomal dominant syndromes like Von Hippel–Lindau (VHL) [29]. Inherited forms of RCC present earlier in life usually have bilateral kidney involvement and have other systemic processes as part of the syndrome. Patients have an inherited defect on one allele and present with symptoms of the disease in organs with a "second hit" on the other allele. Other autosomal dominant conditions related to developing RCC include tuberous sclerosis, Britt Hogg–Dube syndrome, and hereditary papillary RCC [30].

Histopathology and Molecular Pathology of RCC

Clear cell RCC accounts for 75% of RCC; papillary (10–15%) and chromophobe (5%) are the second and third most common RCC types [29, 31]. Most of the understanding of the molecular basis for RCC comes from knowledge of VHL syndrome. Patients with VHL have a mutation on the short arm of chromosome 3 (3p25-26). The protein coded for by *VHL* is involved in ubiquination and degradation of hypoxia inducible factor (HIF). HIF is an oxygen concentration controlled transcription factor and thus plays a role in gene expression. Increased activity by HIF is shown among other things to promote vascular endothelial growth factor (VEGF) expression and angiogenesis. Most patients with sporadic (noninherited) clear cell RCC acquire defects in both *VHL* alleles with 3p deletion and inactivation of VHL [32]. Besides alteration in 3p, alterations in chromosomes 6, 8, 9, and 14 are also seen [31]. Most papillary RCC have genetic alterations that include trisomy of chromosome 7, 17, and loss of the Y chromosome [31, 33]. In hereditary papillary RCC, the *MET* proto-oncogene on 7q is altered [31]. Chromophobe RCC has the best prognosis with a low tendency to progress and metastasize. Genetic alterations seen in chromophobe RCC include monosomies of chromosomes 1, 2, 6, 10, 13, and 17 [31].

Clinical Presentation

The median age at diagnosis of RCC is approximately 60. Patients can present with localized or systemic symptoms. Very few patients currently present with the classic triad of flank pain, hematuria, and abdominal pain. Hematuria is seen in about 10% of patients, the triad is even rarer [34]. Systemic symptoms can be attributed to paraneoplastic syndromes associated with this disease. Hypercalcemia, hypertension, polycythemia, and Stauffer syndrome (liver dysfunction) are some of the paraneoplastic syndromes associated with RCC [35]. However, most patients are asymptomatic and most present with an incidental finding on CT scan or other imaging modality.

Imaging

With an increase in the use of medical imaging, incidental discovery of renal masses is more common. Multidetector CT is the gold standard in imaging small renal masses with sensitivities >90%. MRI can be used for patients with allergies to iodinated contrast and where CT imaging is indeterminate (Figure 17.1). Current imaging standards involve precontrast and postcontrast acquisitions looking for presence of renal lesions and assessing their enhancement. Arterial and urographic phases can help with surgical planning to determine involvement of vasculature and the urinary collecting system. CT scans can also help detect degree of invasiveness, lymph node involvement, and regional or distant metastases. Enhancement is defined as an attenuation increase of at least 15–20 Hounsfield Units (HU) [36].

Around 20% of renal masses surgically removed are benign. The incidence of benign tumors increases with smaller size [37]. These benign tumors are most commonly angiomyolipomas and oncocytomas [32]. Oncocytomas are hypervascular and are radiographically similar to RCC; angiomyolipomas can be distinguished from RCC by the presence of gross fat on CT.

Staging and Grading

Clinical staging is determined by imaging and is based on the American Joint Committee on Cancer TNM system (see Table 17.1). The 8th edition of the American Joint Cancer Committee Staging manual takes into account mortality findings based on observed tumor characteristics including tumor size, local invasiveness, spread to regional lymph nodes, and venous involvement [38].

(a)

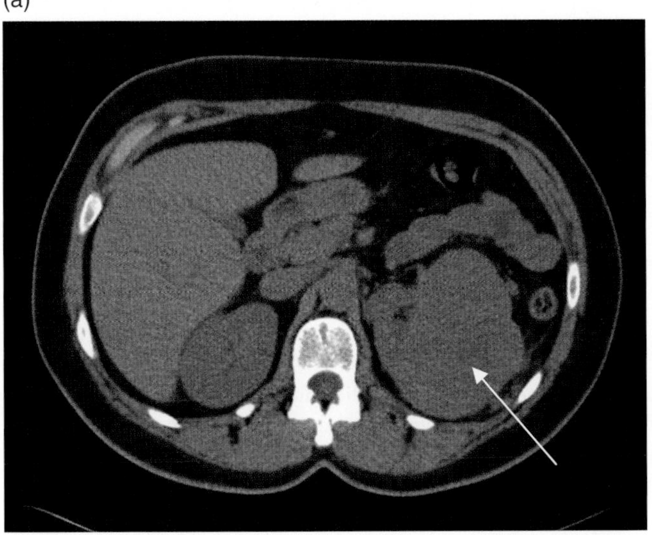

(b)

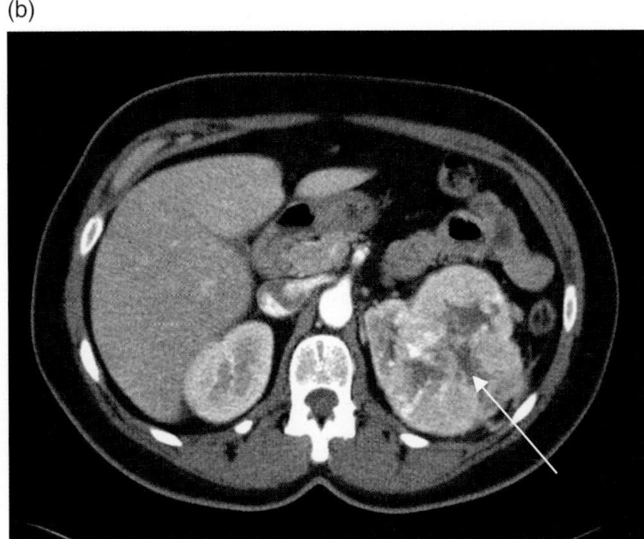

Figure 17.1 Computed tomography scan of a patient with clear cell renal cell carcinoma. Left renal mass before (a) and after (b) intravenous contrast. Enhancement of the mass after intravenous contrast makes it highly suggestive of renal cell carcinoma.

Grading of RCC is based on Fuhrman nuclear grade which takes into account size and shape of the nucleus [39]. The number of nucleoli and chromatin clumping also influence the grade. Cells are graded 1–4, and this grade is of important prognostication value with higher grades carrying a worse prognosis [39, 40].

Management of RCC

Localized Disease

Most RCC are diagnosed as small renal masses (SRMs), classified as those <4.0 cm [41]. Historically, these lesions were treated surgically with a radical nephrectomy [42]. The most serious side effect of radical nephrectomy is the development of chronic kidney disease [43, 44]. Besides the potential for progression to ESRD, there is also a presumed increased risk of cardiovascular events [43, 45]. However, with the advent of nephron-sparing modalities such as partial nephrectomy and ablative procedures, there has been a move towards nephron-sparing modalities especially in patients with a need to preserve renal function. Indications could be relative as in chronic kidney disease, or absolute as in patients with a solitary kidney, bilateral tumors, or a transplanted kidney.

Current guidelines point to partial nephrectomy being the standard of care for stage 1 tumors when surgically feasible [46]. While the prevalence of partial nephrectomies has been increasing, it is still underutilized. There is an equivalent or better survival with a partial nephrectomy for tumors <4.0 cm when compared to radical nephrectomy in retrospective series [47]. However, a recently reported randomized trial did not show a benefit to partial nephrectomy, leading to uncertainty as to the optimal surgical approach in SRMs to balance risk and benefit [48]. The cancer-specific and survival benefits are equal with either a laparoscopic or an open surgical approach.

Cryoablation and radiofrequency ablation are two options used in the treatment of SRMs when a patient is a poor surgical candidate and wishes for active treatment. These approaches use a probe inserted into the renal mass to heat or cool the mass and thus kill the cancer cells. There is a higher risk of local recurrence than in surgical procedures [49]. There is a need for long-term surveillance after treatment and biopsies need to be performed before the tumor is ablated to ensure an RCC diagnosis. Surgical intervention is complicated in the event of a recurrence due to fibrosis and scar formation. There are also not well-defined radiographic parameters for ablation success. Finally, for tumors with irregular borders and/or size >3.5 cm, there are increased risks for recurrence [46].

Active surveillance is another modality which is an alternative for patients with short life expectancies or high-risk surgical candidates due to extensive comorbidities. Some retrospective studies have shown active surveillance to have an equivalent efficacy to surgical resection and a viable alternative in the initial and intermediate term [50]. In these studies, SRMs were followed with imaging every 3–6 months. Interventions if needed were delayed and based on the linear and volumetric growth of masses [50, 51]. Tumors showing rapid growth and tumors which grew to be >3.5 cm needed intervention [50]. Patients undergoing active surveillance need to be informed about the risks of progression to incurable metastatic disease, although this has only been reported in a handful of cases [50].

Larger Renal Tumors

Tumors >7 cm and those which are locally invasive have a higher malignant potential. Radical nephrectomy is the gold standard and can be curative in 40–60% of these patients [52, 53]. Risk factors for recurrence include higher grade and stage, presence of tumor necrosis or tumor-related symptoms, worse performance status, and laboratory parameters such as anemia or a high lactate dehydrogenase [54].

Table 17.1 Staging of renal cell carcinoma AJCC prognostic stage groups.

Primary tumor (T)	
T1a	Tumor ≤4.0 cm; confined to the kidney
T1b	Tumor >4.0 cm but ≤7.0 cm; confined to the kidney
T2a	Tumor >7.0 cm but not >10.0 cm and confined to the kidney
T2b	Tumor >10.0 cm and confined to the kidney
T3a	Tumor extends into the renal vein or its segmental branches, or perirenal fat and/or renal sinus fat but not beyond Gerota fascia
T3b	Tumor extends into the vena cava below the diaphragm
T3c	Tumor extends into the vena cava above the diaphragm, or into the wall of the vena cava
T4	Tumor invades beyond Gerota fascia
Regional lymph nodes (N)	
N1	Metastasis in regional lymph nodes
Distant metastasis (M)	
M1	Distant metastasis

When T is...	And N is...	And M is...	Then the stage group is...
T1	N0	M0	I
T1	N1	M0	III
T2	N0	M0	II
T2	N1	M0	III
T3	N0	M0	III
T3	N1	M0	III
T4	Any N	M0	IV
Any T	Any N	M1	IV

Source: adapted from AJCC Cancer staging manual, 8th edition [38]. Used with permission of the American College of Surgeons, Chicago, Illinois. The original source for this information is the AJCC Cancer Staging Manual, 8th edition (2017), which is published by Springer Science + Business Media.

Locally advanced disease includes patients who have invasion through the renal capsule, invasion into perinephric fat, adrenal involvement, venous tumor thrombus, and invasion into the wall of the vena cava. An aggressive surgical approach with locoregional control offers the best chance of a cure. Radical nephrectomy is the treatment of choice. There are no convincing data about survival benefit from extensive lymphadenectomy. Palpable lymph nodes during surgery and those seen on imaging should be resected [55]. Ipsilateral adrenal resection is not indicated if CT imaging is normal and perioperative findings are not suspicious for direct extension or metastases to the adrenal gland [55, 56].

There are no convincing data for the role of neoadjuvant therapy in RCC. However, neoadjuvant therapy is being explored investigationally is some neoadjuvant settings to shrink masses that are otherwise unresectable and thereby make patients initially denied surgery surgical candidates [57, 58]; and to preserve renal function and allow nephron-sparing surgery in patients who require it but are not currently candidates due to tumor anatomy. However, one must balance the risk of deferring surgery and potential disease spread in the time taken to see radiographic improvement, which is usually 2 months [59].

Even with good surgical margins and locoregional control certain patients have a risk for tumor recurrence. Up to 40% of patients can develop recurrent disease [60–64]. Different adjuvant therapies – immunotherapy [65–68], radiation, and hormonal therapy [71] have not historically been found to be helpful. Recent data regarding the role of VEGF-targeting therapy has emerged with conflicting results [72, 73]. One large study did not show benefit of adjuvant therapy, while a more recent, smaller study showed prolongation of disease-free survival with sunitinib. Other ongoing studies will report out soon to hopefully provide further clarity regarding the potential role of adjuvant VEGF-targeted therapy in RCC. Models with prognostic risk factors which predict recurrence risk have been also been established. The most widely used models are the revised Memorial Sloan Kettering Cancer Center nomogram and the modified UCLA Integrated staging system [74]. Predictive models like these take into account factors like pathologic stage, grade, symptoms, performance status, node positivity, vascular invasion, and risk stratify/predict survival.

In metastatic RCC, a multimodal approach which considers cytoreductive nephrectomy, metastatectomy in very select patients, and systemic treatment is the best approach. Randomized trials have shown the benefit of cytoreductive nephrectomy (removing the primary renal tumor in the face of metastatic disease) versus immunotherapy alone in the metastatic setting [75–77]. Those most likely to benefit from cytoreductive nephrectomy include patients with most of the disease burden in the affected kidney, good performance status, good cardiac function, good pulmonary function, and no liver metastases. It is hypothesized that the improved outcomes could be attributed to a decrease in growth factors and cytokines released from the tumor or by decreasing tumor burden, although the exact mechanism of benefit is uncertain [78]. Patient selection for debulking nephrectomy is critical to deliver the benefits of this approach balanced against inherent surgical risks and the resulting delay of initiation of systemic therapy. Ongoing clinical trials are examining the benefits of debulking nephrectomy in the era of modern targeted therapy.

The most common sites of metastases are the lungs (60–75%). regional lymph nodes (60–65%) skeletal (39–40%), and brain (5–7%) [79]. Patients with limited metastases can undergo metasatectomy, although they represent a small minority of cases. Metastatic sites more amenable to resection include solitary lesions, lesions completely resectable, metachronous presentation, a disease-free interval >12 months, and younger age [80].

Systemic Therapy

Patients who present with metastatic disease or who have recurrent metastases and in whom surgery is not an option will generally undergo systemic treatment. Systemic therapy in metastatic RCC is not generally curative and, given the very diverse and sometime indolent nature of RCC, observation of patients with low-volume, indolent metastatic disease can be considered given the balance of risks and benefits [81]. Prior to 2005, immunotherapy including interferon and interleukin-2 was the standard of care even though response rates and progression- free survival (PFS) were modest. Since 2005, there have been multiple therapies that have been developed that target the VEGF pathway that have improved outcomes

Certain factors have been shown to independently prognosticate poor outcomes in advanced disease. These are performance status (Karnofsky performance status <80), high lactate dehydrogenase, low hemoglobin, high corrected serum calcium, and time from initial diagnosis to start of therapy <1 year [82]. In addition, an increased platelet count and an increased absolute neutrophil count have also shown to better prognosticate poor outcomes [83]. Individuals are classified as having favorable risk (0 risk factors), intermediate risk (1–2 factors), and poor risk (>2 risk factors). Most of the trials with advanced therapy were performed with patients from the favorable or intermediate risk groups.

Immunotherapy

Interferon alpha (IFN-α) and interleukin-2 (IL-2) had been the standard of care until the advent of targeted therapies. IFN-α has been shown to be superior to hormonal therapy [84], chemotherapy [85], and placebo. It has response rates of 6–15% with survival benefit of 3–5 months. It is not used as monotherapy and its current use is limited to first-line therapy in combination with bevacizumab (anti-VEGF antibody). High-dose IL-2 has response rates around 20% with PFS around 3 months. In 7–8% of patients, a durable complete response has been seen [86]. This durable complete response in a small fraction of patients results in occasional high-dose IL-2 use for good/intermediate prognosis patients with clear cell histology. Otherwise, most other patients receive targeted therapy in the first-line setting. The most common toxicity of high-dose IL-2 is capillary leak syndrome which can result in severe pulmonary, cardiac, and renal toxicity. Because concern regarding risk of capillary leak syndrome limits use of high-dose IL-2 to younger, fitter patients, it is not a viable treatment option for most metastatic RCC patients [87].

A newer therapeutic target is the programmed cell death protein 1 (PD-1) which is a T-cell negative regulator expressed by activated cells. When bound to its receptor, it attenuates the cytotoxic T-cell response. Nivolumab (Opdivo), a monoclonal antibody to PD-1, was shown to improve overall survival when compared to everolimus, in patients who had received prior treatment. Nivolumab also had fewer grade 3 or 4 toxicities and fatigue was its most common adverse effect [88]. Ongoing clinical trials include combination immunotherapy approaches.

Targeted Therapy

Targeting the VEGF Pathway (Figure 17.2)

As noted above, the inherent biology of clear cell RCC includes VHL inactivation, which leads to overexpression of VEGF, thereby driving tumor angiogenesis. Sunitinib was one of the first agents in a family of drugs that target different aspects of the VEGF pathway (Table 17.2). It is a tyrosine kinase inhibitor (TKI) that inhibits the tyrosine kinase portion of VEGF-Receptor (VEGF-R) and platelet-derived growth factor (PDGF)-Receptor (PDGF-R). Sunitinib was Food and Drug Administration (FDA) approved in 2006 after showing significant improvement in response rates and later PFS when compared to interferon [89]. Severe side effects include fatigue, diarrhea, hypertension, hand-foot syndrome, neutropenia, and thrombocytopenia. Retrospective analyses have showed that patients who developed hypertension while on sunitinib had better response rates, PFS, and overall survival [90].

Sorafenib is a multiple kinase receptor inhibitor working on VEGF-R and related receptors. It was FDA approved in December 2005, for treatment of patients with advanced RCC. In a phase 3 trial, it was found to increase PFS in patients who had failed previous therapy [91, 92]. Toxicities are similar to those of sunitinib with less fatigue but an increased incidence of hand-foot syndrome.

Pazopanib is a TKI which targets VEGF-R, PDGF-R alpha, and c-KIT. It has been shown to be effective as a first-line agent with clear cell metastatic RCC [93] and was FDA approved in 2009. It was shown to be noninferior in a phase 3 head-to-head trial versus sunitinib and was noted to have lesser incidences of hand-foot syndrome and fatigue. However, there were more liver function test abnormalities seen with pazopanib [94]. The relative risks and benefits of specific drugs for specific patients is not well characterized in metastatic RCC.

Axitinib is a TKI which is an inhibitor of VEGFR1, 2, and 3. Approved by the FDA in 2012, it has been shown to have an improved objective response rate and PFS compared to sorafenib as a second-line therapy for patients who have failed previous therapy [95].

Cabozantinib is a newer TKI which targets VEGFR, MET, and AXL. It has shown to have an improved PFS when compared to everolimus in patients who had disease progression after prior VEGFR-targeted therapy [96].

Bevacizumab is a monoclonal antibody which targets circulating VEGF protein. It has shown to be effective as first-line therapy in combination with IFN-α [97] and was approved by the FDA in 2009. However, the combination of these drugs has side effects including severe fatigue and asthenia, and must be administered parenterally.

Mammalian Target of Rapamycin Inhibition

Mammalian Target of Rapamycin (mTOR) is a key component of intracellular signaling pathways related to cell growth, proliferation, and angiogenesis. In tumorigenesis, the signaling pathways with increased mTOR activity include the phosphoinositide 3 < prime > ' kinase/protein kinase B (PI3K/Akt) pathway. When a cell is stimulated, activated mTOR phosphorylates p70S6 kinase and 4E binding protein. This leads to downstream production of messenger RNAs leading to the production of HIF, c-myc and cyclin D1.

mTOR-inhibiting drugs prevent activation of a multiprotein complex mTORC1 by binding to an intracellular protein FK506 which forms an mTOR inhibitor complex. This prevents the kinase activity of mTORC1. Drugs like temsirolimus and everolimus are similar to rapamycin in that they bind to FK506 thus inhibiting mTORC1.

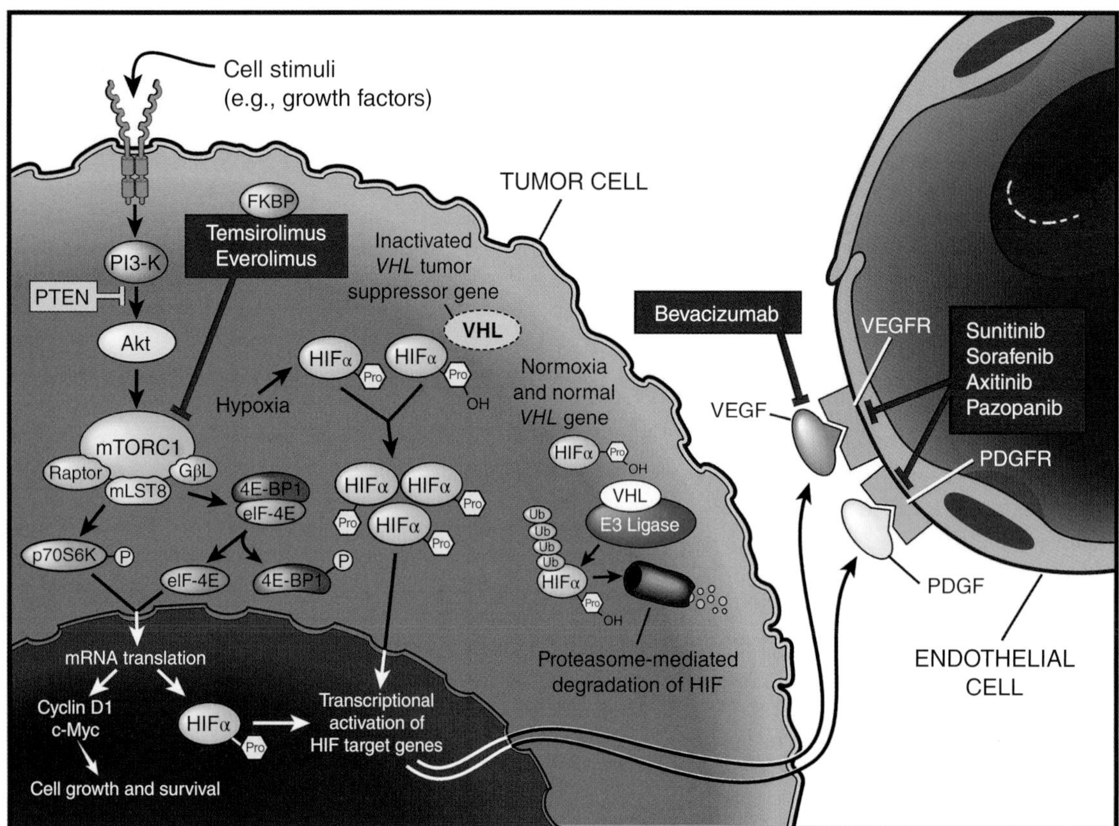

Figure 17.2 Biological pathways and the resulting therapeutic targets in renal cell carcinoma. In conditions of normoxia and normal *VHL* gene function, von Hippel–Landau protein is the substrate recognition component of an E3 ubiquitin ligase complex that targets hypoxia-inducible factor α (HIFα) for proteolysis. In cellular hypoxia or with an inactivated *VHL* gene, the VHL protein–HIF interaction is disrupted, leading to stabilization and accumulation of HIF transcription factors. HIF accumulation can also result from activation of the mammalian target of rapamycin (mTOR) through cellular stimuli and the phosphoinositide 3-kinase (PI3K)/Akt (protein kinase) pathway. mTOR phosphorylates and activates p70S6 kinase (p70S6K) leading to enhanced translation of certain proteins, including HIF. Activated mTOR also phosphorylates 4E binding protein-1 (4E-BP1), promoting dissociation of this complex and allowing eukaryotic initiation factor-4 subunit E (eIF-4E) to stimulate an increase in the translation of mRNAs that encode cell-cycle regulators such as c-myc and cyclin D1. Activated HIF translocates into the nucleus and leads to transcription of a large range of hypoxia-inducible genes, including vascular endothelial growth factor (VEGF) and platelet-derived growth factor (PDGF). These ligands bind to their cognate receptors present on the surface of endothelial cells, leading to cell migration, proliferation, and permeability. Temsirolimus/everolimus bind to FK506-binding protein (FKBP), and the resultant protein–drug complex inhibits the kinase activity of the mTOR complex 1 (mTORC1). Bevacizumab is a VEGF ligand-binding antibody. Sunitinib, sorafenib, pazopanib, and axitinib are small molecule inhibitors of the VEGF receptor (VEGFR) and PDGF receptor (PDGFR) tyrosine kinases. PTEN, phosphatase and tensin homologue. Pro, proline. Ub, ubiquitin. *Source:* Rini *et al.* [104]. Reproduced with permission of Elsevier.

Temsirolimus is used as first-line therapy in poor prognosis RCC including nonclear cell phenotypes [98]. It is a prodrug that gets converted to rapamycin *in vivo*. Temsirolimus demonstrated a PFS and an overall survival advantage compared to interferon as front-line therapy in patients with multiple poor risk features. Known side effects include rash, peripheral edema, hyperglycemia, and hyperlipidemia. Interstitial pneumonitis has also been seen with this drug.

Everolimus is an oral mTOR inhibitor that is used in refractory patients who have failed prior VEGF directed therapy. It was FDA approved in 2009 after showing an improvement in PFS compared to placebo [99].

Palliative Therapy

Radiation therapy, while not of widespread utility in RCC, can play a role in the management of brain metastases, cord compression, and symptomatic bone metastases. Zoledronic acid (a bisphosphonate) has been shown to reduce incidence and delay the onset of skeletal-related events like spinal cord compression and pathologic bone fractures in solid tumors, although only a small cohort of RCC patients were included in the initial trials [100]. Denosumab, a monoclonal antibody inhibiting RANK-ligand, has also been shown to be as effective in the treatment of skeletal metastases [101, 102]. The clinical utility of bone-targeted therapy and the safety of combination therapy with targeted agents requires further study.

Follow-Up and Survivorship

Using data from SEER, patients with kidney cancer have a 5-year survivability of 91.7% for localized disease, 64.2% for regional disease, and 12.3% for distant disease [1]. While no follow-up plan can be generalized to every individual, National

Table 17.2 Summary of phase 3 trials leading to the approval of targeted therapies for renal cell carcinoma.

Drug class	Drug investigated	Control arms	Primary outcomes	Adverse effects
VEGF-R Inhibitor	Sorafenib [72]	Sorafenib vs placebo	PFS 5.5 months vs 2.8 months	Hypertension, ischemic events, diarrhea, rash, HFS
	Sunitinib [89]	Sunitinib vs IFNα	PFS 11 months vs 5 months	Diarrhea, fatigue, vomiting, HFS, neutropenia, thrombocytopenia, hypothyroidism
	Pazopanib [93]	Pazopanib vs placebo	PFS 9.2 months vs 4.2 months	Diarrhea, hypertension, hair color changes, nausea, anorexia, LFT abnormalities, hypothyroidism
	Axitinib [95]	Axitinib vs Sorafenib	PFS 6.7 months vs 4.7 months	Diarrhea, hypertension, fatigue, hypothyroidism
	Cabozantinib [96]	Cabozantinib vs Everolimus	PFS 7.4 months vs 3.8 months	Hypertension, diarrhea, fatigue, HFS
Anti-VEGF antibody	Bevacizumab + IFNα [97]	Bevacizumab + IFNα vs IFNα	PFS 18.3 months vs 17.4 months	Hypertension, anorexia, fatigue, proteinuria
Anti-PD-1 antibody	Nivolumab [88]	Nivolumab vs Everolimus	OS 25.0 months vs 19.6 months	Fatigue, nausea, pruritis
mTOR Inhibitor	Temsirolimus [98]	Temsirolimus vs Temsirolimus + IFN α vs IFNα	OS 10.9 vs 8.4 vs. 7.3 months; PFS 3.8 months vs 3. 7 months vs 1.9 months	Anemia, asthenia, rash, hyperglycemia, pneumonitis
	Everolimus [99]	Everolimus vs placebo	PFS 4.9 months vs 1.9 months	Stomatitis, rash, fatigue, pneumonitis

HFS, hand-foot syndrome; LFT, liver function test; OS, overall survival; PFS, progression-free survival.

Comprehensive Cancer Network guidelines suggest that post initial treatment, patients with RCC stage 1–3 follow up at least every 6 months for the first 2 years and then annually for 5 years. Imaging can be performed at 2–6 month intervals and should include scans of the chest, abdomen +/- pelvis [103]. For metastatic disease no guidelines exist on follow-up protocols and as such, follow-up has to be individualized based on therapy and response to therapy.

In limited disease, long-term side effects of therapy are related to radical nephrectomy. The development of chronic kidney disease and an increased risk of ESRD are the most serious long-term side effects. In metastatic disease, the mainstay of therapy is targeted therapies. Since targeted therapies have only been around for the past decade, there is a paucity of data on their long-term effects.

Future Directions

At present, the appropriate initial therapy and sequence of therapy has not been identified due to the general lack of comparative data and prospective trials. Finding better therapeutic targets in nonclear cell RCC is also a challenge. Identifying biomarkers which will help better risk-stratify patients and predict response to certain therapies could pave the way for 'personalized medicine' and ensure better outcomes.

References

1 Howlader N, Noone AM, Krapcho M, *et al.* (eds) SEER Cancer Statistics Review, 1975–2013, National Cancer Institute. Bethesda, MD. http://seer.cancer.gov/csr/1975_2013/, based on November 2015 SEER data submission, posted to the SEER web site, April 2016.

2 Siegel RL, Miller KD, Jemal A. Cancer statistics, 2017. *CA Cancer J Clin* 2017;67(1):1–24.

3 McLaughlin JK, Lindblad P, Mellemgaard A, *et al.* International renal-cell cancer study. *I. Tobacco use. Int J Cancer* 1995;60(2):194–8.

4 Lipworth L, Tarone RE, McLaughlin JK. The epidemiology of renal cell carcinoma. *J Urol* 2006;176(6):2353–8.

5 Hunt JD, van der Hel OL, McMillan GP, Boffetta P, Brennan P. Renal cell carcinoma in relation to cigarette smoking: meta-analysis of 24 studies. *Int J Cancer* 2005;114(1):101–8.

6 Theis RP, Dolwick Grieb SM, Burr D, Siddiqui T, Asal NR. Smoking, environmental tobacco smoke, and risk of renal cell cancer: a population-based case-control study. *BMC Cancer* 2008;8:387–2407–8–387.

7 Hu J, Ugnat AM, Canadian Cancer Registries Epidemiology Research Group. Active and passive smoking and risk of renal cell carcinoma in Canada. *Eur J Cancer* 2005;41(5):770–8.

8 Renehan AG, Tyson M, Egger M, Heller RF, Zwahlen M. Body-mass index and incidence of cancer: a systematic review and meta-analysis of prospective observational studies. *Lancet* 2008;371(9612):569–78.

9 Adams KF, Leitzmann MF, Albanes D, *et al.* Body size and renal cell cancer incidence in a large US cohort study. *Am J Epidemiol* 2008;168(3):268–77.

10 Bergström A, Hsieh C, Lindblad P, *et al.* Obesity and renal cell cancer – a quantitative review. *Br J Cancer* 2001;85(7):984–90.

11 Leiba A, Kark JD, Afek A, *et al.* Adolescent obesity and paternal country of origin predict renal cell carcinoma: a cohort study of 1.1 million 16 to 19-year-old males. *J Urol* 2013;189(1):25–9.

12 Chow WH, Gridley G, Fraumeni JF, Jr, Jarvholm B. Obesity, hypertension, and the risk of kidney cancer in men. *N Engl J Med* 2000;343(18):1305–11.

13 Shapiro JA, Williams MA, Weiss NS, *et al.* Hypertension, antihypertensive medication use, and risk of renal cell carcinoma. *Am J Epidemiol* 1999;149(6):521–30.

14 Stewart JH, Buccianti G, Agodoa L, *et al.* Cancers of the kidney and urinary tract in patients on dialysis for end-stage renal disease: analysis of data from the United States, Europe, and Australia and New Zealand. *J Am Soc Nephrol* 2003;14(1):197–207.

15 Wong G, Hayen A, Chapman JR, *et al.* Association of CKD and cancer risk in older people. *J Am Soc Nephrol* 2009;20(6):1341–50.

16 Weng PH, Hung KY, Huang HL, *et al.* Cancer-specific mortality in chronic kidney disease: longitudinal follow-up of a large cohort. *Clin J Am Soc Nephrol* 2011;6(5):1121–8.

17 Truong LD, Krishnan B, Cao JT, Barrios R, Suki WN. Renal neoplasm in acquired cystic kidney disease. *Am J Kidney Dis* 1995;26(1):1–12.

18 Satoh S, Tsuchiya N, Habuchi T, *et al.* Renal cell and transitional cell carcinoma in a Japanese population undergoing maintenance dialysis. *J Urol* 2005;174(5):1749–53.

19 Lipworth L, McLaughlin JK, Tarone RE, Blot WJ. Renal cancer paradox: higher incidence but not higher mortality among African-Americans. *Eur J Cancer Prev* 2011;20(4):331–3.

20 Rashidkhani B, Lindblad P, Wolk A. Fruits, vegetables and risk of renal cell carcinoma: a prospective study of Swedish women. *Int J Cancer* 2005;113(3):451–5.

21 Daniel CR, Park Y, Chow WH, *et al.* Intake of fiber and fiber-rich plant foods is associated with a lower risk of renal cell carcinoma in a large US cohort. *Am J Clin Nutr* 2013;97(5):1036–43.

22 Weikert S, Boeing H, Pischon T, *et al.* Fruits and vegetables and renal cell carcinoma: findings from the European prospective investigation into cancer and nutrition (EPIC). *Int J Cancer* 2006;118(12):3133–9.

23 Lee JE, Hunter DJ, Spiegelman D, *et al.* Alcohol intake and renal cell cancer in a pooled analysis of 12 prospective studies. *J Natl Cancer Inst* 2007;99(10):801–10.

24 Laucks SP, Jr, McLachlan MS. Aging and simple cysts of the kidney. *Br J Radiol* 1981;54(637):12–14.

25 Tada S, Yamagishi J, Kobayashi H, Hata Y, Kobari T. The incidence of simple renal cyst by computed tomography. *Clin Radiol* 1983;34(4):437–9.

26 Eknoyan G. A clinical view of simple and complex renal cysts. *J Am Soc Nephrol* 2008;20(9):1874–6.

27 Israel GM, Bosniak MA. An update of the Bosniak renal cyst classification system. *Urology* 2005;66(3):484–8.

28 Gabow PA, Bennett WM. Renal manifestations: complication management and long-term outcome of autosomal dominant polycystic kidney disease. *Semin Nephrol* 1991;11(6):643–52.

29 Linehan WM, Walther MM, Zbar B. The genetic basis of cancer of the kidney. *J Urol* 2003;170(6):2163–72.

30 Choyke PL, Glenn GM, Walther MM, Zbar B, Linehan WM. Hereditary renal cancers. *Radiology* 2003;226(1):33–46.

31 Zambrano NR, Lubensky IA, Merino MJ, Linehan WM, Walther MM. Histopathology and molecular genetics of renal tumors toward unification of a classification system. *J Urol* 1999;162(4):1246–58.

32 Cairns P. Renal cell carcinoma. *Cancer Biomark* 2010;9(1–6):461–73.

33 Kovacs G, Fuzesi L, Emanual A, Kung HF. Cytogenetics of papillary renal cell tumors. *Genes Chromosomes Cancer* 1991;3(4):249–55.

34 Jayson M, Sanders H. Increased incidence of serendipitously discovered renal cell carcinoma. *Urology* 1998;51(2):203–5.

35 Palapattu GS, Kristo B, Rajfer J. Paraneoplastic syndromes in urologic malignancy: the many faces of renal cell carcinoma. *Rev Urol* 2002;4(4):163–70.

36 Kang SK, Chandarana H. Contemporary imaging of the renal mass. *Urol Clin North Am* 2012;39(2):161–70.

37 Schachter LR, Cookson MS, Chang SS, *et al.* Second prize: frequency of benign renal cortical tumors and histologic subtypes based on size in a contemporary series: what to tell our patients. *J Endourol* 2007;21(8):819–23.

38 Amin M, Greene FL, Edge S, *et al.* (eds) *AJCC Cancer Staging Manual*, 8th edn. New York: Springer, 2017.

39 Fuhrman SA, Lasky LC, Limas C. Prognostic significance of morphologic parameters in renal cell carcinoma. *Am J Surg Pathol* 1982;6(7):655–63.

40 Bretheau D, Lechevallier E, de Fromont M, *et al.* Prognostic value of nuclear grade of renal cell carcinoma. *Cancer* 1995;76(12):2543–9.

41 Kane CJ, Mallin K, Ritchey J, Cooperberg MR, Carroll PR. Renal cell cancer stage migration. *Cancer* 2008;113(1):78–83.

42 Robson CJ, Churchill BM, Anderson W. The results of radical nephrectomy for renal cell carcinoma. *J Urol* 1969;101(3):297–301.

43 Huang WC, Levey AS, Serio AM, *et al.* Chronic kidney disease after nephrectomy in patients with renal cortical tumours: a retrospective cohort study. *Lancet Oncol* 2006;7(9):735–40.

44 McKiernan J, Simmons R, Katz J, Russo P. Natural history of chronic renal insufficiency after partial and radical nephrectomy. *Urology* 2002;59(6):816–20.

45 Go AS, Chertow GM, Fan D, McCulloch CE, Hsu C. Chronic Kidney Disease And The Risks Of Death, Cardiovascular Events, *And Hospitalization. N Engl J Med* 2004;351(13):1296–305.

46 Campbell SC, Novick AC, Belldegrun A, *et al.* Guideline for management of the clinical T1 renal mass. *J Urol* 2009;182(4):1271–9.

47 Weight CJ, Lieser G, Larson BT, *et al.* Partial nephrectomy is associated with improved overall survival compared to radical nephrectomy in patients with unanticipated benign renal tumours. *Eur Urol* 2010;58(2):293–8.

48 Van Poppel H, Da Pozzo L, Albrecht W, *et al.* A prospective, randomised EORTC Intergroup Phase 3 Study comparing the oncologic outcome of elective nephron-sparing surgery and

radical nephrectomy for low-stage renal cell carcinoma. *Eur Urol* 2011;59(4):543–52.
49 Kunkle DA, Egleston BL, Uzzo RG. Excise, ablate or observe: the small renal mass dilemma—a meta-analysis and review. *J Urol* 2008;179(4):1227–34.
50 Patel N, Cranston D, Akhtar MZ, *et al.* Active surveillance of small renal masses offers short-term oncological efficacy equivalent to radical and partial nephrectomy. *BJU Int* 2012;110(9):1270–5.
51 Smaldone MC, Kutikov A, Egleston BL, *et al.* Small renal masses progressing to metastases under active surveillance. *Cancer* 2012;118(4):997–1006.
52 Blute ML, Leibovich BC, Lohse CM, Cheville JC, Zincke H. The Mayo Clinic experience with surgical management, complications and outcome for patients with renal cell carcinoma and venous tumour thrombus. *BJU Int* 2004;94(1):33–41.
53 Margulis V, Sánchez-Ortiz RF, Tamboli P, *et al.* Renal cell carcinoma clinically involving adjacent organs. *Cancer* 2007;109(10):2025–30.
54 Lane BR, Kattan MW. Prognostic models and algorithms in renal cell carcinoma. *Urol Clin North Am* 2008;35(4):613–25.
55 Ljungberg B, Cowan NC, Hanbury DC, *et al.* EAU guidelines on renal cell carcinoma: the 2010 update. *Eur Urol* 2010;58(3):398–406.
56 Lane BR, Tiong HY, Campbell SC, *et al.* Management of the adrenal gland during partial nephrectomy. *J Urol* 2009;181(6):2430–6; discussion 2436–7.
57 Thomas AA, Rini BI, Stephenson AJ, *et al.* Surgical resection of renal cell carcinoma after targeted therapy. *J Urol* 2009;182(3):881–6.
58 Rini BI, Garcia J, Elson P, Wood L, *et al.* The effect of sunitinib on primary renal cell carcinoma and facilitation of subsequent surgery. *J Urol* 2012;187(5):1548–54.
59 Timsit M, Albiges L, Méjean A, Escudier B. Neoadjuvant treatment in advanced renal cell carcinoma: current situation and future perspectives. *Exp Rev Anticancer Ther* 2012;12(12):1559–69.
60 Zisman A, Pantuck AJ, Chao D, *et al.* Reevaluation of the 1997 TNM classification for renal cell carcinoma: T1 and T2 cutoff point at 4.5 rather than 7 cm better correlates with clinical outcome. *J Urol* 2001;166(1):54–8.
61 Sorbellini M, Kattan MW, Snyder ME, *et al.* A postoperative prognostic nomogram predicting recurrence for patients with conventional clear cell renal cell carcinoma. *J Urol* 2005;173(1):48–51.
62 Kim SP, Crispen PL, Thompson RH, *et al.* Assessment of the pathologic inclusion criteria from contemporary adjuvant clinical trials for predicting disease progression after nephrectomy for renal cell carcinoma. *Cancer* 2012;118(18):4412–20.
63 Levy DA, Slaton JW, Swanson DA, Dinney CP. Stage specific guidelines for surveillance after radical nephrectomy for local renal cell carcinoma. *J Urol* 1998;159(4):1163–7.
64 Crispen PL, Boorjian SA, Lohse CM, Leibovich BC, Kwon ED. Predicting disease progression after nephrectomy for localized renal cell carcinoma: the utility of prognostic models and molecular biomarkers. *Cancer* 2008;113(3):450–60.
65 Atzpodien J, Schmitt E, Gertenbach U, *et al.* Adjuvant treatment with interleukin-2- and interferon-alpha2a-based chemoimmunotherapy in renal cell carcinoma post tumour nephrectomy: results of a prospectively randomised trial of the German Cooperative Renal Carcinoma Chemoimmunotherapy Group (DGCIN). *Br J Cancer* 2005;92(5):843–6.
66 Clark JI, Atkins MB, Urba WJ, *et al.* Adjuvant high-dose bolus interleukin-2 for patients with high-risk renal cell carcinoma: a cytokine working group randomized trial. *J Clin Oncol* 2003;21(16):3133–40.
67 Messing EM, Manola J, Wilding G, *et al.* Phase III study of interferon alfa-NL as adjuvant treatment for resectable renal cell carcinoma: an Eastern Cooperative Oncology Group/Intergroup trial. *J Clin Oncol* 2003;21(7):1214–22.
68 Pizzocaro G, Piva L, Colavita M, *et al.* Interferon adjuvant to radical nephrectomy in Robson stages II and III renal cell carcinoma: a multicentric randomized study. *J Clin Oncol* 2001;19(2):425–31.
69 Peeling WB, Mantell BS, Shepheard BGF. Post-operative irradiation in the treatment of renal cell carcinoma. *Br J Urol* 1969;41(1):23–30.
70 Kjaer M, Frederiksen PL, Engelholm S. Postoperative radiotherapy in stage II and III renal adenocarcinoma. A randomized trial by the Copenhagen renal cancer study group. *Int J Radiat Oncol Biol Phys* 1987;13(5):665–72.
71 Pizzocaro G, Piva L, Di Fronzo G, *et al.* Adjuvant medroxyprogesterone acetate to radical nephrectomy in renal cancer: 5-year results of a prospective randomized study. *J Urol* 1987;138(6):1379–81.
72 Haas NB, Manola J, Uzzo RG, *et al.* Adjuvant sunitinib or sorafenib for high-risk, non-metastatic renal-cell carcinoma (ECOG-ACRIN E2805): a double-blind, placebo-controlled, randomised, phase 3 trial. *Lancet* 2016;387(10032):2008–16.
73 Ravaud A, Motzer RJ, Pandha HS, *et al.* Adjuvant sunitinib in high-risk renal-cell carcinoma after nephrectomy. *N Engl J Med* 2016;375(23):2246–54.
74 Zisman A, Pantuck AJ, Wieder J, *et al.* Risk group assessment and clinical outcome algorithm to predict the natural history of patients with surgically resected renal cell carcinoma. *J Clin Oncol* 2002;20(23):4559–66.
75 Flanigan RC, Mickisch G, Sylvester R, *et al.* Cytoreductive nephrectomy in patients with metastatic renal cancer: a combined analysis. *J Urol* 2004;171(3):1071–6.
76 Flanigan RC, Salmon SE, Blumenstein BA, *et al.* Nephrectomy followed by interferon alfa-2b compared with interferon alfa-2b alone for metastatic renal-cell cancer. *N Engl J Med* 2001;345(23):1655–9.
77 Mickisch G, Garin A, van Poppel H, de Prijck L, Sylvester R. Radical nephrectomy plus interferon-alfa-based immunotherapy compared with interferon alfa alone in metastatic renal-cell carcinoma: a randomised trial. *Lancet* 2001;358(9286):966–70.
78 Rini BI, Campbell SC. The evolving role of surgery for advanced renal cell carcinoma in the era of molecular targeted therapy. *J Urol* 2007;177(6):1978–84.
79 Ljungberg B, Landberg G, Alamdari FI. Factors of importance for prediction of survival in patients with metastatic renal cell carcinoma, treated with or without nephrectomy. *Scand J Urol Nephrol* 2000;34(4):246–51.

80 Kavolius JP, Mastorakos DP, Pavlovich C, *et al.* Resection of metastatic renal cell carcinoma. *J Clin Oncol* 1998;16(6):2261–6.

81 Rini BI, Dorff TB, Elson P, *et al.* Active surveillance in metastatic renal-cell carcinoma: a prospective, phase 2 trial. *Lancet Oncol* 2016;17(9):1317–24.

82 Motzer RJ, Bacik J, Murphy BA, Russo P, Mazumdar M. Interferon-alfa as a comparative treatment for clinical trials of new therapies against advanced renal cell carcinoma. *J Clin Oncol* 2002;20(1):289–96.

83 Heng DY, Xie W, Regan MM, *et al.* Prognostic factors for overall survival in patients with metastatic renal cell carcinoma treated with vascular endothelial growth factor-targeted agents: results from a large, multicenter study. *J Clin Oncol* 2009;27(34):5794–9.

84 Interferon-alpha and survival in metastatic renal carcinoma: early results of a randomised controlled trial. *Lancet* 1999;353(9146):14–17.

85 Pyrhonen S, Salminen E, Ruutu M, *et al.* Prospective randomized trial of interferon alfa-2a plus vinblastine versus vinblastine alone in patients with advanced renal cell cancer. *J Clin Oncol* 1999;17(9):2859–67.

86 McDermott DF, Regan MM, Clark JI, *et al.* Randomized phase III trial of high-dose interleukin-2 versus subcutaneous interleukin-2 and interferon in patients with metastatic renal cell carcinoma. *J Clin Oncol* 2005;23(1):133–41.

87 Escudier B, Albiges L, Sonpavde G. Optimal management of metastatic renal cell carcinoma: current status. *Drugs* 2013;73(5):427–38.

88 Motzer RJ, Escudier B, McDermott DF, *et al.* Nivolumab versus everolimus in advanced renal-cell carcinoma. *N Engl J Med* 2015;573(19):1803–13.

89 Motzer RJ, Hutson TE, Tomczak P, *et al.* Sunitinib versus interferon alfa in metastatic renal-cell carcinoma. *N Engl J Med* 2007;356(2):115–24.

90 Rini BI, Cohen DP, Lu DR, *et al.* Hypertension as a biomarker of efficacy in patients with metastatic renal cell carcinoma treated with sunitinib. *J Natl Cancer Inst* 2011;103(9):763–73.

91 Escudier B, Eisen T, Stadler WM, *et al.* Sorafenib in advanced clear-cell renal-cell carcinoma. *N Engl J Med* 2007;356(2):125–34.

92 Szcylik C, Demkow T, Staehler M. Randomized phase II trial of first-line treatment of sorafenib versus interferon in patients with advanced renal cell carcinoma: final results. *J Clin Oncol* 2007;25:5025.

93 Sternberg CN, Davis ID, Mardiak J, *et al.* Pazopanib in locally advanced or metastatic renal cell carcinoma: results of a randomized phase III trial. *J Clin Oncol* 2010;28(6):1061–8.

94 Randomized, open label, phase III trial of pazopanib versus sunitinib in first-line treatment of patients with metastatic renal cell carcinoma (mRCC), results of the COMPARZ trial. European Society of Medical Oncology Congress, September 28–October 2, Vienna, Austria, 2012.

95 Rini BI, Escudier B, Tomczak P, *et al.* Comparative effectiveness of axitinib versus sorafenib in advanced renal cell carcinoma (AXIS): a randomised phase 3 trial. *Lancet 201*;378(9807):1931–9.

96 Choueiri TK, Escudier B, Powles T, *et al.* Cabozantinib versus everolimus in advanced renal-cell carcinoma. *N Engl J Med* 2015;373(19):1814–23.

97 Rini BI, Halabi S, Rosenberg JE, *et al.* Bevacizumab plus interferon alfa compared with interferon alfa monotherapy in patients with metastatic renal cell carcinoma: CALGB 90206. *J Clin Oncol* 2008;26(33):5422–8.

98 Hudes G, Carducci M, Tomczak P, *et al.* Temsirolimus, interferon alfa, or both for advanced renal-cell carcinoma. *N Engl J Med* 2007;356(22):2271–81.

99 Motzer RJ, Escudier B, Oudard S, *et al.* Efficacy of everolimus in advanced renal cell carcinoma: a double-blind, randomised, placebo-controlled phase III trial. *Lancet* 2008;372(9637):449–56.

100 Saad F, Lipton A. Zoledronic acid is effective in preventing and delaying skeletal events in patients with bone metastases secondary to genitourinary cancers. *BJU Int* 2005;96(7):964–9.

101 Henry DH, Costa L, Goldwasser F, *et al.* Randomized, double-blind study of denosumab versus zoledronic acid in the treatment of bone metastases in patients with advanced cancer (excluding breast and prostate cancer) or multiple myeloma. *J Clin Oncol* 2011;29(9):1125–32.

102 Lipton A, Fizazi K, Stopeck AT, *et al.* Superiority of denosumab to zoledronic acid for prevention of skeletal-related events: a combined analysis of 3 pivotal, randomised, phase 3 trials. *Eur J Cancer* 2012;48(16):3082–92.

103 NCCN Clinical Practice Guidelines in Oncology (NCCN Guidelines®) Kidney Cancer. Available at: http://www.nccn.org/professionals/physician_gls/pdf/kidney.pdf (accessed 5 October 2017).

104 Rini BI, Campbell SC, Escudier B. Renal cell carcinoma. *Lancet* 2009;373(9669):1119–32.

18

Bladder Cancer and Other Urothelial Sites

Michael C. Risk[1,2], *Ayman Soubra*[1], *and Badrinath R. Konety*[1]

[1] *University of Minnesota, Minneapolis, Minnesota, USA*
[2] *Minneapolis VA Medical Center, Minneapolis, Minnesota, USA*

Urothelial Cell Carcinoma of the Bladder

Introduction

The urinary bladder is the most common site of origin for urothelial cell carcinoma (UCC), although other sites may also develop urothelial tumors including the prostatic urethra, renal pelvis, and ureter. The most common histology of bladder cancer is UCC, formerly referred to as transitional cell carcinoma, but other histologies also exist with both common and unique risk factors. The initial portion of this chapter will focus on UCC of the bladder, with other histologic variants of bladder cancer and other urothelial sites described thereafter.

Incidence and Mortality

The American Cancer Society estimates 79,030 new cases of urinary bladder cancer will be diagnosed in the United States (US) during 2017, and in the same year this disease will cause an estimated 16,870 deaths [1]. Bladder cancer is more than four times as more common in men than in women, with incidence rates of 35.3 and 8.6 cases per 100,000 individuals per year, respectively. Incidence also increases with age, being rare before age 40 and having a median age at diagnosis of 73 years. Non-Hispanic whites are at higher risk of bladder cancer when compared to other racial/ethnic groups in the US [2]. In addition to the human burden of bladder cancer, the financial burden is high; of all malignant diseases, bladder cancer has been estimated to have the highest lifetime cost per patient diagnosed [3].

Risk Factors and Prevention

A variety of genetic and environmental factors have been linked to the development of UCC, the foremost being tobacco. It has been estimated that smoking has led to 50% of cases in men and 35% in women [4]. Cigarette smoking increases the risk of bladder cancer about threefold, and former smokers are still at increased, albeit lower risk. There also appears to be a relationship to both dose (number of cigarettes per day) and duration (number of years smoked) [5]. Pipe and cigar smokers are also at risk though less so than cigarette smokers. Secondhand smoke may slightly increase the risk [6, 7].

A variety of occupational exposures also increase the risk of UCC. In 1954, Case and Hosker demonstrated a 20-fold increased risk of bladder cancer in chemical dye and rubber workers [8], and since then other occupations have also been identified including leather manufacture, aluminum workers, commercial painters, truck drivers, and hairdressers. The agents used in these industries such as aniline dyes, hair dyes, and fossil fuels, all expose workers to arylamines.

Arylamines generate metabolites capable of inducing DNA mutations. A number of genes related to DNA repair and detoxification have been implicated to modify individual risk related to arylamine exposure. The most studied are *N-acetyltransferase 2* (*NAT2*) and *glutathione S-transferase M1* (*GSTM1*), both involved in detoxification. *NAT2* is responsible for N-acetylation of arylamines in the liver, and this gene is known to exhibit polymorphism which affects activity. Decreased activity is associated with slowed clearance of arylamines, and smokers expressing *NAT2* with a slower rate of acetylation have been shown to have increased risk of bladder UCC. *GSTM1* is similarly thought to have a role in detoxification, and one study demonstrated about half of the US White population lacks both copies of this gene [9]. The *GSTM1* null phenotype has been associated with increased risk of bladder cancer in some studies.

Arsenic exposure, mainly through drinking water, is associated with cancers of the bladder, lung, and skin. In Taiwan, regional differences in water arsenic levels correlate with bladder UCC incidence. Risk is clearly increased at levels above 100 μg/L. Recent studies suggest increased risk at lower levels as well [10]. Private wells in certain parts of the US have been found to contain elevated levels, and thus some populations are at risk [11] As with arylamines, there is evidence that genetic susceptibility has a role in arsenic-induced malignancies. Some drugs have been demonstrated to increase the risk of bladder cancer, including phenacetin and cyclophosphamide.

The American Cancer Society's Oncology in Practice: Clinical Management, First Edition. Edited by The American Cancer Society.

More recently, pioglitazone has been associated with increased risk of bladder cancer, although in positive studies the excess risk appears to be small (20% higher) and increases with higher doses and with greater than 2 years of use [12].

As noted above, smoking is a major contributor to the burden of bladder cancer. Evidence suggests that smoking cessation decreases the risk of developing bladder cancer, particularly after 5 years, although the risk continues to remain elevated compared to never smokers [13]. Additionally, there is some evidence suggesting that smoking cessation following the diagnosis of bladder cancer is associated with decreased disease recurrence [14]. Non-steroidal anti-inflammatory use, aside from phenacetin, has been associated with decreased bladder cancer risk [15]. Total fluid intake has also been linked with a decreased risk of bladder cancer in some series, although the effect is not found uniformly across studies. The effect of dietary factors and vitamin supplementation on the development of UCC appears to be minimal [16].

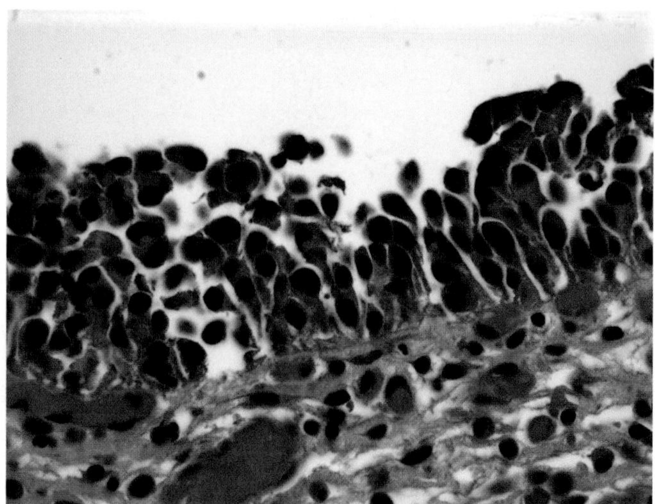

Figure 18.1 Carcinoma *in situ*. *Source:* J.C. Manivel, University of Minnesota and Minneapolis VA Medical Center. Reproduced with permission from Dr Manivel.

Pathology

UCC is the most common histology of bladder cancer in the US, accounting for over 90% of cases. Nonurothelial histologies include squamous cell carcinoma and adenocarcinoma; these rarer histologies will be discussed later in this chapter. Most urothelial tumors demonstrate a papillary growth pattern which is appreciable on cystoscopic examination. Some tumors, particularly high-grade tumors, may be sessile with a solid growth pattern, and carcinoma *in situ* (CIS) is flat with an erythematous or velvety appearance on cystoscopy. The most important pathologic tumor characteristics in UCC are tumor grade and depth of invasion. Invasion can be seen microscopically as nests, clusters, or single cells within the lamina propria or deeper, and often there is an associated desmoplastic or inflammatory response. Most tumors at initial presentation (75–80%) do not invade the detrusor muscle, and are referred to as non-muscle- invasive bladder cancer (NMIBC). This distinction is important as treatment options change dramatically once the tumor invades the detrusor muscle. Invasion of detrusor muscle should be established by histologic evidence of tumor infiltrating thick bundles of smooth muscle, as opposed to involvement of the muscularis mucosa, a thin muscular layer present in the subepithelial connective tissue of some regions of the bladder.

UCC is now graded on a two-tiered system and reported as low grade and high grade per the World Health Organization (WHO). Differences between the two are based on architectural and cytologic changes when compared to normal urothelium. Low-grade urothelial tumors are characterized by ordered cell layers with minimal loss of polarity, and the cells have slight variation in size and shape with occasional mitoses. Low-grade tumors are almost uniformly non-invasive, with invasion only reported rarely into the superficial lamina propria. In contrast, high-grade cancers demonstrate disordered cell layers with frequent loss of polarity, marked cellular pleomorphism, prominent nucleoli and frequent mitoses (Figure 18.1). High-grade tumors are responsible for the majority of muscle-invasive tumors, and thus this finding increases the risk of disease progression. An additional WHO category, papillary urothelial neoplasm of low malignant potential (PUNLMP), has an appearance between normal urothelium and low-grade carcinoma and is by definition noninvasive [17].

An additional pathologic finding important in characterizing invasive urothelial tumors is lymphovascular invasion (LVI). Although not included in bladder cancer staging, LVI is predictive of outcomes in patients with urothelial carcinoma. LVI can be seen in both transurethral resection (TUR) and cystectomy specimens, although there is some interobserver variability in recognizing as well as reporting this finding. In prior studies, LVI is reported in 10–28% of TUR specimens for T1 UCC, and is seen in 30–50% of radical cystectomy specimens [18]. A number of investigators have found that LVI is predictive of pathologic lymph node involvement, disease recurrence, and progression following cystectomy and nephroureterectomy for UCC of the bladder and upper urinary tract, respectively. In patients with clinical stage T1 bladder UCC, LVI independently predicts disease progression and metastases [18]. Thus, LVI may not only help with prognostication, but help identify candidates for neoadjuvant or adjuvant chemotherapy, as well as consideration for early cystectomy.

Some variant histologies of UCC have prognostic and therapeutic implications. These generally represent about 7% of bladder tumors obtained by TUR, although a recent multi-institutional cystectomy database found variant histology in 24.6% of specimens [19]. This disparity is because tumors with variant histology generally present with more advanced stage, warranting more aggressive surgical therapy. UCC with squamous or glandular differentiation is the most common variant histology (Figure 18.2), particularly in those with muscle-invasive bladder carcinoma (MIBC). Thought to be chemoresistant, reanalysis of a Southwest Oncology Group neoadjuvant MVAC (methotrexate, vinblastine, doxorubicin and cisplatin) trial found that UCC with squamous or glandular differentiation were more responsive to MVAC and in fact may be an indication for neoadjuvant chemotherapy [20]. In other aspects as well, these histologies are treated similarly to conventional UCC.

Micropapillary bladder cancer is another histologic variant of UCC, found in about 1% of bladder tumors, although its

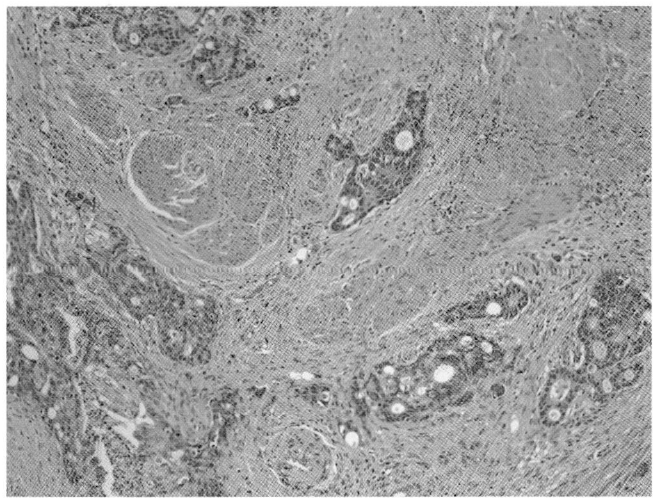

Figure 18.2 High grade, muscle invasive urothelial carcinoma with glandular differentiation *Source:* J.C. Manivel, University of Minnesota and Minneapolis VA Medical Center. Reproduced with permission from Dr Manivel.

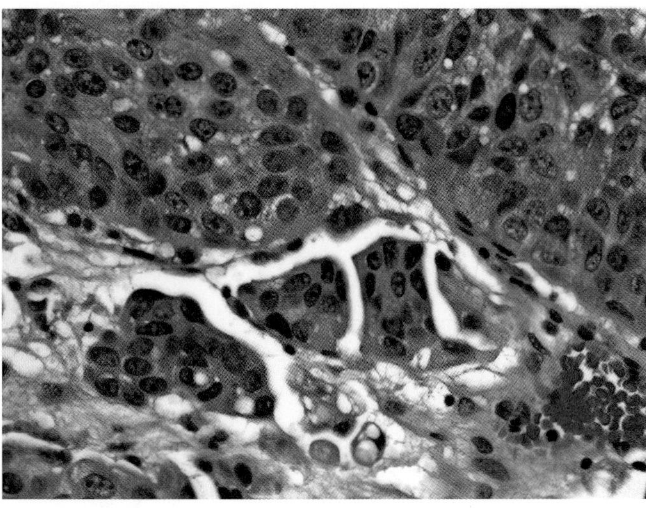

Figure 18.3 Micropapillary variant of high-grade urothelial carcinoma. *Source:* J.C. Manivel, University of Minnesota and Minneapolis VA Medical Center. Reproduced with permission from Dr Manivel.

incidence may be underreported (Figure 18.3). As with many variant histologies, these tumors present more often in advanced stage and evidence suggests worse outcomes following treatment. In a series of 100 patients with micropapillary bladder tumors, Kamat *et al.* found that only 44 had NMIBC at presentation, and 67% of the 27 who attempted bladder preservation with intravesical therapy following TUR developed disease progression [21]. They also noted a high incidence of pathologic upstaging in those undergoing immediate cystectomy (75%) and neoadjuvant chemotherapy did not appear to have any benefit in this series. Despite this aggressive course, outcomes by stage appear similar to conventional UCC [22], and more recent studies demonstrated a good pathologic response to neoadjuvant chemotherapy, with 13/29 (45%) found to be pT0 at cystectomy [23].

Sarcomatoid carcinoma of the bladder, also known as carcinosarcoma, is another rare histologic variant (<1%) of bladder UCC. Similar to sarcomatoid carcinomas of other organs, it contains elements with mesenchymal-appearing morphology in addition to the epithelial (urothelial) elements. The mesenchymal portion can appear as undifferentiated spindle cells, or have other histologic components such as bone, muscle, or cartilage. Molecular studies suggest these cancers are of monoclonal origin, and the component with mesenchymal differentiation is derived from the epithelial component. In comparison with conventional UCC, these tumors present with more advanced stage and have poorer survival even when controlling for stage. Although limited numbers have been reported, these tumors appear to be responsive to similar chemotherapeutic regimens as UCC. Numerous other histologic variants of UCC have been identified [24], some with variations in their management relative to conventional UCC [25], but their description is beyond the scope of this chapter.

Staging

As with any cancer, appropriate staging assists in determining the next step in treatment. The TNM staging system of the American Joint Committee on Cancer and the Union for International Cancer Control for bladder cancer is shown in Table 18.1 [26]. Ta, Tis, and T1 constitute NMIBC, and encompass 70–80% of bladder cancer at diagnosis, with the remainder being T2–T4. It should be noted that prostatic involvement as part of T4 specifically means bladder tumor which has grown to the point where it invades the prostatic stroma, as opposed to an independent prostatic urothelial cancer which would be staged separately. Nodal regions within the true pelvis include the external iliac, obturator, hypogastric, and presacral areas. It should also be noted that involvement of the common iliac nodes is considered N3 disease, and nodal spread beyond this is considered metastatic disease (M1). The M1 category has been divided into M1a (metastasis to nodes beyond the common iliac nodes) and M1b (nonlymph node distant metastases).

Pathologic staging occurs after radical cystectomy, and the specimen allows for more accurate staging and assessment of the risk of recurrence and progression. Clinical staging occurs through the combined findings of transurethral resection of the bladder tumor (TURBT), bimanual examination under anesthesia and cross-sectional imaging (computed tomography (CT) or magnetic resonance imaging (MRI)). The TURBT specimen obtained is evaluated by a pathologist to determine grade and stage, including evidence of invasion. As the resected tumor is obtained in pieces and may contain cautery artifact, depth of tumor invasion in various layers can be difficult to determine. Examination under anesthesia is typically performed before and after TURBT, mainly to determine if the mass is palpable, and if so, if it is still palpable after resection. Masses which are palpable prior to resection are considered at least T2b, and those which are still palpable after resection or are fixed are considered to be locally advanced, T3b–T4 disease. CT or MRI can be used to evaluate the primary tumor as well as to detect evidence of lymphadenopathy or metastatic disease. CT is more

Table 18.1 American Joint Committee on Cancer (AJCC) TNM staging system for bladder cancer.

Primary tumor (T)		
	TX	Primary tumor cannot be assessed
	T0	No evidence of primary tumor
	Ta	Noninvasive papillary carcinoma
	Tis	Carcinoma *in situ*
	T1	Tumor invades subepithelial connective tissue
	T2	Tumor invades muscularis propria
	pT2a	Tumor invades superficial muscularis propria (inner half)
	pT2b	Tumor invades deep muscularis propria (outer half)
	T3	Tumor invades perivesical tissue
	pT3a	Tumor invades perivesical tissue microscopically
	pT3b	Tumor invades perivesical tissue macroscopically
	T4	Tumor invades surrounding organs/ body wall
	T4a	Tumor invades prostatic stroma, uterus, vagina
	T4b	Tumor invades pelvic wall, abdominal wall
Regional lymph nodes (N)		
	NX	Lymph nodes cannot be assessed
	N0	No lymph node metastasis
	N1	Single regional lymph node metastasis in true pelvis
	N2	Multiple regional lymph node metastases in true pelvis
	N3	Lymph node metastasis to the common iliac nodes
Distant metastasis (M)		
	M0	No distant metastasis
	M1	Distant metastasis
	M1a	Distant metastasis limited to lymph nodes beyond the common iliacs
	M1b	Non-lymph node distant metastasis

When T is...	And N is...	And M is...	Then the stage group is...
Ta	N0	M0	0a
Tis	N0	M0	0is
T1	N0	M0	I
T2a	N0	M0	II
T2b	N0	M0	II
T3a, T3b, T4a	N0	M0	IIIA
T1–T4a	N1	M0	IIIA
T1–T4a	N2, N3	M0	IIIB
T4b	N0	M0	IVA
Any T	Any N	M1a	IVA
Any T	Any N	M1b	IVB

Source: Amin MB *et al.* (eds) AJCC Cancer Staging Manual, 8th edn. New York: Springer, 2017. Reproduced with permission of Springer.

commonly used, and can determine tumors with extension into perivesical fat, with sensitivity and specificity ranging from 60 to 96% in various series [27, 28]. MRI appears to have similar results [27], although technological advances in MRI have led to improving capabilities in determining muscle invasion, extravesical extension, and lymph node involvement [29]. In addition to CT and MRI, positron emission tomography (PET)/CT has been demonstrated to improve nodal and metastatic staging [30].

Diagnosis

Bladder cancer presents most commonly as painless gross or microscopic hematuria. Among patients with gross hematuria, about 15% will have bladder cancer found on subsequent evaluation, while in those with microscopic hematuria, bladder cancer is found in about 4% [31]. Other symptoms suggestive of UCC include irritative voiding symptoms such as urinary urgency and frequency, which may be caused by CIS. More advanced disease may present with pelvic, hip, or low back pain, renal insufficiency from obstruction, or symptomatic metastases.

Those who present with hematuria undergo an evaluation which includes cystoscopy, upper urinary tract imaging and voided urine cytology. CT with intravenous contrast including delayed images to evaluate the renal pelvis and ureters (CT urogram) has supplanted excretory urography as the method of upper urinary tract imaging most commonly used for the evaluation of hematuria. This provides evaluation of other potential causes of hematuria, such as kidney stones or renal cell carcinoma, as well as an evaluation of the renal pelvis and ureters for filling defects suggestive of upper urinary tract UCC. Some larger bladder tumors can also be visualized on CT. However, complete hematuria evaluation also requires cystoscopy for bladder evaluation due to sensitivity of 79% for tumors ≤1 cm and 58% when ≤5 mm [32].

Cystoscopy is the gold standard for the detection of bladder tumors, and typically bladder tumors are seen as a papillary or sessile mass within the bladder, or flat erythematous or velvety areas in the case of CIS. A common problem in bladder cancer is recurrence, and while some of this is due to *de novo* formation of new tumors, there is also evidence that some tumors already present are incompletely detected and treated. In recent years some adjunctive technologies have been studied to improve the visualization of tumors and provide better endoscopic treatment. Hexaminolevulinate (HAL) cystoscopy or photodynamic diagnosis is one method shown to improve bladder tumor detection. HAL is an ester of 5-aminolevulinic acid, and when instilled into the bladder it causes protoporphyrin accumulation which can be visualized pink under blue light (around 400 nm). This accumulation occurs preferentially in tumors, and a recent meta-analysis of multiple studies confirms higher detection rates of Ta and Tis tumors when compared with standard white light cystoscopy [33]. Additionally, recurrence rates following TURBT assisted by HAL cystoscopy were lower at 12 months than standard cystoscopy (34.5% vs 45.4%) [33]. More recently narrow-band imaging has been utilized increasingly and shows promise in improving bladder tumor detection. This technology again takes advantage of the higher blood flow within tumor tissues, and uses two light wavelengths (415 and 540 nm) which are absorbed by hemoglobin. It allows better differentiation between surface capillaries and tumors. Tumors continue to appear red against a background of green. Many studies have found improved tumor detection rates with this technology, and two prospective, randomized trials have been able to demonstrate decreased recurrence rates following narrow-band imaging- based tumor resection as well [34, 35].

Urinary cytology is also typically performed as part of the workup of hematuria and in monitoring patients with a history of UCC. The results are reported at most institutions as negative, atypical, suspicious, or positive. Voided urine is typically collected for this test, although some use bladder barbotage at the same time as cystoscopy in an attempt to improve sensitivity. This is because cytology has poor sensitivity for UCC, particularly for low-grade tumors. Reported sensitivity rates for cytology range from 20 to 70%, but typically for high- grade tumors and CIS the sensitivity is 40–60% [36]. The main benefit of cytology is its specificity, which is 90–100% in most series, thus making it useful to identify patients in need of biopsy to look for CIS in the absence of abnormalities on cystoscopy. A number of other urinary markers have been developed and still more are in the investigational stage, mainly in the interest of foregoing cystoscopy in bladder cancer diagnosis or follow-up, or in an attempt to replace urine cytology. The NMP22 BladderChek, Urovysion (FISH), ImmunoCyt and BTA test are Food and Drug Administration approved tests for use in the US. While many have improved sensitivity relative to cytology, as yet none has proven sufficient to supplant cystoscopy [37]. For this reason, the American Urologic Association, National Comprehensive Cancer Network, and European Urologic Association guidelines do not have recommended use of these markers in the diagnosis and treatment of bladder cancer at this time. There are special circumstances where some of these tests may be valuable [38–40], and this was the subject of a recent review [41].

Once a bladder tumor is diagnosed on cystoscopy, the next step in diagnosis and first step in treatment is a TURBT. This is an endoscopic procedure performed under regional or general anesthesia, and the tumor is removed in a piecemeal fashion with the use of monopolar or bipolar electrocautery. Once the tumor is completely resected, an additional specimen of the tumor base is usually obtained to ensure accurate staging in case of invasion. Any additional areas of abnormality should also be biopsied or resected. A final step which can be considered following TURBT is perioperative instillation of mitomycin C (MMC). Immediate or early (within 24 h) administration of intravescial chemotherapy following TURBT has been evaluated in a number of trials, with MMC being the most common agent used for this purpose. A large meta-analysis of various perioperative chemotherapy agents demonstrated decreased recurrence in those who received a single dose of intravesical chemotherapy (odds ratio 0.61) [42]. The benefit is more definitive in those with single, low-grade bladder tumors, with uncertain benefit in the setting of multiple tumors or high-grade disease. MMC is cytotoxic, and if there is any evidence of bladder perforation from the TURBT then MMC should be withheld.

Those with a positive cytology but no evidence of bladder tumor also require an endoscopic procedure to localize the source of the positive cytology. In these cases, random bladder biopsies are performed as well as a prostatic urethral biopsy in males, and upper urinary tract washings are also obtained for cytology. The pathologic results of the TURBT or biopsies, as well as findings on CT and examination under anesthesia, allow for appropriate pathologic staging of the patient with newly diagnosed bladder cancer and assist in decisions regarding the next stage in treatment.

Treatment

The treatment of bladder cancer depends mainly on the pathologic stage and grade. As stated above, a significant threshold exists at the level of muscle invasion which completely alters the treatment algorithm, as does the development of metastatic disease. We will therefore examine treatment for NMIBC (Ta, Tis and T1), MIBC (T2–4, N1–3, M0) and metastatic bladder cancer separately.

NMIBC

This group represents roughly 70–80% of bladder cancer cases at diagnosis. The first step in treatment is that already mentioned – TURBT with or without perioperative instillation of intravesical chemotherapy. The next step depends on a number of factors which all relate to the risk of tumor recurrence and progression. Established risk factors include tumor grade, presence of invasion (T1), presence of concomitant CIS, tumor size ≥3 cm, number of tumors and, in those with a history of bladder tumors, frequency of recurrence [43]. Among those with NMIBC, about 70% are low grade and noninvasive (PUNLMP or low-grade Ta). For most of these patients, no further treatment is required, but surveillance is needed to monitor for recurrence (see Follow-Up). A caveat to this generalization applies to patients with multiple and/or recurrent low-grade Ta tumors, in whom further intravesical therapy may be considered to slow the rate of recurrence.

Repeat TURBT about 6 weeks following initial resection is indicated in those who did not undergo complete tumor resection at initial TURBT, as well as those with invasive disease (T1) found at TURBT. The risk of residual disease and pathologic understaging in those with T1 tumors has been studied by a number of groups. In a large series of suspected T1 tumors, 48% had residual NMIBC (Ta, Tis, or T1) on repeat TURBT, and 30% upstaged to T2 disease [44]. The rate of upstaging on repeat TURBT is higher in those without detrusor muscle present in the initial specimen. Additionally, upstaging at cystectomy for clinical T1 disease has been reported to be as high at 50%, and a randomized controlled trial demonstrated decreased risk of recurrence and progression following repeat TURBT for those with T1 disease on initial resection [45]. Thus, those with T1 disease require repeat resection, and some would argue those with high-grade Ta disease should also undergo repeat TUR, as recurrence rates are lower in retrospective series [46]. The American Urologic Association and European Association of Urology guidelines recommend repeat resection for those with T1 disease.

Patients with NMIBC can be divided into three risk groups – low, intermediate, and high – based on tumor size, number, level of invasion, presence or absence of CIS, and recurrence history. Sylvester *et al.* [43] have developed a mathematical model for prediction of the risk of recurrence and progression using data from a large group of patients who had previously been treated on several clinical trials. These models are represented in the form of tables available in an electronic and paper format that allow for easy calculation of risk of recurrence and progression. The one issue with this prediction model is that most of the patients were treated with intravesical chemotherapy, not immunotherapy such as bacillus Calmette–Guérin (BCG), and hence any advantage that immunotherapy holds over chemotherapy may not be considered. Stratification in this manner can help identify patients who may benefit from further treatment, such as intravesical therapy or early cystectomy, or closer surveillance, as discussed under Follow-Up.

Intravesical therapy is administered in a variety of situations, some of which have been outlined. A variety of agents are used for this purpose, most commonly chemotherapeutic agents such as MMC, gemcitabine, epirubicin, doxorubicin, valrubicin, and thiotepa. The side effects of these agents are mainly due to local toxicity, with the exception of thiotepa, which can cause myelosuppression. Immunotherapeutic agents have also been administered intravesically, such as BCG and interferon. BCG, as an attenuated mycobacterium, can result in systemic side effects including disseminated infection. The two most studied and utilized intravesical agents are MMC and BCG. Postoperative instillation of intravesical chemotherapy, as discussed above, is one common use of intravesical agents, although immunotherapy is not used for this purpose. Intravesical agents are also typically given as an induction course about 2–6 weeks following complete TURBT, and in some cases with an additional maintenance schedule for up to 3 years. The induction course is typically delivered intravesically once per week for 6 weeks. Indications for an induction course of intravesical therapy include multiple, large, or recurrent low-grade Ta tumors, or those with high-grade tumors (Ta, T1, or Tis). For those with extensive or recurrent low-grade disease, in whom the risk of recurrence is high but the risk of progression is low, BCG or MMC can be used to prevent recurrence. There is some evidence that BCG, particularly with maintenance therapy, is more effective in preventing recurrence although at the cost of increased urinary adverse effects [47]. For those with high-grade disease, BCG should be used unless contraindicated, and evidence suggests that maintenance therapy results in greater reduction in disease progression compared to induction alone [48].

For some patients with high-grade NMIBC, radical cystectomy is indicated due to the high risk of occult progression and death from disease. Those with high-grade T1 tumors are particularly at risk for occult muscle invasive disease due to the potential for clinical understaging. In a multicenter study of 1136 patients who underwent cystectomy for high-grade T1 bladder UCC, 50% were ≥ T2 on final pathology and 16% had nodal metastases [49]. For those who initially undergo intravesical BCG instillation following TURBT, approximately 35% of those with high-grade T1 will progress to T2 disease, and this is despite optimized initial staging with repeat TURBT [50]. Additionally, those who present with NMIBC and undergo cystectomy at progression to T2 fare worse than those who present initially with T2 disease with a 3-year cancer-specific survival of 37% versus 67% [51]. Thus, as many will progress and risk poor outcomes with deferring of definitive local therapy, early cystectomy should be considered in some NMIBC patients at high risk of progression. Early cystectomy should be offered to those with high-grade T1 disease and risk factors for recurrence and progression including multifocal disease, difficult resection site hindering complete resection, LVI, tumor within a diverticulum or prostatic urethra, or associated CIS. Another population with NMIBC who should strongly consider cystectomy is patients with high-grade recurrence (including CIS) following BCG, termed BCG failures. Treatment alternatives in this group include repeat BCG induction with or without interferon, intravesical chemotherapy with gemcitabine or other agents, or cystectomy. Response rates for repeat induction BCG with or without interferon are worse than those without prior treatment (15–35%), although this depends on time from initial BCG to recurrence [52]. Gemcitabine has improved activity compared to repeat BCG induction in this population [53], although the progression rate in this small study was similar between the two treatments at around 35%. Thus, for those with early recurrence after induction BCG, termed BCG-refractory, cystectomy should be offered for the increased risk of occult disease progression, similar to those with high-grade T1.

MIBC

Approximately 20% of patients will present with muscle-invasive disease, and others with NMIBC will progress to muscle-invasive disease. Radical cystectomy is the gold standard for obtaining local control in this setting. Prior to consideration for cystectomy, staging is needed in these patients to confirm that there is no evidence of metastatic disease, as this would dramatically alter management. Typically, this involves CT of the abdomen and pelvis including delayed images to examine for upper urinary tract disease, chest X-ray or CT, and bone scan for those with bone pain or elevated alkaline phosphatase. FDG-PET has also been shown to have a potential role in finding nodal or visceral metastases (which can alter management) before cystectomy [54]. Candidates for radical cystectomy also require a thorough preoperative evaluation, as short-term complication rates are reported as high as 60% and perioperative death rates around 2%. Once radical cystectomy is indicated, timely evaluation and treatment are needed as evidence suggests worse outcomes in those with delays greater than 12 weeks from diagnosis [55].

Radical cystectomy in males includes removal of the bladder, prostate, seminal vesicles, and distal ureters. For men interested in orthotopic urinary diversion, the bladder neck and prostatic urethra should be free from tumor, and a frozen section of the urethral margin should confirm this. Nerve-sparing techniques are also performed in select patients to attempt to maintain erectile function, with variable results published to date. Radical cystectomy in females classically involves the removal of the bladder, uterus, adjacent anterior vaginal wall, urethra, and distal ureters. For those concerned with sexual function, the anterior vaginal wall and/or uterus may be spared in cases without extensive posterior wall involvement with invasion of these structures. Additionally, in women interested in orthotopic diversion, the urethra may be spared in the absence of bladder neck and urethral UCC similar to men. While classically radical cystectomy is an open procedure, robot-assisted laparoscopic radical cystectomy is gaining popularity in recent years. While the technique is performed to mimic the open procedure, the results of ongoing clinical trials will help determine the safety and oncologic efficacy of this approach.

Pelvic lymph node dissection is included as a standard part of the surgery, and the nodes include those of the external iliac, obturator, internal iliac, and common iliac vessels. Extent of lymphadenectomy has been associated with increased likelihood of finding positive lymph nodes, as well as a potential therapeutic benefit in lymph node positive and negative patients [56–59]. While attempts have been made to standardize a lymph node count sufficient for prognostic and therapeutic benefit, many patient, surgeon, and pathologist variables have been demonstrated to affect lymph node counts. The template of dissection is likely more important than any actual number [60], and ongoing clinical trials are examining the extent of dissection (standard described above compared to extended dissection up to the inferior mesenteric artery) as it relates to cancer-specific survival.

Table 18.2 Reported 5-year recurrence-free survival (RFS) rates following radical cystectomy for urothelial carcinoma of the bladder [61, 103].

Pathologic stage	5-year RFS (%)
≤pT1	81–88
pT2	70–81
pT3	44–68
pT4	16–44
N+	29–35

Outcomes following radical cystectomy vary based on pathologic stage. Reported 5-year recurrence-free survival rates as related to pathologic stage are listed in Table 18.2. Patients with nonorgan confined disease and positive lymph nodes have worse outcomes overall. In a cohort of 1,054 patients undergoing cystectomy, 558 (53%) had ≥ T3 disease and/or positive lymph nodes at the time of cystectomy, suggesting many patients undergoing cystectomy are at high risk of disease recurrence and death [61]. A recent series of 447 recurrences postcystectomy reveal that most patients (65%) recur at distant sites exclusively, and another 16% recur concomitantly at local and distant sites [62]. Thus, improving outcomes in these patients at high risk of recurrence requires systemic therapy. Neoadjuvant and adjuvant chemotherapy address this need in MIBC, although some controversy exists regarding the optimal timing of delivery of such chemotherapy.

Neoadjuvant chemotherapy for bladder cancer currently consists of cisplatin-based combination therapy, most commonly gemcitabine and cisplatin (GC). A meta-analysis of 11 randomized trials including 3,005 patients demonstrated a 5% improvement in 5-year overall survival (OS) and 9% improvement in 5-year disease-free survival (DFS) with neoadjuvant cisplatin-based combination chemotherapy [63]. Based on phase 2 data and the Southwest Oncology Group trial, a combination of methotrexate, vinblastine, doxorubicin, and cisplatin (MVAC) was initially the most common regimen used, although toxicity limited its utility in the elderly and those with excessive comorbidity. A trial comparing MVAC with GC in the setting of metastatic disease demonstrated relatively equivalent efficacy with reduced toxicity in the latter [64], and this has been extrapolated to the neoadjuvant setting in the absence of level 1 evidence. This is an important point as the GC regimen is better tolerated, potentially allowing better functional status at the time of the subsequent cystectomy. One problem with cisplatin-based regimens is the requirement for adequate renal function and good functional status, which preclude delivery in as many as 40% of patients with MIBC [65]. Alternatives in these patients include carboplatin-based regimens, which have less activity in UCC. Additionally, up to 40% of UCC is resistant to cisplatin-based combinations, thus in many patients the time allotted for chemotherapy is only a delay and chance for disease progression. This is compounded by inaccuracies in clinical staging, which, assuming only those with nonorgan-confined disease benefit from chemotherapy, means overtreatment if all patients with MIBC are given neoadjuvant chemotherapy. This has led to use of adjuvant chemotherapy in selected patients based on their cystectomy pathology (pT3–4 or node-positive disease). Unfortunately, there is less robust data to support the use of adjuvant chemotherapy in MIBC. A meta-analysis of six adjuvant trials with 491 patients demonstrated a 25% reduction in risk of death with adjuvant chemotherapy, although the authors concluded that there was insufficient numbers to make this evidence strong enough to guide clinical practice [66]. Unfortunately, no well-designed trials compare adjuvant and neoadjuvant chemotherapy at this time, and, despite level 1 evidence demonstrating the efficacy of neoadjuvant chemotherapy, it currently has a low level of acceptance. Future studies on molecular markers of treatment susceptibility and improvements in clinical staging may help determine patients appropriate for neoadjuvant therapy and improve usage of this modality.

Radical cystectomy and urinary diversion is an extensive procedure, with a high risk of complications as well as resultant changes in lifestyle from the urinary diversion. Some patients are not candidates for cystectomy due to frailty or extensive comorbidity, and others simply refuse the procedure. Thus, bladder sparing options are available for these patients who have reasonable outcomes with appropriate selection. TURBT alone is capable of completely treating some MIBC, as evidenced by a pT0 rate of about 16% at cystectomy in the absence of neoadjuvant chemotherapy. Selection criteria include T2 disease based on clinical evaluation including examination under anesthesia and imaging, size ≤3 cm and no CIS. Patients considering this treatment need repeat TURBT with no residual tumor on the second resection. Safety of this approach has been verified in small series, with only 18% dying of disease at >10 years of follow-up if no tumor was found at the repeat resection [67]. Partial cystectomy can be offered to a similar patient population with the added benefit of better staging of the local tumor as well as the lymph nodes. One caveat is that the tumor must be in a location amenable to partial cystectomy, such as at the dome or in a diverticulum, and away from the ureteral orifices. Similar outcomes can be found in these patients, and some have used this in patients with a good response to neoadjuvant therapy to ensure complete pathologic response. Lastly, combinations of TURBT, chemotherapy, and radiation have been used in select patients with MIBC who are medically unfit or refuse cystectomy. Best responses are seen in those with solitary cT2–T3a tumors amenable to complete TURBT, no hydronephrosis, no CIS, and adequate renal function for chemotherapy. Five-year survival rates in various trials are around 50%, which is similar to those found in neoadjuvant chemotherapy and cystectomy trials, although no trials directly compare the two modalities in this highly selected patient population. Of note, in one large series about 30% required cystectomy due to incomplete response to therapy or recurrent invasive tumor on follow-up [68], thus close surveillance is required as some patients will fail early or late with persistent or recurrent disease.

Metastatic Bladder Cancer

Patients who have developed metastatic bladder cancer carry a poor prognosis overall. Despite reported response rates to first-line chemotherapy as high as 70% in some series, median overall survival in these trials is in the range of 10–15 months. Prognostic indicators in these patients were analyzed in a large group who received MVAC at Memorial Sloan-Kettering Cancer Center [69]. Karnofsky performance score <80% and presence of visceral metastases were predictors of poorer survival in this population. Patients with neither of these risk factors had a median survival of 33 months, while those with one or two of these factors had a median survival of 13.4 and 9.3 months, respectively.

First-line chemotherapy in these patients is similar to that used in the neoadjuvant setting, with GC and MVAC used most commonly in those with adequate renal function and performance status. In the randomized trial of GC versus MVAC, median OS was 14.8 months for MVAC and 13.8 months for GC ($P = 0.746$) [66]. Response rates were 46% and 49% for MVAC and GC, respectively, with similar complete response rates at 12%. Cisplatin is replaced with carboplatin in some patients with poor renal function or in elderly/frail patients, although response rates for carboplatin are lower. Until recently, second-line therapies for those that failed prior platinum-based regimens included gemcitabine and taxanes either alone or in combination, with a reported median OS in this setting of 7–10 months. While not approved in the US, vinflunine was approved in Europe in 2009 based on a phase 3 randomized trial demonstrating a 2.6 month OS benefit in the population which met all eligibility criteria (6.9 vs 4.3 months, $P = 0.040$), although the intent-to-treat population which included 13 ineligible patients did not reach statistical significance [70]. In May 2016, the Food and Drug Administration approved atezolizumab, a PD-L1 antibody, in those with disease progression following platinum-based chemotherapy based on a single arm, phase 2 trial in 310 patients. Among all patients, 15% had an objective response and in those with higher PD-L1 expression the response rate was higher (26%) [71]. These responses appear durable, as 84% of responders continued to respond at median follow-up of 11.7 months. Since atezolizumab, other PD-L1 inhibitors (durvalumab, avelumab) as well as PD-1 inhibitors (nivolumab, pembrolizumab) have been FDA approved for use in those with locally advanced and metastatic urothelial carcinoma. Future directions include targeted molecular therapies, which are currently in clinical trials.

Follow-Up

Follow-up for patients with NMIBC at some institutions is similar for all patients, without stratification based on risk. Typical follow-up schedules would involve cystoscopy and urinary cytology every 3 months for 2 years, then every 6 months for 2 years and then annually. This presumes no bladder recurrence, but should the patient recur the process starts again. The risk of upper urinary tract cancer in general is low, so upper tract imaging is repeated every 2 years. This does take into account the fact that recurrences are more common in the first 2 years and then recedes thereafter, but it assumes the risk is approximately the same in all patients with NMIBC.

Others have adopted a stratified approach based on the risk of recurrence in certain subgroups. Those with PUNLMP have a

25–50% risk of recurrence and very low risk of progression. For those with low-grade Ta lesions, the risk of recurrence is approximately 50–70% and the risk of progression is approximately 5%. Additionally, the risk of upper tract recurrence is less than 1% in this population. The EAU has adopted surveillance programs based on risk, and this is increasingly being accepted in the US. In these patients, cystoscopy and cytology can be performed at 3 months and, if negative, repeated at 9 months and then annually. Upper tract surveillance is not routinely performed in this group, but rather based on symptoms. The intensity of this regimen increases in those with intermediate risk disease (multifocal, large, or recurrent low-grade Ta UCC), and is further intensified in those at high risk (high-grade disease). Those with high-risk disease are recommended to have cystoscopy and cytology every 3 months for 2 years, then every 6 months until 5 years, then annually. Additionally, due to an up to 20–25% risk in upper tract recurrence, annual or at least biennial upper tract imaging is recommended.

Follow-up after cystectomy is also based on the risk of recurrence at most institutions, although there is debate on the utility of various components. The risks of recurrence include local or distant recurrent disease, as well as risk of upper tract recurrence and urethral recurrence for those with the urethra left *in situ*. General guidelines include routine chest X-ray and cross-sectional imaging of the abdomen and pelvis to examine for local, nodal, and visceral metastases as well as upper urinary tract disease. Urine cytology is also usually performed to examine for upper tract recurrence as well. Urethral surveillance with washings or voided cytology in those with an orthotopic diversion is debated, as some have shown similar outcomes in patients with recurrence detected via surveillance as those with symptomatic presentation (i.e., blood per urethra). This can be stratified based on risk of recurrence determined by pathologic stage, and with decreasing intensity as most local and distant recurrences occur in the first 2–3 years following cystectomy [72].

Upper Urinary Tract Urothelial Carcinoma

UCC of the renal pelvis makes up around 10% of all renal tumors and 5% of all urothelial tumors. Upper urinary tract urothelial carcinoma (UUT-UCC) is much less common than UCC of the bladder, thought to be due to decreased exposure times to the same carcinogens. Exceptions with a higher incidence of UUT-UCC than bladder are in cases of Balkan nephropathy and phenacetin abuse. Balkan nephropathy is a chronic tubulointerstitial disease associated with a high frequency of urothelial atypia. In these cases the tumors are mainly in the upper tract, low grade and often bilateral [73]. Lynch syndrome II of hereditary nonpolyposis colorectal cancers is associated with extracolonic cancer sites, especially UUT-UCC, and in these cases tumors are usually bilateral as well. Aristolochic acid, often ingested in herbal medicines, is a risk factor for UUT-UCC, and is also a potent nephrotoxin. Other risk factors for UUT-UCC are male gender, white race, history of bladder UCC, arsenic exposure, and cigarette smoking.

While most UUT-UCC occur in the renal pelvis, when it occurs in the ureter it is typically in the distal portion. With high-grade UUT-UCC, the disease is often multifocal and associated with CIS. Bladder UCC patients have a low lifetime risk (2–4%) of UUT-TCC. However, UUT-UCC patients have a 25–75% risk of developing a bladder cancer [74] and bladder surveillance is needed in these patients. Most UUT tumors are identified on investigation for sources of hematuria, and larger, obstructing tumors may present with hydronephrosis and renal failure. Staging of UUT-UCC is similar to bladder UCC.

Treatment decisions can be complicated in UUT-UCC for a variety of reasons. Clinical staging is difficult – imaging studies can help although biopsies are usually too small to determine invasion adequately, unlike TURBT. Tumor grade has been shown to correlate directly with tumor stage. Thus, tumor grade often dictates the aggressiveness of therapy, and overall renal function also contributes to treatment decisions. The gold standard in the treatment of UUT-UCC is radical nephroureterectomy, which provides effective local tumor control and is the treatment of choice for high-grade, potentially invasive tumors except in patients with significant morbidity and renal impairment. Nephron-sparing procedures include partial ureterectomy in those with disease confined to the distal ureter and endoscopic management. Endoscopic procedures are performed either through a percutaneous approach or retrograde via the ureter, and can provide local control for lower stage and grade tumors, although it has higher rate of recurrence (up to 25–44%) when compared to extirpative surgeries [75]. Although some high-grade, Ta tumors would likely respond to endoscopic treatment, clinical staging is inaccurate thus depth of invasion is often unknown. This difficulty in clinical staging translates into difficulties in determining appropriate use of nephron-sparing surgery, as well as lymphadenectomy and neoadjuvant chemotherapy. Although there is some data on landing sites for nodal disease based on location of tumor [76], there are mixed results in retrospective studies on the potential therapeutic impact of lymph node dissection. The use of adjuvant chemotherapy is also debatable as there are no randomized trials and the results of retrospective studies are mixed [77, 78]. Another obstacle to the use of adjuvant therapy in UUT-UCC is that the regimens are usually cisplatin-based and contraindicated in those with renal insufficiency that can occur following nephroureterectomy. This makes neoadjuvant delivery an attractive option. However, there are no randomized trials specific to UUT-UCC and there are the same issues with clinical staging and determination of benefit as discussed in bladder UCC. Metastatic disease is treated in a fashion similar to metastatic bladder UCC.

Prostatic Urothelial Carcinoma

Urothelial carcinoma of the prostate can result from direct extension or indirect seeding from bladder UCC, and can also develop from the urothelium of the prostatic urethra. The incidence of primary prostatic UCC is estimated to be 1–4% of all prostate malignancies, whereas the incidence of involvement of the prostate with primary bladder UCC ranges from 12 to 48%. Risk factors for prostatic involvement include CIS of the bladder, multifocal disease, high-stage bladder cancer, lesions located in the trigone or bladder neck, and multiple courses of intravesical therapy. The staging system for primary prostatic UCC is different than staging of bladder UCC with prostatic extension (pT4a). This distinction is important as it correlates with the prognosis. Rather than pT4a and thus poor prognosis, a primary prostate lesion has a prognosis dependent on the depth of invasion of this lesion. Stromal invasion is classified as pT2, with similar implications as muscle involvement regarding need for cystoprostatectomy.

Identification of prostate involvement is crucial but challenging. Lesions may be easily be missed during cystoscopy. In one study 26.5% of patients with NMIBC without known prostatic involvement were found to have UCC in the prostate on biopsy, and 18% of them had CIS [79]. Different methods for the detection of prostate involvement have been examined, and TUR biopsies have better accuracy than prostate needle biopsy and fine needle aspiration. Treatment options for prostatic urothelial tumors depend on the depth of invasion. Superficial lesions can be treated with TUR and BCG with good results. Ductal involvement is still not an absolute indication for radical cystoprostatectomy, whereas stromal invasion is an indication as it is associated with a high nodal metastasis rate and poorer prognosis.

Non-Urothelial Tumors of the Bladder

Adenocarcinoma

Primary adenocarcinoma accounts for 0.5–2% of primary bladder malignancies [80, 81]. It can be classified into urachal and nonurachal adenocarcinoma, where the former is much less common, accounting for 0.35–0.7% of all bladder malignancies [82]. For the sake of simplicity, primary adenocarcinoma of the bladder usually refers to the malignant neoplasm derived from urothelium (the non-urachal subtype). By definition, bladder adenocarcinoma has purely glandular differentiation and should be distinguished from mixed histology with UCC. Secondary adenocarcinoma of the bladder can result from direct extension or metastatic spread. The most frequent origins of secondary adenocarcinoma are colon, prostate, breast, endometrium, and lung [80, 83]. In addition to excluding secondary sources, the diagnosis of primary adenocarcinoma requires the exclusion of benign lesions of the bladder that have glandular histology such as cystitis cystica, cystitis glandularis, von Brunn nests, nephrogenic adenoma (nephrogenic metaplasia), and urachal remnant.

This tumor occurs more commonly in males and people in their sixth decade. Predisposing factors include bladder extrophy, where 90% of tumors arising there are adenocarcinoma, vesical schistosomiasis [81], chronic irritation, infection, and cystitis glandularis [84]. Nonurachal adenocarcinomas are most commonly found in the trigone or posterior bladder wall, and unlike UCC they are often solitary lesions [83]. The most common presentations are hematuria and irritative voiding symptoms.

Due to its rarity and poor prognosis, treatment data is limited to mainly small retrospective studies. Bladder adenocarcinoma generally is very aggressive, with metastatic disease reported in up to 40% of patients at the time of diagnosis and with a reported 5-year DFS rate of 55% (95% CI 50.3–59.3) [81]. The most important prognostic factor is tumor stage, and outcomes are similar to UCC when compared by stage. As most are at an advanced stage at diagnosis, radical cystectomy is the primary option for therapy [85]. Adjuvant radiation or chemotherapy may be considered in some cases. Several studies looked at the effect of 5-fluorouracil as an adjuvant or palliative treatment with good response in some subjects [86].

Urachal adenocarcinoma arises most often at the junction of the urachal ligament and bladder dome. It is believed that these tumors originate either from enteric rests during embryological development or from metaplasia of the urachal ligament [87]. There are still no clear diagnostic criteria for urachal adenocarcinoma, but some suggest that any adenocarcinoma arising at the dome of the bladder should be considered urachal until proven otherwise, often with a sharp demarcation between the tumor and surface epithelium. As with bladder adenocarcinoma, a separate primary adenocarcinoma needs to be excluded [88]. Sheldon *et al.* proposed a staging system that was followed by most reported case series [89], and others utilize the Mayo staging system (Table 18.3). Urachal adenocarcinoma affects younger people when compared with other bladder cancers, and many patients present with locally advanced disease that is not reliably cured with surgery. Treatment for clinically localized disease is partial cystectomy with a 5-year DFS of 44% [87]. There was no benefit of radical versus partial cystectomy in retrospective series. As the majority of survivors had the urachal ligament resected at surgery, it is recommended to remove the urachal ligament via *en bloc* resection of the bladder dome, urachal ligament, posterior rectus fascia, and umbilicus. There appears to be no role for adjuvant therapy at present, although salvage surgery for local recurrence has demonstrated good results [88].

Squamous Cell Carcinoma

The worldwide prevalence of bladder squamous cell carcinoma (SCC) varies by region from 1 to 75% of bladder cancers, and in the US it is about 3–7%. The incidence of this tumor is highest in areas of the Middle East and East Africa where bilharziasis is endemic. In these areas, SCC is the most common tumor of the bladder, and SCC of the bladder is the most common cancer in male patients [90]. Patients at risk for SCC of the bladder include smokers, those with occupational exposures to aromatic amines, *Schistosoma haematobium* (bilharzial) infections, and

Table 18.3 Staging systems for urachal carcinoma [89, 90].

Stage	Sheldon staging system	Mayo staging system
I	Confined to urachal mucosa	Confined to urachus and/or bladder
II	Invasion confined to urachus	Extension beyond muscular layer of urachus or bladder
III A	Extension to bladder	Regional lymph node invasion
III B	Extension to abdominal wall	
III C	Extension to peritoneum	
III D	Extension to viscera other than bladder	
IV A	Metastatic to lymph nodes	Metastatic to nonregional lymph nodes or other distant sites
IV B	Distant metastases	

with long-standing cystitis[91].Chronic bladder infection and inflammation are believed to cause squamous metaplasia and leukoplakia of the urothelium, which are considered precancerous lesions [92]. The presence of a chronic urinary catheter as well as recurrent infections poses risk of this tumor in neuropathic bladder patients, especially in those with spinal cord injury, where the risk goes up to 2.5–10% after 10 years or more although more recent studies suggest a risk of 0.38% [82]. Patients being treated with cyclophosphamide for various malignancies have a 1.8% risk of developing SCC. This risk correlates well with the presence of hemorrhagic cystitis which develops usually after a year of treatment. Other possible risk factors are pelvic irradiation and immunosuppression in transplant patients [90]. There is no notable gender predilection in SCC, unlike urothelial carcinoma [91]. Most US patients with squamous cell carcinoma present in their sixth or seventh decade of life while patients with bilharzial SCC present earlier [93]. Some studies have reported an increased risk of SCC in patients treated with intravesical BCG in the presence of squamous dysplasia [89]. The role of high risk human papillomavirus is unknown [92].

Bilharzial SCC is usually a well-differentiated tumor with exophytic, nodular, fungating lesions and a relatively low prevalence of nodal and distant metastases. Patients with nonbilharzial squamous cell carcinomas usually have advanced stage disease at presentation. The cancer is usually diffusely spread with muscle invasion in more than 80%. Metastases are identified in at least 10% of cases at the time of diagnosis [95] and are associated with a poor prognosis. Common sites for metastases include regional lymph nodes, bone, lung, and bowel.

The clinical presentation is hematuria with or without lower urinary tract symptoms. Diagnosis is usually with cystoscopy and biopsies. SCC is by definition made up entirely of squamous cells with intracellular bridges, pearls and keratohyalin granules, and should be distinguished from urothelial cancer with squamous differentiation [90].

Treatment of SCC mainly depends on the stage of disease at presentation. Superficial cancers are treated like UCC, with endoscopic resection. For muscle invasion, radical cystectomy remains the most effective treatment option where the 5-year survival rate ranges between 23 and 48% [96]. The lower survival rate for SCC as compared to UCC may be contributed to by the fact that patients usually present in advanced stages. Some recommend routine urethrectomy along with radical cystectomy, as urethral recurrence rates are reported to be as high as 40%. Radiotherapy failed to be effective as sole therapy with a reported 5-year survival rate of 5–18%. As for chemotherapy, some studies showed promising results with the adjuvant use of agents such as epirubicin, with a 50–60% response rate being observed in patients with locally advanced and metastatic disease [90]. In cases of advanced disease with nodal or distant metastases, palliative chemotherapy or radiation therapy is used.

Small Cell Carcinoma

Small cell carcinoma (SmCC) is a neuroendocrine tumor, with an estimated incidence of 0.3–1% of all primary bladder cancers [97]. Most affected patients are in the fifth and sixth decade of life, and males are three times more likely to be affected than females [93]. SmCC of the bladder is associated with smoking in about 70% of cases [98] Other risk factors include recurrent or long-standing cystitis, bladder calculi, and augmented cystoplasty. Cases have also been related to pelvic irradiation and occupational chemical exposure [99].

The typical presentation is gross hematuria. Some patients will have symptoms of paraneoplastic syndromes including hypophosphatemia, elevated corticotrophin, and sensory neuropathy similar to pulmonary SmCC. Nephrotic syndrome due to secondary systemic amyloidosis, hypercalcemia, and elevated serum alpha-fetoprotein (AFP) have been also reported with bladder SmCC [97].

When compared to stage-matched bladder UCC, SmCC is more aggressive. SmCC has a tendency to invade adjacent organs, including the ureter, prostate, and ovaries. Bladder SmCC is associated with a high frequency of distant metastases and poor survival. Most patients (94%) with bladder SmCC present with muscle invasion, and approximately 67% of patients develop systemic metastases during the disease course. Metastases most commonly involve the liver, brain, lung, bone, and lymph nodes [100].

Due to the low incidence and the late presentation of the disease, only small retrospective studies are available. Transurethral resection of the bladder tumor as the sole treatment modality is not favored because the tumor is usually muscle invasive with poor 3–6 month survival rates [100]. Cystectomy alone is also usually not curative because of the high rate of systemic recurrence. This prompted the use of neoadjuvant chemotherapy or chemoradiotherapy with bladder-sparing protocols [101]. The most commonly used regimens are cisplatin and etoposide, carboplatin and etoposide, and cyclophosphamide, doxorubicin, and vincristine [97]. Bladder SmCC responds to the same chemotherapy regimens used in pulmonary SmCC, and some patients have durable complete remissions. The overall 5-year survival ranges from 8–40%[100].

References

1 Siegel RL, Miller KD, Jemal A. Cancer Statistics, 2017. *Ca Cancer J Clin* 2017;67(1):7–30.

2 Howlader N, Noone AM, Krapcho M, *et al.* (eds) SEER Cancer Statistics Review, 1975–2013, National Cancer Institute. Bethesda, MD. http://seer.cancer.gov/csr/1975_2013/, based on November 2015 SEER data submission, posted to the SEER web site, April 2016.

3 Botteman MF, Pashos CL, Redaelli A, *et al.* The health economics of bladder cancer: a comprehensive review of the published literature. *Pharmacoeconomics* 2003;21(18):1315–30.

4 Zeegers MP, Tan FE, Dorant E, *et al.* The impact of characteristics of cigarette smoking on urinary tract cancer risk: a meta-analysis of epidemiologic studies. *Cancer* 2000;89(3):630–9.

5 Brennan P, Bogillot O, Cordier S, *et al.* Cigarette smoking and bladder cancer in men: a pooled analysis of 11 case-control studies. *Int J Cancer* 2000;86(2):289–94.

6 Alberg AJ, Kouzis A, Genkinger JM, *et al.* A prospective cohort study of bladder cancer risk in relation to active cigarette smoking and household exposure to secondhand cigarette smoke. *Am J Epidemiol* 2007;165(6):660–6.

7 Zeegers MP, Goldbohm RA, van den Brandt PA. A prospective study on active and environmental tobacco smoking and bladder cancer risk (The Netherlands). *Cancer Causes Control* 2002;13(1):83–90.

8 Case RA, Hosker ME. Tumour of the urinary bladder as an occupational disease in the rubber industry in England and Wales. *Br J Prev Soc Med* 1954;8(2):39–50.

9 Yuan JM, Chan KK, Coetzee GA, *et al.* Genetic determinants in the metabolism of bladder carcinogens in relation to risk of bladder cancer. *Carcinogenesis* 2008;29(7):1386–93.

10 Mendez WM, Eftim S, Cohen J, *et al.* Relationships between arsenic concentrations in drinking water and lung and bladder cancer incidence in US counties. *J Expo Sci Environ Epidemiol* 2017;27(3):235–43.

11 Baris D, Waddell R, Freeman LE, *et al.* Elevated bladder cancer in northern New England: the role of drinking water and arsenic. *J Natl Cancer Inst* 2016;108(9):djw099.

12 Barbalat Y, Dombrovskiy VY, Weiss RE. Association between pioglitazone and urothelial bladder cancer. *Urology* 2012;80(1):1–4.

13 Baris D, Karagas MR, Verrill C, *et al.* A case-control study of smoking and bladder cancer risk: emergent patterns over time. *J Natl Cancer Inst* 2009;101(22):1553–61.

14 Lammers RJ, Witjes WP, Hendricksen K, *et al.* Smoking status is a risk factor for recurrence after transurethral resection of non-muscle-invasive bladder cancer. *Eur Urol* 2011;60(4):713–20.

15 Fortuny J, Kogevinas M, Zens MS, *et al.* Analgesic and anti-inflammatory drug use and risk of bladder cancer: a population based case control study. *BMC Urol* 2007;7:13.

16 Burger M, Catto JW, Dalbagni G, *et al.* Epidemiology and risk factors of urothelial bladder cancer. *Eur Urol* 2013;63(2):234–41.

17 Montironi R, Lopez-Beltran A. The 2004 WHO classification of bladder tumors: a summary and commentary. *Int J Surg Pathol* 2005;13(2):143–53.

18 Cho KS, Seo HK, Joung JY, *et al.* Lymphovascular invasion in transurethral resection specimens as predictor of progression and metastasis in patients with newly diagnosed T1 bladder urothelial cancer. *J Urol* 2009;182(6):2625–30.

19 Xylinas E, Rink M, Robinson BD, *et al.* Impact of histological variants on oncological outcomes of patients with urothelial carcinoma of the bladder treated with radical cystectomy. *Eur J Cancer* 2013;49(8):1889–97.

20 Scosyrev E, Ely BW, Messing EM, *et al.* Do mixed histological features affect survival benefit from neoadjuvant platinum-based combination chemotherapy in patients with locally advanced bladder cancer? A secondary analysis of Southwest Oncology Group-Directed Intergroup Study (S8710). *BJU Int* 2011;108(5):693–9. Epub 2010/11/26.

21 Kamat AM, Dinney CP, Gee JR, *et al.* Micropapillary bladder cancer: a review of the University of Texas M. D. Anderson Cancer Center experience with 100 consecutive patients. *Cancer* 2007;110(1):62–7. Epub 2007/06/02.

22 Wang JK, Boorjian SA, Cheville JC, *et al.* Outcomes following radical cystectomy for micropapillary bladder cancer versus pure urothelial carcinoma: a matched cohort analysis. *World J Urol* 2012;30(6):801–6. Epub 2012/11/08.

23 Meeks JJ, Taylor JM, Matsushita K, *et al.* Pathological response to neoadjuvant chemotherapy for muscle-invasive micropapillary bladder cancer. *BJU Int* 2013;111(8):E325–30.

24 Eble JN, Sauter G, Epstein JI, Sesterhenn IA. *Pathology and Genetics of Tumours of the Urinary System and Male Genital Organs.* Lyon: IARC Press, 2004.

25 Willis DL, Porten SP, Kamat AM. Should histologic variants alter definitive treatment of bladder cancer? *Curr Opin Urol* 2013;23(5):435–43.

26 Amin M, Edge S, Greene R, Byrd D, *Brookland R (eds) Cancer Staging Manual*, 8th Edition. American Joint Committee on Cancer. New York: Springer, 2017.

27 Kim B, Semelka RC, Ascher SM, *et al.* Bladder tumor staging: comparison of contrast-enhanced CT, T1- and T2-weighted MR imaging, dynamic gadolinium-enhanced imaging, and late gadolinium-enhanced imaging. *Radiology* 1994;193(1):239–45.

28 Kim JK, Park SY, Ahn HJ, *et al.* Bladder cancer: analysis of multi-detector row helical CT enhancement pattern and accuracy in tumor detection and perivesical staging. *Radiology* 2004;231(3):725–31.

29 Raza SA, Jhaveri KS. MR imaging of urinary bladder carcinoma and beyond. *Radiol Clin North Am* 2012;50(6):1085–110.

30 Kibel AS, Dehdashti F, Katz MD, *et al.* Prospective study of [18F]fluorodeoxyglucose positron emission tomography/computed tomography for staging of muscle-invasive bladder carcinoma. *J Clin Oncol* 2009;27(26):4314–20.

31 Sutton JM. Evaluation of hematuria in adults. *JAMA* 1990;263(18):2475–80.

32 Jinzaki M, Tanimoto A, Shinmoto H, *et al.* Detection of bladder tumors with dynamic contrast-enhanced MDCT. *Am J Roentgenol* 2007;188(4):913–8.

33 Burger M, Grossman HB, Droller M, *et al.* Photodynamic diagnosis of non-muscle-invasive bladder cancer with hexaminolevulinate cystoscopy: a meta-analysis of detection and recurrence based on raw data. *Eur Urol* 2013;64(5):846–54.

34 Naselli A, Introini C, Timossi L, *et al.* A randomized prospective trial to assess the impact of transurethral resection in narrow band imaging modality on non-muscle-invasive bladder cancer recurrence. *Eur Urol* 2012;61(5):908–13.

35 Geavlete B, Multescu R, Georgescu D, *et al.* Narrow band imaging cystoscopy and bipolar plasma vaporization for large nonmuscle-invasive bladder tumors–results of a prospective, randomized comparison to the standard approach. *Urology* 2012;79(4):846–51.

36 Yafi FA, Brimo F, Auger M, *et al.* Is the performance of urinary cytology as high as reported historically? A contemporary analysis in the detection and surveillance of bladder cancer. *Urol Oncol* 2014:32(1):27.

37 Kamat AM, Karam JA, Grossman HB, *et al.* Prospective trial to identify optimal bladder cancer surveillance protocol: reducing costs while maximizing sensitivity. *BJU Int* 2011;108(7):1119–23.

38 Gayed BA, Seideman C, Lotan Y. Cost effectiveness of fluorescence in situ hybridization in patients with atypical cytology for the detection of urothelial carcinoma. *J Urol* 2013;190(4):1181–6.

39 Kamat AM, Dickstein RJ, Messetti F, *et al.* Use of fluorescence in situ hybridization to predict response to bacillus Calmette-Guerin therapy for bladder cancer: results of a prospective trial. *J Urol* 2012;187(3):862–7.

40 Whitson J, Berry A, Carroll P, *et al.* A multicolour fluorescence in situ hybridization test predicts recurrence in patients with high-risk superficial bladder tumours undergoing intravesical therapy. *BJU Int* 2009;104(3):336–9.

41 Tomasini JM, Konety BR. Urinary markers/cytology: what and when should a urologist use. *Urol Clin North Am* 2013;40(2):165–73.

42 Sylvester RJ, Oosterlinck W, van der Meijden AP. A single immediate postoperative instillation of chemotherapy decreases the risk of recurrence in patients with stage Ta T1 bladder cancer: a meta-analysis of published results of randomized clinical trials. *J Urol* 2004;171(6):2186–90, quiz 435.

43 Sylvester RJ, van der Meijden AP, Oosterlinck W, *et al.* Predicting recurrence and progression in individual patients with stage Ta T1 bladder cancer using EORTC risk tables: a combined analysis of 2596 patients from seven EORTC trials. *Eur Urol* 2006;49(3):466–5; discussion 75–7.

44 Herr HW, Donat SM. Quality control in transurethral resection of bladder tumours. *BJU Int* 2008;102(9):1242–6.

45 Divrik RT, Sahin AF, Yildirim U, *et al.* Impact of routine second transurethral resection on the long-term outcome of patients with newly diagnosed pT1 urothelial carcinoma with respect to recurrence, progression rate, and disease-specific survival: a prospective randomised clinical trial. *Eur Urol* 2010;58(2):185–90.

46 Herr HW. Restaging transurethral resection of high risk superficial bladder cancer improves the initial response to bacillus Calmette-Guerin therapy. *J Urol* 2005;174(6):2134–7.

47 Malmstrom PU, Sylvester RJ, Crawford DE, *et al.* An individual patient data meta-analysis of the long-term outcome of randomised studies comparing intravesical mitomycin C versus bacillus Calmette-Guerin for non-muscle-invasive bladder cancer. *Eur Urol* 2009;56(2):247–56.

48 Sylvester RJ, van der MA, Lamm DL. Intravesical bacillus Calmette-Guerin reduces the risk of progression in patients with superficial bladder cancer: a meta-analysis of the published results of randomized clinical trials. *J Urol* 2002;168(5):1964–70.

49 Fritsche HM, Burger M, Svatek RS, *et al.* Characteristics and outcomes of patients with clinical T1 grade 3 urothelial carcinoma treated with radical cystectomy: results from an international cohort. *Eur Urol* 2010;57(2):300–9.

50 Herr HW, Donat SM, Dalbagni G. Can restaging transurethral resection of T1 bladder cancer select patients for immediate cystectomy? *J Urol* 2007;177(1):75–9; discussion 9.

51 Schrier BP, Hollander MP, van Rhijn BW, *et al.* Prognosis of muscle-invasive bladder cancer: difference between primary and progressive tumours and implications for therapy. *Eur Urol* 2004;45(3):292–6.

52 Gallagher BL, Joudi FN, Maymi JL, *et al.* Impact of previous bacille Calmette-Guerin failure pattern on subsequent response to bacille Calmette-Guerin plus interferon intravesical therapy. *Urology* 2008;71(2):297–301.

53 Di Lorenzo G, Perdona S, Damiano R, *et al.* Gemcitabine versus bacille Calmette-Guerin after initial bacille Calmette-Guerin failure in non-muscle-invasive bladder cancer: a multicenter prospective randomized trial. *Cancer* 2010;116(8):1893–900.

54 Mertens LS, Fioole-Bruining A, Vegt E, *et al.* Impact of F-fluorodeoxyglucose (FDG)-positron-emission tomography/computed tomography (PET/CT) on management of patients with carcinoma invading bladder muscle. *BJU Int* 2013;112(6):729–34.

55 Gore JL, Lai J, Setodji CM, *et al.* Mortality increases when radical cystectomy is delayed more than 12 weeks: results from a Surveillance, Epidemiology, and End Results-Medicare analysis. *Cancer* 2009;115(5):988–96.

56 Wright JL, Lin DW, Porter MP. The association between extent of lymphadenectomy and survival among patients with lymph node metastases undergoing radical cystectomy. *Cancer* 2008;112(11):2401–8.

57 Konety BR, Joslyn SA, O'Donnell MA. Extent of pelvic lymphadenectomy and its impact on outcome in patients diagnosed with bladder cancer: analysis of data from the Surveillance, Epidemiology and End Results Program data base. *J Urol* 2003;169(3):946–50.

58 Skinner DG. Management of invasive bladder cancer: a meticulous pelvic node dissection can make a difference. *J Urol* 1982;128(1):34–6.

59 May M, Herrmann E, Bolenz C, *et al.* Association between the number of dissected lymph nodes during pelvic lymphadenectomy and cancer-specific survival in patients with lymph node-negative urothelial carcinoma of the bladder undergoing radical cystectomy. *Ann Surg Oncol* 2011;18(7):2018–25.

60 Leissner J, Ghoneim MA, Abol-Enein H, *et al.* Extended radical lymphadenectomy in patients with urothelial bladder cancer: results of a prospective multicenter study. *J Urol* 2004;171(1):139–44.

61 Stein JP, Lieskovsky G, Cote R, *et al.* Radical cystectomy in the treatment of invasive bladder cancer: long-term results in 1,054 patients. *J Clin Oncol* 2001;19(3):666–75.

62 Mitra AP, Quinn DI, Dorff TB, *et al.* Factors influencing post-recurrence survival in bladder cancer following radical cystectomy. *BJU Int* 2012;109(6):846–54.

63 Neoadjuvant chemotherapy in invasive bladder cancer: update of a systematic review and meta-analysis of individual patient data advanced bladder cancer (ABC) meta-analysis collaboration. *Eur Urol* 2005;48(2):202–5; discussion 5–6.

64 von der Maase H, Sengelov L, Roberts JT, *et al.* Long-term survival results of a randomized trial comparing gemcitabine plus cisplatin, with methotrexate, vinblastine, doxorubicin, plus cisplatin in patients with bladder cancer. *J Clin Oncol* 2005;23(21):4602–8.

65 Canter D, Viterbo R, Kutikov A, *et al.* Baseline renal function status limits patient eligibility to receive perioperative chemotherapy for invasive bladder cancer and is minimally affected by radical cystectomy. *Urology* 2011;77(1):160–5.

66 Adjuvant chemotherapy in invasive bladder cancer: a systematic review and meta-analysis of individual patient data

Advanced Bladder Cancer (ABC) Meta-analysis Collaboration. *Eur Urol* 2005;48(2):189–99; discussion 99–201.

67 Herr HW. Transurethral resection of muscle-invasive bladder cancer: 10-year outcome. *J Clin Oncol* 2001;19(1):89–93.

68 Efstathiou JA, Spiegel DY, Shipley WU, *et al.* Long-term outcomes of selective bladder preservation by combined-modality therapy for invasive bladder cancer: the MGH experience. *Eur Urol* 2012;61(4):705–11.

69 Bajorin DF, Dodd PM, Mazumdar M, *et al.* Long-term survival in metastatic transitional-cell carcinoma and prognostic factors predicting outcome of therapy. *J Clin Oncol* 1999;17(10):3173–81.

70 Bellmunt J, Theodore C, Demkov T, *et al.* Phase III trial of vinflunine plus best supportive care compared with best supportive care alone after a platinum-containing regimen in patients with advanced transitional cell carcinoma of the urothelial tract. *J Clin Oncol* 2009;27(27):4454–61.

71 Rosenberg JE, Hoffman-Censits J, Powles T, *et al.* Atezolizumab in patients with locally advanced and metastatic urothelial carcinoma who have progressed following treatment with platinum-based chemotherapy: a single-arm, multicentre, phase 2 trial. *Lancet* 2016;387(10031):1909–20.

72 National Comprehensive Cancer Network. NCCN Clinical Practice Guidelines in Oncology. Bladder Cancer. V.1.2017 December 21, 2016. Accessed at www.nccn.org, January 11, 2017.

73 Radovanovic Z, Krajinovic S, Jankovic S, *et al.* Family history of cancer among cases of upper urothelial tumours in a Balkan nephropathy area. *J Cancer Res Clin Oncol* 1985;110(2):181–3.

74 Huben RP, Mounzer AM, Murphy GP. Tumor grade and stage as prognostic variables in upper tract urothelial tumors. *Cancer* 1988;62(9):2016–20.

75 Messer J, Lin YK, Raman JD. The role of lymphadenectomy for upper tract urothelial carcinoma. *Nat Rev Urol* 2011;8(7):394–401.

76 Kondo T, Nakazawa H, Ito F, *et al.* Primary site and incidence of lymph node metastases in urothelial carcinoma of upper urinary tract. *Urology* 2007;69(2):265–9.

77 Lee SE, Byun SS, Park YH, *et al.* Adjuvant chemotherapy in the management of pT3N0M0 transitional cell carcinoma of the upper urinary tract. *Urol Int* 2006;77(1):22–6.

78 Kwak C, Lee SE, Jeong IG, *et al.* Adjuvant systemic chemotherapy in the treatment of patients with invasive transitional cell carcinoma of the upper urinary tract. *Urology* 2006;68(1):53–7.

79 Rikken CH, van Helsdingen PJ, Kazzaz BA. Are biopsies from the prostatic urethra useful in patients with superficial bladder carcinoma? *Br J Urol* 1987;59(2):145–7.

80 Bates AW, Baithun SI. Secondary neoplasms of the bladder are histological mimics of nontransitional cell primary tumours: clinicopathological and histological features of 282 cases. *Histopathology* 2000;36(1):32–40.

81 el-Mekresh MM, el-Baz MA, Abol-Enein H, *et al.* Primary adenocarcinoma of the urinary bladder: a report of 185 cases. *Br J Urol* 1998;82(2):206–12.

82 Wilson TG, Pritchett TR, Lieskovsky G, *et al.* Primary adenocarcinoma of bladder. *Urology* 1991;38(3):223–6.

83 Melicow MM. Tumors of the urinary bladder: a clinico-pathological analysis of over 2500 specimens and biopsies. *J Urol* 1955;74(4):498–521.

84 Abenoza P, Manivel C, Fraley EE. Primary adenocarcinoma of urinary bladder. Clinicopathologic study of 16 cases. *Urology* 1987;29(1):9–14.

85 Kaufman DS, Shipley WU, Feldman AS. Bladder cancer. *Lancet* 2009;374(9685):239–49.

86 Logothetis CJ, Samuels ML, Ogden S. Chemotherapy for adenocarcinomas of bladder and urachal origin: 5-fluorouracil, doxorubicin, and mitomycin-C. *Urology* 1985;26(3):252–5.

87 Siefker-Radtke AO, Gee J, Shen Y, *et al.* Multimodality management of urachal carcinoma: the M. D. Anderson Cancer Center experience. *J Urol* 2003;169(4):1295–8.

88 Ashley RA, Inman BA, Sebo TJ, *et al.* Urachal carcinoma: clinicopathologic features and long-term outcomes of an aggressive malignancy. *Cancer* 2006;107(4):712–20.

89 Sheldon CA, Clayman RV, Gonzalez R, *et al.* Malignant urachal lesions. *J Urol* 1984;131(1):1–8.

90 Manunta A, Vincendeau S, Kiriakou G, *et al.* Non-transitional cell bladder carcinomas. *BJU Int* 2005;95(4):497–502.

91 Kantor AF, Hartge P, Hoover RN, *et al.* Epidemiological characteristics of squamous cell carcinoma and adenocarcinoma of the bladder. *Cancer Res* 1988;48(13):3853–5.

92 Rausch S, Lotan Y, Youssef RF. Squamous cell carcinogenesis and squamous cell carcinoma of the urinary bladder: a contemporary review with focus on nonbilharzial squamous cell carcinoma. *Urol Oncol* 2014;32(1):32.

93 Wong JT, Wasserman NF, Padurean AM. Bladder squamous cell carcinoma. *Radiographics* 2004;24(3):855–60.

94 Brenner DW, Yore LM, Schellhammer PF. Squamous cell carcinoma of bladder after successful intravesical therapy with Bacillus Calmette-Guerin. *Urology* 1989;34(2):93–5.

95 Tekes A, Kamel IR, Chan TY, *et al.* MR imaging features of non-transitional cell carcinoma of the urinary bladder with pathologic correlation. *Am J Roentgenol* 2003;180(3):779–84. E

96 Ghoneim MA, el-Mekresh MM, el-Baz MA, *et al.* Radical cystectomy for carcinoma of the bladder: critical evaluation of the results in 1,026 cases. *J Urol* 1997;158(2):393–9.

97 Shahab N. Extrapulmonary small cell carcinoma of the bladder. *Semin Oncol* 2007;34(1):15–21.

98 Cheng L, Pan CX, Yang XJ, *et al.* Small cell carcinoma of the urinary bladder: a clinicopathologic analysis of 64 patients. *Cancer* 2004;101(5):957–62.

99 Nejat RJ, Purohit R, Goluboff ET, *et al.* Cure of undifferentiated small cell carcinoma of the urinary bladder with M-VAC chemotherapy. *Urol Oncol* 2001;6(2):53–5.

100 Zhao X, Flynn EA. Small cell carcinoma of the urinary bladder: a rare, aggressive neuroendocrine malignancy. *Arch Pathol Lab Med* 2012;136(11):1451–9.

101 Mukesh M, Cook N, Hollingdale AE, *et al.* Small cell carcinoma of the urinary bladder: a 15-year retrospective review of treatment and survival in the Anglian Cancer Network. *BJU Int* 2009;103(6):747–52.

102 Manoharan M, Ayyathurai R, Soloway MS. Radical cystectomy for urothelial carcinoma of the bladder: an analysis of perioperative and survival outcome. *BJU Int* 2009;104(9):1227–32.

Section 5

Female Reproductive Cancer

19

Ovarian, Fallopian Tube, and Primary Peritoneal Cancer

Michael L. Pearl[1], *Erin E. Stevens*[2], *and Joyce Varughese*[1]

[1] Stony Brook Medicine, Stony Brook, New York, USA
[2] Billings Clinic Cancer Center, Billings, Montana, USA

Introduction

Ovarian cancer encompasses approximately 3% of cancer diagnoses and 5% of cancer deaths among women in the United States (US) [1]. Five broad categories of ovarian cancers exist: epithelial, germ cell, sex cord–stromal, nonspecific mesenchymal tumors, and metastases. The majority (~90%) of these cancers are epithelial in origin [2]. Additionally, fallopian tube and primary peritoneal carcinomas share similar histology, patterns of spread, and treatment modalities as epithelial ovarian cancer and are therefore often considered together in discussions of ovarian cancer.

The purpose of this chapter is to discuss the incidence, mortality, risk factors, and the role of screening and early detection of all types of ovarian cancer. The histopathology of the multiple subtypes of ovarian cancer will be discussed. Following this, a detailed discussion on epithelial ovarian cancer, including clinical presentation, surgical management, and systemic chemotherapy is included. Finally, germ cell and sex cord–stromal tumors, the most common of the rarer ovarian cancers are discussed in brief.

Incidence and Mortality

Ovarian cancer accounts for 51% of all deaths from gynecologic cancers among women in the US. An estimated 22,440 ovarian cancer cases (3% of cancer diagnoses among women) and 14,080 deaths (5% of cancer deaths among women) occurred in the US in 2017 [1]. The age-adjusted incidence and mortality rates, based on data from 2009 to 2013, is 11.9/100,000 women per year and 7.5/100,000 women per year, respectively. The approximate lifetime risk of a woman developing ovarian cancer is 1.28% and the lifetime risk of dying from ovarian cancer is 0.94%. The age-adjusted incidence decreased by an average of 1.1% per year from 1975 to 2010. Despite substantial advances in treatment, the survival for women with ovarian cancer has improved only modestly in the past 40 years. Overall, the 5-year relative survival increased from 36.6% from 1975 to 1977 to 46.4% from 2006 to 2012 [3]. These data concerning cases, deaths, incidence and mortality rates, and survival consider ovarian cancer overall, but largely reflect the predominant forms of epithelial ovarian cancers.

Fallopian tube cancer has traditionally been thought to be very rare (<1% of all gynecologic cancers). However, increasing evidence suggests that many serous ovarian cancers originate in the fimbriated end of the fallopian tube. Most patients with fallopian tube cancer are over the age of 50 and 5-year survival rates are difficult to estimate due to the limited number of cases, but are thought to be similar to ovarian cancer (~90% at stage I disease with a decline to 40% for stage IV disease) [4].

Risk Factors for Epithelial Ovarian Cancer and Fallopian Tube Cancer

Age

Aside from those with a genetic predisposition to ovarian cancer, age is the most important risk factor for ovarian cancer with half of all cases in the US occurring in women over the age of 65 [3].

Reproductive Factors

The most strongly associated risk factors for the development of epithelial ovarian and fallopian tube cancers are prior reproductive history and length of reproductive years. Early age at menarche and late age at menopause, as well as nulliparity and infertility, increase the risk of epithelial ovarian cancer, which is thought to be secondary to incessant ovulation [5]. Conversely, those factors that reduce the number of lifetime ovulations are thought to be protective. For example, women with a single pregnancy have a relative risk of 0.6–0.8 compared to nulligravid women and each additional pregnancy further decreases risk [6].

The American Cancer Society's Oncology in Practice: Clinical Management, First Edition. Edited by The American Cancer Society.

Similarly, many studies have shown a 40–50% risk reduction of epithelial ovarian cancer among women who use oral contraceptives [7]. Breastfeeding for more than 18 months also confers some protection against epithelial ovarian cancer with a 2% decreased relative risk with each month of breastfeeding [8].

Obesity

One large Norwegian study found that women who were obese in adolescence and childhood had a relative risk of 1.56 of developing ovarian cancer compared to women of normal weight [9]. This finding was confirmed in a meta-analysis of 28 studies which showed an odds ratio of 1.3–1.5 in obese women versus normal weight women [10].

Hormone Replacement Therapy

A recent meta-analysis of 52 epidemiologic studies conducted in the US, Europe, Australia, China, and Israel concluded that ovarian cancer risk was greater in ever-users of hormone replacement therapy compared to never-users (relative risk 1.20, $P < 0.0001$ for prospective studies and relative risk 1.14, $P < 0.0001$ for all studies) [11]. The meta-analysis also found that risk of ovarian cancer decreases after cessation of HRT use. Large cohort studies in the US and United Kingdom also found increased risk of ovarian cancer in HRT users [12, 13]. These results can be used to inform discussions between physicians and their patients.

Genetic Predisposition

A germline mutation in *BRCA1* or *BRCA2* is found in 10–15% of women with epithelial ovarian cancer. Most hereditary ovarian cancer is seen in patients with *BRCA1* mutations. Please refer to Chapter 5 (Counseling and Testing for Inherited Predisposition to Cancer) in *The American Cancer Society's Principles of Oncology: Prevention to Survivorship* for a more extensive discussion of hereditary ovarian cancer.

Other Factors

There is an increased incidence of epithelial ovarian cancer in the US and Europe, compared to Asia. In addition, endometriosis is well established as a risk factor for ovarian cancers of endometrioid and clear cell histologies.

Risk Factors for Ovarian Stromal and Germ Cell Tumors

While germ cell tumors comprise less than 5% of all ovarian cancers in Western countries, they represent up to 15% of ovarian cancers in Asia. Younger age is a risk factor for germ cell tumors which are rare after the third decade of life. No definitive risk factors for sex cord–stromal tumors have yet been identified.

Screening and Early Detection

Advanced stage at diagnosis and high mortality in ovarian, fallopian tube, and primary peritoneal cancers are due to a lack of effective screening tests for the general population. While cancer antigen 125 (CA-125) is used as a marker of treatment response and post-treatment surveillance in patients already diagnosed with malignancy, it is not effective as a screening test due to its lack of sensitivity and specificity for early-stage disease [14]. Statistical models have been developed to evaluate the utility of serial CA-125 levels in women without ovarian cancer. The risk of ovarian cancer algorithm is a screening algorithm that defines risk based on an individual's sequential CA-125 levels in comparison to the patterns seen in women with and without ovarian cancer. The UK Collaborative Trial of Ovarian Cancer Screening recently reported results of a randomized controlled trial that enrolled 202,638 postmenopausal women randomized to annual screening with serum CA-125 using the risk of ovarian cancer algorithm with transvaginal ultrasound (TVUS) as a second-line test, annual TVUS alone, or no screening. At a median followup of 11.1 years, no mortality benefit was seen in primary analysis. However, a significant reduction in mortality was noted in the group randomized to multimodal screening when prevalent cases were excluded. Further follow-up and research is needed to confirm these findings and evaluate the cost-effectiveness of multimodal ovarian cancer screening [15]. The Prostate, Lung, Colorectal and Ovarian Cancer Screening Trial looked at the mortality benefit in using a combination of CA-125 and TVUS and did not show any benefit with a median follow-up of 14.7 years [16].

Another area of active research is in using serum human epididymal protein 4 (HE4) levels in combination with CA-125 to increase the sensitivity and specificity of the tests. One small study of 108 women undergoing surgery for a pelvic mass showed that the combination of both HE4 and CA-125 increased the sensitivity of detecting malignancy to 68.9% in contrast to 65.5% (HE4 alone) and 58.6% (CA-125 alone) [17]. An Australian study showed that in patients with isolated pelvic masses, the combination of HE4, CA-125, and age had greater diagnostic value in differentiating benign tumors from early-stage epithelial ovarian cancers than CA-125 alone [18].

OVA-1 is a commercially available blood test that combines five immunoassays. This test may be useful, in conjunction with a standard preoperative evaluation and clinical impression, for nongynecologic oncology providers in assessing when a patient with an adnexal mass should be referred to a gynecologic oncologist for further management prior to surgical intervention, although the cost–benefit of this expensive test should be part of the decision-making process [19].

While the above research is promising, no screening test or combination of tests has yet shown sufficient sensitivity/specificity and/or survival benefit to be routinely recommended for the general population currently [20]. Please refer to Chapter 5 (Counseling and Testing for Inherited Predisposition to Cancer) in *The American Cancer Society's Principles of Oncology: Prevention to Survivorship* for management recommendations in high-risk individuals.

Epithelial Ovarian Cancer, Fallopian Tube Cancer, and Primary Peritoneal Cancer

Clinical Presentation

Symptoms

The high proportion of women presenting with advanced stage disease and the consequent high mortality rate are not only due to the lack of screening tests but also because of the vague and nonspecific nature of symptoms of epithelial ovarian, fallopian tube, and primary peritoneal cancers, which include abdominal, pelvic, and menstrual complaints. Specifically, symptoms of abdominal or pelvic pain, abdominal bloating, early satiety, or urinary frequency/urgency for less than a year should be thoroughly evaluated [21].

Older texts describe a classic triad of symptoms and signs for fallopian tube cancer (watery vaginal discharge (hydrops tubae profluens), pelvic pain, and a pelvic mass). However, <15% of patients present with this triad. Fallopian tube cancers more commonly present with vaginal discharge or bleeding or vague abdominopelvic symptoms.

Signs

The presence of a solid, irregular, fixed pelvic mass on physical examination is most suggestive of an ovarian malignancy. Occasionally, an upper abdominal mass or ascites is also present.

Imaging

Diagnostic imaging does not confirm the diagnosis of epithelial ovarian cancer, as tissue diagnosis is required. However, many patients with an adnexal mass or clinical symptoms do undergo ultrasound and those ultrasonographic findings that suggest malignancy include irregular borders, irregular septae, size >8 cm, and the presence of solid components. It is not recommended to biopsy or aspirate masses that are concerning for malignancy due to the likelihood of capsular rupture leading to upstaging of the tumor and possible worse prognosis for the patient.

Computed tomographic (CT) scans can also be useful in advanced-stage disease in determining whether a patient should be offered primary cytoreductive surgery or neoadjuvant chemotherapy (after confirmation of diagnosis by positive biopsy results). See Primary Management section for further discussion.

Staging and Grading

Epithelial ovarian, fallopian tube, and primary peritoneal malignancies are staged according to the Féderation Internationale de Gynécologie et d'Obstétrique [22] system based on findings at surgical exploration performed by a gynecologic oncologist (see Table 19.1 for complete staging of epithelial ovarian, fallopian tube, and primary peritoneal cancers). For details on the surgical staging procedure, please refer to the Primary Management – Surgery section of this chapter. While the FIGO staging system is primarily used by gynecologic oncologists, complementary staging systems (e.g., AJCC) are also acceptable.

Although histologic grade is considered an important prognostic factor in epithelial ovarian cancer, no universal grading system exists for ovarian serous carcinoma. The FIGO grading system is a grade 0–3 scale, with grade 0 being borderline (low malignant potential) tumors, grade 1 well-differentiated tumors, grade 2 moderately differentiated cells, and grade 3 poorly differentiated tumors. Recently, however, a two-tiered system (low grade versus high grade) has been proposed and has quickly gained wide acceptance and usage [23, 24]. This two-tiered system is based less on differentiation of the cells and more on nuclear atypia and mitotic rate. Many studies have shown that low-grade and high-grade serous carcinomas differ in their molecular genotypes and clinical phenotypes, with low-grade carcinomas resembling borderline serous tumors.

Pathology

Epithelial neoplasms comprise 65–70% of ovarian tumors. The main cell types of epithelial ovarian neoplasms are serous and mucinous. Less common epithelial ovarian tumors are of endometrioid (less than 10%) and clear cell (3%) histologies. Serous tumors are, by far, the most common epithelial ovarian tumors and can be characterized as benign, borderline, or malignant (Table 19.2).

Serous tumors can vary greatly in their histologic appearance but are characterized by columnar cells with pink cytoplasm that resemble those of normal tubal epithelium, as well as papillary and micropapillary architecture. Borderline serous tumors have no areas of stromal invasion >5 mm. Most borderline serous tumors are diagnosed as stage I and carry an excellent prognosis. If surgical staging is complete, no further therapy is needed for borderline serous tumors.

Much of what is known regarding the origin of serous ovarian carcinoma comes from data obtained from preoperatively presumed benign fallopian tubes and ovaries in patients with *BRCA* mutations. A noninvasive, but potentially lethal, form of tubal carcinoma termed tubal intraepithelial carcinoma has been found in up to 10% of *BRCA* mutation-positive women undergoing risk-reducing bilateral salpingo-oophorectomy. After this observation was made, it was also noticed that up to 60% of women diagnosed with high-grade serous ovarian cancer or primary peritoneal cancer also had tubal intraepithelial carcinoma in their surgical specimens. Emerging research strongly suggests that high-grade serous "ovarian" cancer may actually arise in the fimbriated end of the fallopian tube [25]. For this pathologic reason, cancers of the ovary and fallopian tubes, as well as primary peritoneal cancer, are all managed in a similar fashion. This concept is also the reason why prophylactic salpingectomy at the time of hysterectomy in women who are at low risk for ovarian cancer is now becoming part of the preoperative discussion for women undergoing surgery for benign disease [26].

The molecular signature of high-grade serous carcinomas is notable for WT1 positivity and almost universal mutations in the *TP53* gene which encodes for a tumor-suppressor protein. Ongoing research suggests that *p53* mutation seems to be an early event in disease progression [27]. Approximately 20–40% of low-grade serous carcinomas (<10% of serous carcinomas) exhibit mutations in *K-RAS* [28].

Mucinous tumors are also classified as benign, borderline, or carcinoma. Mucinous tumors appear microscopically as columnar cells with pale-staining intracellular mucin that resembles endocervical or gastric-type epithelium. Borderline mucinous tumors can be divided into two groups: gastrointestinal type (more common) and endocervical type. Similar to serous borderline tumors, the majority of these tumors are also stage 1 and carry an excellent prognosis. Primary ovarian mucinous carcinomas are rare (most malignant mucinous tumors in the ovary are metastases from the appendix and elsewhere in the gastrointestinal tract). Grossly, these tumors tend to be large, unilateral masses (cystic or solid) with smooth capsules filled with thick, mucinous material and an average size of 18 cm.

Table 19.1 Staging of ovarian, fallopian tube, and primary peritoneal cancer. The Féderation Internationale de Gynécologie et d'Obstétrique (FIGO) and the American Joint Committee on Cancer (AJCC) have defined staging systems for ovarian cancer; the FIGO system is most commonly used.

AJCC	FIGO	Definition
T1	I	Tumor confined to varies or fallopian tubes[1]
T1a, N0, M0	IA	Tumor limited to one ovary (capsule intact) or fallopian tube; no tumor on ovarian or fallopian tube surface; no malignant cells in the ascites or peritoneal washings
T1b, N0, M0	IB	Tumor limited to both ovaries (capsules intact) or fallopian tubes; no tumor on ovarian or fallopian tube surface; no malignant cells in the ascites or peritoneal washings
T1c, N0, M0	IC	Tumor limited to one or both ovaries or fallopian tubes, with any of the following:
T1c1, N0, M0	1C1	Surgical spill
T1c2, N0, M0	1C2	Capsule ruptured before surgery or tumor on ovarian or fallopian tube surface
T1c3, N0, M0	1C3	Malignant cells in the ascites or peritoneal washings
T2, N0, M0	II	Tumor involves one or both ovaries or fallopian tubes with pelvic extension (below pelvic brim) or primary peritoneal cancer[2]
T2a, N0, M0	IIA	Extension and/or implants on uterus and/or fallopian tubes and/or ovaries
T2b, N0, M0	IIB	Extension to other pelvic intraperitoneal tissues
T3, N0-1, M0 or T1–T2, N1, M0	III	Tumor involves one or both ovaries or fallopian tubes, or primary peritoneal cancer, with cytologically or histologically confirmed spread to the peritoneum outside the pelvis and/or metastasis to the retroperitoneal lymph nodes
Any T, N1, M0	IIIA1	Positive retroperitoneal lymph nodes only (cytologically or histologically proven)
Any T, N1a, M0	IIIA1(i)	Metastasis up to 10 mm in greatest diameter
Any T, N1b, M0	IIIA1(ii)	Metastasis greater than 10 mm in greatest diameter
T3a, N0-1, M0	IIIA2	Microscopic extrapelvic (above the pelvic brim) peritoneal involvement with or without positive retroperitoneal lymph nodes
T3b, N0-1, M0	IIIB	Macroscopic peritoneal metastasis beyond the pelvis up to 2 cm in greatest dimension, with or without metastasis to the retroperitoneal lymph nodes
T3c, N0-1, M0	IIIC	Macroscopic peritoneal metastasis beyond the pelvis more than 2 cm in greatest dimension, with or without metastasis to the retroperitoneal lymph nodes (includes extension of tumor to capsule of liver and spleen without parenchymal involvement of either organ)
Any T, any N, M1	IV	Distant metastasis excluding peritoneal metastases
Any T, any N, M1a	IVA	Pleural effusion with positive cytology
Any T, any N, M1b	IVB	Parenchymal metastases and metastases to extra-abdominal organs (including inguinal lymph nodes and lymph nodes outside of the abdominal cavity)

Source: adapted from Prat [22].

[1] It is not possible to have Stage I primary peritoneal cancer.

[2] Dense adhesions with *histologically proven tumor cells* justify upgrading to stage II.

Pseudomyxoma peritonei is a clinicopathologic syndrome most commonly associated with tumors of primary appendiceal origin (ovarian involvement is secondary) with findings of mucinous ascites and extracellular mucin and fibrosis. For this reason, appendectomy is recommended in patients with pseudomyxoma peritonei.

Primary Management

Primary treatment for epithelial ovarian, fallopian tube, and primary peritoneal cancer includes appropriate surgical staging and cytoreductive surgery, followed by systemic cytotoxic platinum- and taxane-based chemotherapy for advanced stages. In some instances, neoadjuvant chemotherapy may be administered prior to cytoreductive surgery.

Surgery

Surgery for ovarian cancer serves multiple purposes. It allows for determination of stage and thereby prognosis. It also decreases the patient's individual tumor burden to allow for more successful treatment with chemotherapy. Recommendations from the National Comprehensive Cancer Network (NCCN) as well as a meta-analysis of published studies conclude that surgery should be performed by a fellowship-trained gynecologic oncologist because of a significant survival benefit to the patient [29, 30].

Surgery is performed via laparotomy through a vertical midline incision. Pelvic washings or aspiration of ascites are obtained upon entry into the abdomen and sent for cytology. If the cancer appears to be confined to the ovary, a total abdominal hysterectomy, bilateral salpingo-oophorectomy, omentectomy, and comprehensive staging is performed. Comprehensive staging includes pelvic and para-aortic lymph node dissection, systematic peritoneal biopsies throughout the pelvic and abdominal cavity, and diaphragm scraping. All peritoneal surfaces throughout the abdominopelvic cavity should be visualized and/or palpated. Any suspicious areas, including adhesions and small implants, should be excised and sent for pathology. Comprehensive surgical staging for presumed early ovarian cancer is important because approximately 30% of patients

Table 19.2 WHO classification of tumors of the ovary.

Epithelial tumors

Serous tumors

Benign
- Serous cystadenoma
- Serous cystadenofibroma
- Serous surface papilloma

Borderline
- Serous borderline tumor/atypical proliferative serous tumor
- Serous borderline tumor–micropapillary variant/noninvasive low-grade serous carcinoma

Malignant
- Low-grade serous carcinoma
- High-grade serous carcinoma

Mucinous tumors

Benign
- Mucinous cystadenoma
- Mucinous adenofibroma

Borderline
- Mucinous borderline tumor/atypical proliferative mucinous tumor

Malignant
- Mucinous carcinoma

Endometrioid tumors

Benign
- Endometriotic cyst
- Endometrioid cystadenoma
- Endometrioid adenofibroma

Malignant
- Endometrioid carcinoma

Clear cell tumors

Benign
- Clear cell cystadenoma
- Clear cell adenofibroma

Borderline
- Clear cell borderline tumor/atypical proliferative clear cell tumor

Malignant
- Clear cell carcinoma

Brenner tumors

Benign
- Brenner tumor

Borderline
- Borderline Brenner tumor/atypical proliferative Brenner tumor

Malignant
- Malignant Brenner tumor

Mesenchymal tumors

Low-grade endometrioid stromal sarcoma

High-grade endometrioid stromal sarcoma

Mixed epithelial and mesenchymal tumors

Adenosarcoma

Carcinosarcoma

Sex cord–stromal tumors

Pure stromal tumors

Fibroma

Cellular fibroma

Thecoma

Luteinized thecoma associated with sclerosing peritonitis

Fibrosarcoma

Sclerosing stromal tumor

Signet ring stromal tumor

Microcystic stromal tumor

Leydig cell tumor

Steroid cell tumor

Steroid cell tumor, malignant

Pure sex cord tumors

Adult granulosa cell tumor

Juvenile granulosis cell tumor

Sertoli cell tumor

Sex cord tumor with annular tubules

Mixed sex cord–stromal tumor

Sertoli–Leydig cell tumors
- Well-differentiated
- Moderately differentiated
  - With heterologous elements
- Poorly differentiated
  - With heterologous elements
- Retiform

With heterologous elements

Sex cord–stromal tumors, NOS

Miscellaneous tumors

Tumors of rete ovarii

Adenoma of rete ovarii

Adenocarcinoma of rete ovarii

Wolffian tumor

Small cell carcinoma, hypercalcaemic type

Small cell carcinoma, pulmonary type

Wilms tumor

(*Continued*)

Table 19.2 (Continued)

Seromucinous tumors	Paraganglioma
Benign	Solid pseudopapillary neoplasm
Seromucinous cystadenoma	
Seromucinous adenofibroma	**Mesothelial tumors**
Borderline	Adenomatoid tumor
Seromucinous borderline tumor/atypical proliferative seromucinous tumor	Mesothelioma
Malignant	
Seromucinous carcinoma	**Soft tissue tumors**
	Myxoma
Undifferentiated carcinoma	Others
Germ cell tumors	**Tumor-like lesions**
Dysgerminoma	Follicle cyst
Yolk sac tumor	Corpus luteum cyst
Embryonal carcinoma	Large solitary luteinized follicle cyst
Nongestational choriocarcinoma	Hyperreactio luteinalis
Mature teratoma	Pregnancy luteoma
Immature teratoma	Stromal hyperplasia
Mixed germ cell tumor	Stromal hyperthecosis
	Fibromatosis
Monodermal teratoma and somatic-type tumors arising from a dermoid cyst	Massive edema
	Leydig cell hyperplasia
Struma ovarii, benign	Others
Struma ovarii, malignant	
Carcinoid	
Strumal carcinoid	**Lymphoid and myeloid tumors**
Mucinous carcinoid	Lymphomas
Neuroectodermal-type tumors	Plasmacytoma
Sebaceous tumors	Myeloid neoplasm
Sebaceous adenoma	
Sebaceous carcinoma	**Secondary tumors**
Other rare monodermal teratomas	
Carcinomas	
Squamous cell carcinoma	
Others	
Germ cell–sex cord–stromal tumors	
Gonadoblastoma, including gonadoblastoma with malignant germ cell tumor	
Mixed germ cell–sex cord–stromal tumor, unclassified	

Source: adapted from Kurman *et al.* [61]. Reproduced with permission of the International Agency for Research on Cancer.
NOS, not otherwise specified.

undergoing staging surgery are upstaged due to microscopic disease [31]. In young patients who desire future fertility, a unilateral salpingo-oophorectomy with comprehensive staging can be performed if the disease is clinically confined to one ovary. Additionally, minimally invasive techniques may be considered in selected early-stage patients when performed by an experienced gynecologic oncologist [29].

In patients where disease has already spread from the ovary, cytoreductive (or debulking) surgery is performed in addition to the comprehensive surgery described above. This may involve radical pelvic dissection and extensive upper abdominal surgery, including splenectomy, distal pancreatectomy, segmental liver resection, diaphragm and peritoneal stripping and resection, as well as bowel resections. The goal of cytoreductive surgery is to remove the bulk of disease the patient harbors at the time of diagnosis. Optimal cytoreduction is defined as less than 1 cm of residual disease. However, maximal surgical effort should be made to remove all visible disease [32, 33]. Patients who have been optimally cytoreduced have a significant survival benefit over those who have not [32, 33]. In those patients who have undergone incomplete surgery initially by another provider, a gynecologic oncologist may perform a completion surgery with the intent of optimal cytoreduction.

Chemotherapy

Chemotherapy for epithelial ovarian, fallopian tube, and primary peritoneal cancer is recommended for all patients with stage II–IV disease. Patients with stage I disease should be comprehensively staged, and recommendation for chemotherapy depends on sub-stage and grade of tumor. Patients with stage IA and IB, grade 1 tumors should be observed, while those with stage IA and IB, grade 2 tumors can also be considered for observation. For all other patients, platinum- and taxane-based chemotherapy has been the standard first-line chemotherapy since the late 1990s [34, 35]. Outside of variation in dose and route of administration of these drugs, there has been little change in primary classes of chemotherapeutic drugs used for first-line treatment of ovarian cancer in the last 20 years.

Standard intravenous (IV) chemotherapy is an every 3-week regimen of paclitaxel and carboplatin for six cycles following comprehensive surgical staging. In the noninferiority trial comparing cisplatin/paclitaxel to carboplatin/paclitaxel, the carboplatin regimen had a 20.7 month progression-free survival (PFS) and a 57.4 month overall survival (OS) in patients optimally cytoreduced stage III disease [36]. No studies have found any OS benefit from addition of a third cytotoxic drug in frontline treatment. There may be some benefit of adding newer biologic therapies to this regimen, as is discussed later. The major side effect of standard IV carboplatin/paclitaxel is sensory peripheral neuropathy. Docetaxel may be substituted for patients who are at high risk for neuropathy. However, these patients often experience more hematologic toxicities, especially neutropenia [37]. Paclitaxel and carboplatin has also been studied on a weekly basis at lower doses for patients with poor performance status or significant comorbidities. This regimen was associated with fewer systemic side effects compared to every 3-week dosing with a similar PFS as standard every 3-week IV regimens [38].

A variation of the standard IV regimen uses paclitaxel in a weekly fashion combined with 3-week carboplatin. The dose-dense regimen was selected based on preclinical data suggesting that duration of exposure to paclitaxel is important in the drug's cytotoxicity and that lower doses of paclitaxel may result in enhanced antiangiogenic activity. Both the initial report of improved PFS (28.2 vs 17.5 months) [39] and the recent updated OS data (100.5 vs 62.2 months) [40] suggest that this regimen offers a superior survival benefit to standard 3-week IV chemotherapy. Neuropathy remains a problem with this regimen and hematologic toxicities are also commonly encountered with dose-dense treatment. Less than half of the subjects enrolled in the trial completed the dose-dense regimen as prescribed, yet there was still a striking OS benefit. However, a recent American study of dose-dense versus standard every 3-week dosing did not find a difference in PFS between the regimens [41]. This study allowed use of bevacizumab at the investigator's discretion and 84% elected to do so. When subanalyses were performed, the dose-dense regimen was associated with a 3.9 month longer PFS compared to every 3-week when bevacizumab was not administered.

Intraperitoneal (IP) chemotherapy allows for a high concentration and long duration of treatment directed at the peritoneal surface epithelium. IV paclitaxel in combination with IP cisplatin/paclitaxel increased OS by 16 months (65.6 vs 49.7 months) and is a recommended regimen for optimally cytoreduced stage II and III patients [29, 42]. Many gynecologic oncologists have extrapolated this regimen to optimally cytoreduced stage II patients as well as stage IV patients after an optimal intra-abdominal cytoreductive surgery has been achieved. IP chemotherapy has the most side effects, including leukopenia, infection, fatigue, renal toxicity, abdominal discomfort, and neurotoxicity, with initial studies showing that only 42% of women were able to complete all six cycles [42]. Despite this, there was still a significant OS benefit, and the NCI issued a clinical announcement that all women undergoing surgery for ovarian cancer should be counseled preoperatively about the benefits associated with combined IV/IP regimen if optimal cytoreduction is achieved [43].

A recent study of dose-dense carboplatin/paclitaxel versus dose-dense IV paclitaxel/IP carboplatin or reduced dose IV paclitaxel/IP cisplatin/paclitaxel revealed no difference in PFS amongst the regimens (26.8 vs 28.7 vs 27.8 months, respectively) [44]. This study also utilized bevacizumab in all arms. It is unclear if the lack of difference in PFS is due to use of bevacizumab, reduced dosing of IP chemotherapy, or other factors.

The following options are category 1 recommendations in the NCCN Guidelines for primary therapy for stage II–IV disease: 3-week IV, weekly IV, dose-dense IV, and IV/IP. A category I is based on high-level evidence and uniform NCCN consensus that the intervention is appropriate.

Neoadjuvant Chemotherapy

Patients with bulky stage III/IV disease or those patients who are poor surgical candidates due to multiple comorbid medical conditions may be considered for neoadjuvant chemotherapy followed by interval cytoreductive surgery. Initial reports of retrospective studies evaluating the use of neoadjuvant chemotherapy found inferior outcomes when compared to primary cytoreductive surgery followed by chemotherapy [45]. A prospective, randomized trial performed in Europe found that there was no difference in OS between the neoadjuvant and the surgical groups and maintained that neoadjuvant chemotherapy is not inferior to primary surgical management [46]. However, the survival in both arms of this study was worse than is typically seen in US trials. It was recommended that patients be reassessed for surgical cytoreductive surgery after three cycles of neoadjuvant chemotherapy.

The Society of Gynecologic Oncology and the American Society of Clinical Oncology jointly issued a Clinical Practice Guideline in 2016 [47]. According to the guideline, "All women with suspected stage IIIC or IV invasive epithelial ovarian cancer should be evaluated by a gynecologic oncologist prior to initiation of therapy. The primary clinical evaluation should include a CT of the abdomen and pelvis, and chest imaging (CT preferred). Women with a high perioperative risk profile or a low likelihood of achieving cytoreduction to <1 cm of residual disease (ideally to no visible disease) should receive neoadjuvant chemotherapy. Women who are fit for primary cytoreductive surgery, and with potentially resectable disease, may receive either neoadjuvant chemotherapy or primary cytoreductive surgery. However, primary cytoreductive surgery is preferred if there is a high likelihood of achieving cytoreduction to <1 cm (ideally to no visible disease) with acceptable morbidity. Before neoadjuvant chemotherapy is delivered, all patients should have confirmation of an invasive ovarian, fallopian tube, or peritoneal cancer".

Future Directions: Targeted Therapies and Maintenance Chemotherapy

Bevacizumab is a monoclonal antibody with anti-VEGF activity that has been studied in the frontline setting in combination with carboplatin/paclitaxel. A small benefit in PFS of 2–4 months was identified in patients who continued to use bevacizumab as a maintenance agent after completion of chemotherapy [48, 49]. However, the minimum dose and duration of treatment needed to provide a clinical benefit has not been determined. Side effects of bevacizumab include hypertension, proteinuria, and bowel perforation. The high cost and the lack of OS benefit has not led to the wide adoption of bevacizumab in the primary setting.

The role of maintenance chemotherapy after achieving a complete clinical response continues to be examined. A previous study investigating paclitaxel monthly did find a PFS advantage but it increased toxicity and therefore has not been widely adopted by gynecologic oncologists. Pazopanib, an oral VEGF inhibitor, has been shown to increase PFS from 12.3 to 17.9 months when used as a maintenance therapy in patients who achieve a complete clinical response after primary therapy [50]. However, the FDA has not yet approved pazopanib for this indication. Currently, studies are underway comparing taxane-based compounds to heightened surveillance in the year after completion of chemotherapy.

Post-Treatment Surveillance

After completion of chemotherapy, most patients will achieve a clinical response/remission. Complete clinical response may be defined as no definitive evidence of disease (i.e., a normal physical examination, normal CA-125 levels, and a negative CT scan with lymph nodes measuring <1 cm in the longest dimension) [29]. Second-look surgeries, once routinely performed, have fallen out of favor with the accessibility of advanced imaging modalities and the lack of benefit in OS [51].

Despite achieving a complete clinical response initially, recurrence rates remain high. Patients should be followed by a gynecologic oncologist for a minimum of the first 5 years after surgery. The Society of Gynecologic Oncology released surveillance (Table 19.3) guidelines for women with gynecologic malignancies and readers should refer to that article for a more detailed discussion [52]. In the first 2 years after completion of treatment, the patient is seen every 3 months and should have a review of symptoms and physical examination, including a bimanual and rectovaginal examination. Up to half of the recurrences will occur in the pelvis and may be identified on palpation of tumor by an experienced provider [53]. After the first 2 years, patients are seen every 4–6 months in the third year and then every 6 months until they have reached a disease-free interval of 5 years. Patients should be educated about the

Table 19.3 Society of Gynecologic Oncology recommendations for ovarian cancer surveillance after completion of treatment.

	Months			Years	
Variable	**0–12**	**12–24**	**24–36**	**3–5**	**>5**
Review of symptoms and physical examination	Every 3 months	Every 3 months	Every 4–6 months	Every 6 months	Yearly[a]
Papanicolaou test/ cytologic evidence	Not indicated	Not indicated	Not indicated	Not indicated	Not indicated
Cancer antigen 125	Optional	Optional	Optional	Optional	Optional
Radiographs imaging (chest x-ray. positron emission tomography/ computed tomography, magnetic resonance imaging)	Insufficient data to support routine use	Insufficient data to support routine use	Insufficient data to support routine use	Insufficient data to support routine use	Insufficient data to support routine use
Recurrence suspected	Computed tomography and/or positron emission tomography scan Cancer antigen 125	Computed tomography and/or positron emission tomography scan Cancer antigen 125	Computed tomography and/or positron emission tomography scan Cancer antigen 125	Computed tomography and/or positron emission tomography scan Cancer antigen 125	Computed tomography and/or positron emission tomography scan Cancer antigen 125

Source: Salani *et al.* [52]. Reproduced with permission of Elsevier.
[a] May be followed by a generalist or gynecologic oncologist

symptoms suggestive of recurrence, including pelvic pain, bloating, changes in bowel or bladder habits, early satiety, obstructive symptoms, weight loss, and fatigue. If patients experience any of these symptoms regularly over a period of weeks, or if tumor is palpated on examination, imaging studies such as a CT or positron emission tomography/CT could be performed to assess for recurrent disease [52].

If the CA-125 level was initially elevated, the measurement of CA-125 at each follow-up evaluation is recommended. However, a multi-institutional European trial assessing the use of CA-125 in monitoring for recurrence after primary therapy found that treating recurrences based on a detectable CA-125 level in asymptomatic patients is not associated with an increase in survival and is associated with a decrease in quality of life [54]. Providers should discuss the pros and cons of routine CA-125 monitoring with their patients. After a documented rise in the CA-125, the median time to clinical relapse is 2–6 months. Data suggest that immediate treatment with cytotoxic chemotherapy is not beneficial for OS, but some patients and physicians chose this route [54].

Recurrent Disease

Although cytotoxic chemotherapy may be initially successful, most patients eventually experience relapse and die of disease [1]. Prognosis is poor for refractory patients, described as those who progress without ever sustaining a clinical response in the frontline setting of carboplatin/paclitaxel. Progression is defined by RECIST criteria of >20% increase in tumor diameter. Platinum-resistant patients, who recur within the first 6 months after completion of frontline chemotherapy, also have a poor prognosis. Platinum refractory and resistant patients are often poorly responsive to common second-line chemotherapy options, with response rates in the 20–27% range (Table 19.4). Enrollment in clinical trials is encouraged for these patients with platinum refractory or resistant disease.

Patients who develop recurrent disease more than 6 months after completion of chemotherapy are considered platinum sensitive. These patients may be candidates for secondary cytoreductive surgery and should be prescribed a secondary regimen that contains a platinum-based chemotherapy (Table 19.4). Evaluation

Table 19.4 Recommended cytotoxic systemic therapy regimens for recurrent ovarian cancer* (NCCN).[1–3] Referenced with permission from the NCCN Clinical Practice Guidelines in Oncology (NCCN Guidelines®) for Ovarian Cancer V.1.2017. © National Comprehensive Cancer Network, Inc. 2017. All rights reserved. To view the most recent and complete version of the guideline, go online to www.NCCN.org.

Preferred agents for platinum sensitive disease[4,5]	Preferred agents for platinum resistant or refractory regimens	Other active agents[10]
Carboplatin	Docetaxel	Altretamine
Carboplatin/docetaxel	Oral etoposide	Capecitabine
Carboplatin/gemcitabine	Gemcitabine	Cyclophosphamide
Carboplatin/gemcitabine/bevacizumab[6,7]	Liposomal doxorubicin	Duxorubicin
Carboplatin/liposomal doxorubicin (category I)	Liposomal doxorubicin/bevacizumab[6,7]	Ifosfamide
Carboplatin/paclitaxel, albumin bound (for patients with confirmed taxane hypersensitivity)	Paclitaxel (weekly)	Irinotecan
Carboplatin/paclitaxel (category I)	Paclitaxel (weekly)/bevacizumab[6,7]	Melphalan
Carboplatin/paclitaxel (weekly)	Tototecan	Oxaliplatin
Cisplatin	Paclitaxel/pazopanib	Paclitaxel
Cisplatin/gemcitabine	Bevacizumab[6,7]	Paclitaxel, albumin bound
Bevacizumab[6,7]	Olaparib[8]	Pemetrexed
Olaparib[8]	Rucaparib[9]	Carboplatin/paclitaxel/bevacizumab (platinum-sensitive disease)
		Vinorelbine
		Rucaparib (for platinum-sensitive disease)[9]

* These agents may also be used for fallopian tube cancer and primary peritoneal cancer.
[1] See NCCN Guidelines for a complete list of acceptable recurrence therapy options, including those for less common ovarian histologies.
[2] Chemotherapy has not been shown to be beneficial in ovarian borderline epithelial tumors (low malignant potential).
[3] Patients who progress on two consecutive regimens without evidence of clinical benefits have diminished likelihood of benefitting from additional therapy. Decisions to offer clinical trials, supportive care, or additional therapy should be made on a highly individual basis.
[4] In general, the panel would recommend combination regimens based on randomized trial data, especially first relapses.
[5] Platinum-based combination therapy should be considered for platinum-sensitive recurrences.
[6] In patients who have not previously received bevacizumab.
[7] Contraindicated for patients at increased risk of gastrointestinal perforation.
[8] For patients with deleterious germline *BRCA*-mutated (as detected by an Food and Drug Administration-approved test or other validated test performed in a Clinical Laboratory Improvement Amendments-approved facility) advanced ovarian cancer who have been treated with three or more lines of chemotherapy.
[9] For patients with deleterious germline and/or somatic *BRCA*-mutated (as detected by a Food and Drug Administration-approved test or other validated test performed in a Clinical Laboratory Improvement Amendments-approved facility) advanced ovarian cancer who have been treated with two or more lines of chemotherapy.
[10] Many of these agents have not been tested in patients who have been treated with modern chemotherapy regimens.

of response should be performed after 2–4 cycles to determine if the patient is benefitting from the additional treatment. It is possible that retreatment with platinums will result in another extended disease-free interval. Additional agents, including liposomal doxorubicin, gemcitabine, and topotecan are nonplatinum agents that have also shown clinical benefit (Table 19.4). However, patients with progression on two consecutive chemotherapy regimens without clinical benefit are unlikely to respond to additional treatments [55]. Decisions regarding additional regimens, clinical trials, or palliative care should be made after an open and candid discussion with the patient.

Novel targeted agents are currently being explored in phase II trials in both platinum-sensitive and platinum-resistant ovarian cancer. These include poly-ADP ribose polymerase inhibitors, tyrosine kinase inhibitors, and other anti-angiogenic drugs. Olaparib, a poly-ADP ribose polymerase inhibitor, has been approved in patients with *BRCA* mutations who have received three or more lines of chemotherapy [56]. For the most part, results from targeted therapies have been disappointing. But as the ability to select the patients who are most likely to respond to a particular drug improves, so should outcomes.

Palliative and End-of-Life Care

According to the Centers for Medicare and Medicaid Services (CMS), "palliative care means patient and family-centered care that optimizes quality of life by anticipating, preventing and treating suffering. Palliative care throughout the continuum of illness involves addressing physical, intellectual, emotional, social and spiritual needs and to facilitate patient autonomy, access to information and choice" [57]. Palliative care is appropriate at any time during management of a serious illness. It can be provided at the same time as, and in addition to, life-prolonging treatment. There are no prognostic requirements and no need to choose between management approaches (palliative care vs curative/life-prolonging care). Contemporary multidisciplinary palliative programs improve patient satisfaction and survival while reducing cost [58, 59].

Unfortunately, despite high rates of initial response to treatment, most women with advanced ovarian cancer will develop recurrent, progressive disease that is ultimately fatal. Typically, the disease recurs within the abdominal cavity, leading to bowel compromise, ascites, and pain. Management should be individualized, multidisciplinary, directed by an experienced gynecologic oncologist and focused on relief of suffering rather than prolonging life.

Hospice care is a form of palliative care that provides care for those at the end of their life. Enrollment in hospice requires two physicians to certify that the patient's life expectancy is less than 6 months and patients must choose to forego life-prolonging care. Although hospice services are widely available, most women with terminal ovarian cancer continue to receive anticancer treatment and have repeated hospital admissions during the last 6 months of their life [60]. Earlier referral to hospice would provide higher quality and more satisfactory care in more appropriate and, often, less costly settings.

Germ Cell Tumors

Clinical Presentation

Ovarian germ cell tumors (OGCTs) account for 2–3% of all ovarian cancers, occurring primarily in younger women. The median age at diagnosis is 16–20 years depending upon histologic type (range 6–40 years). For women in their first two decades, OGCTs account for two-thirds of ovarian malignancies. In contrast to epithelial ovarian cancer, OGCTs grow rapidly. The clinical presentation is comparable for the OGCTs; most patients present with a palpable abdomino-pelvic mass and pain. Approximately 10% of patients present with an acute abdomen from torsion, spontaneous tumor rupture, or hemorrhage. Isosexual precocity from ectopic β-human chorionic gonadotrophin production occurs rarely. Bilateral ovarian involvement occurs extremely rarely except for dysgerminoma (20%); a benign cystic teratoma may occur in the ipsilateral or contralateral ovary in 5–10% of the cases and mimic bilateral involvement. Approximately 70% of cases are stage I, 30% are stage III, and stage II and IV cases are rare.

The initial evaluation of a patient suspected of having an OGCT includes a thorough history and physical examination, preoperative blood work, serum tumor markers and imaging studies (chest X-ray, CT scan of abdomen and pelvis, pelvic ultrasound). These patients should be referred to a gynecologic oncologist or a pediatric surgeon for management as soon as possible.

Pathology

OGCTs are classified by the World Health Organization as benign and malignant tumors [61] (Table 19.2). Benign OGCTs are primarily mature teratomas (dermoid cysts) and their variants. The OGCTs arise from primordial germ cells and recapitulate embryonic and extraembryonic differentiation. Malignant OGCTs can be divided into dysgerminomas and nondysgerminomas. Dysgerminomas are the most common malignant OGCTs (40%); up to 10% develop in phenotypic girls with dysgenetic gonads, including pure (46XY) and mixed gonadal dysgenesis (45X/46XY), and the androgen insensitivity syndrome (46XY) [62]. Consequently, if possible, the karyotype should be determined preoperatively in premenarchal girls with a pelvic mass.

The OGCTs produce serum tumor markers (alpha-fetoprotein and β-human chorionic gonadotrophin) that are useful for diagnosis, treatment monitoring, and surveillance after treatment (Table 19.5). Lactate dehydrogenase and placental alkaline phosphatase are elevated in most women with dysgerminomas. CA-125 is frequently elevated but is nonspecific. In addition, many OGCTs are mixed, making it difficult to interpret the tumor marker panel.

Surgery

Contemporary management of OGCTs begins with surgery; for most patients, surgery is followed by multiagent chemotherapy. As the overwhelming majority of patients with OGCTs are reproductive age, fertility-preserving surgical management is crucial.

Table 19.5 Serum tumor markers for malignant germ cell tumors.

Histology	AFP	βhCG
Dysgerminoma	–	±
Endodermal sinus tumor	+	–
Polyembryoma	±	+
Nongestational choriocarcinoma	–	+
Immature teratoma	±	
Embryonal carcinoma	±	+
Mixed germ cell tumor	±	±

AFP, alpha-fetoprotein. βhCG, beta-human chorionic gonadotropin.

For patients without clinical evidence of extraovarian spread, comprehensive surgical staging includes assessment of peritoneal cytology, unilateral salpingo-oophorectomy, omentectomy, bilateral pelvic and para-aortic lymph node sampling, and multiple peritoneal biopsies. Unless the contralateral ovary appears abnormal, it should be left alone. Comprehensive surgical staging may decrease the need for adjuvant chemotherapy; in a recent review of surgery followed by observation alone, no stage IA patients recurred, compared to 40% of patients with clinical stage I disease [63]. However, lack of comprehensive surgical staging does not appear to worsen prognosis if contemporary adjuvant chemotherapy is administered [64]. Based on these data, it has been suggested that the extent of surgical staging be limited to unilateral oophorectomy with biopsy/excision of any masses, and that reoperation solely for comprehensive surgical staging can be avoided. However, selected patients may choose to undergo comprehensive surgical staging in an attempt to avoid chemotherapy. It is worth noting that conservative surgery does not imply ovarian cystectomy; the safety of ovarian cystectomy rather than oophorectomy remains to be determined and cannot be recommended at this time. In general, the uterus can be preserved even for those patients requiring bilateral salpingo-oophorectomy because assisted reproductive technology with ovum donation could permit future pregnancy. Complete hysterectomy with bilateral salpingo-oophorectomy may be warranted for patients who have completed childbearing. It is unclear whether primary cytoreductive surgery is as important for OGCTs as it is for epithelial ovarian cancers. Although there is a paucity of supportive data, resection of all gross disease seems reasonable, taking into consideration the exquisite chemosensitivity of the OGCTs [65].

Chemotherapy

Currently, the recommended postoperative adjuvant chemotherapy regimen for all OGCTs is bleomycin, etoposide, and cisplatin administered on schedule with hemotologic support [66, 67]. Patients without gross residual disease and negative tumor markers receive three to four cycles; those with measurable disease or elevated tumor markers are treated for two cycles past normalization of tumor markers, disappearance of measurable disease, or six cycles.

Historically, the only exceptions to this approach were patients with comprehensively staged IA grade 1 immature teratoma and stage IA dysgerminoma. Several contemporary reports raise the possibility that postoperative surveillance without adjuvant chemotherapy may be feasible for a broader range of patients with stage I OGCTs [68–72]. In these studies, the relapse rate with surveillance alone approached 50%; however, the salvage rate with chemotherapy ranged from 91 to 100%. Although encouraging, the safety and efficacy of postoperative surveillance without adjuvant chemotherapy in this population remains to be determined.

In an attempt to reduce the toxicity associated with bleomycin, etoposide, and cisplatin, carboplatin may be used in lieu of cisplatin [73]. However, widespread adoption of this regimen awaits the development and completion of a randomized, controlled trial. Targeted therapies of potential interest include tyrosine kinase inhibitors (imatinib and sunitinib) and VEGF inhibitors (bevacizumab). Their role awaits evaluation in prospective studies.

Surveillance

Patients with OGCTs should undergo surveillance visits every 3 months for 2 years and every 6 months for an additional 3 years following treatment, including thorough history and physical examinations, imaging studies and assessment of appropriate tumor markers. The few patients who develop recurrent disease after contemporary treatment generally do so within the first year; recurrences after the second year are extremely rare. Elevated tumor markers are sensitive indicators of progressive or recurrent OGCTs and dictate further evaluation with imaging studies. A mass detected on examination or an imaging study must be adequately biopsied since immature teratoma may recur with nonmalignant mature elements or gliosis. positron emission tomography/CT may be useful to distinguish malignant from nonmalignant masses.

Persistence, Progression, or Recurrence

Given the rarity of persistent, progressive, or recurrent OGCTs, management of these patients has been extrapolated from management of patients with testicular cancer. These patients should be referred to specialized centers. Treatment failures are classified as platinum-refractory (progression during or persistence following primary treatment), platinum-resistant (progression with 6 weeks of primary treatment), or platinum-sensitive (recurrence beyond 6 weeks after primary treatment). Platinum-refractory disease is incurable and the cure rate for platinum-resistant disease is low; ifosphamide-based combination chemotherapy has some activity [74]. Approximately 50% of patients with platinum-sensitive disease may be salvaged with second-line ifosphamide-based high-dose chemotherapy with stem cell rescue and this approach is preferred [75].

Selected patients may benefit from secondary cytoreductive surgery, particularly those with immature teratoma and isolated foci of recurrent tumor that appear resectable on imaging study [76]. Occasionally, persistence of mature tissue elements can occur with immature teratomas, mimicking persistent disease, but there is no benefit to resecting these lesions.

Late Effects

The most feared late effect of etoposide-based chemotherapy is the development of acute myeloid leukemia. Fortunately, the incidence appears quite low (<1%) in this population [67].

Chemotherapy may affect ovarian function, leading to premature ovarian failure. Factors associated with chemotherapy-associated premature ovarian failure include age, cumulative dose, and duration of therapy. Women treated with contemporary fertility-sparing surgery and chemotherapy appear to have a very low risk of premature ovarian failure and have normal fecundity [77]. Women successfully treated for ovarian germ cell tumors are comparable to matched controls except for several chemotherapy-associated sequelae, including peripheral neuropathy, tinnitus, and Raynaud Syndrome [78]. In addition, chemotherapy appeared to have minimal or no effect upon ovarian function for those women who underwent fertility-sparing surgery [79].

Sex Cord–Stromal Tumors

Clinical Presentation

Sex cord–stromal tumors (SCSTs) account for 5–8% of all ovarian cancers and occur in all ages [62]. These tumors arise from the sex cords (granulosa and Sertoli cells) or the stroma (fibroblasts, theca, and Leydig cells) (Table 19.2). Although the peak incidence occurs during the perimenopause, a substantial proportion occurs in women under 40 years old. Approximately 5–7% of childhood or adolescent ovarian tumors are SCSTs.

The SCSTs account for the overwhelming majority of the hormonally active ovarian tumors, although non-SCTS ovarian tumors may be hormonally active if the stroma is luteinized. To a great degree, the clinical presentation of a SCST is determined by its hormonal activity, either estrogenic or androgenic. Typically, the granulosa, Sertoli and theca cell tumors are estrogenic, whereas the Sertoli–Leydig and steroid cell tumors are androgenic. Excess estrogen production results in age-dependent effects ranging from isosexual precocious puberty to menstrual irregularities to postmenopausal bleeding, as well as development of endometrial hyperplasia or endometrial cancer. Excess androgen production results in virilization ranging from oligomenorrhea to frank masculinization.

In addition to the hormonal effects, most patients present with abdominal pain, abdominal distention, and a mass. Spontaneous rupture or torsion may result in a surgical emergency. The tumors vary in size from microscopic to over 40 cm, are nearly always unilateral, and over 90% are stage I.

Most SCSTs are benign or indolent low-grade malignancies with an excellent prognosis. A few, including fibrosarcomas, intermediate and poorly differentiated Sertoli–Leydig cell tumors, and steroid cell tumors not otherwise specified, as well as those with advanced disease, are clinically aggressive with rapid progression and poor outcomes. Late recurrence, often more than a decade after initial treatment, is an unusual feature of adult-type granulosa cell tumors. Similarly, 22% of recurrences of steroid cell tumors not otherwise specified occur after 5 years [80].

Several of the SCSTs are associated with congenital disorders, including sex cord tumors with annular tubules and an occasional Sertoli cell tumor with Peutz–Jeghers syndrome, juvenile granulosa cell tumors with Ollier disease, leprechaunism and Maffucci syndrome, and Sertoli–Leydig cell tumors with Ollier disease [81–86].

The initial evaluation of a patient suspected of having an SCST includes a thorough history and physical examination, preoperative blood work, and imaging studies (chest X-ray, CT scan of abdomen and pelvis, pelvic ultrasound). These patients should be referred to a gynecologic oncologist for management.

Surgery

Contemporary management of most patients with SCSTs is surgical, with systemic therapy reserved for those rare patients with metastatic or recurrent disease. The extent of surgery depends upon a variety of factors, including the patient's age, desire for fertility, apparent extent of disease, and the histology of the SCST. Similar to the management of ovarian germ cell tumors, fertility-sparing surgery appears to be safe and efficacious [87]. Complete hysterectomy with bilateral salpingo-oophorectomy is warranted for those patients who have completed childbearing or those with extraovarian disease.

For those patients with functionally benign SCSTs (Table 19.2) and no evidence of extraovarian disease, unilateral salpingo-oophorectomy is sufficient surgical therapy. Due to the potential for development of endometrial hyperplasia or carcinoma, a thorough curettage must be performed to assess the endometrium in all patients with estrogen-producing tumors undergoing fertility-sparing surgery [88].

Patients with SCSTs with malignant potential (Table 19.2) and no evidence of extraovarian disease should undergo comprehensive surgical staging, including assessment of peritoneal cytology, unilateral salpingo-oophorectomy, omentectomy, and multiple peritoneal biopsies. Routine lymph node sampling is not warranted [89]. Despite a paucity of supportive data, aggressive surgical resection of all extraovarian disease appears warranted.

Secondary, and even repetitive, cytoreductive surgery may be beneficial for patients with recurrent SCSTs, especially those with indolent tumors such as granulosa cell tumors and sex cord tumors with annular tubules not associated with Peutz–Jeghers Syndrome.

Chemotherapy

There are no data demonstrating reduction in recurrence or survival benefit with systemic therapy for patients with stage I SCSTs. In addition, the rarity of advanced stage or recurrent SCSTs has made it difficult to conduct prospective, randomized clinical trials in this population. Currently, the most active and widely used chemotherapy regimen is bleomycin, etoposide, and cisplatin [90]. Taxane-based chemotherapy appears to be active and less toxic than bleomycin, etoposide, and cisplatin [91]. Hormonal therapy is an option for patients with recurrent granulosa cell tumors, including progestins, gonadotropin-releasing hormone agonists and aromatase inhibitors [92–94]. Targeted therapy with agents such as bevacizumab is promising and awaits further evaluation [95].

References

1 Siegel RL, Miller KD, Jemal A. Cancer statistics, 2017. *CA Cancer J Clin* 2017;67(1):7–30.

2 Koonings PP, Campbell K, Mishell DR Jr, Grimes DA. Relative frequency of primary ovarian neoplasm; a 10 year review. *Obstet Gynecol* 1989;74(6):921–6.

3 Howlader N, Noone AM, Krapcho M, *et al.* (eds) *SEER Cancer Statistics Review*, 1975–2013, National Cancer Institute. Bethesda, MD. http://seer.cancer.gov/csr/1975_2013/ based on November 2015 SEER data submission, posted to the SEER web site, April 2016.

4 Ries LAG, Young JL, Keel GE, *et al.* (eds) *SEER Survival Monograph: Cancer Survival Among Adults: U.S. SEER Program*, 1988–2001, *Patient and Tumor Characteristics*. National Cancer Institute, SEER Program, NIH Pub. No. 07-6215, Bethesda, MD, 2007.

5 Casagrande JT, Pike MC, Ross RK, *et al.* "Incessant ovulation" and ovarian cancer. *Lancet* 1979;314(8135):170–3.

6 Risch HA. Marrett LD. Howe GR. Parity, contraception, infertility, and the risk of epithelial ovarian cancer. *Am J Epidemiology* 1994;140(7):585–97.

7 LaVecchia C. Oral contraceptives and ovarian cancer: an update, 1998–2004. *Eur J Cancer Prev* 2006;15(2):117–24.

8 Danforth KN, Tworoger SS, Hecht JL, *et al.* Breastfeeding and risk of ovarian cancer in two prospective cohorts. *Cancer Causes Control* 2007;18(5):517–23.

9 Engeland A, Tretli S, Bjorge T. Height, body mass index, and ovarian cancer: a follow-up of 1.1 million Norwegian women. *J Natl Cancer Inst* 2003;95(16):1244–8.

10 Olsen CM. Green AC. Whiteman DC, *et al.* Obesity and the risk of epithelial ovarian cancer: a systematic review and meta-analysis. *Eur J Cancer* 2007;43(4):690–709.

11 Collaborative Group On Epidemiological Studies Of Ovarian Cancer, Beral V, Gaitskell K, Hermon C, *et al.* Menopausal hormone use and ovarian cancer risk: individual participant meta-analysis of 52 epidemiological studies. *Lancet* 2015;385(9980):1835–42.

12 Lacey JV, Mink PJ, Lubin JH, *et al.* Menopausal hormone replacement therapy and risk of ovarian cancer. *JAMA* 2002;288(3):334–41.

13 Beral V, Million Women Study Collaborators, Bull D, Green J, Reeves G. Ovarian cancer and hormone replacement therapy in the Million Women Study. *Lancet* 2007;369(9574):1703–10.

14 Skates SJ. OCS: Development of the Risk of Ovarian Cancer Algorithm (ROCA) and ROCA Screening Trials. *Int J Gyn Cancer* 2012:22(Suppl 1):S24–26.

15 Jacobs I, Menon U, Ryan A, *et al.* Ovarian cancer screening and mortality in the UK Collaborative Trial of Ovarian Cancer Screening (UKCTOCS): a randomised controlled trial. *Lancet* 2016; 387(10022):945–56.

16 Pinsky PF, Yu K, Kramer BS, *et al.* Extended mortality results for ovarian cancer screening in the PLCO trial with median 15 years follow-up. *Gynecol Oncol* 2017;123(4):592–9.

17 Kadija S. Stefanovic A. Jeremic K, *et al.* The utility of human epididymal protein 4, cancer antigen 125, and risk for malignancy algorithm in ovarian cancer and endometriosis. *Int J Gyn Cancer* 2012;22(2):238–44.

18 Kondalsamy-Chennakesavan S, Hackethal A, Bowtell D. Australian Ovarian Cancer Study Group, Obermair A. Differentiating stage 1 epithelial ovarian cancer from benign ovarian tumours using a combination of tumour markers HE4, CA125, and CEA, and patient's age. *Gynecol Oncol* 2013;129(3):467–71.

19 Bristow RE, Smith A, Zhang Z, *et al.* Ovarian malignancy risk stratification of the adnexal mass using a multivariate index assay. *Gynecol Oncol* 2013;128(2):252–9.

20 Clarke-Pearson DL. Screening for ovarian cancer. *N Engl J Med* 2009;361(2):170–7.

21 Lim AW, Mesher D, Gentry-Maharaj A, *et al.* Predictive value of symptoms for ovarian cancer: comparison of symptoms reported by questionnaire, interview, and general practitioner notes. *J Natl Cancer Inst* 2012;104(2):114–24.

22 Prat J for the FIGO Committee on Gynecologic Oncology. FIGO Guidelines: staging classification for cancer of the ovary, fallopian tube and peritoneum. *Int J Gyn Obstet* 2014;124(1):1–5.

23 Malpica A, Deavers MT, Lu K, *et al.* Grading ovarian serous carcinoma using a two-tier system. *Am J Surg Pathol* 2004;28(4):496–504.

24 Bodurka DC, Deavers MT, Tian C, *et al.* Reclassification of serous ovarian carcinoma by a 2-tier system. *Cancer* 2012;118:3087–94.

25 Tone AA, Salvador S, Finlayson SJ, *et al.* The role of the fallopian tube in ovarian cancer. *Clin Adv Hematol Oncol* 2012;10(5):296–306.

26 Morelli M, Venturella R, Mocciaro R, *et al.* Prophylactic salpingectomy in premenopausal low-risk women for ovarian cancer: primum non nocere. *Gynecol Oncol* 2013;129(3):448–51.

27 Gardi NL, Deshpande TU, Kamble SC, Budhe SR, Bapat SA. Discrete molecular classes of ovarian cancer suggestive of unique mechanisms of transformation and metastases. *Clin Cancer Res* 2014;20(1):87–99.

28 Romero I, Sun CC, Wong KK, Bast RC, Gershenson DM. Low-grade serous carcinoma: new concepts and emerging therapies. *Gynecol Oncol* 2013;130(3):660–6.

29 Referenced with permission from the NCCN Clinical Practice Guidelines in Oncology (NCCN Guidelines®) for Ovarian Cancer V.1.2017. © National Comprehensive Cancer Network, Inc 2013. All rights reserved. Accessed 18 April 2017. To view the most recent and complete version of the guideline, go online to www.nccn.org. NCCN makes no warranties of any kind whatsoever regarding their content, use or application and disclaims any responsibility for their application or use in any way.

30 Giede KC, Lieser L, Dodge J, Rosen B. Who should operate on patients with ovarian cancer? An evidence-based review. *Gynecol Oncol* 2005;99:447–61.

31 Bristow RE, Tomacruz RS, Armstrong DK, *et al.* Survival effect of maximal cytoreductive surgery for advanced ovarian carcinoma during the platinum era: a meta-analysis. *J Clin Oncol* 2002;20:1248–59.

32 Aletti GD, Dowdy SC, Gostout BS, *et al.* Aggressive surgical effort and improved survival in advanced-stage ovarian cancer. *Obstet Gynecol* 2006;107:77–85.

33 Elattar A, Bryant A, Winter-Roach BA, *et al.* Optimal primary surgical treatment for advanced epithelial ovarian cancer. Cochrane Database Syst Rev 2011:CD007565.

34 Thigpen T, Vance R, Puneky L, Khansur T. Chemotherapy in advanced ovarian carcinoma: current standards of care based on randomized trials. *Gynecol Oncol* 1994;55(3):S97–107.

35 McGuire WP, Ozols RF. Chemotherapy of advanced ovarian cancer. *Semin Oncol* 1998;25(3):340–8.

36 Ozols RF, Bundy BN, Greer BE, *et al.* Phase III trial of carboplatin and paclitaxel compared with cisplatin and paclitazel in patients with optimally resected stage III ovarian cancer: a Gynecologic Oncology Group study. *J Clin Oncol* 2003;21:3194–200.

37 Vasey PA, Jayson GC, Gordon A, *et al.* Phase III randomized trial of docetaxel-carboplatin versus paclitaxel-carboplatin as first-line chemotherapy for ovarian carcinoma. *J Natl Cancer Inst* 2004;96:1682–91.

38 Pignata S, Scambia G, Katsaros D, *et al.* Carboplatin plus paclitaxel once a week versus ever 3 weeks in patients with advanced ovarian cancer (MITO-7): a randomized, multicenter, open-label, phase 3 trial. *Lancet Oncol* 2014;15:396–405.

39 Katsumata N, Tasuda M, Takahashi F, *et al.* Dose-dense paclitaxel once a week in combination with carboplatin every 3 weeks for advanced ovarian cancer: an open-label, randomized controlled trial. *Lancet* 2009;374(9698):1331–8.

40 Katsumata N, Yasuda M, Isonishi S, *et al.* Long-term results of dose-dense paclitaxel and carboplatin versus conventional paclitaxel and carboplatin treatment of advanced epithelial ovarian, fallopian tube, or primary peritoneal cancer (JGOG 3016): a randomized, controlled, open-label trial. *Lancet* 2013;14(10):1020–6.

41 Chan JK, Brady MF, Penson RT, *et al.* Weekly vs. every-3-week paclitaxel and carboplatin for ovarian cancer. *N Engl J Med* 2016;374:738–48.

42 Armstrong DK, Bundy B, Wenzel L, *et al.* Intraperitoneal cisplatin and paclitaxel in ovarian cancer. *N Engl J Med* 2006;354(1):34–43.

43 NCI clinical announcement: Intraperitoneal chemotherapy for ovarian cancer. Issued January 2006. http://ctep.cancer.gov/highlights/docs/clin_annc_010506.pdf (accessed 9 October 2017).

44 Walker J, Brady MF, DiSilvestro PA, *et al.* A phase III trial of bevacizumab with IV versus IP chemotherapy for ovarian, fallopian tube, and peritoneal carcinoma: an NRG Oncology Study. Gynecol Oncol 2016;SGO Annual Meeting Late-Breaking Abstract Session.

45 Bristow RE, Chi DS. Platinum-based neoadjuvant chemotherapy and interval surgical cytoreduction for advanced ovarian cancer: a meta-analysis. *Gynecol Oncol* 2006;103:1070–6.

46 Vergote I, Trope CG, Amant F, *et al.* Neoadjuvant chemotherapy or primary surgery in stage IIIC or IV ovarian cancer. *N Engl J Med* 2010;363(10):943–53.

47 Wright AA, Bohlke K, Armstrong DK, *et al.* Neoadjuvant chemotherapy for newly diagnosed, advanced ovarian cancer: Society of Gynecologic Oncology and American Society of Clinical Oncology Clinical Practice Guideline. *Gynecol Oncol* 2016;143(1):3–15.

48 Burger RA, Brady MF, Bookman MA, *et al.* Incorporation of bevacizumab in the primary treatment of ovarian cancer. *N Engl J Med* 2011;365:2473–83.

49 Perren TJ, Swart AM, Pfisterer J, *et al.* A phase 3 trial of bevacizumab in ovarian cancer. *N Engl J Med* 2011;365:2484–96.

50 duBois A, Floquet A, Kim JW, *et al.* Incorporation of pazopanib in maintenance therapy of ovarian cancer. *J Clin Oncol* 2014; 32:3374–82.

51 Vaidya AP, Curtin JP. The follow-up of ovarian cancer. *Semin Oncol* 2003;30:401–12.

52 Salani R, Backes FJ, Fung Kee Fung M, *et al.* Posttreatment surveillance and diagnosis of recurrence in women with gynecologic malignancies: Society of Gynecologic Oncologists recommendations. *Am J Obstet Gynecol* 2011;204(6):466–78.

53 Gadducci A, Cosio S, Zola P, *et al.* Surveillance procedures for patients treated for epithelial ovarian cancer: a review of the literature. *Int J Gynecol Cancer* 2007;17:21–31.

54 Rustin GJ, van der Burg ME; on behalf of MRC and EORTC collaborators. A randomized trial in ovarian cancer (OC) of early treatment of relapse based on CA125 level alone versus delayed treatment based on conventional clinical indicators (MRC OV05/EORTC 55955 trials). *J Clin Oncol* 2009;27:18 s.

55 Griffiths RW, Zee YK, Evans S, *et al.* Outcomes after multiple lines of chemotherapy for platinum-resistant epithelial cancers of the ovary, pertioneum and fallopian tube. *Int J Gynecol Cancer* 2011;21:58–65.

56 Deeks ED. Olaparib: first global approval. *Drugs* 2015;75:231–40.

57 Department of Health and Human Services. Centres for Medicare and Medicaid Services. Medicare and Medicaid Programs: Hospice Conditions of Participation – Final Rule. *Federal Register* 2008;73(109). 42 CFR Part 418.

58 Casarett D, Pickard A, Bailey FA, *et al.* Do palliative care consultations improve patient outcome? *J Am Geriatr Soc* 2008;56(4):593–9.

59 Temel JS, Greer JA, Muzikansky A, *et al.* Early palliative care for patients with metastatic non-small-cell lung cancer. *N Eng J Med* 2010;363(8):733–42.

60 Fauci J, Schneider K, Walters C, *et al.* The utilization of palliative care in gynecologic oncology patients near the end of life. *Gynecol Oncol* 2012;127(1):175–9.

61 Tumours of the Ovary. In: Kurman RJ, Carcanigiu ML, Herrington CS, Young RH, eds. *WHO/IARC Classification of Tumours of Female Reproductive Organs, 4th edn*. Lyon: International Agency for Research on Cancer, 2014.

62 Scully R, Young R, Clement P. *Tumors of the Ovary, Maldeveloped Gonads, Fallopian Tube, and Broad Ligament: Atlas of Tumor Pathology*. American Registry of Pathology, 1999.

63 Palenzuela G, Martin E, Meunier A, *et al.* Comprehensive staging allows for excellent outcome in patients with localized malignant germ cell tumors. *Ann Surg* 2008;248(5):836–41.

64 Billmire D, Vinocur C, Rescorla F, *et al.* Children's Oncology Group (COG). Outcome and staging evaluation in malignant germ cell tumors of the ovary in children and adolescents: an intergroup study. *J Pediatr Surg* 2004;39(3):424–9; discussion 424–9.

65 Williams SD, Blessing JA, Moore DH, Homesley HD, Adcock L. Cisplatin, vinblastine, and bleomycin in advanced and recurrent ovarian germ cell tumors: a trial of the Gynecologic Oncology Group. *Ann Int Med* 1989;111(1):22–7.

66 Gershenson DM, Morris M, Cangir A, *et al.* Treatment of malignant gern cell tumors of the ovary with belomycin, etoposide and bleomycin. *J Clin Oncol* 1990;8(4):715–20.

67 Williams S, Blessing JA, Liao SY, Ball H, Hanjani P. Adjuvant therapy of ovarian germ cell tumors with cisplatin, etoposide and bleomycin: a trial of the Gynecologic Oncology Group. *J Clin Oncol* 1994;12(4):701–6.

68 Dark GG, Bower M, Newlands ES, Paradinas F, Rustin GJ. Surveillance policy for Stage I ovarian germ cell tumors. *J Clin Oncol* 1997;15(2):620–4.

69 Mitchell PL, Al-Nasiri N, A'Hern R, *et al.* Treatment of non-dysgerminomatous ovarian germ cell tumors; an analysis of 69 cases. *Cancer* 1999;85(10):2232–44.

70 Baranzelli MC, Bouffet E, Quintana E, *et al.* Non-seminomatous ovarian germ cell tumors in children. *Eur J Cancer* 2000;36(3):376–83.

71 Gobel U, Schneider DT, Calaminus G, *et al.* Germ cell tumors in children and adolescents. GPOH, MAKEI and the MAHO study groups. *Ann Oncol* 2000;11(3):263–71.

72 Patterson DM, Murugaesu N, Holden L, Seckl MJ, Rustin GJ. A review of the close surveillance policy for Stage I female germ cell tumors of the ovary and other sites. *Int J Gynecol Cancer* 2008;18(1):43–50.

73 Hale J, Olsen TA, Nichelson J, *et al.* Carboplatin (CBP) versus cisplatin (CP) within prognostic troups in pediatric extracranial malignant germ cell tumors (MGCTs). *J Clin Oncol* 2012;30 suppl; abstr 9539.

74 Kondagunta GV, Bacik J, Donadio A, *et al.* Combination of paclitaxel, iphosphamide and cisplatin is an effective second-line therapy of patients with relapsed testicular germ cell tumors. *J Clin Oncol* 2005;23(27):6549–55.

75 Einhorn LH, Williams SD, Chamness A, *et al.* High dose chemotherapy and stem cell rescue for metastatic germ cell tumors. *N Engl J Med* 2007;357(4):340–8.

76 Munkarah A, Gershenson DM, Levenback C, *et al.* Salvage chemotherapy for chemorefractory ovarian germ cell tumors. *Gynecol Oncol* 1994;55(2):217–23.

77 Zanetta G, Bonazzi C., Cantu M, *et al.* Survival and reproductive function after treatment of malignant germ cell tumors. *J Clin Oncol* 2001;19(4):1015–20.

78 Champion V, Williams SD, Miller A, *et al.* Quality of life in long-term survivors of ovarian germ cell tumors: a Gynecologic Oncology Group study. *Gynecol Oncol* 2007;105(3):687–94.

79 Gershenson DM, Miller AM, Champion VL, *et al.* Reproductive and sexual function after platinum-based chemotherapy in long-term germ cell tumor survivors. *J Clin Oncol* 2007;25(19):2792–7.

80 Hayes MC, Scully RE. Ovarian steroid cell tumors (not otherwise specified). A clinicopathological analysis of 63 cases. *Am J Surg Pathol* 1987;11(11):835–45.

81 Young RH, Welch WR, Dickersin GR, Scully RE. Ovarian sex cord tumors with annular tubules: review of 74 cases including 27 with Peutz-Jeghers syndrome and four with adenoma malignum of the cervix. *Cancer* 1982;50(7):1384–402.

82 Ferry JA, Young RH, Engel, Scully RE. Oxyphilic Sertoli cell tumor of the ovary: a report of three cases, in two patients with the Peutz-Jeghers syndrome. *Int J Gynecol Pathol* 1994;13(3):259–66.

83 Tamimi HK, Bolen JW. Endochondromatosis (Ollier's disease) and ovarian juvenile granulosa cell tumor. *Cancer* 1984;53(7):1605–8.

84 Brisgotti M, Fabbretti G, Pesce F, *et al.* Congenital bilateral juvenile granulosa cell tumor of the ovary in leprechaunism: a case report. *Pediatr Pathol* 1993;13(5):549–58.

85 Tanaka Y, Sasaki Y, Nishihira H, Izawa T. Nishi T. Ovarian juvenile granulosa cell tumor associated with Maffucci's syndrome. *Am J Clin Pathol* 1992;97(4):523–7.

86 Weyl-Ben Arush M, Oslander M. Ollier's disease associated with ovarian Sertoli-Leydig cell tumor and breast adenoma. *Am J Pediatr Hematol Oncol* 1991;13(1):49–51.

87 Zhang M, Cheung MK, Shin JY, *et al.* Prognostic factors responsible for survival in sex cord stromal tumors of the ovary-an analysis of 376 women. *Gynecol Oncol* 2007;104(2):396–400.

88 Segal R, DePetrillo AD, Thomas G. Clinical review of adult granulosa cell tumors of the ovary. *Gynecol Oncol* 1995;56(3):338–44.

89 Thrall MM, Paley P, Pizer E, Garcia R, Goff BA. Patterns of spread and recurrence of sex cord-stromal tumors of the ovary. *Gynecol Oncol* 2011;122(2):242–5.

90 Homesley HD, Bundy BN, Hurteau JA, Roth LM. Bleomycin, etoposide, and cisplatin combination therapy of ovarian granulosa cell tumors and other stromal malignancies: a Gynecologic Oncology Group study. *Gynecol Oncol* 1999;72:131–7.

91 Brown J, Shvartsman HS, Deavers MT, *et al.* The activity of taxanes compared with bleomycin, etoposide and cisplatin in the treatment of sex cord-stromal ovarian tumors. *Gynecol Oncol* 2005;97(2):489–96.

92 Hardy RD, Bell JG, Nicely CJ, Reid GC. Hormonal treatment of a recurrent granulosa cell tumor of the ovary: case report and review of the literature. *Gynecol Oncol* 2005;96(3):865–9.

93 Fishman A, Kudelka AP, Tresukosol D, *et al.* Leuprolide acetate for treating refractory or persistent ovarian granulosa cell tumor. *J Repro Med* 1996;41(6):393–6.

94 Freeman SA, Modesitt SC. Anastrazole therapy in recurrent adult granulosa cell tumors: a report of 2 cases. *Gynecol Oncol* 2006;103(2):755–8.

95 Brown J, Brady W, Schink J, Van Le L, *et al.* Bevacizumab shows activity in treating recurrent sex cord stromal ovarian tumors: results of a phase II trial of the Gynecologic Oncology Group. *Gynecol Oncol* 2012;125:771–3(Abstract).

20

Uterine Corpus Cancer

Mario Javier Pineda and John R. Lurain

Northwestern University Feinberg School of Medicine, Robert H. Lurie Comprehensive Cancer Center, Chicago, Illinois, USA

Introduction

This chapter reviews the epidemiology, prevention, early detection, diagnosis, staging, treatment, and follow-up of uterine corpus cancers. Most of these cancers are endometrial carcinomas, which are the primary focus of this chapter. Less common cancers of this site, including endometrial stromal neoplasms, carcinosarcomas, and leiomyosarcomas, are also included.

Endometrial Carcinoma

Incidence and Mortality

Worldwide, the uterine corpus is the second most common site of malignancy in the female reproductive system. In developed countries, uterine corpus cancer occurs more frequently than any other female reproductive malignancy; among women in these countries, only one reproductive system cancer (ovarian) causes more deaths [1]. In the United States, approximately 61,380 women are diagnosed with cancer of the uterine corpus and approximately 10,920 die from this disease each year. [2]. Endometrial adenocarcinomas (and their subtypes) comprise approximately 90.6% of uterine corpus cancers; other types of carcinoma (such as squamous and "not otherwise specified") represent another 1.5% [3].

Etiology and Risk Factors

There appear to be two pathogenetic types of endometrial cancer [4]. Type I, accounting for 75–85% of cases, occurs in younger, perimenopausal women with a history of excess endogenous or exogenous estrogen relative to progesterone. In these women, it is classically thought that tumors begin as hyperplastic endometrium and progress to carcinoma. These "estrogen-dependent" tumors tend to be better differentiated and have a more favorable prognosis than tumors that are not associated with estrogen excess. Type I cancers are associated with factors including menopausal hormone therapy with estrogen only (without progestin), obesity, nulliparity, early menarche, and late menopause. Type II endometrial carcinoma occurs in women without excess estrogenic stimulation of the endometrium. These spontaneously occurring cancers are not as commonly associated pathologically with endometrial hyperplasia, but usually arise in a background of atrophic endometrium. They are less differentiated and associated with poorer prognosis than estrogen-dependent tumors. These "estrogen-independent" tumors tend to occur in older, postmenopausal, thinner women and are present disproportionately in African American women [5, 6]. Molecular genetic studies show that these two tumor types evolve via distinct pathogenetic pathways [7–9].

The most frequent genetic alterations of endometrioid (type I) carcinomas are microsatellite instability and mutations in *PTEN, PIK3CA,* K-RASs, and *CTNNBI* (β-catenin), whereas nonendometrioid (type II, predominantly serous and clear cell) tumors often exhibit *p53* mutations, *HER2/neu* amplification, and chromosomal instability. Approximately 80% of newly diagnosed endometrial carcinomas in the Western world are endometrioid in type [10]. Any factor that increases exposure to unopposed estrogen (e.g., estrogen-replacement therapy, obesity, anovulatory cycles, estrogen-secreting tumors) increases the risk of these tumors, whereas factors that decrease exposure to estrogens or increase progesterone levels (e.g., oral contraceptives or smoking) tend to be protective [11]. Several risk factors for the development of endometrial cancer have been identified (Table 20.1) [12–14].

The average age of women with endometrioid cancers is approximately 62 years, about 70% of these cancers are confined to the corpus at the time of diagnosis, and the 5-year survival is approximately 83% [15]. By contrast, the average age of women with nonendometrioid cancers is 67 years, at least half of the cancers have already spread beyond the corpus at the time of diagnosis, and the 5-year survival is approximately 62% for clear cell carcinomas and 53% for papillary serous cancers [15]. Endometrial cancer may occasionally develop after radiation treatment for cervical cancer [16].

The American Cancer Society's Oncology in Practice: Clinical Management, First Edition. Edited by The American Cancer Society.

Table 20.1 Risk factors for endometrial cancer.

Characteristic	Relative risk
Nulliparity	2–3
Late menopause	2.4
Obesity	
21–50 lb overweight	3
>50 lb overweight	10
Diabetes mellitus	3
Unopposed estrogen therapy	1.5–8
Tamoxifen therapy	2–7
Atypical endometrial hyperplasia	29
Lynch syndrome	20

Endometrial Hyperplasia and Intraepithelial Neoplasia

Classic teaching has been that endometrial hyperplasia represents a spectrum of morphologic and biologic alterations of the endometrial glands and stroma displaying a variety of cytological and architectural alterations. Endometrial hyperplasias are important clinically because they may cause abnormal bleeding, be associated with estrogen-producing ovarian tumors, result from hormonal therapy, and precede or occur simultaneously with endometrial cancer [12, 17].

The World Health Organization (WHO) in 1994 established a widely implemented classification scheme for endometrial hyperplasia, with four categories based on architectural derangement and cytological atypia [12]. In 2014, the WHO revised this classification, recommending only two categories – endometrial hyperplasia without atypia and atypical hyperplasia/endometrial intraepithelial neoplasia [10, 18]. Features of endometrial hyperplasia without atypia include proliferation glands with variable size and irregular shape, formed by cells without significant nuclear atypia. Approximately 1–3% of these lesions progress to endometrial carcinoma. In contrast, in atypical hyperplasia/endometrial intraepithelial neoplasia, cells with significant atypia (large nuclei of variable size and shape that have lost polarity, increased nuclear-to-cytoplasmic ratios, prominent nucleoli, and irregularly clumped chromatin) form very crowded glands with highly irregular shape, including some back-to-back glands without intervening stroma. Women with atypical hyperplasia/endometrial intraepithelial neoplasia face a 25–43% risk of being diagnosed with endometrial carcinoma following immediate hysterectomy or within the following year [10, 19].

For women who have completed childbearing, definitive treatment for hyperplastic lesions with atypia is hysterectomy with consideration of removal of both fallopian tubes and ovaries. This allows intra- and postoperative evaluation and treatment of concurrent adenocarcinoma. Younger patients with endometrial cancer and hyperplastic changes of the endometrium tend to have disorders such as polycystic ovarian syndrome, chronic anovulation, and infertility, indicative of exposure to intrinsic estrogen excess [20]. Lesions in this age group are usually well differentiated and of endometrioid subtype with the potential to regress with progestational therapy [21]. Patients who have multiple medical comorbidities and who are at high risk for surgical complications are another group in whom nonsurgical management may be indicated.

Although, progestational therapy can successfully treat disease while preserving fertility for women with atypical hyperplasia and well-differentiated presumed stage I endometrial cancer, there is no consensus on the treatment protocol. Women must be counseled that failure to identify recurrence or extension of disease during progestational treatment may lead to a delay in definitive surgery and ultimately a compromised prognosis [22] as well as the low likelihood of achieving a live birth upon completion of successful treatment. Imaging (transvaginal ultrasound and pelvic magnetic resonance imaging (MRI)) should be performed in an effort to exclude women with more advanced-stage disease. Continuous progestin therapy with megestrol acetate (40–160 mg per day) or the levonorgestrel intrauterine contraceptive device are probably the most reliable treatments for reversing complex or atypical hyperplasia. The main side effects of systemic treatment are weight gain, edema, thromboembolism, and occasionally hypertension. Short interval endometrial sampling (every 3–6 months) should be performed to evaluate treatment response. Once having achieved a complete response, surveillance should continue as these women are at high risk for disease recurrence.

Endometrial Cancer Screening in the General Population

Screening asymptomatic women for endometrial cancer should not be undertaken because of the lack of an appropriate, cost-effective and acceptable test that reduces mortality [23–25].

Studies and recommendations for the routine screening of women taking tamoxifen with transvaginal ultrasonography or endometrial biopsy are conflicting but generally screening is not considered clinically useful in the absence of symptoms [24, 25]. The American Cancer Society (ACS) considers evidence insufficient to recommend screening for endometrial cancer in women at average risk or at increased risk because of a history of unopposed estrogen therapy, tamoxifen therapy, late menopause, nulliparity, infertility or failure to ovulate, obesity, diabetes, or hypertension. However, the ACS recommends that women at average and increased risk should be informed about endometrial cancer symptoms such as unexpected bleeding and spotting at the onset of menopause and should be strongly encouraged to report these symptoms promptly to their physicians [24]. Screening for endometrial cancer or its precursors may be justified for certain high-risk women, such as members of families with Lynch syndrome [24, 25].

Surveillance and Prevention in Patients at High Risk

Women with Lynch syndrome (previously referred to as hereditary nonpolyposis colorectal cancer syndrome, or HNPCC), a cancer susceptibility syndrome with germline mutations in one of the DNA mismatch repair genes *MLH1*, *MSH2*, *MSH6*, *PMS2*, *EPCAM*, have a 30–60% age-specific cumulative risk by age 70 for endometrial and colon cancer [13, 26, 27]. The majority of studies have focused on the increased incidence of endometrial cancer associated with Lynch syndrome, a highly penetrant disorder (32–42%) that is responsible for 2–4% of all endometrial cancers [13, 28–30]. With regard to endometrial cancer, the disorder is characterized by early age (average age of diagnosis is 49 years). Lynch syndrome mutation carriers are at increased risk for neoplastic lesions in a variety of organs, including the colon, uterus, ovaries, stomach, urinary tract, small bowel, pancreas, gallbladder, prostate, and skin [26, 31, 32]. In a study of 10,283 patients from 537 Lynch syndrome families, the cumulative incidence of all Lynch syndrome cancers was 54% by age 70 years [13]. The lifetime risk of endometrial cancer is 32–42% and the lifetime risk of ovarian cancer is 10–12%, although there are differences in specific risks dependent upon the specific affected gene [13, 33, 34].

Although these data appear to support the use of endometrial cancer surveillance strategies for women with Lynch syndrome, a specific algorithm is not defined [33, 35, 36]. The ACS recommends that women at very high risk for endometrial cancer because of (i) known Lynch syndrome genetic mutation carrier status, (ii) substantial likelihood of being a mutation carrier (i.e., a mutation is known to be present in the family), or (iii) absence of genetic testing results in families with suspected autosomal dominant predisposition to colon cancer should consider beginning annual testing for early endometrial cancer detection at age 35 years [24].

Clinical Features

Approximately 90% of women with endometrial carcinoma have abnormal uterine bleeding as their only presenting symptom [37, 38]. Some women experience pelvic pressure or discomfort indicative of uterine enlargement or extrauterine disease spread. Bleeding may not be noted because of cervical stenosis, especially in older patients, and may be associated with hematometra or pyometra, causing a purulent vaginal discharge; this finding is often associated with a poor prognosis [39]. Fewer than 5% of women diagnosed with endometrial cancer are asymptomatic [40]. In the absence of symptoms, endometrial cancer is detected in some patients as the result of investigation of abnormal Pap test results, discovery of cancer in a uterus removed for some other reason, or evaluation of an abnormal finding on pelvic ultrasonography examination or computed tomography (CT) scan obtained for an unrelated reason. Women who are found to have malignant cells on Pap test are more likely to have more advanced stage disease and non-endometrioid histologies [41].

Abnormal perimenopausal and postmenopausal vaginal bleeding should always be properly investigated, no matter how minimal or nonpersistent. Causes may be nongenital, genital extrauterine, or uterine [42]. Nongenital tract sites should be considered based on the history or examination, including testing for blood in the urine and stool. Invasive tumors of the cervix, vagina, and vulva are usually evident on examination, and any tumors discovered should be biopsied. Traumatic bleeding from an atrophic vagina may account for up to 15% of all causes of postmenopausal vaginal bleeding. This diagnosis can be considered if inspection reveals a thin, friable vaginal wall, but the possibility of a uterine source of bleeding must first be eliminated. Possible uterine causes of perimenopausal or postmenopausal bleeding include endometrial atrophy, endometritis, endometrial polyps, estrogen therapy, endometrial hyperplasia, and carcinoma or sarcoma [42–44]. It is important to recognize that the workup of abnormal uterine bleeding should include endometrial biopsy even in premenopausal patients, as 5% of newly diagnosed endometrial cancers are in women under the age of 40.

Physical examination seldom reveals any evidence of endometrial carcinoma. Abdominal examination is usually unremarkable, except in advanced cases in which ascites or hepatic or omental metastases may be palpable.

Diagnosis

Office endometrial aspiration biopsy is the accepted first step in evaluating a woman with abnormal uterine bleeding or suspected endometrial pathology [45]. The diagnostic accuracy of office-based endometrial biopsy is 90–92% when compared with subsequent findings at hysterectomy [46]. The narrow plastic cannulas are relatively inexpensive, often can be used without a tenaculum, cause less uterine cramping (resulting in increased patient acceptance), and are successful in obtaining adequate tissue samples in more than 95% of cases. A Pap test is an unreliable diagnostic test because only about 30% of women with endometrial cancer have abnormal conventional Pap test results [47].

Hysteroscopy and dilatation and curettage should be reserved for situations in which cervical stenosis or patient tolerance does not permit adequate evaluation by aspiration biopsy, bleeding recurs after a negative endometrial biopsy, or the specimen obtained is inadequate to explain the abnormal bleeding [48–50].

Transvaginal ultrasonography may be a useful adjunct to endometrial biopsy for evaluation of abnormal uterine bleeding and for selecting women for additional testing [46]. The finding of an endometrial thickness greater than 3–5 mm, a polyploidy endometrial mass, or a collection of fluid within the uterus requires further evaluation [51–53].

Pathology

The histologic classification of carcinoma arising in the endometrium and relative frequencies of each type is shown in Table 20.2.

Endometrioid Adenocarcinoma

These tumors are composed of glands that resemble normal endometrial glands; they have pseudostratified columnar cells, little or no intracytoplasmic mucin, and smooth intraluminal surfaces. As tumors become less differentiated, they contain more solid areas, less glandular formation, and more cytologic atypia. The well-differentiated lesions may be difficult to separate from atypical hyperplasia. Tumors are grouped into three grades. The histologic grade is based primarily upon an evaluation of the tumor architecture, and modified by nuclear atypia. About 15–25% of endometrioid carcinomas have areas of squamous differentiation.

Mucinous Carcinoma

In these endometrial carcinomas, more than one-half of the tumor is composed of cells with intracytoplasmic mucin [55–57]. Most of these tumors have a well-differentiated

Table 20.2 Histologic classification of endometrial carcinomas.

Endometrioid adenocarcinoma	75–80%
Ciliated adenocarcinoma	
Secretory adenocarcinoma	
Papillary or villoglandular	
With squamous differentiation	
Papillary serous	<10%
Clear cell	4%
Carcinosarcoma	3%
Mucinous	1%
Squamous cell	<1%
Mixed	10%
Undifferentiated	<1%

Source: Data taken from National Cancer Institute [54].

glandular architecture. Their behavior is similar to that of common endometrioid carcinomas and the prognosis is good. It is important to distinguish mucinous carcinoma of the endometrium as an entity from endocervical adenocarcinoma.

Serous Carcinoma

The morphology of these endometrial carcinomas resembles serous carcinoma of the ovary and fallopian tube [58, 59]. Most often, these tumors are composed of papillae having broad fibrovascular stalks lined by highly atypical cells with tufted stratification. Psammoma bodies may be observed in 30% of cases.

Serous carcinomas, also referred to as uterine papillary serous carcinomas, are considered high-risk lesions. Compared to endometrioid type tumors, serous carcinomas are more likely to present with metastatic disease at first diagnosis and have a less favorable prognosis accounting for up to one-half of the deaths from endometrial carcinoma [58]. They are commonly admixed with other histologic patterns, but even tumors with a small proportion of serous features remain at high risk of recurrence [60]. Serous carcinomas are often associated with lymph-vascular space and deep myometrial invasion. The presence of lymph node metastases, positive peritoneal cytology, and intraperitoneal tumor does not necessarily correlate with increasing myometrial invasion; suggesting that surgical staging should be performed regardless of traditional endometrioid risk factors [61]. Even when these tumors appear to be confined to the endometrium or endometrial polyps without myometrial or lymphvascular invasion, they behave more aggressively than endometrioid carcinomas and have a propensity to spread intra-abdominally, simulating the behavior of ovarian carcinoma [62].

Clear Cell Carcinoma

The cells of clear cell carcinoma have highly atypical nuclei and abundant clear or eosinophilic cytoplasm. The cells often have a hobnail shape with apical rather than basal nuclei, and can be arranged in papillary, tubulocystic, glandular, and solid patterns. Clear cell carcinoma characteristically occurs in older women and like serous carcinoma is considered aggressive, with overall survival rates varying from 33 to 64% [63–65].

Squamous Cell Carcinoma

Squamous cell carcinoma of the endometrium is rare, although other types of endometrial carcinoma may contain foci of squamous differentiation. To establish primary origin of squamous cell carcinoma within the endometrium, there must be no connection with or spread from cervical squamous epithelium. This tumor has a poor prognosis, with an estimated 36% survival rate in patients with clinical stage I disease [66].

Carcinosarcoma

Carcinosarcoma is a morphologically heterogeneous malignancy with some foci displaying the histological appearance of carcinoma and others having the histological characteristics of a sarcoma. The carcinomatous element typically shows glandular histology, whereas the sarcomatous element may be homologous (resembling an endometrial stromal sarcoma), or heterologous (resembling sarcomas with differentiation toward tissues foreign to the uterus, such as rhabdomyosarcoma, chondrosarcoma, osteosarcoma, or liposarcoma). These tumors have historically been classified with uterine sarcomas and in the 2014 WHO classification are in a category of mixed epithelial and mesenchymal tumors that is distinct from carcinomas and sarcomas. However, recent biological and clinical evidence supports the view that carcinomas are high-grade carcinomas with sarcomatous metaplasia. For these reasons, carcinosarcomas are staged in the FIGO system as endometrial carcinomas, and their treatment is similar to that of type II endometrial carcinomas such as serous and clear cell carcinomas [67–69].

The tumor typically grows as a large, soft, polypoid mass that can fill and distend the uterine cavity; necrosis and hemorrhage are prominent features. The myometrium is invaded to various degrees in almost all cases. The most frequent areas of spread are the pelvis, lymph nodes, peritoneal cavity, lungs, and liver. This metastatic pattern suggests that these neoplasms spread by local extension and regional lymph node metastasis in a manner similar to that of endometrial adenocarcinoma. In a significant number of patients, lymph node metastases and positive peritoneal cytology are found with early-stage carcinosarcoma [70].

Simultaneous Tumors of the Endometrium and Ovary

Synchronous endometrial and ovarian cancers are the most frequent synchronous genital malignancies, with a reported incidence of 1.4–3.8% [71, 72]. Most commonly, both the ovarian and endometrial tumors are well-differentiated endometrioid adenocarcinomas of low stage, resulting in an excellent prognosis. Patients are often premenopausal and present with abnormal uterine bleeding. The ovarian cancer usually is discovered as an incidental finding and is diagnosed at an earlier stage because of the symptomatic endometrial tumor, leading to a more favorable outcome.

Pretreatment Evaluation

After establishing the diagnosis of endometrial carcinoma, the next step is to evaluate the patient thoroughly to determine the best and safest approach to management of the disease. A complete history and physical examination are of utmost importance. Patients with endometrial carcinoma are often elderly and obese with a variety of medical problems, such as diabetes mellitus and hypertension, which complicate surgical management. Any abnormal symptoms, such as bladder or intestinal symptoms, should be evaluated. On physical examination, attention should be directed to enlarged or suspicious lymph nodes, including the inguinal area, abdominal masses, and possible areas of cancer spread within the pelvis. Evidence of distant metastasis or locally advanced disease in the pelvis, such as gross cervical involvement or parametrial spread, may alter the treatment approach. The vaginal introitus and suburetheral area, and the entire vagina and cervix, should be carefully inspected and palpated. Bimanual rectovaginal examination should be performed specifically to evaluate the uterus for size and mobility, the adnexa for masses, the parametria for induration, and the cul-de-sac for nodularity.

Chest imaging should be performed to exclude pulmonary metastasis and to evaluate the cardiorespiratory status of the patient, and complete blood and platelet counts should be done. Other preoperative studies may include electrocardiography and serum chemistries (including renal and liver function tests). Studies such as cystoscopy, colonoscopy, and barium enema are not indicated unless dictated by patient symptoms, physical findings, or other laboratory tests [73]. CT scanning of the abdomen and pelvis may be considered in patients with type II uterine cancer to determine if minimally invasive surgery (MIS) is appropriate. Stage IV disease is usually clinically evident based on patient symptomatology and clinical examination. Ultrasonography and MRI can be used to assess myometrial invasion preoperatively with a fairly high degree of accuracy [74]. This information may be of use in planning the surgical procedure with regard to whether lymph node sampling should be undertaken.

Serum CA-125 levels are elevated in most patients with advanced or metastatic endometrial cancer [75]. Preoperative measurement of serum CA-125 may help determine the extent of surgical staging and, if elevated, may be useful as a tumor marker in assessing response to subsequent therapy [76–78].

Staging

Clinical Staging

Clinical staging, according to the 1971 FIGO system, should be performed only in patients who are deemed not to be surgical candidates because of their poor medical condition or the degree of disease spread [79]. The current FIGO staging is surgical, as discussed below, and has supplanted the old clinical system. With improvements in preoperative and postoperative care, anesthesia administration, and surgical techniques, almost all patients are medically suitable for operative therapy. A small percentage of patients will not be candidates for surgical staging because of gross cervical involvement, parametrial spread, invasion of the bladder or rectum, or distant metastasis.

Surgical Staging

Surgical staging for endometrial cancer, consists of hysterectomy, removal of the adnexal structures, peritoneal cytology, and lymph node sampling where appropriate (Table 20.3) [80, 81]. Surgical staging not only identifies most patients with extrauterine disease, but also identifies patients with uterine risk factors for recurrence, including large tumor size, deep myometrial invasion, lymphvascular space invasion, and cervical extension, thereby allowing for a more informed approach to postoperative adjuvant therapy. Lymph node dissections as part of surgical staging is not required in patients assessed intraoperatively to be at low risk for lymph node metastasis (<2 cm, grade 1–2 tumors with superficial myometrial invasion), whereas systematic lymph node dissection should be performed in most other patients with endometrial cancer (Table 20.4) [81].

Table 20.3 Endometrial Cancer Staging.

Stage I[1]	Tumor confined to the corpus uteri
IA[1]	No or less than half myometrial invasion
IB[1]	Invasion equal to or more than half of the myometrium
Stage II[1]	Tumor invades cervical stroma, but does not extend beyond the uterus[2]
Stage III[1]	Local and/or regional spread of the tumor
IIIA[1]	Tumor invades the serosa of the corpus uteri and/or adnexae[3]
IIIB[1]	Vaginal and/or parametrial involvement[3]
IIIC[1]	Metastases to pelvic and/or para-aortic lymph nodes[3]
IIIC1[1]	Positive pelvic nodes
IIIC2[1]	Positive para-aortic lymph nodes with or without positive pelvic lymph nodes
Stage IV[1]	Tumor invades bladder and/or bowel mucosa, and/or distant metastases
IVA[1]	Tumor invasion of bladder and/or bowel mucosa
IVB[1]	Distant metastases, including intra-abdominal metastases and/or inguinal lymph nodes

Source: adapted from FIGO Committee on Gynecologic Oncology. Revised FIGO staging for carcinoma of the vulva, cervix, and endometrium. Int J Gynecol Obstet 2009; 105:103–104.

[1] Either G1, G2, or G3.

[2] Endocervical glandular involvement only should be considered as Stage I and no longer as Stage II.

[3] Positive cytology should be reported separately without changing the stage.

Table 20.4 Surgically staged endometrial cancer: actuarial 5-year survival rate (%) by histologic grade and stage (1988 staging criteria).

	Grade		
Stage	1	2	3
Ia	93.4	91.3	79.5
Ib	91.6	93.4	82.0
Ic	90.6	86.3	74.9
IIa	89.9	83.7	68.3
IIb	81.2	76.9	64.9
IIIa	82.5	71.1	45.1
IIIb	75.0	64.6	30.6
IIIc	66.9	61.0	51.4
IVa	–	32.4	20.9
IVb	48.3	24.1	12.1

Source: adapted from Creasman *et al.* [81].

Table 20.5 Surgical-pathologic findings in clinical stage in endometrial cancer.

Surgical-pathologic findings	Percentage of patients
Histology	
Adenocarcinoma	80
Adenosquamous	16
Other (papillary serous, clear cell)	4
Grade	
1	29
2	46
3	25
Myometrial invasion	
None	14
Inner third	45
Middle third	19
Outer third	22
Positive peritoneal cytology	12
Lymphvascular space invasion	15
Isthmic involvement	16
Adnexal involvement	5
Pelvic lymph node metastasis	9
Aortic lymph node metastasis	6
Other extrauterine metastasis	6

Source: adapted from Creasman *et al.* [86].

Prognostic Variables

Although disease stage is the most significant variable affecting survival, a number of other individual prognostic factors for disease recurrence or survival are known.

Age

In general, younger women with endometrial cancer have a better prognosis than older women. Increased risk for recurrence in older patients is related to a higher incidence of grade 3 tumors or unfavorable histologic subtypes; however, increasing patient age has been shown to be independently associated with disease recurrence. In one study, for every 1-year increase in age, the estimated rate of recurrence increased 7% [82].

Histologic Type

Nonendometrioid histologic subtypes carry an increased risk for recurrence and distant spread [83, 84].

Histologic Grade

Histologic grade of the endometrial tumor is strongly associated with prognosis (Table 20.5) [85–87]. In one study, recurrence developed in 7.7% of grade 1 tumors, 10.5% of grade 2 tumors, and 36.1% of grade 3 tumors. Patients with grade 3 tumors were more than five times more likely to have a recurrence than were patients with grades 1 and 2 tumors. The 5-year disease-free survival rates for patients with grades 1 and 2 tumors were 92% and 86%, respectively, compared with 64% for patients with grade 3 tumors [82].

Tumor Size

Tumor size is a significant prognostic factor for lymph node metastasis and survival in patients with endometrial cancer [88, 89]. One report determined tumor size in 142 patients with clinical stage I endometrial cancer and found lymph node metastasis in 4% of patients with tumors 2 cm or smaller, in 15% of patients with tumors larger than 2 cm, and in 35% of patients with tumors involving the entire uterine cavity [90]. Tumor size better defined an intermediate risk group for lymph node metastasis (i.e., with grade 2 tumors with less than 50% myometrial invasion). Overall, these patients had a 10% risk for lymph node metastasis, but there were no nodal metastases associated with tumors 2 cm or smaller, compared with 18% when tumors were larger than 2 cm. Five-year survival rates were 98% for patients with tumors 2 cm or smaller, 84% for patients with tumors larger than 2 cm, and 64% for patients with tumors involving the whole uterine cavity [89, 91].

Hormone Receptor Status

Patients whose carcinomas are positive for estrogen receptor and/or progesterone receptors have longer survival times than patients whose carcinomas lack these receptors. Even patients with metastases have an improved prognosis with receptor-positive tumors [92–94]. Progesterone receptor levels appear to be stronger predictors of survival than estrogen receptor levels, and the higher absolute levels of the receptors the better the prognosis.

Myometrial Invasion

Because access to the lymphatic system increases as cancer invades into the outer one-half of the myometrium, increasing depth of invasion is associated with increasing likelihood of extrauterine spread, including lymph node metastasis and recurrence [87, 95, 96]. Of patients without demonstrable myometrial invasion, only 1% had pelvic lymph node metastasis, compared with patients with outer one-third myometrial invasion of whom 25% had pelvic and 17% had aortic lymph node metastases. Deep myometrial invasion is the strongest predictor of hematogenous recurrence [97]. Patients with noninvasive or superficially invasive tumors have an 80–90% 5-year survival rate, whereas those with deeply invasive tumors have a 60% survival rate [98, 99].

Lymphvascular Space Invasion

Lymphvascular space invasion (LVSI) appears to be an independent risk factor for recurrence and death from all types of endometrial cancer [100, 101]. LVSI was demonstrated to be a strong predictor of lymphatic dissemination and lymphatic recurrence [102]. Another study reported an 83% 5-year survival rate for patients without demonstrable LVSI, compared with a 64.5% survival rate for those in whom LVSI was present [101].

Isthmus and Cervix Extension

The location of the tumor within the uterus is important. Involvement of the uterine isthmus, cervix or both is associated with an increased risk for extrauterine disease, lymph node metastasis, and recurrence. Cervical stromal invasion (stage II) is a strong predictor of lymphatic dissemination and lymphatic recurrence, especially for pelvic lymph nodes [102]. One study reported that if the fundus of the uterus alone was involved with tumor, there was a 13% recurrence rate, whereas if the lower uterine segment or cervix was involved with occult tumor, there was a 44% recurrence rate [84]. A subsequent Gynecological Oncology Group (GOG) study found that tumor involvement of the isthmus or cervix without evidence of extrauterine disease was associated recurrence rate of a 16% and a relative risk of 1.6 [85].

Peritoneal Cytology

Reports regarding the prognostic relevance of positive peritoneal cytology have been inconsistent, due at least in part to differences in use of multivariate analyses. Patients with positive peritoneal cytology as the only site of extrauterine disease (i.e., no adnexal or uterine serosal invasion) and without poor prognosticators (i.e., myometrial invasion more than 50%, nonendometrioid histologic subtype, grade 3, LVSI, cervical invasion) have very favorable outcomes with an absence of extra-abdominal recurrences [103]. These patients have an associated 5-year survival of 98– 100% even when not treated with adjuvant therapy [104–106]. On the other hand, patients with positive cytology in addition to poor prognostic factors demonstrate a high rate (47%) of distant extra-abdominal failure and may potentially benefit from systemic chemotherapy. Positive peritoneal cytology seems to have an adverse effect on survival only if the endometrial cancer has spread to the adnexa, peritoneum, or lymph nodes, not if the disease is otherwise confined to the uterus [105, 107, 108]. These considerations led to the omission of cytology as a factor impacting stage in the FIGO 2009 staging criteria.

Adnexal or Uterine Serosal Involvement (Stage IIIA)

Most patients with stage IIIA disease have other poor prognostic factors that place them at high risk for recurrence. One series described treatment of all patients with serosal or adnexal invasion (or both) with whole-abdomen radiotherapy. Failures were observed outside the abdomen in 100% of patients with full thickness myometrial invasion or uterine serosal invasion, and in 20–25% of cases in the presence of isolated adnexal invasion [85, 109]. These patients may benefit from postoperative systemic chemotherapy.

Lymph Node Metastasis

Lymph node metastasis is a very important prognostic factor in clinical early-stage endometrial cancer. Of patients with clinical stage I disease, about 10% will have pelvic and 6% will have para-aortic lymph node metastases. Patients with lymph node metastases have almost a sixfold higher likelihood of developing recurrent cancer than patients without lymph node metastasis. One study reported a recurrence rate of 48% among patients with positive pelvic nodes, including 45% with positive pelvic nodes and 64% with positive aortic nodes, compared to 8% for patients with negative nodes. The 5-year disease-free survival rate for patients with lymph node metastases was 54% compared to 90% for patients without lymph metastases [104]. The GOG found that 58% of patients with para-aortic lymph node metastasis developed progressive or recurrent cancer, and only 36% of these patients were alive at 5 years, compared to 85% of patients without para-aortic node involvement [110]. One series examined patients with lymph node metastases in addition to other extrauterine sites of disease (vagina, uterine serosa, positive peritoneal cytology, adnexal invasion). The recurrence rates were 67% (41% extranodal) for those with lymphatic dissemination versus 32% (5% extranodal) for those with other sites of extrauterine disease spread [105].

Intraperitoneal Metastases

Extrauterine metastasis, excluding peritoneal cytology and lymph node metastasis, occurs in about 4–6% of patients with clinical stage I endometrial cancer. Gross intraperitoneal spread is highly associated with lymph node metastases; one study noted that 51% of patients with intraperitoneal tumor had positive lymph nodes, whereas only 7% of patients without gross peritoneal spread had positive nodes [86]. Extrauterine spread other than lymph node metastasis is significantly associated with tumor recurrence. Another study found that 50% of patients with extrauterine disease developed recurrence, compared with 11% of patients without extrauterine disease. The 5-year disease-free survival rate for patients with nonlymphatic extrauterine disease was 50%, compared with 88% in other patients [104]. Predictors of peritoneal relapse include stage IV disease, or stage II or III disease with two or more of the following risk factors: cervical invasion, positive peritoneal cytology, positive lymph nodes, and nonendometrioid histology [111].

Surgical Treatment

The most common current protocol for surgical management of endometrial cancer includes peritoneal cytology, hysterectomy, bilateral salpingo-oophorectomy, and surgical staging. In patients with nonendometrioid cancer, omentectomy and peritoneal biopsies may be performed. The need to perform lymph node sampling or lymphadenectomy is based on the type and grade of endometrial cancer, the tumor size and extent of myometrial invasion, and the presence of extrauterine disease determined during the surgery (see Surgical Staging). The decision to administer postoperative radiation, chemotherapy, or both is predicated on the final results of pathologic examination of the surgical specimen and cytology [112] (Figure 20.1).

Vaginal Hysterectomy

Vaginal hysterectomy may be considered for selected patients who are extremely obese and have a poor medical status or for patients with extensive uterovaginal prolapse. Vaginal hysterectomy with bilateral salpingo-oophorectomy may be considered adequate treatment for patients with low-risk tumors (endometrioid histology, grade 1 or 2, <50% myometrial invasion, and tumor diameter <2 cm). Vaginal hysterectomy is particularly suitable for patients who are at low risk for extrauterine spread of disease (i.e., those with clinical stage I, well-differentiated tumors). In one report, a 94% survival rate was observed among 56 patients with clinical stage I (mostly grade 1) endometrial carcinoma treated by vaginal hysterectomy, with or without postoperative radiotherapy (mostly brachytherapy) [113]. Vaginal hysterectomy is preferable to radiation therapy alone, but should be reserved for specific patients.

Minimally Invasive Surgery: Laparoscopic or Robotic

Advances in endoscopic technologies and power sources have allowed application of laparoscopic/robotic approaches to the management of endometrial cancer [114–116]. A large prospective study by GOG randomized patients to laparoscopy versus laparotomy for primary treatment of endometrial cancer [117]. Consistent with early reports, patients randomized to laparoscopy had shorter hospital stays (52% more than 2 days vs 94% in the laparotomy group), less blood loss, and fewer postoperative complications (14% vs 21%). The rate of intraoperative complications was similar, and the operative time was longer in the laparoscopy cohort. There was no difference in lymph node counts, and stage distribution was identical between groups. A follow-up quality-of-life investigation of the same cohorts revealed better physical functioning, better body image, less pain and its interference with quality of life, and an earlier resumption of normal activities and return to work over the 6-week recovery period in the laparoscopic group [118]. Of concern was the 24% rate of conversion in the laparoscopic cohort; only 4% were converted because of advanced disease. Furthermore, the conversion rate increased dramatically with body mass index. This implied a limitation of the surgical technique in obese patients. Recent longitudinal data from this study demonstrated that laparoscopic

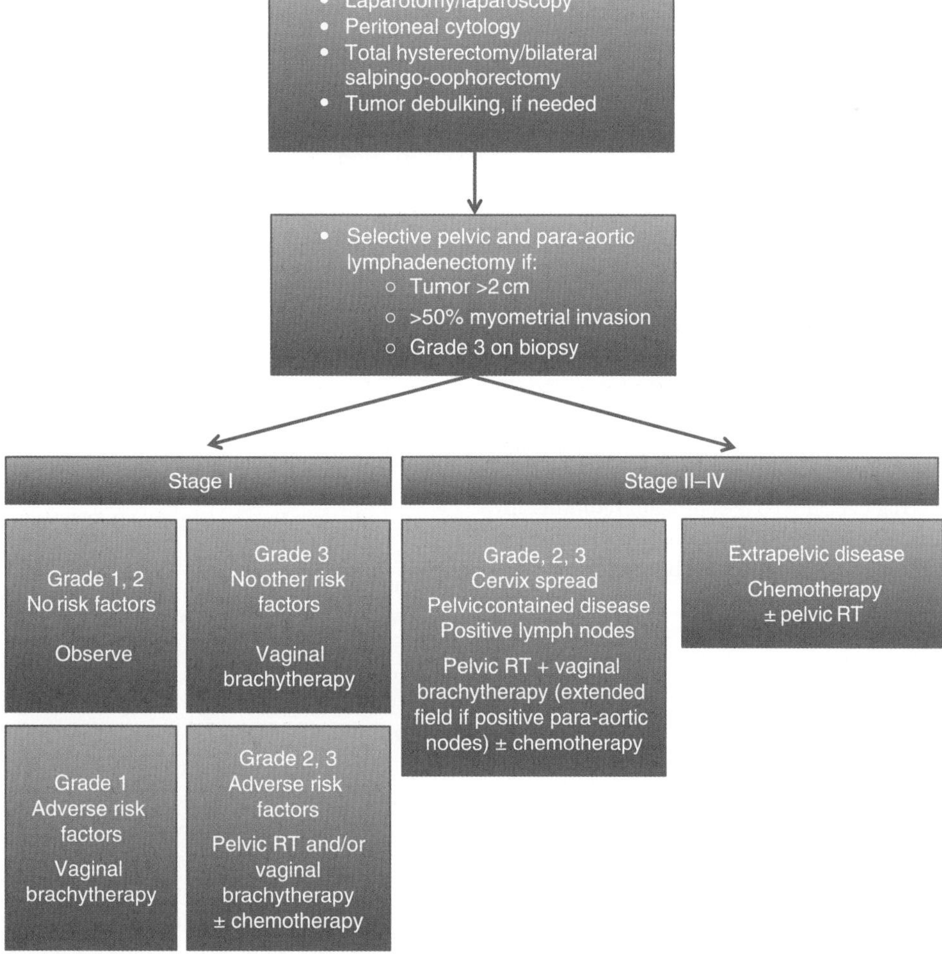

Figure 20.1 Management of patients with endometrial carcinoma. Risk factors: age >60 years, grade 2/3, lymphvascular space invasion, outer half myometrial invasion, histologic subtype serous or clear cell.

staging was associated with a 3-year recurrence rate of 11.4% compared with 10.2% with laparotomy and did not adversely affect overall survival or recurrence patterns [119].

Robotic Surgery

Robotic-assisted surgery has gained popularity for endometrial cancer treatment. Improved instrumentation and visualization allow MIS to be performed by surgeons with less laparoscopic experience, and in patients, particularly obese patients, who otherwise might not be candidates for MIS [120]. In 2010, a systematic review summarized most of the comparative studies on endometrial cancer at that time. The perioperative outcomes were similar for robotic and laparoscopic procedures with decreased blood loss and shorter hospital stays but longer operative times compared with laparotomy. The proportion of MIS cases converted to laparotomy were lower in the robotic group compared with laparoscopy (4.9% vs 9.9%; $P = 0.06$), but all approaches had equivalent rates of cuff dehiscence, vascular complications, and bowel or bladder injuries [121].

Radiation Therapy as Primary Treatment

Primary surgery followed by individualized radiation therapy is the most widely accepted treatment for early-stage endometrial cancers. However, about 5–15% of endometrial cancer patients have severe medical conditions that render them unsuitable for surgery [122]. Several series show that radiotherapy is effective treatment for patients with inoperable endometrial cancer [123–125]. Although radiation alone can produce excellent survival and local control, it should be considered for definitive treatment only if the operative risk is estimated to exceed the 10–15% risk for uterine recurrence that is expected with radiation treatment alone.

Patterns of Metastatic Dissemination: Implications for Postoperative Disease-Based Adjuvant Treatment

Approximately one of every three women who dies of endometrial cancer was considered to have early locoregional disease at primary diagnosis. Most treatment failures and the accompanying compromised longevity probably result from failure to recognize sites of occult extrauterine dissemination at primary diagnosis. Traditional postoperative therapy (modality-based) for high-risk endometrial cancer is external-beam radiotherapy that is frequently supplemented with vaginal brachytherapy [126]. This approach improves local control but not survival in early-stage disease [127–129].

Understanding the different pathways of metastatic dissemination of endometrial cancer and their predictive factors allows the development of an individualized model for target-based therapeutic approaches to the predicted site(s) of failure. The natural history of epithelial corpus cancer includes four potential routes of metastasis: (i) contiguous extension (mainly to the vagina), (ii) hematogenous dissemination, (iii) lymphatic embolization, and (iv) exfoliation with intraperitoneal spread. Independent pathologic risk factors predictive of the four routes of metastatic spread are:

1) Contiguous extension: histologic grade 3 and lymphovascular space invasion are proven predictors of vaginal relapse in stage I endometrial cancer [130].
2) Hematogenous: deep myometrial invasion is the strongest predictor of hematogenous recurrence (>50% for all stages and >66% for stage I) [97, 131].
3) Lymphatic: lymphatic failure (defined in this study as a relapse occurring on the pelvic sidewall, para-aortic area, or other node-bearing area) is more likely to occur when cervical stromal involvement or positive lymph nodes are present at initial surgery [102].
4) Peritoneal: predictors of peritoneal relapse are: (i) stage IV disease or (ii) stage II or III disease with two or more of the following risk factors: cervical invasion, positive peritoneal cytology, lymph node metastasis, and nonendometrioid histology [111].

Patients with the risk factors previously discussed account for 35% of all the overall population with endometrial cancer, but 89% of the observed hematogenous, lymphatic, and peritoneal relapses. Importantly, 46% of the patients considered at risk subsequently experience a recurrence in one or more of the three sites, compared with only 2% of patients not judged to be at risk based on these criteria ($P < 0.001$). The identification of subgroups of patients at risk for the different patterns of recurrence would allow postoperative treatment targeted to the predicted areas of tumor dissemination. Patients at risk for hematogenous or peritoneal recurrence would potentially benefit from systemic cytotoxic treatment, whereas patients at risk for lymphatic or vaginal recurrence would potentially benefit from radiation treatment directed to areas at risk.

Postoperative Treatment

Observation

Patients with grade 1 and 2 lesions, with no or minimal myometrial invasion, and without any of the above risk factors have an excellent prognosis (disease-free 5-year survival rate approaching 100%) and require no postoperative therapy [85, 132, 133].

Vaginal Vault Radiation

Vaginal brachytherapy (VBT) is an attractive alternative to external radiation therapy (ERT). High-dose rate (HDR) VBT is well tolerated with low rates of severe or chronic complications. Vaginal control rates with more convenient, better-tolerated HDR VBT are comparable to control rates with lengthier low-dose rate (LDR) VBT. The standard HDR VBT dosing of 21 Gy to 5 mm depth in three fractions provides local control rates of 98–100% [134, 135]. Retrospective data suggest that the vaginal relapse rate after VBT averages 4–5% and this is similar to the 5-year vaginal failure rate of 3.5% reported among the highest-risk patients who received ERT in PORTEC-1 [129, 132, 133, 136–138].

PORTEC-2 randomized patients with apparent uterine-confined endometrial cancer at high risk for recurrence (>60 years of age with grade 1 or 2, stage IB and grade 3, stage IA; or any age, any grade IIA with <50% myometrial invasion) to pelvic ERT (46 Gy, in 23 fractions) versus VBT (21 Gy in three HDR fractions or 30 Gy LDR, to a depth of 0.5 cm). At 3 years, there was no difference in vaginal failure rates (0.9% for VBT, 2% for pelvic ERT; $P = 0.97$). There was a higher rate of nonvaginal pelvic relapse in the brachytherapy group (3.6%) compared to the ERT group (0.7%). However, the absolute difference was small and there was no difference in overall survival [139]. The difference between nonvaginal pelvic recurrence may be a reflection of unrecognized lymph node metastases at the time of initial surgery treated with ERT. One concern regarding PORTEC-2 is that there was not a surgery-only control in the study. However, the highest risk endometrial cancer subgroup in PORTEC-1 (patients >60 years of age with grade 3 or deeply invasive grade 1 or 2, all stage I) was similar to the cohort included in PORTEC-2 and the locoregional recurrence rate in patients who did not receive adjuvant ERT in PORTEC-1 was 18% [129].

Grade 3 histology and LVSI are proven predictors of vaginal relapse in stage I endometrial cancer. Patients with these risk factors are the most likely group to benefit from VBT [130]. Although vaginal recurrences can be successfully treated and controlled in up to 80% of cases, the addition of VBT to the initial surgical intervention can significantly reduce the risk of such recurrences [140].

External Pelvic Radiation

Radiation therapy traditionally was suggested to patients who were deemed to have an intermediate or high risk of recurrence, according to grade and depth of myometrial invasion. Several retrospective studies and large, randomized trials did not show an overall survival benefit for intermediate- and high-risk patients with stage I endometrial cancer (or occult IIA endometrial cancer according to the 1988 FIGO staging) who received adjuvant pelvic radiotherapy.

The PORTEC trial tested the role of postoperative pelvic radiation therapy for presumed stage I endometrial cancer. Eligibility criteria were stage IB, grades 1 to 2, and stage IA, grades 2 to 3; patients with stage IA, grade 3, were only 10% of the study population, and lymph node biopsies and peritoneal cytology were not required. Local-regional recurrences developed in 14% of the surgery group, compared with 4% of the postoperative pelvic radiation group. The 5-year survival rates were not different between the two groups (85% vs 81%, respectively) [129]. These results were confirmed by GOG99, a prospective, randomized investigation of surgery alone (including lymphadenectomy) versus surgery plus adjuvant pelvic radiation in intermediate-risk endometrial cancer (stages IA to IIB occult). After 2 years, the cumulative recurrence rate was 12% in the group with no postoperative treatment compared with 3% in the group that received pelvic radiation. The pelvic failure rate was 8.9% in the surgery-alone group compared with 1.6% in the postoperative pelvic radiation group. Overall survival rates were not significantly improved, however (92% vs 86%, respectively) [127]. The ASTEC/EN.5 trial provided further confirmation that external-beam radiation therapy in patients at intermediate to high risk of recurrence had no significant effect on overall survival [141].

Postoperative whole-pelvis ERT usually involves the delivery of 4,500–5,040 cGy in 180 cGy daily fractions over 5–6 weeks to a field encompassing the upper one-half of the vagina inferiorly, the lower border of the L4 vertebral body superiorly, and 1 cm lateral to the margins of the bony pelvis. The dose of radiation at the surface of the vaginal apex usually is boosted to 6,000 to 7,000 cGy by a variety of techniques. The most frequently reported side effects are gastrointestinal, usually abdominal cramps and diarrhea, although more serious complications such as bleeding, proctitis, bowel obstruction, and fistula can occur and may require surgical correction. The urinary system may be affected in the form of hematuria, cystitis, or fistula. The overall complication rate ranges from 25 to 40%; and the rate of serious complications requiring surgical intervention is about 1.5–3%.

External-beam pelvic radiation does not appear to impact survival in patients with high-risk stage I endometrial cancer. Patients with extrauterine pelvic disease, including adnexal spread, parametrial involvement, and pelvic lymph node metastases, in the absence of extrapelvic disease, are most likely to benefit from postoperative pelvic radiation.

Extended-Field Radiation

Patients with histologically proven para-aortic node metastases and no other evidence of disease spread outside the pelvis should be treated with extended-field radiation. The entire pelvis, common iliac lymph nodes, and para-aortic lymph nodes are included within the radiation field. The para-aortic radiation dose is limited to 4,500–5,000 cGy. Extended-field radiotherapy appears to improve survival in patients with endometrial cancer who have positive para-aortic lymph nodes [129, 142].

Five-year survival rates of 47% and 43% are reported for patients with surgically confirmed isolated para-aortic lymph node metastases and for those with para-aortic and pelvic lymph node metastases, respectively, using postoperative extended-field radiation. Severe enteric morbidity is uncommon (2%, in one report) [143]. In a GOG study, 37 of 48 patients with positive para-aortic nodes received postoperative para-aortic radiation, 36% of whom remained tumor free at 5 years [85]. A comparison of patients with positive para-aortic nodes treated with megestrol acetate alone versus extended-field radiation showed that survival rate in patients receiving extended-field radiation was significantly better: 53% vs 12.5%, respectively. In another study of 18 patients with positive para-aortic nodes, 5-year survival rates were 67% for those with microscopic nodal disease and 17% with gross nodal disease [144].

Whole-Abdomen Radiation

Whole-abdomen radiation therapy was occasionally used for patients with stage III–IV endometrial cancer or for patients who had stage I–II carcinomas, such as serous, that have a propensity for upper-abdominal recurrence [145–147]. Since the publication of GOG122, demonstrating the superiority of chemotherapy over whole-abdominal radiotherapy in advanced endometrial cancer, the utilization of whole-abdominal radiotherapy in advanced endometrial cancer has been uncommon (see Chemotherapy section) [148].

Progestins

Because most endometrial cancers have both estrogen and progesterone receptors and progestins have been used successfully to treat metastatic endometrial cancer, postoperative adjuvant progestin therapy attempted to reduce the risk of recurrence. This therapy seemed attractive because it provides systemic treatment and has few side effects. Unfortunately, several large randomized, placebo-controlled studies failed to identify a benefit for adjuvant progestin therapy [149, 150].

Chemotherapy

In cases of advanced disease, chemotherapy is now standard treatment. The GOG 122 trial compared whole-abdominal radiotherapy versus systemic chemotherapy in patients with stage III or IV disease who underwent maximal surgical resection of disease to less than 2 cm. Patients who received chemotherapy had a 13% improvement in 2-year progression-free survival (50% vs 46%) and an 11% improvement in overall 2-year survival (70% vs 59%) compared to patients treated with whole-abdomen radiation [148]. However, toxicity was more prevalent with chemotherapy. Despite this improvement with chemotherapy, the proportion of patients with pelvic failure was 18%, suggesting the need for local control. GOG 177 randomized 263 women with advanced or recurrent endometrial cancer to paclitaxel, doxorubicin, and cisplatin (TAP) vs doxorubicin and cisplatin (AP). Despite an increase in toxicity, there was an increase in response rates in patients receiving the three-agent chemotherapy TAP (57% vs 34%, P <0.001) and increased median overall survival (15.3 months for TAP vs 12.3 months for AP, P = 0.037). In a study comparing TAP to the popular two drug regimen, carboplatin and paclitaxel, interim analysis suggested comparable progression-free (14 months vs 14 months, respectively) and overall survival (38 months vs 32 months, respectively) [151, 152].

Other GOG studies and the PORTEC-3 trial are investigating the combination of chemotherapy and radiotherapy in advanced or high-risk endometrial cancer. Results of these trials await maturation. GOG 249 is comparing whole pelvic ERT with or without vaginal cuff boost versus vaginal cuff brachytherapy followed by three cycles of paclitaxel and carboplatin in patients with uterine-confined endometrial cancer at high risk for recurrence. GOG 258 is comparing chemoradiation followed by chemotherapy versus chemotherapy alone in advanced endometrial cancer. PORTEC-3 is investigating overall survival and failure-free survival of patients with high-risk and advanced stage endometrial carcinoma treated after surgery with chemoradiation followed by chemotherapy versus pelvic radiation alone.

Clinical Stage II

Endometrial cancer involving the cervix either contiguously or by lymphatic spread has a poorer prognosis than disease confined to the corpus [153–155]. Preoperative assessment of cervical involvement is difficult. Endocervical curettage has relatively high false-positive (50–80%) and false-negative rates. Histologic proof of cancer infiltration of the cervix or presence of obvious tumor on the cervix is the only reliable method to diagnose cervical involvement, although ultrasonography, hysteroscopy, or MRI may show cervical invasion.

The relatively small number of true stage II cases in reported series and the lack of randomized, prospective studies preclude formulation of a definitive treatment plan. Three areas must be addressed in any treatment plan:

1) For optimal results, the uterus should be removed in all patients.
2) Because the incidence of pelvic lymph node metastases is about 36% in stage II endometrial cancer, any treatment protocol should include treatment of these lymph nodes.
3) Because the incidence of disease spread outside the pelvis to the para-aortic lymph nodes, adnexal structures, and upper abdomen is higher than in stage I disease, attention should be directed to evaluating and treating extrapelvic disease.

Two approaches had been used in the past for treatment of clinical stage II disease:

1) Radical hysterectomy, bilateral salpingo-oophorectomy, and pelvic and para-aortic lymphadenectomy.
2) Combined radiation and surgery (external pelvic radiation and intracavitary radium or cesium followed in 6 weeks by total abdominal hysterectomy and bilateral salpingo-oophorectomy).

The method of management of clinical stage II endometrial cancer that has gained favor is an initial surgical approach followed by radiation. This method is based on the difficulty in establishing the preoperative diagnosis of cervical involvement in the absence of a gross cervical tumor, the evidence that radiation is equally effective when given after hysterectomy, and the high incidence of extrapelvic disease when the cervix is involved. An extrafascial hysterectomy or modified radical hysterectomy, bilateral salpingo-oophorectomy, peritoneal washings for cytology, and resection of grossly enlarged lymph nodes are performed. These procedures are followed by appropriate pelvic or extended-field external and intravaginal radiation, depending on the results of surgical staging. Excellent results are reported using this treatment scheme [69, 156].

Clinical Stages III and IV

Clinical stage III disease accounts for about 7–10% of all endometrial carcinomas [157, 158]. Patients usually have clinical evidence of disease spread to the parametria, pelvic sidewall, or adnexal structures; less frequently, there is spread to the vagina or pelvic peritoneum. Treatment for stage III endometrial carcinoma must be individualized, but initial operative evaluation and treatment should be considered because of the high risk for occult lymph node metastases and intraperitoneal spread when disease is known to extend outside of the uterus into the pelvis. In the presence of an adnexal mass, the initial impetus for surgery is to determine the nature of the mass. Surgery is performed to determine the extent of disease and to remove the bulk of the disease if possible. This procedure should include peritoneal washings for cytologic examination, para-aortic and pelvic lymphadenectomy, biopsy or excision of any suspicious areas within the peritoneal cavity, and omentectomy and peritoneal biopsies. Except in patients with bulky parametrial disease, hysterectomy and bilateral salpingo-oophorectomy should be performed. The goal of surgery is eradication of all macroscopic disease because this finding is one of major prognostic importance in the management of patients with clinical stage III disease. Despite the small number of patients included in the studies examining cytoreduction, it appears that optimal cytoreduction may be associated with improved survival [159]. Postoperative therapy can be tailored to the extent of disease.

Results of therapy depend on the extent and nature of disease. A 5-year survival rate of 54% is reported for all patients with stage III disease; however, the survival is 80% when only adnexal metastases are present, compared with 15% when other extrauterine pelvic structures are involved [160]. Patients with surgical-pathologic stage III disease have a much better survival rate (40–54%) than those with clinical stage III disease (16–36%) [158, 161]. Patients who are treated with combined surgery and radiation fare better than patients who receive radiation therapy alone [158].

Stage IV endometrial adenocarcinoma, in which tumor invades the bladder or rectum or extends outside the pelvis, makes up about 3% of cases [162]. Treatment of stage IV disease is patient dependent but usually involves a combination of surgery, radiation therapy, and systemic hormonal therapy or chemotherapy. One objective of surgery and radiation therapy is to achieve local disease control in the pelvis to provide palliative relief of bleeding, discharge, and complications involving the bladder and rectum. In one report, control of pelvic disease was achieved in 28% patients with stage IV disease treated with radiation alone or in combination with surgery, progestins, or both [163]. Several reports have noted a positive impact of cytoreductive surgery on survival, the median survival being about three times greater with optimal cytoreduction (18–34 months vs 8–11 months, respectively) [163–165]. Pelvic exenteration may be considered in the very rare patient in whom disease is limited to the bladder, rectum, or both [166].

Follow-Up after Treatment

History and physical examination remain the most effective methods of follow-up in patients treated for endometrial cancer [167–169]. Patients should be examined every 3–6 months during the first 2 or 3 years and every 6–12 months thereafter. Physical examination should include a speculum and pelvic examination. Serum CA-125 determinations are considered an optional component of follow-up. Vaginal bleeding is a common symptom consistent with local recurrence; other common symptoms include abdominal and/or pelvic pain, changes in bowel or bladder habits, lethargy, and weight loss. These or related symptoms are reported by 41–83% of patients and more than 80% of recurrences are detected by a combination of physical examination and symptoms. Very few asymptomatic recurrences are detected by vaginal cytology (0–7%) and fewer than 20% of asymptomatic recurrences are detected by annual chest X-ray. Because of the low rates of detection of these screening modalities, many gynecologic oncologists have challenged their use [170]. The most recent National Comprehensive Cancer Network (NCCN) guideline does not specify vaginal cytology and recommends imaging only as clinically indicated. In addition to examinations and tests as surveillance for recurrent disease, the NCCN recommends patient education regarding symptoms of recurrence and health promotion (weight control, nutrition, physical activity, tobacco cessation), and consideration of genetic counseling [69].

Recurrent Disease

About 15% of patients treated for early (stage I–II) endometrial cancer develop recurrent disease [127, 171]. In contrast, recurrent disease is detected in up to 50% of patients with advanced (stage III–IV) endometrial cancer [148]. More than 50% of the recurrences develop within 2 years, and about 75% occur within 3 years of initial treatment. The distribution of recurrences is dependent in large part on the type of primary therapy: surgery alone versus surgery plus local or regional radiotherapy. In a GOG study of 390 patients with surgical stage I disease, vaginal and pelvic recurrences were noted to comprise 53% of all recurrences in the group treated with surgery alone, whereas only 30% of recurrences were vaginal or pelvic in the group treated with combined surgery and radiotherapy. Therefore, after combined surgery and radiotherapy (vaginal or external beam), 70% or more of patients with treatment failures have distant metastases, and most of these patients do not have evidence of local or pelvic recurrence [85]. The most common sites of extrapelvic metastases are lung, abdomen, lymph nodes (aortic, supraclavicular, inguinal), liver, brain, and bone. Patients with isolated vaginal recurrences fare better than those with pelvic recurrences, who in turn have a better chance of cure than those with distant metastases [172]. Patients who initially have well-differentiated tumors or who develop recurrent cancer more than 3 years after the primary therapy also tend to have an improved prognosis.

Hormonal Therapy

Progestins are recommended as initial treatment for all patients with recurrent low-grade endometrioid tumors with hormone receptor-positive tumors. Radiation therapy, surgery or both should be used whenever feasible for treatment of localized recurrent cancer such as vaginal, pelvic, bone, and peripheral lymph node disease; however, these patients should also be given long-term progestin therapy unless they are known to have a progesterone-receptor-negative tumor. Patients with nonlocalized recurrent tumors, especially if progesterone receptors are known to be positive, are candidates for progestin therapy, either megestrol acetate, 80 mg twice daily, or medroxyprogesterone acetate, 50–100 mg three times daily. These commonly used progestins have response rates ranging from 15 to 25% [172]. Higher response rates are observed in patients with well-differentiated tumors and a longer disease-free interval. Progestin therapy should be continued for at least 2–3 months before assessing response. If a response is obtained, the progestin should be continued for as long as the disease is static or in remission. In the presence of a relative contraindication to high-dose progestin therapy (e.g., prior or current thromboembolic disease, severe heart disease, or inability of the patient to tolerate progestin therapy), tamoxifen, 20 mg twice daily, is recommended. Aromatase inhibitors have been used in metastatic or recurrent disease. Failure to respond to hormonal therapy is an indication for initiation of chemotherapy [173].

Radiation Therapy

Radiotherapy is the best treatment option for patients with isolated local-regional recurrences [174, 175]. The best local control and subsequent cure are usually achieved by a combination of ERT followed by VBT boost to deliver a total tumor dose of at least 6,000 cGy. Women with low-volume disease limited to the pelvis (most of which is contained in the vagina) have the best outcome. Retrospective studies showed complete remission rates after salvage therapy for isolated vaginal relapse to be 40–80% in previously unirradiated patients, compared to

10–25% in those who had previously been irradiated [171]. Conversely, for those patients who undergo radiation for pelvic extension of their disease, lower survival rates (0–26%) are reported. Factors associated with improved survival and control of pelvic disease in patients with locally recurrent endometrial cancer include initial low-grade and endometriod histology, younger age at recurrence, recurrent tumor size 2 cm or less, time from initial treatment to recurrence of more than 1 year, vaginal versus pelvic disease, and use of VBT.

Chemotherapy

Chemotherapy with a platinum agent and a taxane has become the standard adjuvant treatment setting for advanced endometrial cancer [152]. Individually, the response rates of platinum agents and paclitaxel range from 20 to 36% [176]. In one retrospective study, the overall response rate to combination carboplatin and paclitaxel in patients with either advanced or recurrent endometrial cancer was 43%, but only 5% achieved a complete response [177]. There are no randomized control trials comparing carboplatin and paclitaxel in the recurrent setting; however, GOG 209 demonstrated carboplatin and paclitaxel to be not inferior to the combination of paclitaxel, doxorubicin, and cisplatin [151]. There are no effective single agents for disease recurrence after treatment with first-line platinum/taxane combinations [172]. Molecularly targeted therapies such as mTOR inhibitors and antiangiogenic agents including bevacizumab are in clinical trials.

Surgery

A small subset of patients with isolated recurrent endometrial cancer may benefit from surgical intervention. A search for distant recurrences prior to treatment is obligatory as such patients are best treated with chemotherapy. In one small series, upper abdominal disease was found at laparotomy in three (37.5%) of eight patients with presumed localized pelvic recurrence. Presence of subclinical extrapelvic metastases was associated with large pelvic tumor size (>2 cm) and elevated serum CA-125 [178]. Isolated vaginal recurrence in patients who have not received prior pelvic radiation is best treated with external radiation plus some type of brachytherapy.

Treatment of patients with pelvic recurrence (generally located on the pelvic sidewall secondary to lymphatic failure) is more complex. Although one study [166] showed no survivors among patients with pelvic recurrences, there is some evidence that a multimodality approach consisting of radiotherapy followed by radical surgical resection and intraoperative radiotherapy may cure some patients, albeit with a higher complication rate [179]. Of 36 patients with isolated central pelvic recurrence who underwent pelvic exenteration for recurrent endometrial carcinoma, 75% died of their cancer within 1 year of operation, and only 14% were alive after 5 years [180].

Estrogen Replacement Therapy after Treatment

Most endometrial cancers are associated with excess estrogen exposure, calling into question the appropriateness of estrogen therapy for women with a history of endometrial cancer following hysterectomy and bilateral salpingo-oophorectomy. Several nonrandomized and cohort retrospective studies have reported that estrogen therapy appears safe with no documented increase in the risk of recurrence following surgical treatment for endometrial carcinoma [181–183]. However, these are small retrospective nonrandomized studies. Some investigations reported higher intercurrent death rates, such as from myocardial infarction, in the group in which estrogen was withheld [181, 184]. A randomized, double-blind, placebo-controlled study designed to determine whether estrogen therapy increased rates of disease recurrence in women with stage I or II endometrial cancer closed early because of a fall-off in accrual after the findings of the Women's Health Initiative were made public in 2002. Although the safety of estrogen therapy in patients with endometrial cancer was not verified with level 1 evidence, this investigation provided sufficient reassurance to justify the practice of offering estrogen therapy to patients with low-grade, FIGO 2009 stage IA disease in the absence of other contraindications. The American College of Obstetricians and Gynecologists issued a committee opinion recommending that providers should take into consideration prognostic indicators, such as depth of invasion, grade, and stage when deciding to administer estrogen therapy to these patients [185]. Similarly, the NCCN guideline also considers estrogen as a reasonable option for symptomatic women with low risk of recurrence, but notes the importance of individualizing decisions after detailed discussion with the patient [69]. For women who decline systemic estrogen therapy, symptoms of vaginal dryness and dyspareunia may be judiciously treated with topical estrogen alone. Symptomatic relief of hot flashes can be achieved by prescribing progestins or nonhormonal agents such as clonidine and venlafaxine.

Uterine Sarcoma

Uterine sarcomas constitute approximately 7.7% of uterine malignancies [3, 186]. There is an increased incidence of uterine sarcomas after radiation therapy to the pelvis for either carcinoma of the cervix or a benign condition. The relative risk of uterine sarcoma after pelvic radiotherapy is estimated to be 5.38, with an interval of 10–20 years [186]. Uterine sarcomas are, in general, the most malignant group of uterine tumors and differ from endometrial cancer with regard to diagnosis, clinical behavior, pattern of spread, and management.

Classification and Staging

The two most common histologic types of uterine sarcoma are leiomyosarcoma (1.9% of uterine corpus cancers) and endometrial stromal sarcoma (1.3% of uterine corpus cancers). Less common types, such as "uterine tumor resembling ovarian sex cord tumor" are included in the WHO classification but are not discussed in this chapter [187]. Carcinosarcoma, also known as malignant mixed mullerian tumor or MMMT, have been classified as sarcomas in the past but are a distinct category (separate from carcinomas and sarcomas) in the current WHO classification, and are currently thought to represent high-grade carcinomas with mesenchymal metaplasia [67, 68].

Staging of uterine sarcomas is based on the FIGO system [188, 189].

Endometrial Stromal Tumors

Stromal tumors occur primarily in perimenopausal and postmenopausal women. There is no apparent relationship to parity, associated disease, or prior pelvic radiotherapy. The most frequent symptom is abnormal uterine bleeding; abdominal pain and pressure caused by an enlarging pelvic mass occur less often, and some patients do not have symptoms. Pelvic examination usually reveals regular or irregular uterine enlargement, sometimes associated with rubbery parametrial induration. The diagnosis may be determined by endometrial biopsy, but the usual preoperative diagnosis is uterine leiomyoma.

Endometrial stromal tumors are composed of cells with morphological and histochemical features resembling normal endometrial stroma. They are divided into three types: endometrial stromal nodule, low-grade endometrial stromal sarcoma, and high-grade endometrial stromal sarcoma. Additionally, undifferentiated uterine sarcoma is grouped in the same category as endometrial stromal sarcomas [18, 68].

Endometrial stromal nodule is an expansile, noninfiltrating, solitary lesion confined to the uterus with well-circumscribed or minimally irregular margins, no lymphatic or vascular invasion, and usually less than five mitotic figures per 10 high-power microscopic fields (5 MF/10 HPF). These tumors should be considered benign because there are no recurrences or tumor-associated deaths reported after surgery [190, 191].

Low-grade endometrial stromal sarcoma is distinguished from high-grade endometrial stromal sarcoma (and with undifferentiated uterine sarcoma) microscopically by mitotic rates of less than 10 MF/10 HPF and more protracted clinical course. The distinction between an endometrial stromal nodule and low-grade endometrial stromal sarcoma is based on prominent myometrial, lymphatic, and in some cases venous invasion. These sarcomas display slight nuclear atypia or little or no necrosis. Recurrences typically occur late, and local recurrence is more common than distant metastases [192, 193].

Optimum initial therapy for patients with low-grade endometrial stromal sarcoma consists of surgical excision of all grossly detectable tumor. Total hysterectomy should be performed. The fallopian tubes and ovaries should usually be removed as well because of the propensity for tumor extension into the parametria, broad ligaments, and adnexal structures and the possible stimulating effect of estrogen on tumor cells if the ovaries are retained. The relatively low rate of lymph node metastasis in the absences of gross lymph node involvement or extrauterine disease suggests that a lymph node sampling or lymphadenectomy is not necessary [194]. Postoperative pelvic radiation is recommended for inadequately excised or locally recurrent pelvic disease. Recurrence occurs in almost 50% of cases at an average interval of 5 years after initial therapy. Owing to the indolent nature of the disease, cytotoxic chemotherapy is unlikely to be beneficial; however, hormonal treatment with progestins appears to have some efficacy, with reported response rates close to 50%. Prolonged survival and cure are common even after development of recurrent or metastatic disease. Five-year overall survival may exceed 90% [195].

High-grade endometrial stromal sarcoma and undifferentiated uterine sarcoma are highly malignant neoplasms although prognosis is poorer for the latter. Histologically, both exhibit greater than 10 MF/10 HPF, foci of necrosis, significant cytological pleomorphism, and prominent myometrial and lymphatic invasion. Undifferentiated uterine sarcomas, by definition, lack recognizable morphological or immunohistochemical evidence of smooth muscle differentiation or endometrial stromal differentiation [68]. This tumor has a much more aggressive clinical course and poorer prognosis than low-grade endometrial stromal sarcoma [187, 191–193]. The 5-year disease-free survival is about 25%. Treatment of high-grade endometrial stromal sarcoma and undifferentiated uterine sarcoma should consist of total hysterectomy and bilateral salpingo-oophorectomy. The poor therapeutic results suggest that radiation therapy, chemotherapy, or both should be used in combination with surgery. These tumors, unlike low-grade endometrial stromal sarcoma, are not responsive to progestin therapy.

Leiomoyosarcoma

The median age for women with leiomyosarcoma is 43–53 years, and premenopausal women have a better chance of survival. This malignancy has no relationship with parity, and the incidence of associated disease is not as high as in carcinosarcoma or endometrial adenocarcinoma. African American women have a higher incidence and a poorer prognosis than women of other races. A history of prior pelvic radiation therapy can be elicited in about 4% of patients with leiomyosarcoma. The incidence of sarcomatous change in benign uterine leiomyomas is reported to be between 0.13 and 0.81%. Survival rates for patients with uterine leiomyosarcoma range from 20 to 63% (mean 47%) [3, 196–198].

Presenting symptoms, which are of short duration (mean 6 months) and not specific to the disease, include vaginal bleeding, pelvic pain or pressure, and awareness of an abdominopelvic mass. The principal finding is the presence of a pelvic mass. The diagnosis should be suspected if severe pelvic pain accompanies a pelvic tumor, especially in a postmenopausal woman. Endometrial biopsy, although not as useful as in other sarcomas, may establish the diagnosis in as many as one-third of cases when the lesion is submucosal.

The number of mitosis in the uterine smooth muscle tumors traditionally was considered the most reliable microscopic indicator of malignant behavior. Tumors with less than 5 MF/10 HPF behave in a benign fashion, and tumors with more than 10 MF/10 HPF are frankly malignant with a poor prognosis. Tumors with 5–10 MF/10 HPF, termed smooth muscle tumors of uncertain malignant potential (STUMP), are less predictable. In addition to a mitotic index greater than 10, other histologic indicators used to classify uterine smooth muscle tumors as malignant are severe cytologic atypia, infiltrating borders, and coagulative tumor necrosis. However, assessment of uterine smooth muscle neoplasms based on a single risk factor can be misleading, and the totality of histological and clinical features should be considered. For example, symplastic leiomyomas typically have prominent nuclear atypia but are clinically benign. Conversely, the deceptively low mitotic rate and minimal nuclear atypia of epithelioid leiomyosarcomas and myxoid leiomyosarcomas is discordant with their malignant behavior [68, 199]. Gross presentation of the tumor at the time of surgery is an important unfavorable prognostic indicator. Tumors with infiltrating tumor margins or extension beyond the uterus are associated with poor prognosis, whereas tumors less than 5 cm, originating within leiomyomas, or with pushing margins are associated with prolonged survival.

The pattern of tumor spread is to the myometrium, pelvic blood vessels and lymphatics, contiguous pelvic structures, abdomen and then distantly, most often the lungs. The recommended treatment is total hysterectomy; bilateral salpingo-oophorectomy is recommended in postmenopausal women and in women with gross extrauterine disease. Preservation of ovaries does not increase risk of recurrence. Retroperitoneal disease and lymphatic disease spread is rare in women with early-stage disease; therefore, routine lymphadenectomy or lymph node sampling is not recommended except with grossly involved nodes or other extrauterine disease [68, 194].

Adjuvant chemotherapy is indicated in patients with advanced leiomyosarcoma. In a phase III trial that included women with uterine leiomyosarcoma, carcinosarcoma, or other uterine sarcoma, doxorubicin 60 mg/m^2 was compared with doxorubicin plus the addition of dacarbazine (DTIC), achieving an objective response in 16% of all women enrolled, with a response of 25% among those with uterine leiomyosarcoma [200]. Ifosfamide as a single-agent for the treatment of leiomyosarcoma demonstrated a 17.2% response rate in a phase II trial [201]. Combining ifosfamide with doxorubicin achieved an objective response of 30% in advanced leiomyosarcoma; the incidence of grade 3 or 4 neutropenia was 48% [202]. Gemcitabine combined with docetaxel for treatment of metastatic leiomyosarcoma yielded an overall response rate of 53%, including patients previously treated with doxorubicin [203]. Median time to progression was 5.6 months. Despite the high recurrence rate (50–70%) in early-stage uterine leiomyosarcoma that has been treated surgically, there is limited experimental data to suggest adjuvant postoperative chemotherapy or radiation affects overall survival; therefore, GOG is conducting a trial of gemcitabine/docetaxel followed by doxorubicin versus observation.

References

1 Torre LA, Bray F, Siegel RL, *et al.* Global cancer statistics, 2012. *CA Cancer J Clin* 2015;65(2):87–108.
2 Siegel RL, Miller KD, Jemal A. Cancer statistics, 2017. *CA Cancer J Clin* 2017;67(1):7–30.
3 Ries LAG, Young JL, Keel GE, *et al.* (eds) SEER Survival Monograph: Cancer Survival Among Adults: U.S. SEER Program, 1988–2001, Patient and Tumor Characteristics. National Cancer Institute, SEER Program, NIH Pub. No. 07-6215, Bethesda, MD, 2007.
4 Bokhman, JV. Two pathogenetic types of endometrial carcinoma. *Gynecol Oncol* 1983;15(1):10–7.
5 Setiawan VW, *et al.* Type I and II endometrial cancers: have they different risk factors? *J Clin Oncol* 2013;31(20):2607–18.
6 Yang HP, *et al.* Endometrial cancer risk factors by 2 main histologic subtypes: the NIH-AARP Diet and Health Study. *Am J Epidemiol* 2013;177(2):142–51.
7 Yeramian A, *et al.* Endometrial carcinoma: molecular alterations involved in tumor development and progression. *Oncogene* 2013;32(4):403–13.
8 Prat J, *et al.* Endometrial carcinoma: pathology and genetics. *Pathology* 2007;39(1):72–87.
9 Prat J. Pathology of cancers of the female genital tract. *Int J Gynecol Obstet* 2015;131:S132–45
10 MacMahon B. Risk factors for endometrial cancer. *Gynecol Oncol* 1974;2(2–3):122–9.
11 Siegel R, *et al.* Cancer statistics, 2011: the impact of eliminating socioeconomic and racial disparities on premature cancer deaths. *CA Cancer J Clin* 2011;61(4): 212–36.
12 Kurman RJ, Kaminski PF, Norris HJ. The behavior of endometrial hyperplasia. A long-term study of "untreated" hyperplasia in 170 patients. *Cancer* 1985;56(2):403–12.
13 Bonadona V, *et al.* Cancer risks associated with germline mutations in MLH1, MSH2, and MSH6 genes in Lynch syndrome. *JAMA* 2011;305(22):2304–10.
14 Beral V, *et al.* Endometrial cancer and hormone-replacement therapy in the Million Women Study. *Lancet* 2005;365 (9470):1543–51.
15 Parazzini F, *et al.* The epidemiology of endometrial cancer. *Gynecol Oncol* 1991;41(1):1–16.
16 Parazzini F, *et al.* Reproductive factors and risk of endometrial cancer. *Am J Obstet Gynecol* 1991;164(2):522–7.
17 Norris HJ, Tavassoli FA, Kurman RJ. Endometrial hyperplasia and carcinoma. *Diagnostic considerations. Am J Surg Pathol* 1983;7(8):839–47.
18 Kurman RJ, Carcangiu ML, Herrington CS, Young RH (eds) *WHO Classification of Tumours of Female Reproductive Organs.* Lyon: IARC, 2014.
19 Trimble CL, *et al.* Concurrent endometrial carcinoma in women with a biopsy diagnosis of atypical endometrial hyperplasia: a Gynecologic Oncology Group study. *Cancer* 2006;106(4):812–9.
20 Ota T, *et al.* Clinicopathologic study of uterine endometrial carcinoma in young women aged 40 years and younger. *Int J Gynecol Cancer* 2005;15(4):657–62.
21 Randall TC, Kurman RJ. Progestin treatment of atypical hyperplasia and well-differentiated carcinoma of the endometrium in women under age 40. *Obstet Gynecol* 1997;90(3):434–40.
22 Huang SY, *et al.* Ovarian metastasis in a nulliparous woman with endometrial adenocarcinoma failing conservative hormonal treatment. *Gynecol Oncol* 2005;97(2):652–5.
23 Sams SB, Currens HS, Raab SS. Liquid-based Papanicolaou tests in endometrial carcinoma diagnosis. Performance, error root cause analysis, and quality improvement. *Am J Clin Pathol* 2012;137(2):248–54.
24 Smith RA, *et al.* Cancer screening in the United States, 2016: A review of current American Cancer Society guidelines and current issues in cancer screening. CA: a cancer journal for clinicians. 2016. *CA Cancer J Clin* 2016;66(2):95–114.

25 National Cancer Institute. Endometrial Cancer Screening (PDQ®)–Health Professional Version. Updated: March 4, 2016, https://www.cancer.gov/types/uterine/hp/endometrial-screening-pdq (accessed 24 October 2016).
26 Vasen HF, *et al.* Revised guidelines for the clinical management of Lynch syndrome (HNPCC): recommendations by a group of European experts. *Gut* 2013;62(6):812–23.
27 Lynch HT, de la Chapelle A. Hereditary colorectal cancer. *N Engl J Med* 2003;348(10):919–32.
28 Parc YR, *et al.* Microsatellite instability and hMLH1/hMSH2 expression in young endometrial carcinoma patients: associations with family history and histopathology. *Int J Cancer* 2000;86(1):60–6.
29 Resnick KE, *et al.* Current and emerging trends in Lynch syndrome identification in women with endometrial cancer. *Gynecol Oncol* 2009;114(1):128–34.
30 Leenen CH, *et al.* Prospective evaluation of molecular screening for Lynch syndrome in patients with endometrial cancer </= 70 years. *Gynecol Oncol* 2012;125(2):414–20.
31 Aarnio M. Clinicopathological features and management of cancers in lynch syndrome. *Patholog Res Int* 2012;2012:350309.
32 Barrow E, Hill J, Evans DG. Cancer risk in Lynch Syndrome. *Fam Cancer* 2013;12(2):229–40.
33 Renkonen-Sinisalo L, *et al.* Surveillance for endometrial cancer in hereditary nonpolyposis colorectal cancer syndrome. *Int J Cancer* 2007;120(4):821–4.
34 Schmeler KM, *et al.* Prophylactic surgery to reduce the risk of gynecologic cancers in the Lynch syndrome. *N Engl J Med* 2006;354(3):261–9.
35 Lindor NM, *et al.* Recommendations for the care of individuals with an inherited predisposition to Lynch syndrome: a systematic review. *JAMA* 2006;296(12):1507–17.
36 Vasen HF, *et al.* Guidelines for the clinical management of Lynch syndrome (hereditary non-polyposis cancer). *J Med Genet* 2007:44(6);353–62.
37 Kimura T, *et al.* Abnormal uterine bleeding and prognosis of endometrial cancer. *Int J Gynaecol Obstet* 2004:85(2);145–50.
38 Seebacher V, *et al.* The presence of postmenopausal bleeding as prognostic parameter in patients with endometrial cancer: a retrospective multi-center study. *BMC Cancer* 2009;9:460.
39 Smith M, McCartney AJ. Occult, high-risk endometrial cancer. *Gynecol Oncol* 1985;22(2):154–61.
40 Barak F, *et al.* The influence of early diagnosis of endometrioid endometrial cancer on disease stage and survival. *Arch Gynecol Obstet* 2013;288(6):1361–4.
41 DuBeshter B, *et al.* Endometrial carcinoma: the relevance of cervical cytology. *Obstet Gynecol* 1991;77(3):458–62.
42 Choo YC, *et al.* Postmenopausal uterine bleeding of nonorganic cause. *Obstet Gynecol* 1985;66(2):225–8.
43 Pacheco JC, Kempers RD. Etiology of postmenopausal bleeding. *Obstet Gynecol* 1968;32(1):40–6.
44 Fortier KJ. Postmenopausal bleeding and the endometrium. *Clin Obstet Gynecol* 1986;29(2):440–5.
45 Chambers JT, Chambers SK. Endometrial sampling: when? where? why? with what? *Clin Obstet Gynecol* 1992;35(1):28–39.
46 Dreisler E, *et al.* EMAS clinical guide: assessment of the endometrium in peri and postmenopausal women. *Maturitas* 2013;75(2):181–90.
47 Mitchell H, Giles G, Medley G. Accuracy and survival benefit of cytological prediction of endometrial carcinoma on routine cervical smears. *Int J Gynecol Pathol* 1993;12(1):34–40.
48 Stelmachow J. The role of hysteroscopy in gynecologic oncology. *Gynecol Oncol* 1982;14(3):392–5.
49 Gimpelson RJ, Rappold HO. A comparative study between panoramic hysteroscopy with directed biopsies and dilatation and curettage. A review of 276 cases. *Am J Obstet Gynecol* 1988;158(3):489–92.
50 Clark TJ, *et al.* Evaluation of outpatient hysteroscopy and ultrasonography in the diagnosis of endometrial disease. *Obstet Gynecol* 2002;99(6):1001–7.
51 Tabor A, Watt HC, Wald NJ. Endometrial thickness as a test for endometrial cancer in women with postmenopausal vaginal bleeding. *Obstet Gynecol* 2002;99(4):663–70.
52 Smith-Bindman R, *et al.* Endovaginal ultrasound to exclude endometrial cancer and other endometrial abnormalities. *JAMA* 1998;280(17):1510–7.
53 Timmermans A, *et al.* Endometrial thickness measurement for detecting endometrial cancer in women with postmenopausal bleeding: a systematic review and meta-analysis. *Obstet Gynecol* 2010;116(1):160–7.
54 National Cancer Institute. Endometrial Cancer Treatment (PDQ®). Health Professional Version. https://www.cancer.gov/types/uterine/hp/endometrial-treatment-pdq#section/_9 (accessed 15 December 2017).
55 Ross JC, *et al.* Primary mucinous adenocarcinoma of the endometrium. A clinicopathologic and histochemical study. *Am J Surg Pathol* 1983;7(8):715–29.
56 Jalloul RJ, *et al.* Mucinous adenocarcinoma of the endometrium: case series and review of the literature. *Int J Gynecol Cancer* 2012;22(5):812–8.
57 Melhem MF, Tobon H. Mucinous adenocarcinoma of the endometrium: a clinico-pathological review of 18 cases. *Int J Gynecol Pathol* 1987;6(4):347–55.
58 Hendrickson M, *et al.* Uterine papillary serous carcinoma: a highly malignant form of endometrial adenocarcinoma. *Am J Surg Pathol* 1982;6(2):93–108.
59 del Carmen MG, Birrer M, Schorge JO. Uterine papillary serous cancer: a review of the literature. *Gynecol Oncol* 2012;127(3):651–61.
60 Fader AN, *et al.* An updated clinicopathologic study of early-stage uterine papillary serous carcinoma (UPSC). *Gynecol Oncol* 2009;115(2):244–8.
61 Goff BA, *et al.* Uterine papillary serous carcinoma: patterns of metastatic spread. *Gynecol Oncol* 1994;54(3):264–8.
62 Slomovitz BM, *et al.* Uterine papillary serous carcinoma (UPSC): a single institution review of 129 cases. *Gynecol Oncol* 2003;91(3):463–9.
63 Christopherson WM, Alberhasky RC, Connelly PJ. Carcinoma of the endometrium: I. A clinicopathologic study of clear-cell carcinoma and secretory carcinoma. *Cancer* 1982;49(8):1511–23.
64 Abeler VM, Kjorstad KE. Clear cell carcinoma of the endometrium: a histopathological and clinical study of 97 cases. *Gynecol Oncol* 1991;40(3):207–17.
65 Abeler VM, *et al.* Clear cell carcinoma of the endometrium. Prognosis and metastatic pattern. *Cancer* 1996;78(8):1740–7.

66 Abeler V, Kjorstad KE. Endometrial squamous cell carcinoma: report of three cases and review of the literature. *Gynecol Oncol* 1990;36(3):321–6.
67 McCluggage WG. A practical approach to the diagnosis of mixed epithelial and mesenchymal tumours of the uterus. *Mod Pathol* 2016;29:S78–91.
68 Prat J, Mbatani N. Uterine sarcomas. *Int J Gynecol Obst* 2015;131:S105–10.
69 National Comprehensive Cancer Network. Endometrial Carcinoma. Version 2.2016. www.nccn.org. (accessed 18 October 2016).
70 Clement PB, Scully RE. Mullerian adenosarcoma of the uterus: a clinicopathologic analysis of 100 cases with a review of the literature. *Hum Pathol* 1990;21(4):363–81.
71 Kline RC, *et al.* Endometrioid carcinoma of the ovary: retrospective review of 145 cases. *Gynecol Oncol* 1990;39(3):337–46.
72 Prat J, Matias-Guiu X, Barreto J. Simultaneous carcinoma involving the endometrium and the ovary. A clinicopathologic, immunohistochemical, and DNA flow cytometric study of 18 cases. *Cancer* 1991;68(11):2455–9.
73 Zerbe MJ, *et al.* Inability of preoperative computed tomography scans to accurately predict the extent of myometrial invasion and extracorporal spread in endometrial cancer. *Gynecol Oncol* 2000;78(1):67–70.
74 Gordon AN, *et al.* Preoperative assessment of myometrial invasion of endometrial adenocarcinoma by sonography (US) and magnetic resonance imaging (MRI). *Gynecol Oncol* 1989;34(2):175–9.
75 Niloff JM, *et al.* Elevation of serum CA125 in carcinomas of the fallopian tube, endometrium, and endocervix. *Am J Obstet Gynecol* 1984;148(8):1057–8.
76 Dotters DJ. Preoperative CA 125 in endometrial cancer: is it useful? *Am J Obstet Gynecol* 2000;182(6):1328–34.
77 Jhang H, *et al.* CA 125 levels in the preoperative assessment of advanced-stage uterine cancer. *Am J Obstet Gynecol* 2003;188(5):1195–7.
78 Nicklin J, *et al.* The utility of serum CA-125 in predicting extra-uterine disease in apparent early-stage endometrial cancer. *Int J Cancer* 2012;131(4):885–90.
79 Classification and staging of malignant tumours in the female pelvis. Acta Obstet Gynecol Scand 1971;50(1): 1–7.
80 Mutch DG. The New FIGO staging system for cancers of the vulva, cervix, endometrium, and sarcomas. *Gynecol Oncol* 2009;115:325–8.
81 Creasman WT, *et al.* Carcinoma of the corpus uteri. FIGO 26th Annual Report on the Results of Treatment in Gynecological Cancer. *Int J Gynaecol Obstet* 2006:95(Suppl 1):S105–43.
82 Lurain JR, *et al.* Prognostic factors associated with recurrence in clinical stage I adenocarcinoma of the endometrium. *Obstet Gynecol* 1991;78(1):63–9.
83 Wilson TO, *et al.* Evaluation of unfavorable histologic subtypes in endometrial adenocarcinoma. *Am J Obstet Gynecol* 1990;162(2):418–23; discussion 423–6.
84 Fanning J, *et al.* Endometrial adenocarcinoma histologic subtypes: clinical and pathologic profile. *Gynecol Oncol* 1989;32(3):288–91.
85 Morrow CP, *et al.* Relationship between surgical-pathological risk factors and outcome in clinical stage I and II carcinoma of the endometrium: a Gynecologic Oncology Group study. *Gynecol Oncol* 1991;40(1):55–65.
86 Creasman WT, *et al.* Surgical pathologic spread patterns of endometrial cancer. *A Gynecologic Oncology Group Study. Cancer* 1987;60(8 Suppl):2035–41.
87 Sutton GP, *et al.* Features associated with survival and disease-free survival in early endometrial cancer. *Am J Obstet Gynecol* 1989;160(6):1385–91; discussion 1391–3.
88 Schink JC, *et al.* Tumor size in endometrial cancer: a prognostic factor for lymph node metastasis. *Obstet Gynecol* 1987;70(2):216–9.
89 Schink JC, *et al.* Tumor size in endometrial cancer. *Cancer* 1991;67(11):2791–4.
90 Aalders J, *et al.* Postoperative external irradiation and prognostic parameters in stage I endometrial carcinoma: clinical and histopathologic study of 540 patients. *Obstet Gynecol* 1980;56(4):419–27.
91 Mariani A, *et al.* Low-risk corpus cancer: is lymphadenectomy or radiotherapy necessary? *Am J Obstet Gynecol* 2000;182(6):1506–19.
92 Martin JD, *et al.* The effect of estrogen receptor status on survival in patients with endometrial cancer. *Am J Obstet Gynecol* 1983;147(3):322–4.
93 Creasman WT, *et al.* Influence of cytoplasmic steroid receptor content on prognosis of early stage endometrial carcinoma. *Am J Obstet Gynecol* 1985;151(7):922–32.
94 Liao BS, *et al.* Cytoplasmic estrogen and progesterone receptors as prognostic parameters in primary endometrial carcinoma. *Obstet Gynecol* 1986;67(4):463–7.
95 Boronow RC, *et al.* Surgical staging in endometrial cancer: clinical-pathologic findings of a prospective study. *Obstet Gynecol* 1984;63(6):825–32.
96 Rotman M, *et al.* Endometrial carcinoma. Influence of prognostic factors on radiation management. *Cancer* 1993;71(4 Suppl):1471–9.
97 Mariani A, *et al.* Hematogenous dissemination in corpus cancer. *Gynecol Oncol* 2001;80(2):233–8.
98 Lutz MH, *et al.* Endometrial carcinoma: a new method of classification of therapeutic and prognostic significance. *Gynecol Oncol* 1978;6(1):83–94.
99 Kaku T, *et al.* Reassessment of myometrial invasion in endometrial carcinoma. *Obstet Gynecol* 1994;84(6):979–82.
100 Hanson MB, *et al.* The prognostic significance of lymph-vascular space invasion in stage I endometrial cancer. *Cancer* 1985;55(8):1753–7.
101 Abeler, VM, Kjorstad KE, Berle E. Carcinoma of the endometrium in Norway: a histopathological and prognostic survey of a total population. *Int J Gynecol Cancer* 1992;2(1):9–22.
102 Mariani A, *et al.* Predictors of lymphatic failure in endometrial cancer. *Gynecol Oncol* 2002;84(3):437–42.
103 Mariani A, *et al.* Stage IIIC endometrioid corpus cancer includes distinct subgroups. *Gynecol Oncol* 2002;87(1): 112–7.
104 Zaino RJ, *et al.* Pathologic models to predict outcome for women with endometrial adenocarcinoma: the importance of the distinction between surgical stage and clinical stage—a

Gynecologic Oncology Group study. *Cancer* 1996;77(6):1115–21.
105 Takeshima N, *et al.* Positive peritoneal cytology in endometrial cancer: enhancement of other prognostic indicators. *Gynecol Oncol* 2001;82(3):470–3.
106 Ebina Y, *et al.* Peritoneal cytology and its prognostic value in endometrial carcinoma. *Int Surg* 1997;82(3):244–8.
107 Kadar N, Homesley HD, Malfetano JH. Positive peritoneal cytology is an adverse factor in endometrial carcinoma only if there is other evidence of extrauterine disease. *Gynecol Oncol* 1992;46(2):145–9.
108 Milosevic MF, Dembo AJ, Thomas GM. The clinical significance of malignant peritoneal cytology in stage I endometrial carcinoma. *Int J Gynecol Cancer* 1992;2(5):225–35.
109 Mariani A, *et al.* Assessment of prognostic factors in stage IIIA endometrial cancer. *Gynecol Oncol* 2002;86(1):38–44.
110 Moore DH, *et al.* Morbidity of lymph node sampling in cancers of the uterine corpus and cervix. *Obstet Gynecol* 1989;74(2):180–4.
111 Mariani A, *et al.* Endometrial cancer: predictors of peritoneal failure. *Gynecol Oncol* 2003;89(2):236–42.
112 Mariani A, *et al.* High-risk endometrial cancer subgroups: candidates for target-based adjuvant therapy. *Gynecol Oncol* 2004;95(1):120–6.
113 Peters WA, 3rd, *et al.* The selective use of vaginal hysterectomy in the management of adenocarcinoma of the endometrium. *Am J Obstet Gynecol* 1983;146(3):285–9.
114 Eltabbakh GH, *et al.* Laparoscopy as the primary modality for the treatment of women with endometrial carcinoma. *Cancer* 2001;91(2):378–87.
115 Obermair A, *et al.* Total laparoscopic hysterectomy for endometrial cancer: patterns of recurrence and survival. *Gynecol Oncol* 2004;92(3):789–93.
116 Malur S, *et al.* Laparoscopic-assisted vaginal versus abdominal surgery in patients with endometrial cancer—a prospective randomized trial. *Gynecol Oncol* 2001;80(2):239–44.
117 Walker JL, *et al.* Laparoscopy compared with laparotomy for comprehensive surgical staging of uterine cancer: Gynecologic Oncology Group Study LAP2. *J Clin Oncol* 2009;27(32):5331–6.
118 Kornblith AB, *et al.* Quality of life of patients with endometrial cancer undergoing laparoscopic international federation of gynecology and obstetrics staging compared with laparotomy: a Gynecologic Oncology Group study. *J Clin Oncol* 2009;27(32):5337–42.
119 Walker JL, *et al.* Recurrence and survival after random assignment to laparoscopy versus laparotomy for comprehensive surgical staging of uterine cancer: Gynecologic Oncology Group LAP2 Study. *J Clin Oncol* 2012;30(7):695–700.
120 Krill LS, Bristow RE. Robotic surgery: gynecologic oncology. *Cancer J* 2013;19(2):167–76.
121 Gaia G, *et al.* Robotic-assisted hysterectomy for endometrial cancer compared with traditional laparoscopic and laparotomy approaches: a systematic review. *Obstet Gynecol* 2010;116(6):1422–31.
122 Marziale P, *et al.* 426 cases of stage I endometrial carcinoma: a clinicopathological analysis. *Gynecol Oncol* 1989; 32(3):278–81.
123 Abayomi O, *et al.* Treatment of endometrial carcinoma with radiation therapy alone. *Cancer* 1982;49(12):2466–9.
124 Jones DA, Stout R. Results of intracavitary radium treatment for adenocarcinoma of the body of the uterus. *Clin Radiol* 1986;37(2):169–71.
125 Wang ML, *et al.* Inoperable adenocarcinoma of endometrium: radiation therapy. *Radiology* 1987; 165(2):561–5.
126 Podczaski ES, *et al.* Stage II endometrial carcinoma treated with external-beam radiotherapy, intracavitary application of cesium, and surgery. *Gynecol Oncol* 1989;35(2):251–4.
127 Keys HM, *et al.* A phase III trial of surgery with or without adjunctive external pelvic radiation therapy in intermediate risk endometrial adenocarcinoma: a Gynecologic Oncology Group study. *Gynecol Oncol* 2004;92(3):744–51.
128 Kadar N, Malfetano JH, Homesley HD. Determinants of survival of surgically staged patients with endometrial carcinoma histologically confined to the uterus: implications for therapy. *Obstet Gynecol* 1992;80(4):655–9.
129 Creutzberg CL, *et al.* Surgery and postoperative radiotherapy versus surgery alone for patients with stage-1 endometrial carcinoma: multicentre randomised trial. PORTEC Study Group. Post Operative Radiation Therapy in Endometrial Carcinoma. *Lancet* 2000;355(9213):1404–11.
130 Mariani A, *et al.* Predictors of vaginal relapse in stage I endometrial cancer. *Gynecol Oncol* 2005;97(3):820–7.
131 Mariani A, *et al.* Surgical stage I endometrial cancer: predictors of distant failure and death. *Gynecol Oncol* 2002;87(3):274–80.
132 Orr JW Jr., Holimon JL, Orr PF. Stage I corpus cancer: is teletherapy necessary? *Am J Obstet Gynecol* 1997;176(4): 777–88; discussion 788–9.
133 Straughn JM, *et al.* Stage IC adenocarcinoma of the endometrium: survival comparisons of surgically staged patients with and without adjuvant radiation therapy. *Gynecol Oncol* 2003;89(2):295–300.
134 Pearcey RG, Petereit DG. Post-operative high dose rate brachytherapy in patients with low to intermediate risk endometrial cancer. *Radiother Oncol* 2000;56(1):17–22.
135 Creutzberg CL, van Stiphout RG, Nout RA, *et al.* Nomograms for prediction of outcome with or without adjuvant radiation therapy for patients with endometrial cancer: a pooled analysis of PORTEC-1 and PORTEC-2 trials. *Int J Radiat Oncol Biol Phys* 2015;91:530–9.
136 Horowitz NS, *et al.* Adjuvant high dose rate vaginal brachytherapy as treatment of stage I and II endometrial carcinoma. *Obstet Gynecol* 2002;99(2):235–40.
137 Mohan DS, *et al.* Long-term outcomes of therapeutic pelvic lymphadenectomy for stage I endometrial adenocarcinoma. *Gynecol Oncol* 1998;70(2):165–71.
138 Chadha M, *et al.* Patterns of failure in endometrial carcinoma stage IB grade 3 and IC patients treated with postoperative vaginal vault brachytherapy. *Gynecol Oncol* 1999;75(1): 103–7.
139 Nout RA, *et al.* Vaginal brachytherapy versus pelvic external beam radiotherapy for patients with endometrial cancer of

high-intermediate risk (PORTEC-2): an open-label, non-inferiority, randomised trial. *Lancet* 2010;375(9717):816–23.
140 Huh WK, *et al.* Salvage of isolated vaginal recurrences in women with surgical stage I endometrial cancer: a multiinstitutional experience. *Int J Gynecol Cancer* 2007;17(4):886–9.
141 Blake P, *et al.* Adjuvant external beam radiotherapy in the treatment of endometrial cancer (MRC ASTEC and NCIC CTG EN.5 randomised trials): pooled trial results, systematic review, and meta-analysis. *Lancet* 2009;373(9658):137–46.
142 Corn BW, *et al.* Endometrial cancer with para-aortic adenopathy: patterns of failure and opportunities for cure. *Int J Radiat Oncol Biol Phys* 1992;24(2):223–7.
143 Potish RA, *et al.* Paraaortic lymph node radiotherapy in cancer of the uterine corpus. *Obstet Gynecol* 1985;65(2):251–6.
144 Feuer GA, Calanog A. Endometrial carcinoma: treatment of positive paraaortic nodes. *Gynecol Oncol* 1987;27(1):104–9.
145 Greer BE, Hamberger AD. Treatment of intraperitoneal metastatic adenocarcinoma of the endometrium by the whole-abdomen moving-strip technique and pelvic boost irradiation. *Gynecol Oncol* 1983;16(3):365–73.
146 Loeffler JS, *et al.* Whole abdominal irradiation for tumors of the uterine corpus. *Cancer* 1988;61(7):1332–5.
147 Small W, Jr, *et al.* Whole-abdominal radiation in endometrial carcinoma: an analysis of toxicity, patterns of recurrence, and survival. *Cancer J* 2000;6(6):394–400.
148 Randall ME, *et al.* Randomized phase III trial of whole-abdominal irradiation versus doxorubicin and cisplatin chemotherapy in advanced endometrial carcinoma: a Gynecologic Oncology Group Study. *J Clin Oncol* 2006;24(1):36–44.
149 Lewis GC, Jr, *et al.* Adjuvant progestogen therapy in the primary definitive treatment of endometrial cancer. *Gynecol Oncol* 1974;2(2–3):368–76.
150 Vergote I, *et al.* A randomized trial of adjuvant progestagen in early endometrial cancer. *Cancer* 1989;64(5):1011–6.
151 Miller D, *et al.* Randomized phase III noninferiority trial of first line chemotherapy for metastatic or recurrent endometrial carcinoma: A Gynecologic Oncology Group study. *Gynecologic Oncology* 2012;125:771.
152 Bestvina CM, Fleming GF. Chemotherapy for endometrial cancer in adjuvant and advanced disease settings. *Oncologist* 2016;21(10):1250–9.
153 Larson DM, *et al.* Prognostic factors in stage II endometrial carcinoma. *Cancer* 1987;60(6):1358–61.
154 Larson DM, *et al.* Stage II endometrial carcinoma. Results and complications of a combined radiotherapeutic–surgical approach. *Cancer* 1988;61(8):1528–34.
155 Sartori E, *et al.* Clinical behavior of 203 stage II endometrial cancer cases: the impact of primary surgical approach and of adjuvant radiation therapy. *Int J Gynecol Cancer* 2001;11(6):430–7.
156 Andersen ES. Stage II endometrial carcinoma: prognostic factors and the results of treatment. *Gynecol Oncol* 1990;38(2):220–3.
157 Grigsby PW, *et al.* Results of therapy, analysis of failures, and prognostic factors for clinical and pathologic stage III adenocarcinoma of the endometrium. *Gynecol Oncol* 1987;27(1):44–57.
158 Aalders JG, Abeler V, Kolstad P. Stage IV endometrial carcinoma: a clinical and histopathological study of 83 patients. *Gynecol Oncol* 1984;17(1):75–84.
159 van Wijk FH, *et al.* Management of surgical stage III and IV endometrioid endometrial carcinoma: an overview. *Int J Gynecol Cancer* 2009;19(3):431–46.
160 Aalders JG, Abeler V, Kolstad P. Clinical (stage III) as compared to subclinical intrapelvic extrauterine tumor spread in endometrial carcinoma: a clinical and histopathological study of 175 patients. *Gynecol Oncol* 1984;17(1):64–74.
161 Greven KM, *et al.* Analysis of failure patterns in stage III endometrial carcinoma and therapeutic implications. *Int J Radiat Oncol Biol Phys* 1989;17(1):35–9.
162 Creasman WT, *et al.* Carcinoma of the corpus uteri. FIGO 26th Annual Report on the Results of Treatment in Gynecological Cancer. *Int J Gynaecol Obstet* 2006;95 Suppl 1:S105–43.
163 Goff BA, *et al.* Surgical stage IV endometrial carcinoma: a study of 47 cases. *Gynecol Oncol* 1994;52(2):237–40.
164 Chi DS, *et al.* The role of surgical cytoreduction in Stage IV endometrial carcinoma. *Gynecol Oncol* 1997;67(1):56–60.
165 Rutledge FN, *et al.* Pelvic exenteration: analysis of 296 patients. *Am J Obstet Gynecol* 1977;129(8):881–92.
166 Aalders JG, Abeler V, Kolstad P. Recurrent adenocarcinoma of the endometrium: a clinical and histopathological study of 379 patients. *Gynecol Oncol* 1984;17(1):85–103.
167 Shumsky AG, *et al.* An evaluation of routine follow-up of patients treated for endometrial carcinoma. *Gynecol Oncol* 1994;55(2):229–33.
168 Berchuck A, *et al.* Postsurgical surveillance of patients with FIGO stage I/II endometrial adenocarcinoma. *Gynecol Oncol* 1995;59(1):20–4.
169 Reddoch JM, *et al.* Surveillance for recurrent endometrial carcinoma: development of a follow-up scheme. *Gynecol Oncol* 1995;59(2):221–5.
170 Salani R, *et al.* Posttreatment surveillance and diagnosis of recurrence in women with gynecologic malignancies: Society of Gynecologic Oncologists recommendations. *Am J Obstet Gynecol* 2011;204(6):466–78.
171 Creutzberg CL, *et al.* Survival after relapse in patients with endometrial cancer: results from a randomized trial. *Gynecol Oncol* 2003;89(2):201–9.
172 Bradford LS, *et al.* Advances in the Management of Recurrent Endometrial Cancer. *Am J Clin Oncol* 2015;38(2): 206–12.
173 Gao C, Wang Y, Tian W, Xue F The therapeutic significance of aromatase inhibitors in endometrial carcinoma. *Gynecol Oncol* 2014;134:190–5.
174 Jhingran A, Burke TW, Eifel PJ. Definitive radiotherapy for patients with isolated vaginal recurrence of endometrial carcinoma after hysterectomy. *Int J Radiat Oncol Biol Phys* 2003;56(5):1366–72.

175 Sears JD, *et al.* Prognostic factors and treatment outcome for patients with locally recurrent endometrial cancer. *Cancer* 1994;74(4):1303–8.

176 Akram T, Maseelall P, Fanning J. Carboplatin and paclitaxel for the treatment of advanced or recurrent endometrial cancer. *Am J Obstet Gynecol* 2005;192(5):1365–7.

177 Sovak MA, *et al.* Paclitaxel and carboplatin in the treatment of advanced or recurrent endometrial cancer: a large retrospective study. *Int J Gynecol Cancer* 2007;17(1):197–203.

178 Dowdy SC, Mariani A. Lymphadenectomy in endometrial cancer: when, not if. *Lancet* 2010;375(9721):1138–40.

179 Angel C, *et al.* Recurrent stage I endometrial adenocarcinoma in the nonirradiated patient: preliminary results of surgical "staging". *Gynecol Oncol* 1993;48(2):221–6.

180 Garton GR, *et al.* Intraoperative radiation therapy in gynecologic cancer: the Mayo Clinic experience. *Gynecol Oncol* 1993;48(3):328–32.

181 Lee TS, *et al.* Feasibility of ovarian preservation in patients with early stage endometrial carcinoma. *Gynecol Oncol* 2007;104(1):52–7.

182 Creasman WT, *et al.* Estrogen replacement therapy in the patient treated for endometrial cancer. *Obstet Gynecol* 1986;67(3):326–30.

183 Suriano KA, *et al.* Estrogen replacement therapy in endometrial cancer patients: a matched control study. *Obstet Gynecol* 2001;97(4):555–60.

184 Levenback C, *et al.* Resection of pulmonary metastases from uterine sarcomas. *Gynecol Oncol* 1992;45(2):202–5.

185 Committee on Gynecologic Practice. ACOG committee opinion. Hormone replacement therapy in women treated for endometrial cancer. Number 234, May 2000 (replaces number 126, August 1993). *Int J Gynaecol Obstet* 2001;73(3):283–4.

186 Brooks SE, *et al.* Surveillance, epidemiology, and end results analysis of 2677 cases of uterine sarcoma 1989–1999. *Gynecol Oncol* 2004;93(1):204–8.

187 Kempson RL, Bari W. Uterine sarcomas. Classification, diagnosis, and prognosis. *Hum Pathol* 1970;1(3):331–49.

188 Prat J. FIGO staging for uterine sarcomas. *Int J Gynaecol Obstet* 2009;104(3):177–8.

189 Dizon DS, *et al.* Corpus Uteri – Sarcoma. In: M Amin, S Edge, R Greene, D Byrd, R Brookland (eds) *Cancer Staging Manual, 8th Edition American Joint Committee on Cancer*. New York: Springer, 2017.

190 Dionigi A, *et al.* Endometrial stromal nodules and endometrial stromal tumors with limited infiltration: a clinicopathologic study of 50 cases. *Am J Surg Pathol* 2002;26(5):567–81.

191 Norris HJ, Taylor HB. Mesenchymal tumors of the uterus. I. A clinical and pathological study of 53 endometrial stromal tumors. *Cancer* 1966;19(6):755–66.

192 Yoonessi M, Hart WR. Endometrial stromal sarcomas. *Cancer* 1977;40(2):898–906.

193 Chang KL, *et al.* Primary uterine endometrial stromal neoplasms. A clinicopathologic study of 117 cases. *Am J Surg Pathol* 1990;14(5):415–38.

194 Nam JH. Surgical treatment of uterine sarcoma. *Best Pract Res Clin Obstet Gynaecol* 2011;25(6):751–60.

195 Hensley ML. Role of chemotherapy and biomolecular therapy in the treatment of uterine sarcomas. *Best Pract Res Clin Obstet Gynaecol* 2011;25(6):773–82.

196 Christopherson WM, Williamson EO, Gray LA. Leiomyosarcoma of the uterus. *Cancer* 1972;29(6): 1512–7.

197 Giuntoli RL, 2nd, *et al.* Retrospective review of 208 patients with leiomyosarcoma of the uterus: prognostic indicators, surgical management, and adjuvant therapy. *Gynecol Oncol* 2003;89(3):460–9.

198 Dinh TA, *et al.* The treatment of uterine leiomyosarcoma. Results from a 10-year experience (1990–1999) at the Massachusetts General Hospital. *Gynecol Oncol* 2004;92(2):648–52.

199 Bell SW, Kempson RL, Hendrickson MR. Problematic uterine smooth muscle neoplasms. A clinicopathologic study of 213 cases. *Am J Surg Pathol* 1994;18(6):535–58.

200 Omura GA, *et al.* A randomized study of adriamycin with and without dimethyl triazenoimidazole carboxamide in advanced uterine sarcomas. *Cancer* 1983;52(4):626–32.

201 Sutton GP, *et al.* Phase II trial of ifosfamide and mesna in leiomyosarcoma of the uterus: a Gynecologic Oncology Group study. *Am J Obstet Gynecol* 1992;166(2):556–9.

202 Sutton G, Blessing JA, Malfetano JH. Ifosfamide and doxorubicin in the treatment of advanced leiomyosarcomas of the uterus: a Gynecologic Oncology Group study. *Gynecol Oncol* 1996;62(2):226–9.

202 Hensley ML, *et al.* Gemcitabine and docetaxel in patients with unresectable leiomyosarcoma: results of a phase II trial. *J Clin Oncol* 2002;20(12):2824–31.

203 National Cancer Institute. Endometrial Cancer Treatment (PDQ®). Health Professional Version. https://www.cancer.gov/types/uterine/hp/endometrial-treatment-pdq#section/_9 (accessed 15 December 2017).

21

Cervical Cancer

Merieme Klobocista[1], Mark H. Einstein[2], and Carolyn D. Runowicz[3]

[1] John Theurer Cancer Center, Hackensack University Medical Center, Hackensack, New Jersey, USA
[2] Rutgers New Jersey Medical School, Newark, New Jersey, USA
[3] Florida International University Herbert Wertheim College of Medicine, Miami, Florida, USA

Incidence and Mortality

There will be an estimated 12,820 new cases of cervical cancer and 4,210 deaths attributable to cervical cancer in the United States (US) in 2017 [1]. The incidence and death rates have remained stable in the US for more than a decade [1]. It is the second most common cancer-related death in women between ages 20 and 39 in the US [1]. The incidence rates in the US are highest among Hispanics/Latinas (9.4 per 100,000 per year) and African Americans (8.9 per 100,000 per year); the mortality rates are highest among African Americans (3.9 per 100,000 per year) and American Indians/Alaska Natives (3.2 per 100,000 per year) [2]. It is the fourth most common cancer diagnosis in women worldwide and the second most common malignancy among women in developing countries Over half a million women are diagnosed annually with cervical cancer and more than half of these women die from their cancer worldwide [3]. The vast burden of death from cervical cancer is in low-resourced countries [3]. The lowest burden of cervical cancer is in Australia/New Zealand, North America and Western Europe, where there is widespread access to and use of screening, whereas the highest burden is found in sub-Saharan Africa [3]. New methods for screening and point of care treatment, especially in regions of the world with limited resources, have resulted in a decreased incidence of and mortality from advanced cervical cancer [4].

Etiology, Risk Factors, and Prevention

The majority of risk factors are surrogate markers for human papillomavirus (HPV) infection and persistence of oncogenic HPV types. These include sexual risk factors such as early age of coitarche, multiple sexual partners, and history of sexually transmitted infections [5–9]. Immunosuppression (e.g., human immunodeficiency virus, chronic steroid use) [10], low socioeconomic status, and smoking are additional risk factors even when controlling for other relevant factors [11–13]. Incidence is increased in current smokers, with increasing number of cigarettes smoked per day, and with younger age at initiation of smoking [12–14]. Oral contraceptive use has been shown to increase risk of high-grade cervical intraepithelial neoplasia (CIN) and cervical cancer [13, 14]. While there is no evidence of a genetic link to cervical cancer, there may be some susceptibility genes related to HPV persistence and cervical cancer [15–17]. Vaccines that prevent HPV 16 and 18 and other high-risk types are an important strategy for prevention. With early vaccination and use of widespread screening, cervical cancer can be a largely preventable cancer.

HPV

An overwhelming majority of cervical cancer is due to an infection from an oncogenic ('high risk') HPV type. These include types that have been associated with malignant transformation of cervical cancers including 16, 18, 31, 33, 35, 39, 45, 51, 52, 56, 58, 59, and 68 [18]. Up to 80% of sexually active individuals will have an infection with some type of HPV in their lifetime [19]. Most, however, will never get any clinically relevant HPV-associated disease. The HPV types that cause most preinvasive disease and cervical cancer are HPV 16 and 18. HPV 16 is found in 20% of HPV infections, but accounts for 40% of high-grade CIN and most cervical cancer. HPV 16 is the most common HPV type found in squamous cell carcinoma, accounting for up to 60%, and is the second most common type found in adenocarcinoma, accounting for 36% of cases [20, 21]. HPV 18 accounts for 10–20% of cervical cancer and is the most common type found in adenocarcinoma (37%), and adenocarcinoma *in situ* (AIS) (43%) [20–22]. HPV 16 is the most frequent type detected in all preinvasive cervical disease, but HPV 18 is more common in AIS as compared to CIN or CIN associated with AIS [22].

Natural History of Cervical Cancer

The natural history of HPV infection from intraepithelial neoplasia to cervical cancer has been well documented. Most HPV infections will regress within a year; persistent HPV infections

The American Cancer Society's Oncology in Practice: Clinical Management, First Edition. Edited by The American Cancer Society.

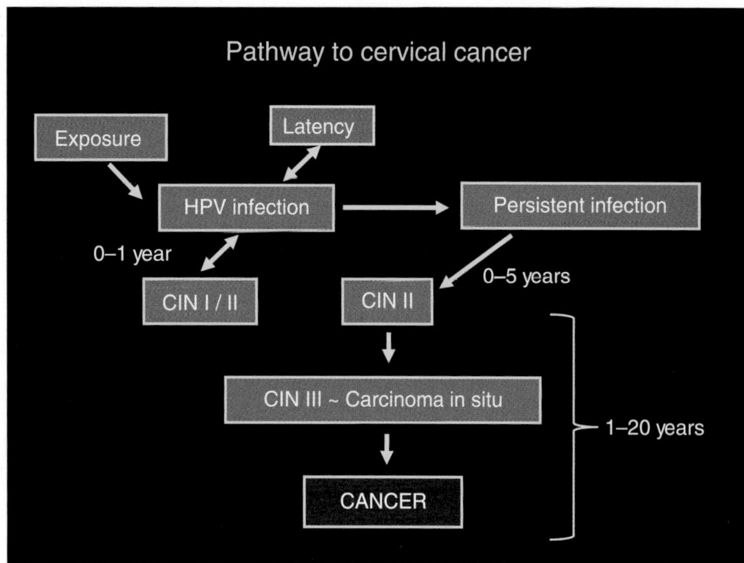

Figure 21.1 Natural history model of cervical cancer showing the time line between exposure, dysplasia, and ultimately cancer. *Source:* Einstein and Burke [192].

can progress to preinvasive cervical disease [23–26]. In organized screening programs, the goal is to identify precancerous lesions that can be treated before they progress. If not treated, some may progress to invasive cervical cancer (Figure 21.1) [23–25, 27, 28]. This process from infection to preinvasive disease and ultimately invasive disease takes an average of 10–15 years, although there have been reports of cancers that have developed in a much shorter period of time [26, 29].

Prevention

The time required to develop an invasive cancer from an HPV infection allows screening to significantly impact the early diagnosis and treatment of preinvasive disease, and thus reducing the incidence of invasive cervical cancer. The routine use of the Papanicolaou (Pap) test as a primary screening method has led to a decrease in the incidence as well as death from cervical cancer [30–33]. The overall incidence of invasive cervical cancer has decreased approximately 53% over the last 35 years and the mortality rate has decreased nearly 60% in the US [34]. The performance of the Pap test can be affected, for example, by inadequate sampling, obscuring blood or mucous from the cervix, and human error. While liquid-based cytology improves many of the sampling issues, diagnostic yields of conventional Pap smears compared with liquid-based cytology are similar [35]. Implementation of clinically validated high-risk HPV testing improves risk stratification of equivocal Pap tests such as atypical squamous cell of unknown significance [36–38]. In 2012, the American Cancer Society, American Society for Colposcopy and Cervical Pathology, and American Society for Clinical Pathology jointly released updated guidelines for cervical cancer screening [38]. During that same year, the US Preventive Service Task Force released a recommendation statement for screening for cervical cancer [39] and The American Congress of Obstetricians and Gynecologists issued a practice bulletin with their recommendations for cervical cancer screening [40]. HPV testing is not recommended for women under the age of 30 due to the high prevalence of HPV among sexually active young women, which is likely due to transient HPV infections [36, 41]. Refer to Chapter 11 in *The American Cancer Society's Principles of Oncology: Prevention to Survivorship* for additional information on early detection of cervical cancer.

Currently there are three Food and Drug Administration approved vaccines: the quadrivalent vaccine (Gardasil®), the bivalent vaccine (Cervarix®), and the nine valent vaccine (Gardasil 9®). These vaccines protect against oncogenic types HPV 16 and 18, which account for over 70% of cervical cancer and 50% of CIN [42]. The quadrivalent vaccine also protects against HPV 6 and 11, which account for approximately 90% of genital warts. Clinical trials in essentially HPV naïve young women demonstrate 93–98% efficacy rates at preventing high-grade CIN related to HPV 16 and 18. However, with prior HPV exposure, the efficacy is less, as expected [43–47]. These vaccines have some crossprotective efficacy with closely related oncogenic HPV types, thus providing additional protection against cervical cancers caused by HPV other than 16 or 18 [48–51]. Gardasil 9®, approved in December 2014, protects against HPV 6, 11, 16, 18, 31, 33, 45, 52, and 58. The vaccines have been well tolerated with few side effects, with the most common side effect being injection site pain. Further study of men, with a specific cohort of men who have sex with men, also showed efficacy at prevention of *in situ* lesions of the anus and other external genital lesions, such as genital warts [52]

The US Federal Advisory Committee on Immunization Practices recommends routine vaccination of all girls and boys ages 11 and 12. The vaccine series can be started as young as age 9 and can be administered in a catch-up population up to age 26. The initial recommendation was for a series of three vaccinations on day 0, 1–2 months later, and 6 months after the first dose. The latest recommendation by the Advisory Committee on Immunization Practices is to use a two-dose schedule for girls and boys who initiate the vaccination series at ages 9–14 years. Three doses remain recommended for person who initiate the vaccination series at ages 15–26 years [52, 53] In addition to prophylactic vaccination, there are ongoing investigations of therapeutic vaccines for high-grade CIN and invasive cervical cancer [54–59].

Clinical Presentation/Diagnosis

Early-stage cervical cancer is often asymptomatic, detected by an abnormal Pap test and most commonly diagnosed after pathologic evaluation of a cervical biopsy. The most commonly reported symptom is abnormal vaginal bleeding, which can include heavy vaginal bleeding, bleeding between menses, postcoital bleeding, and postmenopausal bleeding. Other symptoms of more advanced disease include copious vaginal discharge or odor, pelvic pain or pressure, low back pain that may radiate down the leg, urinary symptoms such as urgency or hematuria, and bowel symptoms such as constipation or hematochezia. The commonly cited triad of symptoms associated with advanced cervical cancer is pelvic pain, sciatica, and lower extremity lymphedema, which is often a sign of pelvic side wall involvement.

Diagnosis

While cytology (Pap test) is helpful as a screening test for CIN and early-stage cervical cancer, a definitive diagnosis requires histology. Patients who present with abnormal bleeding should be evaluated with a pelvic examination, which includes a speculum examination to visualize the cervix and vagina. A biopsy of any abnormal appearing lesion on the cervix should be performed regardless of the Pap test results. Abnormal lesions can range from a small condylomatous type lesion, to an exophytic tumor that completely replaces the cervix and protrudes into the vagina (Figure 21.2). These masses tend to be friable and in some cases can cause significant bleeding when examined or biopsied. On the other hand, the tumor may be endophytic, and may remain mostly in the cervical canal, causing expansion of the cervix as compared to an exophytic growth into the vagina. These endophytic tumors, also known as "barrel shaped" tumors are a common appearance of locally advanced cervical cancers.

Patients who are asymptomatic but present with an abnormal Pap smear and no visible lesion will undergo further workup with colposcopic directed biopsies [60]. If biopsies return as insufficient to assess for invasion, CIN III/carcinoma *in situ* or microinvasive disease, an excisional biopsy with a loop electrosurgical excision procedure (LEEP) or cold knife cone (CKC) is performed to assess for depth of invasion.

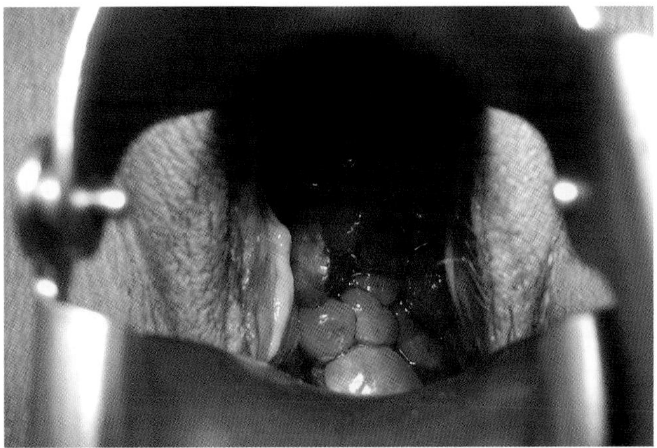

Figure 21.2 A 28-year-old presented with recurrent cervical polyps. She was diagnosed with stage IB1 adenosarcoma of the cervix. She was treated with radical hysterectomy and lymph node dissection followed by chemoradiotherapy.

Histopathology

Squamous cell carcinoma accounts for approximately 60% of all cervical cancer cases [34]. It is most commonly associated with HPV 16, followed by HPV 18. About 10% of cervical cancers can be attributed to more than one HPV type [20, 61, 62]. The incidence of adenocarcinoma (and adenosquamous carcinoma) relative to all cancers of the cervix has increased from 12.4% from 1973 to 1977 to 27.3% from 2006 to 2010 [34, 63]. Some factors that might be associated with this increase include use of exogenous hormones such as oral contraceptives or menopausal hormonal therapy, as well as an increased prevalence of obesity which increases levels of endogenous estrogens [64]. A rare histology, clear cell adenocarcinoma, is associated with diethylstilbesterol exposure *in utero* [65, 66]. Small cell carcinoma accounts for 2% of cervical cancers [67] and is strongly associated with HPV 18 [68, 69]. Up to 33% of small cell carcinomas express neuroendocrine features and are associated with a higher frequency of lymphovascular invasion (LVI), higher rate of recurrence and overall poor prognosis [70]. Other rare histologic subtypes of cervical cancer include sarcoma, carcinosarcoma, lymphoma, and melanoma. Metastasis to the cervix is rare [71].

Staging/Workup

The main staging system used in cervical cancer is the International Federation of Gynecology and Obstetrics (FIGO). Another staging system that can be used is the TNM system developed by the American Joint Committee on Cancer (AJCC) and the Union for International Cancer Control (UICC). In 2009, the FIGO committee on Gynecologic Oncology released a revision of the FIGO staging system [72]. Prior to its release, the document was reviewed by the UICC and the AJCC and was affirmed. The two staging systems are listed in Table 21.1 [73]. In both systems, clinical criteria are used to assign stage of disease. With the TNM classification, there is a category for other pathologic and lymph node findings, which do not change the assigned clinical stage of the disease.

Clinical staging of cervical cancer is uniform worldwide. In addition to a thorough physical examination, a pelvic examination should include a speculum examination, and bimanual and rectovaginal examination to evaluate tumor size, extension of disease to the vagina, the parametria, and pelvic sidewalls (Figure 21.3) [74]. The remainder of the physical examination helps to identify local or distant metastasis. A thorough evaluation for enlarged lymph nodes in the groin, cervical, and supraclavicular area is important as treatment will change if metastatic disease is identified in these areas. If there is evidence of enlarged or fixed lymph nodes, a fine-needle aspiration or biopsy can be performed in the office. If the office pelvic examination is limited due to tumor size or patient discomfort, then

Table 21.1 Cervical cancer staging (TNM and FIGO) [73]. The definitions of the T categories correspond to the stages accepted by the Fédération Internationale de Gynécologie et d'Obstétrique (FIGO). Both systems are included for comparison.

Definition of primary tumor (T)

T category	FIGO stage	T criteria
TX		Primary tumor cannot be assessed
T0		No evidence of primary tumor
T1	I	Cervical carcinoma confined to the uterus (extension to corpus should be disregarded)
T1a	IA	Invasive carcinoma diagnosed only by microscopy. Stromal invasion with a maximum depth of 5.0 mm measured from the base of the epithelium and a horizontal spread of 7.0 mm or less. Vascular space involvement, venous or lymphatic, does not affect classification.
T1a1	IA1	Measured stromal invasion of 3.0 mm or less in depth and 7.0 mm or less in horizontal spread
T1a2	IA2	Measured stromal invasion of more than 3.0 mm and not more than 5.0 mm, with a horizontal spread of 7.0 mm or less
T1b	IB	Clinically visible lesion confined to the cervix or microscopic lesion greater than T1a/IA2. Includes all macroscopically visible lesions, even those with superficial invasion.
T1b1	IB1	Clinically visible lesion 4.0 cm or less in greatest dimension
T1b2	IB2	Clinically visible lesion more than 4.0 cm in greatest dimension
T2	II	Cervical carcinoma invading beyond the uterus but not to the pelvic wall or to lower third of the vagina
T2a	IIA	Tumor without parametrial invasion
T2a1	IIA1	Clinically visible lesion 4.0 cm or less in greatest dimension
T2a2	IIA2	Clinically visible lesion more than 4.0 cm in greatest dimension
T2b	IIB	Tumor with parametrial invasion
T3	III	Tumor extending to the pelvic sidewall[1] and/or involving the lower third of the vagina and/or causing hydronephrosis or nonfunctioning kidney
T3a	IIIA	Tumor involving the lower third of the vagina but not extending to the pelvic wall
T3b	IIIB	Tumor extending to the pelvic wall and/or causing hydronephrosis or nonfunctioning kidney
T4	IVA	Tumor invading the mucosa of the bladder or rectum and/or extending beyond the true pelvis (bullous edema is not sufficient to classify a tumor as T4)

[1] The pelvic sidewall is defined as the muscle, fascia, neurovascular structures, and skeletal portions of the bony pelvis. On rectal examination, there is no cancer-free space between the tumor and pelvic sidewall.

Table 21.1 (Continued)

Definition of regional lymph node (N)

N category	FIGO stage	N criteria
NX		Regional lymph nodes cannot be assessed
N0		No regional lymph node metastasis
N0(i+)		Isolated tumor cells in regional lymph node(s) no >0.2 mm
N1		Regional lymph node metastasis

Definition of distant metastasis (M)

M category	FIGO stage	M criteria
M0		No distant metastasis
M1	IVB	Distant metastasis (including peritoneal spread or involvement of the supraclavicular, mediastinal, or distant lymph nodes; lung; liver; or bone)

AJCC prognostic stage groups

When T is...	And N is...	And M is...	Then the stage group is...
T1	Any N	M0	I
T1a	Any N	M0	IA
T1a1	Any N	M0	IA1
T1a2	Any N	M0	IA2
T1b	Any N	M0	IB
T1b1	Any N	M0	IB1
T1b2	Any N	M0	IB2
T2	Any N	M0	II
T2a	Any N	M0	IIA
T2a1	Any N	M0	IIA1
T2a2	Any N	M0	IIA2
T2b	Any N	M0	IIB
T3	Any N	M0	III
T3a	Any N	M0	IIIA
T3b	Any N	M0	IIIB
T4	Any N	M0	IVA
Any T	Any N	M1	IVB

Source: Erickson *et al.* [73]. Used with permission of the American College of Surgeons, Chicago, Illinois. The original source for this information is the AJCC Cancer Staging Manual, 8th edn (2017), which is published by Springer Science+Business Media.

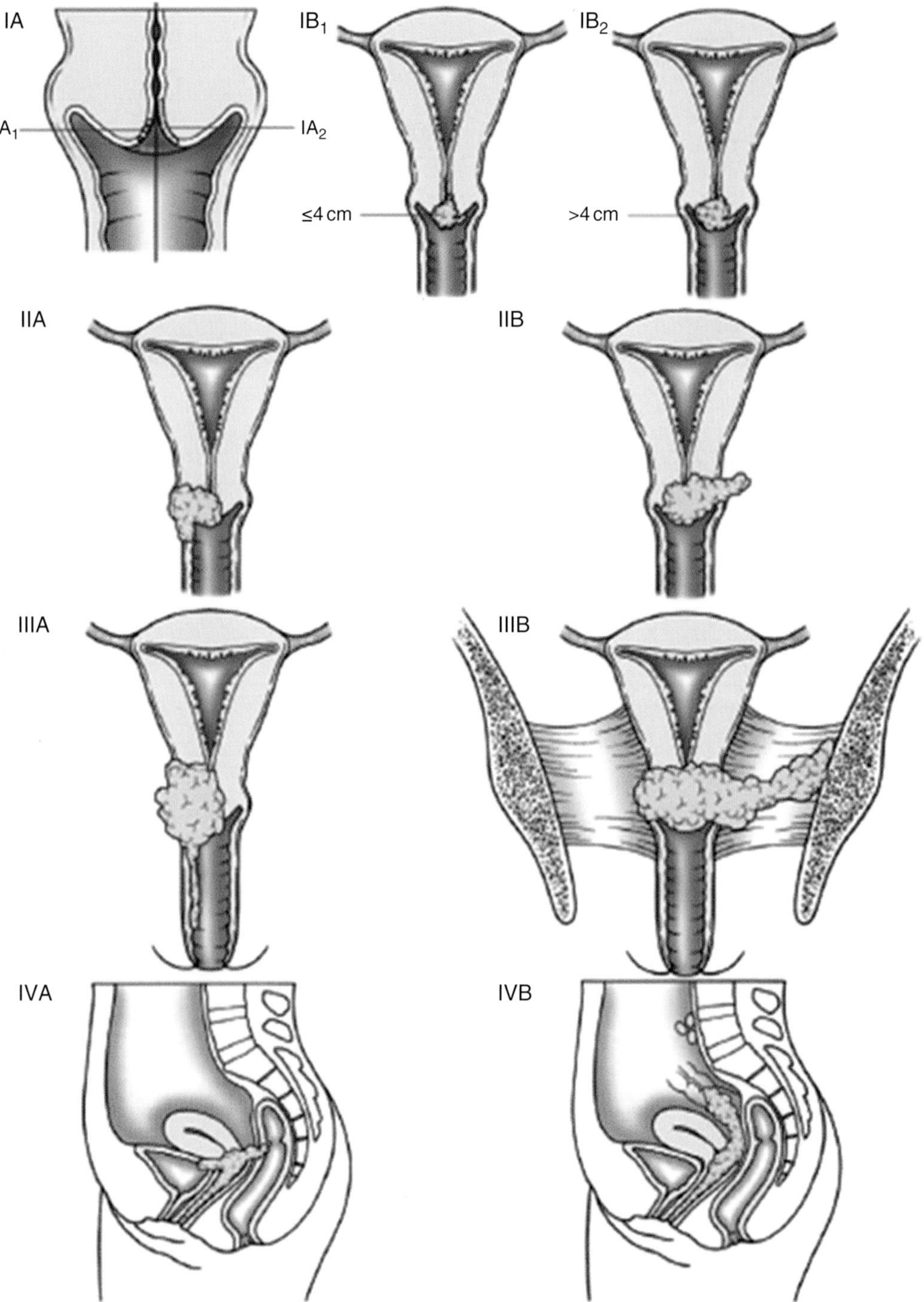

Figure 21.3 Staging of cervical cancer. *Source:* Quinn *et al.* [74]. Reproduced with permission of John Wiley & Sons.

an examination under anesthesia is performed. In addition, a cystoscopy and proctoscopy should be performed in advanced disease to assess bladder and/or rectal involvement, which should be confirmed with biopsies. Additional studies that are allowable under FIGO guidelines to stage cervical cancer clinically include intravenous pyelogram to evaluate for hydronephrosis, chest X-ray (CXR) to evaluate for lung metastasis, and bone X-ray to evaluate for bone metastasis.

Workup

The limitations of clinical staging include subjective evaluation of the size of the tumor and parametrial involvement, and inability to assess adequately if there is lymph node metastasis. Due to these shortcomings of imaging such as intravenous pyelogram, clinicians in high resource regions of the world, including the US, often use additional comprehensive body imaging tools to evaluate for extent of disease such as computed tomography scan (CT), magnetic resonance imaging (MRI), positron emission tomography (PET) or PET/CT fusion scans. The additional information offered by these tools will not change the clinical stage of the disease, but may impact the choices of treatment modality and prognosis.

If a CT scan shows evidence of metastatic disease, the patient is not a candidate for surgery and will undergo radiation therapy (RT) or concomitant chemoradiotherapy. If there are enlarged or suspicious lymph nodes, then either image-guided biopsy or PET can be utilized. PET/CT has a very good performance (sensitivity) for detecting metastasis that are >1 cm [75]. Identification of lymph node metastasis typically allows for tailored treatment planning for RT. Surgical resection of lymph nodes is usually reserved for diagnostic purposes, if imaging modalities fail to achieve a definitive diagnosis [76]. MRI can be used for evaluation of the depth of invasion of the cervical tumor and parametrial involvement. This information can be important in patients who desire fertility-preserving treatment (see section 'Fertility Sparing Surgery') [77, 78]. For locally advanced cervical cancers, evaluation of kidney function and imaging to detect tumor obstructing the ureters is important, because this might prompt the need for diversion through percutaneous nephrostomies. If the renal function is normal and there is concern for obstruction, a renal scan can be helpful in determining if the affected obstructed kidney is still functional. Pretreatment blood work includes a complete blood count (CBC), liver function tests including transaminases, and renal function tests to assess for anemia, hepatitis, and other liver dysfunction. Human immunodeficiency virus testing is recommended since cervical cancer is an autoimmune deficiency syndrome-defining illness and this diagnosis can affect dosing for treatment as well as prompt immediate management in a patient who might not have been on antiretroviral therapy [79].

Treatment/Prognosis

Treatment options for cervical cancer range from minimal surgery, to radical surgery, fertility-sparing surgery, and chemotherapy with radiation. Treatment is dependent on the stage of disease, comorbidities, performance status, and age of the patient. Hysterectomy and trachelectomy can be performed through laparotomy, laparoscopy, robotically, and with either a vaginal or abdominal approach.

Stage IA1

Prior to embarking on treatment pathways, information regarding the presence of LVI and margin status on CKC or LEEP is important. For select patients, less radical and fertility-sparing surgery are potential options. The presence of LVI increases the risk of lymph node metastasis from 0.5 to 4.7% and recurrence from 0.6 to 4.6% [80].

Patients with a negative endocervical margin and negative endocervical curettage after CKC or LEEP can be managed conservatively with a simple, extrafascial hysterectomy if they have completed childbearing or with just a CKC for those who desire fertility preservation [81, 82]. In patients with evidence of LVI, a pelvic lymphadenectomy to assess for lymph node metastasis is performed in combination with a modified radical hysterectomy or a fertility-preserving surgery, which is discussed later in this chapter [81, 83]. Historically, adenocarcinoma of the cervix was thought to behave more aggressively and had a worse prognosis than squamous cell carcinoma, thus treatment was typically more radical [84]. However, careful assessment of well-documented histology controlled for stage and treated similarly has shown that there is no difference in prognosis in patients with squamous cell as compared to adenocarcinoma [85–88].

Patients who have undergone radical hysterectomy for early-stage disease (stage IA1), and lymphadenectomy without evidence of parametrial invasion in the hysterectomy specimen or lymph node involvement did not demonstrate ovarian involvement [89–91]. These data suggest ovarian conservation is an option in this group of early-stage patients. Furthermore, it is suggested that less radical hysterectomy may have the same results as the traditional radical hysterectomy in patients with early-stage cervical cancer. The prognosis for early-stage cervical cancer with appropriate less radical surgery by a trained gynecologic oncology surgeon is excellent, with >95% 5-year overall survival (OS) [74]. In summary, microinvasive squamous cell carcinoma and adenocarcinoma have an excellent prognosis with recent trends showing that we can perform less radical procedures than historically thought without compromising patient survival.

Stage IA2

With increasing depth of invasion, there is an increased risk of lymph node metastasis. In one review, up to 10% of patients with stage IA2 cervical cancer had positive lymph nodes [74]. The risk of lymph node metastasis ranges from 0 to 14% [80, 92–97]. The presence of LVI increases the risk of lymph node metastasis to 11–25% [80, 94, 95]. The primary treatment of choice is surgery with a modified radical hysterectomy or radical trachelectomy, both with a pelvic lymphadenectomy. The prognosis is excellent with 5-year OS at 95% [74, 95].

Stage IB1–IIA

Treatment options include radical hysterectomy or radical trachelectomy (in a subgroup of patients), with pelvic lymph node dissection. However, if medically inoperable, for tumors >4 cm, or other clinical risk factors, concomitant chemoradiotherapy is also an option as outcomes are similar. One prospective randomized trial of radical hysterectomy versus RT for stage IB1–IIA cervical cancer noted no difference in 5-year disease-free survival (DFS) and OS with a median follow-up of 87 months [98]. Patient selection is important when deciding on a treatment modality. Radical surgery provides the ability to remove the primary tumor, ovarian preservation in premenopausal patients, and to assess lymph node involvement. Surgery also avoids radiation-related side effects such as radiation cystitis, proctitis, fistula formation, ovarian failure, and vaginal dryness and sexual dysfunction [99–102]. Acute complications of radical surgery include bleeding, infection, and injury to nearby structures such as bladder, ureter, and bowel. Later complications include vesicovaginal and ureterovaginal fistula, stricture, and bladder atony. The overall incidence of major complications is <5% in experienced hands [103, 104].

Patients with stage IB2 have a higher rate of local, regional, and distant failures than stage IB1. The pelvic failure rate with pelvic radiation can be as high as 50% and the 10-year DFS survival is 47–60% [105]. Proponents for RT argue that the central tumor control in tumors <8 cm is up to 97%, but pelvic tumor control and disease-specific survival is poorer when compared to tumors <5 cm [106]. Doses of up to 85 Gy to the parametria are required and even with such high doses, there is a 35–50% pelvic failure rate [105]. The complication rate with such a high dose of RT needed to treat these tumors is higher than complications in RT-treated smaller cervical cancers. Grade 3 morbidity of the rectum and bladder, which include fistula formation, are up to 10% [107].

Concomitant chemoradiotherapy followed by extrafascial hysterectomy has been studied with the rationale to reduce central pelvic recurrences by performing an extrafascial hysterectomy after RT. There were two studies undertaken by the Gynecologic Oncology Group (GOG) that evaluated the use of extrafascial hysterectomy after RT [108] and concomitant chemoradiotherapy [109, 110]. Patients who underwent RT followed by extrafascial hysterectomy showed a trend towards improvement in the rate of pelvic relapse compared to patients who were treated with RT alone (no surgery) but there was no difference in OS with the addition of extrafascial hysterectomy [109]. In the other GOG study, patients were randomized to cisplatin RT followed by extrafascial hysterectomy or RT followed by extrafascial hysterectomy [110]. There was a significant improvement in progression-free and OS in the patients randomized to concomitant chemoradiotherapy as compared to the group who were treated with radiation alone. Based on these data, the authors concluded that the addition of cisplatin alone, without an extrafascial hysterectomy, should be adequate and that concomitant chemoradiotherapy should be considered the standard of care.

Another study noted that up to 44% of patients with stage IB2 carcinoma have positive pelvic nodes and up to 6% have positive para-aortic nodes [111]. In one report, performance of radical hysterectomy in women with tumor size 4–6 cm was associated with a 49% reduction in mortality rate compared with primary radiation. However, they also noted that 49% of patients in their cohort who underwent radical hysterectomy required postoperative RT due to high risk features [102]. In another study, over 80% of patients with tumor size >4 cm who underwent radical hysterectomy were treated with postoperative RT for high risk features (positive margins, positive lymph nodes, LVI) and the morbidity of the combined treatment was higher than either surgery or RT alone [63].

There is no one standard method of treatment for patients with stage IB2 cancers and the trend is toward multimodality treatment based on results from advanced cervical cancer trials. The 5-year survival is 73–75% [74].

Stage IIB–IVA

Concomitant chemoradiotherapy is the treatment of choice for patients with locally advanced cervical cancer based on three landmark studies and emphasized in a National Cancer Institute clinical alert [108, 112–114]. Due to these results, concomitant chemoradiation is being used in stage IB tumors. The GOG randomized 526 patients with stage IIB, III, and IVA cervical cancer with surgically confirmed negative para-aortic lymph nodes into three groups: weekly cisplatin versus 5-flurouracil (5-FU)/cisplatin/hydroxyurea versus hydroxyurea. All patients received simultaneous external and intracavitary pelvic radiation. The regimens containing cisplatin showed an improved progression-free survival (PFS) as compared to hydroxyurea alone. OS was higher in the groups that received cisplatin containing regimens when compared to hydroxyurea. There was no improvement in survival, but there were higher grade 3 and 4 hematologic toxicities and grade 4 gastrointestinal toxicity in the cisplatin, 5-FU, hydroxyurea regimen as compared to cisplatin alone. The conclusion was that weekly cisplatin is more efficacious than hydroxyurea, and more tolerable than cisplatin/5-FU/hydroxyurea when given concomitantly with RT for locally advanced cervix cancer [114, 115]. Another study randomized 388 patients with stage IIB–IVA cervical cancer, with negative para-aortic lymph nodes sampled at the time of surgical staging into two groups: hydroxyurea versus cisplatin and 5-FU. Both groups received standard pelvic radiation. PFS and OS were statistically better in the cisplatin containing regimen [113]. One other study reported by the Radiation Therapy Oncology Group randomized 403 patients with stage IIB–IVA cervical cancer to receive pelvic and para-aortic radiation or pelvic radiation with concurrent cisplatin/5-FU. The rate of locoregional recurrence and distant metastasis was higher in the group that received radiation alone. The 5-year survival was statistically better in the group that received both chemotherapy and RT. Adverse events were similar in both groups but an increased rate of reversible hematologic toxicity was noted in the group that received chemotherapy [112]. Currently, concomitant chemoradiotherapy with cisplatin is the standard of care for advanced-stage cervical cancer (stage IIB–IVA). Due to the ease of outpatient administration, weekly cisplatin is the commonly used schedule of administration. However, there is improved symptom control and even suggestions of improved survival with 5-day regimens given every 3 weeks [116]. There is a higher completion rate and fewer grade 3 and 4 hematologic toxicity with no difference in OS or PFS with weekly cisplatin with radiation when compared to cisplatin/5-FU with radiation [117]. A Cochrane meta-analysis on the efficacy of concomitant chemoradiotherapy in cervical cancer confirmed that the addition of chemotherapy to radiation improved 5-year survival, reduced local and distant recurrence and progression and improved DFS. A larger survival benefit was noted in two trials that included additional chemotherapy after concomitant chemoradiotherapy in select subjects with lymph node metastasis and other high risk features [118, 119]. A phase III randomized trial comparing concomitant gemcitabine and cisplatin and radiation followed by adjuvant gemcitabine and cisplatin versus concomitant cisplatin and radiation in patients with stage IIB–IVA cervical cancer reported a significant improvement in PFS and OS in the gemcitabine with cisplatin arm [120]. There was an increase in grade 3 and 4 toxicities in the gemcitabine with cisplatin arm. Despite improvement in disease status with the administration of cisplatin with radiation, there continues to be failures within the radiated field. Alternative chemotherapeutic agents in combination with cisplatin given concurrently with RT have been investigated [120–123]. Some combinations such as topotecan and cisplatin, although feasible, were associated with increased toxicity and treatment delay. Trials investigating optimal chemotherapy regimens given concurrently with RT are ongoing [124]. With increasing stage of disease, the survival decreases. The 5-year survival ranges from 66% for stage IIB to 22% for stage IVA [74].

Treatment for Stage IVB, Persistent or Recurrent Cervical Cancer

The prognosis for metastatic cervical cancer is poor with an overall 2-year survival of approximately 20% [74]. The treatment of choice is systemic chemotherapy. Common sites of extrapelvic distant metastasis include lung (33–38%), liver (33%), peritoneum (5–27%), adrenal gland (14–16%), bowel (12%), and skin (10%) [125]. Cisplatin has the most activity in cervical cancer and the response rate ranges from 20 to 31% [126–129]. Combination chemotherapy has been shown to have improved response rates and PFS than single agent cisplatin but was associated with higher grade 3 and 4 toxicity [128–130]. The GOG conducted a trial comparing various cisplatin-based chemotherapy combinations in cervical cancer. The combinations include cisplatin/paclitaxel, cisplatin/gemcitabine, cisplatin/vinorelbine, and cisplatin/topotecan [131]. There was no difference in response rate and risk of death among the four arms with a trend towards improved response rate, PFS and OS in the cisplatin/paclitaxel arm. Toxicity was similar in all arms except the cisplatin/gemcitabine arm that had less febrile neutropenia and the cisplatin/paclitaxel arm had lower grade 3 and 4 thrombocytopenia. Other platinum agents have been investigated to substitute cisplatin [132, 133]. The Japanese Clinical Oncology Group conducted a trial comparing carboplatin/paclitaxel to cisplatin/paclitaxel in patients with stage IVB, persistent, or recurrent cervical cancer [134]. There were similar response rates between the two groups, improved OS in the carboplatin/paclitaxel arm in patients previously treated with cisplatin and a lower OS in the carboplatin/paclitaxel arm in patients not previously treated with cisplatin. The carboplatin/paclitaxel arm had overall lower toxicity (neutropenia, renal insufficiency, gastrointestinal) but higher neuropathic events when compared to cisplatin/paclitaxel. Carboplatin is a reasonable alternative in patients who are unable to receive cisplatin. Another platinum agent that has been shown to have activity in cervical cancer is oxaliplatin. In a phase II study, paclitaxel and oxaliplatin was found to be effective in patients with recurrent or metastatic cervical cancer with a response rate of 22% and overall clinical benefit of 47% [135]. Preliminary results of GOG 240 evaluating the efficacy of bevacizumab in addition to platinum-based chemotherapy in patients with recurrent or metastatic cervical cancer showed an improved overall response rate of 48% compared to 36% ($P = 0.0078$) in the arm with platinum-based chemotherapy alone. Also, the median OS in the bevacizumab containing arm was 17 months compared to 13 months ($P = 0.0035$), respectively [136]. Due to this data showing a high magnitude of significant effect, the National Cancer Institute issued a clinical alert stating bevacizumab significantly improves survival for patients with recurrent or metastatic cervical cancer [137]. Despite combination chemotherapy and the addition of bevacizumab, the prognosis remains poor with a life expectancy on average of less than a year after a diagnosis of recurrence and only with systemic chemotherapy. Palliative care interventions are important options, with a focus on symptom management and quality of life.

Fertility-Preserving Treatment

Cervical cancer is the second most common cancer-related death in women between the ages of 20 and 39 [1]. These women may be candidates for fertility-preserving treatment since the majority are diagnosed at an early stage when survival is over 90%. Fertility-preserving surgery includes cervical conization and radical trachelectomy. Patient criteria include desire to preserve fertility, stage IA1–IB1, tumor lesion ≤2 cm with limited endocervical extension, squamous or adenocarcinoma histology, and negative lymph nodes [138]. Preoperative assessment includes colposcopy to evaluate for tumor extension into the endocervical canal and MRI of the pelvis to asses for tumor size, location, degree of extension into the endocervical canal, cervical length, and the distance between the upper extent of the lesion and the uterine isthmus [77]. At the time of the procedure, a pelvic lymphadenectomy is performed, if indicated. If there is presence of lymph node metastasis, then the radical trachelectomy is contraindicated. At the end of the procedure, a permanent abdominal cerclage is placed at the level of the isthmus. The morbidity of this procedure is similar to that of radical hysterectomy with an intraoperative complication rate of 2.5% and postoperative complication rate of 21% [139]. Up to 15% of patients develop cervical stenosis which can cause dysmenorrhea, hematometria, hematosalpinx, and endometriosis which result in infertility [140–142]. Cervical stenosis makes it difficult to perform intrauterine insemination or embryo transfer in patients undergoing *in vitro* fertilization. The recurrence rate after this procedure ranges from 0 to 7.5% with a mean of 4% [143]. Risk factors for recurrence include large tumor size (>2 cm), LVI and nonsquamous histology [139]. A review of the literature on pregnancy outcome reported that 42% of pregnancies resulted in a full-term delivery. The rate of preterm delivery was 25% but only half of these deliveries ended with significant prematurity [144]. Another retrospective review of 31 pregnancies after a radical abdominal trachelectomy documented a pregnancy rate of 36.2% for those patients that wished to conceive, 11.8% preterm birth between 29 and 32 weeks, 64.7% preterm birth between 32 and 37 weeks, and 23.5% delivery at full term [145].

Cervical Cancer in Pregnancy

Cervical cancer is the second most common solid tumor diagnosed in pregnancy with an incidence of 1 in 1,000 to 1 in 2,500 pregnancies [146, 147]. Most patients are diagnosed at an early stage and the prognosis is similar to their nonpregnant counterparts [148]. Symptomatology is similar to that of nonpregnant patients. Most patients are asymptomatic and are diagnosed at the time of prenatal evaluation, given a Pap test is a routine test if not recently done prior to the pregnancy. The diagnosis is established with a colposcopically-directed cervical biopsy following the receipt of an abnormal Pap test report.

Counseling, balancing the need for treatment and continuation of pregnancy, is discussed with the patient when a diagnosis of invasive cervical cancer occurs during pregnancy. Treatment varies depending on gestational age, stage of disease, and maternal wishes regarding the pregnancy. CKC can be performed in pregnancy. If CKC is to be performed during pregnancy, the ideal time is during the early second trimester between 14 and 20 weeks, often with a cerclage at the same procedure [149, 150]. As in the nonpregnant patient, the clinical stage of disease is determined. For patients with grossly visible tumors, additional imaging with MRI of abdomen and pelvis and CXR with abdominal shielding is performed.

All patients, except for stage IA1 cervical cancer, should be delivered via cesarean section. Patients with stage IA1 cervical cancer diagnosed on CKC with negative margins and negative LVI can safely be observed during pregnancy with pelvic examinations and colposcopy every trimester until delivery [151]. At 6–8 weeks postpartum, a repeat Pap test, colposcopy with biopsy, and endocervical curettage is performed. Patients who have completed child bearing can undergo an extrafascial hysterectomy; if fertility conservation is desired, observation with serial Pap test is performed.

Patients with positive margins on CKC have a 22% risk of residual disease in the uterus [82]. These patients should be followed closely with clinical examination and colposcopy and delivered via cesarean section.

Definitive treatment follows the same standards as in nonpregnant patients and is based on stage. A cesarean radical hysterectomy can be performed at delivery. Cesarean radical hysterectomy is associated with higher intraoperative blood loss when compared to a radical hysterectomy in a nongravid uterus but other perioperative morbidities such as hospital stay, return of bladder function, wound infection, are not different between the two groups [152, 153].

Patients with an early gestation who desire to terminate the pregnancy can undergo a radical hysterectomy with the fetus *in situ* if indicated or as allowable by treatment location. For gestations under 20 weeks, radiation is an option. With pelvic radiation, the pregnancy is terminated in up to 70% of patients [147]. For gestational age over 20 weeks, pregnancy loss is less reliable and prolonged and can result in significant bleeding, therefore evacuation of the fetus prior to definitive radiation treatment is recommended [154]. Neoadjuvant chemotherapy is an option for patients who wish to delay definitive therapy for fetal lung maturity. Cisplatin, used in the second and third trimester of pregnancy, is efficacious and safe and is an option for patients who desire to delay definitive treatment until fetal lung maturity. A meta-analysis of platinum in pregnant patients with cervical cancer reported that 93.5% of patients were stage I–II, and 6.5% were advanced stage. Squamous cell carcinoma was the most common histology. The mean gestational age at diagnosis was 19.5 weeks and the mean gestational age at initiation of chemotherapy was 23.9 weeks [155]. The chemotherapy agents used were cisplatin, as monotherapy or in combination with bleomycin, 5-FU, paclitaxel, or vincristine, and carboplatin with paclitaxel. Response rates included 10% complete response, 63.4% partial response and 23.3% stable disease. Progression of disease occurred in 3.3% of patients. There was minimal toxicity to the mother and over 65% of neonates were completely healthy. Median PFS in this cohort was 48.5 months [155]. Fetal toxicities associated with administration of cisplatin include intrauterine growth restriction, hearing loss, and transient neutropenia in the newborn. The latter can be prevented by avoiding cisplatin within 3 weeks of anticipated delivery [156, 157]. The overall prognosis of cervical cancer during pregnancy is good with a 5-year survival rate of 80% [158, 159].

Neoadjuvant Chemotherapy

Neoadjuvant chemotherapy followed by radical surgery in women with locally advanced cervical cancer has been investigated. The benefits of neoadjuvant chemotherapy include treatment of micrometastasis, tumor reduction to allow for resectability of disease, especially as an alternative to chemoradiotherapy in areas where there is limited access to radiotherapy. Chemotherapy prior to RT has been shown to achieve a pathologic as well as a clinical response, improvement in OS and PFS and a significant reduction in need for postoperative RT [160–162]. Currently the European Organization for Research and Treatment of Cancer is undergoing a phase III randomized trial comparing chemotherapy followed by surgery to chemotherapy plus radiotherapy in patients with stage IB or II cervical cancer [163]. In the US, concomitant chemoradiotherapy continues to be the preferred treatment for locally advanced cervical cancer.

Postoperative Treatment

The requirement of additional treatment after completion of radical hysterectomy with lymphadenectomy is based on criteria associated with increased risk of recurrence, including: LVI, tumor size, depth of stromal invasion, lymph node involvement, positive margins, and parametrial involvement. One study compared radical hysterectomy and lymph node dissection to radical hysterectomy and lymph node dissection followed by RT in patients who exhibit two or more of the following: LVI, greater than one-third cervical stromal invasion, and large tumor diameter [164]. There was a 47% reduction in risk of recurrence in the RT group but an increase in grade 3/4 toxicity of 6% in the RT group compared to the observation group. A follow-up evaluation noted a decreased risk of progression and death ($P = 0.009$) in the RT group but no statistically significant improvement in OS ($P = 0.07$) [165]. However, the group that received postoperative RT were high risk and thus would be expected to have a poorer 5-year survival.

In one study, patients with high-risk features were randomized to concomitant chemoradiotherapy with cisplatin and 5-FU and pelvic RT, versus pelvic RT only [166]. The PFS and OS were significantly improved in the chemotherapy and RT group when compared to the RT group. There were more grade 3 and 4 toxicities, which were mostly hematologic, in the chemoradiotherapy group. The authors concluded that the addition of chemotherapy to RT improved PFS and OS and was well tolerated. Concomitant chemoradiotherapy is the current standard for adjuvant treatment in patients who have completed radical hysterectomy and pelvic lymph node dissection who are at risk for recurrence.

For patients with small cell/neuroendocrine histology, if not treated with primary chemotherapy and radiation, additional treatment with systemic chemotherapy with cisplatin and etoposide is recommended due to the overall poor prognosis of these patients and the propensity for early systemic spread [167].

Recurrence

Recurrent cervical cancer is classified as local–regional recurrence or distant recurrence. The most common sites for local–regional recurrence are the cervix, vaginal cuff, and pelvis. The most common sites for distant recurrence include the lung (21%), para-aortic nodes (11%), abdominal cavity (8%), and supraclavicular lymph nodes (7%) [168]. Risk factors for recurrence include lymph node involvement, parametrial involvement, surgical margin involvement, deep stromal invasion, large tumor size, and LVI [169–171]. The risk of pelvic failure alone or with distant metastasis increases with the stage of disease. For stage IB, IIA, IIB, III, and IVA disease, the risk of recurrence is 13–16%, 22–31%, 22–26%, 32–39%, and 75% respectively [168].The majority of recurrences occur within 2 years from the time of diagnosis [172]. The treatment of choice for recurrent cervical cancer depends on the location of the recurrence, the type of primary therapy, the disease-free interval and medical comorbidities.

Local–Regional Recurrence

Single local or central recurrences may be curable with surgery or radiation or a combination, depending on the initial therapy. Candidates for surgical resection include patients with a central pelvic recurrence, small tumor size, and long disease-free interval [173]. Patients with stage IB–IIA who have undergone primary RT or concomitant chemoradiotherapy for their primary treatment, who have recurrent tumor size <4 cm are candidates for radical hysterectomy for the management of their central recurrence [174]. The 5-year survival rate for patients treated with radical hysterectomy after recurrence ranges from 49 to 84% [174, 175]. Tumor size <2 cm is associated with a 90% 5-year survival rate [170]. The complication rate ranges from 31 to 50% with a fistula rate of 26% and recurrences up to 59% [174, 176].

Patients who have not been exposed to previous RT or who decline to proceed with pelvic exenteration can be treated with RT, with or without chemotherapy. RT can obtain a pelvic control rate of 62–66% and a 5-year survival of 43% in patients with recurrent cervical cancer after prior surgery [177].

For patients that have had a previous hysterectomy or a large central pelvic recurrence, with or without radiation, the treatment of choice for recurrent disease is a pelvic exenteration. Pelvic exenteration involves the removal of the uterus (if present), bladder if involved, rectum if involved, parametria, vagina and vulva if involved. Urinary diversion is necessary if the bladder is removed and can be performed as a continent or incontinent conduit. If the rectosigmoid is removed, a low rectal reanastomosis is an option if the anus is intact; otherwise a sigmoid end colostomy is performed. Reconstruction of the vagina can be performed using various procedures including myocutaneous flaps [178–180]. Pelvic exenteration is associated with up to 70% morbidity and includes complications from the surgical procedure such as hemorrhage, sepsis, thromboembolic events as well as late complications such as fistula, chronic urinary tract infection, obstruction, and renal insufficiency [181, 182]. The perioperative mortality ranges from 2 to 4.5% and the 5-year survival is 47% [178, 183]. Patient selection is important as well as extensive patient counseling prior to surgery.

Distant Recurrences

For patients with single site distant recurrences such as isolated lung recurrence or para-aortic lymph nodes, surgical resection followed by chemotherapy and/or RT is an option. Recurrence in the lymph nodes carries with it a poor prognosis with a 5-year survival rate of <25% [184]. If, however, there is an isolated pulmonary recurrence, generally there is a better prognosis after resection followed by chemotherapy [185]. For patients who are not candidates for surgical excision or RT, then chemotherapy is the only option and prognosis is very poor.

Surveillance

The goal for surveillance after primary therapy is early detection of recurrent disease. Surveillance can help identify early signs of late treatment-related toxicities. The following should be performed in follow up for patients with cervical cancer [186]:

1) History and physical examination including a pelvic and rectovaginal examination should be performed by an experienced clinician every 3–4 months for the first 2 years, then every 6 months for the next 3 years, then annually. This examination alone detected a median of 52% of asymptomatic recurrences.
2) Cervical and/or vaginal cytology does not significantly add to clinical examination in detecting recurrences. A median of 6% of asymptomatic recurrences were detected on cervico-vaginal cytology. However, it might be of help as an adjunct test, given its ease of performance and can be performed annually. There can be false positive results with prior pelvic radiation.
3) Imaging: CXR detected asymptomatic recurrences in 20–47% of patients. Early detection allows for potential resection of isolated nodules followed by chemotherapy for curative intent. CT scan detected recurrences in 0–34% of asymptomatic patients. Although PET was not addressed in this study, it has a sensitivity of 85% in detecting recurrences in patients with an abnormal finding [187].

Serum tumor marker squamous cell antigen has not been shown to be a sensitive marker for early recurrence and does not alter survival [188]. For low-risk patients (early-stage disease treated with surgery alone, no adjuvant treatment, history and physical examination every 6 months for the first 2 years, then annually is recommended. Imaging such as CT or PET should be performed if recurrence is suspected [189, 190].

Conclusion

Cervical cancer screening is very effective and allows for the prevention, early diagnosis, and treatment of cervical cancer with high cure rates. Tragically, cervical cancer remains the second most common cause of cancer-related death in women aged 20–39 years in the US, the third most common cancer among women worldwide, and the fourth ranking cause of death from cancer worldwide among women [1]. The implementation of prophylactic vaccination against HPV will reduce cervical cancer in the US and worldwide [191]. Despite advances in surgical techniques, chemotherapy agents and radiation delivery, mortality from recurrent cervical cancer is high. Further research to identify those patients at risk for recurrence, and further development of novel cytotoxic and targeted biologic agents with minimal toxicity, are needed to impact mortality.

References

1 Siegel RL, Miller KD, Jemal A. Cancer statistics, 2017. *CA Cancer J Clin* 2017;67(1):7–30.

2 Howlader N, Noone AM, Krapcho M, *et al.* (eds) SEER Cancer Statistics Review, 1975–2013, National Cancer Institute. Bethesda, MD. http://seer.cancer.gov/csr/1975_2013/, based on November 2015 SEER data submission, posted to the SEER web site, April 2016.

3 Torre LA, Bray F, Siegel RL, *et al.* Global cancer statistics, 2012. *CA Cancer J Clin* 2015;65(2):87–108.

4 Sankaranarayanan R, Nene BM, Shastri SS, *et al.* HPV screening for cervical cancer in rural India. *N Eng J Med* 2009;360(14):1385–94.

5 Burk RD, Ho GY, Beardsley L, *et al.* Sexual behavior and partner characteristics are the predominant risk factors for genital human papillomavirus infection in young women. *J Infect Dis* 1996;174(4):679–89.

6 Murthy NS, Mathew A. Risk factors for pre-cancerous lesions of the cervix. *Eur J Cancer Prev* 2000;9(1):5–14.

7 Winer RL, Lee SK, Hughes J, *et al.* Genital human papillomavirus infection: incidence and risk factors in a cohort of female university students. *Am J Epidemiol* 2003;157(3):218–26.

8 Schiffman M, Castle PE. Human papillomavirus: epidemiology and public health. *Arch Pathol Lab Med* 2003;127(8):930–4.

9 Svare EI, Kjaer SK, Worm AM, *et al.* Risk factors for genital HPV DNA in men resemble those found in women: a study of male attendees at a Danish STD clinic. *Sex Transm Infect* 2002;78(3):215–8.

10 Strickler HD, Burk RD, Fazzari M, *et al.* Natural history and possible reactivation of human papillomavirus in human immunodeficiency virus-positive women. *J Natl Cancer Inst* 2005;97(8):577–86.

11 International Collaboration of Epidemiological Studies of Cervical Cancer. Cervical carcinoma and reproductive factors: collaborative reanalysis of individual data on 16,563 women with cervical carcinoma and 33,542 women without cervical carcinoma from 25 epidemiological studies. *Int J Cancer* 2006;119(5):1108–24.

12 Appleby P, Beral V, Berrington de González A, *et al.* Carcinoma of the cervix and tobacco smoking: collaborative reanalysis of individual data on 13,541 women with carcinoma of the cervix and 23,017 women without carcinoma of the cervix from 23 epidemiological studies. *Int J Cancer* 2006;118(6):1481–95.

13 International Collaboration of Epidemiological Studies of Cervical Cancer. Comparison of risk factors for invasive squamous cell carcinoma and adenocarcinoma of the cervix: collaborative reanalysis of individual data on 8,097 women with squamous cell carcinoma and 1,374 women with adenocarcinoma from 12 epidemiological studies. *Int J Cancer* 2007;120(4):885–91.

14 Luhn P, Walker J, Schiffman M, *et al.* The role of co-factors in the progression from human papillomavirus infection to cervical cancer. *Gynecol Oncol* 2013;128(2):265–70.

15 Einstein MH, Leanza S, Chiu LG, *et al.* Genetic variants in TAP are associated with high-grade cervical neoplasia. *Clin Cancer Res* 2009;15(3):1019–23.

16 Safaeian M, Hildesheim A, Gonzalez P, *et al.* Single nucleotide polymorphisms in the PRDX3 and RPS19 and risk of HPV persistence and cervical precancer/cancer. *PloS one* 2012;7(4):e33619.

17 Hildesheim A, Wang CP. Genetic predisposition factors and nasopharyngeal carcinoma risk: a review of epidemiological association studies, 2000–2011: Rosetta Stone for NPC: genetics, viral infection, and other environmental factors. *Semin Cancer Biol* 2012;22(2):107–16.

18 Cogliano V, Baan R, Straif K, *et al.* Carcinogenicity of human papillomaviruses. *Lancet Oncol* 2005;6(4):204.

19 Manhart LE, Holmes KK, Koutsky LA, *et al.* Human papillomavirus infection among sexually active young women in the United States: implications for developing a vaccination strategy. *Sex Transm Dis* 2006;33(8):502–8.

20 Li N, Franceschi S, Howell-Jones R, Snijders PJ, Clifford GM. Human papillomavirus type distribution in 30,848 invasive cervical cancers worldwide: Variation by geographical region, histological type and year of publication. *Int J Cancer* 2011;128(4):927–35.

21 Munoz N, Bosch FX, de Sanjosé S, *et al.* Epidemiologic classification of human papillomavirus types associated with cervical cancer. *N Eng J Med* 2003;348(6):518–27.

22 Hariri S, Unger ER, Powell SE, *et al.* Human papillomavirus genotypes in high-grade cervical lesions in the United States. *J Infect Dis* 2012;206(12):1878–86.

23 Schlecht NF, Platt RW, Duarte-Franco E, *et al.* Human papillomavirus infection and time to progression and regression of cervical intraepithelial neoplasia. *J Natl Cancer Inst* 2003;95(17):1336–43.

24 McCredie MR, Paul C, Sharples KJ, *et al.* Consequences in women of participating in a study of the natural history of cervical intraepithelial neoplasia 3. *Aust NZ J Obstet Gynaecol* 2010;50(4):363–70.

25 Rapiti E, Usel M, Neyroud-Caspar I, *et al.* Omission of excisional therapy is associated with an increased risk of invasive cervical cancer after cervical intraepithelial neoplasia III. *Eur J Cancer* 2012;48(6):845–52.

26 Hildesheim A, Hadjimichael O, Schwartz PE, *et al.* Risk factors for rapid-onset cervical cancer. *Am J Obstet Gynecol* 1999;180(3):571–7.

27 Moscicki AB, Shiboski S, Hills NK, *et al.* Regression of low-grade squamous intra-epithelial lesions in young women. *Lancet* 2004;364(9446):1678–83.
28 McCredie MR, Sharples KJ, Paul C, *et al.* Natural history of cervical neoplasia and risk of invasive cancer in women with cervical intraepithelial neoplasia 3: a retrospective cohort study. *Lancet Oncol* 2008;9(5):425–34.
29 Schwartz PE, Hadjimichael O, Lowell DM, Merino MJ, Janerich D. Rapidly progressive cervical cancer: the Connecticut experience. *Am J Obstet Gynecol* 1996;175(4):1105–9.
30 Duguid HL, Duncan ID, Currie J. Screening for cervical intraepithelial neoplasia in Dundee and Angus 1962–81 and its relation with invasive cervical cancer. *Lancet* 1985;2(8463):1053–6.
31 Nieminen P, Kallio M, Hakama M. The effect of mass screening on incidence and mortality of squamous and adenocarcinoma of cervix uteri. *Obs Gynecol* 1995;85(6):1017–21.
32 Parkin DM, Nguyen-Dinh X, Day NE. The impact of screening on the incidence of cervical cancer in England and Wales. *Br J Obstet Gynaecol* 1985;92(2):150–7.
33 Quinn M, Babb P, Jones J, Allen E. Effect of screening on incidence of and mortality from cancer of cervix in England: evaluation based on routinely collected statistics. *BMJ* 1999;318(7188):904–8.
34 Howlader N, Noone AM, Krapcho M, Garshell J, *et al.* (eds). SEER Cancer Statistics Review, 1975–2010, 2013 National Cancer Institute. Bethesda, MD. http://seer.cancer.gov/csr/1975_2010/, based on November 2012 SEER data submission, posted to the SEER web site, April 2013.
35 ACOG Practice Bulletin no. 109: Cervical cytology screening. *Obs Gynecol* 2009;114(6):1409–20.
36 Kulasingam SL, Hughes JP, Kiviat NB, *et al.* Evaluation of human papillomavirus testing in primary screening for cervical abnormalities: comparison of sensitivity, specificity, and frequency of referral. *JAMA* 2002;288(14):1749–57.
37 Franco EL. Chapter 13: Primary screening of cervical cancer with human papillomavirus tests. *J Natl Cancer Inst Monograph* 2003(31):89–96.
38 Saslow D, Solomon D, Lawson HW, *et al.* American Cancer Society, American Society for Colposcopy and Cervical Pathology, and American Society for Clinical Pathology screening guidelines for the prevention and early detection of cervical cancer. *CA Cancer J Clin* 2012;62(3):147–72.
39 Moyer VA. Screening for cervical cancer: U.S. Preventive Services Task Force recommendation statement. *Ann Intern Med* 2012;156(12):880–91, W312.
40 ACOG Practice Bulletin Number 131: Screening for cervical cancer. *Obs Gynecol* 2012;120(5):1222–38.
41 Cuzick J, Szarewski A, Cubie H, *et al.* Management of women who test positive for high-risk types of human papillomavirus: the HART study. *Lancet* 2003;362(9399):1871–6.
42 Smith JS, Lindsay L, Hoots B, *et al.* Human papillomavirus type distribution in invasive cervical cancer and high-grade cervical lesions: a meta-analysis update. *Int J Cancer* 2007;121(3):621–32.
43 FUTURE II Study Group. Quadrivalent vaccine against human papillomavirus to prevent high-grade cervical lesions. *N Eng J Med* 2007;356(19):1915–27.
44 Kahn JA, Burk RD. Papillomavirus vaccines in perspective. *Lancet* 2007;369(9580):2135–7.
45 FUTURE II Study Group. Prophylactic efficacy of a quadrivalent human papillomavirus (HPV) vaccine in women with virological evidence of HPV infection. *J Infect Dis* 2007;196(10):1438–46.
46 Hildesheim A, Herrero R, Wacholder S, *et al.* Effect of human papillomavirus 16/18 L1 viruslike particle vaccine among young women with preexisting infection: a randomized trial. *JAMA* 2007;298(7):743–53.
47 Paavonen, J, Naud P, Salmerón J, *et al.* Efficacy of human papillomavirus (HPV)-16/18 AS04-adjuvanted vaccine against cervical infection and precancer caused by oncogenic HPV types (PATRICIA): final analysis of a double-blind, randomised study in young women. *Lancet* 2009;374(9686):301–14.
48 Wheeler CM, Castellsagué X, Garland SM, *et al.* Cross-protective efficacy of HPV-16/18 AS04-adjuvanted vaccine against cervical infection and precancer caused by non-vaccine oncogenic HPV types: 4-year end-of-study analysis of the randomised, double-blind PATRICIA trial. *Lancet Oncol* 2012;13(1):100–10.
49 Kahn JA, Brown DR, Ding L, *et al.* Vaccine-type human papillomavirus and evidence of herd protection after vaccine introduction. *Pediatrics* 2012;130(2):e249–56.
50 Malagon T, Drolet M, Boily MC, *et al.* Cross-protective efficacy of two human papillomavirus vaccines: a systematic review and meta-analysis. *Lancet Infect Dis* 2012;12(10):781–9.
51 Einstein MH, Baron M, Levin MJ, *et al.* Comparison of the immunogenicity of the human papillomavirus (HPV)-16/18 vaccine and the HPV-6/11/16/18 vaccine for oncogenic non-vaccine types HPV-31 and HPV-45 in healthy women aged 18–45 years. *Hum Vaccin* 2011;7(12):1359–73.
52 Saslow D, Andrews KS, Manassaram-Baptiste D, *et al.* Human papillomavirus vaccination guideline update: American Cancer Society guideline endorsement. *CA Cancer J Clin* 2016;66(5):375–85.
53 Meites E, Kempe A, Markowitz LE. Use of a 2-dose schedule for human papillomavirus vaccination – updated recommendations of the Advisory Committee on Immunization Practices. *MMWR Morb Mortal Wkly* 2016;65:1405–8.
54 Einstein MH, Kadish AS, Burk RD, *et al.* Heat shock fusion protein-based immunotherapy for treatment of cervical intraepithelial neoplasia III. *Gynecol Oncol* 2007;106(3):453–60.
55 Kadish AS, Einstein MH. Vaccine strategies for human papillomavirus-associated cancers. *Curr Opin Oncol* 2005;17(5):456–61.
56 Trimble CL, Peng S, Kos F, *et al.* A phase I trial of a human papillomavirus DNA vaccine for HPV16+ cervical intraepithelial neoplasia 2/3. *Clin Cancer Res* 2009;15(1):361–7.
57 Stern PL, van der Burg SH, Hampson IN, *et al.* Therapy of human papillomavirus-related disease. *Vaccine* 2012;30 Suppl 5:F71–82.
58 Daayana S, Elkord E, Winters U, *et al.* Phase II trial of imiquimod and HPV therapeutic vaccination in patients with vulval intraepithelial neoplasia. *Br J Cancer* 2010;102(7):1129–36.

59 Winters U, Daayana S, Lear JT, *et al.* Clinical and immunologic results of a phase II trial of sequential imiquimod and photodynamic therapy for vulval intraepithelial neoplasia. *Clin Cancer Res* 2008;14(16):5292–9.
60 Massad LS, Einstein MH, Huh WK, *et al.* 2012 updated consensus guidelines for the management of abnormal cervical cancer screening tests and cancer precursors. *J Lower Genit Tract Dis* 2013;17(5 Suppl 1):S1–S27.
61 Forman D, de Martel C, Lacey CJ, *et al.* Global burden of human papillomavirus and related diseases. *Vaccine,* 2012;30(Suppl 5):F12–23.
62 Kasamatsu E, Cubilla AL, Alemany L, *et al.* Type-specific human papillomavirus distribution in invasive cervical carcinomas in Paraguay. A study of 432 cases. *J Med Virol* 2012;84(10):1628–35.
63 Smith HO, Tiffany MF, Qualls CR, Key CR. The rising incidence of adenocarcinoma relative to squamous cell carcinoma of the uterine cervix in the United States – 24-year population-based study. *Gynecol Oncol* 2000;78(2):97–105.
64 Ursin G, Peters RK, Henderson BE, *et al.* Oral contraceptive use and adenocarcinoma of cervix. *Lancet* 1994;344 (8934):1390–4.
65 Herbst AL, Kurman RJ, Scully RE, Poskanzer DC. Clear-cell adenocarcinoma of the genital tract in young females. *Registry report. N Eng J Med* 1972;287(25):1259–64.
66 Kaminski PF, Maier RC. Clear cell adenocarcinoma of the cervix unrelated to diethylstilbestrol exposure. *Obs Gynecol* 1983;62(6):720–7.
67 Albores-Saavedra J, Gersell D, Gilks CB, *et al.* Terminology of endocrine tumors of the uterine cervix: results of a workshop sponsored by the College of American Pathologists and the National Cancer Institute. *Arch Pathol Lab Med* 1997;121(1):34–9.
68 Ambros RA, Park JS, Shah KV, Kurman RJ. Evaluation of histologic, morphometric, and immunohistochemical criteria in the differential diagnosis of small cell carcinomas of the cervix with particular reference to human papillomavirus types 16 and 18. *Mod Pathol* 1991;4(5):586–93.
69 Stoler MH, Mills SE, Gersell DJ, Walker AN. Small-cell neuroendocrine carcinoma of the cervix. A human papillomavirus type 18-associated cancer. *Am J Surg Pathol* 1991;15(1):28–32.
70 van Nagell, JR, Jr, Powell DE, Gallion HH, *et al.* Small cell carcinoma of the uterine cervix. *Cancer* 1988;62(8):1586–93.
71 Lemoine NR, Hall PA. Epithelial tumors metastatic to the uterine cervix. A study of 33 cases and review of the literature. *Cancer* 1986;57(10):2002–5.
72 Pecorelli S. Revised FIGO staging for carcinoma of the vulva, cervix, and endometrium. *Int J Gynaecol Obstet* 2009;105(2):103–4.
73 Erickson, BA, Olawaiye AB, Bermudez A, *et al.* (eds). Cancer Staging Manual, 8th edn. American Joint Committee on Cancer editor. New York: Springer, 2017.
74 Quinn MA, Benedet JL, Odicino F, *et al.* Carcinoma of the cervix uteri. FIGO 26th Annual Report on the Results of Treatment in Gynecological Cancer. Int J Gynaecol Obstet 2006;95 Suppl 1:S43–103.
75 Patel CN, Nazir SA, Khan Z, Gleeson FV, Bradley KM. 18F-FDG PET/CT of cervical carcinoma. *Am J Roentgenol* 2011;196(5):1225–33.
76 Cosin JA, Fowler JM, Chen MD, *et al.* Pretreatment surgical staging of patients with cervical carcinoma: the case for lymph node debulking. *Cancer* 1998;82(11):2241–8.
77 Peppercorn PD, Jeyarajah AR, Woolas R, *et al.* Role of MR imaging in the selection of patients with early cervical carcinoma for fertility-preserving surgery: initial experience. *Radiology* 1999;212(2):395–9.
78 Sahdev A, Sohaib SA, Wenaden AE, Shepherd JH, Reznek RH. The performance of magnetic resonance imaging in early cervical carcinoma: a long-term experience. *Int J Gynecol Cancer* 2007;17(3):629–36.
79 Einstein MH, Phaeton R. Issues in cervical cancer incidence and treatment in HIV. *Curr Opin Oncol* 2010;22(5):449–55.
80 Ostor AG. Pandora's box or Ariadne's thread? Definition and prognostic significance of microinvasion in the uterine cervix. *Squamous lesions. Pathol Ann* 1995;30(2):103–36.
81 Mota F. Microinvasive squamous carcinoma of the cervix: treatment modalities. *Acta Obstet Gynecol Scand* 2003; 82(6):505–9.
82 Roman LD, Felix JC, Muderspach LI, *et al.* Risk of residual invasive disease in women with microinvasive squamous cancer in a conization specimen. *Obs Gynecol* 1997;90(5):759–64.
83 Benedet JL, Anderson GH. Stage IA carcinoma of the cervix revisited. *Obs Gynecol* 1996;87(6):1052–9.
84 Berek JS, Castaldo TW, Hacker NF, *et al.* Adenocarcinoma of the uterine cervix. *Cancer* 1981;48(12):2734–41.
85 Kilgore LC, Soong SJ, Gore H, *et al.* Analysis of prognostic features in adenocarcinoma of the cervix. *Gynecol Oncol* 1988;31(1):137–53.
86 Balega, J, Michael H, Hurteau J, *et al.* The risk of nodal metastasis in early adenocarcinoma of the uterine cervix. *Int J Gynecol Cancer* 2004;14(1):104–9.
87 Bisseling KC, Bekkers RL, Rome RM, Quinn MA. Treatment of microinvasive adenocarcinoma of the uterine cervix: a retrospective study and review of the literature. *Gynecol Oncol* 2007;107(3):424–30.
88 Kasamatsu T, Okada S, Tsuda H, *et al.* Early invasive adenocarcinoma of the uterine cervix: criteria for nonradical surgical treatment. *Gynecol Oncol* 2002;85(2):327–32.
89 Ostor AG. Early invasive adenocarcinoma of the uterine cervix. *Int J Gynecol Pathol* 2000;19(1):29–38.
90 Reynolds EA, Tierney K, Keeney GL, *et al.* Analysis of outcomes of microinvasive adenocarcinoma of the uterine cervix by treatment type. *Obs Gynecol* 2010;116(5):1150–7.
91 Hou J, Goldberg GL, Qualls CR, *et al.* Risk factors for poor prognosis in microinvasive adenocarcinoma of the uterine cervix (IA1 and IA2): a pooled analysis. *Gynecol Oncol* 2011;121(1):135–42.
92 Hasumi K, Sakamoto A, Sugano H. Microinvasive carcinoma of the uterine cervix. *Cancer* 1980;45(5):928–31.
93 van Nagell, JR, Jr, Greenwell N, Powell DF, *et al.* Microinvasive carcinoma of the cervix. *Am J Obstet Gynecol* 1983; 145(8):981–91.
94 Maiman MA, Fruchter RG, DiMaio TM, Boyce JG. Superficially invasive squamous cell carcinoma of the cervix. *Obs Gynecol* 1988;72(3):399–403.
95 Buckley SL, Tritz DM, Van Le L, *et al.* Lymph node metastases and prognosis in patients with stage IA2 cervical cancer. *Gynecol Oncol* 1996;63(1):4–9.

96 Creasman WT, Zaino RJ, Major FJ, *et al.* Early invasive carcinoma of the cervix (3 to 5 mm invasion): risk factors and prognosis. A Gynecologic Oncology Group study. *Am J Obstet Gynecol* 1998;178(1):62–5.

97 Takeshima N, Yanoh K, Tabata T, *et al.* Assessment of the revised International Federation of Gynecology and obstetrics staging for early invasive squamous cervical cancer. *Gynecol Oncol* 1999;74(2):165–9.

98 Landoni F, Maneo A, Colombo A, *et al.* Randomised study of radical surgery versus radiotherapy for stage Ib-IIa cervical cancer. *Lancet* 1997;350(9077):535–40.

99 Hacker NF. Clinical and operative staging of cervical cancer. *Bailliere's Clin Obstet Gynecol* 1988;2(4):747–59.

100 Hacker NF, Wain GV, Nicklin JL. Resection of bulky positive lymph nodes in patients with cervical carcinoma. *Int J Gynecol Cancer* 1995;5(4):250–6.

101 Allen HH, Nisker JA, Anderson RJ. Primary surgical treatment in one hundred ninety-five cases of stage IB carcinoma of the cervix. *Am J Obstet Gynecol* 1982;143(5):581–4.

102 Bansal N, Herzog TJ, Shaw RE, *et al.* Primary therapy for early-stage cervical cancer: radical hysterectomy vs radiation. *Am J Obstet Gynecol* 2009;201(5):485 e1–9.

103 Pikaart DP, Holloway RW, Ahmad S, *et al.* Clinical-pathologic and morbidity analyses of Types 2 and 3 abdominal radical hysterectomy for cervical cancer. *Gynecol Oncol* 2007;107(2):205–10.

104 Sivanesaratnam V, Sen DK, Jayalakshmi P, Ong G. *et al.* Radical hysterectomy and pelvic lymphadenectomy for early invasive cancer of the cervix – 14-year experience. *Int J Gynecol Cancer* 1993;3(4):231–8.

105 Perez CA, Grigsby PW, Chao KS, *et al.* Tumor size, irradiation dose, and long-term outcome of carcinoma of uterine cervix. *Int J Radiat Oncol Biol Phys* 1998;41(2):307–17.

106 Eifel PJ, Morris M, Wharton JT, Oswald MJ. The influence of tumor size and morphology on the outcome of patients with FIGO stage IB squamous cell carcinoma of the uterine cervix. *Int J Radiat Oncol Biol Phys* 1994;29(1):9–16.

107 Montana GS, Fowler WC, Varia MA, *et al.* Analysis of results of radiation therapy for stage IB carcinoma of the cervix. *Cancer* 1987;60(9):2195–200.

108 Cancer: NCAoC and Chemotherapy Plus Radiation Improves Survival. http://www.nih.gov/news/pr/feb99/nci-22.htm.

109 Keys HM, Bundy BN, Stehman FB, *et al.* Radiation therapy with and without extrafascial hysterectomy for bulky stage IB cervical carcinoma: a randomized trial of the Gynecologic Oncology Group. *Gynecol Oncol* 2003;89(3):343–53.

110 Keys HM, Bundy BN, Stehman FB, *et al.* Cisplatin, radiation, and adjuvant hysterectomy compared with radiation and adjuvant hysterectomy for bulky stage IB cervical carcinoma. *N Eng J Med* 1999;340(15):1154–61.

111 Finan MA, DeCesare S, Fiorica JV, *et al.* Radical hysterectomy for stage IB1 vs IB2 carcinoma of the cervix: does the new staging system predict morbidity and survival? *Gynecol Oncol* 1996;62(2):139–47.

112 Morris M, Eifel PJ, Lu J, *et al.* Pelvic radiation with concurrent chemotherapy compared with pelvic and para-aortic radiation for high-risk cervical cancer. *N Eng J Med* 1999;340(15):1137–43.

113 Whitney CW, Sause W, Bundy BN, *et al.* Randomized comparison of fluorouracil plus cisplatin versus hydroxyurea as an adjunct to radiation therapy in stage IIB-IVA carcinoma of the cervix with negative para-aortic lymph nodes: a Gynecologic Oncology Group and Southwest Oncology Group study. *J Clin Oncol* 1999;17(5):1339–48.

114 Rose PG, Bundy BN, Watkins EB, *et al.* Concurrent cisplatin-based radiotherapy and chemotherapy for locally advanced cervical cancer. *N Eng J Med* 1999;340(15):1144–53.

115 Rose PG, Ali S, Watkins E, *et al.* Long-term follow-up of a randomized trial comparing concurrent single agent cisplatin, cisplatin-based combination chemotherapy, or hydroxyurea during pelvic irradiation for locally advanced cervical cancer: a Gynecologic Oncology Group Study. *J Clin Oncol* 2007;25(19):2804–10.

116 Einstein MH, Novetsky AP, Garg M, *et al.* Survival and toxicity differences between 5-day and weekly cisplatin in patients with locally advanced cervical cancer. *Cancer* 2007;109(1):48–53.

117 Kim YS, Shin SS, Nam JH, *et al.* Prospective randomized comparison of monthly fluorouracil and cisplatin versus weekly cisplatin concurrent with pelvic radiotherapy and high dose rate brachytherapy for locally advanced cervical cancer. *Gynecol Oncol* 2008;108(1):195–200.

118 Peters WA, 3rd, Liu PY, Barrett RJ 2nd, *et al.* Concurrent chemotherapy and pelvic radiation therapy compared with pelvic radiation therapy alone as adjuvant therapy after radical surgery in high-risk early-stage cancer of the cervix. *J Clin Oncol* 2000;18(8):1606–13.

119 Kantardzi N, Beslija S, Begic D. [Comparative parameters of myelotoxicity in patients treated with simultaneous chemotherapy and radiotherapy or only radiotherapy]. *Medicinski Arhiv* 2004;58(1):19–22.

120 Duenas-Gonzalez A, Zarbá JJ, Patel F, *et al.* Phase III, open-label, randomized study comparing concurrent gemcitabine plus cisplatin and radiation followed by adjuvant gemcitabine and cisplatin versus concurrent cisplatin and radiation in patients with stage IIB to IVA carcinoma of the cervix. *J Clin Oncol* 2011;29(13):1678–85.

121 Rao GG, Rogers P, Drake RD, Nguyen P, Coleman RL. Phase I clinical trial of weekly paclitaxel, weekly carboplatin, and concurrent radiotherapy for primary cervical cancer. *Gynecol Oncol* 2005;96(1):168–72.

122 Rose PG, Sill MW, McMeekin DS, *et al.* A phase I study of concurrent weekly topotecan and cisplatin chemotherapy with whole pelvic radiation therapy in locally advanced cervical cancer: a gynecologic oncology group study. *Gynecol Oncol* 2012;125(1):158–62.

123 Gatcliffe TA, Tewari KS, Shah A, *et al.* A feasibility study of topotecan with standard-dose cisplatin and concurrent primary radiation therapy in locally advanced cervical cancer. *Gynecol Oncol* 2009;112(1):85–9.

124 Moore K. Cisplatin and Radiation Therapy With or Without Carboplatin and Paclitaxel in Patients With Locally Advanced Cervical Cancer (cited 25 June 2013). Available from: http://clinicaltrials.gov/show/NCT01414608.

125 Fulcher AS, O'Sullivan SG, Segreti EM, Kavanagh BD. Recurrent cervical carcinoma: typical and atypical manifestations. *Radiographics* 1999;19:S103–16; quiz S264–5.

126 Thigpen T, Shingleton H, Homesley H, Lagasse L, Blessing J. Cis-platinum in treatment of advanced or recurrent squamous cell carcinoma of the cervix: a phase II study of the Gynecologic Oncology Group. *Cancer* 1981;48(4):899–903.

127 Bonomi P, Blessing JA, Stehman FB, *et al.* Randomized trial of three cisplatin dose schedules in squamous-cell carcinoma of the cervix: a Gynecologic Oncology Group study. *J Clin Oncol* 1985;3(8):1079–85.

128 Moore DH, Blessing JA, McQuellon RP, *et al.* Phase III study of cisplatin with or without paclitaxel in stage IVB, recurrent, or persistent squamous cell carcinoma of the cervix: a gynecologic oncology group study. *J Clin Oncol* 2004;22(15):3113–9.

129 Scatchard K, Forrest JL, Flubacher M, Cornes P, Williams C. Chemotherapy for metastatic and recurrent cervical cancer. *Cochrane Database Syst Rev* 2012;10:CD006469.

130 Long HJ, 3rd, Bundy BN, Grendys EC Jr, *et al.* Randomized phase III trial of cisplatin with or without topotecan in carcinoma of the uterine cervix: a Gynecologic Oncology Group Study. *J Clin Oncol* 2005;23(21):4626–33.

131 Monk BJ, Sill MW, McMeekin DS, *et al.* Phase III trial of four cisplatin-containing doublet combinations in stage IVB, recurrent, or persistent cervical carcinoma: a Gynecologic Oncology Group study. *J Clin Oncol* 2009;27(28):4649–55.

132 Hirte H, Kennedy EB, Elit L, Fung Kee Fung, M. Systemic therapy for recurrent, persistent, or metastatic cervical cancer: a clinical practice guideline. *Curr Oncol* 2015; 22:211–19

133 Pfaendler KS, Tewari KS. Changing paradigms in the systemic treatment of advanced cervical cancer. *Am J Obstet Gynecol* 2016;214:22–30

134 Kitagawa R, Katsumata N, Shibata T, *et al.* A randomized, phase III trial of paclitaxel plus carboplatin (TC) versus paclitaxle plus cisplatin (TP) in stage IVb, persistent or recurrent cervical cancer: Japan Clinical Oncology Group Study (JCOG0505). J Clin Oncol 2012;30(Abstr 500).

135 Kuo DY, Blank SV, Christos PJ, *et al.* Paclitaxel plus oxaliplatin for recurrent or metastatic cervical cancer: a New York Cancer Consortium Study. *Gynecol Oncol* 2010;116(3):442–6.

136 Tewari, K. Incorporation of bevacizumab in the treatment of recurrent and metastatic cervical cancer: a phase III randomized trial of the Gynecologic Oncology Group. 2013 ASCO Annual Meeting. J Clin Oncol 2013;31(suppl; abstr 3).

137 http://www.cancer.gov/newscenter/newsfromnci/2013/GOG240 (accessed 11 October 2017).

138 Roy M, Plante M. Pregnancies after radical vaginal trachelectomy for early-stage cervical cancer. *Am J Obstet Gynecol* 1998;179(6):1491–6.

139 Marchiole P, Benchaib M, Buenerd A, *et al.* Oncological safety of laparoscopic-assisted vaginal radical trachelectomy (LARVT or Dargent's operation): a comparative study with laparoscopic-assisted vaginal radical hysterectomy (LARVH). *Gynecol Oncol* 2007;106(1):132–41.

140 Boss EA, van Golde RJ, Beerendonk CC, Massuger LF. Pregnancy after radical trachelectomy: a real option? *Gynecol Oncol* 2005;99(3 Suppl 1):S152–6.

141 Alexander-Sefre, F, Chee N, Spencer C, Menon U, Shepherd JH. Surgical morbidity associated with radical trachelectomy and radical hysterectomy. *Gynecol Oncol* 2006;101(3):450–4.

142 Selo-Ojeme DO, Ind T, Shepherd JH. Isthmic stenosis following radical trachelectomy. *J Obstet Gynaecol* 2002;22(3):327–8.

143 Sonoda Y, Chi DS, Carter J, Barakat RR, Abu-Rustum NR. Initial experience with Dargent's operation: the radical vaginal trachelectomy. *Gynecol Oncol* 2008;108(1):214–9.

144 Jolley JA, Battista L, Wing DA. Management of pregnancy after radical trachelectomy: case reports and systematic review of the literature. *Am J Perinatol* 2007;24(9):531–9.

145 Nishio H, Fujii T, Sugiyama J, *et al.* Reproductive and obstetric outcomes after radical abdominal trachelectomy for early-stage cervical cancer in a series of 31 pregnancies. *Hum Reprod* 2013;28(7):1793–8.

146 Pavlidis NA. Coexistence of pregnancy and malignancy. *Oncologist* 2002;7(4):279–87.

147 Sood AK, Sorosky JI. Invasive cervical cancer complicating pregnancy. How to manage the dilemma. *Obstet Gynecol Clin North Am* 1998;25(2):343–52.

148 Zemlickis D, Lishner M, Degendorfer P, *et al.* Maternal and fetal outcome after invasive cervical cancer in pregnancy. *J Clin Oncol* 1991;9(11):1956–61.

149 Muller CY, Smith HO. Cervical neoplasia complicating pregnancy. *Obstet Gynecol Clin North Am* 2005;32(4):533–46.

150 Goldberg G, Altaras MM, Block B. Cone cerclage in pregnancy. *Obs Gynecol* 1991;77(2):315–7.

151 Takushi M, Moromizato H, Sakumoto K, Kanazawa K. Management of invasive carcinoma of the uterine cervix associated with pregnancy: outcome of intentional delay in treatment. *Gynecol Oncol* 2002;87(2):185–9.

152 Sood AK, Sorosky JI, Krogman S, *et al.* Surgical management of cervical cancer complicating pregnancy: a case-control study. *Gynecol Oncol* 1996;63(3):294–8.

153 Monk BJ, Montz FJ. Invasive cervical cancer complicating intrauterine pregnancy: treatment with radical hysterectomy. *Obstet Gynecol* 1992;80(2):199–203.

154 Prem KA, Makowski EL, McKelvey JL. Carcinoma of the cervix associated with pregnancy. *Am J Obstet Gynecol* 1966;95(1):99–108.

155 Zagouri F, Sergentanis TN, Chrysikos D, Bartsch R. Platinum derivatives during pregnancy in cervical cancer: a systematic review and meta-analysis. *Obstet Gynecol* 2013;121(2): 337–43.

156 Caluwaerts S, VAN Calsteren K, Mertens L, *et al.* Neoadjuvant chemotherapy followed by radical hysterectomy for invasive cervical cancer diagnosed during pregnancy: report of a case and review of the literature. *Int J Gynecol Cancer* 2006;16(2):905–8.

157 Weisz B, Meirow D, Schiff E, Lishner M. Impact and treatment of cancer during pregnancy. *Expert Rev Anticancer Ther* 2004;4(5):889–902.

158 Karam A, Feldman N, Holschneider CH. Neoadjuvant cisplatin and radical cesarean hysterectomy for cervical cancer in pregnancy. *Nat Clin Pract Oncol* 2007;4(6):375–80.

159 van der Vange, N, Weverling GJ, Ketting BW, *et al.* The prognosis of cervical cancer associated with pregnancy: a matched cohort study. *Obstet Gynecol*, 1995;85(6):1022–6.

160 Dottino PR, Segna RA. Neoadjuvant chemotherapy in cervix cancer. *Cancer Treat Res* 1994;70:63–71.

161 Rydzewska L, Tierney J, Vale CL, Symonds PR. Neoadjuvant chemotherapy plus surgery versus surgery for cervical cancer. *Cochrane Database Syst Rev* 2012;12:CD007406.

162 Katsumata N, Yoshikawa H, Kobayashi H, *et al.* Phase III randomised controlled trial of neoadjuvant chemotherapy plus radical surgery vs radical surgery alone for stages IB2, IIA2, and IIB cervical cancer: a Japan Clinical Oncology Group trial (JCOG 0102). *Br J Cancer* 2013;108(10):1957–63.

163 http://clinicaltrials.gov/ct2/show/NCT00039338 (accessed 11 October 2017).

164 Sedlis A, Bundy BN, Rotman MZ, *et al.* A randomized trial of pelvic radiation therapy versus no further therapy in selected patients with stage IB carcinoma of the cervix after radical hysterectomy and pelvic lymphadenectomy: a Gynecologic Oncology Group Study. *Gynecol Oncol* 1999;73(2):177–83.

165 Rotman M, Sedlis A, Piedmonte MR, *et al.* A phase III randomized trial of postoperative pelvic irradiation in Stage IB cervical carcinoma with poor prognostic features: follow-up of a gynecologic oncology group study. *Int J Radiat Oncol Biol Phys* 2006;65(1):169–76.

166 Peters WA, 3rd, Liu PY, Barrett RJ 2nd, *et al.* Concurrent chemotherapy and pelvic radiation therapy compared with pelvic radiation therapy alone as adjuvant therapy after radical surgery in high-risk early-stage cancer of the cervix. *J Clin Oncol* 2000;18(8):1606–13.

167 Gardner GJ, Reidy-Lagunes D, Gehrig PA. Neuroendocrine tumors of the gynecologic tract: A Society of Gynecologic Oncology (SGO) clinical document. *Gynecol Oncol* 2011;122(1):190–8.

168 Fagundes H, Perez CA, Grigsby PW, Lockett MA. Distant metastases after irradiation alone in carcinoma of the uterine cervix. *Int J Radiat Oncol Biol Phys* 1992;24(2):197–204.

169 Morley GW, Seski JC. Radical pelvic surgery versus radiation therapy for stage I carcinoma of the cervix (exclusive of microinvasion). *Am J Obstet Gynecol* 1976;126(7):785–98.

170 Hopkins MP, Morley GW. Radical hysterectomy versus radiation therapy for stage IB squamous cell cancer of the cervix. *Cancer* 1991;68(2):272–7.

171 Estape RE, Angioli R, Madrigal M, *et al.* Close vaginal margins as a prognostic factor after radical hysterectomy. *Gynecol Oncol* 1998;68(3):229–32.

172 Webb MJ, Symmonds RE. Site of recurrence of cervical cancer after radical hysterectomy. *Am J Obstet Gynecol* 1980;138(7):813–7.

173 Friedlander M, Grogan M, USPST Force. Guidelines for the treatment of recurrent and metastatic cervical cancer. *Oncologist* 2002;7(4):342–7.

174 Rutledge S, Carey MS, Prichard H, *et al.* Conservative surgery for recurrent or persistent carcinoma of the cervix following irradiation: is exenteration always necessary? *Gynecol Oncol* 1994;52(3):353–9.

175 Coleman RL, Keeney ED, Freedman RS, *et al.* Radical hysterectomy for recurrent carcinoma of the uterine cervix after radiotherapy. *Gynecol Oncol* 1994;55(1):29–35.

176 Maneo A, Landoni F, Cormio G, Colombo A, Mangioni C. Radical hysterectomy for recurrent or persistent cervical cancer following radiation therapy. *Int J Gynecol Cancer* 1999;9(4):295–301.

177 Haasbeek CJ, Uitterhoeve AL, van der Velden J, González DG, Stalpers LJ. Long-term results of salvage radiotherapy for the treatment of recurrent cervical carcinoma after prior surgery. *Radiother Oncol* 2008;89(2):197–204.

178 Goldberg GL, Sukumvanich P, Einstein MH, *et al.* Total pelvic exenteration: the Albert Einstein College of Medicine/Montefiore Medical Center Experience (1987 to 2003). *Gynecol Oncol* 2006;101(2):261–8.

179 Goldberg GL. Total pelvic exenteration: the reconstructive phase. *Gynecol Oncol* 2005;99(3 Suppl 1):S149.

180 Smith HO, Genesen MC, Runowicz CD, Goldberg GL. The rectus abdominis myocutaneous flap: modifications, complications, and sexual function. *Cancer* 1998;83(3):510–20.

181 Fotopoulou C, Neumann U, Kraetschell R, *et al.* Long-term clinical outcome of pelvic exenteration in patients with advanced gynecological malignancies. *J Surg Oncol* 2010;101(6):507–12.

182 Maggioni A, Roviglione G, Landoni F, *et al.* Pelvic exenteration: ten-year experience at the European Institute of Oncology in Milan. *Gynecol Oncol* 2009;114(1):64–8.

183 Peiretti M, Zapardiel I, Zanagnolo V, *et al.* Management of recurrent cervical cancer: a review of the literature. *Surg Oncol* 2012;21(2):e59–66.

184 Hong JH, Tsai CS, Lai CH, *et al.* Recurrent squamous cell carcinoma of cervix after definitive radiotherapy. *Int J Radiat Oncol Biol Phys* 2004;60(1):249–57.

185 Shiromizu K, Kasamatsu T, Honma T, *et al.* Clinicopathological study of recurrent uterine cervical squamous-cell carcinoma. *J Obstet Gynaecol Res* 1999;25(6):395–9.

186 Elit L, Fyles AW, Oliver TK, *et al.* Follow-up for women after treatment for cervical cancer. *Curr Oncol* 2010;17(3):65–9.

187 Chung HH, Kim SK, Kim TH, *et al.* Clinical impact of FDG-PET imaging in post-therapy surveillance of uterine cervical cancer: from diagnosis to prognosis. *Gynecol Oncol* 2006;103(1):165–70.

188 Esajas MD, Duk JM, de Bruijn HW, *et al.* Clinical value of routine serum squamous cell carcinoma antigen in follow-up of patients with early-stage cervical cancer. *J Clin Oncol* 2001;19(19):3960–6.

189 Salani R, Backes FJ, Fung MF, *et al.* Posttreatment surveillance and diagnosis of recurrence in women with gynecologic malignancies: Society of Gynecologic Oncologists recommendations. *Am J Obstet Gynecol* 2011;204(6):466–78.

190 www.nccn.org. Cervical Cancer, 2013 (cited 2013 9 July 2013). Version 2.2013.

191 Markowitz LE, Hariri S, Lin C, *et al.* Reduction in human papillomavirus (HPV) prevalence among young women following HPV vaccine introduction in the United States, National Health and Nutrition Examination Surveys, 2003–2010. *J Infect Dis* 2013;208(3):385–93.

192 Einstein MH, Burk RD. Persistent human papillomavirus infection: definitions and clinical implications. *Papillomavirus Rep* 2001;12:119–23.

22

Vaginal Cancer

Christina Gauthreaux[1], *Anna Kuan-Celarier*[2], *and Carolyn D. Runowicz*[3]

[1] *Washington University School of Medicine/Barnes Jewish Hospital, St Louis, Missouri, USA*
[2] *Louisiana State University Health Sciences Centre, New Orleans, Louisiana, USA*
[3] *Florida International University Herbert Wertheim College of Medicine, Miami, Florida, USA*

Incidence and Mortality

The incidence rate of primary vaginal cancer in the United States is 0.7 cases out of every 100,000 women per year and the corresponding mortality rate is 0.2 deaths per 100,000 women per year. The median age at diagnosis is 67 years [1]. Vaginal cancer comprises 4.5% of all malignant neoplasms of the female genital tract. Approximately 4,810 new cases will be diagnosed in 2017, and account for approximately 1,240 deaths [2]. Although primary malignancies of the vagina are rare, direct extension from involvement of the vagina by other pelvic tumors (e.g., cervix, vulva, rectum) is more common. Metastatic disease from the endometrium, breast, and kidney can also occur.

Vaginal intraepithelial neoplasia (VAIN) represents an asymptomatic lesion of the vagina that is estimated to progress to invasive vaginal cancer in 2–7% of cases [3, 4]. The age at diagnosis is related to the degree of VAIN, with an average of 60 years for VAIN 3 and 45 years for VAIN 1/2 [5]. VAIN often accompanies or follows a diagnosis of carcinoma *in situ* of the cervix.

Etiology

In general, cancer of the vagina is associated with the same risk factors as cervical cancer: infection with human papillomavirus (HPV), immunodeficiencies, and history of smoking [6, 7]. Surrogate markers for HPV infection are often cited as risk factors including multiple lifetime sexual partners and early age at first intercourse. HPV is detected in 100%, 90.1%, and 69.9% VAIN 1, VAIN 2/3, and invasive vaginal cancer cases, respectively [6].

VAIN may be associated with concomitant cervical intraepithelial neoplasia or vulvar intraepithelial neoplasia due to the shared HPV etiology.

Vaginal clear cell adenocarcinomas occur in young women exposed *in utero* to diethylstilbestrol (DES). DES exposure can result in cervical and vaginal clear cell adenocarcinomas [7]. In females exposed to DES *in utero*, the risk of developing a clear cell adenocarcinoma is low (one in 1000 by age 34). A recent update confirmed that the risk of clear cell adenocarcinoma of the vagina and cervix was highest in the 1951–1956 birth cohort. By age 50, the cumulative risk of clear cell adenocarcinoma was 1 per 750 exposed women [8].

Prevention

The HPV vaccine, Gardasil®, a quadrivalent vaccine containing virus-like particles of types 6, 11, 16 and 18, and the 9-valent vaccine (Gardasil 9®), have demonstrated strong protection against cervical intraepithelial neoplasia, genital warts, and vulvar and vaginal neoplasia associated with the HPV types in the vaccine [9–11]. Although there are no published studies to date, it is reasonable to expect a similar protection from the bivalent vaccine (Cervirax®).

Clinical Presentation and Diagnosis: VAIN and Vaginal Cancer

Most women with VAIN have no symptoms. As many as 20% of women diagnosed with vaginal cancer are also asymptomatic with the lesions detected during a routine pelvic examination and Papanicolaou (Pap) test [12]. However, most women with vaginal cancer present with symptoms of vaginal bleeding unrelated to menses. In more advanced stages, urinary retention, hematuria, and urinary frequency can occur. Lesions occurring in the posterior vaginal wall can be associated with gastrointestinal complaints such as tenesmus, constipation, melena, or blood in the stool. Pelvic pain can be present in women in whom the disease has extended beyond the vagina. The most common site of VAIN and primary invasive vaginal cancer is the posterior wall of the upper one-third of the vagina, although lesions do also occur in the middle and lower third of the vagina.

The American Cancer Society's Oncology in Practice: Clinical Management, First Edition. Edited by The American Cancer Society.

The diagnosis is confirmed by punch biopsy and histologic examination.

With VAIN, the diagnosis and site of biopsy can be guided by the application of acetic acid and the use of a colposcope. When acetic acid is applied, VAIN becomes more distinct from the surrounding unaffected vagina. VAIN is often multifocal [3]. With invasive vaginal cancer, there may be raised, thickened, or ulcerated areas.

The diagnostic workup for invasive vaginal cancer includes a complete history and thorough pelvic examination. Significant historical factors include a previous diagnosis of HPV infection, *in utero* exposure to DES, and a history of cervical intraepithelial neoplasia or vulvar intraepithelial neoplasia. The lesion can be missed upon initial examination, especially if it is small or located in the lower one-third of the vagina. Because the two blades of the speculum obscure the anterior and posterior walls of the vagina, the vagina should be carefully inspected while the speculum is being removed, as well as palpated for any lesions during the bimanual examination [13].

Pathology

VAIN

VAIN is defined by the presence of squamous cell atypia without stromal invasion and classified according to the thickness of epithelial involvement: VAIN 1 and 2 involve the lower one-third and two-thirds of the vaginal epithelium, respectively, and VAIN 3 (vaginal carcinoma *in situ*) involves the entire thickness (Figure 22.1). The progression of VAIN to invasive vaginal carcinoma has not been well studied, though several retrospective studies have shown an association. Importantly, VAIN is consistently associated with prior or concurrent neoplasia elsewhere in the lower genital tract, specifically the cervix and vulva.

Squamous Cell Carcinoma

Squamous cell carcinoma of the vagina presents grossly as nodular, ulcerating, indurated, endophytic, or exophytic tumors. Histologically, these tumors are similar to squamous cell tumors from other sites.

Verrucous carcinoma is a rare variant of vaginal squamous cell carcinoma that is well differentiated and has low potential for malignancy. Grossly, it presents as a large, wart-like, fungating mass that is locally aggressive, but rarely metastasizes. Histologically, it is composed of large papillary fronds covered by dense layers of keratin. Its deep margin creates a pushing border of well-oriented rete ridges which help differentiate it from benign condyloma acuminatum.

Adenocarcinoma

Adenocarcinomas may arise in areas of vaginal adenosis, Wolfian remnants, periurethral glands, and foci of endometriosis.

Clear cell carcinoma is the most well-known variant of adenocarcinoma because of its association with *in utero* exposure to DES, and is mostly found in young women aged 7–33 years. Grossly, vaginal clear cell carcinoma presents as polypoid masses, usually on the anterior wall. Of patients with DES-related clear cell carcinoma, 70% are diagnosed at stage I and have good outcomes with surgery, or wide local excision with localized radiation [14].

Sarcoma

Sarcomas of the vagina include leiomyosarcoma, endometrial stromal sarcoma, malignant mixed Mullerian tumors composed of carcinoma and sarcomatous elements, and rhabdomyosarcoma.

Embryonal rhabdomyosarcoma, also known as sarcoma botyroides, is the most common of the vaginal sarcomas (Figure 22.2). Grossly, it presents as soft nodules that fill and sometimes protrude from the vagina, resembling bunches of grapes.

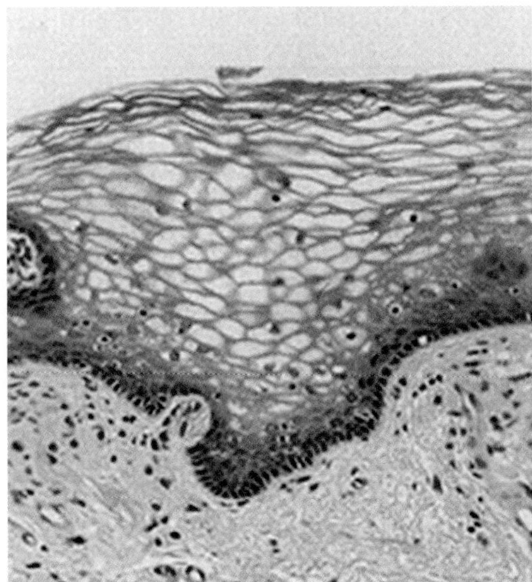

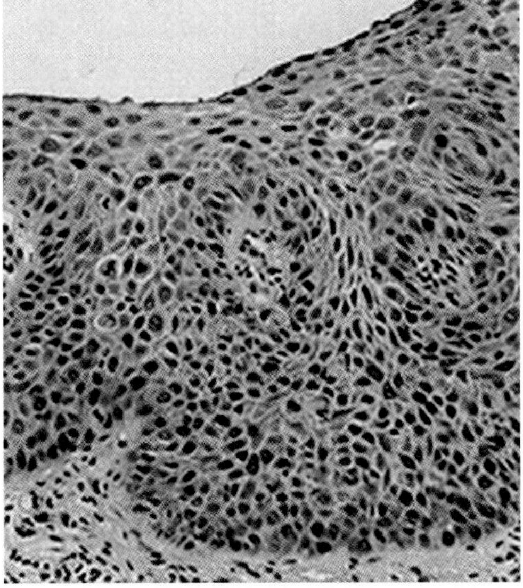

Figure 22.1 Non-neoplastic vaginal epithelium (left) and VAIN 2 (right). In VAIN 2, note the basal cells extend to two-thirds of the thickness of the epithelium. *Source:* Holschneider and Berek [12]. Copyright © 2013 UpToDate, Inc. Reproduced with permission of Wolters Kluwer Health.

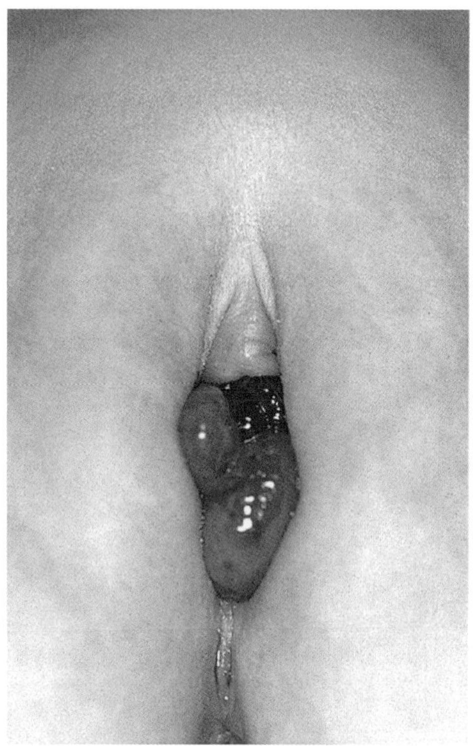

Figure 22.2 Grapelike clusters of tumor project out of vagina. *Source:* Crum *et al.* [26]. Reproduced with permission of Elsevier.

The prognosis for patients with this disease has improved with the use of multiple modalities of therapy, including surgery, chemotherapy, and radiation [14].

Melanoma

Primary melanoma of the vaginal mucosa is relatively rare, and is thought to originate from mucosal melanocytes in areas of melanosis or from atypical melanocytic hyperplasia. Vaginal melanomas have quite different demographic, clinical, and survival characteristics as compared with cutaneous melanoma [15]. Ultraviolet light is not a risk factor for vaginal melanoma. In an updated review of the SEER database, 3.6% of patients with vulvar/vaginal melanomas and 0.6% of those with cutaneous melanoma were Black. The median age at diagnosis of vaginal melanoma was 70.5 years in the SEER analysis, but have been reported in younger women [15, 16]. Vaginal bleeding is often present. Grossly, they appear as blue–black, black–brown, or nonpigmented masses, plaques, or ulcerations, often on the distal third of the anterior wall of the vagina (Figure 22.3). They are often aggressive, with little local response to treatment, and frequently metastasize. Lymph node metastasis is one of the single most important prognostic determinants. Most patients will undergo radical surgery, depending on the location and stage of disease. Radiation therapy is used for disease that is locally advanced and not amenable to radical surgery (hysterectomy/vaginectomy) or as an adjuvant therapy. The 5-year survival rate for primary vaginal melanoma is less than 14% [17]. In the SEER database review for vaginal melanoma, the overall survival was 8.5 months for Black women and 19 months for non-Black women [15].

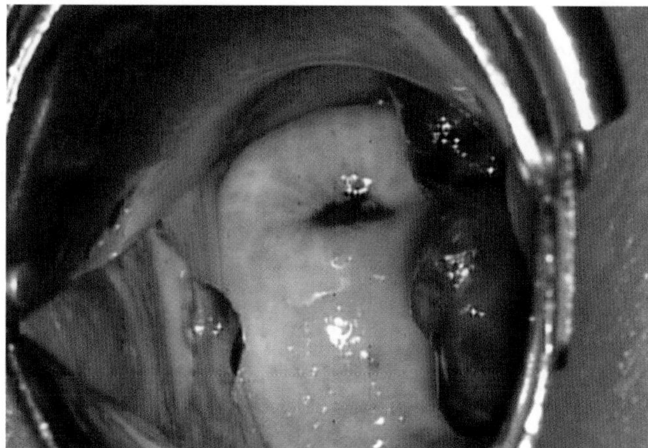

Figure 22.3 Using a speculum, the melanoma is visualized as a pigmented lesion on the left and right vaginal walls. *Source:* Cheon *et al.* [16]. Reproduced with permission of Korean Society of Obstetrics and Gynecology.

Routes of Spread

Vaginal tumors may invade locally and disseminate to other tissues of the true pelvis, as well as distantly. Direct extension to neighboring soft tissue structures may occur, including to the parametria, bladder, urethra, and rectum, and even the bony pelvis. Lymphatic spread is to the internal and external iliac nodes, obturator, common iliac nodes, and the para-aortic lymph nodes for malignancies of the upper vagina (Figure 22.4).

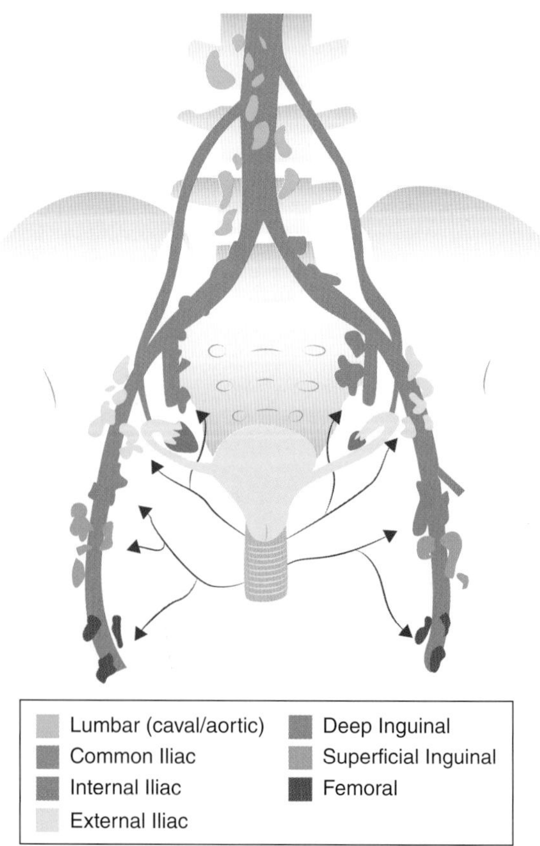

Figure 22.4 Lymphatic drainage. *Source:* Christina Gauthreaux. Reproduced with permission of Christina Gauthreaux.

Lesions in the distal vagina spread to the inguinal and femoral lymph nodes, then to the pelvic and para-aortic nodes. Rarely, hematogenous dissemination may occur to distant organs, particularly the lungs, liver, and bone.

Staging

The purpose of staging is to estimate prognosis and guide treatment. Vaginal cancer is clinically staged using the International Federation of Gynecology and Obstetrics (FIGO) staging system, revised in 2009, and/or the TNM staging system of the American Joint Committee on Cancer and the Union for International Cancer Control (Table 22.1) [18, 19]. These staging systems are based on the tumor size, spread to regional contiguous organs (cervix, urethra/bladder, perineum, rectum), to the regional (pelvic, inguinal, and femoral) lymph nodes, or to distant sites [18, 19]. Radiologic testing such as preoperative computed tomography (CT) scans or positron emission tomography (PET)/CT scans are often used to determine the extent of disease but are not formally used in determining the clinical stage of disease. Findings at surgery do not alter the clinical stage, but are used to determine prognosis and treatment.

In early stage I disease for tumors ≤2 cm, staging, and primary surgical treatment are usually performed as a single procedure. The exact dimensions of the lesion, depth of invasion, and final histopathology are determined during the pathologic examination of the surgical specimen. The status of the lymph nodes is determined at surgery or preoperatively by image-guided needle aspiration/biopsy. Following surgery and pathologic examination, the clinical stage of disease is confirmed and a treatment strategy is developed, which may be influenced by pathologic findings. If more extensive disease is found at surgery or by radiologic testing, the clinical stage is not changed (although the TNM clinical and pathologic stages would differ).

The staging workup for those with >2 cm lesions and advanced stage (higher than stage II) usually includes a bimanual pelvic/rectal examination, with or without anesthesia. A biopsy of the lesion is done to determine the histopathology. A cystoscopy and sigmoidoscopy may be performed if invasion of the bladder or rectum is suspected by examination or symptoms. Fine-needle aspiration/biopsy of lymph nodes may be performed if there are palpable inguinal/femoral nodes. A chest X-ray is performed.

Table 22.1 International Federation of Gynecology and Obstetrics (FIGO) nomenclature for carcinoma of the vagina.

Stage I	The carcinoma is limited to the vaginal wall
Stage II	The carcinoma has involved the subvaginal tissue but has not extended to the pelvic wall
Stage III	The carcinoma has extended to the pelvic wall
Stage IV	The carcinoma has extended beyond the true pelvis or has involved the mucosa of the bladder or rectum; bullous edemas as such does not permit a case to be allotted to stage IV
	IVa – Tumor invades bladder and/or rectal mucosa and/or direct extension beyond the true pelvis
	IVb – Spread to distant organs

Source: adapted from FIGO Committee on Gynecologic Oncology 2009 [18].

A CT scan or MRI is carried out to evaluate the extent of disease, but as noted, is not a formal part of the clinical staging process. Gross and microscopic findings in the resected specimen, including pelvic and para-aortic lymph nodes, are the basis of the TNM pathologic stage.

Stage I (T1, N0, M0) disease is confined to the vaginal wall. Stage II (T2, N0, M0) disease has invaded the subvaginal tissue but has not yet invaded the pelvic wall. Stage III tumor has spread to the pelvic wall (T3) or is a T1 or T2 lesion (spread beyond the vaginal mucosa to the subvaginal tissue) and has spread to regional lymph nodes. Stage IVA disease has spread to bladder or rectum (T4) and Stage IVB cancer has spread to distant organs (M1).

A study using the SEER database revealed that the majority (36%) of patients presented with early-stage disease (Stage I/II) and most (65%) had squamous histology [20]. This review reported 5-year disease specific survival for women with stage I of 84%, stage II of 75%, and 57% for women with advanced disease (stage III or IV).

Treatment

VAIN

Treatment is individualized based on the patient's characteristics, extent of disease, and prior therapy, if any. The management of VAIN varies based on the grade of the lesion. VAIN 1 is usually conservatively managed with cytologic follow-up at 6–12 months, until three consecutive negative results are obtained. A colposcopic examination is performed if indicated by high-grade cytology (VAIN 2–3). VAIN 2–3 should be treated [20]. The treatments can be ablative (CO_2 laser), excisional (loop electrosurgical excision therapy, partial vaginectomy, or wide local excision) or medical (5-fluorouracil, tricholoroacetic acid) [20]. The results of treatments vary depending on the extent of disease, with reported recurrence rates of 5–34%. Imiquimod, an immune response modifier which is locally applied, should only be used in clinical trials.

Invasive Vaginal Cancer

Treatment of vaginal cancer is typically tailored to the stage of disease and site of vaginal involvement, and may involve surgery, radiotherapy, and chemotherapy, or a combination of these treatment modalities. The patient's desire to maintain function of the vagina, the patient's desire to maintain fertility, and concerns about psychosexual identity are important in the treatment planning.

FIGO Stage I

Treatment for FIGO stage I vaginal carcinomas that are ≤2 cm in diameter and involving the upper vagina may be treated with either surgery or intracavitary radiation therapy, with or without external beam radiation (EBRT). The surgical approach usually includes a radical hysterectomy, upper vaginectomy and bilateral pelvic lymphadenectomy. In a patient who has had a hysterectomy, the procedure would be a radical partial or complete vaginectomy, with bilateral pelvic lymphadenectomy. However, in the elderly patient or in a patient with co-morbidities, or with lesions >2 cm, primary radiation therapy is the mainstay of treatment. Radiation is also usually used with lesions in the mid to lower vagina. The most common radiotherapeutic strategy is a combination of intracavitary therapy and EBRT. Lesions in the lower third of the vagina may require vulvovaginectomy in addition to dissection of inguinofemoral nodes. However, the use of such radical surgery appears to have decreased over time and radiation has become the mainstay of treatment. Chemotherapy with cisplatin-based therapy may be incorporated into the treatment plan for lesions >2 cm [21].

FIGO Stage II/III

For FIGO stage II and III vaginal cancer, radiotherapy has been the standard of care. Vaginal brachytherapy and EBRT are most commonly used. Based on the improved results of concomitant cisplatin-based chemotherapy and radiation in cervical cancer, these modalities have been combined in vaginal cancer [22]. A review of the SEER database suggested an improvement in mortality in women with vaginal cancer diagnosed after 2000 and suggested it may reflect the combination of radiation and chemotherapy [21]. However, due to the rarity of this cancer, there have not been any randomized studies comparing radiation with or without chemotherapy. The optimum regimen and therapeutic efficacy of chemotherapy have yet to be determined.

FIGO Stage IV

Patients with FIGO stage IV vaginal cancer are usually treated with EBRT and intracavitary or interstitial brachytherapy. As noted above, concomitant chemoradiation has begun to be utilized in these patients. Pelvic exenteration (removal of the vagina, bladder, and rectum) may be offered to patients with stage IV disease that is invading the bladder or rectum, once metastatic disease has been ruled out by radiologic evaluation, for example by PET/CT. Vaginal reconstruction may also be offered to these patients. For patients with stage IVb disease that has spread to distant organs beyond the true pelvis, radiation for palliation of symptoms is used, sometimes with concurrent chemotherapy with agents such as platinum agents.

Post-Treatment Complications and Follow-Up Surveillance

Approximately 10–15% of patients treated for vaginal cancer will develop treatment-related complications, which may include rectovaginal fistula, vesicovaginal fistula, radiation cystitis or proctitis, rectal and vaginal strictures, and, rarely, vaginal necrosis [23].

To reduce the degree of vaginal stenosis, vaginal dilators and topical estrogen can be helpful during treatment. Women can continue sexual activity after treatment. Those who are not sexually active or for whom intercourse is too painful should use a vaginal dilator with topical estrogen. Maintenance of vaginal patency is important in the clinical follow-up of these patients.

Women who have undergone radiation therapy, surgery, and/or chemotherapy may have sexual complaints that include changes in sexual desire, arousal, orgasmic intensity, and latency [24]. In women under 40 who receive radiation, the risk for radiation-induced menopause is substantial.

An optimal surveillance strategy for survivors has yet to be established, and practices vary. The Society for Gynecologic Oncology released the following set of guidelines in 2011: for low-risk disease (early stage, treated with surgery alone, no adjuvant therapy) a history and physical examination are recommended every 6 months for the first 2 years, then annually. For high-risk disease (advanced stage, treated with primary chemotherapy/radiation therapy or surgery, adjuvant therapy), a history and physical examination are recommended every 3 months for the first 2 years, every 6 months for years 3–5, then annually. Cervical cytology, or vaginal cytology if the cervix is absent, are recommended annually. Vaginal colposcopy is recommended if cytology reveals an abnormality consistent with recurrent disease. A biopsy is recommended if a palpable or grossly visible abnormality is noted on physical examination. Imaging, such as CT and PET scan, are recommended only if recurrence is suspected [25].

Conclusion

The rarity of vaginal cancer has proven to be the greatest challenge in establishing widely accepted guidelines for treatment. Treatment is best performed by a multidisciplinary team of physicians, including a gynecologic oncologist, and is tailored to the stage of disease and patient characteristics (e.g., performance status). It is anticipated that the HPV vaccination program will help to reduce the incidence of this disease further, and that improved strategies to treat other similar neoplasms, such as cervical cancer, will be applied to vaginal cancer and help to improve treatment outcomes, survival, and quality of life.

References

1 Howlader N, Noone AM, Krapcho M, *et al.* (eds). SEER Cancer Statistics Review, 1975–2013, National Cancer Institute. Bethesda, MD. http://seer.cancer.gov/csr/1975_2013/, based on November 2015 SEER data submission, posted to the SEER web site, April 2016.

2 Siegel RL, Miller KD, Jemal A. Cancer statistics, 2017. *CA Cancer J Clin* 2017;67:7–30.

3 Frega A, Sopracordevole F, Assorgi C, *et al.* Vaginal intraepithelial neoplasia: a therapeutic dilemma. *Anticancer Res* 2013;33:29–38.

4 Sopracordevole F, Barbero M, Clemente N, *et al.* High-grade vaginal intraepithelial neoplasia and risk of progression to vaginal cancer: a multicentre study of the Italian Society of Colposcopy and Cervico-Vaginal Pathology (SICPCV). *Eur Rev Med Pharmacol Sci* 2016;20(5):818–24.

5 Diakomanolis E, Stefanidids K, Rodolakis A, *et al.* Vaginal intraepithelial neoplasia: report of 102 cases. *Eur J Gynaecol Oncol* 2002;23:457–9.

6 Daling JR, Madeleine MM, Schwartz SM, *et al.* A population-based study of squamous cell vaginal cancer: HPV and cofactors. *Gynecol Oncol* 2002;84:263–70

7 Laronda MM, Unno K, Butler LM, Kurita T. The development of cervical and vaginal adenosis as a result of diethylstilbestrol exposure in utero. *Differentiation* 2012;84:252–60.

8 Huo D, Anderson D, Palmer JR, Herbst AL. Incidence rates and risks of diethylstilbestrol-related clear-cell adenocarcinoma of the vagina and cervix: update after 40-year follow-up. *Gynecol Oncol* 2017;146:566–71.

9 Joura EA, Garland SM, Paavonen J, *et al.* Effect of the human papillomavirus (HPV) quadrivalent vaccine in a subgroup of women with cervical and vulvar disease: retrospective pooled analysis of trial data. *BMJ* 2012;344:e1401.

10 Joura EA, Giuliano AR, Iversen OE, *et al.* A 9-valent HPV vaccine against infection and intraepithelial neoplasia in women. *N Engl J Med* 2015;372:711–23.

11 Saslow D, Andrews KS, Manassaram-Baptiste D, *et al.* Human papillomavirus vaccination guideline update: American Cancer Society guideline endorsement. *CA Cancer J Clin* 2016;66:375–85.

12 Holschneider C, Berek J. Vaginal intraepithelial neoplasia. UpToDate. http://www.uptodate.com/contents/vaginal-intraepithelial-neoplasia?source=search_result&search=vain&selectedTitle=1~17 (accessed 12 October 2017).

13 Elkas J, Berek J. Vaginal cancer. UpToDate. http://www.uptodate.com/contents/vaginal-cancer?source=search_result&search=vaginal+cancer&selectedTitle=1~31 (accessed 12 October 2017).

14 Hicks ML, Piver MS. Conservative surgery plus adjuvant therapy for vulvovaginal rhabdomyosarcomas, diethylstilbestrol clear cell adenocarcinomas of the vagina and unilateral germ cell tumors of the ovary. *Obstet Gynecol Clin North Am* 1992;19:219–33

15 Mert I, Semaan A, Winer I, *et al.* Vulvar/vaginal melanoma. An updated Surveillance Epidemiology and End Results database review, comparison with cutaneous melanoma and significance of racial disparities. *Int J Gynecol Cancer* 2013;23:1118–25.

16 Cheon J, Lee SJ, Kim SA, *et al.* Two cases of primary malignant melanoma of the vagina. *Korean J Obstet Gynecol* 2012;55:1020–5.

17 Creasman WT, Phillips JL, Menck HR. The National Cancer Data Base report on vaginal cancer. *Cancer* 1998;83:1033–40.

18 FIGO Committee on Gynecologic Oncology: Current FIGO staging for cancer of the vagina, fallopian tube, ovary, and gestational trophoblastic neoplasia. *Int J Gynecol Obstet* 2009;105:3–4.

19 Gibb RK, Olawaiye AB, Chen LM, *et al.* Vagina. In: Amin MB, Edge SB, Greene FL (eds). *AJCC Cancer Staging Manual*, 8th edn. New York: Springer Nature, 2017.

20 Frega A, Sopracordevole F, Assorgi C, *et al.* Vaginal intraepithelial neoplasia: a therapeutic dilemma. *Anticancer Res* 2013;33:29–38.

21 Shah CA, Goff BA, Lowe K, *et al.* Factors affecting risk of mortality in women with vaginal cancer. *Obstet Gynecol* 2009;113:1038–45.

22 Rose PG, Bundy BN, Watkins EB, *et al.* Concurrent cisplatin-based radiotherapy and chemotherapy for locally advanced cervical cancer. *N Engl J Med* 1999;340:1144–53.

23 Rubin SC, Young J, Mikuta JJ. Squamous carcinoma of the vagina: treatment, complication and long-term follow-up. *Gynecol Oncol* 1985;20:346.

24 Krychman M, Millheiser LS. Sexual health issues in women with cancer. *J Sex Med* 2013 (Suppl 1):5–15.

25 Salani R, Backes FJ, Fung MF, *et al.* Posttreatment surveillance and diagnosis of recurrence in women with gynecologic malignancies: Society of Gynecologic Oncologists recommendations. *Am J Obstet Gynecol* 2011;204:466–78.

26 Crum CP, Nucci MR, Lee KR. *Diagnostic Gynecologic and Obstetric Pathology*, 2nd edn. Philadelphia: Saunders, 2011.

23

Vulvar Cancer

Carolyn D. Runowicz

Florida International University Herbert Wertheim College of Medicine, Miami, Florida, USA

Incidence and Mortality

Vulvar cancer is the fourth most common gynecologic cancer and accounts for about 5.1% of cancers of the female reproductive organs and 0.6% of all cancers in women [1]. In 2017, in the United States (US), there will be an estimated 6,020 new cases and 1,150 deaths from this disease [1]. The incidence rate of invasive vulvar cancer, based on cases diagnosed between 2009 and 2013, was approximately 2.4 per 100,000 women per year. During the same time period, the age-adjusted death rate was 0.5 per 100,000 women per year. Incidence rates and death rates in the US were highest among White and American Indian/Alaska Native women, lowest for Asian American/Pacific Islander women, and intermediate for other racial and ethnic groups. Incidence increased by average of 0.6% per year from 2004 to 2013, and death rates increased by an annual average of 0.7% during this period. In the US, approximately 0.3% of women will develop vulvar cancer at some point during their life [2].

Vulvar intraepithelial neoplasia (VIN), a precursor lesion of some types of invasive vulvar cancer, accounts for 57% of vulvar neoplasia. In the US, between 1973 and 2000, the incidence of VIN increased by more than 400% [3]. In comparison with invasive vulvar cancer, VIN occurs in younger women, increasing in incidence until the age of 40–49 and then decreasing. Among women with VIN, the risk of squamous cell carcinoma (SCC) is higher in postmenopausal than in premenopausal women [4].

Etiology

There are likely two independent pathways of vulvar squamous cell carcinogenesis (Table 23.1) [5]. The basaloid type and the warty type of vulvar SCC are typically preceded by the usual type of VIN and commonly contain integrated human papillomavirus (HPV) DNA, usually subtypes 16 and 18. It is diffusely positive for p16, a molecular marker for HPV. The VIN tends to be multifocal, more common in younger women, with a low risk of progression to invasive SCC. In contrast, well-differentiated keratinizing vulvar SCC is preceded by differentiated VIN, vulvar dystrophy, and chronic inflammation [6, 7, 8].

Vulvar carcinoma is encountered most frequently in postmenopausal women, with a median age of 68 [2]. However, age at diagnosis varies substantially with histological/pathologic types.

About half of all vulvar SCCs are linked to high-risk HPV infection (e.g., HPV-16, -18 and -31). Incident infection and risk for progression to VIN 2/3 has been reported to be highest for HPV-16 infections. In one study, the mean time from incident infection to the development of VIN 1–3 was 18.5 months. HPV-16 was observed in 6.5% of VIN 1 and 64.5% of VIN 2/3 lesions [6]. Although treatment may eradicate a VIN caused by HPV, the HPV may persist leading to chronic infection and recurrent disease [7, 8, 9]. A prior history of other HPV-related cancers (e.g., cervical cancer) is positively associated with vulvar cancer incidence.

Immunodeficiency (due to HIV infection or to iatrogenic immunosuppression of transplant recipients) also increases vulvar cancer risk, presumably by blunting the immune response to HPV infection and/or diminishing immune surveillance of early malignancy [9, 10].

Cigarette smoking increases the risk of vulvar cancer, especially in women with a history of HPV infection [11].

Prevention

The HPV vaccine, Gardasil®, a quadrivalent vaccine containing virus-like particles of types 6, 11, 16, and 18 has demonstrated strong protection against genital warts and vulvar neoplasia associated with the HPV types in the vaccine [12]. Although there are no published studies to date, it is reasonable to expect a similar protection from the bivalent vaccine (Cervirax®) and 9-valent vaccine (Gardasil 9®). Thus, prophylactic vaccines have the potential to decrease the incidence of vulvar neoplasia in vaccinated women.

The American Cancer Society's Oncology in Practice: Clinical Management, First Edition. Edited by The American Cancer Society.

Table 23.1 Models of vulvar cancer.

Characteristics	Type 1	Type 2
Age	Younger (35–65 years old)	Older (55–85 years old)
Cervical neoplasia	High association	Low association
Cofactors	Age, immune status, HPV	Vulvar atypia, possibly mutated host genes
Histopathology of tumor	Intraepithelial-like (basaloid), poorly differentiated	Keratinizing squamous cell carcinoma, well differentiated
HPV DNA	Frequent (>60%)	Seldom (<15%)
Pre-existing lesion	VIN ("usual (warty-basaloid) VIN")	(Chronic) vulvar inflammation, lichen sclerosus, squamous cell hyperplasia and differentiated (simplex) VIN
History of condyloma	Strong association	Rare association
History of STD	Strong association	Rare association
Cigarette smoking	High prevalence	Low prevalence

Source: Crum [5].
HPV, human papillomavirus; STD, sexually transmitted disease; VIN, vulvar intraepithelial neoplasia.

Clinical Presentation and Diagnosis

VIN and Vulvar Cancer

Most women with VIN have no symptoms. Patients with invasive vulvar cancer will often present with a visible and palpable lesion (Figure 23.1) [13]. The lesions can be multifocal. Patients with type II (keratinizing) vulvar cancer may present with pruritus, often secondary to the associated lichen sclerosus or squamous hyperplasia. The most common sites for vulvar cancer are the labia (80%), the clitoris (10%), and the perineum (10%) [14].

The diagnosis is confirmed by biopsy and histologic examination. With VIN, the diagnosis and site of biopsy can be guided by the application of acetic acid and the use of a colposcope or handheld magnifying glass. VIN can grossly appear as a greyish-brown area of discoloration or hyperpigmentation. When acetic acid is applied, the area may become more distinct from the surrounding unaffected vulvar skin. With invasive vulvar cancer, there may be a raised, thickened, ulcerated, or cauliflower-like growth (Figure 23.1) [13]. After application of local anesthesia, a punch biopsy (including dermis and subcutis to assess depth of invasion) can be used to sample the lesion(s).

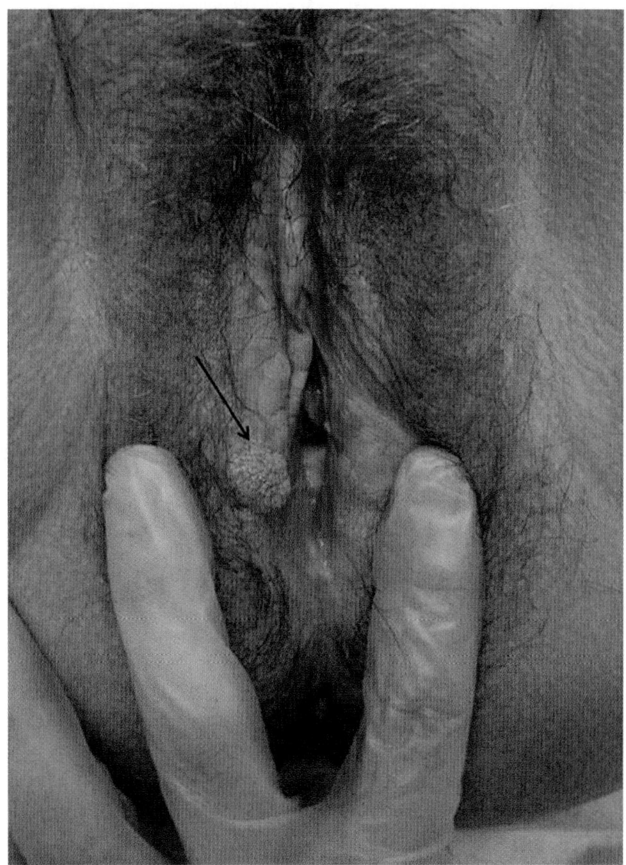

Figure 23.1 Verrucous lesion on the right labium minus, later diagnosed as Langerhans cell histiocytosis. *Source:* Simons *et al.* [13]. Reproduced with permission of Elsevier.

Pathology

VIN

As noted in Table 23.1, there are two main types of VIN, each associated with distinct forms of invasive cancer, and each having distinct epidemiological associations [5]. The usual (warty-basaloid) type comprises 98% of VIN lesions. It is HPV-related and is characterized by immature basaloid cells occupying at least one-third and as much as the full thickness of the epithelium. The proportion of epithelial thickness containing these cells determines the grade (VIN 1, 2, or 3; or low vs high grade VIN). Differentiated (simplex) VIN is characterized by basal and parabasal layers of the epithelium in which the cells show prominent nuclear atypia and abundant keratinized cytoplasm, and form abortive pearls [14].

Invasive SCC

Over 90% of invasive vulvar cancer is SCC. SCCs can present with many clinical patterns, including nodules, ulcerations, and flat, more infiltrating, lesions. The two main types of vulvar SCC are contrasted in Table 23.1 [5]. The warty–basaloid lesions are HPV-related.

The lymph node status and FIGO stage (Table 23.2) are the main predictors of recurrence and survival for vulvar SCC [15, 16].

Table 23.2 Staging for carcinoma of the vulva, (a) AJCC and (b) FIGO.

(a)

Stage I	T1	N0	M0
Stage IA	T1a	N0	M0
Stage IB	T1b	N0	M0
Stage II	T2	N0	M0
Stage IIIA	T1, T2	N1a, N1b	M0
Stage IIIB	T1, T2	N2a, N2b	M0
Stage IIIC	T1, T2	N2c	M0
Stage IVA	T1, T2	N3	M0
	T3	Any N	M0
Stage IVB	Any T	Any N	M1

Source: Gibb [15]. Reproduced with permission of Springer.
Note: FIGO no longer includes Stage 0 (Tis).
Source: reprinted from Pecorelli [16] with permission from Elsevier.

(b)

Stage I	Tumor confined to the vulva
IA	Lesions ≤2 cm in size, confined to the vulva or perineum and with stromal invasion ≤1.0 mm*, no nodal metastasis
IB	Lesions >2 cm in size or with stromal invasion >1.0 mm*, confined to the vulva or perineum, with negative nodes
Stage II	Tumor of any size with extension to adjacent perineal structures (one-third lower urethra, one-third lower vagina, anus) with negative nodes
Stage III	Tumor of any size with or without extension to adjacent perineal structures (one-third lower urethra, one-third lower vagina, anus) with positive inguino-femoral lymph nodes
IIIA	(i) With 1 lymph node metastasis (≥5 mm), or (ii) 1–2 lymph node metastasis(es) (<5 mm)
IIIB	(i) With 2 or more lymph node metastases (≥5 mm), or (ii) 3 or more lymph node metastases (<5 mm)
IIIC	With positive nodes with extracapsular spread
Stage IV	Tumor invades other regional (two-thirds upper urethra, two-thirds upper vagina) or distant structures
IVA	Tumor invades any of the following: (i) upper urethral and/or vaginal mucosa, bladder mucosa, rectal mucosa, or fixed to pelvic vone, or (ii) fixed or ulcerated inguino-femoral lymph nodes
IVB	Any distant metastasis including pelvic lymph nodes

* The depth of invasion is defined as the measurement of the tumor from the epithelial-stromal junction of the adjacent most superficial dermal papilla to the deepest point of invasion.

The presence of inguinofemoral lymph node metastases is the most important prognostic factor for survival. Five-year survival rates range from 70 to 90% for patients with negative inguinofemoral lymph nodes and 25–55% for those with positive nodes [2].

Biological variables do not yet have a clinical relevance and their prognostic role is still investigational. Most studies have focused on HPV and *TP53*, and have identified HPV infection and *TP53* mutations as frequent events in vulvar cancer. The identification of other molecular events in vulvar cancer is limited, but has included alterations in p16, p15, and cyclin D in limited studies. *PTEN* mutations have been identified in VIN and vulvar cancer with a similar frequency as *TP53*, but the studies have involved only small numbers of vulvar cancers [17, 18].

Verrucous Carcinoma

Verrucous carcinoma is a distinct variant of SCC (Figure 23.1) [13]. It is cauliflower-like in appearance. The lesion grows slowly and rarely metastasizes. Although "verruca" is Latin for "wart", vulvar verrucous carcinoma and the warty type of vulvar SCC are histologically and clinically distinct entities. Despite its warty name and clinical appearance, recent studies indicate that vulvar verrucous carcinoma is rarely, if ever, HPV-related [19].

Melanoma

The second most common cancer of the vulva is melanoma, accounting for up to 7–10% of vulvar malignancies. However, melanoma has been reclassified as a cutaneous melanoma and has been removed as a histologic type of vulvar cancer in the 8th edition American Joint Committee on Cancer staging manual [15]. Melanomas occur more frequently in postmenopausal women, with a median age of 62 years. Vulvar melanomas are usually pigmented lesions, but amelanotic melanomas can occur. Pruritus and bleeding may be presenting symptoms. Melanomas usually arise *de novo*, but can be associated with existing junctional or compound nevi. There are three histologic subtypes including superficial spreading melanoma, mucosal lentiginous melanomas, and nodular melanomas [20, 21]. Melanoma is more fully discussed in Chapter 34.

Uncommon Vulvar Cancers

The remaining histopathologic types of vulvar cancer include adenocarcinoma (e.g. Bartholin gland), Paget disease, and basal cell carcinoma.

Bartholin Gland Cancer

Primary carcinoma of the Bartholin gland is rare, accounting for 2–7% of all vulvar carcinoma. The most common finding is a painless mass in the posterior labium majus. The most frequent histologic types are adenocarcinoma and SCC, each accounting for approximately 40% of all cases of Bartholin gland carcinoma. Adenosquamous carcinoma is a rarely encountered histologic subtype of Bartholin gland carcinoma. The remaining cases include adenoid cystic carcinoma, undifferentiated carcinoma, and transitional cell carcinomas.

A delay in appropriate management of Bartholin gland carcinoma is frequently due to its misdiagnosis as a cyst or an abscess when it is small, and a primary vulvar carcinoma when it is large. A definitive diagnosis of a Bartholin gland neoplasm is made only when an area of transition from normal gland to neoplastic tissue is identified. However, it may be impossible to determine the exact origin of extensive, deeply invasive lesions, as the residual normal gland may be completely obliterated. In women over age 40 with a Bartholin cyst abscess, it is generally recommended that a biopsy is performed to exclude an underlying carcinoma [22].

Bartholin gland carcinoma, as a vulvar cancer, is surgically staged as described above for SCCs. Surgical staging includes assessment of the tumor size and depth of invasion, pathologic status of the inguinal lymph nodes, and presence of distant metastases. Treatment of Bartholin gland carcinoma is tailored to the stage of disease. The primary treatment is surgery. Radiation and chemotherapy may be used in advanced disease. There are no standard treatment options for patients with advanced, recurrent, or metastatic disease [23].

Basal Cell Carcinoma

Basal cell carcinomas are relatively innocuous, usually asymptomatic lesions treated with simple wide local excision. As in skin elsewhere in the body, these lesions can have a central ulceration, rolled edges and appear pearly or gray in color. They can also be ill-defined, scaly erythematous lesions with telangiectasias, present as well-circumscribed skin-colored nodules, or as a nondescript ulcerated plaque [24]. Pruritus, irritation, soreness, pain, and rarely bleeding may occur. In a small series of vulvar basal cell cancers, the average age was 76 years [24]. The histological appearance of vulvar basal cell carcinomas are similar to those on sun-exposed skin. Like basal cell carcinoma elsewhere, these tumors have an extremely good prognosis.

Extramammary Paget Disease

Paget disease of the vulva is a rare form of intraepithelial neoplasia characterized by adenocarcinomatous cells and accounts for approximately 2% of vulvar neoplasms. It presents as moist, eczematoid, erythematous, white plaques, characteristically a "cake icing" appearance. It affects mainly postmenopausal women, with a median age of 72 years. The most common signs and symptoms are pruritus, irritation, burning, and bleeding. It is usually multifocal. There may be a delay in diagnosis due to this nonspecific appearance and subsequent misdiagnosis. Although most cases of extramammary vulvar Paget disease are primary rather than associated with underlying adenocarcinoma, approximately 25% of cases are associated with neoplastic disease [25–27]. When associated disease is present, it is typically local (adenocarcinoma in the skin adnexa or Bartholin gland) but also may be distant (most commonly, of the breast, but also of the genital, urinary, or intestinal tract). In contrast, perianal extramammary Paget disease is associated with underlying colorectal adenocarcinoma in up to 80% of cases [25–27]. Thus, when Paget disease is confirmed by biopsy, evaluation including breast, genitourinary tract, and gastrointestinal tract should be considered [25–27].

The treatment is a surgical wide local excision. Local recurrence rates are high despite aggressive surgeries. If an underlying carcinoma is discovered, a more radical surgical treatment is required as discussed for Bartholin gland and SCCs.

Staging

Vulvar cancer is surgically and pathologically staged using the FIGO staging system, revised in 2009, and/or the TNM staging system of the American Joint Committee on Cancer and the Union for International Cancer Control (Table 23.2) [15, 16]. These staging systems are based on the size, spread to regional contiguous organs (vagina, urethral, perineum, anus), or to the regional (inguinal and femoral) lymph nodes. Distant metastases are unusual. Table 23.2 compares the FIGO staging system with the TNM staging system [15, 16].

Staging and primary surgical treatment are usually performed as a single procedure. The exact dimensions of the lesion, depth of invasion and final histopathology are determined during the pathologic examination of the surgical specimen. The status of the lymph nodes is determined at surgery, initially with a sentinel lymph node (SLN) biopsy when indicated (see section on surgical procedures) and if that is positive, a more extensive lymphadenectomy [28]. If the SLNs do not show cancer, further lymph node sampling or dissection is probably not warranted. Following surgery and pathologic examination, the stage of disease is determined and a treatment strategy is developed.

Staging for vulvar melanoma uses the same TNM system as cutaneous melanoma, which is described in Chapter 34.

Treatment of VIN

Preoperative Workup

For VIN, treatment is usually performed in the office or outpatient ambulatory surgical setting under local anesthesia, which typically requires minimal preoperative evaluation. A pelvic examination should be performed and cervical cytology obtained prior to treatment of the VIN. As noted above, at the pretreatment examination, a punch biopsy of the lesion is obtained.

Surgical and Medical Treatment of VIN

The treatment options for VIN include laser ablation, laser excision, wide local excision and rarely, skinning vulvectomy, for multifocal or very large lesions. In excisional procedures, the specimen should be clearly oriented and can be inked to assist the pathologist in assessing whether the lesion has been completely excised. Several small studies have reported the use of imiquimod, a topical immune response modifier that acts by binding on Toll-like receptor 7 on the cell surface of dendritic cells resulting in the secretion of proinflammatory cytokines. Complete and durable responses have been reported [29]. The Food and Drug Administration has not approved the use of imiquimod for VIN. Excisional treatment has diagnostic and treatment advantages in VIN lesions. The goal of treatment is to detect any areas of invasive cancer, prevent progression to invasive cancer, while preserving vulvar anatomy and function [30, 31].

Treatment of Invasive SCC

Preoperative Workup

For patients with an invasive vulvar cancer, a thorough history and physical examination, including a comprehensive pelvic examination and cervical cytology, is performed. This evaluation will determine the extent of workup needed to clear a patient medically for surgery. With current anesthesia techniques and less radical procedures, most patients with lesions confined to the vulva are candidates for surgery. The extent of the preoperative workup is dependent on the findings on the pelvic examination and on examination of the inguinal lymph nodes. A chest X-ray is standard, along with laboratory work (complete blood count with diff and platelets, electrolytes, creatinine, liver enzymes (metabolic panel)). A computed tomography scan, magnetic resonance imaging or positron emission tomography/computed tomography are not routinely obtained, except in patients with large lesions (>2 cm) or suspected metastatic/advanced disease, including involved lymph nodes or extension to the urethra, vagina, paravaginal tissues, or anus. A cystoscopy may be needed if there is disease extending into the urethra or along the anterior vaginal wall. A proctoscopy/sigmoidoscopy may be needed if there is disease extension to the anus [31]. These studies will be helpful in planning treatment, but do not alter the surgical stage of disease.

Surgical Procedures

Historically, for invasive squamous vulvar cancer, a radical vulvectomy was performed which included removal of the entire vulva, to the level of the deep fascia, and included an *en bloc* bilateral radical inguinal/femoral lymphadenectomy. Although the survival was excellent, the acute and chronic morbidity was substantial. Wound disruption, infections, lymphedema, and cellulitis were acute and chronic complications associated with these radical surgical procedures. During the last decades, there has been a continuing evolution in the surgical approach of SCC of the vulva. Patients with T1 tumors are usually treated with a partial radical vulvectomy (radical wide local excision), if the lesion is unifocal and the remainder of the vulva is normal (Figure 23.2(a)) [32]. The surgical planes extend to the urogenital diaphragm and include a tumor-free margin of at least 1 cm. Radical wide local excision may also be an option for patients with involvement of the lower urethra, vagina, or anus (T2), depending on the extent of disease. Radical wide local excision differs from the “traditional” radical vulvectomy by the amount of surrounding normal tissue, with the traditional radical procedure removing the entire vulva. Radical wide local excision removes the entire lesion with a margin of normal tissue (at least 1 cm), sparing the uninvolved areas.

Patients with T1a disease (stage IA) have no risk of lymph node metastases and do not need a surgical evaluation of their

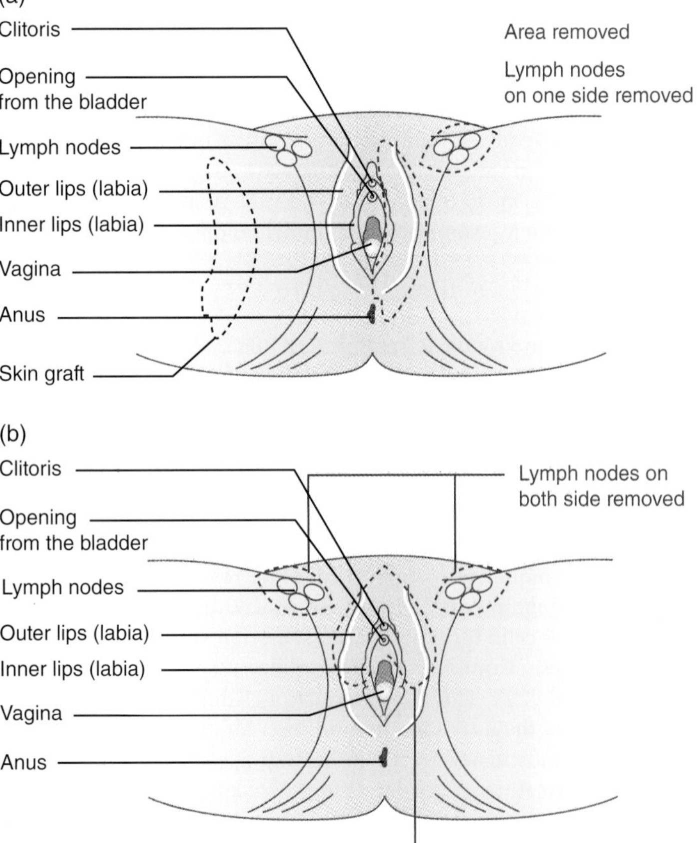

Figure 23.2 (a) A partial or simple vulvectomy on one side of the vulva. (b) A partial or simple vulvectomy affecting the top area of the vulva. *Source*: CancerHelp UK [32]. Reproduced with permission of Cancer Research UK.

inguinal/femoral lymph nodes. Those patients with T1b (stage IB) lesions require evaluation of the inguinal/femoral lymph nodes. In patients with lateral lesions <4 cm, an SLN biopsy can be offered as an alternative to ipsilateral inguinal–femoral lymphadenectomy. A recent randomized study from the Gynecologic Oncology Group reported a less than 2% risk of a groin relapse due to a false-negative SLN procedure in such patients [28]. If positive SLNs are detected, most surgeons would proceed with a unilateral inguinal femoral lymphadenectomy performed through a separate groin incision. If the lesion is ≥4 cm, an inguinal femoral lymphadenectomy is preferred, until more experience is reported for SLN procedures in this group of patients. If the lesion is midline, a bilateral SLN procedure or bilateral inguinal femoral lymphadenectomy is performed, depending on the size and stage of the vulvar cancer (Figure 23.2(b)) [31]. Bilateral inguinal femoral lymphadenectomy through separate groin incisions is performed for stage II or greater disease. Postoperative adjuvant pelvic and ipsilateral groin irradiation is warranted for patients with two or more microscopically involved groin nodes or one or more macroscopically involved lymph nodes, or any evidence of extracapsular spread.

Treatment for advanced disease (stage II, (selected) III and IV) is individualized depending on the size, location, and lymph node status. Chemotherapy may be administered with pelvic radiation (chemoradiation) followed by tailored surgery in advanced disease, which avoids the need for more radical surgical procedures (e.g., pelvic exenterations).

Chemotherapy and Radiation Therapy

There is no standard approach for treating locally advanced primary vulvar cancer (FIGO stages III/IV). Studies using primary chemoradiation or neoadjuvant chemoradiation have been reported. Neoadjuvant chemoradiation has been used to achieve resectability of the tumor and to decrease the radicality of the surgery. A recent Cochrane review concluded that there were no significant differences in overall survival or treatment-related adverse events when chemoradiation (primary or neoadjuvant) was compared with primary surgery. However, the studies reviewed were small and mostly retrospective, with methodological limitations [33]. A Gynecologic Oncology Group Phase II study using primary chemoradiation, with weekly cisplatin, followed by surgical resection reported a less radical surgical resection following chemoradiation [34].

Radiation, as a single modality, has a limited role in vulvar cancer. It can be used as primary treatment for advanced stage vulvar cancer in a patient who is not a surgical candidate or a candidate for combined chemoradiation. Data from the Surveillance, Epidemiology and End Results was reviewed over a 10-year period (1998–2008) and the authors concluded that the use of primary radiation for locally advanced vulvar cancer is limited but has increased over time. In this review, the authors report that most patients with Stage II–IVA vulvar cancer treated with primary radiation therapy did not undergo surgical resection [35].

Following radical vulvectomy and inguinal lymphadenectomy, there is a survival benefit of adjuvant radiation to the groins and pelvis as compared to surgical pelvic lymphadenectomy if there is tumor involvement of the inguinal–femoral nodes (two or more affected lymph nodes or one with extracapsular spread) [36, 37].

Surgical Treatment of Vulvar Melanoma

The primary treatment is a surgical resection of the primary lesion (wide radical local excision) and assessment of the lymph nodes, by SLN procedures or inguinal–femoral lymph node dissection. Involvement of regional lymph nodes, depth of invasion of the lesion, and lesion ulceration are widely accepted prognostic factors. SLN biopsy is recommended for patients with intermediate-thickness melanomas (Breslow thickness, 1–4 mm) of any anatomic site; use of SLN biopsy in this population provides accurate staging. Although there are few studies focusing on patients with thick melanomas (T4; Breslow thickness, >4 mm), SLN biopsy may be recommended for staging purposes and to facilitate regional disease control. There is insufficient evidence to support routine SLN biopsy for patients with thin melanomas (T1; Breslow thickness, <1 mm), although it may be considered in selected patients with high-risk features when staging benefits outweigh risks of the procedure. Completion lymph node dissection is recommended for all patients with a positive SLN biopsy and achieves good regional disease control. Whether completion lymph node dissection after a positive SLN biopsy improves survival is the subject of the ongoing Multicenter Selective Lymphadenectomy in melanoma trial [38].

The systemic therapies for advanced stage melanomas are addressed in the Chapter 34.

Follow-Up and Surveillance

As noted, survival of patients with vulvar cancer correlates with the stage of disease (Table 23.3) [39]. The prognosis for patients with early-stage disease is generally good. Lymph node status is the single most important prognostic factor. Patients with negative lymph nodes have a 5-year survival rate of >70–80%, which falls to <50% for patients with positive lymph nodes and to as low as 13% for those with four or more positive nodes [40]. Although patients with local recurrences may be salvageable, groin or distant recurrences generally are fatal.

The Society of Gynecologic Oncology consensus recommendations for post-treatment follow-up of patients with vulvar cancer are based on expert opinion [41]. Although most recurrences

Table 23.3 Survival rates for carcinoma of the vulva by FIGO Stage [39].

FIGO stage	5-year overall survival (%)
I	84.0
II	74.6
III	47.8
IV	9.4

Source: Zhou and Shan [39].

will occur within 2 years, one-third of relapses have been reported after 5 years [35, 42]. Many of these recurrences are in the vulva and groin. Thus, careful inspection and palpation of the vulva, skin bridges, and groin nodal region is recommended every 3 months for 2 years for patients with advanced disease and then every 6 months for 5 years and every 6 months for patients with early stage disease for 5 years. Because these patients are at risk for other HPV-related cancers, they should be screened for cervical and vaginal cancers. There are no data to recommend routine radiologic testing in the follow-up of asymptomatic patients. For patients with symptoms, the workup will depend on the symptoms, and may include computed tomography, possibly positron emission tomography or magnetic resonance imaging.

The Society of Gynecologic Oncology has developed a survivorship summary for patients with vulvar cancer, which records their treating medical/surgical team, treatment, a list of common symptoms, and a follow-up schedule. This form can be downloaded from the website: www.sgo.org.

Women who undergo surgical treatment for vulvar cancer may be at risk for postoperative sexual dysfunction depending on their age, performance status, mental status, and excisional size of the vulvar malignancy [43]. In the past, with radical vulvectomies, the clitoris was routinely removed. With radical wide local excision procedures, the clitoris can often be spared.

Lower extremity lymphedema and wound infections and breakdowns were commonly associated with radical vulvectomy and bilateral inguinal–femoral lymph node dissections. The addition of pelvic radiation in women with involved groin nodes also increased the risk of these complications. With the increasing use of SLN procedures and radical wide local excisions, these complications have been dramatically decreased [44].

Conclusion

There are likely two independent pathways of vulvar carcinogenesis. The pre-existing lesion in type I is likely HPV-positive warty/basaloid VIN and in type II, chronic inflammation, lichen sclerosus, squamous cell hyperplasia, and differentiated VIN. Type II vulvar SCCs have a significantly worse prognosis than the type I vulvar SCCs.

For VIN, treatment is usually performed in the office or outpatient ambulatory surgical setting under local anesthesia.

During the last decades, there has been a continuing evolution in the surgical approach of SCC of the vulva. The surgical approach includes a radical wide excision of the vulvar cancer, with node sampling using an SLN technique or in more advanced disease an inguinofemoral lymphadenectomy through a separate incision. These radical procedures are performed by gynecologic oncologists.

The HPV vaccine will likely result in a reduction of type I vulvar preinvasive and invasive cancer.

References

1 Siegel RL, Miller KD, Jemal A. Cancer statistics, 2017. *CA Cancer J Clin* 2017;67:7–30.
2 National Cancer Institute. SEER Cancer Stat Facts: Vulvar Cancer. National Cancer Institute. Bethesda, MD. http://seer.cancer.gov/statfacts/html/vulva.html (accessed 12 October 2017).
3 Akerman G, Dussour C, Haddad B, *et al.* Epidemiology of vulvar intra-epithelial neoplasias. *Gynecol Obstet Fertil* 2007;35:1251–6.
4 Nugent EK, Brooks RA, Barr CD, *et al.* Clinical and pathologic features of vulvar intraepithelial neoplasia in premenopausal and postmenopausal women. *J Low Genit Tract Dis* 2011;15:15–19.
5 Crum CP. Carcinoma of the vulva: epidemiology and pathogenesis. *Obstet Gynecol* 1992;79:448–54.
6 Jones RW, Rowan DM, Stewart AW. VIN: aspects of the natural history and outcome in 405 women. *Obstet Gynecol* 2005;106:1319–26.
7 Heller DS, van Seters M, Marchitelli C, *et al.* Update on intraepithelial neoplasias of the vulva: Proceedings of a workshop at the 2009 World Congress of the International Society for the Study of vulvovaginal diseases, Edinburgh, Scotland, September 2009. *J Low Genit Tract Dis* 2010;14:363–73.
8 van de Nieuwenhof HP, van Kempen LCLT, de Hullu JA. The etiologic role of HPV in vulvar squamous cell carcinoma fine tuned. *Cancer Epidemiol Biomarkers Prev* 2009;18:2061–7.
9 Grulich AE, van Leeuwen MT, Falster MO, *et al.* Incidence of cancers in people with HIV/AIDS compared with immunosuppressed transplant recipients: a meta-analysis. *Lancet* 2007;370:59–67.
10 Engels EA, Pfeiffer RM, Fraumeni JF Jr, *et al.* Spectrum of cancer risk among US solid organ transplant recipients. *JAMA* 2011;306:1891–901.
11 Madeleine MM, Daling JD, Carter JJ, *et al.* Cofactors with human papillomavirus in a population-based study of vulvar cancer. *J Natl Cancer Inst* 1997;89:1516–23.
12 Joura EA, Garland SM, Paavonen J, *et al.* Effect of the human papillomavirus (HPV) quadrivalent vaccine in a subgroup of women with cervical and vulvar disease: retrospective pooled analysis of trial data. *BMJ* 2012;344:e1401.
13 Simons M, Van De Nieuwenhof HP, Van Der Avoort IAM, *et al.* A patient with lichen sclerosus, Langerhans cell histiocytosis, invasive squamous cell carcinoma of the vulva. *Am J of Obstet Gynecol* 2010;203:e7–e10.
14 Taube JM, Badger J, Kong CS, *et al.* Differentiated (simplex) vulvar intraepithelial neoplastic: a case report and review of the literature. *Am J Dermatopathol* 2011;33:e27–e30.
15 Gibb RK, Olawaiye AB, Chen LM, *et al.* Vulva. Amin MB, Edge SB, Greene FL (eds). *AJCC Cancer Staging Manual*, 8th edn. New York: Springer Nature, 2017
16 Pecorelli S, Chairman, FIGO Committee on Gynecological Oncology. Revised FIGO staging for carcinoma of the vulva, cervix and endometrium. *Int J Gynaecol Obstet* 2009;105:103–4.

17 Gadducci A, Tana R, Barsotti C, *et al.* Clinico-pathological and biological prognostic variables in squamous cell carcinoma of the vulva. *Crit Rev Oncol Hematol* 2012;83:71–83.

18 Knopp S, Trope C, Nesland JM, *et al.* A review of molecular pathological markers in vulvar carcinoma: lack of application in clinical practice. *J Clin Pathol* 2009;62:212–18.

19 del Pino M, Bleeker MC, Quint WG, *et al.* Comprehensive analysis of human papillomavirus prevalence and the potential role of low-risk types in verrucous carcinoma. *Mod Pathol* 2012;25:1354–63.

20 Sugiyama VE, Chan JK, Kapp DS. Management of melanoma of the female genital tract. *Curr Opin Oncol* 2008;20:565–9

21 Moxley KM, Fader AN, Rose PG, *et al.* Malignant melanoma of the vulva: an extension of cutaneous melanoma. *Gynecol Oncol* 2011;122:612–17.

22 Copeland LJ, Sneige N, Gershenson DM, *et al.* Bartholin gland carcinoma. *Obstet Gynecol* 1986;67:794–801.

23 Ouldamer L, Chraibi Z, Arbion F, *et al.* Bartholin's gland carcinoma: epidemiology and therapeutic management. *Surg Oncol* 2013;22:117–22.

24 Mulvany NJ, Rayoo M, Allen DG. Basal cell carcinoma of the vulva: a case series. *Pathology* 2012;44:528–33.

25 Delport ES. Extramammary Paget's disease of the vulva: an annotated review of the current literature. *Australas J Dermatol* 2013;54:9–21.

26 Cai Y, Sheng W, Xiang L, *et al.* Primary extramammary Paget's disease of the vulva: the clinicopathological features and treatment outcomes in a series of 43 patients. *Gynecol Oncol* 2013;129:412–16.

27 Lloyd J, Flanagan AM. Mammary and extramammary Paget's disease. *J Clin Pathol* 2000;53:742–9.

28 Levenback CF, Ali S, Coleman RL, *et al.* Lymphatic mapping and sentinel lymph node biopsy in women with squamous cell carcinoma of the vulva: a Gynecologic Oncology Group study. *J Clin Oncol* 2012;30:3786–91.

29 van Seters M, van Beurden M, ten Kate FJ, *et al.* Treatment of vulvar intraepithelial neoplasia with topical imiquimod. *N Engl J Med* 2008;358:1465–73.

30 Ribeiro F, Figueiredo A, Paula T, *et al.* Vulvar intraepithelial neoplasia: evaluation of treatment modalities. *J Low Genit Tract Dis* 2012;16:313–17.

31 Fuh KC, Berek JS. Current management of vulvar cancer. *Hematol Oncol Clin North Am* 2012;26:45–62.

32 CancerHelp UK, the patient information website of Cancer Research UK: http://www.cancerresearchuk.org/cancer-help/type/vulval-cancer/treatment/surgery/diagrams/diagrams-of-partial-vulvectomy-operations (accessed 12 October 2017).

33 Shylasree TS, Bryant A, Howelss REJ. Chemoradiation for advanced primary vulval cancer. *Cochrane Database Syst Rev* 2011;April 13(4):CD0003752.

34 Moore DH, Ali S, Koh WJ, *et al.* A phase II trial of radiation therapy and weekly cisplatin for the treatment of locally-advanced squamous cell carcinoma of the vulva: a gynecologic oncology study. *Gynecol Oncol* 2012;124:529–33

35 Sharma C, Deutsch I, Herzog TJ, *et al.* Patterns of care for locally advanced vulvar cancer. *Am J Obstet Gynecol* 2013;209:60e.1–5.

36 Homesley H, Bundy B, Sedlis A, *et al.* Radiation therapy versus pelvic node resection for carcinoma of the vulva with positive groin nodes. *Obstet Gynecol* 1986;68:733–40.

37 Parthasarathy A, Cheung M, Osann, *et al.* The benefit of adjuvant radiation therapy in single-node positive squamous cell vulvar carcinoma. *Gynecol Oncol* 2006;103:1095–9.

38 Morton DL. Overview and update of the phase III Multicenter Selective Lymphadenectomy Trials (MSLT-I and MSLT-II) in melanoma. *Clin Exp Metastasis* 2012;29:699–706.

39 Zhou J, Shan G. The prognostic role of FIGO stage in patients with vulvar cancer: a systematic review and meta-analysis. *Curr Med Res Opin* 2016;32:1121–30.

40 Beller U, Quinn MA, Benedet JL, *et al.* Carcinoma of the vulva. FIGO 26th annual report on the results of treatment in gynecological cancer. *Int J Gynaecol Obstet* 2006;95:S7–27.

41 Salani R, Backes FJ, Fung MF, *et al.* Posttreatment surveillance and diagnosis of recurrence in women with gynecologic malignancies: Society of Gynecologic Oncologists recommendations. *Am J Obstet Gynecol* 2011;204:466–78.

42 Gonzalez Bosquet J, Magrina JF, Gaffey TA, *et al.* Long-term survival and disease recurrence in patients with primary squamous cell carcinoma of the vulva. *Gynecol Oncol* 2005;97:828–33.

43 Aerts L, Enzlin P, Vergote I, *et al.* Sexual, psychological, and relational functioning in women after surgical treatment for vulvar malignancy: a literature review. *J Sex Med* 2012;9:361–71.

44 de Melo Ferreira AP, de Figueuredo EM, Lima RA. Quality of life in women with vulvar cancer submitted to surgical treatment: a comparative study. *Eur J Obstet Gynecol Repro Biol* 2012;165:91–5.

24

Gestational Trophoblastic Disease

Alok Pant[1] and John R. Lurain[2]

[1] John I Brewer Trophoblastic Disease Center, Northwestern University Feinberg School of Medicine, Chicago, Illinois, USA
[2] Northwestern University Feinberg School of Medicine, Robert H. Lurie Comprehensive Cancer Center, Chicago, Illnois, USA

Introduction

Gestational trophoblastic disease (GTD) describes four interrelated forms of growth disturbance of the placental trophoblast (complete and partial hydatidform mole, invasive mole, choriocarcinoma, placental site trophoblastic tumor/epithelioid trophoblastic tumor). Gestational trophoblastic neoplasia (GTN) encompasses the latter three disease states. GTN most commonly arises after a molar pregnancy, but it can develop after other pregnancy events.

GTD was historically associated with high morbidity and mortality. Hydatidiform moles were often accompanied by serious bleeding and medical complications prior to the development of early detection and effective uterine evacuation techniques. While the overall cure rate for GTN now exceeds 90%, before the advent of effective chemotherapy, more than 15% of patients with invasive mole died, as did nearly all patients who had metastatic choriocarcinoma. The marked improvement in treatment of GTN relates to the inherent sensitivity of trophoblastic diseases to chemotherapy, the effective use of sensitive assays for the tumor marker human chorionic gonadotropin (hCG), the development of specialized treatment centers, identification of predictive factors that enhance individualization of therapy, and the use of combined aggressive therapy including multiagent chemotherapy, surgery, and radiation in the highest risk patients [1–3].

Incidence and Etiology

The epidemiology of GTD has been difficult to define strictly because of the rare nature of the disease, variable definitions of different disease states, and lack of centralized databases. Determining the specific populations at risk for the development of GTD and the contributing risk factors has proven difficult because of similar issues and the lack of control groups [1]. Varying incidence rates of hydatidiform mole have been reported in different parts of the world. A rate of 0.6–1.1 hydatidiform moles per 1000 pregnancies has been reported in North America, Europe, and Australia, as compared to rates as high as 2.0 per 1000 pregnancies in Southeast Asia and Japan [4]. Even though a variation in incidence based on geographical location has been reported, no specific genetic or cultural differences have been identified among different ethnic groups that would contribute to the different rates in different parts of the world. Several reports have demonstrated a link between higher rates of molar pregnancy and decreased intake of animal fat and vitamin A (carotene). Infertility and a history of spontaneous abortion have also been linked to a higher rate of complete and partial mole. Women with a history of miscarriage have a two- to threefold higher risk of molar pregnancy compared to women who have never had a miscarriage [1].

The two most significant risk factors for the development of complete hydatidiform molar pregnancy are extremes of maternal reproductive age and prior history of molar pregnancy. Along with very young women, women over the age of 40 have an increased risk of molar pregnancy. Compared to women aged 21–35, women over the age of 40 have a 7.5-fold higher rate of molar pregnancy [5]. After one prior molar pregnancy, the risk of a second subsequent molar pregnancy is 1%, which is 10–20-fold higher than the risk of molar pregnancy in the general population. After two prior molar pregnancies, the risk of a third molar pregnancy jumps to 15–20%, regardless of a change in partner [6]. Increased risk of partial molar pregnancy is not linked to increased maternal age or vitamin A deficiency, but is associated with the use of oral contraceptive pills with high estrogen content and a history of irregular menstruation [7].

A novel missense mutation in the NLRP7 locus on chromosome 19 has been linked to a familial predisposition to hydatidiform mole with one study reporting a 60% rate of this mutation in patients with two molar pregnancies. This gene mutation is involved in maternal imprinting and is seen in clusters of complete moles of biparental origin as opposed to paternal origin [8].

Choriocarcinoma is 1000 times more likely following a complete mole compared to another pregnancy event. Risk factors associated with the development of choriocarcinoma are advanced maternal age, menarche after age 12, light menstrual

The American Cancer Society's Oncology in Practice: Clinical Management, First Edition. Edited by The American Cancer Society.

flow, prior complete hydatidiform mole, or Asian American, Native American, or African American race [9]. Long-term oral contraceptive use and presence of blood group A appear to confer an increased risk of development of choriocarcinoma [10]. Fifteen percent of patients will develop locally invasive gestational trophoblastic neoplasia following evacuation of molar pregnancy. One in 50,000 pregnancy events will result in choriocarcinoma. Half of all cases of choriocarcinoma arise from complete moles.

Insufficient data exist regarding placental site trophoblastic tumor (PSTT), and its variant epithelioid trophoblastic tumor (ETT), to characterize their epidemiology and risk factors adequately. However, 95% of all cases of PSTT and ETT develop following term pregnancy or nonmolar abortion and may develop after several months or years [1].

Pathology

Molar pregnancies and gestational trophoblastic neoplasms take their origin from the placental trophoblast. Following fertilization, the zygote transforms into a morula, which, in turn, evolves into a blastocyst that houses an inner layer called the embryoblast and an outer cell layer known as the trophoblast. The trophoblast begins to proliferate after the blastocyst has attached to the uterine wall and differentiates into the cytotrophoblast and the syncytiotrophoblast. The syncytiotrophoblast extends into the endometrial stroma with no discernable cell boundaries and plays an important role in blastocyst implantation. The syncytiotrophoblast produces the biochemical marker of pregnancy, hCG. The cytotrophoblast forms the chorionic sac as it continues to supply the growing syncytiotrophoblast with cells. The chorionic sac becomes covered with branching villi, outpouchings of the cytotrophoblast cells, carrying blood vessels with fetal blood. The chorionic sac contains the amniotic sac and the fetal embryo. The villous chorion combines with the basalis layer of the endometrium to form the placenta where the maternal and fetal units exchange nutrients and waste products. The three placental cellular elements, the cytotrophoblast, the syncytiotrophoblast, and the intermediate trophoblast, are the basis for molar pregnancies and gestational trophoblastic neoplasms. All three types of trophoblast can differentiate into GTD lesions [11].

Complete Hydatidiform Moles

Complete hydatidiform moles are characterized by the absence of fetal tissue. The vast majority of complete moles have a 46, XX karyotype. Usually, a haploid (23X) sperm fertilizes an ovum and then duplicates its own chromosomes. The maternal component is either absent or inactive. Approximately 10% of complete moles have a 46, XY karyotype, where, once again, all the genetic material is of paternal origin. These moles result when an empty ovum is fertilized by two separate sperm. The chorionic villi are grossly and uniformly edematous with central cisterns of fluid and the presence of diffuse trophoblastic hyperplasia. Initial villous cisterns disappear as cisterns form so that complete moles lack intrinsic vascularity. Trophoblastic neoplasia (invasive mole or choriocarcinoma) follows complete mole in 15–20% of cases [12].

Partial Hydatidiform Moles

Partial hydatidiform moles demonstrate identifiable fetal tissue and consist of chorionic villi with focal villous edema and some persistently immature, unaffected villi. The villi vary in size and shape and display scalloping and prominent trophoblastic inclusions along with a functional villous circulation and focal trophoblastic hyperplasia with only mild atypia. Most partial moles are triploid, most often 69, XXY, with two sets of paternal chromosomes resulting from either dispermic fertilization of a normal egg or duplication of chromosomes in a single sperm after fertilization of a normal egg. Fewer than 5% of partial moles will develop postmolar GTN [13].

Invasive Mole

Invasive mole is a benign tumor resulting from a hydatidiform mole displaying myometrial invasion via venous channels or direct extension through tissue. Approximately 10–17% of hydatidiform moles will result in invasive moles and, of these, approximately 15% will metastasize to the lungs or vagina [14].

Choriocarcinoma

Choriocarcinoma is a malignant condition characterized by abnormal trophoblastic hyperplasia and anaplasia, absence of chorionic villi, hemorrhage, and necrosis with direct invasion into the myometrium and vasculature that allows for metastasis to lungs, brain, liver, pelvis, vagina, intestines, and spleen. The tumor tends to elicit minimal surrounding tissue inflammation. The presence of syncytiotrophoblast confers the ability to secrete hCG. Approximately 2–3% of women with complete moles develop choriocarcinoma. However, 50% of choriocarcinomas are associated with other pregnancy events [15–19].

Placental Site Trophoblastic Tumor

PSTT usually develops from placental implantation site intermediate trophoblast after a normal or aborted uterine pregnancy. These lesions contain mononuclear intermediate trophoblasts without chorionic villi that infiltrate the uterine wall in sheets between myometrial fibers. PSTT do have potential for locally aggressive behavior and metastasis via lymphatic channels. Most tumors have fewer than five mitoses per ten high power fields. Immunohistochemical staining reveals the diffuse presence of low molecular weight cytokeratins, inhibin, CD10, HLA-G, and human placental lactogen (hPL), only focal expression of hCG, a Ki-67 proliferation rate of more than 10%, and the absence of nuclear p63. The tumor is usually grossly confined to the uterus [20, 21].

Epithelioid Trophoblastic Tumor

ETT is a rare variant of PSTT that simulates carcinoma. ETT is a malignant tumor arising from the neoplastic transformation of chorion-type intermediate trophoblast. Immunohistochemical staining typically demonstrates expression of inhibin, cytokeratin 18, and (nuclear) p63, with only focal, if any, reactivity for hPL or hCG. Most ETTs present years after a full-term delivery [21–23].

Clinical Presentation

Complete hydatidiform mole most commonly presents with vaginal bleeding, occurring in at least 90% of cases between 6 and 16 weeks' gestation (Table 24.1). Other classical clinical signs and symptoms are excessive uterine size (28%), hyperemesis (8%), and pregnancy-induced hypertension or other medical complications such as hyperthyroidism and trophoblastic embolization (1%). Serum hCG levels are often >100,000 mIU/mL, and fetal heart tones are absent. Theca lutein ovarian cysts are seen in association with molar pregnancies in approximately 15% of cases. These cysts are frequently 6–12 cm in size, bilateral, and result from ovarian hyperstimulation by high serum levels of hCG. The mean time to resolution of these cysts following evacuation of molar pregnancy is 8 weeks and complications, such as ovarian torsion, are uncommon. Hyperthyroidism is associated with high levels of circulating hCG. Hyperthyroidism that is poorly controlled at presentation may result in the development of thyroid storm at the time of anesthesia induction. Beta-adrenergic blocking agents are instrumental in preventing and reversing this condition. The acute onset of respiratory insufficiency after evacuation of a large molar pregnancy (>16 weeks) is rare, but has been attributed to embolization of trophoblastic tissue, along with complications from pre-eclampsia, thyroid storm or large fluid volume replacement. Earlier diagnosis of complete molar pregnancy is much more common now due to widespread use of ultrasound and sensitive hCG assays, resulting in a lower frequency of these classic signs and symptoms [24].

Partial molar pregnancy does not have the same presentation as a complete mole. More than 90% of patients with partial moles present with signs or symptoms of a missed or incomplete abortion, and the diagnosis is usually made after histologic review of curettage specimens. While vaginal bleeding does occur in 75% of patients, uterine enlargement, hyperemesis, hypertension, hyperthyroidism, and theca lutein cysts are rare in partial moles. Pre-evacuation hCG levels are >100,000 mIU/mL in <10% of patients with partial moles [25].

Gestational trophoblastic neoplasia has a varied presentation depending on the antecedent pregnancy event, extent of disease, and histopathology. Postmolar GTN (invasive mole or choriocarcinoma) most commonly presents as irregular bleeding following evacuation of a hydatidiform mole. Signs suggestive of postmolar GTN are an enlarged, irregular uterus and persistent bilateral ovarian enlargement. Occasionally, a metastatic vaginal lesion may be noted on evaluation, disruption of which may cause uncontrolled bleeding. Choriocarcinoma associated with a nonmolar gestation has no characteristic symptoms or signs, which are mostly related to invasion of tumor in the uterus or at metastatic sites. PSTTs and ETTs almost always cause irregular uterine bleeding often distant from a preceding nonmolar

Table 24.1 Clinicopathologic features of gestational trophoblastic disease.

Disease	Pathologic features	Clinical factors
Complete mole	Diploid (46,XX, rarely 46,XY) Absent fetus/embryo Diffuse swelling of villi Diffuse trophoblastic hyperplasia	Vaginal bleeding Large for dates uterine size Bilateral theca lutein cysts Medical complications hCG often >100,000 mIU/mL 15–20% postmolar GTN
Partial mole	Triploid (69,XXY;69,XYY; 69,XXX) Abnormal fetus/embryo Focal swelling of villi Focal trophoblastic hyperplasia	Pre-D&C diagnosis usually incomplete or missed abortion Medical complications rare hCG rarely > 100,000 mIU/mL <5% postmolar GTN
Invasive Mole	Swollen villi Hyperplastic trophoblast Myometrial invasion	Irregular postmolar vaginal bleeding Persistent hCG elevation Most often diagnosed clinically, rather than pathologically 15% metastatic – lung/vagina
Choriocarcinoma	Abnormal trophoblastic hyperplasia Absent villi Hemorrhage Necrosis	Irregular vaginal bleeding after any pregnancy event hCG elevation Symptoms associated with vascular spread to distant sites
PSTT	Diploid Intermediate trophoblastic hyperplasia Absent villi Less hemorrhage and necrosis Vascular and lymphatic invasion Tumor cells stain positive for hPL	Enlarged uterus Total hCG low hCG free beta subunit elevated Relatively chemoresistant Mainly surgical treatment
ETT	Rare variant of PSTT Chorionic-type intermediate trophoblast Extensive necrosis Rare hemorrhage	Enlarged uterus Metastases with associated symptoms No or very low elevation of serum hCG Relatively chemoresistant

Source: Lurain [1]. Reproduced with permission of Elsevier.

D&C, dilatation and curettage; ETT, epithelioid trophoblastic tumor; GTN, gestational trophoblastic neoplasia; hCG; human chorionic gonadotropin; hPL, human placental lactogen; PSTT, placental site trophoblastic tumor.

gestation, and rarely virilization or nephrotic syndrome. The uterus is usually symmetrically enlarged and serum hCG levels are only slightly elevated or normal [26].

Diagnosis

Ultrasound

Ultrasound plays a crucial role in the diagnosis of complete and partial molar pregnancy and allows for much earlier diagnosis. The diffuse hydropic swelling of the chorionic villi in complete moles results in a characteristic vesicular pattern on ultrasound with many multiple echos (holes) in the placental mass and usually no fetus. For partial moles, ultrasound can detect focal cystic spaces in the placenta and an enlarged gestational sac [27, 28].

Human Chorionic Gonadotropin

Human chorionic gonadotropin, the disease-specific tumor marker produced by molar pregnancies and gestation trophoblastic neoplasms, can be easily measured in the urine and blood and has been found to correlate with the amount of disease present. It is a placental glycoprotein composed of an alpha and beta subunit. The alpha subunit resembles that of the pituitary glycoprotein hormones and the beta subunit is unique to placental production. Patients with complete moles commonly have markedly elevated levels of hCG, with pre-evacuation levels of >100,000 mIU/mL in approximately 50% of patients. Alternatively, less than 10% of partial moles have such elevated levels of serum hCG. Serum hCG measurements need to be taken at several time intervals to differentiate a complete molar pregnancy from a normal gestation, multiple gestation, or other pregnancy conditions associated with an enlarged placenta [29].

At least six major variants of hCG are detected in serum: hyperglycosylated, nicked, hCG missing the beta subunit C-terminal segment, free beta subunit, nicked free beta subunit, and free alpha subunit. Hyperglycosylated hCG is produced by GTN lesions and promotes growth and invasion of abnormal trophoblasts. In the urine and serum of patients with trophoblastic disease, the hCG molecules are more degraded than those in normal pregnancies. For this reason, it is important that an hCG assay which recognizes all main forms of hCG and its fragments be used when following patients with GTD. Most institutions currently use rapid, automated radiolabeled monoclonal antibody sandwich assays that measure different mixtures of hCG-related molecules [30].

A clinical diagnosis of postmolar GTN is most often made by the finding of rising or plateauing hCG levels following evacuation of a hydatidiform mole. Choriocarcinoma is usually diagnosed by the finding of an elevated hCG level, frequently in conjunction with the discovery of metastases, following other pregnancy events. PSTT and ETT are commonly associated with only slightly raised hCG levels. The hCG free beta subunit is a reliable marker for PSTT [31].

False positive hCG results, sometimes as high as 800 mIU/mL, can be due to the presence of nonspecific, heterophilic antibodies that mimic hCG and can interfere with the hCG sandwich assay. These antibodies are present in 3–4% of people. Since the antibody does not pass into urine, false positive values can be determined by urine hCG testing. Additionally, there is some hCG crossreactivity with pituitary luteinizing hormone (LH) which may lead to falsely elevated low levels of hCG. Measurement of LH to identify this possibility and suppression of LH with oral contraceptive pills will prevent these problems [32, 33].

Quiescent gestational trophoblastic disease is a term applied to presumed inactive form of GTN that is characterized by persistent, relatively unchanging low levels (usually <200 mIU/mL) of "real" hCG for at least 3 months associated with a history of GTN or spontaneous abortion but without clinically detectable disease. The hCG levels do not change with chemotherapy or surgery. Subanalysis of hCG reveals no hyperglycosylated hCG, which is associated with cytotrophoblast invasion. Follow-up of patients with presumed quiescent GTD reveals subsequent development of active GTN in about 25%, which is heralded by an increase in both hyperglycosylated and total hCG [30]. According to the International Society for the Study of Trophoblastic Diseases recommendations for managing a presumptive diagnosis of quiescent GTD are: exclude a false positive hCG resulting from heterophile antibodies or LH interference, thoroughly investigate the patient for evidence of disease, avoid immediate chemotherapy or surgery, and monitor the patient with long term hCG testing while avoiding pregnancy. Treatment should be undertaken only when there is a sustained rise in hCG or the appearance of overt clinical disease [31, 34].

Pathologic Diagnosis

Pathologic diagnosis of complete and partial moles is made by examination of curettage specimens. Immunohistochemical staining for *PHLDA2* (a paternally imprinted, maternally expressed gene) can differentiate absent immunostaining complete moles from hydropic abortuses and partial moles [35]. Analysis by flow cytometry or selective molecular genotyping can distinguish androgenic diploid complete moles from diandrogenic triploid partial moles from biparental diploid hydropic abortuses [15–17]. 34 Additionally, pathologic diagnosis of invasive mole, choriocarcinoma, PSTT and ETT can sometimes be made by curettage, biopsy of metastatic lesions, or examination of hysterectomy specimens or placentas. Biopsy of a vaginal lesion suggestive of a gestational trophoblast tumor is dangerous because of the massive bleeding that may occur [36].

Hydatidiform Mole

Once the diagnosis of molar pregnancy is suspected by history, hCG levels, and ultrasound findings, the patient should be evaluated for the presence of medical complications (anemia, pre-eclampsia, hyperthyroidism) by way of physical examination findings, complete blood count, basic chemistries, hepatic and thyroid panel, blood type and cross match, serum hCG level, and chest X-ray. Suction evacuation and curettage under ultrasound guidance is the preferred treatment for patients who wish to preserve their future fertility. Rh-negative patients should receive Rh immunoglobulin because the Rh D factor is expressed by trophoblastic cells. If childbearing has been completed, then hysterectomy is a potential alternative to suction curettage. Despite the presence of theca lutein cysts, the adnexae may be left intact. While hysterectomy does eliminate the risk of local myometrial invasion, the potential for persistent GTN remains 3–5%, so continued hCG monitoring is still required. Medical induction of labor and hysterotomy are not recommended due to increased maternal morbidity and trophoblastic dissemination resulting in postmolar GTN that may require chemotherapy [37, 38].

Prophylactic chemotherapy, either methotrexate or actinomycin D, administered at the time of molar evacuation or immediately afterwards can reduce the risk of postmolar GTN from 15–20% down to 3–8%. However, due to the otherwise extremely high cure rates, the use of prophylactic chemotherapy should be limited to patients with a greater than normal risk of postmolar GTN or those who are less likely to follow–up [39–42].

To ensure that remission is obtained, serial serum hCG measurements are recommended for all patients following the evacuation of a molar pregnancy. Serum hCG levels should be collected within 48 h of molar evacuation, every 1–2 weeks while elevated, and then at 3-month intervals for 6 months after spontaneous return to normal levels has been reached. Contraception, preferably using oral contraceptive pills, is recommended until 6 months after the first normal hCG result [39]. More than 50% of patients will achieve a normal hCG level within 2 months of evacuation. Approximately 15–20% of patients with complete moles and 1–5% of patients with partial moles will develop persistent disease requiring chemotherapy. The likelihood of persistent disease developing after evacuation of a complete mole is increased in patients older than 40 years of age, pre-evaluation hCG level >100,000 mIU/mL, excessive uterine enlargement, large theca lutein cysts, a repeat molar pregnancy, and medical complications of the molar pregnancy [2]. Women with a history of molar pregnancy also have a higher risk of GTD in subsequent pregnancies. Women should wait to become pregnant for at least 6 months following spontaneous regression of hCG to normal. Pathologic examination of the placenta and other products of conception as well as determination of a 6-week postpartum hCG level is recommended with all future pregnancies [39, 43].

Gestational Trophoblastic Neoplasia

GTN encompasses invasive mole, choriocarcinoma, PSTT, and ETT. The diagnosis of GTN is made when there is clinical, radiologic, pathologic, and/or hormonal evidence of abnormal trophoblastic tissue proliferation [1–3]. GTN most commonly follows molar pregnancy, but it may occur after any pregnancy event. The diagnosis of invasive mole is usually made clinically based on persistently elevated hCG levels. Invasive mole results from invasion of abnormal trophoblasts into myometrium or embolization of molar tissue via the pelvic venous plexus. Approximately 15% of patients with invasive mole will have metastatic disease, most commonly in the lungs or vagina. Choriocarcinoma can occur after any pregnancy event. It can invade early in its disease course and patients may present with widely metastatic disease. The incidence of choriocarcinoma is 1 in 40,000 pregnancies. PSTT and ETT are relatively resistant to chemotherapy, but surgery is usually curative for localized disease. Once a diagnosis of GTN is suspected or established, a workup for metastatic disease and an evaluation for risk factors should take place, including a history, physical examination, complete blood count, serum chemistries, and serum hCG level. Radiographic studies should include chest X-ray and computed tomography (CT) of the chest if negative, CT scan of the abdomen/pelvis, and CT or magnetic resonance imaging of the brain. If the physical examination and chest X-ray are normal in the absence of symptoms, other sites of metastases are uncommon [44–46].

In 2002, the International Federation of Gynecology and Obstetrics (FIGO) proposed a combined anatomic staging (Table 24.2) and modified World Health Organization (WHO) risk-factor scoring system (Table 24.3) for GTN [47]. This system also defined criteria for diagnosing postmolar GTN, which included: (i) hCG plateau for four consecutive values over 3 weeks; (ii) hCG rise of ≥10% for three values over 2 weeks; (iii) hCG persistence 6 months after molar evacuation; (iv) histopathologic diagnosis of choriocarcinoma; or (v) presence of metastatic disease. Treatment of GTN is based on classification into different risk groups. Patients with a risk score of 6 or lower are designated low risk and those with a score of 7 or higher are deemed high risk. Patients with nonmetastatic (FIGO stage I) and low-risk metastatic (FIGO stage II and III; score <7) GTN can be treated with single-agent chemotherapy with survival rates approaching 100%. Patients with high-risk metastatic disease (FIGO stage IV or stages II and III, score ≥7) should be treated more aggressively with multiagent chemotherapy and potentially radiation and/or surgery to achieve cure rates of 80–90%. Use of the FIGO staging system is essential for determining initial therapy to assure best possible outcomes with the least morbidity [47, 48].

Low-Risk Disease

Single-agent chemotherapy, either methotrexate or actinomycin D, is the preferred treatment for patients with nonmetastatic (stage I) and low-risk metastatic (stages II and III, score <7) GTN. Several different outpatient chemotherapy protocols have been shown to be effective in mostly nonrandomized retrospective studies (Table 24.4). The variability in primary remission rates reflects differences in drug dosages, schedules, and routes of administration, as well as patient selection. Also, older patient age, higher hCG levels, nonmolar antecent pregnancy, clinicopathologic diagnosis of choriocarcinoma, presence of metastatic disease, and higher FIGO score have each been associated with an increased risk of initial chemotherapy resistance [49]. In general, one of the multiday methotrexate or actinomycin D protocols are more effective than the weekly intramuscular or intermittent intravenous infusion methotrexate and the biweekly single-dose actinomycin D protocols, especially in the setting of metastatic disease, a FIGO score >4, and/

Table 24.2 FIGO staging for gestational trophoblastic neoplasia.

Stage I	Disease confined to the uterus
Stage II	Disease extends outside the uterus but is limited to the genital structures (adnexa, vagina, broad ligament)
Stage III	Disease extends to the lungs with or without genital tract involvement
Stage IV	Disease involves other metastatic sites

Table 24.3 FIGO (modified World Health Organization) scoring system for gestational trophoblastic neoplasia.

	Score			
Risk factor	**0**	**1**	**2**	**3**
Age	≤39	>39	—	—
Antecedent pregnancy	Mole	Abortion	Term	
Pregnancy event to treatment interval (months)	<4	4–6	7–12	>12
Pretreatment hCG (mIU/mL)	$<10^3$	10^3–10^4	10^4–10^5	$>10^5$
Largest tumor mass, including uterus (cm)	<3	3–4	≥5	—
Site of metastases	—	Spleen, kidney	Gastrointestinal tract	Brain, liver
Number of metastases	—	1–4	5–8	>8
Previous failed chemotherapy	—	—	Single drug	≥2 drugs

The total score for a patient is obtained by adding the individual scores for each prognostic factor: low risk <7; high risk ≥7.

Table 24.4 Chemotherapy regimens for low-risk gestational trophoblastic neoplasia [50].

Chemotherapy regimen	Primary remission rate (%)
1. MTX 0.4 mg/kg (max 25 mg)/day or IM for 5 days. Repeat every 14 days	81–93
2. MTX 1 mg/kg IM days 1, 3, 5, 7; folinic acid 0.1 mg/kg IM or PO days 2, 4, 6, 8. Repeat every 14 days	74–90
3. 2. MTX 30–50 mg/m² IM weekly	49–74
4. MTX 100 mg/m² IVP, then 200 mg/m² in 500 mL D5W over 12 h. Folinic acid 15 mg IM or PO every 12 h for four doses beginning 24 h after the start of MTX. Repeat every 14 days, or as needed	69–90
5. Act-D 10–13 µg/kg IV daily for 5 days. Repeat every 14 days	77–94
6. Act-D 1.25 mg/m² (max 2 mg) IV every 2 weeks	69–90
7. Alternating MTX/Act-D regimens 1 and 5	100

Act-D, actinomycin D; D5W, 5% dextrose in water; IM, intramuscular; IV, intravenous; IVP, intravenous push; MTX, methotrexate; PO, per os.

or a diagnosis of choriocarcinoma [50]. Despite these differences in primary remission rates with initial chemotherapy, almost all patients are eventually cured with most being able to preserve fertility. Common side effects of these chemotherapy regimens are stomatitis, mucositis of the gastrointestinal tract, pleuritis, conjunctivitis and skin rash for methotrexate, and nausea and alopecia for actinomycin D, although toxicity necessitating a change in chemotherapy occurs in only about 10% of patients [51–55].

In 2012 we reported on the results of treatment in 358 FIGO-defined low-risk GTN patients at the Brewer Trophoblastic Disease Center from 1979 to 2009, including an analysis of risk factors for developing methotrexate resistance [56]. Patients initially received methotrexate 0.4 mg/kg (maximum 25 mg) intravenous push daily for 5 days every 14 days. Actinomycin D 0.5 mg intravenous push daily for 5 days every 14 days was used in 64 patients who developed resistance or toxicity to methotrexate, and multiagent chemotherapy regimens were used in 20 patients who failed single-agent therapy. The complete response rate to initial methotrexate chemotherapy was 81% and the complete response rate to actinomycin D as secondary therapy was 75%, making the overall complete response rate to sequential single-agent therapy 94%. The remaining patients all achieved permanent remission with multiagent chemotherapy with or without surgery. Resistance to initial methotrexate chemotherapy was significantly associated with increasing FIGO score, clinicopathologic diagnosis of choriocarcinoma, higher pretreatment hCG level, and presence of metastatic disease [56, 57].

Regardless of the treatment protocol used, chemotherapy should be continued until hCG values have returned to normal and at least one course has been administered after the first normal hCG level is achieved. Chemotherapy is changed to an alternate single agent if the hCG level plateaus above normal during treatment or if toxicity precludes adequate dose or frequency of treatment. Multiagent chemotherapy is indicated in the event of significant elevation in hCG level, development of metastases, or resistance to sequential single-agent chemotherapy [58–60].

Hysterectomy for low-risk GTN may be performed as an adjuvant treatment coincident with the initiation of chemotherapy to shorten the duration of treatment if fertility preservation is not desired. Hysterectomy may also become necessary to eradicate persistent, chemotherapy-resistant disease in the uterus or to remedy uterine tumor hemorrhage. Hysterectomy is the treatment of choice for PSTT and ETT.

In summary, cure rates for both nonmetastatic and metastatic low-risk GTN should approach 100% with the use of initial drug methotrexate or actinomycin D chemotherapy. Approximately 20–30% of low-risk patients will develop resistance to the initial drug, but most of these will be cured by the use of sequential single-agent chemotherapy. Eventually, about 10% of patients will require multiagent chemotherapy with or without surgery to achieve remission [61].

High-Risk Disease

Multiagent chemotherapy with or without adjuvant radiation or surgery is the treatment of choice for patients with high-risk metatstatic GTN (stages II and III, score ≥7 and stage IV). With this aggressive, multimodality treatment approach, cure rates of 80–90% have been achieved [62].

Chemotherapy for the treatment of high-risk GTN has undergone evolution since the late 1960s, when it was first recognized that single-agent chemotherapy followed by multiagent chemotherapy had a much lower cure rate than initial treatment with multiple drug regimens. During most of the 1970s and into the 1980s, the primary multidrug regimen used was MAC (methotrexate, actinomycin D, and cyclophosphamide or chlorambucil), which yielded cure rates of 63–71% [63, 64]. In the early 1980s, the combination regimen of cyclophosphamide, hydroxyurea, actinomycin D, methotrexate with folinic acid, vincristine, and doxorubicin (CHAMOCA) was reported to have a primary remission rate of 82%. However, in a randomized clinical trial of CHAMOCA versus MAC, both the primary remission rate (65% vs 73%) and the ultimate cure rate (70% vs 95%) were inferior for CHAMOCA compared with MAC, and CHAMOCA was more toxic. In the early 1980s, etoposide was discovered to be a very effective agent for treating GTN, and its addition to a multiagent chemotherapy regimen containing high-dose methotrexate with folinic acid, actinomycin D, cyclophosphamide, and vincristine (EMA-CO) resulted in improved primary remission and survival rates with low toxicity [61] (Table 24.5).

Over the last 20 years, the efficiency of the EMA-CO regimen as primary therapy for high-risk GTN has been confirmed by several treatment centers around the world, reporting complete response rates of 71–78% and long-term survival rates of 85–94% [65]. In three reported series from the Brewer Trophoblastic Disease Center, the complete response rates ranged from 54 to 76%, depending on the definition of high-risk disease, and the overall survival rates were 91–93% [66]. The only patients who died had FIGO stage IV disease with scores >12. No treatment-related deaths or life-threatening toxicity occurred. Neutropenia necessitating a one-week delay in treatment, anemia requiring blood transfusion, and grades 3–4 neutropenia without thrombocytopenia were associated with only 14%, 6%, and 2% of treatment cycles, respectively. The EMA-CO protocol, or some variation of it, is currently the initial treatment of choice for high-risk GTN because of low toxicity allowing adherence to treatment schedules, high complete response rates, and overall high resultant survival. Some centers recommend induction chemotherapy with etoposide and cisplatin (EP) followed by EMA-CO or EMA-EP in the highest risk patients (FIGO score >12). Chemotherapy for high-risk disease is continued for at least two to three courses after the first normal hCG level is achieved.

Table 24.5 EMA-CO (etoposide, high-dose methotrexate with folinic acid, actinomycin D, cyclophosphamide and vincristine) chemotherapy for high-risk gestational trophoblastic neoplasia. Repeat cycle on days 15, 16, and 22 (every 2 weeks).

Day	Drug	Dosing
1	Etoposide	100 mg/m^2 IV over 30 min
	Actinomycin D	0.5 mg IVP
	Methotrexate	100 mg/m^2 IVP, then 200 mg/m^2 in 500 mL D5W over 12 h
2	Etoposide	100 mg/m^2 IV over 30 min
	Actinomycin D	0.5 mg IVP
	Folinic acid	15 mg/m^2 IM or PO every 12 h for four doses starting 24 h after the start of MTX
8	Cyclophosphamide	600 mg/m^2 IV
	Vincristine	1.0 mg/m^2 IVP

D5W, 5% dextrose in water; IM, intramuscular; IV, intravenous; IVP, intravenous push; MTX, methotrexate; PO, per os.

When central nervous system metastases are present, whole brain irradiation (3000 cGy in 200 cGy fractions), or surgical excision with stereotactic irradiation in selected patients, is usually given simultaneously with the initiation of systemic chemotherapy to lower the risk of cerebral hemorrhage. During radiotherapy, the EMA-CO regimen is modified such that the methotrexate infusion dose is increased to 1 g/m^2 and 30 mg of folinic acid is given every 12 h for 3 days starting 32 h after the infusion begins. An alternative to brain irradiation is the use of intrathecal as well as high-dose intravenous methotrexate. Reported cure rates with brain metastases are 50–85%, depending on patient symptoms, as well as number, size, and location of the brain lesions [66–71].

Adjuvant surgical procedures, especially hysterectomy and pulmonary resection for chemotherapy-resistant disease as well as procedures to control hemorrhage are important components in the management of high-risk GTN [72]. Approximately 50% of patients with high-risk GTN will require some form of surgical procedure during the course of treatment to effect cure [73]. Imaging with 18FDG-PET combined with CT scanning may help target resistant disease for surgical excision. Selective arterial embolization may be useful in treating bleeding from uterine or vaginal tumors [74]. In a series of 50 high-risk GTN patients treated with EMA-CO as primary or secondary therapy at the Brewer Trophoblastic Disease Center from 1986 to 2005, 24 (48%) underwent 28 adjuvant surgical procedures, 21 (87.5%) of whom were cured. Those patients cured included 15 of 17 who underwent hysterectomy, four of five who had resistant foci of choriocarcinoma in the lung resected, all four who had suturing of the uterus, uterine artery embolization, small bowel resection or salpingectomy for bleeding, and one who had uterine wedge resection for resistant choriocarcinoma [75, 76].

Despite the use of multimodal primary therapy in high-risk GTN, approximately 30% of patients will have an incomplete response to first-line therapy or relapse from remission and will require secondary chemotherapy. Most of these patients with resistant disease will have multiple metastases to sites other than the lungs and vagina and many will have had inadequate initial chemotherapy. Salvage chemotherapy often combined with surgical excision of persistent tumor will result in cure of most of these high-risk patients. The EMA-EP regimen, substituting etoposide and cisplatin for cyclophosphamide and vincristine in the EMA-CO protocol, is considered the most appropriate therapy for patients who have responded to EMA-CO but have plateauing low hCG levels or who have developed re-elevation of hCG levels after a complete response to EMA-CO [77, 78]. In patients who have clearly developed resistance to methotrexate-containing protocols, drug combinations containing etoposide and platinum with bleomycin (BEP), ifosfamide (VIP, ICE), or paclitaxel (TP/TE) have been found to be effective [79–82].

At the Brewer Trophoblastic Disease Center, we initially reported in 2005 on 26 patients with persistent or relapsed high-risk GTN who received secondary platinum-based salvage chemotherapy. The overall survival was 61.5% [78]. In 2012, we reviewed the effect of etoposide/platinum-based salvage therapy in a series of 49 FIGO-defined high-risk GTN patients who were initially treated with EMA-CO [80]. Of the 28 patients who developed resistance to EMA-CO, 82% achieved lasting complete responses to salvage therapy, including three of four patients who received radiation therapy for brain metastases that developed during treatment and nine of 11 patients who had surgical procedures to remove metastases. High hCG level at the start of salvage therapy, greater number of metastatic sites, and metastases to sites other than the lung and vagina were significantly associated with lower survival. Overall, salvage therapy was responsible for the survival of 53% of the high-risk patients who were cured.

In summary, cure rates for high-risk GTN of 80–90% are now achievable with intensive multimodality therapy employing initial EMA-CO chemotherapy, along with adjuvant radiotherapy and surgery when indicated, and salvage therapy with platinum-containing drug combinations often in conjunction with surgical resection of sites of persistent tumor. Even those patients at the highest risk with metastatic disease to the brain, liver, and gastrointestinal tract now have a 75%, 73%, and 50% survival rate, respectively [2].

PSTT and ETT

Because of the relative resistance of PSTT and ETT to chemotherapy and their propensity for lymphatic spread, hysterectomy with lymph node dissection is the recommended treatment. Chemotherapy should be used in patients with metastatic disease and in patients with nonmetatstatic disease who have adverse prognostic factors, such as interval from last known pregnancy to diagnosis >2 years, deep myometrial invasion, tumor necrosis, and mitotic count >5/10 high power fields. Although the optimal chemotherapy regimen for PSTT and ETT remains to be defined, the current clinical impression is that a platinum-containing regimen, such as EMA-EP or TP/TE, is the preferred treatment. Survival rates should approach 100% for nonmetastatic disease and 50–60% for metastatic disease [83, 84].

Reasons for Treatment Failure

In 2008 we reviewed our experience with GTN patients whose care was transferred to the Brewer Trophoblastic Disease Center after treatment failure elsewhere to determine the cause of treatment failure and to compare our results of secondary therapy from 1979 to 2006 with those previously reported from 1962 to 1978 [85]. The most common reasons for unsuccessful GTN treatment before transfer to the Brewer Center were: use of single-agent chemotherapy for patients with high-risk disease and inappropriate use of weekly intramuscular methotrexate for treatment of patients with metastatic disease, FIGO scores ≥7, and/or nonpostmolar choriocarcinoma. Successful secondary chemotherapy in this patient group improved from 59% between 1962 and 1978 to 93% between 1979 and 2006, most likely as a result of more center experience and use of more effective chemotherapy regimens. Request for advice from or referral for treatment to clinicians with expertise in management of GTN is recommended for patients who fail single-agent therapy for low-risk disease and for any patient with high-risk disease.

Follow-up After Treatment for GTN

After hCG has returned to normal levels and treatment has been completed, serum quantitative hCG levels should be obtained at 1-month intervals for 12 months. The risk of relapse is about 3% in the first year after completing therapy and is exceedingly low thereafter. Physical examinations should be performed at 6–12 month intervals. Other testing, such as X-rays or scans, is rarely indicated. Contraception should be maintained during treatment and for 1 year after completion of chemotherapy, preferably using oral contraceptives, to allow for uninterrupted hCG follow-up and to permit the elimination of mature ova that may have been damaged by exposure to cytotoxic drugs [39].

Successful treatment of GTN with chemotherapy has allowed women to preserve their reproductive potential despite exposure to drugs that are toxic to the ovary. Most women resume normal ovarian function after chemotherapy and exhibit no increase in infertility, although menopause may occur earlier [86]. Many successful pregnancies have been reported without an increased rate of abortions, stillbirths, congenital abnormalities, prematurity, or major obstetrical complications. There is no evidence for reactivation of disease with subsequent pregnancies, although patients who have had one trophoblastic disease episode have a 1–2% risk of a second GTD event in a subsequent pregnancy, unrelated to whether they had previously received chemotherapy. Therefore, pelvic ultrasound is recommended in the first trimester of any post-GTD pregnancy to confirm a normal gestation. Also, the products of conception or placentas from future pregnancies should be carefully examined histopathologically and a serum quantitative hCG level should be determined 6 weeks after any pregnancy [87].

Because many anticancer drugs are known carcinogens, there is concern that the chemotherapy used to induce cures of one cancer may induce second malignancies. Due to the relatively short exposure of most GTN patients to intermittent schedules of methotrexate and actinomycin D and the infrequent use of alkylating agents, there were no reports of increased susceptibility to the development of other malignancies related to these drugs. After the introduction of etoposide-containing drug combinations for treatment of high-risk GTN in the 1980s, however, an increased risk of secondary malignancies, including acute myelogenous leukemia, colon cancer, melanoma and breast cancer, was identified [88].

References

1 Lurain JR. Gestational trophoblastic disease I: epidemiology, pathology, clinical presentation and diagnosis of gestational trophoblastic disease, and management of hydatidiform mole. *Am J Obstet Gynecol* 2010;203:531–9.

2 Lurain JR. Gestational trophoblastic disease II: classification and management of gestational trophoblastic neoplasia. *Am J Obstet Gynecol* 2011;204:11–18.
3 Ngan HY, Seckl MJ, Berkowitz RS, *et al.* Update on the diagnosis and management of gestational trophoblastic disease. *Int J Gynecol Obstet* 2015;131:S123–6.
4 Parazzini F, Mangili G, LaVecchia C, *et al.* Risk factors for gestational trophoblastic disease: a separate analysis of complete and partial hydatidiform mole. *Obstet Gynecol* 1991;78:1039–45.
5 Parazzini F, LaVecchia C, Pampallona S. Parental age and risk of complete and partial hydatidiform mole. *BJOG* 1986;93:582–5.
6 Sebire NJ, Foskett M, Fisher RA, *et al.* Risk of partial and complete molar pregnancy in relation to maternal age. *BJOG* 2002;109:99–102.
7 Garrett LA, Garner EI, Feltmate CM, *et al.* Subsequent pregnancy outcomes in patients with molar pregnancy and persistent gestational trophoblastic neoplasia. *J Reprod Med* 2008;53:481–6.
8 Wang CM, Dixon PH, Decordova S, *et al.* Indentification of 13 novel NLRP7 mutations in 2 families with recurrent hydatidiform mole; missense mutations cluster in the leucine-rich region. *J Med Genet* 2009;46:569–75.
9 Smith HO, Qualls CR, Prarie BA, *et al.* Trends in gestational choriocarcinoma: a 27-year perspective. *Obstet Gynecol* 2003;102:978–87.
10 Palmer JR, Driscoll SG, Rosenberg L, *et al.* Oral contraceptive use and risk of gestational trophoblastic tumors. *J Natl Cancer Inst* 1999;91:635–40.
11 Moore KL, Persaud TVN. *The Developing Human – Clinically Oriented Embryology.* Philadelphia: W.B. Saunders, 1993.
12 Bentley RC. Pathology of gestational trophoblastic disease. *Clin Obstet Gynecol* 2003;46:513–22.
13 Szulman AE, Surti U. The syndromes of hydatidiform mole, I: cytogenetic and morphologic correlations. *Am J Obset Gynecol* 1978;131:665–71.
14 Szulman AE, Surti U. The syndromes of hydatidiform mole, II: morphologic evolution of the complete and partial mole. *Am J Obset Gynecol* 1978;132:20–7.
15 Paradinas FJ, Browne P, Fisher RA, *et al.* A clinical, histopathological and flow of cytometric study of 149 complete moles, 146 partial moles, and 107 non-molar hydropic abortions. *Histopathology* 1996;28:101–10.
16 Seibre NJ, Fisher RA, Rees HC. Histopathologic diagnosis of partial and complete hydatidiform mole in the first trimester of pregnancy. *Pediatr Dev Pathol* 2003;6:69–77.
17 Seibre NJ, Makrydimas G, Agnantis NJ, *et al.* Updated diagnostic criteria for partial and complete hydatidiform moles in early pregnancy. *Anticancer Res* 2003;23:1723–8.
18 Lurain JR, Brewer JI. Invasive mole. *Semin Oncol* 1982;9:174–80.
19 Lage JM. Gestational trophoblastic diseases. In: SJ Robboy MC Anderson, P Russell, *et al.* (eds) *Pathology of the Female Reproductive Tract.* Edinburgh: Churchill Livingstone, 2001:759–81.
20 Baergen RN, Rutgers JL, Young RH, *et al.* Placental site trophoblastic tumor: a study of 55 cases and review of the literature emphasizing factors of prognostic significance. *Gynecol Oncol* 2006;100:511–20.
21 Zaloudek CJ. Epithelioid trophoblastic tumor of the uterus: differential diagnosis and a review of gestational trophoblastic tumors. *AJSP* 2016;21:93–102.
22 Shih IM, Kurman RJ. Epithelioid trophoblastic tumor: a neoplasm distinct from choriocarcinoma and placental site trophoblastic tumor simulating carcinoma. *Am J Surg Pathol* 1998;22:1393–403.
23 Allison KH, Love JE, Garcia RL. Epithelioid trophoblastic tumor: Review of a rare neoplasm of the chorionic-type intermediate trophoblast. *Arch Pathol Lab Med* 2006;130:1875–7.
24 Soto-Wright V, Bernstein MR, Goldstein DP, *et al.* The changing clinical presentation of complete molar pregnancy. *Obstet Gynecol* 1995;86:775–9.
25 Hou JL, Wan XR, Xiang Y, *et al.* Changes in clinical features in hydatidiform mole: analysis on 113 cases. *J Reprod Med* 2008;53:629–33.
26 Lurain JR. Gestational trophoblastic tumors. *Semin Surg Oncol* 1990;6:347–53.
27 Santos-Ramos R, Forney JP, Schwarz BE. Sonographic findings and clinical correlations in molar pregnancy. *Obstet Gynecol* 1980;56:186–92.
28 Benson CB, Genest DR, Bernstein MR, *et al.* Sonographic appearance of first trimester complete hydatidiform moles. *Ultrasound Obstet Gynecol* 2000;16:188–91.
29 Berkowitz RS, Ozturk M, Goldstein D, *et al.* Human chorionic gonadotropin and free subunits' serum levels in patient with partial and complete hydatidiform moles. *Obstet Gynecol* 1989;74:212–16.
30 Cole LA, Khanlian SA. Hyperglycosylated hCG: a variant with separate biological functions to regular hCG. *Mol Cell Endocrinol* 2007;260:228–36.
31 Cole LA, Khanlian SA, Muller CY, *et al.* Gestational trophoblastic diseases. 3. Human chorionic gonadotropin-free beta-submit, a reliable marker of placenta site trophoblastic tumors. *Gynecol Oncol* 2006;102:160–4.
32 Palmieri C, Dhillon T, Fisher RA, *et al.* Management and outcome of healthy women with a persistently elevated β-hCG. *Gynecol Oncol* 2007;160:35–43.
33 Hancock BW. hCG measurement in gestational trophoblastic neoplasia: a critical appraisal. *J Reprod Med* 2006;51:859–60.
34 Cole LA, Butler SA, Khanlian SA, *et al.* Gestational trophoblastic diseases: 2. Hyperglycosylated hCG as a tumor marker of active neoplasia. *Gynecol Oncol* 2006;102:151–9.
35 Thaker HM, Berlin A, Tycko B, *et al.* Immunohistochemistry for the imprinted gene product IPL/PHLDA2 for facilitating the differential diagnosis of complete hydatidiform mole. *J Reprod Med* 2004;49:630–6.
36 Berry E, Hagopian GS, Lurain JR. Vaginal metastases in gestational trophoblastic neoplasia. *J Reprod Med* 2008;53:487–92.
37 Fisher RA, Tommasi A, Short D, *et al.* Clinical utility of selective molecular genotyping for diagnosis of partial hydatidiform mole; a retrospective study from a regional trophoblastic disease unit. Journal of clinical pathology. *J Clin Pathol* 2014;67:980–4.
38 Berkowitz RS, Goldstein DS. Clinical practice. Molar pregnancy. *N Engl J Med* 2009;360:1639–45.
39 Hancock BW, Tidy JA. Current management of molar pregnancy. *J Reprod Med* 2002;47:347–54.

40 Tidy JA, Gillespie AM, Bright N, *et al.* Gestational trophoblastic disease: a study of mode of evaluation and subsequent need for treatment with chemotherapy. *Gynecol Oncol* 2000;78:309–12.

41 Kim DS, Moon H, Kim KT, *et al.* Effects of prophylactic chemotherapy for persistent trophoblastic disease in patients with complete hydatidiform mole. *Obstet Gynecol* 1986;67:690–4.

42 Limpongsanurak S. Prophylactic actinomycin D for high-risk complete hydatidiform mole. *J Reprod Med* 2001;46:110–16.

43 Deicas RE, Miller DS, Rademaker AW, *et al.* The role of contraception in the development of postmolar gestational trophoblastic tumor. *Obstet Gynecol* 1991;78:221–6.

44 Feltmate CM, Batorfi J, Fulop V, *et al.* Human chorionic gonadotropin follow-up in patient with molar pregnancy: a time for reevaluation. *Obstet Gynecol* 2003;101:732–6.

45 Hancock BW, Nazir K, Everard JE. Persistent gestational trophoblastic neoplasia after partial hydatidiform mole: incidence and outcome. *J Reprod Med* 2006;51:764–6.

46 Feltmate CM, Growden WB, Wolfberg AJ, *et al.* Clinical characteristics of persistent gestational trophoblastic neoplasia after partial hydatidiform molar pregnancy. *J Reprod Med* 2006;51:902–6.

47 Ngan HYS, Bender H, Benedet JL, *et al.* Gestational trophoblastic neoplasia, FIGO staging and classification. *Int J Gynecol Obstet* 2003;83:175–7.

48 Lurain JR, Casanova LA, Miller DS, Rademaker AW. Prognostic factors in gestational trophoblastic tumors: a proposed new scoring system based on multivariate analysis. *Am J Obstet Gynecol* 1991;164:611–16.

49 Lurain JR. Pharmacotherapy of gestational trophoblastic disease. Expert Opin

50 Alazzam M, Tidy J, Hancock BW, Osborne R. First line chemotherapy in low risk gestational trophoblastic neoplasia. *Cochrane Database Syst Rev* 2009(1):D007102.

51 Roberts JP, Lurain JR. Treatment of low-risk metastatic gestational trophoblastic tumors with single-agent chemotherapy. *Am J Obstet Gynecol* 1996;174:1917–24.

52 Berkowitz RS, Goldstein DS, Bernstein MR. Ten years' experience with methotrexate and folinic acid as primary therapy for gestational trophoblastic disease. *Gynecol Oncol* 1986;23:111–18.

53 Sita-Lumsden A, Short D, Lindsay I, *et al.* Treatment outcomes for 618 women with gestational trophoblastic tumors following a molar pregnancy at the Charing Cross Hospital, 2000–2009. *Br J Cancer* 2012;107:1810–14.

54 Taylor F, Grew T, Everard J, *et al.* The outcome of patients with low risk gestational trophoblastic neoplasia treated with single agent intramuscular methotrexate and oral folinic acid. *Eur J Cancer* 2013;49:3184–90.

55 Yarandi F, Eftekhar Z, Shojaei H, *et al.* Pulse methotrexate versus pulse actinomycin D in the treatment of low-risk gestational trophoblastic neoplasia. *Int J Gynecol Obstet* 2008;103:33–7.

56 Lurain JR, Chapman-Davis E, Hoekstra AV, Schink JC. Actinomycin D for methotrexate-failed low-risk gestational trophoblastic neoplasia. *J Reprod Med* 2012;57:283–7.

57 Bagshawe KD, Dent J, Newlands ES, *et al.* The role of low-dose methotrexate and folinic acid in gestational trophoblastic tumors. *Br J Obstet Gynecol* 1989;96:795–802.

58 Osborne R, Filiaci M, Schink J, *et al.* A randomized phase III trial comparing weekly parenteral methotrexate and "pulsed" actinomycin as primary management for low-risk gestational trophoblastic neoplasia. A Gynecologic Oncology Group study. Gynecol Oncol 2008;108:52(abstract).

59 Lertkhachonsuk A, Isrангura N, Wilailak S, *et al.* Actinomycin D versus methotrexate-folinic acid as the treatment of stage I, low-risk gestational trophoblastic neoplasia. A randomized controlled trial. *Int J Gynecol Cancer* 2009;19:985–8.

60 Abrao RA, de Andrade JM, Tiezzi DG, *et al.* Treatment for low-risk gestational trophoblastic disease: comparison of single-agent methotrexate, dactinomycin and combination regimens. *Gynecol Oncol* 2008;108:149–53.

61 Hoekstra AV, Lurain JR, Rademaker AW, *et al.* Gestational trophoblastic neoplasia: treatment outcomes. *Obstet Gynecol* 2008;112:251–8.

62 Bower M, Newlands ES, Holden L, *et al.* EMA/CO for high-risk gestational trophoblastic disease. Results from a cohort of 272 patients. *J Clin Oncol* 1997;15:2636–43.

63 Kim SJ, Bae SN, Kim JH, *et al.* Risk factors for the prediction of treatment failure in gestational trophoblastic tumors treated with EMA/CO regimen. *Gynecol Oncol* 1998;71:247–53.

64 Lurain JR, Singh DK, Schink JC. Primary treatment of metastatic high-risk gestational trophoblastic neoplasia with EMA-CO chemotherapy. *J Reprod Med* 2006;51:767–72.

65 Turan T, Karacay O, Tulunay G, *et al.* Results with EMA/CO (etoposide, methotrexate, actinomycin D, cyclophosphamide, vincristine) chemotherapy in gestational trophoblastic neoplasia. *Int J Gynecol Cancer* 2006;16:1432–8.

66 Lurain JR, Singh DK, Schink JC. Management of metastatic high-risk gestational trophoblastic neoplasia FIGO stages II–IV: risk factors score ≥7. *J Reprod Med* 2010;55:199–207.

67 Evans AC Jr, Soper JT, Clarke-Pearson DL, *et al.* Gestational trophoblastic disease metastatic to the central nervous system. *Gynecol Oncol* 1995;59:226–30.

68 Rustin GJ, Newlands ES, Begent RH, *et al.* Weekly alternating etoposide, methotrexate and actinomycin D/vincristine and cyclophosphamide chemotherapy for treatment of CNS metastases of choriocarcinoma. *J Clin Oncol* 1989;7:900–4.

69 Newlands ES, Holden L, Seckl MJ, *et al.* Management of brain metastases in patients with high-risk gestational trophoblastic tumors. *J Reprod Med* 2002;47:465–71.

70 Neubauer NL, Latif N, Kalakota K, *et al.* Brain metastasis in gestational trophoblastic neoplasia: an update. *J Reprod Med* 2013;57:288–92.

71 Savage P, Kelpanides I, Tuthill M, Short D, Seckl MJ. Brain metastases in gestational trophoblast neoplasia: an update on incidence, management and outcome. *Gynecol Oncol* 2015;137:73–6.

72 Kanis MJ, Lurain JR. Pulmonary resection in the management of high-risk gestational trophoblastic neoplasia. *Int J Gynecol Cancer* 2016;26:796–800.

73 Pisal N, North C, Tidy J, *et al.* Role of hysterectomy in the management of gestational trophoblastic disease. *Gynecol Oncol* 2002;87:190–2.

74 Newlands ES, Bower M, Holden L, *et al.* Management of resistant gestational trophoblastic tumors. *J Reprod Med* 1998;43:111–18.

75 Lurain JR, Singh DK, Schink JC. The role of surgery in the management of high–risk gestational trophoblastic neoplasia. *J Reprod Med* 2006;51:773–6.

76 Dhillon T, Palmieri C, Sebire NJ, *et al.* Value of whole body 18FDG-PET to identify the active site of gestational trophoblastic neoplasia. *J Reprod Med* 2006;51:879–87.

77 Lim AK, Agarwal R, Seckl MJ, *et al.* Embolization of bleeding residual uterine vascular malformations in patient with treated gestational trophoblastic tumors. *Radiology* 2002;222:640–4.

78 Lurain JR, Nejad B. Secondary chemotherapy for high-risk gestational trophoblastic neoplasia. *Gynecol Oncol* 2005;97:618–23.

79 Yang J, Xiang Y, Wan X, *et al.* Recurrent gestational trophoblastic tumor: management and risk factors for recurrence. *Gynecol Oncol* 2006;103:587–90.

80 Lurain JR, Schink JC. Importance of salvage therapy in the management of high-risk gestational trophoblastic neoplasia. *J Reprod Med* 2012;57:219–24.

81 Mao Y, Wan X, Lv W, *et al.* Relapsed or refractory gestational trophoblastic neoplasia treated with etoposide and cisplatin/etoposide, methotrexate, and actinomycin D (EP-EMA) regimen. *Int J Gynecol Cancer* 2007;98:44–7.

82 Wang J, Short D, Sebire NJ, *et al.* Salvage chemotherapy of relapsed or high-risk gestational trophoblastic neoplasia (GTN) with paclitaxel/cisplatin alternating with paclitaxel/etoposide (TP/TE). *Ann Oncol* 2008;19:1578–83.

83 Hassadia A, Gillespie A, Tidy J, *et al.* Placental site trophoblastic tumor: clinical features and management. *Gynecol Oncol* 2005;99:603–7.

84 Schmid P, Nagai Y, Agarwal R, *et al.* Prognostic markers and long-term outcome of placental-site trophoblastic tumors: a retrospective observational study. *Lancet* 2009;374:48–55.

85 Lurain JR, Hoekstra AV, Schink JC. Results of treatment of patients with gestational trophoblastic neoplasia referred to the Brewer Trophoblastic Disease Center after failure of treatment elsewhere (1979–2006). *J Reprod Med* 2008;53:535–40.

86 Woolas RP, Bower M, Newlands ES, *et al.* Influence of chemotherapy for gestational trophoblastic disease on subsequent pregnancy outcome. *Br J Obstet Gynecol* 1998;105:1032–5.

87 Matsui H, Iitsuka Y, Suzuka K, *et al.* Early pregnancy outcomes after chemotherapy for gestational trophoblastic tumor. *J Reprod Med* 2004;49:531–4.

88 Rustin GJS, Newlands ES, Lutz J-M, *et al.* Combination but not single agent methotrexate chemotherapy for gestational trophoblastic tumors (GTT) increases the incidence of second tumors. *J Clin Oncol* 1996;14:2769–73.

Section 6

Male Reproductive Cancers

25

Testicular Cancer

Costantine Albany, Nasser Hanna, and Lawrence H. Einhorn

Indiana University School of Medicine, Simon Cancer Center, Indianapolis, Indiana, USA

Incidence and Mortality

Approximately 8,850 new testicular cancers are diagnosed (0.5% of cancer diagnoses among men) and approximately 410 deaths from testicular cancers occur (0.13% of cancer deaths among men) annually in the United States (US) [1].

The incidence rate of testicular cancers, based on cases diagnosed between 2009 and 2013, was approximately 5.7 per 100,000 men per year. During the same time period, the age-adjusted death rate was 0.3 per 100,000 men per year. The lifetime risk of developing testicular cancer is approximately 0.39% or one in 256 men. Incidence rates for men in the US is highest among non-Hispanic whites and lowest among African Americans and Asians/Pacific Islanders. In the US, the testicular cancer incidence rate increased by an average of 2.3% per year from 1975 to 1989, and by an average of 0.8% annually from 1989 to 2013 [2]. Testicular cancer is the most common malignancy in men between the ages of 15 and 39 years [3].

The worldwide incidence of germ cell tumors (GCTs) has doubled in the past 40 years with the highest worldwide incidence in Scandinavian countries [4,5]. Most testicular tumors are GCTs (95%); the remaining 5% are non-germ cell tumors such as Sertoli cell and Leydig cell tumors. Extragonadal GCTs are a distinct clinical entity constituting 5–10% of all GCTs [6]. GCTs in adult males have a bimodal age distribution, with nonseminomatous germ cell tumor (NSGCT) most commonly diagnosed between ages 15 and 35 and seminoma in older patients aged 40–60 [7].

Etiology and Tumorigenesis

Cryptorchidism and testicular dysgenesis are risk factors for the development of GCT [8–10]. The risk of developing GCT is 10- to 40-fold higher in an undescended testis. However, both testes are at risk as 25% of testicular cancers in patients with cryptorchidism develop in the normally descended testicle. Of boys with a history of an undescended testicle, 1–5% will develop GCT [11]. Surgical correction of an undescended testis before puberty lowers the risk of testis cancer [12]. Patients with a family history of brothers or fathers with testicular cancer have an increased risk of developing GCT. Brothers of patients with GCT have a relative risk of GCT of 8–10, and for father–son the relative risk is 4–6 [13]. Patients who have been cured of testicular cancer have approximately a 1–3% cumulative risk of developing a cancer in the contralateral testicle during the 15 years after initial diagnosis [14]. Klinefelter syndrome (47 XXY) is a rare disease that affect approximately one in 600 newborn males; there is a high risk of a primary mediastinal NSGCT with Klinefelter syndrome of about 20% [15]. Patients with XY gonadal dysgenesis, testicular feminization, and Down syndrome also have a greatly increased risk of GCTs [16].

Development of GCT is determined by a series of genetic, epigenetic and environmental events that occur mainly during fetal testicular development and continue after birth and puberty. Primordial germ cells are progenitors of the germ cell lineage and express PLAP, NANOG, KIT, SOX2, OCT3/4 and SALL4 [17]. During the differentiation process, the germ cells gradually lose expression of these pluripotency markers and by birth should not have any [18]. The widely accepted theory of GCT tumorigenesis is that development of intratubular germ cell neoplasia (IGCN) starts *in utero*. The disturbance of germ cell development results in arrest of fetal germ cells at the gonocyte stage. Among the first proteins demonstrated to be expressed both by gonocytes and preinvasive neoplastic germ cells is KIT, which involves aberrantly activated KIT ligand (KITLG)/KIT pathway and overexpression of embryonic transcription factors such as NANOG and OCT3/4, which in turn leads to suppression of apoptosis, increased proliferation, and accumulation of mutations in gonocytes [18].

Genome-wide association studies have identified several single nucleotide polymorphisms that are central to normal primordial germ cell biology that predispose to GCT [19–21] (Table 25.1). Polymorphism in KITLG is four times more common in Whites than in Blacks and is associated with a threefold higher risk of developing GCT [22]. Genome-wide association studies also showed a link between a locus on the long arm of the X chromosome (Xq27) and increased risk of familial GCT [8]. In sporadic GCT cases, gr/gr deletion on the Y chromosome

The American Cancer Society's Oncology in Practice: Clinical Management, First Edition. Edited by The American Cancer Society.

Table 25.1 Common genetic single nucleotide polymorphisms that predispose to germ cell tumors, identified by genome-wide association studies [19].

Pathway	Locus	Function
KIT pathway		
KIT/KITLG	12q22	KIT is crucial for survival, proliferation, and migration of germ cells
SPRY4	5q31	Inhibitor of KIT-regulated MAPK signaling
BAK1	6p21	Promotes apoptosis and it is inhibited by KIT
Telomerase pathway		
TERT *ATF7IP*	5p15 12p13	Telomere regulation, Overexpression seen in seminomas
Sex determination pathway		
DMRT1	9P24	Deletion linked to TGCTs
Y Chromosome		
gr/gr del	Yq11	The most common genetic alteration in infertility patients which results into a two-fold increase in risk for TGCT
TSPY1	Yp11	TSPY1 Copy number variation <21 or > 55 linked to spermatogenic failure /infertility and testicular dysgenesis syndrome
X Chromosome		
TGCT1	Xq27	Associated with a risk of familial and bilateral TGCT

has been found to be the most common genetic alteration in infertility patients which results in a twofold increase in risk for GCT [23]. All these studies report relatively weak associations and still await an independent confirmation (Table 25.1).

Invasive GCT consistently show gain of chromosome 12p, typically isochromosome 12p (i12p) which is present in nearly all GCTs. i12p is an early and probably necessary event in the development of invasive GCT and it is a pathognomonic feature of GCT of all histologic types [24]. Although the i12p target genes have not been clearly defined, several candidate genes have been mapped to an amplified region at 12p11 and 12p13 [25]. Several other regions of the genome are also imbalanced, at a lower frequency than i12p.

Some of the most important findings in recent years, is recognizing the role of epigenetics, specifically DNA methylation in the development of GCT. Seminomatous GCT show more global hypomethylation and almost no CpG island methylation, whereas nonseminomas show more methylated DNA, both globally and at CpG islands [26]. Additional research may allow epigenetic profiles to identify risk groups, predict clinical outcomes and allow the development of hypomethylating therapies in patients with poor risk GCT [27,28].

Metastatic Patterns

Regardless of histologic subtype, testicular cancer tends to spread in a predictable and logical fashion through lymphatic drainage and hematogenous spread. Testicular cancer spreads to the ipsilateral retroperitoneal lymph nodes (primary landing zones) followed by retrocrural, posterior mediastinum, and then supraclavicular lymph nodes. A right-sided testicular primary spreads to the interaortocaval lymph nodes. A left testis primary spreads to the left para-aortic and preaortic lymph nodes. Contralateral nodal involvement occurs in 15% of patients especially from right to left [29]. Iliac, pelvic, and inguinal lymph node metastasis can be associated with disruption of normal lymphatic drainage with scrotal violation or prior surgery such as vasectomy or herniorrhaphy. NSGCT tend to spread through hematogenous dissemination to the lung and less commonly to the liver, brain, and bones.

Diagnostic and Staging Workup

The first step in the diagnosis and staging of a testicular mass is physical examination followed by scrotal ultrasound. The physical examination should focus on manual examination of the scrotal contents; testis cancers are firm, hard, or fixed. This finding should be confirmed by scrotal ultrasound. A hypoechoic mass is diagnostic of testicular cancer. This should be followed by measuring preorchiectomy serum tumor markers alpha-fetoprotein (AFP) and human chorionic gonadotropin (hCG). Proper urologic management is radical inguinal orchiectomy. Trans-scrotal biopsy should never be done as this may lead to a violation of scrotal integrity causing aberrant lymphatic drainage from the tumor that increases the possibility of the unusual pattern of metastases to scrotum and inguinal lymph nodes. If serum tumor markers were elevated preorchiectomy, they should be repeated after orchiectomy to see if they normalize. The half-life of AFP is 5 days and hCG 24–48 h. Marker decline in patients with clinical stage I disease should be assessed until normalization. Rising serum tumor markers after orchiectomy indicates the presence of metastatic disease, while normalization of marker levels after orchiectomy does not rule out the presence of metastases. AFP is a glycoprotein derived from yolk sac or embryonal carcinoma. hCG is derived from embryonal carcinoma, seminoma, or choriocarcinoma. False elevations of hCG could be secondary to smoking marijuana or due to crossreactivity with high LH secondary to low testosterone. Elevated AFP level could result from hepatitis or other liver dysfunction.

Computed tomography (CT) scan of the abdomen and pelvis is performed to assess retroperitoneal lymph nodes (RPLN). Interaortocaval or left para-aortic, preaortic lymph nodes more than 1 cm are considered enlarged and suspicious for metastatic disease. Chest CT scan is recommended when abdominal adenopathy is found to rule out metastases within the lungs or mediastinum. Positron emission tomography (PET) imaging is not recommended as part of the initial evaluation for diagnosis or staging of GCT. Head magnetic resonance imaging is only indicated in patients with CNS signs or symptoms at the time of diagnosis. Testicular cancer is staged using the TNM staging system by the American Joint Committee on Cancer (Table 25.2) [30].

Pathology

Intratubular germ cell neoplasia is the common precursor lesion of all GCT except spermatocytic seminoma (Figure 25.1). Seminomas account for 40% of all GCT. NSGCT include the

Table 25.2 Key aspects of TNM staging system for testicular germ cell tumors [30,31].

Stage	TNM	Description	Incidence (%)
I	T1–4, N0, M0, S0	Tumor confined to the testis	74.5
Is	T1–4, N0, M0, S1	Elevated tumor markers post orchiectomy and no evidence of metastatic disease on imaging studies	
II	T1–4, N1–3, M0, S0–3	Metastasis confined to the retroperitoneal lymph nodes	13.3
III	T1–4, N1–3, M1, S0–3	Supradiaphragmatic LN or disseminated disease	12.2

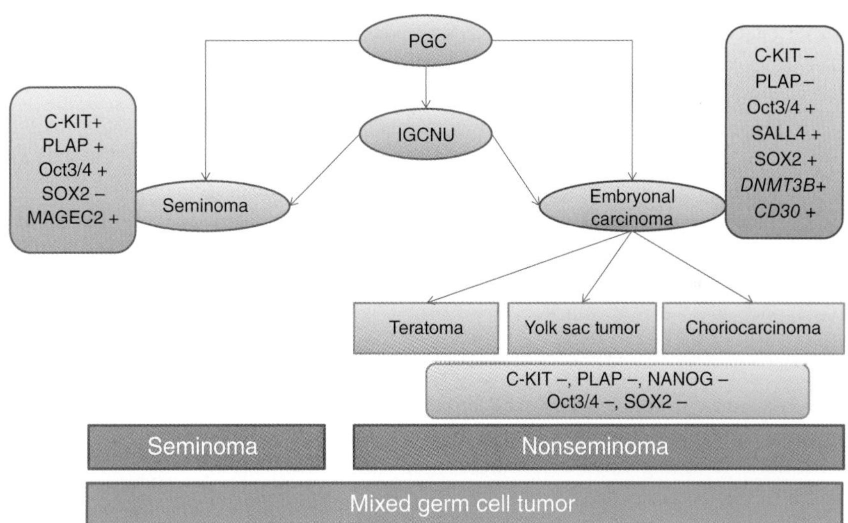

Figure 25.1 Pathology of germ cell tumor by immunohistochemistry.

following subtypes: embryonal carcinoma (EC), yolk sac tumor (YST), teratoma, choriocarcinoma, and tumors with various combinations of these histologies. If seminoma is present with any NSGCT elements it should be treated as NSGCT. Seminomas are classified as classic or spermatocytic. Classic seminomas account for 90% of all seminomas and are characterized by positive staining for placental alkaline phosphatase (PLAP), CD117 (c-Kit), OCT-4, and SALL-4 and are negative for CD30 by immunohistochemistry (Figure 25.1) [32]. Melanoma-associated gene C2 (*MAGEC2*) was recently identified to be expressed in 94% of seminomas [33]. Spermatocytic seminoma doesn't express PLAP or OCT3/4 and are almost always cured by orchiectomy alone. Seminomas can occasionally be confused with sex cord-stromal tumors (SCSTs) [34]. However, the latter are characterized by positive staining for inhibin-alpha on immunohistochemistry and uniformly negative for PLAP, OCT3/4, SALL4, and c-Kit [35]. Distinction of these two entities is important because their clinical management is different.

ECs account for 20% of all testicular GCT. Microscopically, it is the most undifferentiated subtype with the totipotential capacity to differentiate into YST, choriocarcinoma, as well as teratoma. EC show a positive staining for CD30, SOX2, OCT-4, SALL-4, and are negative for PLAP and c-Kit [34]. YST and choriocarcinoma exhibit morphologies resembling extra-embryonically differentiated tissues. YST is positive for AFP, SALL-4 and negative for c-Kit and CD30. Choriocarcinoma is extremely rare in its pure form, constituting fewer than 1% of testicular GCT. More frequently, it is part of mixed GCT in approximately 8–10% of cases [34].

Teratoma is classified as mature and immature. Mature teratoma has elements of one or more of the three germinal layers that are fully differentiated, and a pathologic mix of fully differentiated cartilage, hair, bone, and epithelium is often seen. If a teratoma has areas that resemble embryonic or fetal tissue, it is referred to as immature teratoma. The age of occurrence appears to play a significant role in the behavior of testicular teratomas. It is therefore of crucial importance for the pathologist not to use the term "benign" to a teratoma of the testis in a postpubertal patient [36]. This classification lacks prognostic significance as both mature and immature teratoma can undergo malignant transformation of one of its histologic components to other cancers including sarcoma, adenocarcinoma, primitive neuroectodermal tumor, and leukemia [37]. Mature teratomas are negative for Oct3/4, CD30, and SOX2 [38]. Vimentin expression is limited to mesenchymal components of mature teratoma and interstitial and other support cells. Oct3/4 expression by immunohistochemistry is negative in YST, mature and immature teratoma, and choriocarcinoma [39].

Clinical Presentation

Testicular Germ Cell Tumors

Testicular GCT most commonly present as a painless palpable mass noted incidentally by the patient (up to 90% of cases) [40]. In patients with retroperitoneal metastases or disseminated disease, backache, flank pain, neck mass, malaise, and other systemic features may be the presenting findings. Less commonly, some patients may present with gynecomastia due to high hCG, or with infertility. Patients with extensive pulmonary metastasis may present with shortness of breath, cough, and hemoptysis. Classic seminoma presents most commonly as an enlarging painless testicular mass (stage I) in approximately 70% of patients, metastatic to RPLN (stage II) in 25%, and 5% will present with stage III [41]. Spermatocytic seminoma represents approximately 5–10% of all seminomas and it typically appears after the age of 60 years, is bilateral 10% of the time, and it has an indolent course. Seminoma can cause low level elevation in serum hCG in 5–10% due to the presence of syncytiotrophoblastic elements within the tumor [42]. Seminoma does not secrete AFP. Elevation of AFP denotes the presence of embryonal or yolk sac tumor elements. However, stable low levels of AFP (<25 ng/mL) may be normal for individual patients.

Embryonal carcinoma can behave aggressively and carries a higher risk of lymphovascular invasion and hematogenous spread. Over 60% of patients with EC have metastatic disease on presentation and about 50% of patients presenting with stage I already have micrometastatic disease [43]. EC may contain trophoblastic and yolk sac elements causing elevation of serum hCG and AFP. Tumor markers are normal in about 20% of metastatic ECs.

YST can have hematogenous dissemination. Serologically, patients have elevated levels of AFP and normal hCG in 80–90% of cases. Choriocarcinoma is among the most aggressive GCTs, with early hematogenous dissemination to lungs, liver, brain, and other visceral sites and is characterized serologically by the production of large amounts of hCG. Pure testicular choriocarcinoma is rare, accounting for fewer than 1% of GCTs. Choriocarcinomas tend to be vascular tumors and patients may present with hemoptysis, gastrointestinal bleeding, or hemorrhagic stroke. Widely metastatic choriocarcinoma may manifest as a "burned-out" local testis lesion that consists of a fibrous scar with absent or minute amounts of viable tumor. Patients presenting with diffuse metastatic disease and very high hCG have a choriocarcinoma syndrome and biopsy should be avoided as this clinical presentation is life-threatening and requires immediate treatment.

Sex Cord-Stromal Tumors

SCSTs represent about 5% of all testicular tumors. They can present at any age with a mean age of about 40. These tumors do not secrete AFP or hCG. Leydig cell tumors (LCTs) constitute 75–80% of these tumors, and they are seen three times more frequently than Sertoli cell tumors [44]. LCTs are often associated with an excess of sex steroid production. Leydig cells are the principal testicular source of testosterone and are also capable of producing estrogen. LCTs present often as testicular mass in association with gynecomastia, virilization, and pseudopuberty [45].

Extragonadal Germ Cell Tumors

Extragonadal germ cell tumors represent only 5–10% of adult germ cell malignancies [46]. Their histology is identical to testicular germ cell tumors; however, their biology, especially primary mediastinal NSGCT (PMNSGCT) is substantially different. Extragonadal germ cell tumors are characterized by their location of midline structures from the pineal gland to the coccyx. The most common primary site is the anterior mediastinum followed by retroperitoneum, with rare occurrence in the pineal gland and presacral area.

Benign mature teratoma or seminomas are the most common germ cell tumors in the anterior mediastinum. However, PMNSGCTs represent the most challenging group of malignant germ cell tumors to treat. Survival outcome is dependent on both chemotherapy and a skilled thoracic surgeon. The significant elevation in tumor markers including hCG >1000 U/L and/or any elevation in AFP confirms the diagnosis of NSGCT and no biopsy is needed to make a diagnosis [47]. Patients with normal tumor markers or mild elevation in hCG require a biopsy to establish the diagnosis of pure seminoma versus NSGCT versus other etiology such as thymic malignancy or lymphoma (Figure 25.2).

Treatment of Early Stage Disease

Stage I Seminoma

Seventy-five to eighty percent of seminomas present as clinical stage I (normal serum markers and normal CT scans of the chest and abdomen) (Table 25.2). There is a 15–20% risk of relapse when managed with orchiectomy followed by surveillance with most relapses occurring in the retroperitoneum. Options include surveillance, one or two cycles of carboplatin, or radiation therapy (Figure 25.3). Our preferred option at Indiana University is surveillance. The largest study of surveillance in stage I seminoma followed over 1,800 patients for 15 years. Ten-year cancer specific survival was 99.6%. Relapse rate was 20% [48].

Seminomas are exquisitely sensitive to radiation. This characteristic, combined with their predictable lymphatic spread made adjuvant radiotherapy a standard of care for many years. Typical doses range from 20 to 30 Gy delivered in daily doses of 1.5–2.0 Gy to the para-aortic and ipsilateral iliac lymph nodes. However, more awareness of the late consequences of radiation including the increased risk of secondary malignancy of organs in the radiation field has led many oncologists to avoid radiotherapy for clinical stage I seminoma [49]. A randomized noninferiority trial showed relapse-free rates at 3 years of 96% for patients treated with radiation and 94.7% for a single cycle of carboplatin AUC7 [50,51]. Adjuvant therapy reduces the risk of relapse from 15 to 20% to 4 to 5%.

Surveillance for Stage I Seminoma

The National Comprehensive Cancer Network guidelines recommend that patients with clinical stage I seminoma undergo surveillance every 3–4 months for years 1–3, every 6 months for years 4–7, with abdominal/pelvic CT at each visit, chest X-ray at alternative visits (up to 10 years) [52]. At Indiana University we perform surveillance with history and physical examination, tumor markers, and CT scan of the abdomen and pelvis every 4 months for the first year, every 6 months for the second year, and annually years 3–5. Lifelong follow-up is needed in all patients with history of testicular cancer as there is about a 2% risk of developing a contralateral primary at 15 years [14].

Stage II Seminoma

Radiation therapy continues to be a standard treatment option for stage II seminoma if RPLNs measure less than 3 cm. A curative

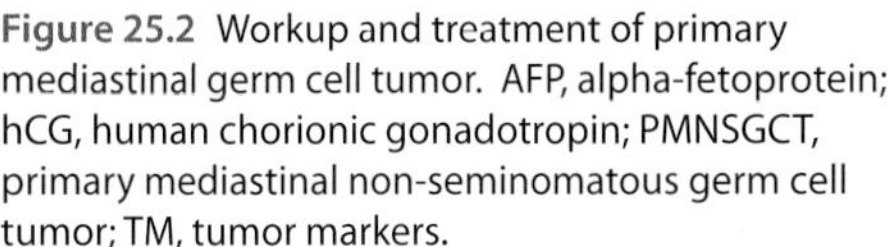

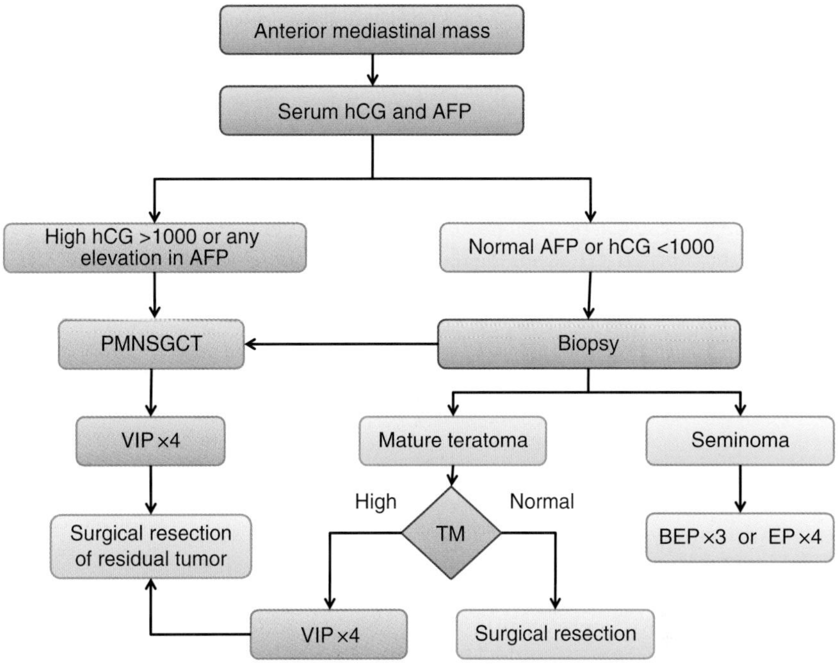

Figure 25.2 Workup and treatment of primary mediastinal germ cell tumor. AFP, alpha-fetoprotein; hCG, human chorionic gonadotropin; PMNSGCT, primary mediastinal non-seminomatous germ cell tumor; TM, tumor markers.

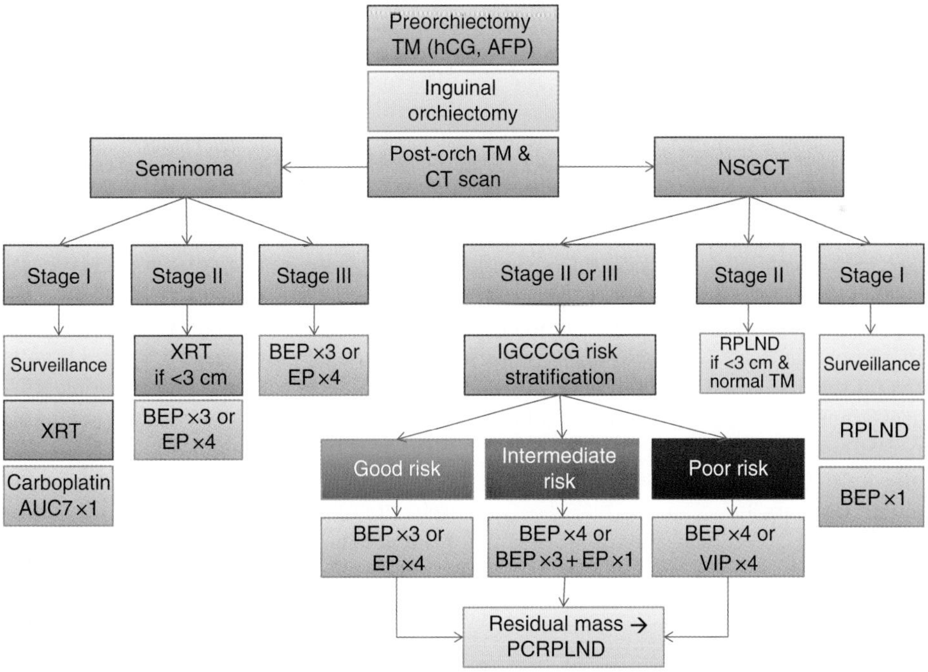

Figure 25.3 Treatment options for germ cell tumor. AFP, alpha-fetoprotein; hCG, human chorionic gonadotropin: TM, tumor markers: CT, computed tomography; IGCCCG, International Germ Cell Cancer Collaborative Group; NSGCT, non-seminomatous germ cell tumor; RPLND, retroperitoneal lymph node dissection; PCRPLND, post chemotherapy retroperitoneal lymph node dissection; XRT, radiation therapy; X, the number of cycles of recommended chemotherapy.

radiation therapy dose between 30 and 36 Gy to the para-aortic and ipsilateral iliac lymph nodes results in a cure rate of 90% [53]. However, for lesions larger than 3 cm or the presence of multiple RPLNs there is a relapse rate up to 40% when patients are treated with radiation [54]. For these patients, three cycles of bleomycin, etoposide, and cisplatin (BEP × 3) or four cycles of EP is advised (Figure 25.3). We recommend BEP × 3 as first choice, unless the patient is older than 50 years, or serum creatinine level >2 [53,55]. Single agent carboplatin chemotherapy is not proven to be effective as compared to combined cisplatin-based chemotherapy [56]. Five-year survival rates for stage II seminoma are 95–100%.

Management of residual masses postchemotherapy is vexing. Continued regression of residual mass is frequent, thus an active surveillance is recommended. Residual masses >3 cm should have a CT/PET scan 6 weeks after finishing chemotherapy. Positive PET (standard uptake value >4) most likely represents active seminoma [57]. The decision to perform surgical resection of the residual mass or salvage chemotherapy should not be based exclusively on a positive PET image since there are false-positive results [58]. Radiation to the residual retroperitoneal seminoma is not recommended in the postchemotherapy setting [59].

Stage I Nonseminomatous GCT

Clinical stage I NSGCT (normal postorchiectomy serum tumor markers and normal CT scans of the chest/abdomen/pelvis) represents about 40% of all NSGCT. Stage I patients are divided into low risk (20% relapse rate) or high risk (40–50% relapse rate) according to the absence or presence of vascular invasion or embryonal carcinoma predominant histology. In a meta-analysis of 23 studies between 1979 and 2001, reporting a total of 2,587 patients, including 1,966 patients on surveillance, the presence of vascular invasion by the primary tumor cells was the strongest predictor for relapse. Intermediate risk was associated with embryonal carcinoma predominance in the primary tumor [60]. The overall relapse rate was about 30%. More than 95% of relapses occur within the first 2 years following orchiectomy. One-half of relapses were in the RPLNs. An additional one-third of all relapses are in the lungs or mediastinum, while about 11% are manifested only by elevated serum tumor markers. With the use of cisplatin-based chemotherapy in the recurrent setting, over 95% of all patients who relapse were alive without disease [60].

Three treatment options are standard, which result in a 98–100% cure rate regardless of which management option is chosen (Figure 25.3) [61]. The options include active surveillance, nerve-sparing retroperitoneal lymph node dissection (RPLND), or primary chemotherapy. Our preferred option at Indiana University is surveillance. Relapses are routinely cured with BEP × 3 or EP × 4 [62].

Surveillance for stage I NSGCT requires history and physical examination, serum tumor markers (hCG and AFP), chest X-ray every 2 months for the first year, every 4 months for the second year, and every 6 months for the third, fourth, and fifth year and annually thereafter. CT scans of the abdomen are performed every 4 months for the first year, every 6 months for the second year, and annually for years 3–5.

The second treatment option for clinical stage I NSGCT is nerve-sparing RPLND. The advantages of RPLND include knowledge about the RPLNs, elimination of further abdominal CT scans, and reduced need for subsequent chemotherapy.

Primary chemotherapy with one or two cycles of BEP in patients with high-risk clinical stage I NSGCT decreases the relapse rate from 40 to 50% down to 1 to 2%. A pooled analysis of 13 studies involving 1043 patients with high risk clinical stage I NSGCT revealed a relapse rate of 1.6% with six patients (0.6%) dying of disease [63]. All but two of these series involved two courses of platinum-based chemotherapy. In a randomized phase III study, 382 patients with clinical stage I NSGCT were randomly assigned to receive either RPLND or BEP × 1 after orchiectomy. After a median follow-up of 4.7 years, two and 15 recurrences were observed with chemotherapy and surgery, respectively ($P = 0.0011$). The 2-year recurrence-free survival rate was 99% for the chemotherapy group and 91% for surgery [64]. A recent phase III study presented at GU ASCO 2017, showed BEP × 1 had similar 2-year recurrence rate to that seen with 2 cycles of BEP [65]. The adoption of BEP × 1 as standard chemotherapy for clinical stage I NSGCT would reduce overall exposure to chemotherapy in this young patient population.

Stage II Nonseminomatous GCT

Patients who present with one or more RPLNs measuring ≤3 cm in greatest dimension on CT and normal tumor markers can be treated with primary RPLND, which offers a 50–80% cure rate. However, the cure rate following RPLND for men with a nodal mass >3 cm is 65% and primary chemotherapy with BEP × 3 or EP × 4 is recommended if RPLNs >3 cm [66,67]. The Testicular Cancer Intergroup Study randomly assigned 195 men with pathologic stage II disease to surveillance or adjuvant chemotherapy (two cycles of a platinum-containing regimen). At a median follow-up of 4 years, there was no statistically significant difference in the survival rates between the two groups with three deaths from testicular cancer in the surveillance arm and one in the chemotherapy arm. However, the recurrence rate was 6 and 49% following adjuvant chemotherapy or surveillance, respectively [67].

Treatment for Advanced Disease

Historical Background

The most important development in the treatment of advanced testicular cancer was the discovery of cisplatin by Rosenberg in 1965 [68]. Cisplatin was established as the essential component for treatment of advanced disease and marked the beginning of the modern era of chemotherapy for GCT. PVB (cisplatin, vinblastine, and bleomycin) was regarded as the standard of care in first-line management of advanced GCT between 1974 and 1984 based upon a landmark study of induction chemotherapy of four cycles of PVB followed by maintenance vinblastine for 21 months [69]. Subsequent studies have focused on reducing the side effects without compromising efficacy by reducing the dose of vinblastine from 0.4 mg/kg to 0.3 mg/kg [70] and eliminating maintenance vinblastine [71].

Etoposide (VP16) was found to have efficacy in patients with refractory GCT as a single agent [72]. Etoposide was synergistic with cisplatin in preclinical models and this was confirmed in a clinical trial of patients with refractory disease [73]. From 1981 through 1984, a randomized study compared cisplatin plus bleomycin and either vinblastine (PVB) or etoposide (BEP) in the first-line setting [74]. Of the patients randomized to the BEP arm, 83% achieved disease-free status versus 74% of patients randomized to the PVB arm. Based on this study, BEP became the standard first-line treatment for patients with metastatic GCT.

In 1997, following a multinational analysis including data from almost 6,000 patients, consensus statement for metastatic GCT was published by the International Germ Cell Cancer Collaborative Group (IGCCCG) [75]. The IGCCCG risk stratification system considers the primary tumor site, metastatic sites, and amplitude of serum tumor marker levels. Based on that, patients with advanced GCT at first diagnosis can be subdivided into three groups: good, intermediate, and poor risk (Table 25.3). This classification allows the study of less toxic regimens in good-risk disease and more aggressive therapy in those with poor-risk cancer.

Table 25.3 International Germ Cells Cancer Collaborative Group (IGCCG) prognostic system for metastatic germ cell tumors [75].

	Description	
IGCCG classification	**NSGCT**	**Seminoma**
Good risk	Requires all of the following: gonadal or retroperitoneal primary tumor, absence of NPVM, hCG <5000 mIU/dL, AFP <1000 ng/dL, and LDH <1.5 × ULN	Absence of NPVM 90% of seminoma are good risk
5-year PFS/OS	89/92	82/86
Intermediate risk	Requires gonadal or retroperitoneal primary tumor, absence of NPVM, and ≥1 of the following: hCG 5,000–50,000 mIU/dL, AFP 1,000–10,000 ng/dL, or LDH 1.5–10.0 × ULN	Presence of NPVM 10% of seminomas are intermediate risk
5-year PFS/OS	75/80	67/72
Poor risk	Requires any of the following: mediastinal primary tumor site, presence of NPVM, HCG >50,000 mIU/dL, AFP >10,000 ng/dL, or LDH 10 × ULN	Seminoma are never poor risk
5-year PFS/OS	41/48	

AFP, alpha-fetoprotein; hCG, human chorionic gonadotropin; LDH, lactate dehydrogenase; NPVM, non-pulmonary visceral metastasis; NSGCT, nonseminoma germ cell tumor; OS, overall survival; PFS, progression free survival.

Good-Risk GCT

Approximately 60% of patients with metastatic GCTs have good-risk disease [75]. A randomized controlled study evaluated the standard four courses of BEP versus three courses (9 weeks). There were 184 patients entered into this study, and 97% achieved a no-evidence-of-disease (NED) status. An identical 92% of patients on each arm are continuously NED [76]. A long-term follow-up of this study showed no significant difference between the two treatment groups in terms of overall ($P = 0.80$) or disease-free ($P = 0.93$) survival [77]. This study established BEP × 3 as standard treatment for good-risk disease.

A randomized trial at Memorial Sloan Kettering Cancer Center (MSKCC) compared cisplatin, vinblastine, bleomycin, dactinomycin, cyclophosphamide (VAB-6) regimen versus etoposide plus cisplatin (EP × 4), finding no difference in efficacy [78]. This study has established EP × 4 as another standard option for good-risk disease. More recently, a European randomized phase III trial compared BEP × 3 versus EP × 4 in good-risk NSGCT [79]. The 4-year event-free survival rates were 91% and 86% for BEP × 3 and EP × 4 respectively ($P = 0.135$). The 4-year overall survival (OS) rates were not significantly different (five deaths in the BEP × 3 arm vs 12 deaths with EP × 4, ($P = 0.096$)).

Studies compared cisplatin-containing regimens versus carboplatin containing regimens in patients with good-risk disease [80,81]; each study reported that carboplatin was inferior to cisplatin. We recommend BEP × 3 as first-line option in patients with good-risk disease. If there is a contraindication to bleomycin, then EP × 4 is recommended.

Intermediate and Poor-Risk GCTs

Approximately 28% of patients with NSGCT have intermediate risk and 16% have poor-risk disease. Seminomas are never poor risk, and only approximately 10% fall into the intermediate-risk category (Table 25.3). The standard of care for these patients is BEP × 4. Etoposide (VP16), ifosfamide, cisplatin (VIP) for four cycles is comparable to BEP × 4. A cooperative group study randomized 304 men with advanced disseminated GCT to BEP × 4 or VIP × 4. Overall complete remission rate (VIP, 37%; BEP, 31%), favorable response rate (VIP, 63%; BEP, 60%), failure-free at 2 years (VIP, 64%; BEP, 60%), and 2-year OS (VIP, 74%; BEP, 71%) were not significantly different between the two treatments. Grade 3 or worse toxicity, particularly hematologic and genitourinary toxicity, was significantly more common in patients who received VIP [82].

Further studies attempted regimen modification or treatment intensification with incorporation of high-dose chemotherapy (HDCT) or the addition of paclitaxel to BEP (T-BEP). Two randomized clinical trials compared BEP × 4 with BEP × 2 followed by HDCT as first-line treatment in patients with poor-risk GCT [83,84] and one trial compared BEP × 4 to VIP × 1 followed by high dose VIP × 3 [85]. All these studies failed to demonstrate any advantage over BEP × 4, and toxicity was more severe with the investigational regimens.

An intergroup phase III trial enrolled 219 patients with intermediate or poor-risk GCT to receive either standard BEP × 4 or BEP × 2, followed by two cycles of HDCT, followed by hematopoietic stem-cell rescue (BEP + HDCT). The 1-year durable complete response rate was 52% after BEP + HDCT and 48% after BEP alone ($P = 0.53$) [83].

Bleomycin should be used with caution, if at all, in patients over age 50 due to increased risk of pulmonary toxicity or those with increased creatinine >2 mg/dL due to increased mucocutaneous toxicity. In patients who need 12 weeks of bleomycin, we recommend baseline pulmonary function tests and then prior to the final course of BEP. If the diffusing capacity of the lung for carbon monoxide is 60% or lower, bleomycin should be discontinued and replaced by ifosfamide.

Postchemotherapy Surgery

Approximately one-third of patients who undergo chemotherapy for metastatic GCTs have residual retroperitoneal abnormalities and require postchemotherapy RPLND [86]. Resection of residual masses (>1 cm) is considered when tumor markers (hCG and AFP) have normalized. Patients with rising markers are generally treated with salvage chemotherapy rather than surgery. Residual masses harbor teratoma in 25–40% of cases and viable GCT in 10–15% [87,88]. If there was teratoma in the orchiectomy, 85% will have teratoma in the postchemotherapy RPLND. However, 48% of patients without teratomas in the orchiectomy specimen will have teratoma in the retroperitoneum [89]. The absence of teratoma in the orchiectomy specimen does not reliably predict the absence of teratoma in the surgical specimen at postchemotherapy RPLND. The pathologic findings after the RPLND help guide further treatment. If teratoma or necrosis is found at the RPLND, no further treatment is recommended. By contrast, when pathology demonstrates viable GCT, two additional cycles of etoposide and cisplatin (EP) chemotherapy should be administered to decrease the chance of relapse [90].

The current recommended procedure for residual retroperitoneal disease is open nerve sparing RPLND. The best outcomes are associated with management at a center of excellence; therefore, patients should be referred to experienced surgeons.

Salvage Therapy for Relapsed GCT

Approximately 20–30% of patients presenting with metastatic GCT are either refractory to or relapse following initial treatment. The IGCCCG risk classification helps us predict that with standard first-line cisplatin-based chemotherapy, approximately 10% of good-risk, 25% of intermediate-risk, and more than 50% of poor-risk patients will progress following first-line treatment [91]. The majority of relapses occur within the first 2 years of completing initial treatment and these cases are classified as early relapses [92]. Patients who relapse after initial chemotherapy can still potentially be cured with second-line and even third-line regimens. In contrast to initial therapy, treatment in the salvage situation after relapse is less well defined and there are different options for treatment.

Conventional Dose Salvage Chemotherapy

The concept for conventional dose salvage chemotherapy (CDCT) has been to use cisplatin plus other active agents not previously used, as long as patients didn't have platinum refractory disease, defined by disease progression during or within 4 weeks after completion of cisplatin-based therapy.

Cisplatin in combination with ifosfamide and etoposide (VIP), vinblastine (VeIP), or paclitaxel (TIP) are commonly used [93–97]. These studies showed durable response rates in patients with recurrent GCT. However, in the absence of randomized controlled trials comparing these regimens, no standard approach has been defined.

Investigators from Indiana University reported on the use of vinblastine, ifosfamide, and cisplatin (VeIP). One-hundred and thirty-five patients with relapsed metastatic GCTs after cisplatin-etoposide-based combination chemotherapy were treated with VeIP × 4. Patients who progressed within 3 weeks of previous cisplatin therapy were excluded. Sixty-seven (50%) patients achieved a disease free status after chemotherapy with or without surgical resection of residual carcinoma or teratoma. Overall, 42 (32%) patients are alive and 32 (23.7%) are continuously free of disease [95] (Table 25.4).

Investigators from MSKCC evaluated the combination of paclitaxel, ifosfamide, and cisplatin (TIP) as second-line therapy for patients with relapsed GCT. Thirty patients with favorable prognostic features (testis primary and complete response to first-line chemotherapy) were treated with TIP × 4 with granulocyte colony-stimulating factor support, followed by resection of residual disease. Twenty-four (80%) of 30 patients achieved a favorable response (complete response (CR) + partial response (PR)). Two patients relapsed, and 22 (73%) of the favorable responses remain durable at a median follow-up duration of 33 months [96] (Table 25.4).

A subsequent phase II study by the same group treated 46 patients with favorable prognostic metastatic GCTs with four

Table 25.4 Summary of selected clinical trials of salvage chemotherapy in relapsed germ cell tumors.

Salvage therapy	Regimen	Phase	No. of patients	FRR (%)	OS (%)	Reference
CDCT	VeIP	II	135	50	24	95
	TIP	I/II	30	80	73	96
	TIP	II	51	60	70	98
HDCT	CE	Retrospective	184	63		100
	TI-CE	II	107	50	52	102

CE, carboplatin and etoposide; CDCT, conventional dose salvage chemotherapy; FRR, favorable response rate; HDCT, high dose chemotherapy; OS, overall survival; TI-CE, paclitaxel, ifosfamide, carboplatin and etoposide; TIP, paclitaxel, ifosfamide, and cisplatin; VeIP, vinblastine, ifosfamide, and cisplatin.

cycles of TIP as second-line therapy. Thirty-two (70%) patients achieved a CR to treatment. Three patients (7%) who achieved a CR relapsed after TIP chemotherapy. Twenty-nine patients are continuously disease free at a median follow-up time of 69 months, resulting in a 63% durable CR rate and a 2-year progression-free survival rate of 65% [97]. Myelosuppression was the major toxicity.

The Medical Research Council (MRC) reported results from a phase II trial of salvage TIP chemotherapy for patients who have progressed following initial BEP. Patients received four courses of TIP at 3-weekly intervals. Of 51 patients, eight (15%) achieved complete remission (CR), and 60% had CR or PR; survival at 1 year was 70% (56–84%) [98].

High-Dose Chemotherapy

HDCT, with carboplatin and etoposide and autologous bone marrow transplant, was initiated at Indiana University in 1986 [99]. Peripheral blood stem cell tandem transplant (SCT) replaced bone marrow transplant in 1996 [100].

One-hundred and eighty-four patients with metastatic GCT that had progressed after first-line cisplatin-based combination chemotherapy were treated with high dose chemotherapy consisting of carboplatin and etoposide for 3 days, and each followed by autologous peripheral-blood SCT; 173 patients received two consecutive transplants. In 110 patients, one or two courses of VeIP preceded the HDCT to reduce tumor bulk and prevent progression prior to high-dose treatment. Of the 184 patients, 116 (63%) had complete remission of disease without relapse during a median follow-up of 48 months. Of the 135 patients who received the treatment as second-line therapy, 94 (69.6%) were disease free during follow-up; 22 of 49 (45%) patients who received treatment as third-line or later therapy were disease free. Of 40 patients with cancer that was platinum refractory, 18 (45%) were disease free. A total of 98 of 144 (68%) patients who had platinum-sensitive disease were disease free, and 26 of 35 (74%) patients with seminoma and 90 of 149 (60%) patients with NSGCT were disease free. Among the 184 patients, there were three drug-related deaths during therapy [100]. HDCT with SCT is our preferred initial salvage chemotherapy in relapsed GCT at Indiana University [101].

Investigators from MSKCC evaluated the TI-CE protocol, incorporating paclitaxel and ifosfamide (TI) as induction chemotherapy and stem cell mobilization, followed by three cycles of high-dose carboplatin and etoposide (HD-CE) and autologous stem cell transplantation. Fifty-four (50%) patients achieved a CR: 45 (42%) to chemotherapy alone and nine (8%) to chemotherapy plus surgery. The 5-year disease-free survival was 47% and OS was 52% (median follow-up, 61 months) [102].

Prognostic Factors at Relapse

The International Prognostic Factors Study Group retrospectively studied nearly 1,600 patients with metastatic GCT who relapsed after first-line chemotherapy and received first-salvage CDCT ($n=773$) or HDCT ($n=821$) in North America and Europe [103]. The patients were divided into five prognostic categories with a 2-year progression-free survival ranging between 75 and 6% (Table 25.5). This retrospective study identified prognostic factors in relapse. There was also a statistical improvement of OS and PFS for patients treated with HDCT over CDCT [104]. These results were consistent within each prognostic category except among low-risk patients, for whom similar OS was observed between the two treatment groups. However, this was not a randomized study.

Further Relapses

Patients who have failed salvage platinum-based regimens or HDCT have an extremely poor prognosis. With the exception of anatomically confined disease, where salvage surgery is an option to achieve long-term survival, there is no standard treatment for patients with multiply relapsed and refractory disease after HDCT. Daily oral etoposide has activity in heavily pretreated patients with response rates of about 20% [105]. Gemcitabine, oxaliplatin, and paclitaxel have shown single-agent activity among patients with cisplatin-refractory disease. The rationale of using oxaliplatin is based on *in vitro* studies

Table 25.5 Prognostic score for patients with relapsed germ cell tumor.

	Score points				
	−1	0	1	2	3
Primary site		Gonadal	Extragonadal	–	PMNSGCT
Prior response		CR/ PR neg TM	PR pos TM/SD	PD	
PFI (months)		>3 months	<3 months	–	
AFP		Normal	≤1000	>1000	
hCG		≤1000	>1000	–	
NPVM		No	Yes	–	
Histology	Seminoma	NSGCT			

Score sum (values from 0 to 10). Regroup score sum into categories: (0) = 0; (1 or 2) = 1; (3 or 4) = 2; (5 or more) = 3. Final prognostic score (−1 = very low risk; 0 = low risk; 1 = intermediate risk; 2 = high risk; 3 = very high risk). AFP, alpha-fetoprotein; CR, complete remission; hCG, human chorionic gonadotrophin; neg TM, negative markers; ; NPVM, nonpulmonary visceral metastasis (liver, bone, brain metastases); PD, progressive disease; PFI, progression-free interval; pos TM, positive markers; PR, partial remission; SD, stable disease; NPVM, nonpulmonary visceral metastasis (liver, bone, brain metastases).

indicating incomplete crossresistance between cisplatin and oxaliplatin. The combination of gemcitabine and oxaliplatin (GEMOX) has shown activity [106]. The overall response rate ranged from 32 to 43% with GEMOX. Toxicities involved mainly myelosuppression and neuropathy. A phase II trial of gemcitabine plus paclitaxel was conducted in patients relapsing after HDCT [107]. Of 28 evaluable patients, six responded, including three who had durable complete responses with overall response rates of 32%.

Late Relapse

Late relapse is defined as a relapse more than 2 years after prior treatment. The incidence is 2–3%. Most late relapses happen after 5 years. Late relapse most often present as elevated AFP. The main treatment is surgical resection. Late relapses respond to standard chemotherapy but they are rarely cured with chemotherapy alone.

Treatment of Sex Cord-Stromal Tumors

Most SCSTs are benign. However, about 10–20% of tumors in adults are malignant and can metastasize and ultimately result in death. Tumor, necrosis (>5 cm), lymphovascular invasion, hemorrhage, nuclear atypia, and high mitotic index are considered malignant criteria with high risk of metastasis. After an inguinal orchiectomy, patients should have a CT scan of the chest, abdomen, and pelvis. For patients with clinical stage I disease with high-risk criteria, RPLND should be considered. Sertoli cell tumors are not curable with chemotherapy or radiation. The incidence of hypogonadism after orchiectomy appears to be higher in men with SCSTs than in those with GCT (42 vs 5–13%). Thus, men with SCSTs are more likely to require testosterone replacement following surgery [108].

Treatment of Mediastinal GCT

Patients with PMNSGCT has extremely poor prognosis and should be treated with four courses of platinum-based triple chemotherapy [109]. We recommend using VIP × 4 as the standard chemotherapy for PMNSGCT [86] followed by surgical resection [110]. We recommend ifosfamide instead of bleomycin to prevent pulmonary complications as these patients require extensive thoracic surgical resection (Figure 25.2). Surgical resection of the residual disease should be considered even if tumor markers have not normalized. Primary mediastinal seminoma represents a good-risk disease with a cure rate near 100% when treated with BEP × 3 or EP × 4. No surgical resection is needed postchemotherapy.

References

1 Siegel RL, Miller KD, Jemal A. Cancer statistics, 2017. *CA Cancer J Clin* 2017;67(1):7–30.
2 Howlader N, Noone AM, Krapcho M, *et al.* (eds). SEER Cancer Statistics Review, 1975–2013, National Cancer Institute. Bethesda, MD. http://seer.cancer.gov/csr/1975_2013/, based on November 2015 SEER data submission, posted to the SEER web site, April 2016.
3 Barr RD, Ries LA, Lewis DR, *et al.* Incidence and incidence trends of the most frequent cancers in adolescent and young adult Americans, including "nonmalignant/noninvasive" tumors. *Cancer* 2016;122(7):1000–8
4 Sokoloff MH, Joyce GF, Wise M. Urologic Diseases in America. *Testis cancer. J Urol* 2007;177(6):2030–41.
5 Huyghe E, Matsuda T, Thonneau P. Increasing incidence of testicular cancer worldwide: a review. *J Urol* 2003;170(1):5–11.
6 Stang A, Trabert B, Wentzensen N, *et al.* Burden of extragonadal germ cell tumours in Europe and the United States. *Eur J Cancer* 2012;48(7):1116–7.
7 Einhorn LH. Treatment of testicular cancer: a new and improved model. *J Clin Oncol* 1990;8(11):1777–81.
8 Lutke Holzik MF, Rapley EA, Hoekstra HJ, *et al.* Genetic predisposition to testicular germ-cell tumours. *Lancet Oncol* 2004;5(6):363–71.
9 Akre O, Pettersson A, Richiardi L. Risk of contralateral testicular cancer among men with unilaterally undescended testis: a meta analysis. *Int J Cancer* 2009;124(3):687–9.
10 Skakkebaek NE, Rajpert-De Meyts E, Main KM. Testicular dysgenesis syndrome: an increasingly common developmental disorder with environmental aspects. *Human Reprod* 2001;16(5):972–8.
11 Swerdlow AJ, Higgins CD, Pike MC. Risk of testicular cancer in cohort of boys with cryptorchidism. *BMJ* 1997;314 (7093):1507–11.
12 Pettersson A, Richiardi L, Nordenskjold A, Kaijser M, Akre O. Age at surgery for undescended testis and risk of testicular cancer. *New Eng J Med* 2007;356(18):1835–41.
13 Chia VM, Li Y, Goldin LR, Graubard BI, *et al.* Risk of cancer in first- and second-degree relatives of testicular germ cell tumor cases and controls. *Int J Cancer* 2009;124(4):952–7.
14 Fossa SD, Chen J, Schonfeld SJ, *et al.* Risk of contralateral testicular cancer: a population-based study of 29,515 U.S. men. *J Natl Cancer Inst* 2005;97(14):1056–66.
15 Nichols CR, Heerema NA, Palmer C, *et al.* Klinefelter's syndrome associated with mediastinal germ cell neoplasms. *J Clin Oncol* 1987;5(8):1290–4.
16 Pleskacova J, Hersmus R, Oosterhuis JW, *et al.* Tumor risk in disorders of sex development. *Sex Dev* 2010;4(4–5):259–69
17 Kerr CL, Hill CM, Blumenthal PD, Gearhart JD. Expression of pluripotent stem cell markers in the human fetal testis. *Stem Cells* 2008;26(2):412–21.
18 Sheikine Y, Genega E, Melamed J, *et al.* Molecular genetics of testicular germ cell tumors. *Am J Cancer Res* 2012;2(2):153–67.
19 Gilbert D, Rapley E, Shipley J. Testicular germ cell tumours: predisposition genes and the male germ cell niche. *Nature Rev Cancer* 2011;11(4):278–88.
20 Rapley EA, Turnbull C, Al Olama AA, *et al.* A genome-wide association study of testicular germ cell tumor. *Nature Genet* 2009;41(7):807–10
21 Kratz CP, Han SS, Rosenberg PS, *et al.* Variants in or near KITLG, BAK1, DMRT1, and TERT-CLPTM1L predispose to

familial testicular germ cell tumour. *J Med Genet* 2011;48(7):473–6.

22 Kanetsky PA, Mitra N, Vardhanabhuti S, *et al.* Common variation in KITLG and at 5q31.3 predisposes to testicular germ cell cancer. *Nature Genet* 2009;41(7):811–5.

23 Nathanson KL, Kanetsky PA, Hawes R, *et al.* The Y deletion gr/gr and susceptibility to testicular germ cell tumor. *Am J Human Genet* 2005;77(6):1034–43.

24 Looijenga LH, Zafarana G, Grygalewicz B, *et al.* Role of gain of 12p in germ cell tumour development. *APMIS* 2003;111(1):161–71; discussion 72–3.

25 Reuter VE. Origins and molecular biology of testicular germ cell tumors. *Mod Pathol* 2005;18 Suppl 2:S51–60.

26 Brait M, Maldonado L, Begum S, *et al.* DNA methylation profiles delineate epigenetic heterogeneity in seminoma and non-seminoma. *Br J Cancer* 2012;106:414–23.

27 Van Der Zwan YG, Stoop H, Rossello F, White SJ, Looijenga LHJ. Role of epigenetics in the etiology of germ cell cancer. *Int J Dev Biol* 2013;57:299–308.

28 Sonnenburg D, Spinella MJ, Albany C. Epigenetic targeting of platinum resistant testicular cancer. *Curr Cancer Drug Targets* 2016;16(9):789–95.

29 Donohue JP, Zachary JM, Maynard BR. Distribution of nodal metastases in nonseminomatous testis cancer. *J Urol* 1982;128(2):315–20.

30 Brimo F, Srigley JR, Ryan CJ, *et al.* Testis. In: Amin MB, Edge SB, Greene FL (eds) *AJCC Cancer Staging Manual*, 8th edn. New York: Springer Nature, 2017.

31 Lerro CC, Robbins AS, Fedewa SA, Ward EM. Disparities in stage at diagnosis among adults with testicular germ cell tumors in the National Cancer Data Base. *Urol Oncol* 2014;32(1):23–e15.

32 Ulbright TM. Germ cell tumors of the gonads: a selective review emphasizing problems in differential diagnosis, newly appreciated, and controversial issues. *Mod Pathol* 2005;18 Suppl 2:S61–79.

33 Bode PK, Barghorn A, Fritzsche FR, *et al.* MAGEC2 is a sensitive and novel marker for seminoma: a tissue microarray analysis of 325 testicular germ cell tumors. *Mod Pathol* 2011;24(6):829–35.

34 Ulbright TM. The most common, clinically significant misdiagnoses in testicular tumor pathology, and how to avoid them. *Adv Anatom Pathol* 2008;15(1):18–27.

35 Ye H, Ulbright TM. Difficult differential diagnoses in testicular pathology. *Arch Pathol Lab Med*2012 Apr;136(4):435–46. PubMed PMID: 22458906. Epub 2012/03/31. eng.

36 Ulbright TM. Gonadal teratomas: a review and speculation. *Adv Anatom Pathol* 2004;11(1):10–23.

37 Motzer RJ, Amsterdam A, Prieto V, *et al.* Teratoma with malignant transformation: diverse malignant histologies arising in men with germ cell tumors. *J Urol* 1998;159(1):133–8.

38 Anuradha G, Deepti D, Semra O, *et al.* Testicular mixed germ cell tumors: a morphological and immunohistochemical study using stem cell markers, OCT3/4, SOX2 and GDF3, with emphasis on morphologically difficult-to-classify areas. *Mod Pathol* 2009;22(8):1066–74.

39 Jones TD, Ulbright TM, Eble JN, Baldridge LA, Cheng L. OCT4 staining in testicular tumors: a sensitive and specific marker for seminoma and embryonal carcinoma. *Am J Surg Pathol* 2004;28(7):935–40.

40 Bosl GJ, Motzer RJ. Testicular germ-cell cancer. *New Eng J Med* 1997;337(4):242–53.

41 Horwich A, Dearnaley DP. Treatment of seminoma. *Semin Oncol* 1992;19(2):171–80.

42 Javadpour N. Current status of tumor markers in testicular cancer. A practical review. *Eur Urol* 1992;21 Suppl 1:34–6.

43 Sweeney CJ, Hermans BP, Heilman DK, *et al.* Results and outcome of retroperitoneal lymph node dissection for clinical stage I embryonal carcinoma–predominant testis cancer. *J Clin Oncol* 2000;18(2):358–62.

44 Dilworth JP, Farrow GM, Oesterling JE. Non-germ cell tumors of testis. *Urology* 1991;37(5):399–417.

45 Suardi N, Strada E, Colombo R, *et al.* Leydig cell tumour of the testis: presentation, therapy, long-term follow-up and the role of organ-sparing surgery in a single-institution experience. *BJU Int* 2009;103(2):197–200.

46 Stang A, Trabert B, Wentzensen N, *et al.* Gonadal and extragonadal germ cell tumours in the United States, 1973–2007. *Int J Androl* 2012;35(4):616–25.

47 Albany C, Einhorn LH. Extragonadal germ cell tumors: clinical presentation and management. *Curr Opin Oncol* 2013;25(3):261–5.

48 Mortensen MS Gundgard MG, Lauritsen J. A nationwide cohort study of surveillance for stage I seminoma. J Clin Oncol 2013;suppl; abstr 4502.

49 Horwich SDF, Stenning SP, Bliss JM, Hall E. Risk of second cancers among a cohort of 2,703 long-term survivors of testicular seminoma treated with radiotherapy. *J Clin Oncol* 2010;28:15s (suppl; abstr 4538).

50 Oliver RT, Mead GM, Rustin GJ, *et al.* Randomized trial of carboplatin versus radiotherapy for stage I seminoma: mature results on relapse and contralateral testis cancer rates in MRC TE19/EORTC 30982 study (ISRCTN27163214). *J Clin Oncol* 2011;29(8):957–62.

51 Mead GM, Fossa SD, Oliver RT, *et al.* Randomized trials in 2466 patients with stage I seminoma: patterns of relapse and follow-up. *J Natl Cancer Inst* 2011;103(3):241–9.

52 Motzer RJ, Agarwal N, Beard C, *et al.* NCCN clinical practice guidelines in oncology: testicular cancer. *JNCCN* 2009;7(6):672–93.

53 Schmoll HJ, Jordan K, Huddart R, *et al.* Testicular seminoma: ESMO Clinical Practice Guidelines for diagnosis, treatment and follow-up. *Ann Oncol* 2010;21 Suppl 5:v140–6.

54 Domont J, Massard C, Patrikidou A, *et al.* A risk-adapted strategy of radiotherapy or cisplatin-based chemotherapy in stage II seminoma. *Urol Oncol* 2013;31(5):697–705.

55 Krege S, Beyer J, Souchon R, *et al.* European consensus conference on diagnosis and treatment of germ cell cancer: a report of the second meeting of the European Germ Cell Cancer Consensus Group (EGCCCG): part II. *Eur Urol* 2008;53(3):497–513.

56 Krege S, Boergermann C, Baschek R, *et al.* Single agent carboplatin for CS IIA/B testicular seminoma. A phase II study of the German Testicular Cancer Study Group (GTCSG). *Ann Oncol* 2006;17(2):276–80.

57 De Santis M, Becherer A, Bokemeyer C, *et al.* 2-18fluoro-deoxy-D-glucose positron emission tomography is a reliable

predictor for viable tumor in postchemotherapy seminoma: an update of the prospective multicentric SEMPET trial. *J Clin Oncol* 2004;22(6):1034–9.

58 Hinz S, Schrader M, Kempkensteffen C, *et al.* The role of positron emission tomography in the evaluation of residual masses after chemotherapy for advanced stage seminoma. *J Urol* 2008;179(3):936–40; discussion 40.

59 Duchesne GM, Stenning SP, Aass N, *et al.* Radiotherapy after chemotherapy for metastatic seminoma–a diminishing role. MRC Testicular Tumour Working Party. *Eur J Cancer* 1997;33(6):829–35.

60 Vergouwe Y, Steyerberg EW, Eijkemans MJ, Albers P, Habbema JD. Predictors of occult metastasis in clinical stage I nonseminoma: a systematic review. *J Clin Oncol* 2003;21(22):4092–9.

61 Schmoll HJ, Jordan K, Huddart R, *et al.* Testicular non-seminoma: ESMO clinical recommendations for diagnosis, treatment and follow-up. *Ann Oncol* 2009;20(Suppl 4):89–96.

62 Chovanec M, Hanna N, Cary KC, Einhorn L, Albany C. Management of stage I testicular germ cell tumours. *Nat Rev Urol* 2016;13(11):663–73.

63 Westermann DH, Studer UE. High-risk clinical stage I nonseminomatous germ cell tumors: the case for chemotherapy. *World J Urol* 2009;27(4):455–61.

64 Albers P, Siener R, Krege S, *et al.* Randomized phase III trial comparing retroperitoneal lymph node dissection with one course of bleomycin and etoposide plus cisplatin chemotherapy in the adjuvant treatment of clinical stage I Nonseminomatous testicular germ cell tumors: AUO trial AH 01/94 by the German Testicular Cancer Study Group. *J Clin Oncol* 2008;26(18):2966–72.

65 Huddart RA, Joffe JK, White JD, *et al.* 111:A single-arm trial evaluating one cycle of BEP as adjuvant chemotherapy in high-risk, stage 1 non-seminomatous or combined germ cell tumors of the testis (NSGCTT). *Journal of Clinical Oncology* 2017;35(suppl 6):400.

66 Donohue JP, Thornhill JA, Foster RS, *et al.* The role of retroperitoneal lymphadenectomy in clinical stage B testis cancer: the Indiana University experience (1965 to 1989). *J Urol* 1995;153(1):85–9.

67 Williams SD, Stablein DM, Einhorn LH, *et al.* Immediate adjuvant chemotherapy versus observation with treatment at relapse in pathological stage II testicular cancer. *New Eng J Med* 1987;317(23):1433–8.

68 Rosenberg B, Vancamp L, Krigas T. Inhibition of Cell Division in Escherichia Coli by Electrolysis Products from a Platinum Electrode. *Nature* 1965;205:698–9.

69 Einhorn LH, Donohue J. Cis-diamminedichloroplatinum, vinblastine, and bleomycin combination chemotherapy in disseminated testicular cancer. *Ann Intern Med* 1977;87(3):293–8.

70 Stoter G, Sleyfer DT, ten Bokkel Huinink WW, *et al.* High-dose versus low-dose vinblastine in cisplatin-vinblastine-bleomycin combination chemotherapy of non-seminomatous testicular cancer: a randomized study of the EORTC Genitourinary Tract Cancer Cooperative Group. *J Clin Oncol* 1986;4(8):1199–206.

71 Einhorn LH, Williams SD, Troner M, Birch R, Greco FA. The role of maintenance therapy in disseminated testicular cancer. *New Eng J Med* 1981;305(13):727–31.

72 Williams SD, Einhorn LH, Greco FA, Oldham R, Fletcher R. VP-16-213 salvage therapy for refractory germinal neoplasms. *Cancer* 1980;46(10):2154–8.

73 Hainsworth JD, Williams SD, Einhorn LH, Birch R, Greco FA. Successful treatment of resistant germinal neoplasms with VP-16 and cisplatin: results of a Southeastern Cancer Study Group trial. *J Clin Oncol* 1985;3(5):666–71.

74 Williams SD, Birch R, Einhorn LH, *et al.* Treatment of disseminated germ-cell tumors with cisplatin, bleomycin, and either vinblastine or etoposide. *New Eng J Med* 1987;316(23):1435–40.

75 International Germ Cell Consensus Classification: a prognostic factor-based staging system for metastatic germ cell cancers. International Germ Cell Cancer Collaborative Group. *J Clin Oncol* 1997;15(2):594–603.

76 Einhorn LH, Williams SD, Loehrer PJ, *et al.* Evaluation of optimal duration of chemotherapy in favorable-prognosis disseminated germ cell tumors: a Southeastern Cancer Study Group protocol. *J Clin Oncol* 1989;7(3):387–91.

77 Saxman SB, Finch D, Gonin R, Einhorn LH. Long-term follow-up of a phase III study of three versus four cycles of bleomycin, etoposide, and cisplatin in favorable-prognosis germ-cell tumors: the Indian University experience. *J Clin Oncol* 1998;16(2):702–6.

78 Bosl GJ, Geller NL, Bajorin D, *et al.* A randomized trial of etoposide + cisplatin versus vinblastine + bleomycin + cisplatin + cyclophosphamide + dactinomycin in patients with good-prognosis germ cell tumors. *J Clin Oncol* 1988;6(8):1231–8.

79 Culine S, Kerbrat P, Kramar A, *et al.* Refining the optimal chemotherapy regimen for good-risk metastatic nonseminomatous germ-cell tumors: a randomized trial of the Genito-Urinary Group of the French Federation of Cancer Centers (GETUG T93BP). *Ann Oncol* 2007;18(5):917–24.

80 Bajorin DF, Sarosdy MF, Pfister DG, *et al.* Randomized trial of etoposide and cisplatin versus etoposide and carboplatin in patients with good-risk germ cell tumors: a multiinstitutional study. *J Clin Oncol* 1993;11(4):598–606.

81 Bokemeyer C, Kohrmann O, Tischler J, *et al.* A randomized trial of cisplatin, etoposide and bleomycin (PEB) versus carboplatin, etoposide and bleomycin (CEB) for patients with 'good-risk' metastatic non-seminomatous germ cell tumors. *Ann Oncol* 1996;7(10):1015–21.

82 Nichols CR, Catalano PJ, Crawford ED, *et al.* Randomized comparison of cisplatin and etoposide and either bleomycin or ifosfamide in treatment of advanced disseminated germ cell tumors: an Eastern Cooperative Oncology Group, Southwest Oncology Group, and Cancer and Leukemia Group B Study. *J Clin Oncol* 199816(4):1287–93.

83 Motzer RJ, Nichols CJ, Margolin KA, *et al.* Phase III randomized trial of conventional-dose chemotherapy with or without high-dose chemotherapy and autologous hematopoietic stem-cell rescue as first-line treatment for patients with poor-prognosis metastatic germ cell tumors. *J Clin Oncol* 2007;25(3):247–56.

84 Droz JP, Kramar A, Biron P, *et al.* Failure of high-dose cyclophosphamide and etoposide combined with double-dose cisplatin and bone marrow support in patients with high-volume metastatic nonseminomatous germ-cell tumours:

mature results of a randomised trial. *Eur Urol* 2007;51(3):739–46.

85 Daugaard G, Skoneczna I, Aass N, *et al.* A randomized phase III study comparing standard dose BEP with sequential high-dose cisplatin, etoposide, and ifosfamide (VIP) plus stem-cell support in males with poor-prognosis germ-cell cancer. An intergroup study of EORTC, GTCSG, and Grupo Germinal (EORTC 30974). *Ann Oncol* 2011;22(5):1054–61.

86 Heidenreich A, Pfister D. Retroperitoneal lymphadenectomy and resection for testicular cancer: an update on best practice. *Ther Adv Urol* 2012;4(4):187–205.

87 Steyerberg EW, Keizer HJ, Fossa SD, *et al.* Prediction of residual retroperitoneal mass histology after chemotherapy for metastatic nonseminomatous germ cell tumor: multivariate analysis of individual patient data from six study groups. *J Clin Oncol* 1995;13(5):1177–87.

88 Oldenburg J, Alfsen GC, Lien HH, *et al.* Postchemotherapy retroperitoneal surgery remains necessary in patients with nonseminomatous testicular cancer and minimal residual tumor masses. *J Clin Oncol* 2003;21(17):3310–7.

89 Beck SD, Foster RS, Bihrle R, *et al.* Teratoma in the orchiectomy specimen and volume of metastasis are predictors of retroperitoneal teratoma in post-chemotherapy nonseminomatous testis cancer. *J Urol* 2002;168(4):1402–4.

90 Fox EP, Weathers TD, Williams SD, *et al.* Outcome analysis for patients with persistent nonteratomatous germ cell tumor in postchemotherapy retroperitoneal lymph node dissections. *J Clin Oncol* 1993;11(7):1294–9.

91 Voss MH, Feldman DR, Bosl GJ, Motzer RJ. A review of second-line chemotherapy and prognostic models for disseminated germ cell tumors. *Hematol Oncol Clin North Am* 2011;25(3):557–76, viii –ix.

92 Koychev D, Oechsle K, Bokemeyer C, Honecker F. Treatment of patients with relapsed and/or cisplatin-refractory metastatic germ cell tumours: an update. *Int J Androl* 2011;34(4):e266–73.

93 Loehrer PJ, Sr., Einhorn LH, Williams SD. VP-16 plus ifosfamide plus cisplatin as salvage therapy in refractory germ cell cancer. *J Clin Oncol* 1986;4(4):528–36.

94 Loehrer PJ, Sr., Lauer R, Roth BJ, *et al.* Salvage therapy in recurrent germ cell cancer: ifosfamide and cisplatin plus either vinblastine or etoposide. *Ann Intern Med* 1988;109(7):540–6.

95 Loehrer PJ, Sr., Gonin R, Nichols CR, Weathers T, Einhorn LH. Vinblastine plus ifosfamide plus cisplatin as initial salvage therapy in recurrent germ cell tumor. *J Clin Oncol* 1998;16(7):2500–4.

96 Motzer RJ, Sheinfeld J, Mazumdar M, *et al.* Paclitaxel, ifosfamide, and cisplatin second-line therapy for patients with relapsed testicular germ cell cancer. *J Clin Oncol* 2000;18(12):2413–8.

97 Kondagunta GV, Bacik J, Donadio A, et al. Combination of paclitaxel, ifosfamide, and cisplatin is an effective second-line therapy for patients with relapsed testicular germ cell tumors. *J Clin Oncol* 2005;23(27):6549–55.

98 Mead GM, Cullen MH, Huddart R, *et al.* A phase II trial of TIP (paclitaxel, ifosfamide and cisplatin) given as second-line (post-BEP) salvage chemotherapy for patients with metastatic germ cell cancer: a medical research council trial. *Br J Cancer* 2005;93(2):178–84.

99 Nichols CR, Tricot G, Williams SD, *et al.* Dose-intensive chemotherapy in refractory germ cell cancer–a phase I/II trial of high-dose carboplatin and etoposide with autologous bone marrow transplantation. *J Clin Oncol* 1989;7(7):932–9.

100 Einhorn LH, Williams SD, Chamness A, *et al.* High-dose chemotherapy and stem-cell rescue for metastatic germ-cell tumors. *New Eng J Med* 2007;357(4):340–8.

101 Adra N, Abonour R, Althouse SK, *et al.* High-dose chemotherapy and autologous peripheral-blood stem-cell transplantation for relapsed metastatic germ cell tumors: the Indiana University Experience. *J Clin Oncol* 2017;35(10):1096–102.

102 Feldman DR, Sheinfeld J, Bajorin DF, *et al.* TI-CE high-dose chemotherapy for patients with previously treated germ cell tumors: results and prognostic factor analysis. *J Clin Oncol* 2010;28(10):1706–13.

103 International Prognostic Factors Study G, Lorch A, Beyer J, Bascoul-Mollevi C, *et al.* Prognostic factors in patients with metastatic germ cell tumors who experienced treatment failure with cisplatin-based first-line chemotherapy. *J Clin Oncol* 2010;28(33):4906–11.

104 Lorch A, Bascoul-Mollevi C, Kramar A, *et al.* Conventional-dose versus high-dose chemotherapy as first salvage treatment in male patients with metastatic germ cell tumors: evidence from a large international database. *J Clin Oncol* 2011;29(16):2178–84.

105 Miller JC, Einhorn LH. Phase II study of daily oral etoposide in refractory germ cell tumors. *Semin Oncol* 1990;17(1 Suppl 2):36–9.

106 Pectasides D, Pectasides M, Farmakis D, *et al.* Gemcitabine and oxaliplatin (GEMOX) in patients with cisplatin-refractory germ cell tumors: a phase II study. *Ann Oncol* 2004;15(3):493–7.

107 Einhorn LH, Brames MJ, Juliar B, Williams SD. Phase II study of paclitaxel plus gemcitabine salvage chemotherapy for germ cell tumors after progression following high-dose chemotherapy with tandem transplant. *J Clin Oncol* 2007;25(5):513–6.

108 Conkey DS, Howard GC, Grigor KM, McLaren DB, Kerr GR. Testicular sex cord-stromal tumours: the Edinburgh experience 1988–2002, and a review of the literature. *Clin Oncol* 2005;17(5):322–7.

109 Adra N, Althouse SK, Liu H, *et al.* Prognostic factors in patients with poor-risk germ-cell tumors: a retrospective analysis of the Indiana University experience from 1990 to 2014. *Ann Oncol* 2016;27(5):875–9.

110 Kesler KA, Rieger KM, Hammoud ZT, *et al.* A 25-year single institution experience with surgery for primary mediastinal nonseminomatous germ cell tumors. *Ann Thorac Surg* 2008;85(2):371–8.

26

Prostate Cancer

Bobby C. Liaw[1] *and William K. Oh*[2]

[1] *Icahn School of Medicine at Mount Sinai, Mount Sinai Downtown Chelsea Center, New York, New York, USA*
[2] *The Tisch Cancer Institute, Icahn School of Medicine at Mount Sinai, New York, New York, USA*

Incidence and Mortality

In the United States (US), an estimated 161,360 new cases of prostate cancer will be diagnosed in 2017, and approximately 26,730 men will die of prostate cancer. Given current screening practices, it is estimated that one in six American males will acquire the diagnosis in their lifetime, and one in 36 will die from the disease [1]. Much of the statistical information regarding prostate cancer in the US is derived from the US National Cancer Institute's Surveillance, Epidemiology, and End Results (SEER) Program.

Incidence rates have fluctuated in the recent past, most significantly affected by the introduction of prostate-specific antigen (PSA) testing in the mid-1980s. As availability and utilization of PSA testing became more widespread, detection of prostate cancer increased, resulting in substantial increases in incidence rates of approximately 16.5% a year between 1988 and 1992. The subsequent decline in incidence of about 1.5% per year until 1995 represented a time when the majority of prevalent detectable cases had already been identified (Figure 26.1).

The small and transient rise in incidence seen around the new millennium is thought to be the result of a combination of increased prostate cancer screening initiatives, and the transition from six-core (sextant) prostate biopsy to the more sensitive extended (10–12) core prostate biopsy as the standard of care. The incidence rate decline of approximately 10.7% annually from 2010 to 2013 is thought to be the result of reduced use of PSA testing [1,2]

Prostate cancer-specific mortality in the US has declined significantly since the early 1990s [1,2], and there are multiple factors likely contributing to its improvement. While large randomized, controlled trials have not shown a significant mortality benefit to PSA screening, some argue that the effects from the early implementation of PSA screening is delayed, and are only starting to become manifest now as mortality reduction. Treatments have also been refined and new therapies realized since the inception and completion of the clinical trials. Changes to the World Health Organization's definition of death attributed to a specific cause, and morbidities such as increased cardiovascular risk secondary to hormonal therapy for prostate cancer treatment, need to be taken into consideration as well.

Worldwide, prostate cancer remains the second most common cancer in men. Incidence rates of prostate cancer vary widely across country borders, with developing countries having lower rates compared to industrialized nations.

Risk Factors

Of all the well-established risk factors for prostate cancer, age is by far the strongest. Prostate cancer is rarely diagnosed in men under the age of 40. Based on data from the SEER database from 2007 to 2009, the probability of prostate cancer diagnosis in American men from birth to age 39 is only 0.01%. The corresponding probabilities for men ages 40–59, 60–69, and 70+ are 2.68%, 6.78%, and 12.06%, respectively.

Ethnic background is an important prostate cancer risk factor. Among different races, African American men have the highest incidence of prostate cancer in the world. They present with higher PSAs, Gleason scores, and stages of disease, even after controlling for socioeconomic, clinical, and pathologic variables [2]. Prostate cancer is more common in Whites from North America and northwestern Europe, and less common in men in Asia and South America.

Family history and genetics are also strong risk factors. A meta-analysis of epidemiological studies found that having a first-degree relative with prostate cancer places a male at over 2.5× relative risk of developing prostate cancer in their lifetime [3]. An even greater risk has been observed in men with multiple relatives with prostate cancer, or a family history of early prostate cancer disease onset [3–5].

Further supporting the hypothesis that genetics is an important factor in driving prostate cancer pathogenesis, a Scandinavian study of male twins found a 21.1% concordance for monozygotic twins as compared to 6.4% for dizygotic twins. Hereditary factors may represent as much as 42% of the risk of prostate cancer, greater than that seen in colorectal (35%) and

The American Cancer Society's Oncology in Practice: Clinical Management, First Edition. Edited by The American Cancer Society.

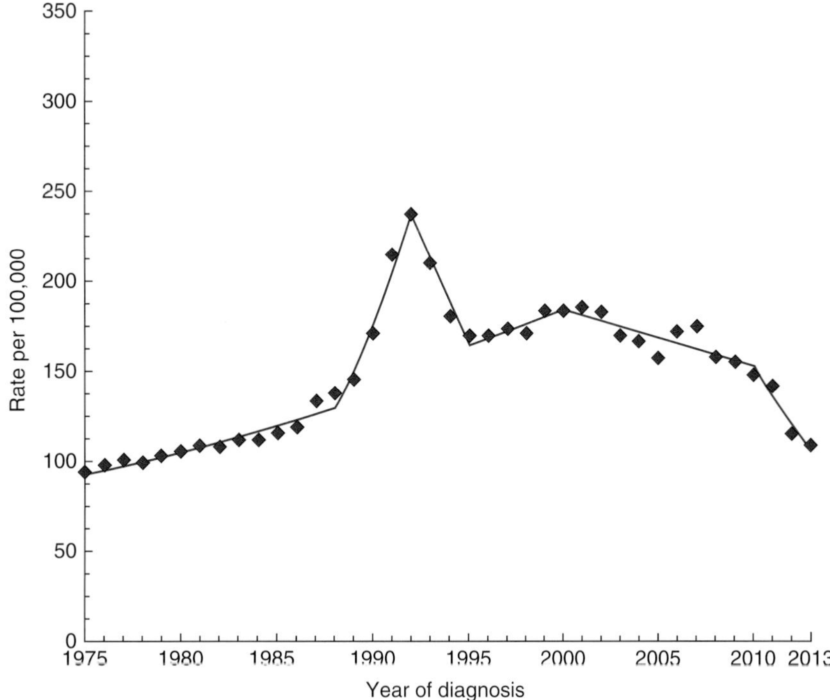

Figure 26.1 Age-Adjusted SEER Incidence Rates of Prostate Cancer. Rates are per 100,000 and age-adjusted to the 2000 US Standard Population. Regression lines are calculated using the Joinpoint Regression Program Version 4.2.0, April 2015, National Cancer Institute. *Incidence source:* SEER 9 areas (San Francisco, Connecticut, Detroit, Hawaii, Iowa, New Mexico, Seattle, Utah, and Atlanta). Adapted from Fast Stats: An interactive tool for access to SEER cancer statistics [149].

breast cancer (27%) [6]. Germline mutations in *BRCA1* and *BRCA2* account for small percentages of prostate cancer, but are associated with higher Gleason scores and overall worse prognosis [7–11].

Through genome-wide association studies, multiple single nucleotide polymorphisms (SNPs) have been identified as markers for prostate cancer risk [12–21]. Many of these SNPs reside in regions of the genome not yet well understood. With further research, these SNPs may help yield further insights into prostate cancer biology, to be used in screening, or become future targets for therapeutics.

Many observations have suggested that environmental factors play a major role in the etiology of prostate cancer. As an example, Japanese immigrants in the US, while at lower risk for prostate cancer as compared to their White American counterparts, have a higher risk than Japanese men who reside in Japan. This and other similar risk patterns may be explained by different dietary habits and other lifestyle attributes.

The effects of dietary intake and nutritional factors on prostate cancer risk have been widely studied although the body of evidence is often difficult to interpret due to differences in individual trial designs and inconsistent tools for measuring intake. Diets high in cruciferous vegetables, such as broccoli and cauliflower, are associated with a decreased risk of aggressive prostate cancer [22]. A similar association has been shown in recent meta-analyses with certain soy products, such as tofu, which is thought to be due to phytoestrogens having an effect on reducing cell proliferation and angiogenesis [23], and decreasing concentrations of dihydrotestosterone via 5a-reductase inhibition. Other foods such as tomatoes, legumes, and fish have also been associated with reduced risk, although the evidence is not as convincing [24].

Dietary fat, particularly alpha-linoleic acids that are commonly found in red meats, has been implicated for increasing prostate cancer risk [25,26]. Increased dairy and calcium intake may also be modestly associated with increased risk of nonaggressive prostate cancer [27].

Selenium and vitamin E, which were initially thought to be protective based on early observational studies and post-hoc analyses of randomized trials evaluating risk of other cancers, was studied in a randomized, prospective chemoprevention trial called SELECT (Selenium and Vitamin E Cancer Prevention Trial); they were found to be not beneficial in reducing prostate cancer risk [28], and are no longer recommended as a preventative supplement.

With regards to dietary intake, the American Cancer Society advises eating at least 2.5 cups of a wide variety of vegetables and fruits each day [24]. No specific recommendations are made for calcium and dairy intake as they may play a role in decreasing colorectal cancer risk, however it is advisable to not exceed recommended daily intake levels [24].

The effects of hormonal factors on prostate cancer was studied in a pooled analysis of 18 prospective studies, which showed that prediagnosis serum androgen and estrogen levels were not associated with an increased risk of disease development [29]. The use of testosterone supplementation for treatment of medical conditions such as hypogonadism, were similarly found not to affect subsequent prostate cancer risk [29].

Metabolic factors affect prostate cancer risk as well. Prospective studies have demonstrated an association between obesity and prostate cancer specific mortality at diagnosis [30], and that it portends a worse prognosis following treatment [31]. These were confirmed in a large meta-analysis which found a 5 kg/m^2 increase in body mass index at diagnosis was associated with a 15% higher risk of dying of prostate cancer (relative risk 1.15, 95% CI 1.06–1.25, P <0.01), as well as a 21% increased risk of biochemical recurrence for the same increase in body mass index following primary treatment (relative risk 1.21, 95% CI 1.11–1.31, P <0.01) [32]. Multiple studies also support a relationship between higher serum insulin levels and insulin resistance with higher prostate cancer risk. High circulating IGF-1 concentrations have been shown in meta-analysis to be associated with a moderately increased risk for prostate cancer, although more positively associated with low-grade than with high-grade disease [33].

Physical activity was demonstrated to have a small inverse association with prostate cancer risk in a meta-analysis of 19 cohort and 24 case-control studies [34]. Since other health benefits are derived from increased physical activity, men should be encouraged to maintain a healthy weight, pursue regular exercise, and stay active in their daily lives [24].

Screening

Although the majority of diagnoses in the US are made by PSA, routine PSA screening remains controversial. It is well established that PSA is an imperfect test for prostate cancer, as benign conditions such as benign prostatic hypertrophy and prostatitis commonly elevate PSA levels. At a PSA level of 4.0 ng/mL, the traditional limit set by laboratories as the upper limit of normal range, the positive predictive value for prostate cancer is only 30%. Attempts at enhancing PSA testing specificity and sensitivity using PSA velocity [35,36], density [37], and fractionation [38], have not consistently outperformed PSA alone when compared in retrospective series. An abnormal finding on digital rectal examination (DRE), however, adds to the positive predictive value of PSA testing [39].

Early PSA screening guidelines were adopted in the absence of prospective randomized data in the hopes that early detection would translate to decreased prostate cancer morbidity and mortality. Unfortunately, routine PSA screening uncovered many low-risk prostate cancers that would otherwise not become clinically meaningful during a man's lifetime. The unnecessary treatment of these "clinically insignificant" cancers exposed men to significant morbidities, such as urinary, bowel, and sexual dysfunction, as well as the psychological distress that comes with a cancer diagnosis.

In 2009, two large randomized PSA screening trials were published, providing for the first time ever, clinical data to help guide prostate cancer screening. Both the European Randomized Study of Screening for Prostate Cancer (ERSPC) and the Prostate, Lung, Colorectal, and Ovarian Cancer (PLCO) Screening Trial found higher incidences of prostate cancer in their PSA screening arms as compared to the control arms. The two trials differed in that ERSPC found some long-term reduction in prostate cancer-specific mortality associated with PSA screening, whereas PLCO did not [40,41]. However, both trials underscored the high rate of false positives and significant risk of overdiagnosis associated with PSA-based screening. Additionally, both commented that the risks patients are subjected to from screening, diagnosis, and overtreatment can considerably compromise quality of life.

Despite data questioning the efficacy of prostate cancer screening and a lack of universally accepted screening guidelines, PSA testing has nevertheless become a standard of care in many medical practices. While different medical organizations have differing recommendations (Table 26.1), they all stress the importance of helping patients make informed personal decisions about whether or not to check screening PSA levels [42–45]. For a more detailed review of prostate cancer screening, please refer to Chapter 11 in the *American Cancer Society's Principles of Oncology: Prevention to Survivorship.*

Diagnosis

A PSA level of 4.0 ng/mL has historically been the accepted cutoff for referral for prostate biopsy, although the optimal threshold remains unclear. Subgroup analysis of the large, phase III,

Table 26.1 Prostate cancer screening guidelines.

Organization	Last revision	Recommendations
American Cancer Society (ACS) [42]	03/03/2010	• Informed decision for men with ≥10-year life expectancy, starting at age 50 if average risk, age 45 if high risk (African American, one first degree relative), age 40 if appreciably higher risk (multiple family members with prostate cancer before age 65) • For men who choose screening, PSA test annually with optional DRE. In men whose PSA is <2.5 ng/mL, screening intervals can be extended to every 2 years
American College of Physicians (ACP) [43]	05/21/2013	• Informed decision for PSA screening in men aged 50–69 • No clear evidence guides the periodicity or frequency of screening • Recommends against PSA screening in men age <50 at average risk, age ≥70, or life expectancy less than 10–15 years
American Urologic Association (AUA) [44]	05/06/2013	• Informed decision for men age 55–69 if average risk, or age 40–54 if higher risk (African American race, positive family history) • For men who choose PSA screening, a routine schedule of 2 years or more may be preferred over annual screening • Recommends against PSA screening in men age <55 at average risk, age ≥70, or life expectancy less than 10–15 years
United States Preventative Services Task Force (USPSTF) [45]	05/22/2012	• Informed decision for all men • Recommends against PSA based screening, regardless of age

DRE, digital rectal examination; PSA, prostate-specific antigen.

randomized Prostate Cancer Prevention Trial in which men underwent routine prostate biopsy at the completion of the trial, found that 26.9% of patients in the placebo arm over the age of 55 and with PSA levels 3.1–4.0 ng/mL, demonstrated prostate cancer on end-of-study biopsy. Even more striking is the fact that 25% of those cases were categorized as high-grade prostate cancer [46]. There continues to be debate whether the PSA cut-off for referral needs to be lowered in order to diagnose this subgroup of high-risk patients at the risk of increasing overdiagnosis.

A definitive diagnosis of prostate cancer is made by transrectal ultrasound-guided prostate biopsy. The procedure is usually performed under local anesthesia in the outpatient setting. The current standard of care is for 10–14 core biopsies to be taken in order to establish diagnosis. In the past, the six-core (sextant) biopsy approach had been the standard; however, sextant biopsies were later shown in a systematic review of 87 studies to miss 31% of clinically significant cancers when compared to extended core (>6) biopsies. It also showed that taking more than 12 cores did not add significant benefit to cancer detection [47].

While generally well tolerated, prostate biopsy is not without its side effects. Many patients report pain and discomfort with the procedure. Local anesthesia reduces patient discomfort during prostate biopsy, and is not associated with an increase in rate of complications [48]. A retrospective review of 5,802 transurethral ultrasound-guided sextant biopsies, found that 22.6% of men had hematuria that lasted longer than 3 days, and 50.4% had hematospermia following biopsy [49]. Major complications were observed in small numbers, but notable for fever (3.5%), rectal bleeding (1.3%), and urinary retention (0.4%). Need for hospitalization due to complications of prostate biopsy was rare (0.5%), with most cases attributed to prostatitis or urosepsis.

More than 95% of prostatic malignancy is accounted for by adenocarcinoma. Other histologic diagnoses are rare, and are not limited to neuroendocrine tumors, sarcomas, lymphomas, small cell carcinomas, and transitional cell carcinomas (Table 26.2).

If prostatic adenocarcinoma is discovered on pathologic review of the core needle biopsy, the pathologist grades the most prevalent pattern of glandular architecture and differentiation on the Gleason scale of 1–5, with 1 being the most differentiated and 5 being the least differentiated. The second most prevalent pattern is similarly graded, with the sum of the two grades comprising the overall Gleason sum or score. While the Gleason score is based solely upon architectural features of prostate cancer cells, it is an important prognostic factor as it closely correlates with clinical behavior. In the most popular risk stratification (D'Amico criteria), a Gleason score of 6 (Gleason 3 + 3) or below is considered low-grade disease, 7 (Gleason 3 + 4 or 4 + 3) is considered intermediate-grade disease, and 8 (Gleason 4 + 4) or above is considered high-grade disease.

Staging

Prostate cancer is staged either clinically or pathologically according to the TNM staging system developed by the American Joint Committee on Cancer. Revised in 2016, the 8th edition combines anatomic (TNM) stage, pretreatment PSA levels, and histologic grade to define different prognostic groups (Tables 26.3 and 26.4).

Table 26.2 Histologic subtypes of prostate cancer.

Epithelial tumors	Acinar adenocarcinoma
	Ductal adenocarcinoma
	Pseudohyperplastic carcinoma
	Foamy gland carcinoma
	Signet ring cell carcinoma
	Lymphoepithelioma-like carcinoma
	Sarcomatoid/spindle cell carcinoma
	Mucinous adenocarcinoma
	Urothelial carcinoma
	Squamous/adenosquamous carcinoma
	Basal cell/adenoid carcinoma
Neuroendocrine tumors	Neuroendocrine differentiation within adenocarcinoma
	Small-cell carcinoma
	Carcinoid tumor
	Paraganglioma
	Neuroblastoma
Stromal tumors	Stromal sarcoma

The clinical stage, PSA level, and biopsy Gleason score are used in combination for risk stratification [50] (Table 26.5). The combination of these clinicopathologic parameters has been demonstrated in multiple studies to strongly predict treatment outcome and risk for recurrence following definitive localized treatment. Low-risk disease is generally characterized by a serum PSA level ≤10 ng/mL, Gleason score ≤6, and clinical stage less than T1c or T2. The disease is more commonly nonpalpable on DRE (T1c), with the only evidence of disease being found pathologically from transurethral resection of the prostate or prostate biopsy. Intermediate-risk disease patients have either PSA levels that range from 10 to ≤20 ng/mL, Gleason score 7, and/or clinical stage T2b. High-risk disease is defined by serum PSA values >20 ng/mL, Gleason score 8–10, and/or clinical stage T2c.

Since prostate cancer metastasizes preferentially to bone, radionuclide bone scans are the most widely used method to evaluate for skeletal metastases. Not all newly diagnosed prostate cancers require a bone scan for workup. A study of 631 prostate cancer patients demonstrated the importance of clinical stage, Gleason score, and PSA, in predicting the likelihood of bony metastasis. Their analysis found that only 1% (3/308) of men with disease stage T2b or less, Gleason score ≤7, and PSA ≤50 ng/mL had a positive bone scan [51]. In the subset of men within the previously defined group except with PSA levels ≤15 ng/mL, none had positive bone scans. This and other similar studies demonstrate that there is a group of low-risk patients that can be easily identified based on the three clinicopathologic factors, in whom bone scan could be omitted.

For patients with higher grade or stage of disease, bone scans and other imaging modalities such as computed tomography and magnetic resonance imaging are indicated for disease staging, and provide guidance for further management. Newer staging modalities such as NaF positron emission tomography

Table 26.3 TNM definitions of the American Joint Committee on Cancer.

Definition of primary tumor (T)	
Clinical T (cT)	
T category	**T criteria**
TX	Primary tumor cannot be assessed
T0	No evidence of primary tumor
T1	Clinically inapparent tumor that is not palpable
T1a	Tumor incidental histologic finding in 5% or less of tissue resected
T1b	Tumor incidental histologic finding in more than 5% of tissue resected
T1c	Tumor identified by needle biopsy found in one or both sides, but not palpable
T2	Tumor is palpable and confined within prostate
T2a	Tumor involves one-half of one side or less
T2b	Tumor involves more than one-half of one side but not both sides
T2c	Tumor involves both sides
T3	Extraprostatic tumor that is not fixed or does not invade adjacent structures
T3a	Extraprostatic extension (unilateral or bilateral)
T3b	Tumor invades seminal vesicle(s)
T4	Tumor is fixed or invades adjacent structures other than seminal vesicles such as external sphincter, rectum, bladder, levator muscles, and/or pelvic wall
Pathological T (pT)[1]	
T category	**T criteria**
T2	Organ confined
T3	Extraprostatic extension
T3a	Extraprostatic extension (unilateral or bilateral) or microscopic invasion of bladder neck
T3b	Tumor invades seminal vesicle(s)
T4	Tumor is fixed or invades adjacent structures other than seminal vesicles such as external sphincter, rectum, bladder, levator muscles, and/or pelvic wall
Definition for regional lymph node (N)	
N category	**N criteria**
NX	Regional nodes were not assessed
N0	No positive regional nodes
N1	Metastases in regional node(s)
Definition for distant metastasis (M)[2]	
M category	**M criteria**
M0	No distant metastasis
M1	Distant metastasis
M1a	Nonregional lymph node(s)
M1b	Bone(s)
M1c	Other site(s) with or without bone disease

Table 26.3 (Continued)

Definition of prostate-specific antigen (PSA)		
PSA values		
<10		
≥10<20		
<0		
≥20		
Any value		
Definition of histologic grade groups (G)		
Grade group	**Gleason score**	**Gleason pattern**
1	≤6	≤3+3
2	7	3+4
3	7	4+3
4	8	4+4
5	9 or 10	4+5, 5+4, or 5+5

Source: adapted from AJCC Cancer Staging Manual, 8th edn (2017) published by Springer New York, Inc. Used with permission of the American College of Surgeons, Chicago, Illinois. The original source for this information is the AJCC Cancer Staging Manual, 8th edn (2017), which is published by Springer Science + Business Media.

[1] There is no pathological T1 classification. Positive surgical margin should be indicated by an R1 descriptor, indicating residual microscopic disease.

[2] When more than one site of metastasis is present, the most advanced category is used. M1c is most advanced.

scans demonstrate some promise for more sensitive detection of metastasis, without loss of specificity.

Treatment of Localized Prostate Cancer

Options for treatment of localized prostate cancer include active surveillance (AS), radical prostatectomy (RP), external beam radiation therapy (EBRT), and brachytherapy.

Active Surveillance

For men with low-risk disease that is unlikely to progress based on their clinicopathologic parameters, and in older men with significant comorbidities and/or limited life expectancies, active surveillance (AS) is a preferred option. AS entails regular office visits with PSA checks and DREs, as well as periodic repeat prostate biopsies to monitor the status of the disease. Optimal frequency for monitoring is not clearly established, but a reasonable surveillance protocol would be PSA evaluations every 6 months, DRE every 12 months, and repeat biopsies every 12–24 months, particularly during the initial monitoring period. Definitive therapy can be initiated only if there are significant laboratory or pathologic changes or clinical symptoms to suggest disease progression.

The comparative effectiveness of AS versus definitive therapy was demonstrated in a large prospective trial that randomized 1,643 men with predominantly Gleason 6 (77%) and T1c disease (76%), to receive either AS, radical prostatectomy, or radical radiotherapy. At a median 10 years of follow-up, no significant difference in prostate cancer-specific mortality was demonstrated between the three treatment arms (1.5 vs 0.9 vs 0.7

Table 26.4 American Joint Committee on Cancer prognostic stage groups.

Tumor (T)	Node (N)	Metastasis (M)	PSA	Grade group (G)	Stage group
cT1a–c, cT2a	N0	M0	<10	1	I
pT2	N0	M0	<10	1	I
cT1a–c, cT2a	N0	M0	≥10 < 20	1	IIA
cT2b–c	N0	M0	<20	1	IIA
T1-2	N0	M0	<20	2	IIB
T1-2	N0	M0	<20	3	IIC
T1-2	N0	M0	<20	4	IIC
T1-2	N0	M0	≥20	1–4	IIIA
T3-4	N0	M0	Any	1–4	IIIB
Any T	N0	M0	Any	5	IIIC
Any T	N1	M0	Any	Any	IVA
Any T	N0	M1	Any	Any	IVB

Source: adapted from AJCC Cancer Staging Manual, 8th edn (2017) published by Springer New York, Inc. Used with permission of the American College of Surgeons, Chicago, Illinois. The original source for this information is the AJCC Cancer Staging Manual, 8th edn (2017), which is published by Springer Science + Business Media. When either prostate-specific antigen (PSA) or grade group is not available, grouping should be determined by T category and/or either PSA or grade group as available.

Table 26.5 Risk stratification for localized prostate cancer.

Risk	PSA level (ng/mL)		Gleason score		Clinical stage
Low	≤10	and	≤6	and	T1c or T2a
Intermediate	>10–20	or	7	or	T2b
High	>20	or	8–10	or	T2c

Source: adapted from Thompson *et al.* [50].
PSA, prostate-specific antigen.

events per 1,000 person-years, respectively, $P = 0.48$) [52]. Higher rates of disease progression and metastases were seen in the AS cohort as compared to prostatectomy and radiotherapy cohorts however (22.9 vs 8.9 vs 9.0 events per 1,000 person-years, respectively, $P < 0.001$) [52].

Subgroup analyses from two older studies, the Scandinavian Prostate Cancer Group Study 4 and the Prostate Cancer Interventions versus Observation Trial (PIVOT) suggest a possible benefit for RP over surveillance in younger men (<65 years old) [53] or those with PSA levels >10 [54], although taking into consideration that 20 RPs would need to be performed in order to prevent one death in 10 years, and the risk for RP-associated erectile dysfunction and urinary leakage, AS may still be favored.

Although AS allows men to avoid or defer the potential significant complications associated with the active treatment of prostate cancer, it can cause significant patient anxiety. The psychological toll of having a cancer diagnosis without receiving cancer treatment may – for some patients – outweigh the benefits that AS may bring to a patient's quality of life. Many patients (and their physicians) opt out of an AS program in favor of starting definitive treatment, despite not having any signs of clinical disease progression.

Definitive Treatment in Low- to Intermediate-Risk Localized Disease

Once the decision is made to treat, there are two broad modalities of treatment that are considered definitive treatment for localized prostate cancer: RP or radiation therapy (RT). Surgical treatment with RP can be performed by either an open or robot-assisted laparoscopic approach, whereas radiation therapy can be delivered as EBRT or brachytherapy (radiation seed implants).

No large randomized clinical trials have directly compared RP and RT, but historically, they have yielded similar outcomes in terms of freedom from local or distant recurrence. An observational study attempted to compare the two modalities of treatment; they retrospectively followed men who were diagnosed in the mid-1990s with localized prostate cancer that underwent subsequent treatment with either RP or EBRT over a follow-up period of 15 years. The study suggested a mortality benefit associated with RP as compared to EBRT [55]. However, these results need to be approached carefully as RT has evolved dramatically since the 1990s. Higher prostate radiation dosing, the advent of three-dimensional radiation therapy techniques, and the current practice of adding androgen deprivation therapy (ADT) to EBRT in high-risk localized prostate cancer, need to be taken into consideration. Residual selection bias in the EBRT group is also a potential confounder in this particular study. More likely, large case series suggest that cancer control and survival is comparable in risk-matched localized prostate cancer patients treated with either surgery or radiation.

Treatment selection is often based on age, patient preference, side effect profiles, and impact on quality of life. A multi-institutional, observational study prospectively measured the outcomes reported by 1,201 patients and 625 spouses or partners before and after RP, brachytherapy, or EBRT. Notably, the use of adjuvant hormone therapy with brachytherapy or EBRT was associated with worse outcomes in multiple quality of life metrics [56]. Overall, both surgical and radiation approaches cause sexual dysfunction, but RP is associated with more urinary incontinence, while RT with more urinary and gastrointestinal irritation.

Radiation Therapy in High-risk Localized Disease

The combination of ADT and EBRT has been shown in randomized trials to confer a benefit in localized high-risk disease. ADT in these studies consisted of chemical castration with a GnRH agonist either alone or in combination with an antiandrogen agent. The purpose behind the antiandrogen is to suppress the testosterone flare that is observed with the initiation of a GnRH agonist, although there is limited data documenting the frequency and clinical consequences of a testosterone flare. Whether an antiandrogen needs to be given adjunctively when starting a GnRH agonist in prostate cancer patients has not been properly addressed in prospective randomized trials. A retrospective study compared metastatic prostate cancer patients who received a GnRH agonist alone or with an oral antiandrogen, and found that antiandrogen use was not associated with any significant differences in fractures, spinal cord compression, bladder outlet obstruction, or narcotic prescriptions [57]. As discussed previously, ADT can significantly impact quality of life, potentially causing fatigue, hot flashes, erectile dysfunction, decreased libido, decreased bone density, and increased risk of cardiovascular events. The side effects are largely reversible upon discontinuation, although there is a moderate age and therapy duration-dependent risk of permanent testosterone suppression.

The RTOG 8610 trial randomized 471 men with bulky tumors with or without pelvic lymph node involvement to treatment with goserelin 2 months prior to and 2 months concurrent with EBRT vs EBRT alone. With median follow-up of 12.5 years, it was found that ADT significantly decreased 10-year prostate cancer mortality (23% vs 36%), distant metastases (23% vs 36%), and biochemical failure rates (65% vs 80%). Ten-year overall survival (OS) and median survival times favored the combination therapy, but did not reach statistical significance ($P = 0.12$) [58]. Similarly, the EORTC 22863 trial randomized 415 poor-risk prostate cancer patients to EBRT vs EBRT with 3 years of goserelin, and found that the 10-year disease-free survival was greatly improved with the prolonged combination treatment (47.7% vs 22.7%). The 10-year OS was also significantly better with ADT (58.1% vs 98.8%), with prostate cancer mortality decreased (10.3% vs 30.4%) [59].

Current standard of care for ADT treatment in high-risk patients receiving RT is a prolonged course of 2–3 years, but the optimal duration of androgen suppression is still being challenged. Prior attempts to minimize the duration of ADT have not definitively shown that a shorter course of ADT is as efficacious as the prolonged courses [60,61]. However, recently presented at the American Society of Clinical Oncology Annual Meeting in 2017, the final results of a trial of 630 men with high-risk, node negative prostate cancer randomized to EBRT with either 36 or 18 months of total ADT, showed similar 10-year OS rates between the 36-month and 18-month arms (62.4% vs 62.0%, respectively). QOL analysis showed a significant difference ($P < 0.001$) in 6 scales and 13 items favoring the 18-month duration of ADT [62]. These results may lead to a shortening of the duration of ADT used in the near future for patients with high-risk disease receiving salvage RT.

In most studies, the current standard of care for neoadjuvant ADT is to start 2 months prior to the initiation of EBRT. Although ADT has been shown to augment EBRT, it has not been shown to have a similar effect in the setting of brachytherapy when used alone. Brachytherapy alone is primarily a treatment for low- and intermediate-risk disease, but it is increasingly being used in combination with ADT and EBRT for intermediate- and high-risk prostate cancer as it allows for an escalation of effective radiation dose delivered to the prostate over what EBRT alone is able to provide. In a study cohort of 1342 men with high-risk prostate cancer who underwent brachytherapy, either alone, with supplemental ADT, with EBRT, or both ADT and EBRT, the prostate cancer-specific mortality rate was significantly decreased in the group that received both ADT and EBRT as compared to brachytherapy alone, but not in any other group [63]. Notably, the risk reduction was significant despite there being a higher proportion of higher grade and more clinically advanced cancers in the group that received both supplemental ADT and EBRT.

Radical Prostatectomy in High-risk Localized Disease

The role of radical prostatectomy as monotherapy for high-risk localized disease is limited given the risk of local recurrence and micrometastasis. Evidence of extraprostatic extension, tumor fixation to adjacent structures, or lymph node involvement, suggests that RP will not be curative, and consideration should be given for treatment with ADT and RT. However, some men are only found to have high-risk disease on pathology after surgery has been performed.

While there is no established role for adjuvant ADT or chemotherapy following RP in a patient with high-risk disease, adjuvant RT appears to favorably influence the course of disease. It has been shown in multiple studies to decrease the risk of biochemical relapse and improve local control rates in men that have extraprostatic extension (stage pT3a), seminal vesicle involvement (stage pT3b), or positive margins following RP [64–66]. Of the three large randomized trials of adjuvant RT versus observation, the SWOG 8794 study found improved metastasis-free survival (hazard ratio (HR) 0.71, 95% CI 0.54–0.94, $P = 0.016$) and OS (HR 0.72, 95% CI 0.55–0.96, $P = 0.023$) in their long-term follow-up [67]. Other studies have not confirmed this, but may require longer follow-up to assess these outcomes accurately. Trials are also currently underway to evaluate the benefit of the combination of adjuvant ADT and RT following RP in high-risk patients.

The use of neoadjuvant ADT is known to reduce overall tumor burden and decrease the rate of positive margins following RP in high-risk localized prostate cancer patients. However, a review of seven prospective randomized trials showed that neoadjuvant ADT does not improve rates of seminal vesicle invasion, rates of lymph node metastasis, PSA-free survival, or OS [68]. The review also found no significant differences in operative time, operative blood loss, transfusion requirements, or length of hospital stay. There is currently no data to support the routine use of neoadjuvant hormonal therapy prior to prostatectomy. Neoadjuvant chemohormonal therapy (chemotherapy and ADT) is currently under investigation in a randomized phase III cooperative group trial.

Treatment of Recurrent and Advanced Prostate Cancer

Unfortunately, definitive local therapy does not guarantee cure, and prostate cancer may recur as often as a third of the time. Recurrence can present either biochemically (rising PSA only), locally, or as disseminated metastatic disease. The approach to treatment depends on the site of recurrence.

Biochemical and Local Recurrence

Following definitive local therapy, serum PSA should be regularly monitored since the first sign of recurrent prostate cancer is usually a rising PSA without any other signs or symptoms. Often in biochemical recurrence, even after detailed evaluation and imaging, no evidence of locally recurrent or metastatic disease can be found, although new diagnostic tools are being explored in this space. Recently approved in patients with rising PSA after definitive therapy, is the PET radiotracer ^{18}F-fluciclovine, which was found to outperform ^{11}C-choline in detection rate of lesions, lymph nodes, bone lesions, and local relapse [69].

While PSA is a controversial test for screening and diagnosis of prostate cancer, it is an effective and highly sensitive biomarker that can be followed during and after treatment as it is elevated in 95% of men with advanced prostate cancer. The time to nadir in serum PSA differs depending on the modality of treatment that was undertaken initially. Patients reach nadir quickly following successful RP during which all prostatic tissue is removed, while the decline in PSA following RT is gradual and more variable, at around 12–18 months.

Local recurrences following definitive RT can be confirmed on prostate biopsy. After RP, recurrence rates in the prostate bed are reported to be anywhere from 20 to 40% in the medical literature, and should be considered in patients who had prostatic disease that extended beyond the prostate capsule or other high-risk features.

Treatment options for PSA-only and local recurrence include observation, salvage RT or RP, or systemic therapy with ADT. There are no randomized trials that directly compare the different modalities of salvage treatment to guide selection, although salvage therapy options depend upon what treatment the patient had initially undergone. Importantly, the disease must have a high likelihood of remaining locally confined for local salvage therapy to have a chance at durable long-term disease control. If clinical and pathologic parameters suggest a high risk of disease dissemination, local salvage therapy is unlikely to succeed. A patient's overall performance status, as well as medical comorbidities, also influences whether aggressive local therapy would be a reasonable option.

Salvage Therapy Following Initial Radiation Therapy

Salvage RP can provide durable disease control in a select group of confirmed, localized patients who recur after radiation therapy. A systematic review performed of the available medical literature showed that salvage RP is associated with significant surgical complications and morbidity, but with careful selection of patients and improvements in modern surgical techniques, outcomes with salvage RP have improved compared to the past. Published rates of positive surgical margins and pathologic organ-confined disease in recent studies show improvement [70]. Ten-year cancer-specific survival and OS with salvage RP ranged from 70 to 83% and 54 to 89%, respectively [70], making it a procedure worth considering in some men with an otherwise good life expectancy.

Quality of life continues to be a major factor, however. Rates of postoperative sexual and urinary dysfunction are significant. While rates of most surgical complications in salvage RP following radiation failure have improved as compared to the past, they are still significantly increased when compared to RPs without prior radiotherapy [71]. Occurrences of late urinary incontinence and anastomotic strictures are acceptable, but have not significantly improved despite better patient selection and advances to surgical techniques [72].

Cryoablation and brachytherapy have also been studied as treatments following RT failure. Efficacy of salvage cryoablation is difficult to ascertain, as only retrospective data is available. In a retrospective study of 98 men, it was found that salvage RP significantly outperformed salvage cryoablation in rates of biochemical disease-free survival (66% vs 42%) and OS (95% vs 85%), but not disease-specific survival at 5 years (98% vs 96%) [73]. Salvage cryoablation can be a consideration in older patients with significant comorbidities or in those unwilling to undergo salvage RP. Brachytherapy currently has limited studies to support its use following initial RT failure, and further studies will be needed to better understand its merits.

Salvage Therapy Following Initial Radical Prostatectomy

In patients with recurrence of disease following RP, salvage RT provides the potential for long-term cancer control. While early retrospective studies presented some conflicting findings, overall it was indicative that salvage RT provides long-term survival benefits, but should be initiated soon after biochemical relapse is found [74–76].

Prospective randomized data soon followed that demonstrated the benefit for concurrent ADT use along with salvage RT. In RTOG 9601, a double-blinded, placebo-controlled trial enrolling patients with pT2 or pT3 disease with a rising PSA ranging 0.2–4.0 after prostatectomy, 760 men received salvage RT with either bicalutamide 150 mg daily or a placebo, for a duration of 24 months. With a median follow up of 12.6 years, the study found that the addition of 24 months of bicalutamide to salvage RT resulted in a significantly higher actuarial rate of OS at 12 years (76.3% vs 71.3%, HR 0.77, 95% CI 0.59–0.99, $P = 0.04$), lower incidence of metastatic disease at 12 years (14.5% vs 23.0%, $P = 0.005$), and a lower 12-year incidence of death from prostate cancer (5.8% vs 13.4%, $P < 0.001$). Notably, incidence of gynecomastia was much higher in the bicalutamide group (69.7% vs 10.9%, $P < 0.001$) [77].

Another prospective study, GETUG-AFU 16, enrolled 743 men with pT2–pT4a prostate cancer with a rising PSA of 0.2–2.0 μg/L following radical prostatectomy, and randomized them to receive salvage RT with or without goserelin for 6 months. Patients receiving concurrent goserelin had a significantly higher rate of progression free survival at 5 years (80% vs 62%, HR 0.50, 95% CI 0.38–0.66, *P* <0.0001) [78]. While this study was not able to demonstrate a statistically significant improvement in its secondary endpoint of 5-year OS with the addition of goserelin (96% vs 95%, HR 0.7, 95% CI 0.4–1.2, *P* = 0.18) [78], the hazard ratio is similar to that of RTOG 9601 for its primary 12-year OS endpoint. Longer follow-up may be enlightening.

Androgen Deprivation Therapy for Biochemical or Local Recurrence

Systemic treatment with ADT can be considered in patients with biochemical or local recurrence, especially in those who have unfavorable disease characteristics such as short PSA doubling times or high initial Gleason scores. While ADT is not considered curative, over 90% of patients respond with decreases in PSA levels.

The optimal timing to initiating ADT after confirmation of biochemical recurrence remains controversial, as it is unclear whether early treatment delays progression to metastatic disease or confers a survival advantage. Practices vary widely, with some practitioners starting treatment immediately, while others defer until there are clinical signs or symptoms of metastatic disease to avoid the adverse effects of a treatment not shown to improve OS. A review of randomized trials in patients with prostate cancer finds that there is a decrease in relative risk for prostate cancer specific mortality, but no OS advantage to early initiation of ADT versus deferral until onset of symptoms [79]. There are limited data to suggest that early ADT may delay the onset of metastases in patients with aggressive high-risk disease. In the absence of more definitive data, most favor early intervention with ADT, especially in patients with long life expectancies, high-grade disease, or other high-risk clinicopathologic features to their disease.

ADT causes a host of side effects that can significantly affect quality of life, prompting the study of intermittent ADT as an alternative treatment option. Intermittent ADT can provide respite from short-term reversible side effects, as well as delay potential long-term complications such as osteoporosis and cardiovascular disease. An international, multicenter, controlled, intent-to-treat phase III study randomized 1,386 men with biochemical recurrence of prostate cancer to receive treatment with either intermittent ADT or continuous ADT. Intermittent ADT consisted of 8-month treatment cycles with a luteinizing hormone releasing hormone agonist and an upfront nonsteroidal antiandrogen for at least 4 weeks. A nontreatment interval was allowed after each 8-month cycle if there was no evidence of clinical disease progression and PSA levels were stably suppressed at <4 ng/mL. While off treatment, PSA levels were monitored every 2 months, with ADT restarted if PSA ≥10 ng/mL, or if there was evidence of disease progression. At a median follow-up of 6.9 years, median OS with intermittent ADT met significance for noninferiority when compared with continuous ADT (8.8 vs 9.1 years, *P* = 0.009) [80]. While the intermittent therapy group saw more disease-specific and treatment-related deaths, it had fewer deaths unrelated to prostate cancer as compared to the continuous arm.

The intermittent therapy arm scored better for overall quality of life than the continuous therapy arm, but the differences were not statistically significant. However, there were some individual aspects of quality of life that were observed. For individual symptoms, intermittent therapy scored significantly better for hot flashes, libido, and urinary symptoms, as well as trended towards significance in fatigue [80]. Testosterone and potency recovery were not universal. Only 35% of the intermittent ADT group had testosterone recovery to pretreatment levels within 2 years after the first period of treatment, with patients older than 75 years of age less likely to achieve pretreatment levels. Only 29% of men who were potent at baseline recovered potency [80].

Nonsteroidal antiandrogen monotherapy, such as with flutamide or bicalutamide, has also been studied as a potential treatment option. A meta-analysis of clinical trials comparing it with other androgen ablating treatments, including orchiectomy, diethylstilbestrol, and GnRH agonists, suggested inferiority of antiandrogen monotherapy, associating it with lower survival rates [81]. It may still be a consideration in selected men who have PSA-recurrence of previously low-risk disease, and who prefer to avoid castration.

The combination of an antiandrogen and a 5-alpha reductase inhibitor has some data supporting its use [82–84]. It is an attractive prospect since the combination works more selectively within the prostate, allowing for serum testosterone levels to be maintained, helping some men retain libido, potency, and muscle mass. Toxicity has been described by uncontrolled trials to be mild [85], and it has been shown in a nonrandomized trial of men with biochemical recurrence to perform better than antiandrogen monotherapy at lowering PSA levels and rates of progression [86]. Further studies will be needed to better validate its efficacy, especially as compared to ADT, the current standard of care.

Metastatic Disease

Prostate cancer has a predilection for bone, with a particular affinity for those in the axial skeleton. Over 90% of patients with metastatic prostate cancer will present with bone metastases, which are predominantly osteoblastic lesions. While initially asymptomatic, bone metastases can cause complications of pain, pathologic fractures, spinal cord compression, and calcium metabolism abnormalities over time. Bone scans are sensitive tests for osteoblastic metastases, but not for osteolytic disease. Plain film, computed tomography, and magnetic resonance imaging are useful modalities in the evaluation of other common sites of metastatic disease, which includes the lymph nodes, lung, liver, and adrenal glands.

Newly diagnosed metastatic prostate cancer in the absence of previous hormonal treatment is considered hormone sensitive, and the standard first-line therapy is continuous ADT. In a phase III noninferiority trial, men with newly diagnosed, metastatic, hormone-sensitive prostate cancer were randomized to receive either intermittent ADT or continuous ADT. The hazard ratio for death was 1.10, favoring the continuous ADT arm. However, the study was statistically inconclusive, unable to rule out a significant inferiority of intermittent therapy as compared to continuous ADT, but also unable to rule out a 20% greater risk of death with intermittent therapy [87]. As with PSA-only recurrence, optimal timing to initiation of continuous ADT in hormone-sensitive metastatic disease is unclear. Immediate ADT is associated with a statistically significant decrease in prostate cancer-related deaths, but no OS benefit as compared to delayed ADT [79].

The benefit of chemohormonal therapy in the upfront management of metastatic hormone-sensitive prostate cancer (mHSPC) was demonstrated in two phase III studies, CHAARTED and STAMPEDE. Study designs differed considerably; CHAARTED randomized 790 men with mHSPC to ADT plus docetaxel (75 mg/m^2 every 3 weeks × 6 cycles) or ADT alone, whereas STAMPEDE randomized 2,962 men with metastatic (61%), node-positive (15%), or high-risk localized (24%) hormone-sensitive prostate cancer to four different treatment arms: ADT alone, ADT plus zoledronic acid, ADT plus docetaxel, or ADT plus zoledronic acid and docetaxel. A consistent OS benefit was seen in both studies with the addition of docetaxel to ADT (CHAARTED: 57.6 vs 44.0 months; HR 0.61; 95% CI 0.47–0.80; $P = 0.001$, STAMPEDE: 77 vs 67 months; HR 0.76; 95% CI 0.63–0.91; $P = 0.003$) [88,89]. Secondary endpoints of time to castration resistance, time to clinical progression, and achieving PSA levels <0.2 ng/mL at 6 and 12 months, all uniformly favored docetaxel in CHAARTED [88], and failure-free survival benefit was demonstrated by STAMPEDE in its overall study population [89].

Planned subgroup analyses of the CHAARTED data at initial interim analysis showed an unprecedented 17-month OS improvement with the addition of docetaxel in patients with high-volume disease (49.2 months vs 32.2 months; HR 0.60; 95% CI 0.45–0.81; $P < 0.001$), but not in low-volume disease [88]. Updated survival data presented at ESMO 2016, suggests that early chemohormonal benefit is limited to high-burden disease (51.2 months vs 34.4 months; HR 0.63; 95% CI 0.50–0.79, $P < 0.0001$), as low-volume patients were still without OS improvement (63.5 vs NR; HR 1.04; 95% CI 0.70–1.55, $P = 0.86$) [90]. There remains controversy whether low-volume patients should be offered early chemohormonal therapy despite the negative subgroup analysis because of the significantly positive overall study. For high-volume patients, early chemohormonal therapy has already been adopted by treatment guidelines, although selection of suitable candidates requires consideration of the inherent toxicities associated with docetaxel therapy.

Recently, two large randomized phase III studies also demonstrated a significant benefit for abiraterone in the management of mHSPC. LATITUDE randomly assigned 1199 men with high-risk mHSPC to receive either abiraterone 1000 mg and prednisone 5 mg daily or dual placebos. Patients were eligible for the study if their disease met at least two of three high-risk features: Gleason score of 8 or more, at least three bone lesions, and the presence of measurable visceral metastasis. At planned interim analysis with a median follow-up of 30.4 months, the addition of abiraterone was associated with significant improvements in the two primary efficacy endpoints of OS (NR vs 34.7 months, HR 0.62, 95% CI 0.51–0.76, $P < 0.001$) and rPFS (33.0 months vs 14.8 months, HR 0.47, 95% CI 95% 0.39–0.55, $P < 0.001$) [91].

Similarly, STAMPEDE randomized 1917 men with metastatic (52%), node-positive (20%), and nonmetastatic disease (28%) hormone sensitive prostate cancer to receive ADT alone or ADT plus abiraterone 1000 mg daily and prednisolone 5 mg daily. With median follow-up of 40 months, a significant advantage was seen in 3-year OS in the abiraterone arm for the overall study population (83% vs 76%, HR 0.63; 95% CI 0.52–0.76; $P < 0.001$). Failure-free survival at 3 years also favored the combination group (75% vs 45%; HR 0.29; 95% CI 0.25–0.34; $P < 0.001$) [92]. In analysis of the metastatic subgroup, OS and FFS benefits were statistically significant (HR 0.61 and 0.31, respectively) [92], consistent with the findings reported in LATITUDE.

Despite the initial effectiveness of ADT, regardless of the addition of docetaxel or abiraterone, the disease eventually progresses, becoming castration-resistant prostate cancer (CRPC). Time to the development of ADT resistance is variable, but the median duration is around 18–24 months in men with metastatic disease. There is a growing arsenal of effective treatments for CRPC, each with distinct mechanisms of actions, but the optimal selection, sequence, and timing are still unknown. In selection of treatment, consideration must be given regarding patient comorbidities, functional status, disease burden, rate of progression, organ functions, and potential adverse effects (Table 26.6).

Cytotoxic Chemotherapy

The early trials of traditional chemotherapeutic agents found poor responses in the treatment of prostate cancer leading to the initial belief that the disease was chemotherapy-resistant.

In the mid-1990s, mitoxantrone demonstrated a palliative benefit in both quality and duration of pain control when used in combination with prednisone compared to prednisone alone. No OS benefit was observed [93]. A second phase III trial randomized both symptomatic and asymptomatic men to mitoxantrone plus hydrocortisone versus hydrocortisone alone. While the addition of mitoxantrone appeared to delay time to treatment failure and disease progression, there was again no difference in OS. However, quality of life and pain control was again improved [94]. Mitoxantrone was thus approved for palliative treatment of CRPC based on the findings of these two randomized trials.

Taxanes, a class of microtubule inhibitors, are the only cytotoxic agents that have been demonstrated in clinical trials to prolong OS in men with CRPC. Multiple phase II trials suggested docetaxel as an active agent in metastatic CRPC [95–97], which led to the design of the pivotal phase III randomized TAX 327 trial comparing docetaxel plus prednisone

Table 26.6 Systemic prostate cancer treatments.

LHRH agonist/antagonist	Leuprolide, goserelin, degarelix
Androgen receptor antagonist	Flutamide, bicalutamide, enzalutamide
Androgen synthesis inhibitors	Ketoconazole, abiraterone
Cytotoxic chemotherapy	Mitoxantrone, estramustine, docetaxel, cabazitaxel
Immunotherapy	Sipuleucel-T
Radionuclide therapy	Samarium-153, strontium-89, radium-223

LHRH, luteinizing hormone releasing hormone.

versus mitoxantrone plus prednisone in the treatment of metastatic CRPC (mCRPC). Docetaxel plus prednisone demonstrated a superior survival compared with prednisone alone; in addition there were improved rates of pain response, serum PSA levels, and quality of life [98]. Final analysis of the TAX 327 study confirmed a significant survival advantage, with a difference in median survival time of 2.9 months ($P=0.004$, HR 0.79), after treatment with docetaxel every 3 weeks as compared with mitoxantrone, across all subgroups of patients studied [99]. On the merits of this study, docetaxel every 3 weeks with prednisone was approved by the Food and Drug Administration (FDA) in 2004 for treatment of mCRPC and remains a standard first-line regimen.

Cabazitaxel is a semisynthetic taxane developed for treatment of patients with docetaxel-refractory disease. It was selected for clinical testing because of its poor affinity for ATP-dependent drug efflux pump P-glycoprotein 1, a known mechanism of taxane resistance, as well as its ability to penetrate the blood–brain barrier. Preclinical and phase I studies demonstrated antitumor activity in various solid tumor types, with promising results in a small cohort of mCRPC patients. The randomized, multinational, open-label, phase III TROPIC trial was launched comparing cabazitaxel with mitoxantrone in men previously treated and progressed on docetaxel. A total of 755 men were randomized 1:1 to each arm and included in the intention-to-treat analysis, the primary outcome of the study being OS. All patients were concurrently treated with prednisone 10 mg daily. After a median follow-up of 12.8 months, cabazitaxel demonstrated superior OS compared with mitoxantrone (15.1 months vs 12.7 months, HR 0.70, $P=0.0001$), as well as superiority in the secondary end points of progression-free survival, PSA response, time to tumor progression, radiographic tumor response, and time to PSA progression [100]. However, cabazitaxel is associated with significant toxicities, most notably hematologic toxicity (80%), febrile neutropenia (7.5%), and treatment-related death (5%). Because of the high incidence of neutropenia, many practitioners commonly use G-CSF support. This study led to the FDA approval of cabazitaxel 25 mg/m^2 every 21 days as a second-line chemotherapeutic agent for treatment of mCRPC after docetaxel. Lower treatment doses and use in combination with other therapies are currently being investigated.

Estramustine phosphate consists of estradiol, an estrogen derivative, and a nitrogen mustard moiety. As a single agent, estramustine demonstrates modest levels of activity in CRPC, but a meta-analysis showed that in combination with other chemotherapies, it significantly improves PSA progression-free survival (HR 0.74, $P=0.01$) and OS (HR 0.77, $P=0.008$) [101]. The combination of docetaxel and estramustine was studied in phase I and II trials in treatment of men with CRPC, and demonstrated significant declines in PSA levels and disease response [102,103]. A phase III trial randomized 674 patients with CRPC to receive docetaxel and estramustine or mitoxantrone and prednisone in an intention-to-treat analysis. Overall survival was significantly longer in the docetaxel/estramustine arm (17.5 months vs 15.6 months, HR 0.80, $P=0.02$). The docetaxel/estramustine combination was also associated with significantly improved time to progression, PSA declines, and objective tumor responses [104]. Although estramustine is FDA approved for use in combination with docetaxel for treatment of CRPC, it is associated with significant toxicity, most notably thromboembolic events. Prophylactic anticoagulation has not proven to be effective, leading to this agent being largely abandoned.

Other classes of cytotoxic chemotherapeutic agents that have been studied in CRPC include epothilones and platinums. Epothilones are a class of microtubule stabilizing drugs that are less susceptible to mechanisms that confer taxane resistance, such as microtubulin mutations and overexpression of P-glycoprotein efflux pumps [105–107]. Data suggests that taxanes and epothilones are not crossresistant, with epothilones still demonstrating efficacy in taxane-refractory prostate, breast, ovarian, and lung cancer [108–110]. Of the epothilones, ixabepilone is arguably the best studied, as it is already FDA approved for treatment of taxane and anthracycline refractory metastatic breast cancer. In phase II studies, ixabepilone has demonstrated modest activity in CRPC in both the chemotherapy naïve and taxane-refractory settings [111,112].

Platinum salts have long been studied in prostate cancer and may have a potential role in treatment of prostate cancer with neuroendocrine features. Hormonally independent neuroendocrine cells, which are classically platinum sensitive, are thought to be selected for by prolonged courses of androgen deprivation [113]. Recent studies show the combination of carboplatin and docetaxel to have significant activity in the first-line setting, and to have additional activity in docetaxel-refractory disease [114–116]. Satraplatin, a fourth generation platinum analogue, has demonstrated activity in cisplatin-resistant prostate cancer. SPARC was a multinational, double-blinded, placebo-controlled, phase III trial comparing satraplatin plus prednisone to prednisone alone. While satraplatin was associated with a 33% reduction in the risk of progression, and higher PSA response rates, there was no difference seen in OS between the two groups [117] and satraplatin is no longer under clinical development.

Phase III trials of cytotoxic chemotherapeutic agents in mCRPC are shown in Table 26.7.

Secondary Hormonal Therapy

Prostate cancers that develop resistance to ADT were historically thought to have become totally independent of the androgen-signaling axis, but a better understanding of the androgen-signaling pathway suggests that the androgen pathway remains an important therapeutic target in CRPC. Targeting mechanisms of castration resistance such as nontesticular androgen production, androgen receptor (AR) binding, AR nuclear translocation, and AR gene amplification, has led to the development of novel therapies in CRPC. Two important new agents, abiraterone acetate and enzalutamide, have been recently approved for use in mCRPC (Table 26.8).

Abiraterone is an orally administered, selective, irreversible inhibitor of CYP17 that catalyzes two essential steps required for androgen biosynthesis in the testes, adrenals, and tumor. It was developed by rational design based on long time understanding that ketoconazole exhibits antitumor activity by inhibiting multiple CYP enzymes required for steroid and testosterone synthesis.

Phase I studies showed that abiraterone is effective at reducing serum testosterone and results in regression of disease,

Table 26.7 Phase III trials of cytotoxic chemotherapeutic agents in metastatic castration resistant prostate cancer (mCRPC).

Treatment	Study arms	Primary outcome	Secondary outcomes	Approval
Mitoxantrone	Mitoxantrone and prednisone vs prednisone alone [93]	Pain palliation: 29% vs 12% ($P = 0.01$) Duration of pain response: 43 weeks vs 18 weeks ($P < 0.0001$)	Improvements in several dimensions of quality of life	Palliative treatment of mCRPC
	Mitoxantrone and hydrocortisone vs hydrocortisone alone [94]	OS: 12.6 months vs 12.3 months ($P = 0.77$)	Time to disease progression and treatment failure: 3.7 months vs 2.3 months ($P = 0.0254$, $P = 0.0218$)	
Docetaxel	Docetaxel q3wk vs docetaxel q1wk vs mitoxantrone (each with prednisone) [99]	OS: 19.2 months vs 17.8 months vs 16.3 months ($P = 0.004$ for D3P vs MP)	–	Treatment of mCRPC
Cabazitaxel	Cabazitaxel and prednisone vs mitoxantrone vs prednisone [100]	OS: 15.1 months vs 12.7 months (HR 0.70, $P < 0.0001$)	PFS: 2.8 months vs 1.4 months (HR 0.74, $P < 0.0001$) Higher rates of tumor and PSA response Improvements in time to tumor and PSA progression	Treatment of mCRPC previously treated with docetaxel
Docetaxel/ estramustine	Docetaxel and estramustine vs mitoxantrone and prednisone [104]	OS: 17.5 months vs 15.6 months ($P = 0.02$)	TTP: 6.3 vs 3.2 ($P < 0.001$) PSA decline: 50% vs 27% ($P < 0.001$) Objective tumor response: 17% vs 11% ($P = 0.30$)	Treatment of mCRPC
Satraplatin	Satraplatin and prednisone vs prednisone alone [117]	OS: 61.3 weeks vs 61.4 weeks (HR 0.98, $P = 0.80$) PFS: 11.1 weeks vs 9.7 weeks ($P < 0.001$)	Tumor response: 8% vs 0.7% ($P = 0.002$) Pain response: 24.2% vs 13.8% ($P = 0.005$) PSA response: 25.4% vs 12.4% ($P < 0.001$)	Not FDA approved

FDA, Food and Drug Administration; HR, hazard ratio; OS, overall survival; PFS, progression-free survival; PSA, prostate-specific antigen; q3wk, every 3 weeks; q1wk, once a week; TTP, time to progression.

Table 26.8 Phase III trials of hormonal therapies in metastatic castration resistant prostate cancer (mCRPC).

Treatment	Study arms	Primary outcome	Secondary outcomes	Approval
Abiraterone	Abiraterone and prednisone vs prednisone alone [121]	OS: 14.8 months vs 10.9 months (HR 0.66, $P < 0.001$)	Time to PSA progression: 10.2 months vs 6.6 months (HR 0.58, $P < 0.001$) Radiographic PFS: 5.6 months vs 3.6 months (HR 0.67, $P < 0.001$) PSA response rate: 29% vs 6% ($P < 0.001$)	Treatment of mCRPC in both pre- and postchemotherapy settings
	Abiraterone and prednisone vs prednisone alone [124]	OS: median not reached vs 8.3 months (HR 0.43, $P < 0.001$) Radiographic PFS: 16.5 months vs 8.3 months (HR 0.53, $P < 0.001$)	Time to PSA progression: 11.1 months vs 5.6 months (HR 0.49, $P < 0.001$) Time to initiation of cytotoxic chemotherapy: 25.2 months vs 16.8 months (HR 0.58, $P < 0.001$) Time to ECOG score decline: 12.3 vs 10.9 (HR 0.82, $P = 0.005$) Time to opiate use: median not reached vs 23.7 months (HR 0.69, $P < 0.001$)	
Enzalutamide	Enzalutamide vs placebo [130]	OS: 18.4 months vs 13.6 months (HR 0.63, $P < 0.001$)	Time to PSA progression: 8.3 months vs 3.0 months (HR 0.25, $P < 0.001$) Radiographic PFS: 8.3 months vs 2.9 months (HR 0.40, $P < 0.001$) Time to first skeletal-related event: 16.7 months vs 13.3 months (HR 0.69, $P < 0.001$) PSA response rate: 54% vs 2% ($P < 0.001$) Soft tissue response rate: 29% vs 4% ($P < 0.001$) FACT-P QOL response: 43% vs 18% ($P < 0.001$)	Treatment of mCRPC previously treated with docetaxel

ECOG, Eastern Cooperative Oncology Group; HR, hazard ratio; OS, overall survival; PFS, progression free survival; PSA, prostate-specific antigen.

even in patients who had previously received ketoconazole [118]. Two phase II studies conducted in chemotherapy-naïve patients again showed significant antitumor activity by virtue of marked PSA declines, observed radiographic response, and delayed time to progression [119,120]. Two phase III randomized trials were subsequently designed to evaluate abiraterone in two different settings: docetaxel-treated mCRPC and chemotherapy-naïve mCRPC.

The COU-AA-301 trial randomized 1,195 patients in a 2:1 ratio to treatment with abiraterone and prednisone versus placebo and prednisone in CRPC patients previously treated with docetaxel. The abiraterone arm showed a statistically significant OS benefit (14.8 months vs 10.9 months, HR 0.65, P <0.0001), as well as significantly improved time to PSA progression, radiographic progression-free survival, and PSA response [121]. Additional analysis of this trial also found that the combination of abiraterone and prednisone resulted in significant improvements in fatigue and pain palliation over prednisone alone [122,123]. The second phase III trial, COU-AA-302, randomized patients with chemotherapy-naïve mCRPC to receive either abiraterone and prednisone or placebo and prednisone. The abiraterone arm showed superiority in terms of radiographic progression-free survival, one of two coprimary endpoints. There was an improvement in OS, although it did not reach the prespecified cut-off for significance, as well as time to initiation of cytotoxic chemotherapy, opiate use for cancer-related pain, PSA progression, and decline in performance status [124]. Based on data from these two large randomized trials, the FDA has approved abiraterone for treatment of mCRPC in both the pre- and postchemotherapy setting, making it another first-line treatment option.

As mentioned previously, optimal sequencing of CRPC therapies remain the subject of further study. Some recent data raises the concern that the activity of docetaxel may be decreased following prior treatment with abiraterone, suggesting some degree of cross resistance [125].

While generally well tolerated, abiraterone can result in mineralocorticoid excess due to its inhibitory effect on steroid metabolism, leading to fluid retention and hypertension. The addition of low dose prednisone in phase II and III studies did not fully eliminate this effect, but the toxicities were mostly low grade and tolerable.

Enzalutamide is an orally administered androgen receptor signaling inhibitor that potently and competitively binds AR, leading to a two- to threefold reduction of binding affinity from the natural ligand dihydrotestosterone. In addition, it also prevents AR nuclear translocations, DNA binding, and coactivator recruitment by the ligand-receptor complex [126]. By inhibiting ligand-bound complex translocation, enzalutamide markedly reduces aberrant recruitment of coactivators to enhancer regions leading to target gene activation.

Its selection for clinical development was based on preclinical demonstration of activity even in the presence of AR amplification, a known mechanism of resistance to antiandrogens in CRPC [127]. It also differs from prior generation AR antagonists, such as bicalutamide, in that it does not confer any degree of agonist activity. Even when complexed with mutant AR protein W741C, which unmasks agonist qualities of bicalutamide [128], enzalutamide remains antagonistic [126].

In early clinical phase I/II trials in men with CRPC, enzalutamide exhibited significant antitumor activity in patients previously treated with docetaxel, ketoconazole, or both [129]. A PSA decline of 50% or more was observed in 56% of men, with radiographic responses in 22%. It also showed a favorable toxicity profile, although associated with small but increased risk for seizures. These results led to two randomized, placebo-controlled, phase III trials studying enzalutamide in the docetaxel-refractory mCRPC (AFFIRM) and chemotherapy-naïve mCRPC (PREVAIL) setting.

In the AFFIRM trial, 1199 men were randomized 2:1 to receive either enzalutamide 160 mg daily or placebo. At a planned interim analysis with median follow-up of 14.4 months, enzalutamide demonstrated superior OS as compared to placebo (18.4 months vs 13.6 months, HR 0.63, P <0.001). Enzalutamide was also associated with higher rates of PSA decline (54% vs 2%, P <0.001), soft-tissue response rate (29% vs 4%, P <0.001), quality-of-life response (43% vs 18%, P <0.001), time to PSA progression (8.3 months vs 3.0 months, HR 0.25, P <0.001), radiographic progression-free survival (8.3 months vs 2.9 months, HR 0.40, P <0.001), and time to first skeletal-related event (16.7 months vs 13.3 months, HR 0.69, P <0.001) [130]. Additionally, subsequent multivariate analysis showed a survival benefit in all studied subgroups of patients.

Similarly, PREVAIL randomized 1717 men with mCRPC to either enzalutamide 160 mg daily or placebo, in the prechemotherapy setting. There was significant improvement in both coprimary endpoints of radiographic PFS at 12 months follow-up (65% vs 14%, HR 0.19, 95% CI 0.15–0.23, P <0.001) and OS (HR 0.71, 95% CI 0.60–0.84, P <0.001) with the use of enzalutamide over placebo [131]. Multiple secondary endpoints of median time until initiation of cytotoxic therapy, time until PSA progression, time until first skeletal related event, and time until decline of quality of life, all favored enzalutamide as well [131]. Based on the merits of AFFIRM and PREVAIL, enzalutamide received FDA indication in both the pre- and post-chemotherapy setting for mCRPC.

Unlike abiraterone and other therapeutic options for CRPC, enzalutamide does not require the concurrent use of corticosteroids. This is an important factor to consider as corticosteroids may be relatively contraindicated in some men owing to its effects on muscle strength, skin integrity, bone density, glycemic control, and weight control. Optimal sequence and combination of the novel secondary hormone therapy agents are not yet defined.

Immunotherapy

Another treatment approach for mCRPC utilizes immunotherapeutic strategies. Sipuleucel-T is an autologous dendritic cell vaccine produced by coculturing antigen-presenting cells, collected by leukapheresis, with a recombinant fusion protein consisting of prostatic acid phosphatase (PAP) and granulocyte macrophage colony-stimulating factor. The end product consists of activated dendritic cells specifically sensitized to the PAP antigen, which is specific to prostate cancer cells. The cells are infused back into the patient where they induce an augmented host antigen-specific cytotoxic T lymphocyte response against prostate cancer cells.

Three randomized phase III trials compared sipuleucel-T against placebo in men with asymptomatic or minimally symptomatic mCRPC. An integrated analysis of two of these trials (D9901 and D9902A) showed that the primary endpoint of improvement in time to disease progression was not met. However, the patients randomized to receive sipuleucel-T demonstrated a survival benefit, with a 33% reduction in the risk of death (HR 1.5, 95% CI 1.10–2.05, $P=0.011$) [132]. The IMPACT study randomized 512 patients in a 2:1 ratio to either three infusions of sipuleucel-T administered every 2 weeks or reinfusion of peripheral blood mononuclear cells alone on the same schedule. With median follow-up of 34.1 months, the sipuleucel-T arm had a relative reduction of 22% in the risk of death (HR 0.78, $P=0.03$), which represented a 4.1 month improvement in median survival (25.8 months vs 21.7 months) [133]. Again, time to objective disease progression did not differ significantly between the two groups. Based on the results of these trials, sipuleucel-T was approved by the FDA for the treatment of asymptomatic or minimally symptomatic mCRPC.

There are no data on the efficacy of sipuleucel-T in men whose only evidence of disease is an elevated PSA or in those with symptomatic metastatic disease. Currently, usage is not indicated in patients on steroids or opioids for cancer-related pain. Additionally, since treatment with sipuleucel-T does not usually affect serum PSA levels, it should not be used in patients with rapidly progressive disease where a brisk response to treatment is needed.

Other novel immunotherapies are being developed and entering advanced stages of clinical testing. Anti-CTLA-4 and anti-PD1/PDL1 antibodies are the subjects of ongoing investigation in CRPC. New viral vector-based vaccines are also under clinical investigation.

Radionuclide Therapy

Prostate cancer is a disease that metastasizes preferentially to bone. Over 90% of patients with mCRPC have radiographic evidence of bony involvement that can often lead to pathologic fractures, functional impairment, pain, decreased quality of life, and bone marrow suppression. Two beta-particle emitting radiopharmaceuticals, strontium-89 chloride (^{89}Sr) and samarium-153 lexidronam (^{153}Sm), were previously approved by the FDA for only palliative management of pain secondary to bony metastases.

There is renewed interest in bone-targeting radionuclides with the introduction of radium-223 dichloride (^{223}Ra). Radium-223 is a next generation, targeted alpha-emitter that selectively binds to areas of increased bone turnover, such as in the environment of bone metastases. It emits high-energy alpha particles that produce high, linear energy transfer with a range of less than 100 μm. Its short half-life (11.4 days) and superficial tissue penetration translates into less toxic effects on adjacent healthy tissue.

Phase I and II trials demonstrated that radium-223 was well tolerated and had a favorable toxicity profile, most notably associated with minimal myelotoxicity [134,135]. Other phase II trials also showed that radium-223 significantly improved pain and decreased disease-related biomarkers, such as bone alkaline phosphatase [136,137].

Data from an initial phase II study suggested a survival advantage with radium-223 [135], which led to the design of the phase III, randomized, double-blinded, multinational ALSYMPCA study. Radium-223 dosed at 50 kBq/kg every 4 weeks for six doses was compared with placebo in 921 men with CPRC with symptomatic bone metastases randomized in a 2:1 ratio. Radium-223 was found to improve OS significantly, with a 30% reduction in the risk of death, as compared to placebo (14.0 months vs 11.2 months, HR 0.70, 95% CI 0.55–0.88, $P=0.002$) [138]. Radium-223 also significantly prolonged the time to the first symptomatic skeletal event, as well as time to alkaline phosphatase and PSA level increase. Based on this study, the FDA approved radium-223 for treatment of mCRPC with symptomatic bone metastases without other visceral metastases.

Table 26.9 summarizes phase III trials of immunotherapy and radionuclide therapy for mCRPC.

Bone-Directed Therapy

Other bone-targeting therapies can palliate pain and delay skeletal-related events (SRE), but do not confer an OS benefit.

For palliation of bone pain that is limited to one or a few discrete metastatic sites, EBRT is a good option. Large randomized trials have found that a single fraction of 8 Gy is as effective at providing pain relief as compared with higher radiation doses divided over multiple fractions [139–141]. Patients treated with a single fraction are more likely to require retreatment than those who were initially treated with a fractionated regimen (20% vs 8%) [142], but the majority can be successfully retreated with a single fraction.

Bisphosphonates, as a class of medications, have demonstrated efficacy in preventing osteoporosis from prolonged

Table 26.9 Phase III trials of immunotherapy and radionuclide therapy for metastatic castration resistant prostate cancer (mCRPC).

Treatment	Study arms	Primary outcome	Secondary outcomes	Approval
Sipuleucel-T	Sipuleucel-T vs placebo [133]	OS: 25.8 months vs 21.7 months (HR 0.78, $P=0.03$)	Time to objective disease progression: 14.6 months vs 14.4 months (HR 0.95, $P=0.63$)	Treatment of asymptomatic or minimally symptomatic mCRPC
Radium-223 dichloride	Radium-223 vs placebo [138]	OS: 14.0 months vs 11.2 months (HR 0.70, $P=0.002$)	Time to first symptomatic skeletal event: 15.6 vs 9.8 months (HR 0.66, $P<0.001$) Time to alkaline phosphatase level increase: 7.4 months vs 3.8 months (HR 0.17, $P<0.001$) Time to PSA level increase: 3.6 months vs 3.4 months (HR 0.64, $P<0.001$)	Treatment of mCRPC with symptomatic bone metastases and no known visceral metastatic disease

HR, hazard ratio; OS, overall survival; PSA, prostate-specific antigen.

ADT use, but are not all equally effective in the management of prostate cancer bone metastases. Zoledronic acid has been well studied in mCRPC, demonstrating the ability to reduce frequency of SRE and improve median time to development of SRE [143], and is also associated with meaningful reductions in pain scores [144]. It is currently the only bisphosphonate approved for use in castrate-resistant disease with bone metastases.

Denosumab, a monoclonal antibody that binds RANK ligand, is also effective at preventing ADT-associated osteoporosis [145,146]. When compared to placebo in a randomized phase III trial of nonmetastatic CRPC patients, denosumab significantly increased bone metastasis-free survival time (29.5 months vs 25.2 months, HR 0.85, 95% CI 0.73–0.98) and time to first bone metastasis (33.2 months vs 29.5 months, HR 0.84, 95% CI 0.71–0.98) [147]. Furthermore, when compared to zoledronic acid in a randomized phase III trial of mCRPC patients, denosumab significantly delayed time to first SRE (20.7 months vs 17.1 months, HR 0.82, 95% CI 0.71–0.95) [148]. No improvements to OS were observed in either trial. While generally well tolerated, hypocalcemia and osteonecrosis of the jaw occur more frequently with denosumab use than with zoledronic acid.

Conclusion

An improved understanding of prostate cancer has paved the way for multiple novel therapies to be developed. However, there is still much that is still not fully understood about the biology of prostate cancer and its management. As drug development continues to accelerate and we acquire a wider breadth of therapy options, clinical trials will be needed to answer questions regarding how best to implement these new treatments in clinical practice. Optimal timing, sequencing, and combination of different treatment modalities need not only to be studied in the advanced metastatic disease setting, but also in the early disease stages where a cure may still be imminently attainable. Further research will also be needed to help clinicians better guide their patients along the fine line between improved survival and quality of life.

References

1 Siegel R, Miller KD, Jemal A. Cancer statistics, 2017. *CA Cancer J Clin* 2017;67(1):7–30.
2 Hoffman RM, *et al.* Racial and ethnic differences in advanced-stage prostate cancer: the Prostate Cancer Outcomes Study. *J Natl Cancer Inst* 2001;93(5):388–95.
3 Zeegers MP, Jellema A, Ostrer H. Empiric risk of prostate carcinoma for relatives of patients with prostate carcinoma: a meta-analysis. *Cancer* 2003;97(8):1894–903.
4 Hemminki K, Czene K. Age specific and attributable risks of familial prostate carcinoma from the family-cancer database. *Cancer* 2002;95(6):1346–53.
5 Valeri A, *et al.* Targeted screening for prostate cancer in high risk families: early onset is a significant risk factor for disease in first degree relatives. *J Urol* 2002;168(2):483–7.
6 Lichtenstein P, *et al.* Environmental and heritable factors in the causation of cancer–-analyses of cohorts of twins from Sweden, Denmark, and Finland. *N Engl J Med* 2000;343(2):78–85.
7 Tryggvadottir L, *et al.* Prostate cancer progression and survival in BRCA2 mutation carriers. *J Natl Cancer Inst* 2007;99(12):929–35.
8 Narod SA, *et al.* Rapid progression of prostate cancer in men with a BRCA2 mutation. *Br J Cancer* 2008;99(2):371–4.
9 Edwards SM, *et al.* Prostate cancer in BRCA2 germline mutation carriers is associated with poorer prognosis. *Br J Cancer* 2010;103(6):918–24.
10 Mitra A, *et al.* Prostate cancer in male BRCA1 and BRCA2 mutation carriers has a more aggressive phenotype. *Br J Cancer* 2008;98(2):502–7.
11 Agalliu I, *et al.* Associations of high-grade prostate cancer with BRCA1 and BRCA2 founder mutations. *Clin Cancer Res* 2009;15(3):1112–20.
12 Amundadottir LT, *et al.* A common variant associated with prostate cancer in European and African populations. *Nat Genet* 2006;38(6):652–8.
13 Eeles RA, *et al.* Multiple newly identified loci associated with prostate cancer susceptibility. *Nat Genet* 2008;40(3):316–21.
14 Freedman ML, *et al.* Admixture mapping identifies 8q24 as a prostate cancer risk locus in African-American men. *Proc Natl Acad Sci USA* 2006;103(38):14068–73.
15 Gudmundsson J, *et al.* Genome-wide association study identifies a second prostate cancer susceptibility variant at 8q24. *Nat Genet* 2007;39(5):631–7.
16 Gudmundsson J, *et al.* Two variants on chromosome 17 confer prostate cancer risk, and the one in TCF2 protects against type 2 diabetes. *Nat Genet* 2007;39(8):977–83.
17 Haiman CA, *et al.* Multiple regions within 8q24 independently affect risk for prostate cancer. *Nat Genet* 2007;39(5):638–44.
18 Thomas G, *et al.* Multiple loci identified in a genome-wide association study of prostate cancer. *Nat Genet* 2008;40(3):310–5.
19 Yeager M, *et al.* Genome-wide association study of prostate cancer identifies a second risk locus at 8q24. *Nat Genet* 2007;39(5):645–9.
20 Zheng SL, *et al.* Association between two unlinked loci at 8q24 and prostate cancer risk among European Americans. *J Natl Cancer Inst* 2007;99(20):1525–33.
21 Zheng SL, *et al.* Cumulative association of five genetic variants with prostate cancer. *N Engl J Med* 2008;358(9):910–9.
22 Kirsh VA, *et al.* Prospective study of fruit and vegetable intake and risk of prostate cancer. *J Natl Cancer Inst* 2007;99(15): 1200–9.
23 Hwang YW, *et al.* Soy food consumption and risk of prostate cancer: a meta-analysis of observational studies. *Nutr Cancer* 2009;61(5):598–606.
24 Kushi LH, *et al.* American Cancer Society Guidelines on nutrition and physical activity for cancer prevention: reducing the risk of cancer with healthy food choices and physical activity. *CA Cancer J Clin* 2012;62(1):30–67.

25 Sinha R, *et al.* Meat and meat-related compounds and risk of prostate cancer in a large prospective cohort study in the United States. *Am J Epidemiol* 2009;170(9):1165–77.

26 Gann PH, *et al.* Prospective study of plasma fatty acids and risk of prostate cancer. *J Natl Cancer Inst* 1994;86(4):281–6.

27 Ahn J, *et al.* Dairy products, calcium intake, and risk of prostate cancer in the prostate, lung, colorectal, and ovarian cancer screening trial. *Cancer Epidemiol Biomarkers Prev* 2007;16(12):2623–30.

28 Klein EA, *et al.* Vitamin E and the risk of prostate cancer: the Selenium and Vitamin E Cancer Prevention Trial (SELECT). *JAMA* 2011;306(14):1549–56.

29 Roddam AW, *et al.* Endogenous sex hormones and prostate cancer: a collaborative analysis of 18 prospective studies. *J Natl Cancer Inst* 2008;100(3):170–83.

30 Wright ME, *et al.* Prospective study of adiposity and weight change in relation to prostate cancer incidence and mortality. *Cancer* 2007;109(4):675–84.

31 Freedland SJ, *et al.* Impact of obesity on biochemical control after radical prostatectomy for clinically localized prostate cancer: a report by the Shared Equal Access Regional Cancer Hospital database study group. *J Clin Oncol* 2004;22(3):446–53.

32 Cao Y, Ma J. Body mass index, prostate cancer-specific mortality, and biochemical recurrence: a systematic review and meta-analysis. *Cancer Prev Res (Phila)* 2011;4(4):486–501.

33 Roddam AW, *et al.* Insulin-like growth factors, their binding proteins, and prostate cancer risk: analysis of individual patient data from 12 prospective studies. *Ann Intern Med* 2008;149(7):461–71, W83–8.

34 Liu Y, *et al.* Does physical activity reduce the risk of prostate cancer? A systematic review and meta-analysis. *Eur Urol* 2011;60(5):1029–44.

35 Vickers AJ, *et al.* Systematic review of pretreatment prostate-specific antigen velocity and doubling time as predictors for prostate cancer. *J Clin Oncol* 2009;27(3):398–403.

36 Pinsky PF, *et al.* Prostate-specific antigen velocity and prostate cancer gleason grade and stage. *Cancer* 2007;109(8):1689–95.

37 Catalona WJ, *et al.* Comparison of prostate specific antigen concentration versus prostate specific antigen density in the early detection of prostate cancer: receiver operating characteristic curves. *J Urol* 1994;152(6):2031–6.

38 Lee R, *et al.* A meta-analysis of the performance characteristics of the free prostate-specific antigen test. *Urology* 2006;67(4):762–8.

39 Catalona WJ, *et al.* Comparison of digital rectal examination and serum prostate specific antigen in the early detection of prostate cancer: results of a multicenter clinical trial of 6,630 men. *J Urol* 1994;151(5):1283–90.

40 Schroder FH, *et al.* Screening and prostate-cancer mortality in a randomized European study. *N Engl J Med* 2009;360(13):1320–8.

41 Andriole GL, *et al.* Mortality results from a randomized prostate-cancer screening trial. *N Engl J Med* 2009;360(13):1310–9.

42 Wolf AM, *et al.* American Cancer Society guideline for the early detection of prostate cancer: update 2010. *CA Cancer J Clin* 2010;60(2):70–98.

43 Qaseem A, *et al.* Screening for prostate cancer: a guidance statement from the Clinical Guidelines Committee of the American College of Physicians. *Ann Intern Med* 2013;158(10):761–9.

44 Carter HB, *et al.* Early detection of prostate cancer: AUA Guideline. *J Urol* 2013;190(2):419–26.

45 Moyer VA. Screening for prostate cancer: U.S. Preventive Services Task Force recommendation statement. *Ann Intern Med* 2012;157(2):120–34.

46 Thompson IM, *et al.* Prevalence of prostate cancer among men with a prostate-specific antigen level < or =4.0 ng per milliliter. *N Engl J Med* 2004;350(22):2239–46.

47 Eichler K, *et al.* Diagnostic value of systematic biopsy methods in the investigation of prostate cancer: a systematic review. *J Urol* 2006;175(5):1605–12.

48 Turgut AT, *et al.* Complications and limitations related to periprostatic local anesthesia before TRUS-guided prostate biopsy. *J Clin Ultrasound* 2008;36(2):67–71.

49 Raaijmakers R, *et al.* Complication rates and risk factors of 5802 transrectal ultrasound-guided sextant biopsies of the prostate within a population-based screening program. *Urology* 2002;60(5):826–30.

50 Thompson I, *et al.* Guideline for the management of clinically localized prostate cancer: 2007 update. *J Urol* 2007;177(6):2106–31.

51 Lee N, *et al.* Which patients with newly diagnosed prostate cancer need a radionuclide bone scan? An analysis based on 631 patients. *Int J Radiat Oncol Biol Phys* 2000;48(5):1443–6.

52 Hamdy FC, *et al.* 10-Year Outcomes after Monitoring, Surgery, or Radiotherapy for Localized Prostate Cancer. *N Engl J Med* 2016;375(15):1415–24.

53 Bill-Axelson A, *et al.* Radical prostatectomy versus watchful waiting in early prostate cancer. *N Engl J Med* 2011;364(18):1708–17.

54 Wilt TJ, *et al.* Radical prostatectomy versus observation for localized prostate cancer. *N Engl J Med* 2012;367(3):203–13.

55 Hoffman RM, *et al.* Mortality after radical prostatectomy or external beam radiotherapy for localized prostate cancer. *J Natl Cancer Inst* 2013;105(10):711–8.

56 Sanda MG, *et al.* Quality of life and satisfaction with outcome among prostate-cancer survivors. *N Engl J Med* 2008;358(12):1250–61.

57 Oh WK, *et al.* Does oral antiandrogen use before leuteinizing hormone-releasing hormone therapy in patients with metastatic prostate cancer prevent clinical consequences of a testosterone flare? *Urology* 2010;75(3):642–7.

58 Roach M, 3rd, *et al.* Short-term neoadjuvant androgen deprivation therapy and external-beam radiotherapy for locally advanced prostate cancer: long-term results of RTOG 8610. *J Clin Oncol* 2008;26(4):585–91.

59 Bolla M, *et al.* External irradiation with or without long-term androgen suppression for prostate cancer with high metastatic risk: 10-year results of an EORTC randomised study. *Lancet Oncol* 2010;11(11):1066–73.

60 Horwitz EM, *et al.* Ten-year follow-up of radiation therapy oncology group protocol 92-02: a phase III trial of the duration of elective androgen deprivation in locally advanced prostate cancer. *J Clin Oncol* 2008;26(15):2497–504.

61 Bolla M, *et al.* Duration of androgen suppression in the treatment of prostate cancer. *N Engl J Med* 2009;360(24):2516–27.
62 Nabid A, *et al.* Duration of androgen deprivation therapy in high-risk prostate cancer: a randomized trial. *J Clin Oncol (Meeting Abstracts)* 2013;31(18_suppl):LBA4510.
63 D'Amico AV, *et al.* Risk of death from prostate cancer after brachytherapy alone or with radiation, androgen suppression therapy, or both in men with high-risk disease. *J Clin Oncol* 2009;27(24):3923–8.
64 Bolla M, *et al.* Postoperative radiotherapy after radical prostatectomy: a randomised controlled trial (EORTC trial 22911). *Lancet* 2005;366(9485):572–8.
65 Wiegel T, *et al.* Phase III postoperative adjuvant radiotherapy after radical prostatectomy compared with radical prostatectomy alone in pT3 prostate cancer with postoperative undetectable prostate-specific antigen: ARO 96-02/AUO AP 09/95. *J Clin Oncol* 2009;27(18):2924–30.
66 Thompson IM, Jr., *et al.* Adjuvant radiotherapy for pathologically advanced prostate cancer: a randomized clinical trial. *JAMA* 2006;296(19):2329–35.
67 Thompson IM, *et al.* Adjuvant radiotherapy for pathological T3N0M0 prostate cancer significantly reduces risk of metastases and improves survival: long-term followup of a randomized clinical trial. *J Urol* 2009;181(3):956–62.
68 Scolieri MJ, Altman A, Resnick MI. Neoadjuvant hormonal ablative therapy before radical prostatectomy: a review. Is it indicated? *J Urol* 2000;164(5):1465–72.
69 Nanni C, *et al.* 18F-Fluciclovine PET/CT for the detection of prostate cancer relapse: a comparison to 11C-Choline PET/CT. *Clin Nucl Med* 2015;40(8):e386–91.
70 Chade DC, *et al.* Cancer control and functional outcomes of salvage radical prostatectomy for radiation-recurrent prostate cancer: a systematic review of the literature. *Eur Urol* 2012;61(5):961–71.
71 Gotto GT, *et al.* Impact of prior prostate radiation on complications after radical prostatectomy. *J Urol* 2010;184(1):136–42.
72 Stephenson AJ, Eastham JA. Role of salvage radical prostatectomy for recurrent prostate cancer after radiation therapy. *J Clin Oncol* 2005;23(32):8198–203.
73 Pisters LL, *et al.* Locally recurrent prostate cancer after initial radiation therapy: a comparison of salvage radical prostatectomy versus cryotherapy. *J Urol* 2009;182(2):517–25; discussion 525–7.
74 Boorjian SA, *et al.* Radiation therapy after radical prostatectomy: impact on metastasis and survival. *J Urol* 2009;182(6):2708–14.
75 Trock BJ, *et al.* Prostate cancer-specific survival following salvage radiotherapy vs observation in men with biochemical recurrence after radical prostatectomy. *JAMA* 2008;299(23):2760–9.
76 Cotter SE, *et al.* Salvage radiation in men after prostate-specific antigen failure and the risk of death. *Cancer* 2011;117(17):3925–32.
77 Shipley WU, *et al.* Radiation with or without antiandrogen therapy in recurrent prostate cancer. *N Engl J Med* 2017;376(5):417–28.
78 Carrie C, *et al.* Salvage radiotherapy with or without short-term hormone therapy for rising prostate-specific antigen concentration after radical prostatectomy (GETUG-AFU 16): a randomised, multicentre, open-label phase 3 trial. *Lancet Oncol* 2016;17(6):747–56.
79 Loblaw DA, *et al.* Initial hormonal management of androgen-sensitive metastatic, recurrent, or progressive prostate cancer: 2006 update of an American Society of Clinical Oncology practice guideline. *J Clin Oncol* 2007;25(12):1596–605.
80 Crook JM, *et al.* Intermittent androgen suppression for rising PSA level after radiotherapy. *N Engl J Med* 2012;367(10):895–903.
81 Seidenfeld J, *et al.* Single-therapy androgen suppression in men with advanced prostate cancer: a systematic review and meta-analysis. *Ann Intern Med* 2000;132(7):566–77.
82 Tay MH, *et al.* Finasteride and bicalutamide as primary hormonal therapy in patients with advanced adenocarcinoma of the prostate. *Ann Oncol* 2004;15(6):974–8.
83 Oh WK, *et al.* Finasteride and flutamide therapy in patients with advanced prostate cancer: response to subsequent castration and long-term follow-up. *Urology* 2003;62(1):99–104.
84 Brufsky A, *et al.* Finasteride and flutamide as potency-sparing androgen-ablative therapy for advanced adenocarcinoma of the prostate. *Urology* 1997;49(6):913–20.
85 Monk JP, *et al.* Efficacy of peripheral androgen blockade in prostate cancer patients with biochemical failure after definitive local therapy: results of Cancer and Leukemia Group B (CALGB) 9782. *Cancer* 2012;118(17):4139–47.
86 Banez LL, *et al.* Combined low-dose flutamide plus finasteride vs low-dose flutamide monotherapy for recurrent prostate cancer: a comparative analysis of two phase II trials with a long-term follow-up. *BJU Int* 2009;104(3):310–4.
87 Hussain M. *et al.* Intermittent versus continuous androgen deprivation in prostate cancer. *N Engl J Med* 2013;368(14):1314–25.
88 Sweeney CJ, *et al.* Chemohormonal therapy in metastatic hormone-sensitive prostate cancer. *N Engl J Med* 2015;373(8):737–46.
89 James ND, *et al.* Addition of docetaxel, zoledronic acid, or both to first-line long-term hormone therapy in prostate cancer (STAMPEDE): survival results from an adaptive, multiarm, multistage, platform randomised controlled trial. *Lancet* 2016;387(10024):1163–77.
90 Sweeney C, *et al.* Long term efficacy and QOL data of chemohormonal therapy (C-HT) in low and high volume hormone naïve metastatic prostate cancer (PrCa): E3805 CHAARTED trial. Abstract 72 OPD, European Society of Medical Oncology meeting, 2016.
91 Fizazi K, *et al.* Abiraterone plus prednisone in metastatic, castration-sensitive prostate cancer. *N Engl J Med* 2017;377(4):352–60.
92 James ND, *et al.* Abiraterone for Prostate cancer not previously treated with hormone therapy. *N Engl J Med* 2017;377(4):338–51.
93 Tannock IF, *et al.* Chemotherapy with mitoxantrone plus prednisone or prednisone alone for symptomatic hormone-resistant prostate cancer: a Canadian randomized trial with palliative end points. *J Clin Oncol* 1996;14(6):1756–64.

94 Kantoff PW, *et al.* Hydrocortisone with or without mitoxantrone in men with hormone-refractory prostate cancer: results of the cancer and leukemia group B 9182 study. *J Clin Oncol* 1999;17(8):2506–13.

95 Beer TM, *et al.* Phase II study of weekly docetaxel in symptomatic androgen-independent prostate cancer. *Ann Oncol* 2001;12(9):1273–9.

96 Berry W, *et al.* Phase II trial of single-agent weekly docetaxel in hormone-refractory, symptomatic, metastatic carcinoma of the prostate. *Semin Oncol* 2001;28(4 Suppl 15):8–15.

97 Friedland D, *et al.* A phase II trial of docetaxel (Taxotere) in hormone-refractory prostate cancer: correlation of antitumor effect to phosphorylation of Bcl-2. *Semin Oncol* 1999;26(5 Suppl 17):19–23.

98 Tannock IF, *et al.* Docetaxel plus prednisone or mitoxantrone plus prednisone for advanced prostate cancer. *N Engl J Med* 2004;351(15):1502–12.

99 Berthold DR, *et al.* Docetaxel plus prednisone or mitoxantrone plus prednisone for advanced prostate cancer: updated survival in the TAX 327 study. *J Clin Oncol* 2008;26(2):242–5.

100 de Bono JS, *et al.* Prednisone plus cabazitaxel or mitoxantrone for metastatic castration-resistant prostate cancer progressing after docetaxel treatment: a randomised open-label trial. *Lancet* 2010;376(9747):1147–54.

101 Fizazi K, *et al.* Addition of estramustine to chemotherapy and survival of patients with castration-refractory prostate cancer: a meta–analysis of individual patient data. *Lancet Oncol* 2007;8(11):994–1000.

102 Petrylak DP, *et al.* Phase I/II studies of docetaxel (Taxotere) combined with estramustine in men with hormone-refractory prostate cancer. *Semin Oncol* 1999;26(5 Suppl 17):28–33.

103 Savarese DM, *et al.* Phase II study of docetaxel, estramustine, and low-dose hydrocortisone in men with hormone-refractory prostate cancer: a final report of CALGB 9780. Cancer and Leukemia Group B. *J Clin Oncol* 2001;19(9):2509–16.

104 Petrylak DP, *et al.* Docetaxel and estramustine compared with mitoxantrone and prednisone for advanced refractory prostate cancer. *N Engl J Med* 2004;351(15):1513–20.

105 Goodin S, Kane MP, Rubin EH. Epothilones: mechanism of action and biologic activity. *J Clin Oncol* 2004;22(10): 2015–25.

106 Kelly WK. Epothilones in prostate cancer. *Urol Oncol* 2011;29(4):358–65.

107 Vahdat L. Ixabepilone: a novel antineoplastic agent with low susceptibility to multiple tumor resistance mechanisms. *Oncologist* 2008;13(3):214–21.

108 Dumontet C, Jordan MA, Lee FF. Ixabepilone: targeting betaIII-tubulin expression in taxane-resistant malignancies. *Mol Cancer Ther* 2009;8(1):17–25.

109 Rosenberg JE, *et al.* Phase I study of ixabepilone, mitoxantrone, and prednisone in patients with metastatic castration-resistant prostate cancer previously treated with docetaxel-based therapy: a study of the department of defense prostate cancer clinical trials consortium. *J Clin Oncol* 2009;27(17):2772–8.

110 Thomas ES, *et al.* Ixabepilone plus capecitabine for metastatic breast cancer progressing after anthracycline and taxane treatment. *J Clin Oncol* 2007;25(33):5210–7.

111 Galsky MD, *et al.* Multi-institutional randomized phase II trial of the epothilone B analog ixabepilone (BMS-247550) with or without estramustine phosphate in patients with progressive castrate metastatic prostate cancer. *J Clin Oncol* 2005;23(7):1439–46.

112 Rosenberg JE, *et al.* Activity of second-line chemotherapy in docetaxel-refractory hormone-refractory prostate cancer patients : randomized phase 2 study of ixabepilone or mitoxantrone and prednisone. *Cancer* 2007;110(3):556–63.

113 Oh WK, Tay MH, Huang J. Is there a role for platinum chemotherapy in the treatment of patients with hormone-refractory prostate cancer? *Cancer* 2007;109(3):477–86.

114 Nakabayashi M. *et al.* Response to docetaxel/carboplatin-based chemotherapy as first- and second-line therapy in patients with metastatic hormone-refractory prostate cancer. *BJU Int* 2008;101(3):308–12.

115 Ross RW, *et al.* A phase 2 study of carboplatin plus docetaxel in men with metastatic hormone-refractory prostate cancer who are refractory to docetaxel. *Cancer* 2008;112(3):521–6.

116 Regan MM, *et al.* Efficacy of carboplatin-taxane combinations in the management of castration-resistant prostate cancer: a pooled analysis of seven prospective clinical trials. *Ann Oncol* 2010;21(2):312–8.

117 Sternberg CN, *et al.* Multinational, double-blind, phase III study of prednisone and either satraplatin or placebo in patients with castrate-refractory prostate cancer progressing after prior chemotherapy: the SPARC trial. *J Clin Oncol* 2009;27(32):5431–8.

118 Attard G, *et al.* Phase I clinical trial of a selective inhibitor of CYP17, abiraterone acetate, confirms that castration-resistant prostate cancer commonly remains hormone driven. *J Clin Oncol* 2008;26(28):4563–71.

119 Attard G, *et al.* Selective inhibition of CYP17 with abiraterone acetate is highly active in the treatment of castration-resistant prostate cancer. *J Clin Oncol* 2009;27(23): 3742–8.

120 Danila DC, *et al.* Phase II multicenter study of abiraterone acetate plus prednisone therapy in patients with docetaxel-treated castration-resistant prostate cancer. *J Clin Oncol* 2010;28(9):1496–501.

121 de Bono JS, *et al.* Abiraterone and increased survival in metastatic prostate cancer. *N Engl J Med* 2011;364(21):1995–2005.

122 Sternberg CN, *et al.* Effect of abiraterone acetate on fatigue in patients with metastatic castration-resistant prostate cancer after docetaxel chemotherapy. *Ann Oncol* 2013;24(4):1017–25.

123 Logothetis CJ, *et al.* Effect of abiraterone acetate and prednisone compared with placebo and prednisone on pain control and skeletal-related events in patients with metastatic castration-resistant prostate cancer: exploratory analysis of data from the COU-AA-301 randomised trial. *Lancet Oncol* 2012;13(12):1210–7.

124 Ryan CJ, *et al.* Abiraterone in metastatic prostate cancer without previous chemotherapy. *N Engl J Med* 2013;368(2):138–48.

125 Mezynski J, *et al.* Antitumour activity of docetaxel following treatment with the CYP17A1 inhibitor abiraterone: clinical evidence for cross-resistance? *Ann Oncol* 2012;23(11):2943–7.

126 Tran C, *et al.* Development of a second-generation antiandrogen for treatment of advanced prostate cancer. *Science* 2009;324(5928):787–90.

127 Scher HI, Sawyers CL. Biology of progressive, castration-resistant prostate cancer: directed therapies targeting the androgen-receptor signaling axis. *J Clin Oncol* 2005;23(32):8253–61.

128 Yoshida T, *et al.* Antiandrogen bicalutamide promotes tumor growth in a novel androgen-dependent prostate cancer xenograft model derived from a bicalutamide-treated patient. *Cancer Res* 2005;65(21):9611–6.

129 Scher HI, *et al.* Antitumour activity of MDV3100 in castration-resistant prostate cancer: a phase 1-2 study. *Lancet* 2010;375(9724):1437–46.

130 Scher HI, *et al.* Increased survival with enzalutamide in prostate cancer after chemotherapy. *N Engl J Med* 2012;367(13):1187–97.

131 Beer TM, *et al. Enzalutamide in metastatic prostate cancer before chemotherapy. N Engl J Med* 2014;371(5):424–33.

132 Higano CS, *et al.* Integrated data from 2 randomized, double-blind, placebo-controlled, phase 3 trials of active cellular immunotherapy with sipuleucel-T in advanced prostate cancer. *Cancer* 2009;115(16):3670–9.

133 Kantoff PW, *et al.* Sipuleucel-T immunotherapy for castration-resistant prostate cancer. *N Engl J Med* 2010;363(5):411–22.

134 Nilsson S, *et al.* First clinical experience with alpha-emitting radium-223 in the treatment of skeletal metastases. *Clin Cancer Res* 2005;11(12):4451–9.

135 Nilsson S, *et al.* Bone-targeted radium-223 in symptomatic, hormone-refractory prostate cancer: a randomised, multicentre, placebo-controlled phase II study. *Lancet Oncol* 2007;8(7):587–94.

136 Parker CC, *et al.* A randomized, double-blind, dose-finding, multicenter, phase 2 study of radium chloride (Ra 223) in patients with bone metastases and castration-resistant prostate cancer. *Eur Urol* 2013;63(2):189–97.

137 Nilsson S, *et al.* A randomized, dose-response, multicenter phase II study of radium-223 chloride for the palliation of painful bone metastases in patients with castration-resistant prostate cancer. *Eur J Cancer* 2012;48(5):678–86.

138 Parker C, *et al.* Alpha emitter radium-223 and survival in metastatic prostate cancer. *N Engl J Med* 2013;369(3):213–23.

139 Steenland E, *et al.* The effect of a single fraction compared to multiple fractions on painful bone metastases: a global analysis of the Dutch Bone Metastasis Study. *Radiother Oncol* 1999;52(2):101–9.

140 Hartsell WF, *et al.* Randomized trial of short- versus long-course radiotherapy for palliation of painful bone metastases. *J Natl Cancer Inst* 2005;97(11):798–804.

141 Bone Pain Trial Working Party. 8 Gy single fraction radiotherapy for the treatment of metastatic skeletal pain: randomised comparison with a multifraction schedule over 12 months of patient follow-up. *Radiother Oncol* 1999;52(2):111–21.

142 Lutz S, *et al.* Palliative radiotherapy for bone metastases: an ASTRO evidence-based guideline. *Int J Radiat Oncol Biol Phys* 2011;79(4):965–76.

143 Saad F, *et al.* Long-term efficacy of zoledronic acid for the prevention of skeletal complications in patients with metastatic hormone-refractory prostate cancer. *J Natl Cancer Inst* 2004;96(11):879–82.

144 Weinfurt KP, *et al.* Effect of zoledronic acid on pain associated with bone metastasis in patients with prostate cancer. *Ann Oncol* 2006;17(6):986–9.

145 Smith MR, *et al.* Denosumab in men receiving androgen-deprivation therapy for prostate cancer. *N Engl J Med* 2009;361(8):745–55.

146 Smith MR, *et al.* Effects of denosumab on bone mineral density in men receiving androgen deprivation therapy for prostate cancer. *J Urol* 2009;182(6):2670–5.

147 Smith MR, *et al.* Denosumab and bone-metastasis-free survival in men with castration-resistant prostate cancer: results of a phase 3, randomised, placebo-controlled trial. *Lancet* 2012;379(9810):39–46.

148 Fizazi K, *et al.* Denosumab versus zoledronic acid for treatment of bone metastases in men with castration-resistant prostate cancer: a randomised, double-blind study. *Lancet* 2011;377(9768):813–22.

149 Surveillance Research Program, N.C.I. Fast Stats: An interactive tool for access to SEER cancer statistics. http://seer.cancer.gov/faststats (accessed 17 October 2017).

27

Penile Cancer

David Bowes[1] *and Juanita Crook*[2]

[1] *Nova Scotia Cancer Center, Dalhousie University, Halifax, Nova Scotia, Canada*
[2] *University of British Columbia, British Columbia Cancer Agency, Cancer Center for the Southern Interior, Kelowna, British Columbia, Canada*

Introduction

Penile cancer is an uncommon malignancy of the male genital tract which has remarkable geographic variation in incidence. It is highly curable in the early stages but because of lack of awareness or access to medical care, often presents in an advanced and highly fatal stage. Poor hygiene and human papilloma (HPV) virus infection play a role in the etiology. Penile-sparing approaches are encouraged where feasible as surgical amputation can have devastating psychosexual consequences.

Incidence and Mortality

The penile cancer incidence and mortality rates in the United States (US) are 0.9 new diagnoses and 0.2 deaths per 100,000 men per year. The incidence rate for men in the US increased by an average of 1.2% per year between 2004 and 2013, and the mortality rate decreased by an average of 0.6% per year during that period. The median age at diagnosis is 68 years [1]. Approximately 2,120 men are diagnosed with penile cancer, and approximately 360 men die of this disease each year in the US [2].

An estimated 22,000 cases of penile cancer occur worldwide [3]. There is wide geographical variation, with penile cancer accounting for 10–20% of cancers of men in parts of Asia, Africa, and South America. This geographic variability is related to circumcision practices and socioeconomic factors [4]. In the developed world, penile cancer is most commonly diagnosed in the sixth decade of life, but occurs earlier in regions where the incidence is higher.

Etiology

Circumcision

Neonatal circumcision is protective against penile cancer, with only rare reports in men circumcised in infancy [5]. The increased risk of penile cancer in uncircumcised men is related to poor hygiene, chronic infections, greater susceptibility to HPV infection and condylomata, and phimosis, the latter being a particularly strong risk factor [6]. Circumcision later in life does not appear to have the same protective effect, and when performed for phimosis in an adult may unmask preinvasive disease.

HPV

HPV is a family of double-stranded DNA viruses which commonly infect the squamous cells of the anogenital and orophayrngeal mucosa. HPV plays an etiologic role in 40–45% of penile cancers. The percentage of cases with detectable HPV DNA is higher among warty and basaloid types, and lower among cancers with keratinizing and verrucous histology [7]. HPV-16 and HPV-18 are the most common subtypes identified by polymerase chain reaction DNA analysis [6,8,9]. An increased rate of penile cancer has been observed in male partners of women with cervical cancer [10,11], likely an effect of HPV.

Men with a history of genital warts have an increased risk of penile cancer, as well as cancers of the anal canal and head and neck. Blomberg *et al.* recently performed a large cohort study in Denmark of individuals with genital warts, and found an approximately eightfold increased risk of penile cancer [12]. It is not clear if this is attributable to HPV subtypes responsible for the genital warts, or to other differences between men with genital warts and the population at large.

Phimosis and Inflammation

Chronic inflammatory conditions also increase the risk of penile cancer, through molecular pathways unique from those associated with HPV. Phimosis often leads to retention of smegma, which is associated with chronic inflammation of the foreskin and glans. Phimosis also increases the likelihood of bacterial or fungal infections that also contribute to inflammation [7]. Balanitis xerotica obliterans, also known as penile lichen sclerosis, is a chronic inflammatory condition that leads to the development of white plaques on the glans and foreskin.

The American Cancer Society's Oncology in Practice: Clinical Management, First Edition. Edited by The American Cancer Society.

This results in difficulty retracting the foreskin and problems with hygiene [13]. The incidence of penile cancer in men with balanitis xerotica obliterans is 4–8% [13].

Immune Disorders

Disorders of the immune system can also promote the development of penile cancer, presumably through the propagation of high risk HPV infection. Men with human immunodeficiency virus infection are at high risk for HPV-associated malignancies. Research is limited examining the link between human immunodeficiency virus infection and penile cancer, though a recent study of men in Brazil has shown a high rate of preinvasive penile lesions [14].

Smoking

Several studies reported that smoking also increases the risk of developing penile cancer, although the mechanism remains uncertain [7,15].

Ultraviolet Radiation

Treatment of psoriasis with photo chemotherapy (PUVA) in case of psoriasis also a risk factor.[7].

Prevention

Given the low incidence, neonatal circumcision is not recommended as an intervention to reduce the risk of penile cancer. Similarly, with such a low burden of penile cancer in the general population, there is no role for regular screening. Rather, emphasis should be placed on education, foreskin hygiene, and management of phimosis. Measures which reduce or prevent transmission of HPV, such as safe sexual practices (including condom use) and HPV vaccination may also reduce the incidence. There is no established role for HPV vaccination for penile cancer prevention but it is reasonable to assume that vaccination programs that reduce the burden of HPV in the population may ultimately reduce the incidence of penile cancer, in addition to cervix cancer and head neck cancers. An advisory panel of the 2009 International Consultation on Urologic Disease Consensus Publishing Group acknowledged HPV infection and lack of circumcision as important factors in the development of penile cancer, but did not recommend routine screening [16].

Histopathology and Molecular Pathology

Penile cancer is characterized using the 2004 World Health Organization classification system [17] which was updated to include several histologic variants [18]. The overwhelming majority of penile cancers are well-differentiated squamous cell carcinomas which originate in the epithelium of the glans, coronal sulcus, and foreskin. Common subtypes of squamous cell carcinoma include verrucous, warty (or verruciform), and basaloid carcinoma. Sarcomatoid tumors are rare, and are typically associated with widespread nodal and distant metastases. Other rare types of carcinoma include small cell neuroendocrine type, clear cell, basaloid, papillary, Merkel cell, and sebaceous. Melanomas, lymphomas, and sarcomas can occur, as can metastases from other sites such as bladder and prostate cancers [19].

Premalignant lesions include Bowen disease, erythroplasia of Queyrat (EQ), and bowenoid papulosis, and are collectively defined as penile intraepithelial neoplasia. Pathologically, Bowen disease and EQ are both squamous cell carcinomas *in situ*; Bowen disease presents as a scaly, plaque-like lesion on the penile shaft, and EQ presents as a red-colored plaque that involves the inner prepuce or glans [16,20]. Bowenoid papulosis is commonly associated with genital HPV infection and/or immune-suppression. EQ is often observed in the setting of lichen sclerosis.

Separate molecular pathways may be responsible for HPV-dependent and HPV-independent penile cancers. The prevalence of HPV DNA in the penile cancer genome, as determined using polymerase chain reaction, has been reported to be 40–45% [21,22]. HPV types 16 and 18 are most commonly associated with penile cancer. The oncogenic effects of HPV in cancer development are primarily the effect of interference with *p53*, a tumor suppressor gene [21].

There is contradictory evidence describing the prognostic effect of the presence of HPV. The presence of *p53* mutations has been associated with an increased risk of nodal metastases [23,24], although other series have shown the presence of *p53* mutations or HPV DNA to be associated with favorable survival outcomes [8,25]. p16 is another marker which has been used as a surrogate for high-risk HPV in other malignancies, and has been associated with improved survival in a series of Canadian men with penile cancer [25].

Diagnosis

Most penile cancers arise on the glans, coronal sulcus, or the prepuce (foreskin). Early recognition and management of suspected penile cancer is important, as early-stage disease is highly curable. However, delayed presentation is common, as patients may be hesitant to seek medical attention. The average delay in seeking medical attention for these lesions is about 2 years. Men with early penile cancer typically present with an area of erythema or induration, or discharge from an unretractable foreskin. More advanced disease presents with larger or ulcerated lesions, and overlying infection is common. Pain at presentation is uncommon. Untreated, penile cancer is characterized by slow local progression to involve the shaft and corpus cavernosum, and eventually the scrotum or even the abdominal wall. Autoamputation by tumor is rare though has been reported.

Although enlarged inguinal lymph nodes as the first presenting symptom are rare, metastases to regional lymph nodes are present in 28–64% of patients at presentation [26]. Clinical evaluation of lymph nodes can be misleading due to local tumor necrosis and infection. Palpable nodes may be histologically negative at resection, while occult metastases may be identified in clinically normal nodes. Inguinal lymph nodes are the first echelon of nodal drainage [27], with involvement of pelvic lymph nodes occurring subsequently. Distant metastases typically occur in patients with locoregionally advanced disease, but patients can die of penile cancer without distant metastases due to infectious complications and involvement of major blood vessels from locoregional extension.

Giant condyloma acuminatum (also known as Buschke–Lowenstein tumor) is a rare, slow-growing, verruciform tumor. It typically presents as a large mass in the anogenital area, and is associated with HPV subtypes 6 and 11. Untreated, it can grow to a very large size, and eventually invades locally. It is treated with radical surgical excision.

Staging

Initial evaluation should include a description of the number, diameter, and location of lesion(s), the morphology, color, boundaries, and relationship to other structures. Penile length and the expected residual length after partial penectomy should also be estimated [28].

Staging uses the system of the American Joint Committee on Cancer 8th Edition (Table 27.1) [29]. In practice, clinical staging is very subjective as evaluation of invasion of the corpora is difficult. Biopsies are often not deep enough to demonstrate corporal involvement. Thus, techniques which do not treat the full thickness of the penis should be used with caution. Magnetic resonance imaging (MRI) with induction of artificial erection using prostaglandin E1 can assess invasion, and shows a high concordance with eventual pathologic stage [30]. Ultrasound may be helpful in settings where MRI is not available.

The presence of nodal metastases is the most powerful predictor of survival. A review of the literature by Ficarra *et al.* showed that 5-year cancer-specific survival for patients with pathologically negative inguinal nodes is 85–100% versus 16–45% [31]. The prognosis depends on the number of positive nodes, unilateral versus bilateral disease, involvement of pelvic nodes, and the presence of capsular invasion [31]. Appropriate evaluation and management of the regional nodes is paramount. Clinical examination should focus on palpable nodes, the number of enlarged nodes, unilateral versus bilateral findings, fixation, size, proximity to surrounding structures, and the presence of lower extremity edema. Computed tomography (CT) imaging should be performed in patients with grade 2 or 3 lesions, or with clinical stage T2 or higher.

For those with clinically and radiographically negative groins, the optimal strategy for inguinal management is controversial. Historically, patients managed with primary radiotherapy have not undergone inguinal node dissection. However, without surgical removal of the primary tumor, pathologic prognosticators of lymph node involvement cannot be fully appreciated.

Approximately 20% of men with clinically negative nodes will have microscopic nodal disease which is curable by lymphadenectomy. Surgical series have demonstrated improved survival for patients with clinically occult but pathologically involved groin nodes, as compared with those undergoing therapeutic lymph node dissection at the time of recurrence [32,33]. However, since lymphadenectomy may represent overtreatment in many men and is associated with substantial risk of complications including lymphedema, wound infection, and

Table 27.1 TNM staging for penile cancer.

Definitions of AJCC TNM	
Definition of primary tumor (T)	
T category	**T criteria**
TX	Primary tumor cannot be assessed
T0	No evidence of primary tumor
Tis	Carcinoma *in situ* (penile intraepithelial neoplasia (PeIN))
Ta	Noninvasive localized squamous cell carcinoma
T1	Glans: tumor invades lamina propria Foreskin: tumor invades dermis, lamina propria, or dartos fascia Shaft: tumor invades connective tissue between epidermis and corpora regardless of location All sites with or without lymphovascular invasion or perineural invasion and is or is not high grade
T1a	Tumor is without lymphovascular invasion or perineural invasion and is not high grade (i.e., grade 3 or sarcomatoid)
T1b	Tumor exhibits lymphovascular invasion and/or perineural invasion or is high grade (i.e., grade 3 or sarcomatoid)
T2	Tumor invades into corpus spongiosum (either glans or ventral shaft) with or without urethral invasion
T3	Tumor invades into corpora cavernosum (including tunica albuginea) with or without urethral invasion
T4	Tumor invades into adjacent structures (i.e., scrotum, prostate, pubic bone)
Definition of regional lymph node (N)	
Clinical N (cN)	
cN category	**cN criteria**
cNX	Regional lymph nodes cannot be assessed
cN0	No palpable or visibly enlarged inguinal lymph nodes
cN1	Palpable mobile unilateral inguinal lymph node
cN2	Palpable mobile ≥2 unilateral inguinal nodes or bilateral inguinal lymph nodes
cN3	Palpable fixed inguinal nodal mass or pelvic lymphadenopathy unilateral or bilateral
Pathological N (pN)	
pN category	**pN criteria**
pNX	Lymph node metastasis cannot be established
pN0	No lymph node metastasis
pN1	≤2 unilateral inguinal metastases, no ENE
pN2	≥3 unilateral inguinal metastases or bilateral metastases
pN3	ENE of lymph node metastases or pelvic lymph node metastases

(Continued)

Table 27.1 (Continued)

Definition of distant metastasis (M)

M category	M criteria
M0	No distant metastasis
M1	Distant metastasis present

AJCC prognostic stage groups

When T is...	And N is...	And M is...	Then the stage group is...
Tis	N0	M0	0is
Ta	N0	M0	0a
T1a	N0	M0	I
T1b	N0	M0	IIA
T2	N0	M0	IIA
T3	N0	M0	IIB
T1-3	N1	M0	IIIA
T1-3	N2	M0	IIIB
T4	Any N	M0	IV
Any T	N3	M0	IV
Any T	Any N	M1	IV

Source: Pettaway *et al.* [29]. Used with permission of the American College of Surgeons, Chicago, Illinois. The original source for this information is the American Joint Committee on Cancer (AJCC) Cancer Staging Manual, 8th edn (2017), which is published by Springer Science+Business Media.

lymphocele formation, lymph node dissection should be selectively applied.

For grade 1, T1 disease, the rate of failure in inguinal lymph nodes after treatment of the primary site is sufficiently low that inguinal nodal dissection is not required [28,34]. For patients with grade 2 or 3 disease, lymphovascular invasion on biopsy, or clinical stage T2 (or higher), prophylactic inguinal node dissection is indicated. Dynamic sentinel lymph node mapping can be considered in high volume centers where expertise exists, with completion inguinal dissection for positive sentinel nodes. The risk of a false negative result with dynamic sentinel lymph node biopsy is about 5%, and the morbidity is sufficiently low compared with modified lymph node dissection that this risk of a false negative result is considered acceptable. In centers where sentinel lymph node biopsy is not available, or when the nodes are clinically positive, bilateral modified inguinal nodal dissection is the appropriate surgical staging. Although approximately 50% of patients with palpable lymph nodes at diagnosis will prove to have benign reactive adenopathy, delayed management with a 6-week course of antibiotics is no longer recommended [35]. CT imaging of the abdomen and pelvis should be performed to determine if there are enlarged pelvic and/or para-aortic lymph nodes. Fine-needle aspiration (FNA) can determine whether clinically suspicious nodes contain malignancy. Clinically suspicious nodes with negative initial FNA should be considered for repeat FNA or excisional biopsy to guide definitive management. Node positive disease is discussed further below.

Management

Biopsy of the primary tumor is required before definitive therapy. This confirms the diagnosis and provides vital information on grade and histology to direct further therapy and assist with evaluation of the risk of lymph node involvement. All patients undergoing penile preserving treatment should undergo circumcision as a first step. This allows complete evaluation of the extent of disease, and reduces complications like balanitis and phimosis after radiotherapy. It also facilitates follow-up as these patients are at risk for local recurrence in the long term. Circumcision may incidentally provide definitive management of small, preinvasive lesions confined to the foreskin.

Early Stage Disease (Tis, T1, T2)

Penile-preserving approaches are recommended for stage Tis, T1a, T1b and T2 lesions <4 cm (Figure 27.1).

Superficial Lesions

Topical therapies, like 5-fluorouracil and imiquod, are commonly used for superficial preinvasive lesions (Tis, Ta, T1a). Evidence is limited to small retrospective series but topical therapies appear to be effective, at least as an initial treatment [36]. The rates of long-term control are not well documented, and patients should be closely monitored.

Although external radiotherapy is not often used for superficial lesions, orthovoltage photon beams have been used for well-lateralized *in situ* lesions. Neither is brachytherapy typically delivered for this stage of disease, except in the setting of recurrence.

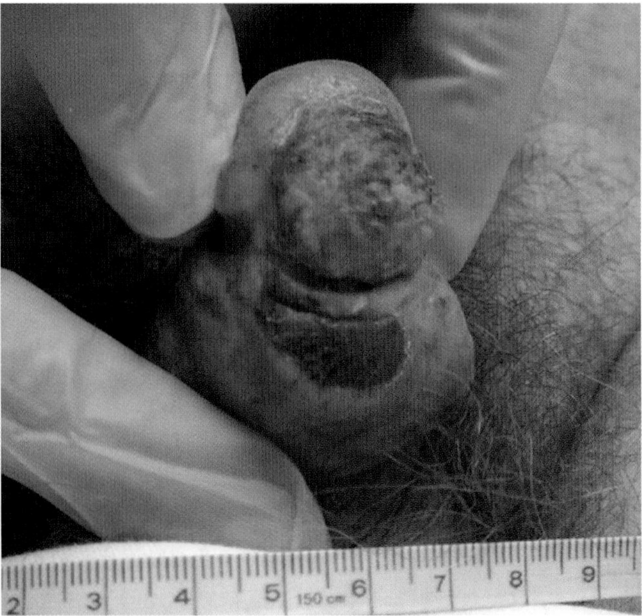

Figure 27.1 Squamous carcinoma of the penis in a 58-year-old male. Clinical stage T2. Involvement of adjacent face of retracted foreskin evident.

Surgery

There are several penile-preserving surgical approaches that can be considered for men with small preinvasive or superficially invasive tumors. Traditionally, the surgical approach aimed for 2 cm resection margins, limiting the likelihood of preserving penile function. More recent reports have shown that this appears unnecessary [37]. Margins of 5–10 mm are now considered adequate [28] as local recurrences can be salvaged with further therapy.

Mohs surgery involves intraoperative assessment of margin status, with removal of successive layers of tissue until clear margins are obtained [38]. Local recurrence rates appear to be higher than with more extensive surgery, though many recurrences can be salvaged with repeat procedures [39]. Thus, survival and regional progression rates are favorable. Resection with carbon dioxide or neodymium:yttrium-aluminum-garnet (Nd:YAG) laser can be considered for small, superficial lesions [39]. As with Mohs surgery, close surveillance is required. Schlenker *et al.* have reported a 42% rate of local recurrence in 54 patients with mostly *in situ* and T1 disease [40]. Meijer *et al.* have also reported a relatively high local recurrence rate in a series of patients with long-term follow-up [41]. For patients with early-stage disease, recurrences may be salvageable with repeat resection, and survival is not likely to be compromised.

Early Stage, Nonsuperficial

For T1b and T2 lesions <4 cm, there are several penile-preserving options. For clinical stage T2 disease and higher, the rates of local and nodal recurrence are sufficiently high that laser therapy is not recommended [28]. Likewise, Mohs surgery is not a suitable approach. Glansectomy is preferable to partial penectomy, and multiple single institution studies have shown the feasibility of this approach [42–46]. Glansectomy appears to provide a better functional and cosmetic result than amputative surgery. This involves stripping of the epithelium of the glans with coverage of the surgical defect with a skin graft. Local recurrences are still possible, though they can often be salvaged with partial or total penectomy without compromising long-term survival. In the series reported by Veeratterapillay *et al.*, 85% of men maintained erectile function at 1 year postsurgery [43]. A small number of patients were noted to develop contacture of the glans in follow-up requiring repeat surgery. Patients with extension onto the penile shaft are not candidates for glansectomy. When glansectomy cannot be performed, a partial penectomy is indicated.

Radiotherapy

Radiotherapy is an organ-preserving approach that provides favorable oncologic and functional outcomes. Radiotherapy can be delivered as external beam radiotherapy (EBRT) or brachytherapy, which involves interstitial placement of radioactive sources into the penis. In suitable patients, brachytherapy provides a high likelihood of local control and maintenance of erectile and urinary function, though it requires considerable specialized expertise. EBRT is more widely available and may be preferred for larger tumors over 4 cm and those extending onto the penile shaft. Published radiotherapy series extend over decades with a variety of treatment techniques and dose prescriptions, which do not reflect recent technical improvements in radiotherapy delivery. Outcomes from selected radiotherapy series are shown in Table 27.2.

External Beam Radiotherapy

EBRT is commonly used in the definitive management of penile cancer. It is widely available and does not require specific technical expertise. As the results for early-stage disease are less favorable for EBRT than for brachytherapy, it is not the preferred option in these patients; however, EBRT is a reasonable alternative where brachytherapy expertise is not available.

EBRT requires the penis to be positioned such that incidental irradiation to the surrounding tissues is avoided. Typically, the patient is treated supine with the penis encased in a 10 × 10 cm block of tissue equivalent material such as wax or Perspex. This allows reproducibility of set up and full radiation dose delivery to the penile surface. A central cylindrical space houses the penis within the block and a "cork" of tissue equivalent material is placed on the distal end to close the cylinder. Over the course of radiotherapy, the central cylinder may need to be enlarged, as edema and skin reaction develop. Perspex has the advantage of being transparent, allowing easy verification of the penile position within the central cylinder. Shielding of the testicles should be considered for patients who wish to maintain fertility.

The most commonly used fractionation schedule is 60–66 Gy in 2 Gy daily fractions, over 6–6.5 weeks. Two opposed low energy photon beams will treat the entire thickness of the penis to a therapeutic dose with full dose to the skin surface.

EBRT is an effective form of penile preservation. Local control rates of 57–62% at 5 years have been reported [47–50], but there are no reports of outcomes after longer follow-up. Cause-specific survival rates are satisfactory as salvage surgery is often effective for local recurrence. This usually involves either partial or total penectomy, depending on the extent of recurrence and length of penile shaft which has been irradiated.

Brachytherapy

Brachytherapy is a highly effective treatment for men with localized penile cancer stageT1b, T2 tumors <4 cm and selected T3 cases. There is limited awareness of this procedure in the uro-oncologic community, given the rarity of penile cancer and the fact that brachytherapy is delivered in specialized centers. There is considerable published experience supporting its use, and referral for an opinion to an appropriate center should be considered.

Brachytherapy delivers a high dose of radiotherapy in a very accurate fashion. Crook *et al.* have described the penile brachytherapy technique in detail [51,52]. It involves the placement of two to three parallel planes of hollow, thin needles within the penis (four to nine needles in total), spaced 12–18 mm apart. The needles are held together with two Lucite plates which "sandwich" the penis (Figure 27.2). The procedure is performed under either general anesthesia or a local penile block with sedation. A radiotherapy plan is generated based on needle position and the size and location of the tumor. As the depth of invasion of the cancer is difficult to assess clinically, sufficient margin is required at a depth to account for potential subclinical invasion. The needles are loaded with the radiation sources

Table 27.2 Selected results from brachytherapy and external beam radiotherapy series (of at least 50 patients).

First author	Patients (*n*)	Dose	Median follow-up	Local control at 5 years	CSS at 5 years	Complications	Penile preservation
Brachytherapy							
Crook [54]	67	60 Gy (LDR)	48 months	87%	84%	12% necrosis 9% stenosis	88% at 5 years 67% at 10 years
de Crevoisier [53]	144	Median dose 65 Gy (LDR)	5.7 years	80%	92% at 10 years	26% ulceration at 10 years 29% stenosis at 10 years	72% avoidance of penile surgery (preservation not reported)
Delannes [55]	51	Mean dose 60 Gy (LDR)	Mean follow-up 5.5 years	86%	85%	23% necrosis 45% stenosis	75%
Mazeron [72]	50	60–70 Gy	Range 36–96 months	78% crude	Not reported	6% necrosis 19% stenosis	74%
Cordoba [74]	71	Median dose 60 Gy (LDR)	51.8 months	74%	91.4%	6.6% stenosis 6.8% necrosis requiring amputation 5.3% dysuria	87.9%
External beam radiotherapy							
Gotsadze [75]	155	40–60 Gy	6.5 years	65%	86% at 5 years 82% at 10 years	2 patients with stenosis 1 with necrosis	65%
Sarin [48]	101	60 Gy	62 months	55%	66%	3% necrosis 9/59 stenosis	50%

CSS, cause-specific survival; LC, local control; LDR, low-dose rate.

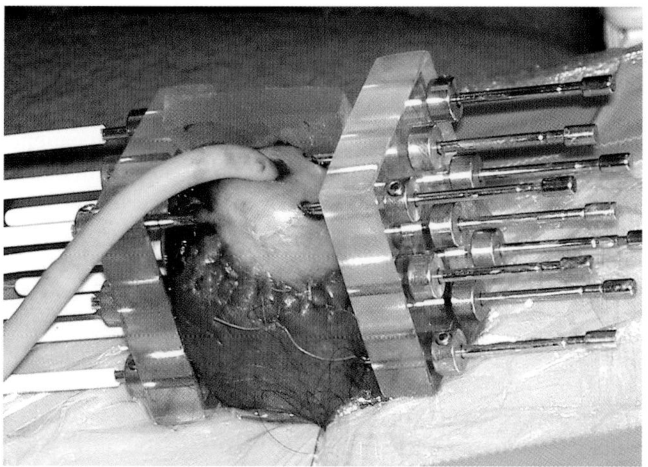

Figure 27.2 Brachytherapy implant. Urinary catheter *in situ*.

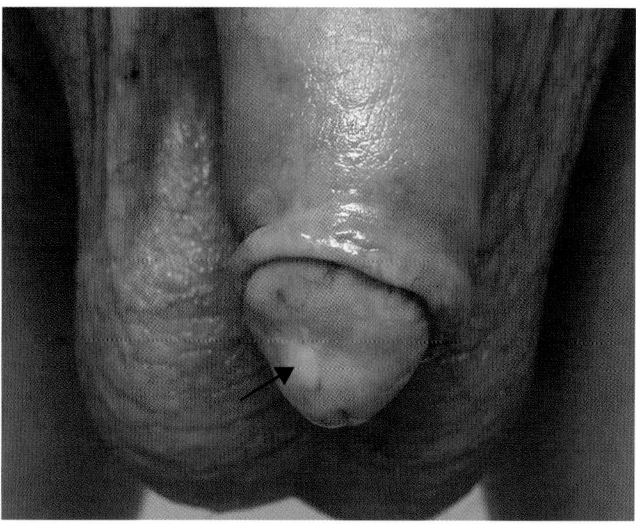

Figure 27.3 Cosmetic result 7 years after brachytherapy showing a pale flat scar and mild telangiectasia

either manually or using an automated afterloading machine commonly available in radiotherapy departments. The appropriate dose of radiation is delivered through the needles over a period of 4–5 days. The patient is hospitalized over the course of treatment, and bed rest is recommended. In general, the treatment is well tolerated and sufficient analgesia is achieved with acetaminophen +/– codeine. At completion of treatment, the needles can be removed at the bedside with appropriate premedication.

The majority of the reported experience for penile brachytherapy has used low-dose rate or pulse-dose rate radiotherapy, delivering 60 Gy over 4–5 days at a rate of 50–60 cGy per hour. High-dose rate treatment is now more commonly available in radiotherapy departments but the total dose and schedule for high-dose rate are not well established. There is little published literature on high-dose rate penile brachytherapy. Unpublished experience suggests that the delivery of 38–45 Gy total dose over multiple fractions (twice daily with a minimum 6 hours between) over 6 days may be effective. Homogeneity and volume considerations still need to be worked out before recommending any prescription as the risk of subsequent soft tissue necrosis is considerable.

Two large series have recently been published on long-term outcomes in patients treated at single institutions with low-dose rate penile brachytherapy. De Crevoisier *et al.* reported the rates of local recurrence-free and cause-specific survival to be 80% and 92% respectively for 144 men [53]. Crook *et al.* reported actuarial local control and penile preservation rates after penile brachytherapy to be 87% and 88% at 5 years, and 72% and 67% at 10 years [54]. Late local recurrence can occur up to 8–10 years after treatment, so prolonged follow-up is mandatory. Local recurrences are highly salvageable with surgery (either partial or total penectomy).

As with other penile-preserving therapies, appropriate patient selection is paramount. Brachytherapy is ideally reserved for men with clinical stage T1, T2, and selected T3 disease, with tumors under 4 cm and located on the glans. This population represents most of those treated in the studies discussed above. Brachytherapy is also effective in moderately- or poorly-differentiated tumors, although these patients also require surgical staging of the inguinal lymph nodes. Size of the primary tumor >4 cm is a relative contraindication imparting an increased risk of recurrence and radiotherapy-related complications.

Patients treated for local disease require appropriate management of the inguinal lymph nodes. In the series by Crook *et al.* tumors with moderate or poor differentiation had a high rate of regional or distant recurrence at 31%, compared to 4% in those that were well differentiated [54]. For this reason patients with moderately or poorly differentiated tumors or T3 disease should undergo surgical staging of the lymph nodes, regardless of whether they are clinically and radiographically (CT staging) node-negative. This is reflected in the 2009 European Association of Urology guidelines for the management of penile cancer [28].

Moist desquamation in the treated area peaks about 2–3 weeks after treatment and takes 2–3 months to resolve. Healing is delayed by smoking, poor hygiene, and diabetes. The most common late sequelae of brachytherapy are soft-tissue ulceration or necrosis, and meatal stenosis. Soft tissue ulceration is reported in 6–26% of patients. The likelihood depends on dose, radiation technique, tumor stage, and treated volume. The peak time for occurrence of soft tissue ulceration is 7–18 months, although it can occur later [55]. Conservative management is recommended, with good hygiene, antibiotic creams, and avoidance of trauma and cold exposure. Hyperbaric oxygen therapy can be effective if conservative measures fail [56]. Debridement should be undertaken cautiously as it can worsen necrosis; amputative surgery should only be performed as a last resort.

Meatal stenosis has been reported in up to 45% of patients, and tends to occur later in follow-up [57]. This can be managed with self-dilatation using a meatal dilator as required. Dilatation is more successful if initiated early, and routine provision of a dilator at the 3-month follow-up visit may prevent subsequent clinical issues. Urethroplasty or meatoplasty may be considered in severe cases but is rarely required.

Cosmesis after brachytherapy is usually good, with some degree of hypopigmentation and telangiectasia in the irradiated area (Figure 27.3). Fibrosis is usually subtle and is limited to the irradiated area. More deeply invading tumors may leave a tissue defect in the treated area which re-epithelializes slowly.

Locally Advanced Disease (T3, T4, node positive, metastatic)

Patients with early-stage primary tumors and clinically involved lymph nodes can still be managed with penile-sparing approaches. In this situation, local control at the primary site can be achieved and the nodes managed surgically. However, for patients with larger tumors or extension on to the shaft, more radical surgery is required. Partial penectomy can be considered if adequate margins can be obtained, leaving enough penile shaft to allow direction of the urinary stream. Otherwise, total penectomy with perineal urethrostomy is recommended. Postoperative radiotherapy should be considered for positive surgical margins.

For clinically negative nodes with high-risk primary tumor features (G2 or 3, T2 or greater disease, and lymphovascular invasion), a superficial inguinal node dissection anterior to the fascia lata of the thigh can be performed with saphenous vein sparing. This is associated with a low risk of chronic lymphedema. These nodes will have to be sampled real time and if positive, one or both sides with superficial positive nodes will have to undergo deep dissection, skeletonizing the anterior surface of the femoral vessel. Lymphedema is almost guaranteed. If the deep nodes are positive, then a pelvic lymph node dissection is indicated. Positive pelvic lymph nodes impart a poor prognosis. Inguinal lymphadenectomy is recommended in all patients with involved lymph nodes. If clinically suspicious nodes are present, ultrasound-guided FNA may precede pathological assessment. A modified inguinal lymphadenectomy reduces the volume of surgical dissection, and is associated with less morbidity than a radical lymphadenectomy but should include the central and superior zones of the inguinal region [58]. Prophylactic radiotherapy for clinically negative groins is not routinely recommended as an alternative for surgical staging, although may be considered in cases where there is an increased risk of nodal involvement, but inguinal lymphadenectomy is not possible.

Direct lymphatic drainage from the penis to pelvic lymph nodes is rare [27]. Pelvic lymphadenectomy is recommended in patients with more than two involved inguinal lymph nodes and/or with extracapsular extension. Postoperative adjuvant radiotherapy to the nodal regions should be considered in patients with more than one positive node or if there is extracapsular extension. There is little direct evidence to guide decisions in this setting but adjuvant radiotherapy is routinely offered to patients with high risk cancers of the anal canal and vulva [22,59,60]. The treatment fields typically include the groins and pelvis bilaterally, treating to a dose of 45–50 Gy over 5 weeks. A boost can be considered for extracapsular disease. The pelvis can be omitted if pelvic lymph node dissection is negative. The primary site is typically not treated postoperatively unless there are positive surgical margins. A recent study by Franks *et al.* suggested a benefit in a small population of men receiving adjuvant radiotherapy, with 8 of 14 patients treated being alive and free of locoregional relapse after a median follow-up of 27 months [61].

Preoperative therapy can be considered for unresectable nodal disease. Various preoperative chemotherapy regimens have been used in the setting of locally advanced disease. A recent phase II study from MD Anderson Cancer Center used a regimen of paclitaxel, ifosfamide, and cisplatin (TIP) in patients with N2 or N3 penile cancer. Twenty-two of 30 patients completed the protocol therapy and went on to receive lymphadenectomy, and nine of 30 were alive without evidence of disease at last follow-up (median follow-up 34 months) [62]. A Southwest Oncology Group study used cisplatin, methotrexate, and bleomycin (BMP), showing encouraging response rates. However, there was a higher rate of toxicity than in the MD Anderson study, with five treatment-related deaths in 40 patients [63]. If chemotherapy does not render surgery possible, palliative radiotherapy can be considered to optimize local control.

There is very little published data on combined chemotherapy and radiotherapy either as an alternative to surgery in locally advanced disease, or as preoperative treatment. The addition of surgery should be considered if chemoradiotherapy renders the disease resectable. Experience in cancer of the vulva and anal canal has demonstrated that long-term local control and survival can be achieved in patients with unresectable, locally advanced disease. Preoperative chemoradiotherapy has also been described in vulvar cancer, and a recent Gynecologic Oncology Group study reported high rates of complete clinical and pathologic response in patients who received preoperative radiotherapy and concurrent weekly cisplatin [64]. A similar approach is under development as an international initiative. The International Penile Advanced Cancer Trial (InPACT: NCT02305654), sponsored by the International Rare Cancers Initiative, the Institute of Cancer Research, Cancer Research UK, and the National Cancer Institute will test this approach in the neoadjuvant scenario against surgery alone or neoadjuvant chemotherapy (TIP regimen: paclitaxel, ifosfamide, and platinum) for men with pathologically involved inguinal nodes, and for those men with high-risk groin pathology in an adjuvant postoperative setting or in place of pelvic node surgery. Four hundred patients are to be randomized in the UK and North America. Results will provide important insights into optimal management of this disease [65].

Men who are symptomatic with locoregionally advanced disease may benefit from palliative radiotherapy for local symptoms such as pain, bleeding, and edema. Those with symptoms from distant metastatic disease to bone, lung, or other sites may also benefit. Typical doses of palliative radiotherapy include 8 Gy in a single fraction, 20 Gy in five fractions, and 30 Gy in 10 fractions.

Palliative chemotherapy can be considered in patients with recurrent or metastatic disease. Cisplatin-based regimens appear to be most effective and are typically used as first-line therapy in medically fit patients. The Southwest Oncology Group study, previously discussed, evaluating BMP chemotherapy included patients with metastatic disease; the toxicity was such that bleomycin should be avoided in palliative regimens. TIP chemotherapy, as described above, is reasonable as first-line treatment for metastatic disease in medically fit patients. Five-fluorouracil and cisplatin have also been used. Paclitaxel may also be of benefit as a second-line agent [66]. Epidermal growth factor receptor activity has been noted in penile cancer, and recent reports have demonstrated activity of anti-epidermal growth factor receptor monoclonal antibodies (including cetuximab) in patients with advanced disease [67,68].

Follow-Up

Patients who have undergone penile-preserving therapies require prolonged follow-up, as local recurrences can be salvaged. At present, there is no clear role for routine imaging investigations; CT, MRI, and PET should be directed at investigating symptoms of disease recurrence. Local recurrence in the penis is best detected on physical examination. Most local recurrences occur in the first 2 years, though recurrences as late as 10 years are reported. Men should be taught to monitor the treated area for erythema, induration, and ulceration. Similarly, most recurrences in inguinal lymph nodes occur within the first 2 years. Biannual CT or ultrasound of the pelvis and inguinal areas may supplement physical examination in the initial follow-up period.

Quality of Life

The impact of penile cancer and its therapies on sexual function has not been well documented. With partial penectomy, many men are able to maintain some degree of sexual function, though in general, achieve less satisfaction from their sexual relationships [69]. Windahl *et al.* conducted face-to-face interviews following laser surgery for penile cancer, reporting that most men who were sexually active prior to therapy maintained function afterwards, and were satisfied with their penile cosmesis [70]. Reconstructive surgery may be considered using skin grafts and tissue flaps, cutting of the suspensory ligament, or removal of fat.

Erectile function after brachytherapy appears to be well maintained. In a series of 49 men undergoing brachytherapy, 22 of 27 who reported normal potency at baseline maintained adequate erectile function in follow-up [71]. Other smaller series have reported similar findings [48,55,72]. There are no prospective studies documenting erectile function after external radiotherapy.

Urinary function can be compromised, particularly in men who have undergone total penectomy. Patients undergoing partial penectomy should have enough residual penis to allow direction of the urinary stream. Men undergoing total penectomy typically have a perineal urethrostomy, which requires one to sit to urinate. Continence should be maintained in all patients. Men who develop meatal stenosis after brachytherapy may require periodic dilatation.

The effects of penile cancer and its treatment on psychological wellbeing are substantial. A recent systematic review of quality of life and psychosexual health reported psychiatric symptoms in about 50% of men, with two-thirds reporting detrimental effects on sexual function [73]. Patients with penile cancer should be screened for depression and offered referral to mental health services for counseling as appropriate.

Men who have undergone inguinal lymph node dissection, with or without EBRT, are at risk for developing lymphedema of the lower extremities. Recurrent disease in the groins should be ruled out. Referral to a lymphedema clinic can be helpful to assist with management.

Conclusion

Penile cancer is a rare and challenging disease to treat. The psychologic and sexual effects of treatment can be devastating, and these potential consequences need to be discussed at the time of initial evaluation in all patients. Early stage disease is highly curable, and all efforts should be made to minimize the potential effects on psychosexual quality of life. Morbidity and mortality are much higher in patients with advanced-stage disease, and cooperative group trials are necessary to evaluate new treatment paradigms in this population.

References

1 Howlader N, Noone AM, Krapcho M, *et al.* (eds). SEER Cancer Statistics Review, 1975–2013, National Cancer Institute. Bethesda, MD. http://seer.cancer.gov/csr/1975_2013/, based on November 2015 SEER data submission, posted to the SEER web site, April 2016.

2 Siegel RL, Miller KD, Jemal A. Cancer statistics, 2017. *CA Cancer J Clin* 2017;67(1):7–30.

3 Detel C, Ferlay J, Franceschi S, *et al.* Global burden of cancers attributable to infections in 2008: a review and synthetic analysis. *Lancet Oncol* 2012;13(6):607–15.

4 Brinton LA, Li JY, Rong SD, *et al.* Risk factors for penile cancer: results from a case-control study in China. *Int J Cancer* 1991;47(4):504–9.

5 Saibishkumar EP, Crook J, Sweet J. Neonatal circumcision and invasive squamous cell carcinoma of the penis: a report of 3 cases and a review of the literature. *Can Urol Assoc J* 2008;2(1):39–42.

6 Daling JR, Madeleine MM, Johnson LG, *et al.* Penile cancer: importance of circumcision, human papillomavirus and smoking in in situ and invasive disease. *Int J Cancer* 2005;116(4):606–16.

7 Bleeker MC, Heideman DA, Snijders PJ, *et al.* Penile cancer: epidemiology, pathogenesis and prevention. *World J Urol* 2009;27(2):141–50.

8 Bezerra AL, Lopes A, Santiago GH, *et al.* Human papillomavirus as a prognostic factor in carcinoma of the penis: analysis of 82 patients treated with amputation and bilateral lymphadenectomy. *Cancer* 2001;91(12):2315–21.

9 Picconi MA, Eijan AM, Distefano AL, *et al.* Human papillomavirus (HPV) DNA in penile carcinomas in Argentina: analysis of primary tumors and lymph nodes. *J Med Virol* 2000;61(1):65–9.

10 Graham S, Priore R, Graham M, *et al.* Genital cancer in wives of penile cancer patients. *Cancer* 1979;44(5):1870–4.

11 Martinez I. Relationship of squamous cell carcinoma of the cervix uteri to squamous cell carcinoma of the penis among Puertorican women married to men with penile carcinoma. *Cancer* 1969;24(4):777–80.

12 Blomberg M, Friis S, Munk C, Bautz A, Kjaer SK. Genital warts and risk of cancer: a Danish study of nearly 50 000 patients with genital warts. *J Infect Dis* 2012;205(10):1544–53.

13 Clouston D, Hall A, Lawrentschuk N. Penile lichen sclerosus (balanitis xerotica obliterans). *BJU Int* 2011;108(Suppl 2): 14–19.

14 Figliuolo G, Maia J, Jalkh AP, Miranda AE, Ferreira LC. Prevalence of and risk factors for penile infection by high-risk human papillomavirus among men infected with HIV. *J Med Virol* 2013;85(3):413–18.

15 Dillner J, von Krogh G, Horenblas S, Meijer CJ. Etiology of squamous cell carcinoma of the penis. *Scand J Urol Nephrol Suppl* 2000;205:189–93.

16 Minhas S, Manseck A, Watya S, Hegarty PK. Penile cancer–prevention and premalignant conditions. *Urology* 2010;76(2 Suppl 1):S24–35.

17 Cubilla AL, Dillner J, Schellhammer P. Tumors of the penis: malignant epithelial tumours. In: JN Eble (ed.) *World Health Organization Classification of Tumours: Pathology & Genetics of Tumours of the Urinary System and Male Genital Organs.* Lyon: International Agency for Research on Cancer, 2004:279–90.

18 Chaux A, Velazquez EF, Barreto JE, Ayala E, Cubilla AL. New pathologic entities in penile carcinomas: an update of the 2004 world health organization classification. *Semin Diagn Pathol* 2012;29(2):59–66.

19 Chaux A, Amin M, Cubilla AL, Young RH. Metastatic tumors to the penis: a report of 17 cases and review of the literature. *Int J Surg Pathol* 2011;19(5):597–606.

20 Porter WM, Francis N, Hawkins D, Dinneen M, Bunker CB. Penile intraepithelial neoplasia: clinical spectrum and treatment of 35 cases. *Br J Dermatol* 2002;147(6):1159–65.

21 Kayes O, Ahmed HU, Arya M, Minhas S. Molecular and genetic pathways in penile cancer. *Lancet Oncol* 2007;8(5):420–9.

22 Longpre MJ, Lange PH, Kwon JS, Black PC. Penile carcinoma: lessons learned from vulvar carcinoma. *J Urol* 2013;189(1):17–24.

23 Zhu Y, Zhou XY, Yao XD, Dai B, Ye DW. The prognostic significance of p53, Ki-67, epithelial cadherin and matrix metalloproteinase-9 in penile squamous cell carcinoma treated with surgery. *BJU Int* 2007;100(1):204–8.

24 Lopes A, Bezerra AL, Pinto CA, *et al.* P53 as a New prognostic factor for lymph node metastasis in penile carcinoma: analysis of 82 patients treated with amputation and bilateral lymphadenectomy. *J Urol* 2002;168(1):81–6.

25 Bethune G, Campbell J, Rocker A, *et al.* Clinical and pathologic factors of prognostic significance in penile squamous cell carcinoma in a North American population. *Urology* 2012;79(5):1092–7.

26 Heyns CF, Mendoza-Valdes A, Pompeo AC. Diagnosis and staging of penile cancer. *Urology* 2010;76(2 Suppl 1):S15–23.

27 Leijte JA, Valdes Olmos RA, Nieweg OE, Horenblas S. Anatomical mapping of lymphatic drainage in penile carcinoma with SPECT-CT: implications for the extent of inguinal lymph node dissection. *Eur Urol* 2008;54(4):885–90.

28 Pizzocaro G, Algaba F, Horenblas S, *et al.* EAU penile cancer guidelines 2009. *Eur Urol* 2010;57(6):1002–12.

29 Pettaway CA, Srigley JR, Brookland RK, *et al.* Penis. In: Amin MB. *AJCC Cancer Staging Manual*, 8th edn. New York: Springer, 2017.

30 Kayes O, Minhas S, Allen C, *et al.* The role of magnetic resonance imaging in the local staging of penile cancer. *Eur Urol* 2007;51(5):1313–8; discussion 1318–9.

31 Ficarra V, Akduman B, Bouchot O, Palou J, Tobias-Machado M. Prognostic factors in penile cancer. *Urology* 2010;76 (2 Suppl 1):S66–73.

32 Ornellas AA, Seixas AL,ota A, *et al.* Surgical treatment of invasive squamous cell carcinoma of the penis: retrospective analysis of 350 cases. *J Urol* 1994;151(5):1244–9.

33 Fraley EE, Zhang G, Manivel C, Niehans GA. The role of ilioinguinal lymphadenectomy and significance of histological differentiation in treatment of carcinoma of the penis. *J Urol* 1989;142(6):1478–82.

34 Crook J, Ma C, Grimard L. Radiation therapy in the management of the primary penile tumor: an update. *World J Urol* 2009;27(2):189–96.

35 Heyns CF, Fleshner N, Sangar V, *et al.* Management of the lymph nodes in penile cancer. *Urology* 2010;76(2 Suppl 1): S43–57.

36 Alnajjar HM, Lam W, Bolgeri M, *et al.* Treatment of carcinoma in situ of the glans penis with topical chemotherapy agents. *Eur Urol* 2012;62(5):923–8.

37 Minhas S, Kayes O, Hegarty P, *et al.* What surgical resection margins are required to achieve oncological control in men with primary penile cancer? *BJU Int* 2005;96(7):1040–3.

38 Mohs FE, Snow SN, Larson PO. Mohs micrographic surgery for penile tumors. *Urol Clin North Am* 1992;19(2):291–304.

39 Shindel AW, Mann MW, Lev RY, *et al.* Mohs micrographic surgery for penile cancer: management and long-term followup. *J Urol* 2007;178(5):1980–5.

40 Schlenker B, Tilki D, Seitz M, *et al.* Organ-preserving neodymium-yttrium-aluminium-garnet laser therapy for penile carcinoma: a long-term follow-up. *BJU Int* 2010;106(6):786–90.

41 Meijer RP, Boon TA, van Venrooij GE, Wijburg CJ. Long-term follow-up after laser therapy for penile carcinoma. *Urology* 2007;69(4):759–62.

42 Smith Y, Hadway P, Biedrzycki O, *et al.* Reconstructive surgery for invasive squamous carcinoma of the glans penis. *Eur Urol* 2007;52(4):1179–85.

43 Veeratterapillay R, Sahadevan K, Aluru P, *et al.* Organ-preserving surgery for penile cancer: description of techniques and surgical outcomes. *BJU Int* 2012;110(11):1792–5.

44 Shabbir M, Muneer A, Kalsi J, *et al.* Glans resurfacing for the treatment of carcinoma in situ of the penis: surgical technique and outcomes. *Eur Urol* 2011;59(1):142–7.

45. Palminteri E, Berdondini E, Lazzeri M, Mirri F, Barbagli G. Resurfacing and reconstruction of the glans penis. *Eur Urol* 2007;52(3):893–8.

46 O'Kane HF, Pahuja A, Ho KJ, *et al.* Outcome of glansectomy and skin grafting in the management of penile cancer. *Adv Urol* 2011;2011:240824.

47 McLean M, Akl AM, Warde P, *et al.* The results of primary radiation therapy in the management of squamous cell carcinoma of the penis. *Int J Radiat Oncol Biol Phys* 1993;25(4):623–8.

48 Sarin R, Norman AR, Steel GG, Horwich A. Treatment results and prognostic factors in 101 men treated for squamous carcinoma of the penis. *Int J Radiat Oncol Biol Phys* 1997 1;38(4):713–22.

49 Azrif M, Logue JP, Swindell R, *et al.* External-beam radiotherapy in T1-2 N0 penile carcinoma. *Clin Oncol (R Coll Radiol)* 2006;18(4):320–5.

50 Ravi R, Chaturvedi HK, Sastry DV. Role of radiation therapy in the treatment of carcinoma of the penis. *Br J Urol* 1994;74(5):646–51.

51 Crook J, Jezioranski J, Cygler JE. Penile brachytherapy: technical aspects and postimplant issues. *Brachytherapy* 2010;9(2):151–8.

52. Crook J. Radiation therapy for cancer of the penis. *Urol Clin North Am* 2010;37(3):435–43.

53 de Crevoisier R, Slimane K, Sanfilippo N, *et al.* Long-term results of brachytherapy for carcinoma of the penis confined to the glans (N- or NX). *Int J Radiat Oncol Biol Phys* 2009 15;74(4):1150 6.

54 Crook J, Ma C, Grimard L. Radiation therapy in the management of the primary penile tumor: an update. *World J Urol* 2009;27(2):189–96.

55 Delannes M, Malavaud B, Douchez J, Bonnet J, Daly NJ. Iridium-192 interstitial therapy for squamous cell carcinoma of the penis. *Int J Radiat Oncol Biol Phys* 1992;24(3):479–83.

56 Gomez-Iturriaga A, Crook J, Evans W, Saibishkumar EP, Jezioranski J. The efficacy of hyperbaric oxygen therapy in the treatment of medically refractory soft tissue necrosis after penile brachytherapy. *Brachytherapy* 2011;10(6):491–7.

57 Rozan R, Albuisson E, Giraud B, *et al.* Interstitial brachytherapy for penile carcinoma: a multicentric survey (259 patients). *Radiother Oncol* 1995;36(2):83–93.

58 Protzel C, Alcaraz A, Horenblas S, *et al.* Lymphadenectomy in the surgical management of penile cancer. *Eur Urol* 2009;55(5):1075–88.

59 Kunos C, Simpkins F, Gibbons H, Tian C, Homesley H. Radiation therapy compared with pelvic node resection for node-positive vulvar cancer: a randomized controlled trial. *Obstet Gynecol* 2009;114(3):537–46.

60 Homesley HD, Bundy BN, Sedlis A, Adcock L. Radiation therapy versus pelvic node resection for carcinoma of the vulva with positive groin nodes. *Obstet Gynecol* 1986;68(6):733–40.

61 Franks KN, Kancherla K, Sethugavalar B, *et al.* Radiotherapy for node positive penile cancer: experience of the Leeds teaching hospitals. *J Urol* 2011;186(2):524–9.

62 Pagliaro LC, Williams DL, Daliani D, *et al.* Neoadjuvant paclitaxel, ifosfamide, and cisplatin chemotherapy for metastatic penile cancer: a phase II study. *J Clin Oncol* 2010 20;28(24):3851–7.

63 Haas GP, Blumenstein BA, Gagliano RG, *et al.* Cisplatin, methotrexate and bleomycin for the treatment of carcinoma of the penis: a Southwest Oncology Group study. *J Urol* 1999;161(6):1823–5.

64 Moore DH, Ali S, Koh WJ, *et al.* A phase II trial of radiation therapy and weekly cisplatin chemotherapy for the treatment of locally-advanced squamous cell carcinoma of the vulva: a gynecologic oncology group study. *Gynecol Oncol* 2012;124(3):529–33.

65 Crook J. Radiotherapy approaches for locally advanced penile cancer: neoadjuvant and adjuvant. *Curr Opin Urol* 2017;27(1):62–7.

66 Di Lorenzo G, Federico P, Buonerba C, *et al.* Paclitaxel in pretreated metastatic penile cancer: final results of a phase 2 study. *Eur Urol* 2011;60(6):1280–4.

67 Di Lorenzo G, Buonerba C, Ferro M, *et al.* The epidermal growth factor receptors as biological agents in penile cancer. *Expert Opin Biol Ther* 2015;15(4):473–6.

68 Brown A, Ma Y, Danenberg K, *et al.* Epidermal growth factor receptor-target therapy in squamous cell carcinoma of the penis: a report of 3 cases. *Urology* 2014;83(1):159–65.

69 Romero FR, Romero KR, Mattos MA, *et al.* Sexual function after partial penectomy for penile cancer. *Urology* 2005;66(6):1292–5.

70 Windahl T, Skeppner E, Andersson SO, Fugl-Meyer KS. Sexual function and satisfaction in men after laser treatment for penile carcinoma. *J Urol* 2004;172(2):648–51.

71 Crook JM, Jezioranski J, Grimard L, Esche B, Pond G. Penile brachytherapy: results for 49 patients. *Int J Radiat Oncol Biol Phys* 2005;62(2):460–7.

72 Mazeron JJ, Langlois D, Lobo PA, *et al.* Interstitial radiation therapy for carcinoma of the penis using iridium 192 wires: the Henri Mondor experience (1970–1979). *Int J Radiat Oncol Biol Phys* 1984;10(10):1891–5.

73 Maddineni SB, Lau MM, Sangar VK. Identifying the needs of penile cancer sufferers: a systematic review of the quality of life, psychosexual and psychosocial literature in penile cancer. *BMC Urol* 2009;9:8-2490-9-8.

74 Cordoba A, Escande A, Lopez S, Mortier L, *et al.* Low-dose brachytherapy for early stage penile cancer: a 20-year single-institution study (73 patients). *Radiat Oncol* 2016;11:96.

75 Gotsadze D, Matveev B, Zak B, Mamaladze V. Is conservative organ-sparing treatment of penile carcinoma justified? *Eur Urol* 2000;38(3):306–12.

Section 7

Breast Cancer

28

Breast Cancer, Including Brief Discussion of Male Breast Cancer

Elisavet Paplomata[1] and Ruth O'Regan[2]

[1] Winship Cancer Institute of Emory University, Atlanta, Georgia, USA
[2] University of Wisconsin School of Medicine and Public Health, Madison, Wisconsin, USA

Incidence, Mortality, and Survival

Breast cancer is the most common malignancy and the leading cause of cancer-related deaths among women worldwide [1]. In the United States (US) and in developed countries overall it is the most common cancer and the second most common cause of cancer-related death [2, 3]. Approximately 252,710 women will be diagnosed and an estimated 40,610 women will die of breast cancer in the US in 2017 [3]. The incidence of breast cancer increased during the 1980s, mainly reflecting increased detection with mammography screening [3]. The incidence of breast cancer declined during the 2000s, despite the more widespread use of screening; this may be due to the reduced use of menopausal hormone therapy [4]. However, it is still estimated one in eight women will be diagnosed with breast cancer sometime in their life. Survival rates have improved in the past decades. The overall 5-year relative survival rate for all stages has improved to 90.6% for women diagnosed during 2008, from 75.2% for those diagnosed during 1975. The 5-year relative survival rate is 98.9% for patients diagnosed with localized disease, however survival drops to 26.9% in patients diagnosed with distant metastases [5].

Risk Factors

Age, Gender, and Race

The risk of breast cancer increases significantly with increasing age and female gender. The median age at diagnosis is 62 years [5]. Approximately 1% of breast cancers occur in men. [3] Male breast cancer is more commonly estrogen receptor positive and is often associated with genetic predisposition, occupational or radiation exposure, and estrogen excess [6].

African American women have a lower incidence of breast cancer than White women, however survival rates are worse among Black women (5-year survival rates 80% versus 91% among White women, from 2005 to 2011). African American women are more likely to be diagnosed at a more advanced stage but they also have poorer survival rates within each stage, possibly due to socioeconomic factors [7]. Cancer at a younger age and triple-negative histology are also more common among African American women [8]. The combination of genetic predisposition and lifestyle is probably contributing to the higher incidence among White women, for example use of hormone replacement therapy, access to screening, older age of first pregnancy, and age of menarche (Table 28.1).

Exogenous and Endogenous Hormones

It has been reported that women who have early age of menarche, late age of menopause, age of first pregnancy older than 35 years, or are nulliparous are at increased risk. All these factors are related to hormonal factors and ovulation.

Preclinical data indicate that a full-term pregnancy leads to differentiation of the mammary glands, decrease of the metabolic rate, and resistance to malignant transformation [9]. The net effect of pregnancy is a short-term increase and long-term decrease in risk [10]. The risk of breast cancer increases with every year of delayed childbirth until the age of 35; it is also reported that the closer timing of subsequent pregnancies can decrease risk [11]. The association between breast cancer risk and infertility or infertility treatments has been unclear [12, 13].

Breastfeeding has been shown to decrease risk due to delayed resumption of ovulation after delivery [14], and delayed menopause has been associated with increased cancer risk of approximately 3% every year [15]. Hormone therapy consisting of a combination of estrogen and progestin is also associated with increased risk of breast cancer and mortality, regardless of menopausal status [16]. The risk is slightly increased (relative rate of 1.6) when taking estrogen-only containing hormonal therapy. The risk decreases after the cessation of treatment and returns to baseline after 5 years [17].

Lifestyle

The role of obesity seems to be related to menopausal status. Postmenopausal women who have gained >10 kg are at increased risk [18]. This may be related to the higher levels of circulating

The American Cancer Society's Oncology in Practice: Clinical Management, First Edition. Edited by The American Cancer Society.

Table 28.1 Risk factors for developing breast cancer.

Nonmodifiable	Modifiable
Age	Exogenous hormones
Female gender	Nulliparity or first full-term pregnancy >35 years old
White race	High-fat diet
Family history	Obesity
Early menarche	Alcohol
Late menopause	Inactive lifestyle
Radiation exposure	Breastfeeding (protective)
BRCA1 and *BRCA2, PTEN, TP53* mutations	
Benign breast disease	
Prior biopsies	
Breast density	

estrogens in women with high body mass index (BMI). Alcohol intake has been strongly associated with the risk of developing breast cancer and higher risk of recurrence. The consumption of one alcoholic drink a day can increase the risk up to 7%, regardless of the type of beverage [15]. Physical inactivity has been associated with increased risk but the role of high-fat diet is less clear.

Radiation

Exposure to ionizing radiation at a young age, such as chest irradiation for the treatment of Hodgkin disease, or surviving a nuclear bombing or nuclear accident, is also associated with a high risk of developing breast cancer.

Genetic Predisposition

Family history of breast cancer, especially in first-degree relatives, strongly affects the risk of breast cancer. The age at diagnosis is also very important. Having a first-degree relative diagnosed under the age of 30 increases the risk by threefold; the risk is only increased 1.5-fold if the relative is diagnosed after the age of 60.

Less than 10% of breast cancers are related to inherited genes, such as the breast cancer susceptibility gene (*BRCA*) 1 or 2, phosphatase and tensin homolog (*PTEN*), and tumor protein 53 (*TP53*). *BRCA1* and *BRCA2* are tumor suppressor genes, which are involved in the maintenance of the integrity of the genome, and their functions include the repair of double-stranded DNA breaks. Over one thousand different mutations of *BRCA 1* and *2* have been reported, thus it is very important to test an afflicted family member prior to screening relatives. Germline mutations of *BRCA 1* and *2* are inherited in an autosomal dominant manner and loss of a wild allele results in genomic instability and tumorigenesis [19]. Carriers are at increased risk of developing breast and ovarian cancer; the overall risk of developing breast cancer for *BRCA1* carriers is 80%, and ovarian cancer 30–40%, while the risk is slightly less with *BRCA2* mutations, 50% and 10–15% respectively. Having a family history of breast cancer is not necessarily associated with an inherited mutation, but it increases the risk of breast cancer by twofold. Patients who are young at diagnosis, who are diagnosed with breast and ovarian malignancies, who have multiple relatives affected at a young age, and patients with a male relative with breast cancer should be referred for genetic counseling [20].

Benign and Noninvasive Breast Disease

The history of benign breast disease, prior breast biopsies, and dense breasts by mammography are also linked to higher risk. Breast density may be genetically determined and is inversely associated with fat content. High density at first screening may be accompanied by an increase of risk up to five times. Having a breast biopsy before the age of 50–55 years increases the risk up to fivefold. Having a benign breast disorder, which includes proliferative changes and/or atypia, further increases the risk of developing breast cancer [21]. A personal history of breast cancer or ductal carcinoma *in situ* (DCIS) increases the risk of having breast cancer in the contralateral breast or a second primary breast cancer in the ipsilateral breast.

Prevention

Lifestyle modifications can decrease a woman's risk of breast cancer. Surgery or chemoprevention can be considered for women at high risk, such as carriers of *BRCA* mutations or as determined by risk determination models.

There are several models that predict the risk of developing breast cancer. The modified Gail model is the most widely used tool to calculate the absolute risk of developing invasive or *in situ* breast cancer. This model includes variables such as age, age at menarche, age at first full-term pregnancy, family history, prior breast biopsies, and history of hyperplasia with atypia [22]. The model has also been validated for African Americans [23].

Carriers of *BRCA* mutations can be counseled on bilateral mastectomy, which decreases the risk of breast cancer by over 90% in these patients. Bilateral salpingo-oophorectomy additionally decreases the risk of ovarian and fallopian tube malignancies. Prophylactic contralateral mastectomy can also decrease the risk of new primary breast cancers in selected patients with sporadic tumors. However, the recognition of the patients who will benefit from a prophylactic mastectomy is challenging, and the discussion should include the absolute risk of cancer involved and the risks associated with the operation [24].

The selective estrogen receptor modulators (SERMs) tamoxifen and raloxifene reduce the incidence of primary invasive breast cancer when taken for 5 years (7–9 cases per 1,000) [25]. These SERMs reduced the risk of hormone receptor-positive breast cancer but did not decrease the risk of hormone receptor-negative or noninvasive cancer and did not reduce mortality. The risk reduction was noted not only during the active treatment period but also during follow-up for up to 10 years. Women with the highest risk and those previously diagnosed with atypical hyperplasia gained the most benefit from chemoprevention. Both drugs increased the risk of thromboembolic events and tamoxifen was also clearly associated with an increased risk of endometrial cancer. Even though a head-to-head comparison of tamoxifen and raloxifene reported that tamoxifen was more effective in preventing the development of breast cancer, raloxifene had less toxicity [26].

Anastrozole was reported to reduce breast cancer risk by 53% compared to placebo in postmenopausal women at high risk. The benefit included invasive disease, estrogen receptor-positive disease, and *in situ* tumors [27]. Exemestane was also shown to be effective as chemoprevention in postmenopausal women [28]. The use of aromatase inhibitors in primary prevention needs to be further evaluated and their use has not yet been established.

Screening

Mammography remains the main modality of screening for breast cancer. Film and digital mammography have similar efficacy but digital mammography may be more accurate in patients who are pre- or peri-menopausal and who have dense breasts. The United States Preventive Services Task Force (USPSTF) recommends biennial screening mammography for women ages 50–74 and also stated that the decision to begin screening before age 50 should be individualized.[29] The ACS recommends that (i) women undergo regular screening mammography starting at age 45 years, (ii) women aged 45–54 years should be screened annually, (iii) women should have the opportunity to begin annual screening between ages 40 and 44 years, (iv) women aged ≥55 years should transition to biennial screening or have the opportunity to continue screening annually, and (v) women should continue screening mammography as long as their overall health is good and they have a life expectancy ≥10 years [30, 31].

Ultrasonography is often used for the evaluation of palpable masses and guidance for core biopsies but it has not been validated as a screening tool alone, or in combination with mammography.

Magnetic resonance imaging (MRI) has been found to be more sensitive but less specific in detecting invasive cancers and is associated with high cost. Studies support that women with high risk for breast cancer (genetic predisposition, history of radiation exposure) should be screened with annual MRI in addition to mammography [32]. Women who are *BRCA* positive should be referred for genetic counseling and educated on options to decrease their risk surgically and also for methods of intensified surveillance. The current screening recommendation for women who are *BRCA* carriers is the combination of annual mammography and annual MRI. Other risk groups who benefit from MRI screening are patients who have received chest radiation before the age of 30, who have genetic mutations of *TP53* and *PTEN*, first-degree relatives of *BRCA* carriers, and women with a lifetime risk of more than 20–25% [31].

Studies on breast self-examination have failed to show a survival benefit; breast self-examination is not currently recommended as a preferred method of breast cancer screening.

Screening can have negative effects, including false positives, unnecessary biopsies, overdiagnosis and overtreatment, which are associated with financial and health outcomes for the patients. For more information refer to *The American Cancer Society's Oncology in Practice: Clinical Management*, Chapter 11.

Pathology of Breast Cancer

Histologic Subtypes

Most breast cancers are carcinomas, which arise from the epithelium. The *in situ* carcinomas are classified as ductal or lobular; most invasive carcinomas are infiltrating ductal, followed by lobular, ductal/lobular, mucinous (colloid), medullary or papillary histologies. Other subtypes are rare and comprise less than 5% of cases (Table 28.2). Infiltrating ductal carcinoma (IDC) comprises 70–80% of invasive breast cancers. IDC can be subdivided into well differentiated (grade 1), moderately differentiated (grade 2), or poorly differentiated (grade 3). Ductal carcinomas are usually firm masses comprising of cells growing in tubules and/or sheets.

Infiltrating lobular carcinoma is the second most common type of breast cancer and accounts for 5–10% of cases. It tends to be multifocal or bilateral and sometimes presents with no evident mass. Prognosis is generally the same as IDC. Lobular carcinomas typically stain negative for E-cadherin; they are more commonly hormone receptor (HR) positive and rarely human epidermal growth factor receptor-2 (HER2) positive [33].

Tubular carcinomas are rare tumors. They are usually HR positive and HER2 negative; they have excellent prognosis and rarely metastasize. Invasive cribriform and mucinous carcinomas are also rare and have a favorable prognosis compared to IDC. Invasive micropapillary carcinoma is seen in less than 2% of cases; it is usually diagnosed at an advanced stage and is associated with a poor prognosis. Metaplastic breast carcinoma is seen in less than 1% of cases and is believed to be a variant of ductal carcinoma. It can consist of matrix-producing, squamous cells, spindle cells, or osteoclastic-like giant cells. Metaplastic carcinoma is most often seen in women over the age of 50; it is usually ER/PR negative and can be HER2 positive in up to 46% of the cases. Prognosis is worse compared to the typical IDC [34]. Inflammatory breast cancer is characterized by inflammatory changes of the skin of the breast and its invasive component microscopically most commonly reveals an IDC [33].

Hormone Receptors

Approximately two-thirds of breast cancers express estrogen and/or progesterone receptors (ER/PR). The most commonly used assay to evaluate ER/PR status is immunohistochemistry (IHC), which can be performed on paraffin-embedded tissues or cytologic preparations; the presence of at least 1% staining nuclei defines HR-positive disease.

The estrogen receptor (ER) belongs to the steroid/thyroid nuclear receptor family and consists of ER-alpha and ER-beta, which are transcribed by different genes and are thought to have distinct functions. ER-alpha was described first, and it is often used interchangeably with ER in the literature, since the functions of ER-beta have not been completely elucidated. The ER is activated when bound to estrogen, and subsequently leads to phosphorylation, dimerization, and activation of estrogen response elements (ERE), which are located on the promoter target genes [35]. The presence of ER is usually associated with slower growing and well-differentiated tumors and it predicts response to hormonal therapy.

Table 28.2 Histologic subtypes of breast cancer and effect on prognosis compared to IDC NOS.

Histologic type (frequency)	Features	Prognosis
Invasive ductal carcinoma (IDC), not otherwise specified (NOS) (70–80%)	Firm mass, cells grow in sheets or trabeculae	
Invasive lobular carcinoma (5–10%)	May be firm, mass may be absent. Negative for E-cadherin. Usually ER/PR+ and HER2−	Same as IDC
Invasive tubular carcinoma (7.7–27%)	Firm mass, tubules with single layer or epithelial cells. Usually ER/PR+ and HER2−	Excellent
Invasive cribriform carcinoma (1–3%)	Mass may be well defined, with stellate/gray surface. Cells in a cribriform structure, occasional giant cells	Favorable
Invasive mucinous carcinoma (2%)	Well-defined mass with soft surface. Nest-forming cells, presence of mucin. Usually ER/PR+ and HER2−. May be associated with neuroendocrine features	Favorable
Invasive medullary (<1%)	Well-defined mass, no glandular structures, presence of lymphoplasmacytic infiltration, usually HR−	Uncertain
Invasive micropapillary carcinoma (<2%)	Cells form tubular nests, common LVI and lymph node metastases	Poor
Invasive metaplastic carcinoma (<1%)	May be associated with necrosis, consists of squamous, osteoclastic, matrix-producing, carcinosarcomatous or spindle cells. Often ER/PR−, up to 46% may express HER2	Worse than IDC
Invasive apocrine carcinoma (<1%)	Cells with abundant eosinophilic cytoplasm, large nuclei, prominent nucleoli. ER/PR−, up to 50% HER2 +	Favorable
Invasive papillary carcinoma (<2%)	Often associated with IDC. Usually ER/PR+, HER2−	Favorable
Invasive adenoid cystic (0.1%)	Well-circumscribed nodular masses. Cells form tubules, nests, or cribriform areas	Excellent

ER/PR, estrogen receptor/progesterone receptor; HER2, human epidermal growth factor receptor 2; IDC, invasive ductal carcinoma; LVI, lymphovascular invasion; NOS, not otherwise specified.

The progesterone receptor (PR) gene is dependent on estrogen and more than 50% of breast cancers are PR positive. It is unclear why the progesterone receptor is lost in some tumors or metastatic sites but there are clinical data suggesting that hormone therapy is less effective in tumors that are ER positive/PR negative. PR-negative tumors may be larger, may exhibit a more aggressive clinical behavior, and can be associated with worse outcomes [36, 37].

HER2 (ERBB2)

HER2 belongs to the family of epidermal growth factor receptors (EGFR), which includes HER1, HER2, HER3, and HER4. The HER2 receptor consists of an extracellular, a transmembrane, and an intracellular tyrosine kinase domain. HER2 does not have an identifiable ligand but it has the tendency to heterodimerize with other growth factor receptors and thus activates intracellular downstream pathways, such as mitogen activating protein kinase (*MAPK*) and phosphatidylinositol 3-kinase (*PI3K*) [38]. HER2 is overexpressed in approximately 20% of breast cancers and it is associated with shorter disease-free survival and overall survival [39]. The use of targeted agents has significantly improved outcomes in patients with HER2-positive breast cancer [40].

All newly diagnosed patients or patients who develop metastatic disease should be tested for HER2. HER2 is reported positive when a specimen has a score of +3 by immunohistochemistry, and negative if the score is 0 or +1. A score of +2 is considered equivocal and requires reflex testing with an alternate test or testing of a new specimen.

The ISH (*in situ* hybridization) score is reported as single-probe average *HER2* copy numbers or dual-probe *HER*/CEP17 ratio (the ratio of *HER2* to the centromeric portion of chromosome 17). A positive result is an average of *HER2* copy number of ≥6 signals/cell or *HER2*/CEP17 ratio of ≥2. A ratio of <2 in the presence of ≥6 signals/cell is also considered positive. A negative result is based on a *HER2* copy number of <4 signals/cell, while an equivocal test is a single-probe average *HER2* copy number of ≥4 but <6 signals/cell [41]. If ISH was performed first and is equivocal, the recommendation is to perform IHC or test a new sample.

All patients with positive HER2 testing should be considered for HER2-directed therapy in the adjuvant and/or metastatic setting.

Intrinsic Molecular Subtypes

Breast tumors are classified into HR-positive, HER2-positive, or triple-negative (no ER, PR, or HER2 expression) based on hormone and HER2 receptor status; however, even within these groups, breast cancer is heterogeneous. As a result of an attempt to decipher breast cancer biology, cDNA microarrays revealed that breast tumors could further be subclassified as basal-like, ERBB2-positive, normal breast-like, and luminal subtype A and B. The basal-like subtype is accompanied by a high rate of *TP53* mutations and mostly overlaps with the triple-negative tumors. *BRCA1*-positive tumors also mostly fall into that subtype. The basal-like subtype is clinically associated with the worst overall and relapse-free survival. The ERBB2 subtype shows a high expression of HER2 and high rate of *TP53* mutations and is also associated with inferior outcomes. The normal breast-like tumors express genes similar to adipose tissue and nonepithelial cell types and they have intermediate prognosis. It is currently unclear if the normal-like subtype exists or if it is a result of contamination from surrounding tissues. The luminal subtypes are hormone receptor positive and they can be further subclassified according to the degree of HR positivity. The luminal A subtype is characterized by strong expression of ER, while the luminal B subtype has low or moderate ER expression. Luminal A tumors are linked to the best outcomes [42–45].

Diagnosis

Most breast cancers will be found during screening with an abnormal mammogram. Rarely, a woman will discover a palpable mass accidentally or during a self-examination.

If a woman less than 30 years old has a palpable mass, it is usually recommended to proceed with an ultrasound, while women over the age of 30 should also have a bilateral mammogram. Ultrasonography will distinguish a solid versus a cystic mass, and simple versus complicated versus complex cysts. In general, simple cysts are followed by imaging and complicated cysts may be followed by imaging or aspirated. Tissue evaluation by core biopsy or fine-needle aspiration (FNA) is recommended for complex cysts and cysts that recur and/or contain hemorrhagic fluid [46]. A solid mass also needs to be evaluated with a biopsy. A core biopsy offers more tissue and is generally preferable to an FNA [46, 47].

Mammographic findings are reported according to the Breast Imaging Reporting and Data System (BI-RADS), which was developed by the American College of Radiology to decrease inconsistency among users. A BI-RADS category 0 means an incomplete evaluation that requires further imaging with additional views. A BI-RADS category 1 or 2 signifies benign or no findings and regular follow-up can resume. A BI-RADS category 3 means that the findings are probably benign but a shorter interval screening is recommended (usually 6 months). BI-RADS category 4 and 5 findings are suspicious or highly suspicious for malignancy, respectively [48]. If an abnormality is found on a screening mammogram in the absence of a palpable mass, additional views and/or an ultrasound are often obtained. Suspicious masses are usually spiculated and poorly defined, and they may be associated with microcalcifications or distorted architecture. A nonpalpable mass is usually biopsied under ultrasound guidance or with a stereotactic biopsy. An axillary ultrasound can also help identify and aid in the biopsy of suspicious lymph nodes [49].

MRI is more sensitive than mammography and it can help identify ipsilateral foci and contralateral synchronous breast tumors. These findings can lead to overestimation of the extent of the disease, more aggressive surgery, and overtreatment of lesions that might have never been clinically significant [50]. MRI has not been shown to impact overall survival and it is thus not routinely recommended. However there are individualized cases where preoperative MRI may prove useful, such as high-risk patients, where the risk of contralateral breast cancer is very high, patients who present with an axillary mass and no palpable breast abnormality, patients who have implants that interfere with conventional imaging, and evaluation of response to neoadjuvant chemotherapy [51].

Staging/Evaluation

After the pathologic diagnosis of breast cancer is established, the clinician should proceed with clinical staging evaluation when indicated. It is always recommended to obtain a history and physical examination, complete blood count, and chemistry for evaluation of liver and renal function. Patients who are at high risk for hereditary cancer should be referred for genetic counseling, and young patients who want to maintain fertility should be referred for fertility counseling. For patients with early-stage disease (I–IIB), additional studies are ordered based on symptoms or laboratory abnormalities. Patients with bone pain or elevated alkaline phosphatase should be evaluated with a bone scan, patients with pulmonary symptoms should have computerized tomography (CT) of the chest, and patients with abdominal symptoms or abnormal liver function tests will get a CT or MRI of the abdomen. The National Comprehensive Cancer Network (NCCN) guidelines recommend against positron emission tomography (PET) or PET-CT imaging in these early-stage patients, as the rate of false negatives is high in patients with small lesions [46]. For patients with locally advanced or metastatic disease, imaging with CT and bone scan (or PET-CT) is indicated to determine the extent of the disease and evaluate response to treatment. All patients should have pathologic evaluation of the tumor including hormone receptor and HER2 status.

PET-CT is generally considered optional by NCCN but is used increasingly in clinical practice. PET-CT is not sensitive for small tumors of less than 1 cm. It has been reported that standardized uptake value (SUV) can correlate with histology (IDC has higher uptake than invasive lobular cancer), grade, tumor proliferation index (Ki-67), and the presence of *TP53* mutations. Imaging cannot substitute for a pathologic diagnosis and all suspicious axillary or distant findings need to be biopsied. PET is especially efficient in diagnosing recurrence in asymptomatic patients and it has been found to be superior to conventional techniques in that setting. The NCCN recommends to monitor patients for recurrence using a consistent technique [52].

The eighth edition of the tumor node metastasis (TNM) system is currently used to determine the clinical and pathologic stage of breast cancer (Table 28.3) [53].The pathologic staging is designated as pTNM and if the patient has received neoadjuvant chemotherapy, the pathologic staging is recorded as ypTNM. The use of the staging system facilitates clinical decision-making, provides an estimate of prognosis, and helps communication between treating physicians and researchers. The most recently proposed staging system includes two separate classifications, the anatomic stage groups and prognostic stage groups. The anatomic stage groups are based on tumor size and extent of disease and the prognostic stage group includes the biomarkers tested, grade, receptor status, and genomic testing. HR-positive, HER2-negative tumors with no lymph node involvement and low risk of recurrence based on genomic testing are classified to the same risk category as T1a-b

Table 28.3 TNM staging for breast cancer (anatomic stage groups).

Primary tumor (T)	
T0	No evidence of primary tumor
Tis	Carcinoma *in situ*
Tis (DCIS)	Ductal carcinoma *in situ*
Tis (Paget's)	Paget's disease not associated with invasive component
T1	Tumor ≤2 cm in greatest dimension
T1mi	Tumor ≤0.1 cm in greatest dimension
T1a	Tumor >0.1 cm but ≤0.5 cm in greatest dimension (round any measurement >1.0 – 1.9 mm to 2 mm)
T1b	Tumor >0.5 cm but ≤1 cm in greatest dimension
T1c	Tumor >1 cm but ≤2 cm in greatest dimension
T2	Tumor >2 cm but ≤5 cm in greatest dimension
T3	Tumor >5 cm in greatest dimension
T4	Tumor of any size with direct extension to the chest wall and/or to the skin (ulceration or macroscopic nodules); invasion of the dermis alone does not qualify as T4
T4a	Extension to the chest wall; invasion or adherence to pectoralis muscle in the absence of invasion of chest wall structures does not qualify as T4
T4b	Ulceration and/or ipsilateral macroscopic satellite nodules and/or edema (including peau d'orange) of the skin that does not meet the criteria for inflammatory carcinoma
T4c	Both T4a and T4b
T4d	Inflammatory carcinoma
Regional lymph nodes (N)	
Clinical	
cN0	No regional lymph node metastases
cN1	Metastasis to movable ipsilateral level I, II axillary lymph node(s)
cN2	Metastasis in ipsilateral level I, II axillary lymph nodes that are clinically fixed or matted; or in clinically detected ipsilateral internal mammary (IM) nodes in the *absence* of clinically evident axillary lymph node metastases
cN2a	Metastasis in ipsilateral axillary lymph nodes fixed to one another (matted) or to other structures
cN2b	Metastasis only in clinically detected IM nodes in the *absence* of clinically detected axillary lymph nodes
cN3	Metastasis in ipsilateral infraclavicular (level III axillary) lymph node(s) with or without level I, II axillary lymph node involvement; or in clinically detected ipsilateral IM lymph nodes with clinically evident level I, II axillary lymph node metastasis; or metastasis in ipsilateral supraclavicular lymph node(s) with or without axillary or IM lymph node involvement
cN3a	Metastasis in infraclavicular lymph node(s)
cN3b	Metastasis in internal mammary lymph node(s) and axillary lymph node(s)
cN3c	Metastasis in supraclavicular lymph node(s)
Pathologic (pN)	
pNx	Regional nodes cannot be assessed (e.g., not removed for pathological study or previously removed)
pN0	No regional lymph node metastasis
pN0(i+)	ITCs only (malignant cell clusters no larger than 0.2 mm) in regional lymph node(s)
pN0(mol+)	Positive molecular findings by reverse transcriptase polymerase chain reaction (RT-PCR); no ITCs detected
pN1	Micrometastasis; or metastasis in 1–3 axillary lymph nodes; and/or in IM nodes with metastasis detected by SLN biopsy but not clinically detected
pN1mi	Micrometastases (approximately 200 cells, larger than 0.2 mm, but none larger than 2.0 mm)
pN1a	Metastasis in 1–3 axillary lymph nodes, at least one metastasis greater than 2 mm
pN1b	Metastases in ipsilateral internal mammary sentinel nodes, excluding ITCs
pN1c	pN1a and pN1b combined
pN2	Metastasis in 4–9 axillary lymph nodes; or in clinically detected IM lymph nodes in the *absence* of axillary lymph node metastasis

Table 28.3 (Continued)

pN2a	Metastasis in 4–9 ipsilateral axillary lymph nodes (at least one >2.0 mm)
pN2b	Metastasis in clinically detected IM lymph nodes in the *absence* of axillary lymph node metastasis
pN3	Metastases in 10 or more axillary lymph nodes; or in infraclavicular (level III axillary) lymph nodes; or positive ipsilateral internal mammary lymph nodes by imaging in the presence of one or more positive level I, II axillary lymph nodes; or in more than three axillary lymph nodes and micrometastases or macrometastases by sentinel lymph node biopsy in clinically negative ipsilateral internal mammary lymph nodes; or in ipsilateral supraclavicular lymph nodes
pN3a	Metastasis in ten or more axillary lymph nodes (at least one greater than 2 mm); or metastasis in infraclavicular (level III axillary lymph) nodes
pN3b	pN1a or pN2a in the presence of cN2b (positive internal mammary nodes by imaging); or pN2a in the presence of pN1b
pN3c	Metastasis in ipsilateral supraclavicular lymph nodes

Note: (sn) and (f) suffixes should be added to the N category to denote confirmation of metastasis by sentinel node biopsy or FNA/core needle biopsy respectively, with NO further resection of nodes.

Distant metastases (M)

M0	No clinical or radiographic evidence of distant metastasis
cM0(i+)	No clinical or radiographic evidence of distant metastases in the presence of tumor cells or deposits no larger than 0.2 mm detected microscopically or by molecular techniques in circulating blood, bone marrow, or other nonregional nodal tissue in a patient without symptoms or signs of metastases
M1	Distant metastases detected by clinical and radiographic means (cM) and/or histologically proven metastases larger than 0.2 mm (pM)

Anatomic stage (TNM)

0	Tis	N0	M0
IA	T1	N0	M0
IB	T0	N1mi	M0
	T1	N1mi	M0
IIA	T0	N1	M0
	T1	N1	M0
	T2	N0	M0
IIB	T2	N1	M0
	T3	N0	M0
IIIA	T0	N2	M0
	T1	N2	M0
	T2	N2	M0
	T3	N1	M0
	T3	N2	M0
IIIB	T4	N0	M0
	T4	N1	M0
	T4	N2	M0
IIIC	Any T	N3	M0
IV	Any T	Any N	M1

Source: Hortobagyi 2017 [53]. Used with permission of the American College of Surgeons, Chicago, Illinois. The original source for this information is the *AJCC Cancer Staging Manual*, Eighth Edition (2016), which is published by Springer Science + Business Media.
Tumors >1 mm and <2 mm should be reported rounding to 2 mm.
With multiple synchronous tumors, only the maximum dimension of the largest tumor is utilized for cT and pT; the size of multiple tumors is not added.
H&E, hematoxylin and eosin; RT/PCR, reverse transcriptase/polymerase chain reaction; SLN, sentinel lymph nodes.

tumors regardless of the T size. Cancer registries in the US will be required to use the prognostic stage groups for case reporting. If biomarkers are not available, the cancer will be reported as unstaged.

Prognostic Factors

Anatomic Factors

The most important prognostic factor in breast cancer is stage and the degree of involvement of the lymph nodes; the prognosis worsens as the positive axillary nodes are increased, especially if more than three nodes are involved. Thus, axillary staging with an FNA or during surgery is very important [54]. The presence of involved internal mammary (IM) nodes is also a bad prognostic indicator and the presence of both IM and axillary nodes is worse than metastases to either site alone. In the absence of lymph node involvement, tumor size is the most important prognostic factor. Larger tumors are associated with shorter relapse-free survival and overall survival. Localized disease with tumors less than 1 cm in diameter have a small risk of recurrence, while tumors larger than 1 cm are usually treated with adjuvant therapy to decrease the risk of recurrence [55].

Biology

IDC and invasive lobular carcinoma are the most common histologic subtypes of breast cancer. Other subtypes are uncommon and are usually associated with a favorable prognosis, except for invasive micropapillary carcinoma, which is associated with a very unfavorable prognosis (Table 28.2).

High nuclear and histologic grade, high Ki-67 index, the presence of lymphovascular invasion, and the presence of necrosis are all associated with worse outcomes [56].

Estrogen and/or progesterone receptor-positive tumors are usually more differentiated, grow slowly, and have better outcomes compared to hormone receptor-negative tumors. HR-positive tumors also respond to hormonal therapy. ER-positive/PR-positive tumors have the best prognosis, ER-negative and PR-negative tumors have the worst prognosis, while ER-positive/PR-negative tumors have intermediate prognosis, as there is evidence that these tumors may show resistance to hormonal therapy [37].

HER2 overexpression and the presence of *TP53* mutation are also associated with poor overall survival [57].

Gene expression profiling has distinguished intrinsic molecular subtypes of breast cancer, which correlate with outcomes. Luminal A tumors, which highly express ER, have the best prognosis, while the basal-like and ERBB2-positive subtypes, which coincide with the triple-negative and HER2-overexpressing tumors respectively, have the worst outcomes.

Gene Expression Signatures

The 21-gene recurrence score (Oncotype DX®) is used to predict the likelihood of developing distant metastases in patients with HR-positive, node-negative breast cancer and, more importantly, can determine a subset of these cancers that obtain minimal to no benefit from systemic chemotherapy. Using specimens from the NSABP B-20 trial, which evaluated the addition of systemic chemotherapy to tamoxifen in patients with HR-positive, node-negative breast cancer, approximately 50% of cancers were designated low risk using the 21-gene recurrence score and obtained no significant benefit from the addition of chemotherapy to tamoxifen. In contrast, cancers designated as high risk by the recurrence score assay obtained a significant benefit in preventing the development of distant metastases when chemotherapy was added prior to tamoxifen. Approximately one-quarter of patients with HR-positive, node-negative breast cancer have recurrence scores in the intermediate range. Overall this group does not appear to obtain a significant benefit from the addition of chemotherapy to tamoxifen, and the cut-off score where patients obtain benefit from chemotherapy is being addressed in the TAILORx trial. There are emerging data that the 21-gene recurrence score is prognostic and potentially predictive of chemotherapy benefit in patients with HR-positive, node-positive breast cancer, and this is being addressed in the ongoing RxPONDER trial, in which patients with HR-positive breast cancers with ≤3 involved lymph nodes and a tumor recurrence score of less than 25 are being randomized to endocrine therapy with or without chemotherapy [58]. Oncotype Dx® can be performed with fixed paraffin-embedded tissues.

The 70-gene prognostic score (MammaPrint®) has been shown to be prognostic of outcome in node-negative and node-positive breast cancers. Tumors are classified as having a good prognostic or poor prognostic signature, offering the possible advantage of no intermediate risk group [59]. Initially, this assay had to be performed in fresh tissue, but it is now available for paraffin-embedded specimens. Nonrandomized data suggest that the 70-gene score is potentially predictive of benefit of chemotherapy in early-stage breast cancers, and this hypothesis is being addressed in the MINDACT trial, in which patients with cancers that are discordant by classic prognostic factors and the 70-gene score are randomized to receive chemotherapy or not, along with endocrine therapy where appropriate.

The Breast Cancer Index (BCI) is a newer assay that may have the potential to predict which patients with HR-positive breast cancers are most likely to develop late (more than 5 years from diagnosis) metastases and potentially benefit from extended adjuvant endocrine therapy.

In addition, the Predictor Analysis of Microarray (PAM) 50 and the Genomic Grade Index (GCI) are gene signatures developed to predict response to hormonal therapy and survival in patients with breast cancer [60].

Even though these gene signatures are expensive, they can be cost-effective. The Oncotype DX® assay may identify patients who will not benefit from chemotherapy, thus reducing the cost of treatment and decreasing the rate of therapy-related toxicities.

Surgical Therapy for Early-Stage Breast Cancer

Multiple trials have validated that mastectomy is equivalent to breast-conserving surgery followed by radiation [61]. Breast-conserving surgery has been established as primary surgical treatment for women with early-stage breast cancer, mainly due to the advantage of better cosmetic results and patient preference. However, women with multicentric tumors, diffuse calcifications, inflammatory cancer, and contraindications to radiation therapy (e.g., prior radiation therapy, pregnancy) should still be treated with mastectomy. The goal of breast-sparing surgery is total excision of the tumor with clear margins. Thus, it is recommended to appropriately orient surgical specimens in order to report the margin status and the distance of the tumor from the closest margin.

The management of the axilla is currently evolving. Clinically positive axillary lymph nodes by examination or ultrasound should be assessed with an FNA, or it is standard practice to evaluate sentinel lymph nodes (SLN) during surgery [62, 63]. Patients with negative SLNs need no further axillary dissection. Patients with only 1–2 involved nodes also may not need a dissection, as this has not been shown to improve survival in the Z11 trial [64].

Radiation Therapy

Radiation therapy plays a very significant role in the treatment of breast cancer and it has been shown to decrease local recurrence rates and improve survival in patients undergoing breast-conserving surgery and also in some patients with positive axillary lymph nodes [65].

Radiotherapy was found to reduce the 10-year risk of recurrence from 35% to 19% and also reduced the 15-year risk of breast cancer-related death from 25% to 21% in a large meta-analysis [66]. However, some patients with low risk of local recurrence may not require additional therapy after breast-conserving surgery. The CALGB 9343 trial demonstrated that in women of at least 70 years of age with clinical stage I ER-positive breast cancer, the addition of radiation decreased locoregional recurrence; however this was not translated in advantage in overall survival, distant disease-free survival, or breast preservation. Thus, in this subset of elderly women, treatment with adjuvant hormonal therapy alone is an acceptable option.

Following a mastectomy, adjuvant radiation therapy of the chest wall and regional lymph nodes is indicated in patients with 4 or more positive axillary lymph nodes, with tumors more than 5 cm, and with T4 tumors regardless of lymph node status. Women with 4 or more lymph nodes have a high risk of local recurrence and should receive radiotherapy post mastectomy as standard of care. Radiation should also be considered in patients with 1–3 positive nodes [67].

Patients with characteristics putting them at higher risk of recurrence, such as age <50 years, positive axillary lymph nodes, lymphovascular invasion, and close resection margins, should also have the opportunity to discuss the addition of boost to the tumor bed following standard whole-breast radiation therapy [68].

Radiation therapy is associated with short-term and long-term toxicities. Acute toxicities mainly involve damage to the skin/bone/connective tissue, infections, nerve damage, lung injury, and fat necrosis. Chronic toxicities can happen years after treatment and include cardiotoxicity, lung toxicity, and secondary malignancies [69].

Systemic Therapy for Breast Cancer

All systemic therapy decisions in breast cancer are based on ER, PR, and HER2. Adjuvant treatment of early-stage breast cancer has been demonstrated to decrease the risk of distant recurrence and improve survival [70]. Although the majority of patients receive adjuvant treatment following surgery, increasingly more patients receive systemic treatment prior to surgery using a neoadjuvant approach. Molecular profiling of breast cancers in the early-stage setting is used to tailor systemic therapy appropriately, allowing the omission of systemic chemotherapy in a large number of patients [58]. The use of endocrine agents and HER2-directed therapies has improved the outcome for metastatic HR-positive and HER2-positive cancers, respectively [71].

Adjuvant Therapies for Early-Stage Breast Cancer

Adjuvant Chemotherapy for HER2-Negative Breast Cancer

The use of adjuvant chemotherapy has improved outcome for patients with early-stage breast cancer and is routine for triple-negative (HR-negative, HER2-negative) and a subset of HR-positive breast cancers [70]. The use of molecular profiling for node-negative HR-positive breast cancer has decreased the use of systemic chemotherapy for a subset of patients with these cancers. Systemic chemotherapy remains the standard of care for all node-positive breast cancers and node-negative breast cancers measuring greater than 1 cm if triple-negative, HER2-positive, and HR-positive, if designated as high risk by molecular profiling [72].

One of the first adjuvant regimens for early-stage breast cancer was cyclophosphamide, methotrexate, and 5-fluorouracil (CMF), which remains an option for patients today. CMF was largely replaced by anthracycline-based regimens, based on studies that demonstrated their superiority [73]. A trial that utilized an epirubicin-based regimen demonstrated the benefit of an anthracycline [74]. A large trial failed to show superiority of Adriamycin–Cytoxan (AC) over CMF, but the duration of treatment was shorter; anthracycline-based treatment is the treatment of choice, at least in the US [75]. Even though anthracyclines carry the risk of cardiomyopathy, anthracycline–taxane-based regimens remain widely used, particularly for patients with triple-negative breast cancers. The most commonly used regimen is AC, followed by paclitaxel or docetaxel–Adriamycin–Cytoxan (TAC). Pivotal randomized trials in patients with node-positive breast cancer have demonstrated that AC followed by paclitaxel is superior to AC alone [76, 77]; AC followed by paclitaxel given in a dose-dense manner every 2 weeks is superior to the 3-weekly schedule [78]; and TAC is superior to 5-fluorouracil–Adriamycin–Cytoxan (FAC) [79]. Based on these trials the most widely used regimens for patients with node-positive breast cancer in the US are: (i) TAC every 3 weeks for 6 cycles; (ii) AC followed by paclitaxel, each for 4 cycles given dose dense every 2 weeks; (iii) AC given every 2 or 3 weeks for 4 cycles followed by paclitaxel weekly for 12 weeks. TC every 3 weeks, given for 4 cycles, has been widely accepted as an option for patients with lower- risk node-positive and node-negative breast cancer [80].

In summary, systemic chemotherapy decisions are made based on breast cancer subtype and nodal status, as well as other issues including the patient's age and general health. Regimens that include an anthracycline and taxane are generally preferred for the majority of patients with node-positive HER2-negative breast cancer, though TC is often used in patients with HR-positive breast cancers deemed lower risk by molecular profiling, especially if they have ≤3 positive lymph nodes. Patients with node-negative triple-negative cancers are generally recommended an anthracycline–taxane-based regimen or TC, depending on the perceived risk of recurrence. Chemotherapy can be avoided in more than 50% of HR-positive node-negative breast cancers, when molecular profiling is utilized. For the remaining HR-positive, node-negative breast cancers with higher risk profiles, TC is commonly used.

Molecular Profiling of HR-Positive Breast Cancers

Historically, systemic chemotherapy was widely used to prevent recurrence in patients with HR-positive breast cancers, regardless of nodal status. However, it was clear from meta-analyses that the benefit of systemic chemotherapy was significantly greater in HR-negative breast cancers. Molecular profiling of early-stage breast cancers has markedly decreased the use of systemic chemotherapy for HR-positive, node-negative breast cancers, and is being investigated in HR-positive, node-positive breast cancers.

The 21-gene recurrence score (Oncotype DX®) is the most commonly used tool that predicts the risk of distant recurrence. Patients with a score ≥31 have lower ER expression and higher proliferation indices and benefit from adjuvant chemotherapy. Patients with a score <18 do not benefit from chemotherapy and are treated with adjuvant hormone therapy alone. The management of patients with intermediate scores is currently under investigation.

Several other assays are in development but the 21-gene recurrence score and 70-gene prognostic score are the most widely used.

Adjuvant Therapy for HER2-Positive Breast Cancers

The use of trastuzumab-based chemotherapy has dramatically improved outcome for patients with HER2-positive, early-stage breast cancers. The addition of trastuzumab to paclitaxel following AC in patients with predominantly node-positive, HER2-positive breast cancer significantly decreased recurrence rate and improved survival [81]. These results were confirmed in the Breast Cancer International Research Group (BCIRG) trial [82], which included both node-positive and node-negative, HER2-positive breast cancers. The trial additionally included a novel regimen comprised of docetaxel, carboplatin, and trastuzumab (TCH), which was as effective, and carried a decreased risk of cardiomyopathy. All of these regimens included the continuation of single-agent trastuzumab after chemotherapy for a total duration of 1 year. The Herceptin Adjuvant (HERA) trial evaluated the addition of trastuzumab after adjuvant chemotherapy in patients with node-positive and node-negative HER2-positive breast cancer [83]. Updated results of the HERA trial continue to demonstrate a superior outcome for patients treated with 1 year of trastuzumab, compared to the control group [84].

The optimal duration of trastuzumab and whether it is necessary to give trastuzumab as a single agent or just concomitantly with chemotherapy is unclear. The FinHER trial evaluated trastuzumab given for only 9 weeks concurrent with chemotherapy, and demonstrated a significant decrease in recurrence in patients with node-positive, HER2-positive breast cancer [85]. A third arm of the HERA trial in which patients received 2 years of trastuzumab following chemotherapy has demonstrated no advantage over 1 year of trastuzumab. However, 6 months of trastuzumab was found not definitively equivalent to 1 year of trastuzumab [86]. In conclusion, 1 year of trastuzumab in the adjuvant setting remains optimal at this time. The results of the FinHER trial can be used, however, to reassure patients who have to stop trastuzumab early for decreases in left ventricular ejection fraction. Despite the positive results of the HERA trial, the majority of patients treated in the US receive trastuzumab concurrent with chemotherapy. This approach is supported by interim results from the Intergroup trial which demonstrated that patients treated with concurrent chemotherapy plus trastuzumab have an improved outcome compared to patients treated with chemotherapy and trastuzumab given sequentially [87].

Another controversy is which patients, if any, require an anthracycline as part of their trastuzumab-based regimen. The BCIRG trial demonstrated equivalent outcomes for patients receiving an anthracycline-based regimen and those receiving TCH, though there were numerically fewer events in the anthracycline-based arm [82]. Both regimens were equally effective in patients with multiple involved lymph nodes, in whom the additional risk of cardiomyopathy could perhaps be justified. Amplification of TOP2, a gene associated with benefit from anthracyclines, was assessed in tumors from patients enrolled in the BCIRG trial in an attempt to identify patients who may benefit from the addition of an anthracycline to trastuzumab-based chemotherapy. In patients whose tumors had HER2 amplification without TOP2 amplification, the anthracycline-containing arm and TCH were equivalent in disease-free survival; in patients with tumors exhibiting co-amplification of HER2 and TOP2, there were fewer recurrences in patients treated with the anthracycline-containing regimen, but the difference was not significant compared to patients on the TCH arm. The final analysis of the BCIRG-006 trial, as presented in the San Antonio Breast Cancer Symposium, confirmed the efficacy of trastuzumab and also confirmed the increased risk of toxicity of anthracyclines, mainly cardiac toxicity and second malignancies [88].

Currently, either an anthracycline-containing regimen or TCH is a reasonable option for patients with early-stage HER2-positive breast cancer. Patients with factors known to be associated with an increased risk of cardiomyopathy, such as coexisting hypertension and borderline baseline ejection fractions, may be best treated with TCH [89].

Lastly there is considerable controversy on how to treat patients with node-negative HER2-positive breast cancers that measure less than 1 cm, particularly when they are HR positive. Retrospective analyses have generally demonstrated that small HER2-positive breast cancers have a worse outcome than small HR-positive breast cancers [90]. However, almost none of the adjuvant trastuzumab trials recruited patients with node-negative breast cancers measuring <1 cm. Extrapolation of results from the adjuvant trials including patients with higher-risk HER2-positive cancers has led to many patients with T1B, stage 1A, HER2-positive breast cancer being recommended or receiving trastuzumab-based chemotherapy.

A single-arm trial of adjuvant paclitaxel and trastuzumab in node-negative, HER2-positive breast cancers measuring 3 cm or less in diameter demonstrated a 3-year survival free from invasive disease of 98.7% (95% CI 97.6–99.8). Even though this was a nonrandomized, single-arm study and the follow-up was only 4 years, it showed that the patients had excellent outcomes with acceptable toxicity and it offers a reasonable option for patients with small HER2-positive breast cancer [91]. A 7-year update of this trial showed that the 7-year disease-free survival (DFS) was 93.3% (95% CI 90.4–96.2), with a 7-year DFS for HR-positive patients of 94.6% (95% CI 91.8–97.5) and for HR-negative patients of 90.7% (95% CI 84.6–97.2). The 7-year overall survival (OS) was 95.0% (95% CI 92.4–97.7). These data confirm the role of adjuvant therapy with paclitaxel and trastuzumab for these patients with early-stage disease [92].

The role of estrogen receptor in HER2-positive breast cancers remains unclear. Historically, HER2-positive breast cancers that express HR have been demonstrated to be intrinsically resistant to endocrine therapy in many cases. However, it seems likely that at least a subset of HR-positive, HER2-positive breast cancers are driven by ER and may, therefore, require less aggressive adjuvant approaches [93]. To date, molecular profiling has not been able to clearly delineate which of HR-positive, HER2-positive breast cancers may potentially not benefit from the addition of chemotherapy to trastuzumab and endocrine therapy. Ongoing trials will hopefully address these questions.

A number of HER2-directed agents, such as lapatinib, pertuzumab, and trastuzumab-DM1, have shown promise and are approved for patients with HER2-positive, advanced breast cancer. These agents are being evaluated in the adjuvant setting. The ALLTO trial is evaluating chemotherapy with trastuzumab alone, lapatinib alone, and the combination of trastuzumab and lapatinib, in patients with early-stage HER2-positive breast cancer. Though final results of this trial are not available, the lapatinib-alone arm was discontinued following an interim analysis.

Adjuvant Endocrine Therapy for HR-Positive Early-Stage Breast Cancer

Multiple studies have demonstrated the benefit of adjuvant endocrine therapy in nonmetastatic, HR-positive breast cancer. Available agents include tamoxifen, a selective estrogen receptor modulator, aromatase inhibitors, and ovarian function suppression (OFS).

Tamoxifen has been the endocrine agent of choice for premenopausal women.

The Early Breast Cancer Trialists have clearly demonstrated the benefit of adjuvant tamoxifen in HR-positive early-stage breast cancer [70]. In postmenopausal women, 5 years of third-generation aromatase inhibitors, which act by preventing the peripheral synthesis of estrogen, improved disease-free survival, compared to 5 years of tamoxifen; there was no improvement in survival when the two were compared [94–96]. Overall, in postmenopausal women, aromatase inhibitors are somewhat safer than tamoxifen and are not associated with endometrial cancer. It is important to remember that women who are premenopausal at diagnosis and undergo temporary cessation of menses from adjuvant chemotherapy are still considered premenopausal. The transition of these women to an aromatase inhibitor should be done only after documentation of menopausal status, by measuring follicle-stimulating hormone (FSH) and estradiol levels, or with the use of surgical or pharmacologic OFS. Aromatase inhibitors have not been demonstrated to be effective in premenopausal women and should not be used in women with intact ovarian function without OFS.

There is now evidence for premenopausal women to be treated with OFS plus endocrine therapy as opposed to tamoxifen alone, and the choice between the two regimens is based on the presence of high-risk factors.

For patients with high-risk features, OFS plus tamoxifen or exemestane is recommended as opposed to tamoxifen alone. This recommendation is based on data from the SOFT trial, which randomized more than 3,000 premenopausal patients to tamoxifen, OFS plus tamoxifen, or OFS plus exemestane [97]. That trial demonstrated that the addition of OFS to tamoxifen resulted in an absolute improvement of DFS of 2% at 5 years. In the higher-risk cohort of patients, tamoxifen plus OFS resulted in an absolute improvement of 4.5% compared to tamoxifen alone; in the patients treated with exemestane plus OFS, the absolute improvement was 7.7%. High-risk features are generally defined as a case in which chemotherapy is indicated, secondary to involved axillary lymph nodes, large tumor size, lymphovascular invasion, high tumor grade, and high recurrence score by Oncotype DX®. In addition, women who are younger than 35 years old also seem to benefit from this more aggressive approach.

Premenopausal patients without high-risk features are treated with tamoxifen for 5–10 years. Two large randomized trials [98] have demonstrated a benefit for continuing tamoxifen for 10 years, rather than stopping at 5 years. Interestingly, the additional benefit in outcome for patients receiving 10 years of tamoxifen is seen more than 10 years following diagnosis. One can hypothesize that patients with luminal A cancers may achieve the greatest benefit from extended adjuvant therapy, since these are the cancers destined to late relapses, whereas luminal B cancers tend to recur early within the first 5 years. Molecular profiling may identify which patients require longer duration of endocrine therapy.

In general, the majority of postmenopausal women are treated with an aromatase inhibitor but sequencing of these agents with tamoxifen can be considered for patients who are unable to tolerate them. Several trials evaluated a sequenced approach of tamoxifen for approximately 2 years followed by an aromatase inhibitor for the remainder of 5 years, compared to 5 years of tamoxifen. These trials demonstrated that patients who switched to an aromatase inhibitor following tamoxifen had an improved disease-free survival, compared to patients treated with tamoxifen alone [99, 100]. The BIG-1-98 trial compared letrozole for 5 years, tamoxifen for 2 years followed by letrozole, letrozole for 2 years followed by tamoxifen, with tamoxifen for 5 years. All three study arms were found to be superior to tamoxifen alone for disease-free survival but, interestingly, there was no significant difference in outcome between the three study arms [101]. Letrozole for 5 years following 5 years of tamoxifen significantly improved outcome, compared to patients who received 5 years of tamoxifen alone [102]. Patients with node-positive breast cancer and those with cancers that expressed both ER and PR achieved the greatest benefit from extended adjuvant letrozole.

A recent study compared extended therapy of aromatase inhibitor for 10 years versus 5 years, in some cases following 5 years of tamoxifen [103]. The 5-year disease-free survival rate was 95% in the letrozole arm, and 91% in the placebo arm (hazard ratio 0.66; $P=0.01$). The 5-year overall survival was 93% with letrozole and 94% with placebo (hazard ratio 0.97; $P=0.83$). Extended endocrine therapy significantly decreased the risk of contralateral breast cancer. Bone-related adverse events occurred more frequently in the patients receiving letrozole for 10 years.

The use of adjuvant bisphosphonates remains controversial in the early-stage setting. The use of upfront zoledronic acid was demonstrated to decrease recurrence, compared to delayed use, with a concomitant increase in bone mineral density [104]. The AZURE trial, which evaluated the addition of zoledronic acid to standard therapy in patients with early-stage breast cancer, did not demonstrate a significant improvement in disease-free survival for patients receiving the bisphosphonate [105]. However, a subset analysis demonstrated a significant benefit for the addition of zoledronic acid in patients in the AZURE trial who were definitely postmenopausal. An Austrian study demonstrated that the addition of zoledronic acid to endocrine therapy plus goserelin in premenopausal patients with HR-positive early-stage breast cancer decreased recurrence risk [106]. A meta-analysis of patients from randomized trials reported that the use of adjuvant bisphosphonates reduces bone recurrence and improves breast cancer survival in postmenopausal women [107]. Taken together, these trials suggest that zoledronic acid is effective primarily in a low-estrogen environment.

In a placebo-controlled, phase 3 trial of postmenopausal women with HR-positive breast cancer, more than 3,000 women were randomly assigned to denosumab 60 mg or placebo administered subcutaneously every 6 months [108]. The study demonstrated that denosumab reduced fractures caused by adjuvant endocrine therapy with aromatase inhibitors by 50%, and in addition to the skeletal benefits, patients who received denosumab had an 18% reduced risk of disease recurrence.

Neoadjuvant Therapy

Neoadjuvant Chemotherapy

The use of preoperative chemotherapy has been demonstrated to down-stage breast cancers, while not impacting long-term outcome, compared to postoperative chemotherapy. The pivotal NSABP B-18 trial demonstrated equivalent outcomes for patients treated with AC for 4 cycles prior to surgery, and patients who had surgery followed by the same chemotherapy [109]. Additionally, a higher percentage of patients treated with neoadjuvant chemotherapy were rendered candidates for breast-conserving surgery. This trial was the first to demonstrate the importance of response to chemotherapy, in particular a pathologic complete response (PCR), defined as an absence of residual invasive cancer in the breast and axillary lymph nodes, as a predictor for long-term outcome. The prognostic value of PCR was confirmed in subsequent trials [110]. Importantly, these NSABP trials recruited patients with cancers unselected for subtype or HR status. It is increasingly apparent that obtaining a PCR is of more prognostic importance in patients with HR-negative breast cancers, compared to HR-positive breast cancers [111]. Patients with triple-negative breast cancers who do not achieve a PCR or near PCR following preoperative chemotherapy are highly likely to relapse within 2–3 years of diagnosis [112]. PCR is prognostic in HER2-positive cancers, but appears to be more important in HER2-positive, HR-negative breast cancers, compared to HER2-positive, HR-positive breast cancers [111].

In general, similar chemotherapeutic regimens are used in the neoadjuvant setting as in the adjuvant setting. The neoadjuvant setting allows an early assessment of chemosensitivity and is a useful area to evaluate new agents. Additionally, the ability to collect cancer tissue following chemotherapy allows an analysis of mechanisms associated with resistance to specific agents.

Neoadjuvant chemotherapy is used as initial therapy for locally advanced breast cancers, including inflammatory breast cancers. Standard adjuvant chemotherapeutic regimens are typically used, though this is an active area for the evaluation of novel agents and approaches.

Neoadjuvant Therapy for HER2-Positive Breast Cancers

Neoadjuvant trastuzumab-based chemotherapy is widely used in patients with early-stage and locally advanced HER2-positive breast cancer. Most commonly patients are treated with standard adjuvant trastuzumab-based regimens, which may or may not include an anthracycline. Novel approaches have been evaluated including the addition of other HER2-directed agents, such as lapatinib and pertuzumab [113–115]. The addition of these agents to trastuzumab has been demonstrated to increase the rate of PCR. Several trials have evaluated the use of HER2-directed agents alone without chemotherapy in the neoadjuvant setting [115, 116]. These trials have demonstrated that a small percentage of patients achieve a PCR without chemotherapy, which supports the concept that not all HER2-positive cancers require chemotherapy in addition to HER2-directed agents. The NCCN guidelines contain a list of regimens, containing HER2-directed agents, from randomized trials. The combination of pertuzumab, trastuzumab, and docetaxel, with or without carboplatin, is among the most commonly used non-anthracycline containing regimens approved for the preoperative treatment of HER2-positive breast cancer [115, 117].

Interestingly, all the randomized trials that have evaluated HER2-directed agents, with or without chemotherapy, consistently demonstrate a lower rate of PCR in HR-positive, HER2-positive breast cancers, compared to HR-negative, HER2-positive breast cancers [93]. ER has been demonstrated to act as an escape mechanism in some HR-positive, HER2-positive cancers, suggesting that in a subset of these cancers inhibition of ER as well as HER2 may be important.

Neoadjuvant Endocrine Therapy

It is clear that HR-positive breast cancers are less likely to achieve a PCR compared to HR-negative cancers following preoperative chemotherapy, though many HR-positive tumors exhibit at least a partial response [111]. This is not surprising given the fact that adjuvant chemotherapy does not improve outcome for a subset of HR-positive cancers. There is, therefore, increasing interest in evaluating preoperative endocrine therapy as a means of down-staging HR-positive breast cancers prior to surgery. The majority of clinical trials utilized 3–4 months of endocrine therapy and demonstrated reasonable partial response rates [118, 119]. A randomized trial that compared preoperative chemotherapy with preoperative endocrine therapy demonstrated equivalent response rates in patients with HR-positive breast cancer [120]. There are emerging data to suggest that longer durations of preoperative endocrine therapy (12 months or longer) are associated with higher response rates, including PCR rates, compared to shorter durations of endocrine therapy [121]. Currently the use of preoperative endocrine therapy is largely reserved for older patients with comorbid illnesses that may preclude the use of chemotherapy.

Some studies have demonstrated that decreases in Ki-67 following the institution of preoperative endocrine therapy may be a surrogate for long-term outcome [122]. There is interest in evaluating Ki-67 decreases by immunostaining of biopsies shortly after commencing endocrine therapy and using this as a means of continuing or stopping endocrine therapy [123].

There is interest in combining novel agents with endocrine therapy in the preoperative setting. The addition of the mechanistic target of rapamycin (mTOR) inhibitor, everolimus, to letrozole in the preoperative setting improved response rate, compared to letrozole alone [124]. The preoperative setting can potentially be used to determine sensitivity to endocrine therapy and gain a better understanding of the mechanisms underlying endocrine resistance.

Treatment of Metastatic Disease

Similar to the early-stage setting, the treatment of metastatic breast cancer is generally dictated by the breast cancer subtype. The use of targeted therapies has improved outcome for patients with HR-positive and HER2-positive breast cancers, with median survivals in the range of 4 and 3 years, respectively. Unfortunately the same is not true for metastatic triple-negative breast cancer, where the absence of targeted agents and inherent chemoresistance result in median survivals of only about 12 months. As with all metastatic cancers, the goals of treatment are improved survival, with as minimal effects on quality of life as possible.

Treatment of HR-Positive Metastatic Breast Cancer

Patients with HR-positive metastatic breast cancer are often treated with sequential lines of endocrine therapy until resistance occurs. This offers patients the highest chance of disease control with the lowest toxicity. However, chemotherapy is indicated if patients have life-threatening visceral metastases, such as lymphangitic carcinomatosis, or eventually when resistance to endocrine agents occurs. The median survival for patients with HR-positive metastatic breast cancer has been demonstrated to be as long as 4 years; factors predictive of a longer survival include long time since initial diagnosis, presence of bone metastases only, older age, postmenopausal status, and presence of both ER and PR.

There are a number of endocrine agents available for postmenopausal patients with HR-positive metastatic breast cancer. Each of the aromatase inhibitors has been compared to tamoxifen in the first-line treatment of HR-positive metastatic breast cancer and found to be superior in most endpoints, though none of these trials demonstrated a clear survival advantage for the aromatase inhibitors [125]. Fulvestrant, an estrogen receptor down-regulator, is approved for patients with HR-positive early-stage breast cancer who have received prior anti-estrogen therapy. Fulvestrant, at 250 mg every 4 weeks, was found to be equivalent to tamoxifen in the first-line treatment of HR-positive metastatic breast cancer [126]. However, fulvestrant at a dose of 500 mg every 4 weeks following a loading dose was found to be superior to the 250 mg dosing schedule, with minimal increase in toxicity, in a randomized trial which accrued patients who had previously received nonsteroidal aromatase inhibitors [127]. This high-dose schedule of fulvestrant was approved by the US Food and Drug Administration (FDA), and is the current optimal dose and schedule of this agent. A randomized trial compared fulvestrant, at the 500 mg dose, to anastrozole in the first-line treatment of HR-positive metastatic breast cancer and demonstrated a highly significant improvement in progression-free survival (PFS) for patients treated with fulvestrant [128]. Lastly, trials that compared a combination of fulvestrant and anastrozole to anastrozole alone in the first-line treatment of HR-positive metastatic breast cancer had conflicting results [129, 130]. The FACT trial did not show an advantage for the combination, while a SWOG trial demonstrated a significant 1.5-month improvement in PFS for the combination, compared to anastrozole. Notably, patients in the SWOG trial were somewhat less likely to have received adjuvant endocrine therapy, and patients in the control arm had a longer PFS than those on the FACT trial, raising the possibility that the combination of fulvestrant and anastrozole may be especially effective in patients previously untreated with endocrine therapy. The FALCON study is a phase 3 randomized, double-blind trial of fulvestrant versus anastrozole in HR-positive patients who were endocrine therapy naïve [131]. Fulvestrant significantly improved PFS compared to the anastrozole group (HR 0.797, 95% CI 0.637–0.999, $P=0.0486$). The median PFS was 16.6 months in the fulvestrant group versus 13.8 months in the anastrozole group. Notably, a subgroup analysis of FALCON showed that patients without visceral involvement benefitted the most, and they had a PFS of >20 months. This makes fulvestrant a very appealing choice as first-line therapy for some patients.

Finally, CDK 4/6 inhibition plays a significant role in the management of HR-positive breast cancer. One of the hallmarks of cancer is the dysregulation of the cell cycle. In order for a cell to divide while avoiding genetic damage, it has to go through strictly predefined stages in a specific fashion, and this process is called the cell cycle. Cyclin-dependent kinases (CDKs) are a large family of kinases; together with their regulatory protein partners, the cyclins, CDKs play a pivotal role in the progression of the cell through the cell cycle, and specifically in the transition of the cell from G0/G1 to S phase [132]. Palbociclib, abemaciclib, and ribociclib are all orally active, potent, and highly selective inhibitors of CDK4 and CDK6.

Palbociclib was the first CDK4/6 inhibitor approved as a first-line therapy for HR-positive HER2-negative metastatic breast cancer. This was based on the PALOMA trials of oral palbociclib in combination with letrozole compared to letrozole alone. PALOMA-1 was a phase 2 trial that demonstrated an improvement in the PFS from 10.2 months (95% CI 5.7–12.6) in the letrozole group to 20.2 months (13.8–27.5) in the palbociclib plus letrozole group (HR 0.488, 95% CI 0.319–0.748; one-sided $P=0.0004$) [133]. PALOMA-2 was a double-blind, phase 3 study that confirmed the findings of PALOMA-1 and showed improvement in the median PFS from 14.5 months in the letrozole group to 24.8 months in the combination arm (hazard ratio for disease progression or death, 0.58; 95% CI, 0.46–0.72; $P<0.001$) [134]. The most common adverse events seen with palbociclib are neutropenia (occurring in up to 66.4% of patients, though febrile neutropenia is uncommon at 1.8%), leukopenia (24.8%), anemia (5.4%), and fatigue (1.8%).

Ribociclib is the second CDK 4/6 inhibitor approved in the first-line setting. In the Monaleesa-2 trial, ribociclib plus letrozole improved the median PFS compared to letrozole alone; median duration of PFS was not reached in the ribociclib group but was reached in the control group in 14.7 months (hazard ratio, 0.56; 95% CI 0.43–0.72; $P=3.29\times10^{-6}$ for superiority) [135]. Ribociclib has a similar structure and similar side effect profile as palbociclib.

Finally, abemaciclib is the third available CDK 4/6 inhibitor, approved in combination with fulvestrant in patients who progressed while on adjuvant endocrine therapy, within 1 year of stopping their endocrine therapy, or during their first-line endocrine therapy for metastatic disease. Abemaciclib plus fulvestrant improved median PFS compared to fulvestrant alone from 9.3 to 16.4 months, with hazard ratio 0.553, 95% CI 0.449–0.681, and $P<0.001$ [136]. Abemaciclib has a different structure and side effect profile compared to the other two CDK 4/6 inhibitors. The most common adverse events in the abemaciclib group were diarrhea (86.4%), neutropenia (46.0%), nausea (45.1%), and fatigue (39.9%).

In summary, there are a number of options for the first-line treatment of HR-positive metastatic breast cancer, and treatment should be based on whether the patient has previously received adjuvant endocrine therapy, which agents the patient was exposed to in the adjuvant setting, and the timing of relapse. Hormone resistance is usually defined as relapse during or within 1 year after the completion of adjuvant endocrine therapy. Beyond that 1-year mark, cancers are considered sensitive. In general, *de novo* metastatic disease is considered hormone sensitive.

The optimal management of patients with HR-positive metastatic breast cancer is the sequential use of endocrine agents. The optimal sequence, as with the optimal first-line choice of endocrine agent, remains undefined. The EFECT trial compared fulvestrant, at the 250 mg dose, to exemestane in patients who had all received prior nonsteroidal aromatase inhibitors and many of whom had received tamoxifen, prior to study entry [137]. The PFS was identical at 3.7 months on each arm, suggesting that the choice of endocrine agent in the second- and third-line setting may not be that important, since most patients will receive most endocrine agents at some point during the course of their disease. Importantly, the nonsteroidal aromatase inhibitors, anastrozole and letrozole, have been demonstrated to be cross-resistant in HR-positive metastatic breast cancer. In contrast, the steroidal aromatase inhibitor, exemestane, exhibits activity after nonsteroidal aromatase inhibitors, and the opposite sequence is also effective.

A key component in the management of HR-positive breast cancer in premenopausal patients is ovarian suppression, using luteinizing hormone releasing hormone (LHRH) agonists or bilateral oophorectomies. A randomized trial, which compared tamoxifen alone, ovarian suppression alone, and the combination of tamoxifen and ovarian suppression, demonstrated a significantly improved PFS and survival for patients treated with both ovarian suppression and tamoxifen, and this combination is the optimal choice in the first-line setting for patients who have not received tamoxifen in the adjuvant setting [138]. Toremifene, a chlorinated derivative of tamoxifen, is approved as an alternative to tamoxifen for patients who cannot tolerate tamoxifen. Once menopause has been induced in premenopausal patients, they can be treated with any of the agents used for postmenopausal patients.

Resistance to endocrine therapy is multifactorial, but activation of growth factor pathways and downstream signaling pathways has been shown to be important. The use of growth factor receptor inhibitors, such as gefitinib and bevacizumab, has shown modest activity at best. This may be because the majority of these trials were performed in the first-line setting when only a subset of breast cancers are likely to be truly resistant to endocrine agents. Inhibition of mTOR was demonstrated to be a rational target in endocrine-resistant preclinical models. The BOLERO2 pivotal trial evaluated the addition of everolimus to exemestane in postmenopausal patients previously treated with nonsteroidal aromatase inhibitors. The addition of everolimus to exemestane significantly improved PFS by 6 months, compared to exemestane alone, and everolimus in combination with exemestane is approved for the treatment of HR-positive metastatic breast cancer in patients who have received prior nonsteroidal aromatase inhibitors [139]. Despite the benefit in the PFS, the combination of everolimus and exemestane did not improve overall survival (31 vs 26.6 months, $P=0.14$) [140]. Everolimus can cause mucositis, hyperglycemia, rash, and rarely noninfectious pneumonitis, thereby increasing the toxicity associated with endocrine therapy [141]. The optimal timing of everolimus remains unclear and is being evaluated in ongoing trials.

CDK 4/6 inhibitors play a significant role in the management of second-line and beyond metastatic breast cancer. The PALOMA-3 trial compared palbociclib plus fulvestrant versus fulvestrant alone in patients with advanced HR-positive HER2-negative breast cancer who had progressed on prior endocrine therapy or within 12 months of adjuvant endocrine therapy [142]. Palbociclib improved the median PFS from 4.6 months to 9.5 months (hazard ratio 0.46, 95% CI 0.36–0.59, $P<0.0001$).

Abemaciclib as single-agent therapy was shown to be effective in patients with breast cancer who had progressed on prior therapies, with an objective response rate of 19.7%, clinical benefit rate of 42.4%, median PFS of 6.0 months, and median overall survival of 17.7 months [143].

In summary, sequential use of endocrine agents or combination of endocrine therapy with cyclin-dependent kinase (CDK) 4/6 inhibitors or everolimus is the treatment of choice for patients with HR-positive metastatic breast cancer. Premenopausal women may be treated with ovarian suppression, in combination with endocrine agents. Chemotherapy is reserved for patients with life-threatening metastatic disease, and when endocrine therapies no longer are effective.

Treatment of HER2-Positive Metastatic Breast Cancer

The use of trastuzumab-based approaches has significantly improved the outcome for patients with HER2-positive metastatic breast cancer, and the median survival is approximately 3 years. The initial pivotal trial that led to the approval of trastuzumab and paclitaxel in the metastatic setting evaluated the addition of trastuzumab to either AC or paclitaxel in the first-line metastatic setting [40]. Due to the unexpected increase in cardiomyopathy in patients treated with AC and trastuzumab, the use of anthracyclines and trastuzumab is generally avoided if possible. Subsequent trials have demonstrated that the addition of trastuzumab to other chemotherapeutic agents is feasible and effective.

Three other HER2-directed agents have been approved for the treatment of patients with metastatic HER2-positive breast cancer. Pertuzumab is a monoclonal antibody that targets the domain of the HER2 receptor, which is involved with dimerization with HER3. The combination of pertuzumab, trastuzumab, and docetaxel improved PFS by 6 months, compared to trastuzumab and docetaxel, in the first-line treatment of patients with HER2-positive metastatic breast cancer, and this regimen is approved in the first-line setting [144], The addition of lapatinib, a tyrosine kinase inhibitor that targets HER1 and HER2, to capecitabine improves outcome compared to capecitabine alone in patients with HER2-positive metastatic breast cancer previously treated with trastuzumab-based chemotherapy, and this combination is approved in this setting [145]. The addition of lapatinib to trastuzumab improves overall survival compared to lapatinib alone in patients with metastatic HER2-positive breast cancer previously treated with multiple prior trastuzumab-based regimens [146]. Trastuzumab-DM1 is a conjugate of trastuzumab and maytansine, which has demonstrated single-agent activity in patients with HER2-positive metastatic breast cancer previously treated with trastuzumab and lapatinib [147]. A randomized trial demonstrated a 3-month improvement in PFS in patients with trastuzumab pretreated HER2-positive metastatic breast cancer, treated with trastuzumab-DM1 compared to lapatinib and capecitabine [148].

Chemotherapy for HER2-Negative Metastatic Breast Cancer

The only available systemic treatment for patients with metastatic triple-negative breast cancer is chemotherapy, which results in median survivals in the range of 12 months. Additionally, the majority of patients with hormone receptor-positive metastatic breast cancer will ultimately receive systemic chemotherapy, once endocrine therapy options have been exhausted. Potential chemotherapeutic regimens can be found at nccn.org. It is currently unclear whether combination therapy offers any advantage over single agents. A randomized trial which compared single-agent paclitaxel, single-agent Adriamycin, and combination paclitaxel and Adriamycin demonstrated an improved response rate and PFS for patients treated with the combination compared to the single agents [149]. However, there was no survival advantage for patients treated with the combination since there was a pre-specified crossover from one single agent to the other at the time of disease progression. The combination arm was associated with increased toxicity compared to the single-agent arms. In general, combination therapy should probably be reserved for patients with large-volume metastatic disease, in whom a response to treatment will likely improve quality of life.

Prevention of Skeletal-Related Events in Patients with Breast Cancer and Bone Metastases

One of the most common sites of metastases in patients with breast cancer is the bones, which can lead to complications including fractures, pain, and hypercalcemia. The bisphosphonate pamidronate has been demonstrated to decrease the risk of skeletal-related complications, compared to placebo, in patients with breast cancer metastatic to bones [150]. Subsequently, zoledronic acid was found to be equivalent to pamidronate in this setting [151]. Intravenous bisphosphonates can result in renal issues and osteonecrosis of the jaw, and the optimal duration of treatment and frequency of dosing remain unclear. Denosumab is a RANK-ligand inhibitor, which is equivalent to zoledronic acid in patients with bone metastases [152]. In contrast to bisphosphonates, denosumab is given subcutaneously and does not cause renal toxicity, though the risk of osteonecrosis of the jaw is similar with all these agents.

Male Breast Cancer

Breast cancer is very rare in males. It is estimated that 2,470 new cases will be diagnosed and 460 men will die with breast cancer in the US during 2017 [3]. Most risk factors are the same as for female breast cancer, such as family history, *BRCA 1* and *2* mutations (risk is higher with *BRCA2* mutations), radiation exposure, benign breast disease, obesity, and inactive lifestyle. Interestingly, the association with alcohol intake is not as strong as with breast cancer in women. However, some factors are unique to men, such as the diagnosis of Klinefelter syndrome, low bone density, gynecomastia, and orchitis/epididymitis, most of which are conditions associated with high estrogen/androgen ratio [153, 154]. Almost 90% of male breast cancers are IDC. The importance of estrogen excess in the risk of developing breast cancer in males is explained by the fact that most male tumors are HR-positive. A population-based epidemiologic study reported that among 829 men diagnosed with breast cancer from 2005 to 2009, 82% were HR positive, 15% were HER2 positive, and 3.6% had triple-negative tumors. HER2-positive cancers occur more commonly in young patients, while Hispanic and non-Hispanic Black patients tend to have ER-positive/PR-negative staining [155].

Most cases present as a painless, palpable mass. The workup involves a mammogram with or without an ultrasound and if imaging findings are suspicious, a biopsy is indicated for pathologic diagnosis. After the pathologic diagnosis is established, the staging and workup is the same as with female cancers. The TNM staging system is used, and the most important prognostic factors are the stage, tumor size, and number of involved lymph nodes. The preferred surgical treatment for men is modified radical mastectomy, however patients with sufficient breast tissue may allow for breast-conserving surgery, followed by radiation. Postmastectomy radiation may be also indicated in patients with locally advanced disease and >4 positive axillary nodes [156, 157]. The same principles of adjuvant and metastatic therapy apply in men as in women; the exception is that tamoxifen is the agent of choice for HR-positive tumors in men [158]. There is currently no specific evidence supporting the use of HER2- directed therapies in men, however all HER2-positive patients should be offered targeted treatment based on female breast cancer studies.

References

1 International Agency for Reasearch on Cancer/World Health Organization. Available at: http://globocan.iarc.fr/ia/world/atlas.html (accessed 1 February 2014).

2 International Agency for Reasearch on Cancer/World Health Organization. Available at: http://globocan.iarc.fr/Pages/fact_sheets_cancer.aspx (accessed 1 February 2014).

3 Siegel RL, Miller KD, Jemal A. Cancer statistics, 2017. *CA Cancer J Clin* 2017;67(1):7–30.

4 Ravdin PM, Cronin KA, Howlader N, *et al.* The decrease in breast-cancer incidence in 2003 in the United States. *New Engl J Med* 2007;356(16):1670–4.

5 SEER Stat Fact Sheets: Breast. Available from: https://seer.cancer.gov/statfacts/html/breast.html (accessed 4 October 2017).

6 Johansen Taber KA, Morisy LR, Osbahr AJ, 3rd, Dickinson BD. Male breast cancer: risk factors, diagnosis, and management (Review). *Oncol Rep* 2010;24(5):1115–20.

7 DeSantis CE, Siegel RL, Sauer AG, *et al.* Cancer statistics for African Americans, 2016: Progress and opportunities in reducing racial disparities. *CA Cancer J Clin* 2016;66(4):290–308.

8 Carey LA, Perou CM, Livasy CA, *et al.* Race, breast cancer subtypes, and survival in the Carolina Breast Cancer Study. *JAMA* 2006;295(21):2492–502.

9 Russo J, Tay LK, Russo IH. Differentiation of the mammary gland and susceptibility to carcinogenesis. *Breast Cancer Res Treat* 1982;2(1):5–73.

10 Rosner B, Colditz GA. Nurses' health study: log-incidence mathematical model of breast cancer incidence. *J Natl Cancer Inst* 1996;88(6):359–64.

11 Trichopoulos D, Hsieh CC, MacMahon B, *et al.* Age at any birth and breast cancer risk. *Int J Cancer* 1983;31(6):701–4.

12 Gammon MD, Thompson WD. Infertility and breast cancer: a population-based case-control study. *Am J Epidemiol* 1990;132(4):708–16.

13 Gennari A CM, Paleari L, Puntoni M, *et al.*, eds. Breast cancer incidence after hormonal infertility treatments: Systematic review and meta-analysis of population based studies. San Antonio Breast Cancer Symposium 2013; S5–08.

14 Collaborative Group on Hormonal Factors in Breast Cancer. Breast cancer and breastfeeding: collaborative reanalysis of individual data from 47 epidemiological studies in 30 countries, including 50302 women with breast cancer and 96973 women without the disease. *Lancet* 2002;360(9328):187–95.

15 Colditz GA, Rosner B. Cumulative risk of breast cancer to age 70 years according to risk factor status: data from the Nurses' Health Study. *Am J Epidemiol* 2000;152(10):950–64.

16 Chlebowski RT, Anderson GL, Gass M, *et al.* Estrogen plus progestin and breast cancer incidence and mortality in postmenopausal women. *JAMA* 2010;304(15):1684–92.

17 Reeves GK, Beral V, Green J, Gathani T, Bull D; Million Women Study Collaborators. Hormonal therapy for menopause and breast-cancer risk by histological type: a cohort study and meta-analysis. *Lancet Oncol* 2006;7(11):910–8.

18 Eliassen AH, Colditz GA, Rosner B, Willett WC, Hankinson SE. Adult weight change and risk of postmenopausal breast cancer. *JAMA* 2006;296(2):193–201.

19 O'Donovan PJ, Livingston DM. BRCA1 and BRCA2: breast/ovarian cancer susceptibility gene products and participants in DNA double-strand break repair. *Carcinogenesis* 2010;31(6):961–7.

20 Pruthi S, Gostout BS, Lindor NM. Identification and management of women with BRCA mutations or hereditary predisposition for breast and ovarian cancer. *Mayo Clin Proc* 2010;85(12):1111–20.

21 Vogel VG. Epidemiology, genetics, and risk evaluation of postmenopausal women at risk of breast cancer. *Menopause* 2008;15(4 Suppl):782–9.

22 NCI, Breast cancer risk assessment tool. Available from: http://www.cancer.gov/bcrisktool/ (accessed 19 May 2013).

23 Gail MH, Costantino JP, Pee D, *et al.* Projecting individualized absolute invasive breast cancer risk in African American women. *J Natl Cancer Inst* 2007;99(23):1782–92.

24 Zakaria S, Degnim AC. Prophylactic mastectomy. *Surg Clin North Am* 2007;87(2):317–31, viii.

25 Nelson HD, Smith ME, Griffin JC, Fu R. Use of medications to reduce risk for primary breast cancer: a systematic review for the U.S. Preventive Services Task Force. *Ann Intern Med* 2013;158(8):604–14.

26 Cuzick J, Sestak I, Bonanni B, *et al.* Selective oestrogen receptor modulators in prevention of breast cancer: an updated meta-analysis of individual participant data. *Lancet* 2013;381(9880):1827–34.

27 Cuzick J, Sestak I, Forbes JF, *et al.* Anastrozole for prevention of breast cancer in high-risk postmenopausal women (IBIS-II): an international, double-blind, randomised placebo-controlled trial. *Lancet* 2014;383(9922):1041–8.

28 Goss PE, Ingle JN, Ales-Martinez JE, *et al.* Exemestane for breast-cancer prevention in postmenopausal women. *N Engl J Med* 2011;364(25):2381–91.

29 Siu AL; U.S. Preventive Services Task Force. Screening for Breast Cancer: U.S. Preventive Services Task Force Recommendation Statement. *Ann Intern Med* 2016;164:279–96.

30 Oeffinger KC, Fontham ET, Etzioni R, *et al.* Breast Cancer Screening for Women at Average Risk: 2015 Guideline Update From the American Cancer Society. *JAMA* 2015;314(15):1599–614.

31 Smith RA, Andrews K, Brooks D, *et al.* Cancer screening in the United States, 2016: A review of current American Cancer Society guidelines and current issues in cancer screening. *CA Cancer J Clin* 2016;66:95–114.

32 Kuhl CK, Schrading S, Leutner CC, *et al.* Mammography, breast ultrasound, and magnetic resonance imaging for surveillance of women at high familial risk for breast cancer. *J Clin Oncol* 2005;23(33):8469–76.

33 Corben AD. Pathology of invasive breast disease. *Surg Clin North Am* 2013;93(2):363–92.

34 Luini A, Aguilar M, Gatti G, *et al.* Metaplastic carcinoma of the breast, an unusual disease with worse prognosis: the experience of the European Institute of Oncology and review of the literature. *Breast Cancer Res Treat* 2007;101(3):349–53.

35 Murphy L, Cherlet T, Lewis A, Banu Y, Watson P. New insights into estrogen receptor function in human breast cancer. *Ann Med* 2003;35(8):614–31.

36 Cui X, Schiff R, Arpino G, Osborne CK, Lee AV. Biology of progesterone receptor loss in breast cancer and its implications for endocrine therapy. *J Clin Oncol* 2005;23(30):7721–35.

37 Arpino G, Weiss H, Lee AV, *et al.* Estrogen receptor-positive, progesterone receptor-negative breast cancer: association with growth factor receptor expression and tamoxifen resistance. *J Natl Cancer Inst* 2005;97(17):1254–61.

38 Nahta R. Molecular mechanisms of trastuzumab-based treatment in HER2-overexpressing breast cancer. *ISRN Oncol* 2012;2012:428062.

39 Slamon DJ, Clark GM, Wong SG, *et al.* Human breast cancer: correlation of relapse and survival with amplification of the HER-2/neu oncogene. *Science* 1987;235(4785):177–82.

40 Slamon DJ, Leyland-Jones B, Shak S, *et al.* Use of chemotherapy plus a monoclonal antibody against HER2 for metastatic breast cancer that overexpresses HER2. *N Engl J Med* 2001;344(11):783–92.

41 Wolff AC, Hammond ME, Hicks DG, *et al.* Recommendations for human epidermal growth factor receptor 2 testing in breast cancer: American Society of Clinical Oncology/College of American Pathologists clinical practice guideline update. *J Clin Oncol* 2013;31(31):3997–4013.

42 Perou CM, Sorlie T, Eisen MB, *et al.* Molecular portraits of human breast tumours. *Nature* 2000;406(6797):747–52.

43 Sorlie T, Perou CM, Tibshirani R, *et al.* Gene expression patterns of breast carcinomas distinguish tumor subclasses with clinical implications. *Proc Natl Acad Sci U S A* 2001;98(19):10869–74.

44 Parker JS, Mullins M, Cheang MC, *et al.* Supervised risk predictor of breast cancer based on intrinsic subtypes. *J Clin Oncol* 2009;27(8):1160–7.

45 Sorlie T, Tibshirani R, Parker J, *et al.* Repeated observation of breast tumor subtypes in independent gene expression data sets. *Proc Natl Acad Sci U S A* 2003;100(14):8418–23.

46 National Comprehensive Cancer Network (NCCN). Clinical Practice Guidelines in Oncology. Breast Cancer Screening and Diagnosis, Version 1.2016.2. Available from: http://www.nccn.org (accessed 14 January 2017).

47 Pisano ED, Fajardo LL, Caudry DJ, *et al.* Fine-needle aspiration biopsy of nonpalpable breast lesions in a multicenter clinical trial: results from the radiologic diagnostic oncology group V. *Radiology* 2001;219(3):785–92.

48 Obenauer S, Hermann KP, Grabbe E. Applications and literature review of the BI-RADS classification. *Eur Radiol* 2005;15(5):1027–36.

49 Smetherman DH. Screening, imaging, and image-guided biopsy techniques for breast cancer. *Surg Clin North Am* 2013;93(2):309–27.

50 Kulkarni S, Singh N, Crystal P. Preoperative breast magnetic resonance imaging: applications in clinical practice. *Can Assoc Radiol J* 2012;63(3):207–14.

51 Solin LJ. Counterview: Pre-operative breast MRI (magnetic resonance imaging) is not recommended for all patients with newly diagnosed breast cancer. *Breast* 2010;19(1):7–9.

52 Groheux D, Espie M, Giacchetti S, Hindie E. Performance of FDG PET/CT in the clinical management of breast cancer. *Radiology* 2013;266(2):388–405.

53 Hortobagyi NG, Connolly JL, D'Orsi CJ, *et al.* Chapter 48, Breast. In: M Amin, S Edge, R Greene, *et al.* (eds) *AJCC Cancer Staging Manual*, 8th edn. New York: Springer, 2017.

54 de Boer M, van Dijck JA, Bult P, Borm GF, Tjan-Heijnen VC. Breast cancer prognosis and occult lymph node metastases, isolated tumor cells, and micrometastases. *J Natl Cancer Inst* 2010;102(6):410–25.

55 Donegan WL. Tumor-related prognostic factors for breast cancer. *CA Cancer J Clin* 1997;47(1):28–51.

56 Esteva FJ, Hortobagyi GN. Prognostic molecular markers in early breast cancer. *Breast Cancer Res* 2004;6(3):109–18.

57 Marks JR, Humphrey PA, Wu K, *et al.* Overexpression of p53 and HER-2/neu proteins as prognostic markers in early stage breast cancer. *Ann Surg* 1994;219(4):332–41.

58 Paik S, Tang G, Shak S, *et al.* Gene expression and benefit of chemotherapy in women with node-negative, estrogen receptor-positive breast cancer. *J Clin Oncol* 2006;24(23):3726–34.

59 van't Veer LJ, Dai H, van de Vijver MJ, *et al.* Gene expression profiling predicts clinical outcome of breast cancer. *Nature* 2002;415(6871):530–6.

60 Zelnak AB, O'Regan RM. Genomic subtypes in choosing adjuvant therapy for breast cancer. *Oncology (Williston Park)* 2013;27(3):204–10.

61 Fisher B, Anderson S, Bryant J, *et al.* Twenty-year follow-up of a randomized trial comparing total mastectomy, lumpectomy, and lumpectomy plus irradiation for the treatment of invasive breast cancer. *N Engl J Med* 2002;347(16):1233–41.

62 Lyman GH, Giuliano AE, Somerfield MR, *et al.* American Society of Clinical Oncology guideline recommendations for sentinel lymph node biopsy in early-stage breast cancer. *J Clin Oncol* 2005;23(30):7703–20.

63 Krag DN, Anderson SJ, Julian T B, *et al.*, eds. Primary outcome results of NSABP B-32, a randomized phase III clinical trial to compare sentinel node resection (SNR) to conventional axillary dissection (AD) in clinically node-negative breast cancer patients. 2010 ASCO Annual Meeting Proceedings (Post-Meeting Edition); 2010.

64 Giuliano AE, Hunt KK, Ballman KV, *et al.* Axillary dissection vs no axillary dissection in women with invasive breast cancer and sentinel node metastasis: a randomized clinical trial. *JAMA* 2011;305(6):569–75.

65 Clarke M, Collins R, Darby S, *et al.* Effects of radiotherapy and of differences in the extent of surgery for early breast cancer on local recurrence and 15-year survival: an overview of the randomised trials. *Lancet* 2005;366(9503):2087–106.

66 Early Breast Cancer Trialists' Collaborative Group, Darby S, McGale P, Correa C, Taylor C, Arriagada R, *et al.* Effect of radiotherapy after breast-conserving surgery on 10-year recurrence and 15-year breast cancer death: meta-analysis of individual patient data for 10,801 women in 17 randomised trials. *Lancet* 2011;378(9804):1707–16.

67 Overgaard M, Nielsen HM, Overgaard J. Is the benefit of postmastectomy irradiation limited to patients with four or more positive nodes, as recommended in international consensus reports? A subgroup analysis of the DBCG 82 b&c randomized trials. *Radiother Oncol* 2007;82(3):247–53.

68 Bartelink H, Horiot JC, Poortmans P, *et al.* Recurrence rates after treatment of breast cancer with standard radiotherapy with or without additional radiation. *N Engl J Med* 2001;345(19):1378–87.

69 Hooning MJ, Botma A, Aleman BM, *et al.* Long-term risk of cardiovascular disease in 10-year survivors of breast cancer. *J Natl Cancer Inst* 2007;99(5):365–75.

70 Early Breast Cancer Trialists' Collaborative Group. Effects of chemotherapy and hormonal therapy for early breast cancer on recurrence and 15-year survival: an overview of the randomised trials. *Lancet* 2005;365(9472):1687–717.

71 Dawood S, Broglio K, Buzdar AU, Hortobagyi GN, Giordano SH. Prognosis of women with metastatic breast cancer by HER2 status and trastuzumab treatment: an institutional-based review. *J Clin Oncol* 2010;28(1):92–8.

72 Carlson RW, Allred DC, Anderson BO, *et al.* Breast cancer. Clinical practice guidelines in oncology. *J Natl Compr Canc Netw* 2009;7(2):122–92.

73 Polychemotherapy for early breast cancer: an overview of the randomised trials. Early Breast Cancer Trialists' Collaborative Group. Lancet 1998;352(9132):930–42.

74 Levine MN, Bramwell VH, Pritchard KI, *et al.* Randomized trial of intensive cyclophosphamide, epirubicin, and fluorouracil chemotherapy compared with cyclophosphamide, methotrexate, and fluorouracil in premenopausal women with node-positive breast cancer. National Cancer Institute of Canada Clinical Trials Group. *J Clin Oncol* 1998;16(8):2651–8.

75 Fisher B, Brown AM, Dimitrov NV, *et al.* Two months of doxorubicin-cyclophosphamide with and without interval reinduction therapy compared with 6 months of

cyclophosphamide, methotrexate, and fluorouracil in positive-node breast cancer patients with tamoxifen-nonresponsive tumors: results from the National Surgical Adjuvant Breast and Bowel Project B-15. *J Clin Oncol* 1990;8(9):1483–96.

76 Henderson IC, Berry DA, Demetri GD, *et al.* Improved outcomes from adding sequential Paclitaxel but not from escalating Doxorubicin dose in an adjuvant chemotherapy regimen for patients with node-positive primary breast cancer. *J Clin Oncol* 2003;21(6):976–83.

77 Mamounas EP, Bryant J, Lembersky B, *et al.* Paclitaxel after doxorubicin plus cyclophosphamide as adjuvant chemotherapy for node-positive breast cancer: results from NSABP B-28. *J Clin Oncol* 2005;23(16):3686–96.

78 Citron ML, Berry DA, Cirrincione C, *et al.* Randomized trial of dose-dense versus conventionally scheduled and sequential versus concurrent combination chemotherapy as postoperative adjuvant treatment of node-positive primary breast cancer: first report of Intergroup Trial C9741/Cancer and Leukemia Group B Trial 9741. *J Clin Oncol* 2003;21(8):1431–9.

79 Mackey JR, Martin M, Pienkowski T, *et al.* Adjuvant docetaxel, doxorubicin, and cyclophosphamide in node-positive breast cancer: 10-year follow-up of the phase 3 randomised BCIRG 001 trial. *Lancet Oncol* 2013;14(1):72–80.

80 Jones S, Holmes FA, O'Shaughnessy J, *et al.* Docetaxel with cyclophosphamide is associated with an overall survival benefit compared with doxorubicin and cyclophosphamide: 7-year follow-up of US Oncology Research Trial 9735. *J Clin Oncol* 2009;27(8):1177–83.

81 Romond EH, Perez EA, Bryant J, *et al.* Trastuzumab plus adjuvant chemotherapy for operable HER2-positive breast cancer. *N Engl J Med* 2005;353(16):1673–84.

82 Slamon D, Eiermann W, Robert N, *et al.* Adjuvant trastuzumab in HER2-positive breast cancer. *N Engl J Med* 2011;365(14):1273–83.

83 Piccart-Gebhart MJ, Procter M, Leyland-Jones B, *et al.* Trastuzumab after adjuvant chemotherapy in HER2-positive breast cancer. *N Engl J Med* 2005;353(16):1659–72.

84 Gianni L, Dafni U, Gelber RD, *et al.* Treatment with trastuzumab for 1 year after adjuvant chemotherapy in patients with HER2-positive early breast cancer: a 4-year follow-up of a randomised controlled trial. *Lancet Oncol* 2011;12(3):236–44.

85 Joensuu H, Kellokumpu-Lehtinen PL, Bono P, *et al.* Adjuvant docetaxel or vinorelbine with or without trastuzumab for breast cancer. *N Engl J Med* 2006;354(8):809–20.

86 Pivot X, Romieu G, Debled M, *et al.* 6 months versus 12 months of adjuvant trastuzumab for patients with HER2-positive early breast cancer (PHARE): a randomised phase 3 trial. Lancet Oncol 2013.

87 Perez EA, Suman VJ, Davidson NE, *et al.* Sequential versus concurrent trastuzumab in adjuvant chemotherapy for breast cancer. *J Clin Oncol* 2011;29(34):4491–7.

88 Slamon DJ, Eiermann W, Robert NJ, *et al.* Ten-year follow-up of BCIRG-006 comparing doxorubicin plus cyclophosphamide followed by docetaxel with doxorubicin plus cyclophosphamide followed by docetaxel and trastuzumab with docetaxel, carboplatin and trastuzumab in HER2-positive early breast cancer patients. San Antonio Breast Cancer Symposium Abstract S5-04 Presented December 11, 2015.

89 Tan-Chiu E, Yothers G, Romond E, *et al.* Assessment of cardiac dysfunction in a randomized trial comparing doxorubicin and cyclophosphamide followed by paclitaxel, with or without trastuzumab as adjuvant therapy in node-positive, human epidermal growth factor receptor 2-overexpressing breast cancer: NSABP B-31. *J Clin Oncol* 2005;23(31):7811–9.

90 Templeton A, Ocana A, Seruga B, *et al.* Management of small HER2 overexpressing tumours. *Breast Cancer Res Treat* 2012;136(1):289–93.

91 Tolaney SM, Barry WT, Dang CT, *et al.* Adjuvant paclitaxel and trastuzumab for node-negative, HER2-positive breast cancer. *N Engl J Med* 2015;372(2):134–41.

92 Tolaney SM, Barry WT, Guo H, *et al.* Seven-year (yr) follow-up of adjuvant paclitaxel (T) and trastuzumab (H) (APT trial) for node-negative, HER2-positive breast cancer (BC). *J Clin Oncol* 2017;35(15) suppl: 511.

93 Nahta R, O'Regan RM. Therapeutic implications of estrogen receptor signaling in HER2-positive breast cancers. *Breast Cancer Res Treat* 2012;135(1):39–48.

94 Baum M, Budzar AU, Cuzick J, *et al.* Anastrozole alone or in combination with tamoxifen versus tamoxifen alone for adjuvant treatment of postmenopausal women with early breast cancer: first results of the ATAC randomised trial. *Lancet* 2002;359(9324):2131–9.

95 Breast International Group 1-98 Collaborative G, Thurlimann B, Keshaviah A, Coates AS, *et al.* A comparison of letrozole and tamoxifen in postmenopausal women with early breast cancer. *N Engl J Med* 2005;353(26):2747–57.

96 van de Velde CJ, Rea D, Seynaeve C, *et al.* Adjuvant tamoxifen and exemestane in early breast cancer (TEAM): a randomised phase 3 trial. *Lancet* 2011;377(9762):321–31.

97 Francis PA, Regan MM, Fleming GF. Adjuvant ovarian suppression in premenopausal breast cancer. *N Engl J Med* 2015;372(17):1673.

98 Davies C, Pan H, Godwin J, *et al.* Long-term effects of continuing adjuvant tamoxifen to 10 years versus stopping at 5 years after diagnosis of oestrogen receptor-positive breast cancer: ATLAS, a randomised trial. *Lancet* 2013;381(9869):805–16.

99 Coombes RC, Hall E, Gibson LJ, *et al.* A randomized trial of exemestane after two to three years of tamoxifen therapy in postmenopausal women with primary breast cancer. *N Engl J Med* 2004;350(11):1081–92.

100 Ingle JN. Adjuvant endocrine therapy for postmenopausal women with early breast cancer. *Clin Cancer Res* 2006;12(3 Pt 2):1031s–6s.

101 Regan MM, Neven P, Giobbie-Hurder A, *et al.* Assessment of letrozole and tamoxifen alone and in sequence for postmenopausal women with steroid hormone receptor-positive breast cancer: the BIG 1-98 randomised clinical trial at 8.1 years median follow-up. *Lancet Oncol* 2011;12(12):1101–8.

102 Goss PE, Ingle JN, Martino S, *et al.* Randomized trial of letrozole following tamoxifen as extended adjuvant therapy in receptor-positive breast cancer: updated findings from NCIC CTG MA.17. *J Natl Cancer Inst* 2005;97(17):1262–71.

103 Goss PE, Ingle JN, Pritchard KI, *et al.* extending aromatase-inhibitor adjuvant therapy to 10 years. *N Engl J Med* 2016;375(3):209–19.

104 Bundred NJ, Campbell ID, Davidson N, *et al.* Effective inhibition of aromatase inhibitor-associated bone loss by zoledronic acid in postmenopausal women with early breast cancer receiving adjuvant letrozole: ZO-FAST Study results. *Cancer* 2008;112(5):1001–10.

105 Coleman RE, Marshall H, Cameron D, *et al.* Breast-cancer adjuvant therapy with zoledronic acid. *N Engl J Med* 2011;365(15):1396–405.

106 Gnant M, Mlineritsch B, Luschin-Ebengreuth G, *et al.* Adjuvant endocrine therapy plus zoledronic acid in premenopausal women with early-stage breast cancer: 5-year follow-up of the ABCSG-12 bone-mineral density substudy. *Lancet Oncol* 2008;9(9):840–9.

107 Coleman R GM, Paterson A, Powles T, *et al*, On Behalf of the Early Breast Cancer Trialists' Collaborative Group (EBCTCG)'s Bisphosphonate Working Group. Sheffield Cancer Research Centre, ed. Effects of bisphosphonate treatment on recurrence and cause-specific mortality in women with early breast cancer: A meta-analysis of individual patient data from randomised trials. San Antonio Breast Cancer Symposium 2013.

108 Gnant M, Pfeiler G, Dubsky PC, *et al.* Adjuvant denosumab in breast cancer (ABCSG-18): a multicentre, randomised, double-blind, placebo-controlled trial. *Lancet* 2015;386(9992):433–43.

109 Wolmark N, Wang J, Mamounas E, Bryant J, Fisher B. Preoperative chemotherapy in patients with operable breast cancer: nine-year results from National Surgical Adjuvant Breast and Bowel Project B-18. *J Natl Cancer Inst Monographs* 2001(30):96–102.

110 Bear HD, Anderson S, Smith RE, *et al.* Sequential preoperative or postoperative docetaxel added to preoperative doxorubicin plus cyclophosphamide for operable breast cancer: National Surgical Adjuvant Breast and Bowel Project Protocol B-27. *J Clin Oncol* 2006;24(13):2019–27.

111 von Minckwitz G, Untch M, Blohmer JU, *et al.* Definition and impact of pathologic complete response on prognosis after neoadjuvant chemotherapy in various intrinsic breast cancer subtypes. *J Clin Oncol* 2012;30(15):1796–804.

112 Esserman LJ, Berry DA, DeMichele A, *et al.* Pathologic complete response predicts recurrence-free survival more effectively by cancer subset: results from the I-SPY 1 TRIAL--CALGB 150007/150012, ACRIN 6657. *J Clin Oncol* 2012;30(26):3242–9.

113 Baselga J, Bradbury I, Eidtmann H, *et al.* Lapatinib with trastuzumab for HER2-positive early breast cancer (NeoALTTO): a randomised, open-label, multicentre, phase 3 trial. *Lancet* 2012;379(9816):633–40.

114 Guarneri V, Frassoldati A, Bottini A, *et al.* Preoperative chemotherapy plus trastuzumab, lapatinib, or both in human epidermal growth factor receptor 2-positive operable breast cancer: results of the randomized phase II CHER-LOB study. *J Clin Oncol* 2012;30(16):1989–95.

115 Gianni L, Pienkowski T, Im YH, *et al.* Efficacy and safety of neoadjuvant pertuzumab and trastuzumab in women with locally advanced, inflammatory, or early HER2-positive breast cancer (NeoSphere): a randomised multicentre, open-label, phase 2 trial. *Lancet Oncol* 2012;13(1):25–32.

116 Rimawi MF, Mayer IA, Forero A, *et al.* Multicenter phase II study of neoadjuvant lapatinib and trastuzumab with hormonal therapy and without chemotherapy in patients with human epidermal growth factor receptor 2-overexpressing breast cancer: TBCRC 006. *J Clin Oncol* 2013;31(14):1726–31.

117 Schneeweiss A, Chia S, Hickish T, *et al.* Pertuzumab plus trastuzumab in combination with standard neoadjuvant anthracycline-containing and anthracycline-free chemotherapy regimens in patients with HER2-positive early breast cancer: a randomized phase II cardiac safety study (TRYPHAENA). *Ann Oncol* 2013;24(9):2278–84.

118 Smith IE, Dowsett M, Ebbs SR, *et al.* Neoadjuvant treatment of postmenopausal breast cancer with anastrozole, tamoxifen, or both in combination: the Immediate Preoperative Anastrozole, Tamoxifen, or Combined with Tamoxifen (IMPACT) multicenter double-blind randomized trial. *J Clin Oncol* 2005;23(22):5108–16.

119 Eiermann W, Paepke S, Appfelstaedt J, *et al.* Preoperative treatment of postmenopausal breast cancer patients with letrozole: A randomized double-blind multicenter study. *Ann Oncol* 2001;12(11):1527–32.

120 Semiglazov VF, Semiglazov VV, Dashyan GA, *et al.* Phase 2 randomized trial of primary endocrine therapy versus chemotherapy in postmenopausal patients with estrogen receptor-positive breast cancer. *Cancer* 2007;110(2):244–54.

121 Allevi G, Strina C, Andreis D, *et al.* Increased pathological complete response rate after a long-term neoadjuvant letrozole treatment in postmenopausal oestrogen and/or progesterone receptor-positive breast cancer. *Br J Cancer* 2013;108(8):1587–92.

122 Anderson H, Bulun S, Smith I, Dowsett M. Predictors of response to aromatase inhibitors. *J Steroid Biochem Mol Biol* 2007;106(1-5):49–54.

123 Ellis MJ, Suman V, McCall L, *et al.* Z1031B Neoadjuvant Aromatase Inhibitor Trial: A Phase 2 study of Triage to Chemotherapy Based on 2 to 4 week Ki67 level > 10%. *Cancer Res* 2012;72(24):Supplement 3. doi: 10.1158/0008. SABCS12-PD07-01.

124 Baselga J, Semiglazov V, van Dam P, *et al.* Phase II randomized study of neoadjuvant everolimus plus letrozole compared with placebo plus letrozole in patients with estrogen receptor-positive breast cancer. *J Clin Oncol* 2009;27(16):2630–7.

125 Riemsma R, Forbes CA, Kessels A, *et al.* Systematic review of aromatase inhibitors in the first-line treatment for hormone sensitive advanced or metastatic breast cancer. *Breast Cancer Res Treat* 2010;123(1):9–24.

126 Howell A, Robertson JF, Abram P, *et al.* Comparison of fulvestrant versus tamoxifen for the treatment of advanced breast cancer in postmenopausal women previously untreated with endocrine therapy: a multinational, double-blind, randomized trial. *J Clin Oncol* 2004;22(9):1605–13.

127 Di Leo A, Jerusalem G, Petruzelka L, *et al.* Results of the CONFIRM phase III trial comparing fulvestrant 250 mg with fulvestrant 500 mg in postmenopausal women with estrogen receptor-positive advanced breast cancer. *J Clin Oncol* 2010;28(30):4594–600.

128 Robertson JF, Lindemann JP, Llombart-Cussac A, *et al.* Fulvestrant 500 mg versus anastrozole 1 mg for the first-line treatment of advanced breast cancer: follow-up analysis from the randomized 'FIRST' study. *Breast Cancer Res Treat* 2012;136(2):503–11.

129 Mehta RS, Barlow WE, Albain KS, *et al.* Combination anastrozole and fulvestrant in metastatic breast cancer. *N Engl J Med* 2012;367(5):435–44.

130 Bergh J, Jonsson PE, Lidbrink EK, *et al.* FACT: an open-label randomized phase III study of fulvestrant and anastrozole in

combination compared with anastrozole alone as first-line therapy for patients with receptor-positive postmenopausal breast cancer. *J Clin Oncol* 2012;30(16):1919–25.

131 Robertson JFR, Bondarenko IM, Trishkina E, *et al.* Fulvestrant 500 mg versus anastrozole 1 mg for hormone receptor-positive advanced breast cancer (FALCON): an international, randomised, double-blind, phase 3 trial. *Lancet* 2016;388(10063):2997–3005.

132 O'Leary B, Finn RS, Turner NC. Treating cancer with selective CDK4/6 inhibitors. *Nat Rev Clin Oncol* 2016;13:417–30.

133 Finn RS, Crown JP, Lang I, *et al.* The cyclin-dependent kinase 4/6 inhibitor palbociclib in combination with letrozole versus letrozole alone as first-line treatment of oestrogen receptor-positive, HER2-negative, advanced breast cancer (PALOMA-1/TRIO-18): a randomised phase 2 study. *Lancet Oncol* 2015;16(1):25–35.

134 Finn RS, Martin M, Rugo HS, *et al.* Palbociclib and letrozole in advanced breast cancer. *N Engl J Med* 2016;375:1925–36.

135 Hortobagyi GN, Stemmer SM, Burris HA, *et al.* Ribociclib as first-line therapy for HR-positive, advanced breast cancer. *N Engl J Med* 2016;375(18):1738–48.

136 Sledge GW, Jr, Toi M, Neven P, *et al.* MONARCH 2: abemaciclib in combination with fulvestrant in women with HR+/HER2– advanced breast cancer who had progressed while receiving endocrine therapy. *J Clin Oncol* 2017;35(25):2875–84.

137 Mauriac L, Romieu G, Bines J. Activity of fulvestrant versus exemestane in advanced breast cancer patients with or without visceral metastases: data from the EFECT trial. *Breast Cancer Res Treat* 2009;117(1):69–75.

138 Klijn JG, Beex LV, Mauriac L, *et al.* Combined treatment with buserelin and tamoxifen in premenopausal metastatic breast cancer: a randomized study. *J Natl Cancer Inst* 2000;92(11):903–11.

139 Baselga J, Campone M, Piccart M, *et al.* Everolimus in postmenopausal hormone-receptor-positive advanced breast cancer. *N Engl J Med* 2012;366(6):520–9.

140 Piccart M, Hortobagyi GN, Campone M, *et al.* Everolimus plus exemestane for hormone-receptor-positive, human epidermal growth factor receptor-2-negative advanced breast cancer: overall survival results from BOLERO-2dagger. *Ann Oncol* 2014;25(12):2357–62.

141 Paplomata E, Zelnak A, O'Regan R. Everolimus: side effect profile and management of toxicities in breast cancer. *Breast Cancer Res Treat* 2013;140(3):453–62.

142 Cristofanilli M, Turner NC, Bondarenko I, *et al.* Fulvestrant plus palbociclib versus fulvestrant plus placebo for treatment of hormone-receptor-positive, HER2-negative metastatic breast cancer that progressed on previous endocrine therapy (PALOMA-3): final analysis of the multicentre, double-blind, phase 3 randomised controlled trial. *Lancet Oncol* 2016;17(4):425–39.

143 Dickler MN, Tolaney SM, Rugo HS, *et al.* MONARCH 1, A Phase II Study of Abemaciclib, a CDK4 and CDK6 Inhibitor, as a Single Agent, in Patients with Refractory $HR^{+}/HER2^{-}$ Metastatic Breast Cancer. *Clin Cancer Res* 2017;23(17):5218–24.

144 Baselga J, Cortes J, Kim SB, *et al.* Pertuzumab plus trastuzumab plus docetaxel for metastatic breast cancer. *N Engl J Med* 2012;366(2):109–19.

145 Geyer CE, Forster J, Lindquist D, *et al.* Lapatinib plus capecitabine for HER2-positive advanced breast cancer. *N Engl J Med* 2006;355(26):2733–43.

146 Blackwell KL, Burstein HJ, Storniolo AM, *et al.* Overall survival benefit with lapatinib in combination with trastuzumab for patients with human epidermal growth factor receptor 2-positive metastatic breast cancer: final results from the EGF104900 Study. *J Clin Oncol* 2012;30(21):2585–92.

147 Burris HA, 3rd, Rugo HS, Vukelja SJ, *et al.* Phase II study of the antibody drug conjugate trastuzumab-DM1 for the treatment of human epidermal growth factor receptor 2 (HER2)-positive breast cancer after prior HER2-directed therapy. *J Clin Oncol* 2011;29(4):398–405.

148 Verma S, Miles D, Gianni L, *et al.* Trastuzumab emtansine for HER2-positive advanced breast cancer. *N Engl J Med* 2012;367(19):1783–91.

149 Sledge GW, Neuberg D, Bernardo P, *et al.* Phase III trial of doxorubicin, paclitaxel, and the combination of doxorubicin and paclitaxel as front-line chemotherapy for metastatic breast cancer: an intergroup trial (E1193). *J Clin Oncol* 2003;21(4):588–92.

150 Lipton A, Theriault RL, Hortobagyi GN, *et al.* Pamidronate prevents skeletal complications and is effective palliative treatment in women with breast carcinoma and osteolytic bone metastases: long term follow-up of two randomized, placebo-controlled trials. *Cancer* 2000;88(5):1082–90.

151 Rosen LS, Gordon D, Kaminski M, *et al.* Zoledronic acid versus pamidronate in the treatment of skeletal metastases in patients with breast cancer or osteolytic lesions of multiple myeloma: a phase III, double-blind, comparative trial. *Cancer J* 2001;7(5):377–87.

152 Stopeck AT, Lipton A, Body JJ, *et al.* Denosumab compared with zoledronic acid for the treatment of bone metastases in patients with advanced breast cancer: a randomized, double-blind study. *J Clin Oncol* 2010;28(35):5132–9.

153 Brinton LA, Carreon JD, Gierach GL, McGlynn KA, Gridley G. Etiologic factors for male breast cancer in the U.S. Veterans Affairs medical care system database. *Breast Cancer Res Treat* 2010;119(1):185–92.

154 Brinton LA, Richesson DA, Gierach GL, *et al.* Prospective evaluation of risk factors for male breast cancer. *J Natl Cancer Inst* 2008;100(20):1477–81.

155 Chavez-Macgregor M, Clarke CA, Lichtensztajn D, Hortobagyi GN, Giordano SH. Male breast cancer according to tumor subtype and race: a population-based study. *Cancer* 2013;119(9):1611–7.

156 Cutuli B, Lacroze M, Dilhuydy JM, *et al.* Male breast cancer: results of the treatments and prognostic factors in 397 cases. *Eur J Cancer* 1995;31A(12):1960–4.

157 Golshan M, Rusby J, Dominguez F, Smith BL. Breast conservation for male breast carcinoma. *Breast* 2007;16(6):653–6.

158 Eggemann H, Ignatov A, Smith BJ, *et al.* Adjuvant therapy with tamoxifen compared to aromatase inhibitors for 257 male breast cancer patients. *Breast Cancer Res Treat* 2013;137(2):465–70.

Section 8

Hematologic Cancers

29

Myeloid Malignancies

Joshua F. Zeidner[1], Darshan Roy[2], Alexander Perl[3], and Ivana Gojo[4]

[1] *Lineberger Comprehensive Cancer Center, University of North Carolina Chapel Hill, North Carolina, USA*
[2] *Rowan School of Medicine, Stratford, New Jersey, USA*
[3] *Perelman Center for Advanced Medicine, University of Pennsylvania, Philadelphia, Pennsylvania, USA*
[4] *Sidney Kimmel Comprehensive Cancer Center, Johns Hopkins University, Baltimore, Maryland, USA*

Overview

Myeloid neoplasms are a heterogeneous group of clonal disorders that arise in hematopoietic precursors or stem cells and disrupt normal myeloid cell production and differentiation. Symptoms in these conditions are commonly due to cytopenias, extramedullary hematopoiesis causing splenomegaly, thrombohemorrhagic complications, or constitutional symptoms. Myeloid neoplasia is organized into four major categories based on a combination of clinical presentation and genetic abnormalities: myelodysplastic syndromes (MDS), myeloproliferative neoplasms (MPN), MDS/MPN overlap syndromes, and acute myeloid leukemia (AML). Chronic myelogenous leukemia (CML) historically has been considered an MPN but will be considered independently, due to its distinct biology and therapy.

Clinically, MDS patients present with cytopenias and dysplasia (i.e., abnormal cellular morphology) while MPNs present with peripheral blood evidence of increased myeloid cell accumulation (leukocytosis, erythrocytosis, or thrombocytosis) and generally show normal cellular morphology. Both MDS/MPN overlap syndromes and AML may present with features of the two conditions (i.e., cytopenias of certain lineages with increases of other lineages as well as dysplasia). A diagnosis of AML, however, is contingent upon demonstration of excess numbers of immature myeloid cells and is made when the percentage of blasts within the peripheral blood or bone marrow (BM) is ≥20%. With two prominent exceptions – hypoplastic MDS and primary myelofibrosis – myeloid neoplasms generally show increased hematopoietic activity, reflected by increased marrow cellularity. In MDS, this is often associated with a marked increase in intramedullary apoptosis.

A diverse number of genetic events underlie myeloid neoplasia. However, individual patients' affected cells typically only show a few discrete recurrent mutations and these arise in genes whose functions can be divided into eight categories [1]. These include transcription factors, signal transduction kinases or phosphatases, genes altering DNA methylation, post-translational chromatin modifiers, RNA splicing machinery genes, the cohesin complex, tumor suppressors, and the gene encoding nucleophosmin-1. Some generalizations can be made for MPNs, which nearly uniformly show mutations in genes that up-regulate signal transduction. However, the mutational complement underlying MDS and AML appears considerably more diverse, with several recurrent mutations cooperating to cause disease phenotype. It is important to note that while some of the genetic changes have strong genotype:phenotypic associations – for example the Philadelphia chromosome in CML (t(9;22)) and t(15;17) in acute promyelocytic leukemia – nearly all genetic abnormalities seen across these neoplasms are closely linked to myeloid neoplasia per se but are *not* specific to a single diagnostic entity. This includes mutations in genes that regulate epigenetic functions (e.g., DNA or histone methylation, lysine acetylation, etc.), receptor tyrosine kinases, RNA splicing machinery, and transcription factors. Accordingly, the contribution of these mutations to altered hematopoiesis is shared across a number of conditions and likely underlies some overlap in presentation and pathogenesis among myeloid neoplasms.

With the increased prevalence of next-generational sequencing, multiple large-scale studies on normal populations have yielded some interesting results. These studies have found that a small portion of the population harbor genetic mutations often seen in those with MDS and AML. Conceptually similar to monoclonal gammopathy of undetermined significance (MGUS) and monoclonal B-cell lymphocytosis (MBL), clonal hematopoiesis with indeterminate prognosis (CHIP) is defined as having at least 2% variant allele frequency of somatic mutations known to be associated with hematopoietic neoplasms without meeting the criteria for MDS or AML [2]. While many do not develop overt MDS or AML, there is a documented increased risk of at least 0.5–1% per year of progressing to MDS or AML, with this rate increasing with the size of the variant clone. The incidence of CHIP is thought to be age-related with greater than 10% of the population over the age of 70 having somatic mutations in relevant genes [3]. The majority of the

The American Cancer Society's Oncology in Practice: Clinical Management, First Edition. Edited by The American Cancer Society.

variant alleles in the population occur in four genes, three of them often seen mutated in hematologic malignancies: *DNMT3A*, *TET2*, and *ASXL1* [4]. As methods progress to identify genetic events before the manifestation of phenotypically identifiable diseases, additional precursor events will be identified; however, the true significance of these precursor mutations is still yet to be determined.

Myelodysplastic Syndromes

Incidence and Etiology

Myelodysplastic syndromes (MDS) are a group of myeloid neoplasms that are characterized by ineffective hematopoiesis and abnormal cytomorphology. MDS incidence rates are higher among males than females and increase substantially with age; incidence rates among individuals aged 60–69, 70–79, and 80+ living in the United States (US) are 9.3, 30.2, and 59.8 new cases per 100,000 persons per year [5]. Although the true incidence and prevalence of MDS may be substantially underestimated due to incomplete reporting to cancer registries, conservative estimates of incidence and prevalence in the US have been reported as more than 10,000 new cases per year and more than 60,000 persons living with MDS [6].

The vast majority of MDS cases have no apparent risk factor. Familial MDS presenting in childhood occurs quite rarely and usually reflects inherited mutations in DNA repair enzymes (e.g., Fanconi anemia pathway genes) or – as in the syndrome dyskeratosis congenita – telomere maintenance [7, 8]. Familial MDS presenting in adulthood is rarer still and may relate to germline mutations in *RUNX1* or *GATA2* [9, 10]. Chronic exposure to certain chemical agents (e.g., benzene and certain pesticides), smoking, as well as previous chemotherapy and/or radiation are the best established risk factors for sporadic MDS. Among cases that follow chemical exposures, a latency of several years but seldom more than a decade between exposure and clinical findings is typically observed.

Pathogenesis and Genetics

The pathogenesis of MDS is thought to relate to acquired mutations in myeloid progenitors and/or stem cells that disturb differentiation, apoptosis/survival, and self-renewal.

The most consistent genetic findings in MDS marrow cells are clonal cytogenetic abnormalities, which are seen in approximately 50% of cases. These abnormalities most commonly represent numeric alterations (monosomies or trisomies) or partial chromosomal deletions, particularly from the long arms of chromosomes 5, 7, or 20. Unlike AML or MPNs, balanced translocations are rare, except in MDS that follows prior radiation [11]. With the notable exception of the chromosome 5q gene RPS14, whose haploinsufficiency is strongly implicated in a discrete subset of MDS cases, the specific genes responsible for disease pathogenesis in most large-scale deletions have not been identified [12].

Next-generation sequencing has allowed characterization of a number of recurrent single gene mutations in MDS [13–15]. While many mutations are shared between AML and MPNs, mutations that activate signal transduction kinases are considerably less frequent in MDS than the other two diseases. Genome-wide studies have shown that marrow cells from patients with MDS show significant epigenetic modification to their DNA, either through methylation of bases or post-translational histone modification [16]. Finally, gene expression in MDS is commonly perturbed by mutations affecting genes that regulate mRNA splicing [15, 17].

Recurrent mutations in genes that regulate DNA methylation, such as *DMNT3A* and *TET2*, occur commonly in MDS [18]. While it is known that promoter methylation at CpG islands impairs gene transcription, the role of hypomethylation on transcription, the functional effects of cytosine hydroxymethylation, and identification of the critical genes and processes targeted by these mutations remain topics of investigation.

Recent studies have shown that the majority of patients with MDS show acquired mutations in genes responsible for RNA processing ("the spliceosome") with the greatest number of cases occurring in *SF3B1*, *U2AF1*, *SRSF2*, and *ZRSR2* [17]. While heterogeneous, these mutations are mutually exclusive, suggesting overlapping cellular effects. How these mutations mechanistically are responsible for disease pathogenesis is still to be determined [18]. It is notable that there is a strong association between the morphologic finding of ring sideroblasts and mutations of *SF3B1* as well as CMML and *SRSF2* mutations.

Clinical Presentation

Patients most commonly present with symptomatic cytopenias (e.g., fatigue, bruising, or recurrent infection), though many cases are noted incidentally on routine laboratory testing. Subsequent bone marrow (BM) studies often find a hypercellular BM with cells containing cytologic atypia (dysplasia).

Classification

The diagnosis of MDS can be made histologically by identifying dysplasia in one or more lineages in the BM aspirate or core biopsy. These abnormalities need to be seen definitively in at least 10% of cells. Dysplastic erythropoiesis manifests as nuclear irregularities, often with nuclear budding or multinucleated erythroid precursors. The granulocytic lineage can show abnormal lobation and reduced granulation. Megakaryocytic dysplasia is seen as small hypo- or abnormally lobated nuclei. A presumptive diagnosis of MDS can also be made in the absence of dysplasia if there is evidence of specific, recurrent chromosomal abnormalities. These include, but are not limited to, monosomy 7, del(7q), monosomy 5, or del(5q) [19]. The current World Health Organization (WHO) classification of MDS is divided into numerous categories based upon the number of lineages showing dysplasia and the presence and number of myeloblasts, with a unique identity for cases of myelodysplasia with an isolated del(5q) (Table 29.1) [20].

Myelodysplasia with isolated del(5q), also called "5q− syndrome," is a unique entity within the subgroup of MDS. It is more prevalent in women and often presents with macrocytic anemia with or without thrombocytosis. These patients by definition have only one cytogenetic abnormality, the deletion of long arm of chromosome 5, and overall have a better prognosis than most MDS patients, due to low leukemic transformation risk. This group of patients preferentially shows clinical response to lenalidomide [21].

Table 29.1 WHO Classification systems for myeloid neoplasms [20].

Acute myeloid leukemia (AML) and related neoplasms
With recurrent genetic abnormalities:
t(8;21) *(RUNX1-RUNX1T1)*
inv(16) or t(16;16) *(CBFB-MYH11)*
APL with *PML-RARA*
t(9;11) *(MLLT3-KMT2A)*
t(6;9) *(DEK-NUP214)*
inv(3q) or t(3;3) *(GATA2, MECOM)*
t(1;22) *(RBM15-MLK1)*
Provisional entity: AML with *BCR-ABL1*
AML with mutated *NPM1*
AML with biallelic mutations of *CEBPA*
Provisional entity: AML with mutated *RUNX1*
AML with myelodysplasia-related changes
Therapy-related myeloid neoplasms
Myeloid sarcoma
Myeloid proliferations related to Down syndrome
Transient abnormal myelopoiesis (TAM)
Myeloid leukemia associated with Down syndrome
AML, not otherwise specified
AML with minimal differentiation
AML without maturation
AML with maturation
Acute myelomonocytic leukemia
Acute monoblastic/monocytic leukemia
Pure erythroid leukemia
Acute megakaryoblastic leukemia
Acute panmyelosis with myelofibrosis
Myelodysplastic syndromes (MDS)
MDS with single lineage dysplasia
MDS with ring sideroblasts (MDS-RS)
MDS-RS and single lineage dysplasia
MDS-RS and multilineage dysplasia
MDS with multilineage dysplasia
MDS with excess blasts
MDS with isolated del(5q)
MDS, unclassifiable
Provisional entity: Refractory cytopenia of childhood
Myeloid neoplasms with germline predisposition

Molecular lesions of myelodysplastic syndrome likely will play an increasing role in classifying MDS, determining prognosis, and perhaps guiding therapy. To date, the prognostic relevance of each of the various mutations has largely been examined in isolation. Similar to AML, it seems likely that detailed classification schemes that incorporate multiple genes will prove necessary to decipher particular mutations' impact upon prognosis [14, 15, 22].

Risk Stratification/Prognosis

MDS is a heterogeneous disease with distinct outcomes based on risk stratification and disease status at the time of diagnosis. The International Prognostic Scoring System (IPSS) was originally published in 1997 and represents the most widely used scoring system for determining risk group, prognosis, and ultimately therapeutic options for patients with MDS [23]. With the IPSS, a patient can be scored into one of four risk (low, intermediate-1, intermediate-2, and poor) groups based on BM blast percentage, cytogenetics, and degree of cytopenias. However, a newer classification, Revised-IPSS (IPSS-R), shown in Table 29.2, has replaced the IPSS score for most clinicians as the IPSS-R has five different risk groups (instead of four), has five cytogenetic risk groups (as opposed to three), and has more additive features that can more accurately predict survival [24].

Therapy of MDS

Overview

The need for therapy is primarily determined based on the disease risk (cytopenias, risk for disease transformation such as presence of blasts and/or poor risk karyotype), patient age, and preference/goals of therapy. Treatment can be divided into three basic categories: supportive care, low-intensity therapies (immunosuppression, lenalidomide, hypomethylating agents), and high-intensity therapies (combination chemotherapy and allogeneic hematopoietic stem cell transplantation, SCT).

Supportive Care

Supportive care is appropriate for patients with low-risk IPSS/IPSS-R scores, patients with poor ECOG performance status (PS: ≥3), or elderly patients in which other therapies may be relatively contraindicated. The main goal of supportive care in this setting is to improve quality of life. Supportive care involves transfusions to maintain platelet and hemoglobin levels (usually hemoglobin ≥ 8 g/dL, and platelets ≥10,000/μL), antibiotics to treat infections, use of erythropoietin-stimulating agents for anemia, correction of superimposed nutritional deficiencies, vaccination (against influenza yearly and pneumococcus every 5 years), and iron chelation when appropriate. Erythropoietin-stimulating agents (ESAs) at doses between 30,000 and 70,000 units/week can improve anemia associated with MDS in up to 30% of cases [25]. Erythropoietin levels should be checked at baseline in patients with MDS; ESAs work best in patients with low erythropoietin (<500 mU/UL) plus low transfusion needs [25]. For patients who do not respond in 4–6 weeks to ESAs, the addition of myeloid growth factors (G-CSF, GM-CSF) may improve responses in 20–30% of cases [26].

Iron overload is a prominent feature of MDS given the high number of red cell transfusions required to maintain hemoglobin levels >7–8 g/dL. Deleterious effects of iron overload affect the heart, liver, and several endocrine organs. Retrospective data suggest that iron overload leads to a poor prognosis in MDS patients [27]. Therefore, ferritin levels should be monitored periodically in patients with MDS receiving chronic red cell transfusions, with a goal of maintaining

Table 29.2 IPSS-R Score for MDS.

Prognostic variable	Score: 0	Score: 0.5	Score: 1	Score: 1.5	Score: 2	Score: 3	Score: 4
Cytogenetics[1]	Very Good	—	Good	—	Intermediate	Poor	Very Poor
BM Blast (%)	≤2%	—	3–4%	—	5–10%	>10%	—
Hemoglobin (g/dL)	≥10	—	8–9	<8	—	—	—
Platelets (/mm^3)	≥100	50–100	<50	—	—	—	—
Absolute neutrophil count (/mm^3)	≥0.8	<0.8	—	—	—	—	—

[1] Cytogenetic definitions:
Very good: −Y, del(11q)
Good: Normal, del(5q), del(12p), del(20q), double including del(5q)
Intermediate: del(7q), +8, +19, i(17q), or any other single or double independent clones
Poor: −7, inv(3)/t(3q)/del(3q), double including −7/del(7q), 3 chromosomal abnormalities
Very poor: Complex: >3 chromosomal abnormalities

Risk group	IPSS-R score	Median overall survival (years)
Very low	≤1.5	8.8
Low	2–3	5.3
Intermediate	3.5–4.5	3.0
High	5–6	1.6
Very high	>6	0.8

ferritin <1000 ng/mL [28]. Based primarily on nonrandomized prospective studies, iron chelators (such as deferoxamine and deferasirox) have been shown to decrease iron overload, and are indicated in patients with iron overload secondary to chronic anemias in order to minimize its adverse effects [27, 29]. There is currently an ongoing randomized phase 3 trial comparing deferasirox with placebo in patients with MDS to determine if iron chelation can improve overall outcomes in MDS. Other clinical trials are addressing whether iron chelation alters the natural history of MDS. Currently, iron chelation is generally recommended in patients with low or intermediate-1 MDS with chronic red cell transfusions with a ferritin >2500 ng/mL [28].

Low-Intensity Therapies

Immunosuppression

Immunosuppressive medications, such as antithymocyte globulin (ATG) or cyclosporine, can lead to hematologic responses in up to one-third of MDS patients with lower-risk IPSS scores [30]. A scoring system was developed by the National Institute of Health to predict which patients would respond to immunosuppressive therapy. Positive predictors of response to immunosuppressive agents include: HLA-DR15 phenotype, presence of a paroxysmal nocturnal hemoglobinuria (PNH) clone, hypoplastic MDS, bone marrow blasts <5%, younger age, shorter duration of red cell transfusion dependence, and normal karyotype or trisomy 8 [31]. A randomized, multicenter, phase 3 trial comparing the combination of ATG and cyclosporine with best supportive care for treatment of MDS found no difference in overall survival (OS), transformation to AML, or toxicities between the two arms, but there was an increased rate of hematologic response (29% vs 9%) with the combination immunosuppressive regimen. Responses with immunosuppressive therapy were seen most commonly in those with hypoplastic MDS and without increased blasts [32].

Lenalidomide

Lenalidomide belongs to a class of immunomodulatory drugs called IMiDs, which are analogs of thalidomide. Lenalidomide is approved for treatment of anemia in low/intermediate-1 IPSS MDS associated with del(5q) with or without additional cytogenetic abnormalities [33]. A pivotal study by List *et al.* [34] evaluated low-dose lenalidomide in 148 patients with MDS in low/intermediate-1 IPSS associated with del(5q) with or without other cytogenetic abnormalities and transfusion dependence. Lenalidomide led to a 64% rate of transfusion independence, the majority remaining transfusion-independent for at least 1 year. Notably, 73% of evaluable patients experienced a cytogenetic response, half of which were complete responses [34]. These high response rates were confirmed in a randomized phase 3 trial of patients with transfusion-dependent lower-risk MDS with del(5q) [35]. There was no OS difference in this trial, but the study was confounded by a large number of crossover patients. Lenalidomide was also shown to improve anemia and reduce red blood cell transfusions in up to 43% of patients with low or intermediate-1 risk MDS without 5q abnormalities, but responses were not durable [36].

Hypomethylating Agents

Azacitidine and decitabine are two hypomethylating agents approved for treatment of MDS. Hypomethylating agents demethylate DNA through inhibition of DNMT, leading to re-expression of tumor suppressor genes that are otherwise silenced in MDS. A pivotal randomized phase 3 trial compared azacitidine with best supportive care in 191 patients with MDS. All patients with MDS were eligible if they had either symptomatic anemia requiring transfusions, thrombocytopenia <50,000/uL, or neutropenia (<1000/μL and/or infection). Patients were allowed to cross over to the treatment arm if their disease was progressing. Azacitidine resulted in a superior response rate (60% vs 5%), increased time to leukemic transformation (median 21 months vs median 12 months), and improved quality of life. Median OS, however, was not significantly different between azacitidine and best supportive care (20 months vs 14 months); however the effect on OS was limited by the proportion of patients who crossed over to azacitidine [37]. A subsequent phase 3 study (AZA-001) randomized higher-risk MDS patients (intermediate-2/high) to azacitidine versus conventional care (best supportive care, low-dose cytarabine, or combination chemotherapy) and found increased median OS (24.5 vs 15 months) and less toxicity in the azacitidine arm [38].

Similar results have been seen with decitabine in the phase 2 and phase 3 setting, demonstrating high response rates (17–49%) and longer time to transformation of AML, but no OS benefit [39, 40]. A subsequent phase 3 study compared three different doses of decitabine (20 mg/m^2 IV daily for 5 days, 20 mg/m^2 subcutaneous daily for 5 days, and 10 mg/m^2 IV daily for 10 days) and found the optimal dose to be 20 mg/m^2 IV daily for 5 days [41].

It is important to note that hypomethylating agents are not curative, and patients with higher-risk MDS warrant curative therapy with an allogeneic SCT, if eligible. Hypomethylating agents are typically recommended in the first-line setting in patients with higher-risk MDS, in order to achieve a response, as a bridge to an SCT. Patients who are not candidates for SCT, or those with lower-risk MDS, should continue to receive hypomethylating agents indefinitely, given the OS advantage, until disease progression or toxicity/intolerability.

High-Intensity Therapies

Combination Chemotherapy

Combination chemotherapy is an option for select patients with high-risk MDS. An AML induction chemotherapy regimen of cytarabine and anthracycline-based chemotherapy is typically recommended when intensive chemotherapy is considered. However, intensive chemotherapy agents have lower response rates in patients with high-risk MDS than in patients with *de novo* AML, with complete remission (CR) rates between 34 and 80% and treatment-related mortality as high as 36% [42]. Patients younger than 65 years may have better outcomes than older patients with intensive chemotherapy. It is important to note, however, that these responses are typically not durable, with >70% of patients achieving a CR ultimately relapsing [43]. Patients with normal karyotype tend to have a better response with intensive chemotherapy agents than patients with cytogenetic abnormalities. This relative chemoresistance of high-risk MDS is likely due to multiple factors such as older age at presentation, poor-risk cytogenetics and molecular mutations, and early primitive stem-cell nature of the disease. Although there have been no randomized comparisons of intensive chemotherapy versus low-intensive therapies in patients with high-risk MDS, it is reasonable to consider combination chemotherapy in younger patients with RAEB-2, as a bridge to an allogeneic SCT, though studies have shown similar outcomes after allogeneic SCT following initial therapy of high-intensity chemotherapy or azacitidine [44]. Thus, individual patient characteristics such as age, ECOG performance status, comorbidities, treatment goal, and patient preference are important when considering high-intensity therapy for MDS. Patients who achieve a CR after induction chemotherapy should receive postremission therapy (i.e., allogeneic SCT or consolidation chemotherapy) in order to improve disease-free survival (DFS).

Allogeneic SCT

MDS is incurable with the conventional therapies listed above. Lower-risk MDS subtypes can behave indolently for many years without progression. However, higher-risk MDS subtypes (such as IPSS intermediate-2/high and high/very high IPSS-R) have an extremely poor prognosis, with median OS 3 months (high risk) to 18 months (intermediate-2) [23] and the treatment options previously discussed are directed at hematologic improvement and symptom control. Allogeneic SCT is the only known curative treatment for MDS; however, its use is limited by donor availability as well as transplant-related morbidity and mortality, which increases with advanced age. The Seattle group published results of post-SCT outcomes in patients with MDS according to IPSS score and demonstrated a 5-year DFS of 60%, 36%, and 28% for low and intermediate-1 risk, intermediate-2 risk, and high risk, respectively [45]. Other groups have published similar results, corroborating a curative allogeneic graft-versus-tumor effect in MDS.

Nonmyeloablative allogeneic SCTs have greatly expanded the number of eligible MDS patients for SCT. Although nonmyeloablative SCTs have not been directly compared with myeloablative SCTs for MDS, a retrospective analysis demonstrated significantly increased relapse rates but significantly decreased nonrelapse mortality in patients undergoing a nonmyeloablative SCT, with similar OS rates to myeloablative SCTs [46]. Thus, nonmyeloablative SCTs remain an attractive option for older patients (>60 years) or patients with significant comorbidities.

The timing of allogeneic SCT in MDS patients remains unclear and controversial. For patients with low or intermediate-1 IPSS scores, delayed transplantation is usually recommended until disease progression [47]. For patients with intermediate-2 or high-risk IPSS scores, allogeneic SCT is recommended early during treatment, if justified by age and overall performance status/comorbidities. Patients without excess blasts can be taken directly to SCT, whereas those with excess blasts (RAEB-1/2) may warrant treatment with either hypomethylating agents or combination chemotherapy prior to undergoing an SCT, as an increased number of BM blasts at the time of SCT significantly worsens outcome [44, 48].

Acute Myeloid Leukemia

Incidence, Mortality, and Etiology

Acute myeloid leukemia (AML) is a hematologic malignancy characterized by rapid expansion of clonal myeloid cells whose maturation is arrested at the myeloblast stage, ultimately leading to ineffective hematopoiesis. In the US, the incidence rate is 4.1/100,000 persons/year and increases with age to 11.9 and 27.0, respectively, for individuals aged 65–69 and 80–84 [5].There are approximately 21,380 new cases of AML (11,960 males and 9.420 females) in the US each year and 10,590 deaths (6,110 males and 4,480 females) from AML [49]. Although the majority of cases arise *de novo*, AML can be preceded by either MDS or MPN. Risk factors include exposure to benzene, cytotoxic chemotherapy, tobacco smoke, or radiation [50]. Familial cases occur only rarely. Childhood-onset familial AML cases relate to inheritance of defective DNA damage repair enzymes (e.g. Bloom syndrome, ataxia telangiectasia, or Fanconi anemia). Adult-onset familial AML can arise from Li–Fraumeni syndrome (inherited p53 mutation), as well as germline *CEBP-α GATA2*, or *RUNX1* mutations. Despite sound evidence for environmental carcinogens and/or impaired host response to DNA damage as etiologic factors, >95% of AML patients have no identifiable risk factor.

Clinical Presentation

The clinical presentation of AML is nonspecific, and occasionally patients can be diagnosed by incidental blood work. However, typical symptoms of AML include bruising/bleeding, fatigue/malaise, infections, and/or symptoms of leukostasis, such as chest pain, shortness of breath, headaches, and confusion. The peripheral smear from patients with AML generally shows circulating myeloblasts. Myeloblasts can be morphologically identified by their larger nuclear size, fine cytoplasmic granulation, and scant cytoplasm. Leukemic myeloblasts sometimes show needle-like azurophilic aggregates of myeloperoxidase called Auer rods, which are pathognomonic of AML. In the absence of Auer rods, myeloblasts cannot be definitively distinguished from lymphoblasts using morphology alone. Therefore, microscopy must always be supplemented with appropriate immunophenotypic, cytochemical, cytogenetic, and molecular diagnostic testing. Current classification requires the presence of ≥20% myeloblasts in the peripheral blood or BM for a diagnosis of AML. A few specific exceptions exist, namely, myeloid sarcoma and AML bearing specific recurrent translocations: t(8;21), t(15;17), or inv(16) [51]. Myeloid sarcomas represent focal collections of leukemic blasts in tissue, sometimes causing demonstrable mass lesions, with or without marrow involvement by tumor cells.

Pathogenesis and Genetics

Recurrent mutations occur in nearly all cases of AML. These mutations arise from a number of genetic events including translocations, chromosomal amplification and deletions, as well as point mutations, insertions, and tandem duplications. An abnormal karyotype is identified in approximately 50% of AML patients. Specific cytogenetic abnormalities can independently predict prognosis and the likelihood of achieving remission in AML [52–54]. Additionally, in the case of *PML-RARA* fusion arising from t(15;17), cytogenetic findings predict responsiveness to particular antileukemic agents (e.g., all-*trans* retinoic acid and/or arsenic trioxide). More recently, molecular abnormalities can be used to provide prognostic information [22]. Thus, understanding the genetic complement of AML is helpful for diagnostics, therapeutics, and prognostics.

Cytogenetic abnormalities in AML commonly include recurrent, balanced translocations, additions, and deletions, with the particular abnormalities found often being similar to those observed in MDS. These include monosomy 5, del(5q), monosomy 7, del(7q), +8, +21, and others. In cases of AML following cytotoxic chemotherapy (particularly alkylating agents) or radiation, complex cytogenetic abnormalities commonly occur, often containing long arm deletions or monosomies of chromosomes 5 or 7, as well as mutation or deletion of the tumor suppressor gene, TP53. The most relevant recurrent translocations (see Table 29.1, AML with recurrent genetic abnormalities) often lead to production of abnormal transcription factors. These translocations are specific for a diagnosis of AML rather than other myeloid neoplasms, and are categorized as unique diagnostic entities as defined by the WHO [20].

Nucleophosmin-1 (NPM1) is a ribosomal shuttling protein often found in the nucleolus of cells. *NPM1* mutations have been identified in approximately 30% of AML cases. In the absence of negative prognostic mutations (e.g., *FLT3-ITD*), an *NPM1* mutation confers a favorable prognosis in patients with AML [55]. *CEBP-α* is involved in cellular proliferation as well as granulocytic differentiation. Cases of AML with *CEBP-α* mutations (particularly when bi-allelic) appear to have a relatively favorable prognosis [56, 57]. Both *NPM1* and *CEBP-α* mutations occur almost exclusively in patients with normal cytogenetics.

Signal transduction-activating gene mutations occur commonly in AML. The most common and prognostically important signaling mutations in AML involve FMS-like tyrosine kinase 3 (*FLT3*). *FLT3* is a hematopoietic cytokine receptor tyrosine kinase that regulates proliferation and differentiation of hematopoietic stem and early progenitor cells. *FLT3* is commonly overexpressed in AML, and mutations are identified in approximately 30% of patients with AML [1, 58]. *FLT3* mutations are more common in patients with normal karyotype, where they commonly coexist with mutations in *NPM1* and/or *DNMT3A*. They also commonly occur in cases with the recurrent translocations t(6;9) and t(15;17). FLT3 kinase activating mutations occur in two hotspots: the juxtamembrane region and tyrosine kinase domain (TKD). Juxtamembrane mutations occur as internal tandem duplications (ITD). *FLT3-ITD* mutations and *FLT3-TKD* mutations both lead to leukocytosis and high BM blast percentage at diagnosis. *FLT3-ITD* mutations confer a high risk of relapse and poor prognosis, whereas the prognostic significance of the *TKD* mutation remains unclear [58, 59]. Small molecules targeting FLT3 are being developed clinically [60].

Mutations leading to *c-KIT* activation also occur in AML, particularly in AML with translocations involving subunits of core binding factor: t(8;21) and inv(16). Mutations generally occur in exon 8, which encodes the extracellular part of the receptor, or exon 17 that encodes the activation loop in the kinase domain. *KIT* mutations, particularly among patients with t(8;21), appear to blunt the otherwise favorable effects of these karyotypes and may confer an intermediate-risk group for prognosis [61].

Classification

One of the older models for classification that is sometimes still used is the French–American–British (FAB) system, which organized the disease based on morphologic and cytochemical features [62]. This system contained eight categories (M0 through M7). Knowledge of pathogenesis and disease development led to reclassification of these diseases in 2001 by the WHO as clinicopathologic entities with the integration of genetic information. The current classification was most recently revised in 2016 (Table 29.1) [20, 51].

Acute Promyelocytic Leukemia

Acute promyelocytic leukemia (APL: t(15;17)(q22;q12); PML-RARA) currently encompasses all cases of the previous FAB classification of AML-M3 (Table 29.3). APL is seen in approximately 8% of all AMLs and has a relatively young median age at diagnosis. Morphologically, APL is characterized by a maturation arrest and proliferation of promyelocytes, rather than myeloblasts. Leukemic promyelocytes have abundant cytoplasm that is densely granulated and often contains multiple Auer rods. A microgranular variant also occurs in approximately one-quarter of cases, in which dense granules are undetectable by light microscopy but can be seen by electron microscopy. Leukemic cells in both variants frequently show bi-lobed nuclei ("cottage-loaf" cell). Although APL represents a distinct morphology and immunophenotype [63, 64], a final diagnosis requires genetic confirmation of t(15;17) or its transcript via cytogenetics, fluorescent *in situ* hybridization (FISH), or reverse transcriptase polymerase chain reaction (RT-PCR).

APL frequently presents with pancytopenia and potentially lethal disseminated intravascular coagulopathy (DIC), making urgent diagnosis and rapid initiation of therapy critical. Blood tests at initial presentation of APL typically show depleted levels of clotting factors as well as evidence of hypofibrinogenemia. The coagulopathy of APL is primarily characterized by profound risk of unprovoked bleeding, which is complicated by thrombocytopenia. The pathogenesis of DIC in APL and involves the presence of prothrombotic proteins within granules (e.g., cancer procoagulant and tissue factor), aberrant expression of the tissue plasminogen activator cofactor annexin II (a cofactor for tissue plasminogen activator), and activation of fibrinolysis [65–67].

Risk Stratification/Prognosis

The most widely used risk stratification of AML patients is that published by the European LeukemiaNet (ELN) International Panel, which includes diagnostic and prognostic cytogenetic and molecular features of AML at diagnosis [68]. As shown in Table 29.4, the ELN classifies patients into four risk groups (favorable, intermediate-1, intermediate-2, adverse). Among 818 younger (age <60 years) patients treated on frontline Cancer

Table 29.3 FAB classification of AML and MDS.

AML
M0 undifferentiated
M1 without differentiation
M2 with differentiation
(*note: many cases have t(8;21) and favorable prognosis*)
M3 promyelocytic differentiation (APL)
(*note: strongly associated with t(15;17) and favorable prognosis*)
M4 myelomonocytic differentiation
M4Eo myelomonocytic with abnormal eosinophils
(*note: strongly associated with inv(16) and favorable prognosis*)
M5 monocytic/monoblastic differentiation
M6 erythroblastic
M7 megakaryoblastic
MDS
Refractory anemia (RA)
Refractory anemia, with ringed sideroblasts (RARS)
Refractory anemia with excess blasts (RAEB)
Refractory anemia with excess blasts in transformation (RAEB-T)
Chronic myelomonocytic leukemia (CMML)

Table 29.4 Risk stratification of AML.

Risk status	Subsets	Postremission therapy
Favorable	CBF AML [t(8;21); inv(16)/t(16;16)] *NPM1* mutation without *FLT3-ITD* mutation (normal karyotype) *CEBPA* mutation (normal karyotype)	Four courses of HiDAC consolidation therapy
Intermediate-1	*NPM1* mutation with *FLT3-ITD* mutation (normal karyotype) Wild-type *NPM1* with *FLT3-ITD* mutation (normal karyotype) Wild-type *NPM1* without *FLT3-ITD* mutation (normal karyotype)	Allogeneic SCT in CR1
Intermediate-2	t(9;11) (*MLL* gene rearrangement) Cytogenetic abnormalities not classified as favorable or poor-risk	Allogeneic SCT in CR1
Poor/adverse	inv(3) t(6;9) t(v;11) (*MLL* gene rearrangement other than t(9;11)) −5 or del(5q); −7; abnl(17p); complex karyotype	Allogeneic SCT in CR1

CR, complete remission; HiDAC, high-dose intermittent ARA-C; SCT, hematopoietic stem cell transplantation.

Table 29.5 Genomic classification of AML.

Genomic subgroup	Frequency
AML with *NPM1* mutation	27%
AML with mutated chromatin, RNA-splicing genes or both	18%
AML with *TP53* mutations, chromosomal aneuploidy, or both	13%
AML with driver mutations but no detected class-defining lesions	11%
AML with inv(16) or t(16;16); *CBFB-MYH11*	5%
AML with biallelic *CEBPA* mutations	4%
AML with t(15;17); *PML-RARA*	4%
AML with t(8;21); *RUNX1-RUNX1T1*	4%
AML with no detected driver genes	4%
AML meeting criteria for ≥2 genomic subgroups	4%
AML with *MLL* fusion genes; t(x;11)	3%
AML with inv(3) or t(3;3); *GATA2, MECOM (EVI1)*	1%
AML with *IDH2*^{R172} mutations and no other class-defining lesion	1%
AML with t(6;9); *DEK-NUP214*	1%

and Leukemia Group B (CALGB) studies, the 3-year DFS was 55%, 23%, 34%, and 10% among patients in the favorable, intermediate-1, intermediate-2, and adverse risk groups according to ELN classification, respectively. In comparison, older patients (age ≥60 years) had distinctively worse outcomes across each subset with a 3-year DFS of 24%, 10%, 11%, and 6% among patients in the favorable, intermediate-1, intermediate-2 and adverse risk groups, respectively [69]. More recently, numerous molecular mutations have been identified that are associated with distinct genomic classes and may elucidate prognosis more accurately than other risk scores. The largest genomic classification of AML, published by Papaemmanuil *et al.* [70], analyzed 1540 patients and 111 cancer genes from three prospective trials of induction chemotherapy. The authors identified >5,000 driver mutations across 76 genes with the majority of patients (86%) having at least two or more driver mutations. Eleven distinct genomic classes were identified with unique biology and prognosis (Table 29.5). Importantly, specific gene–gene interactions appear to display prognostic significance. Ultimately, genomic classification may replace our current outdated risk score stratification models.

Therapy of AML

Overview

The overall therapeutic approach to patients with AML depends on their age, ECOG PS, and comorbidities, as well as molecular and genetic risk factors determined at the time of diagnosis. In general, treatment is divided into induction and postremission (i.e., consolidation) therapies. The purpose of induction therapy is to rapidly debulk the leukemic burden with the goal of achieving a complete remission (CR). CR is defined by <5% blasts in the BM and hematologic recovery (absolute neutrophil count >1000/μL, platelet count >100,000/μL). Once CR is achieved, further postremission therapy is given to eradicate residual leukemic burden and extend DFS, unless prohibited by the clinical condition of the patient. The type of postremission therapy depends on the risk of relapse, patient age, and comorbidities, and consists of either multiple cycles of chemotherapy or an allogeneic SCT.

Induction Therapy

Induction therapy for AML includes two main chemotherapeutic agents, cytarabine and an anthracycline. The regimen known as "7 + 3," standing for 7 days of a continuous infusion (CI) of cytarabine (100 or 200 mg/m^2/day) and 3 days of an anthracycline, has been generally accepted as a "standard" induction therapy for AML, producing CR rates of approximately 70–75% in younger (<60 years old) and 35–55% in older AML patients [71, 72]. Multiple studies have attempted to optimize induction therapy by dose-escalating cytarabine or adding a third conventional chemotherapeutic agent to the standard regimen; unfortunately, these studies have failed to consistently demonstrate improvement in outcomes over conventional 7 + 3 [73]. Substitution of anthracyclines in the induction regimen, such as idarubicin in place of daunorubicin, has led to inconsistent results [73].

Dose intensification of anthracyclines may improve OS in younger and in a select group of older AML patients. The Eastern Cooperative Oncology Group (ECOG) conducted a phase 3 study (E1900) [74] comparing high-dose daunorubicin (90 mg/m^2/day) versus standard-dose daunorubicin (45 mg/m^2/day), given along with cytarabine CI (7 + 3), to 657 younger patients (age <60 years) with newly diagnosed AML. High-dose daunorubicin led to improved CR rates (71% vs 57%) and improved OS (median 23.7 months vs 15.7 months). Patients with favorable and intermediate karyotypes seemed to have the greatest benefit from the high-dose daunorubicin [74]. The benefit of high-dose daunorubicin versus standard-dose daunorubicin (90 mg/m^2/day vs 45 mg/m^2/day) in younger AML patients is further supported by data from a randomized study by the Korean group [75].

The multicenter European study compared the same doses of daunorubicin (90 mg/m^2 vs 45 mg/m^2) in induction in patients 60 years of age and older and showed that high-dose daunorubicin improved CR rates compared to low-dose daunorubicin (52% vs 35%) but improvement in OS was observed only in the subgroup of patients aged 60–65 years (2-year OS 38% vs 23%) [76]. Most importantly, in all of these studies, toxicities were similar between the arms, suggesting that daunorubicin can be safely dose escalated. While these studies support the use of high-dose daunorubicin at 90 mg/m^2 (or idarubicin 12 mg/m^2) in conjunction with cytarabine (100–200 mg/m^2/day CI) as induction therapy in patients up to 65 years of age, particularly if they have intermediate and favorable karyotype, further genomic studies would hopefully help identify the patient population that is most likely to derive benefit from daunorubicin dose escalation. Genetic profiling of patients treated in the E1900 study identified a subset of patients harboring *DNMT3A*, *NPM1* mutations, or *MLL* translocation to preferentially benefit from high-dose daunorubicin [22].

Although high-dose daunorubicin (90 mg/m^2) clearly showed benefit compared with low-dose daunorubicin (45 mg/m^2) in select patient populations, it is unclear if daunorubicin 90 mg/m^2 is equivalent to 60 mg/m^2. The UK National Cancer Research Institute (NCRI) AML17 trial randomized 1206 adults with newly diagnosed AML or high-risk MDS to 90 mg/m^2 of daunorubicin versus 60 mg/m^2 on days 1, 3, and 5 when combined with cytarabine 100 mg/m^2 every 12 hours on days 1–10 [77]. There were no differences in CR rates between both doses of daunorubicin (73% vs 75%) but higher 60 day mortality in the 90 mg/m^2 arm (10% vs 5%). However, all patients on this study received double induction therapy which is not generally utilized in the US. Thus, it remains an unanswered question whether 60 mg/m^2 of daunorubicin is equivalent to 90 mg/m^2 when combined with cytarabine in the 7 + 3 regimen for newly diagnosed AML patients. Both doses are acceptable to use in the front-line setting.

Several novel nucleoside analogs, including fludarabine, clofarabine, and cladribine, have been studied in front-line therapy for AML. The most promising results are from the Polish Adult Leukemia Group (PLAG): a phase 3 study comparing the addition of cladribine or fludarabine to 7 + 3 versus 7+ 3 alone in 652 AML patients less than 60 years of age. The findings showed that the addition of cladribine, but not fludarabine, improved the response rates, DFS, and OS compared with standard 7 + 3 therapy [78]. The 7 + 3 arm on this study, however, utilized cytarabine 200 mg/m^2 CI on days 1–7 and daunorubicin 60 mg/m^2 on days 1–3. Thus, it is unclear if these results are generalizable given the lower doses of daunorubicin in the comparator arms. Nonetheless, cladribine + 7 + 3 (DAC) is a reasonable first-line treatment option for newly diagnosed AML patients <60 years based on the results of this phase 3 study.

In older patients, administration of clofarabine (20 mg/m^2 days 1–5) improved response rates compared with low-dose cytarabine (100 mg/m^2 twice a day on days 1–10), but produced no difference in OS in the Medical Research Council (MRC)/National Cancer Research Institute (NCRI) AML16 study [79]. Additionally, an intergroup randomized phase 3 clinical trial of clofarabine 30 mg/m^2 IV on days 1–5 compared with 7 + 3 in newly diagnosed older (>60 years) AML patients showed no differences in CR rates but improved OS in the 7 + 3 arm [80].

Targeted therapies have been explored in induction regimens for AML. Gemtuzumab ozogamicin (GO), a monoclonal antibody targeting CD33 linked to calicheamicin, received accelerated regulatory approval in the US for the treatment of first relapse in AML patients >60 years of age and unsuitable for intensive therapy, but a follow-up study (S0106) [81] that randomized patients younger than 60 years to GO (6 mg/m^2 on day 4) plus 7 + 3 (daunorubicin 45 mg/m^2) versus 7 + 3 (daunorubicin 60 mg/m^2) induction demonstrated no clinical benefit but increased death rate on the GO arm. Unfortunately, this led to the removal of GO from the market in the US. The results of several large randomized European studies have been reported since, however, showing the OS benefit for lower doses of GO (3 mg/m^2) or fractionated doses (GO 3 mg/m^2 on days 1, 4, and 7) given in conjunction with induction chemotherapy to newly diagnosed patients with AML [82]. These studies have showed no excess in mortality on the GO arm, however, the benefit was confined only to patients with favorable or intermediate-risk karyotypes. GO has since been approved by the US Food and Drug Administration (FDA) in September 2017 for the treatment of adults with newly diagnosed CD33-positive AML in combination with induction chemotherapy or as a single agent in relapsed/refractory disease.

Clinical studies exploring single-agent multitargeted tyrosine kinase inhibitors (TKIs) with FLT3 inhibitory activity in AML have demonstrated very limited clinical activity, likely related to incomplete *in vivo* FLT3 inhibition [83]. Two phase 3 studies exploring such agents (midostaurin and lestaurtinib) in combination with induction chemotherapy in patients with newly diagnosed FLT3-ITD mutated AML have been recently completed. The addition of midostaurin to 7 + 3 induction chemotherapy in newly diagnosed adults with FLT3 mutations showed improved OS and event-free survival (EFS) when compared to 7 + 3 plus placebo [84, 85]. The results of this study led to the FDA approval of midostaurin in combination with induction chemotherapy in newly diagnosed AML patients with an FLT3 mutation, ending a 17-year drought of new agents approved for AML. A randomized, double blind, placebo-controlled phase 2 trial in younger (≤60 years) AML patients was performed in Europe comparing 7 + 3 with the addition of sorafenib (400 mg orally twice daily on days 10–19) versus placebo [86]. The findings from this large 276 patient study revealed an EFS of 21 months in the sorafenib group compared with 9 months in the placebo group. However, the sorafenib group had more toxicity. Quizartinib (AC220), a second-generation FLT3 inhibitor (more potent and selective), showed considerable clinical activity in patients with relapsed/refractory FLT3-ITD AML producing promising CR rates [87].

Postremission Therapy

Consolidation Chemotherapy

After CR has been achieved, further therapy is required to achieve long-term leukemia-free survival (LFS) or cure. The selection of postremission therapy depends on many factors, such as the relapse risk, patient age, comorbidities, overall ECOG PS, and the availability of a donor. Consolidation chemotherapy is generally recommended for patients with favorable-risk AML (Table 29.4); it may also be given for 1–2 cycles in patients in whom an SCT is planned, in order to allow adequate time to prepare for SCT.

For younger patients, high-dose cytarabine (HiDAC) has been considered the consolidation regimen of choice. Three different doses of cytarabine (100 mg/m^2 CI for 5 days, 400 mg/m^2 CI for 5 days, 3 g/m^2 over 3 hours twice a day on day 1, 3, 5) given for 4 cycles were studied as postremission therapy in a CALGB randomized trial, which demonstrated that HiDAC (3 g/m^2 over 3 hours twice a day on day 1, 3, 5) had the best overall outcome, producing 44% 4-year DFS in patients ≤60 years [88]. For older patients, all consolidation regimens produced similar DFS of 16% at 2 years. HiDAC consolidation seems to benefit patients with core binding factor leukemias [89]. Retrospective analysis by CALGB suggested that 4 cycles of HiDAC or 1 cycle of HiDAC followed by autologous SCT produce similar outcome in patients with normal karyotype AML [90]. However, patients with poor-risk features had a relapse-free survival (RFS) of only 15% with HiDAC, and thus these patients warrant therapy with an allogeneic SCT for improved outcome [89].

The MRC/NCRI AML15 study demonstrated equivalent outcomes with cytarabine consolidation at 1.5 g/m^2 and 3 g/m^2 in younger AML patients. However, both HiDAC doses produced inferior outcomes in patients with adverse-risk karyotype in comparison to the mitoxantrone/cytarabine/amsacrine-based consolidation arm [91]. In this study, there was no benefit of extending consolidation beyond 2 cycles after patients received 2 induction cycles. Thus, it is reasonable to consider reducing the dose and duration of HiDAC consolidation, particularly in older patients, those with poor ECOG PS, or those who are at high risk of developing neurologic toxicity.

The ALFA 9803 [92] phase 3 clinical trial randomized patients ≥65 years in CR after intensive induction chemotherapy to ambulatory versus intensive postremission therapy. The ambulatory group received 6 monthly courses of daunorubicin 45 mg/m^2 or idarubicin 9 mg/m^2 IV on day 1 in combination with cytarabine SQ Q12 hours on days 1–5. The intensive group received another cycle of intensive induction chemotherapy analogous to cycle 1 induction therapy. Of the 164 patients randomized in consolidation, there was a significant OS and DFS benefit to ambulatory consolidation when compared to intensive postremission therapy. Thus, ambulatory postremission therapy, as outlined above, is a reasonable option for patients aged ≥65 years in their first CR (CR1) after intensive induction therapy.

Allogeneic SCT

Allogeneic SCT should be strongly considered in AML patients without favorable-risk features (Table 29.4) in CR1, due to poor outcomes associated with conventional chemotherapy. Whether or not consolidation chemotherapy, such as HiDAC, should be given prior to allogeneic SCT is controversial. Allogeneic SCT can improve cure rate in those patients via an immunologic graft-versus-leukemia effect. A variety of SCT sources have been used successfully in AML with comparable outcomes, including matched-related and matched-unrelated donors, as well as newer approaches such as haploidentical donors and cord blood [93, 94]. Nonmyeloablative (NMA) SCT has expanded the availability of allogeneic SCT for older patients and patients who may otherwise not be fit for a myeloablative SCT.

Indications for an SCT in CR1 in AML are shown in Table 29.4 and are based on the cytogenetic and molecular risk status of the patient. A systematic review and meta-analysis of 3,638 AML patients younger than 60 years in CR1 demonstrated an RFS and OS advantage of allogeneic SCT over chemotherapy in patients with intermediate- and poor-risk, but not with favorable-risk karyotypes [95]. Patients with intermediate-risk AML and normal karyotype can be further subclassified as either intermediate-risk or favorable-risk based on three molecular mutations: *FLT3*, *NPM1*, and *CEBP-α*. Patients with a normal karyotype and an *NPM1* or double *CEBP-α* mutation without a *FLT3* mutation are regarded as a favorable-risk subtype, and allogeneic SCT does not seem to benefit this patient group. On the other hand, patients with a normal karyotype having *FLT3-ITD* mutations (with or without *NPM1*) or patients without *FLT3-ITD*, *NPM1*, or *CEBP-α* mutations appear to have an OS advantage with allogeneic SCT over consolidation chemotherapy [55]. Allogeneic SCT can lead to long-term LFS in approximately 50% of patients transplanted in CR1 [96]. However, patients with poor-risk features, such as those having monosomal karyotype or complex cytogenetics have a poor prognosis even after an allogeneic SCT, with OS rates approximately 20–25% after allogeneic SCT [97, 98].

Relapsed and Refractory AML

More than half of patients treated with conventional chemotherapy for AML will either have refractory disease (inability to reach CR after induction therapy) or will relapse after initial achievement of a CR. The duration of the first CR is an important predictor of response to subsequent salvage therapy. Up to 50% of patients with CR1 duration >1 year will respond to reinduction therapy, whereas those having CR1 <6 months have <20% chance of achieving a CR2 [99]. In addition to CR1 duration, several other parameters such as increased age, unfavorable karyotype, *FLT3-ITD* mutation, and prior allogeneic SCT adversely influence the outcome after salvage therapy [99].

Given the extremely poor prognosis among this subgroup of AML patients, allogeneic SCT is the only therapeutic option that provides a chance of long-term LFS, and is strongly recommended in patients who respond to a salvage regimen. Several salvage regimens have been used with response rates ranging from 20 to 50% in different studies [99–102], including HiDAC; mitoxantrone, etoposide, with or without cytarabine (MEC); or using alternative nucleosides such as fludarabine, cladribine, or clofarabine in combination with cytarabine and G-CSF (FLAG, CLAG, GCLAC). Patients with *FLT3-ITD* mutated AML should be treated on clinical studies using targeted agents, when applicable. In general, patients should be encouraged to participate in clinical trials, otherwise any of above regimens can be attempted in order to achieve a CR2. With allogeneic SCT, up to 30–40% of patients may achieve long-term LFS if transplanted in CR2 [99].

IDH2 mutations occur in approximately 8–10% of AML patients. Enasidenib is an oral *IDH2* inhibitor that has demonstrated safety and activity in relapsed/refractory AML patients who harbor an *IDH2* mutation. Overall response rates and CR rates with enasidenib are approximately 38% and 20%, respectively, in patients with relapsed/refractory AML and *IDH2* mutations [103]. Based on these data, enasidenib was FDA approved for the treatment of relapsed/refractory AML patients with *IDH2* mutations in August 2017.

Treatment of Elderly Patients with AML

The majority of patients diagnosed with AML are older than 60 [104]. Conventional chemotherapeutic agents used for treatment of younger AML patients are less effective in older AML patients. Elderly patients tend more frequently to have AML phenotypes that are chemoresistant, such as poor-risk karyotype or AML arising from an antecedent hematologic disorder (secondary AML) or prior chemotherapy/radiation therapy (treatment-related AML). Due to age-associated comorbidities, older AML patients also have an increased risk of treatment-related morbidity and mortality when treated with conventional chemotherapeutics. Retrospective analysis of 968 AML patients treated on five Southwestern Oncology Group (SWOG) protocols demonstrated that death rate following chemotherapy was positively associated with worse ECOG PS and increasing age [105]. Nonetheless, some older patients do in fact benefit from intensive induction chemotherapy. The improved outcomes seen in elderly patients (aged 60–65 years) with favorable and intermediate karyotypes treated with high-dose daunorubicin suggest that this group of patients may benefit from administration of standard chemotherapy [76]. A retrospective analysis by the Swedish Acute Leukemia Registry also demonstrated that early death rates and OS were improved in older patients up to age 79 years who received conventional induction chemotherapy regimens when compared to palliative methods [106]. Several studies have also demonstrated that age up to 70 years may not affect the outcome after NMA allogeneic SCT, extending this potentially curative therapeutic option to elderly AML patients [107].

Different intensity therapies have been studied in elderly AML patients in order to increase response rates and decrease treatment-related mortality. A randomized study demonstrated that low-dose cytarabine (20 mg subcutaneous injection twice daily for 10 days) was superior to hydroxyurea in terms of CR rate (18% vs 1%) and OS when given to elderly AML patients unfit for intensive chemotherapy approach; however, patients with poor-risk karyotype did not benefit from this therapy [108]. The hypomethylating agent, azacitidine, produced similar response rates but improved OS compared to conventional care regimens among patients with AML (20–30% blasts) treated on the original phase 3 study for patients with high-risk MDS, and thus represents an attractive first-line option for elderly patients with AML who cannot withstand intensive induction therapy [38]. Moreover, an international phase 3 study compared azacitidine to physician choice, which included best supportive care, intensive induction chemotherapy, or low-dose cytarabine in newly diagnosed AML patients ≥65 years with bone marrow blasts ≥30% [109]. Median OS was 10.4 months on azacitidine compared with 6.5 months on physician choice ($P = 0.10$). One-year survival rates were still low on both arms (46.5% vs 34.2%, respectively). Importantly, in patients preselected to receive intensive induction chemotherapy, there was no difference in median OS compared with azacitidine (12.2 months vs 13.3 months), suggesting that azacitidine may be a reasonable first-line treatment for newly diagnosed elderly patients with AML (age ≥65 years). Decitabine (20 mg/m^2 × 5 days), another hypomethylating agent, may also be a treatment option for elderly AML patients, though there were no significant improvements in OS when compared with low-dose cytarabine and/or supportive care, and thus decitabine is not FDA approved for AML [110]. Other dosing regimens including decitabine 20 mg/m^2 × 10 days have been explored with promising results [111].

In older patients, administration of clofarabine (20 mg/m^2 on days 1–5) improved response rates compared with low-dose cytarabine (100 mg/m^2 twice a day on days 1–10), but produced no difference in OS in the MRC/NCRI AML16 study [79]. Additionally, an intergroup randomized phase 3 clinical trial of clofarabine 30 mg/m^2 IV on days 1–5 compared with 7 + 3 in newly diagnosed older (>60 years) AML patients showed no differences in CR rates but improved OS in the 7 + 3 arm [80].

CPX-351, a liposomal formulation of cytarabine and daunorubicin in a 5:1 molar ratio, represents a new standard of care first-line treatment regimen for newly diagnosed older (≥60 years) adults with poor-risk features such as secondary AML or adverse-risk cytogenetics. A randomized phase 3 trial of CPX-351 versus 7 + 3 in patients 60–75 years with untreated AML with history of prior cytotoxic therapy, antecedent MDS or CMML, or AML with MDS-related cytogenetic abnormalities was recently completed and reported [112]. CPX-351 was found to have a significant median OS advantage (9.56 vs 5.95 months; $P = 0.005$) when compared with 7 + 3. Based on these data, CPX-351 was FDA approved for the treatment of adults with newly diagnosed therapy-related AML or AML with MDS-related changes.

The management of AML in the elderly remains complex with many unanswered questions regarding the use of intensive induction chemotherapy versus lower-intensity regimens such as hypomethylating agents. Hopefully, future clinical trials will address this patient population to establish a standard of care for the majority of patients.

Treatment of APL

APL is a distinct subset of AML (FAB classification: M3), characterized by a t(15;17) (PML-RARA). Patients with APL tend to present with low white blood cell (WBC) counts and coagulopathy, with hemorrhagic events leading to 10–15% excess early mortality during induction chemotherapy. The incorporation of all-*trans* retinoic acid (ATRA), as a differentiation agent, into the early management of APL has dramatically improved clinical outcomes. Anthracyclines and ATRA represent the backbone of APL induction and consolidation chemotherapy. Several large group studies (French and North American) also included cytarabine during induction and consolidation. All studies (with or without cytarabine) reported >90% CR rates in patients with an initial WBC count <10,000/μL. Thus ATRA represents a breakthrough therapy for APL and should be administered as soon as APL is suspected [104].

Patients with APL can be risk stratified based on WBC and platelet count at the time of presentation into three risk categories: low risk (WBC ≤10,000/μL and platelets >40,000/μL) with DFS of 97%; intermediate risk (WBC <10,000/μL and platelets <40,000/μL) with DFS of 86%; and high risk (WBC >10,000/μL) with DFS of 78% [113]. More recently, platelets have been excluded from the risk stratification and patients are only defined as low risk (WBC ≤10,000/μL) versus high risk (WBC >10,000/μL).

Given the excellent results obtained with arsenic trioxide (ATO) in patients with relapsed APL, several groups introduced ATO in the initial treatment of APL to improve efficacy and to reduce use of chemotherapy. The randomized North American Intergroup study showed improved EFS and DFS when 2 cycles of ATO were added to consolidation chemotherapy. In a single-arm study, the efficacy of ATO plus ATRA therapy in patients presenting with WBC ≤10,000/mm^3 was comparable to previous results with chemotherapy [104]. This led to a phase 3 study in 156 newly diagnosed APL patients <70 years old and with presenting WBC ≤10,000/μL that randomized patients to receive ATRA plus ATO or ATRA plus idarubicin chemotherapy. A CR was achieved in 100% in the ATRA and ATO arm compared with 95% in the ATRA plus chemotherapy arm, and 2-year EFS rates were 97% and 86% for the ATRA plus ATO and ATRA plus chemotherapy arms, respectively. OS was also improved in the ATRA plus ATO arm thus demonstrating that it is possible to eliminate chemotherapy from the induction strategy of low/intermediate-risk APL patients [114]. ATRA and ATO therapy represent a new standard of care for patients with low-risk (WBC ≤10,000/μL) APL.

Chemotherapy in combination with ATRA and/or ATO is still the standard of care for high-risk APL patients. There are a number of evidence-based treatment regimens to consider for patients with high-risk APL incorporating anthracycline ± cytarabine in induction [115].

It is important to note that differentiation syndrome (DS), consisting of fever, weight gain, respiratory distress, and pulmonary infiltrates, can occur in patients with APL treated with ATRA or ATO. Early diagnosis of DS is crucial as these symptoms can lead to high rates of morbidity and mortality. Treatment of DS includes steroids as well as temporarily discontinuing the offending agent (ATRA or ATO) if necessary [116].

Although initial studies suggested that maintenance therapy with ATRA with or without methotrexate and 6-mercaptopurine may be beneficial, several recent studies demonstrated that this strategy may not be helpful in patients who are in complete molecular remission following intensive consolidation [117].

ATO is also effective as a single agent in patients with relapsed APL, and can achieve CR2 rates as high as 90% [104]. GO is also a promising strategy for patients with relapsed APL, demonstrating 100% molecular response rate after 3 doses [118].

Myeloproliferative Neoplasms

Myeloproliferative neoplasms (MPN) are clonal proliferations of myeloid elements leading to the elevation of peripheral blood counts. These include chronic myeloid leukemia (CML) and Philadelphia chromosome-negative MPNs such as polycythemia vera (PV), essential thrombocythemia (ET), primary myelofibrosis (PMF), and mastocytosis. A separate category of myeloid lesions presenting with eosinophilia has also been recently described and defined by mutations in the tyrosine kinases PDGFRA, PDGFRB, or FGFR1. All of these conditions (except mastocytosis) share clinical presenting features, which include elevated peripheral counts and splenomegaly.

Chronic Myeloid Leukemia

Incidence, Mortality, and Etiology

In the US, the CML incidence rate is 1.8/100,000 persons/year, and increases with age to 4.8 and 9.8, respectively, for individuals aged 65–69 and 80–84. The median age at diagnosis is 64 years [5]. In 2017, 8,950 new cases of CML (5,230 males and 3,720 females) are estimated to occur in the US, with 1,080 deaths (610 males and 470 females) from CML [49].

Clinical Presentation

CML typically presents as a marked increase in the granulocytic lineage in the BM and the peripheral blood, with increased numbers of myelocytes, metamyelocytes, and neutrophils, along with eosinophilia and basophilia. Patients sometimes present with symptoms related to splenomegaly, but more commonly are asymptomatic and identified when routine blood work shows left-shifted leukocytosis and thrombocytosis.

Pathogenesis and Genetics

Chronic myeloid leukemia (CML) is defined as an MPN arising from the mutation t(9;22)(q34;q11.2); BCR-ABL1, recognized cytogenetically as the Philadelphia (Ph) chromosome. This translocation fuses the ABL1 kinase domain with the BCR oligomerization domain, leading to constitutive activation of the kinase [119]. The presence of the Ph chromosome is necessary for the diagnosis of CML, though it is not specific for it as the Ph chromosome can be seen in acute lymphoblastic leukemia (ALL) and rarely in *de novo* AML. In nearly all cases of CML (>90%), the Ph chromosome can be seen on conventional karyotype. Additional cases can only be seen by FISH, while the remainder of cases have cryptic translocations and may be found with molecular techniques. In advanced phases of CML, marrow karyotypes may show additional chromosomal abnormalities, most commonly another copy of the Ph chromosome, trisomy 8, or isochromosome 17q, which represents TP53 deletion.

Classification

In the era prior to TKIs (i.e., imatinib), the natural history of CML was one of inexorable progression from a generally asymptomatic and clinically indolent period in early disease toward eventual and generally abrupt clinical decompensation in advanced disease, characterized by blast phase transformation. Transformation to "blast crisis" usually occurred within 3–5 years from diagnosis and was rapidly progressive and generally fatal. CML has three clinical phases: chronic phase (CP), accelerated phase (AP), and blast crisis (BC). In AP and BC, additional mutations are acquired and cooperate with *BCR-ABL1* to impair differentiation and generally increase aggressiveness of the disease. Experimental data suggest that in CP CML, the *BCR-ABL1* mutation occurs in a hematopoietic stem cell and thus affects all lineages, while BC arises in a slightly more mature clone and generally shows maturation arrest and proliferation of blasts from myeloid (70–80% of cases) or lymphoid lineages (20–30% of cases) [120, 121].

CML patients in CP typically have peripheral leukocytosis, immature circulating myeloid cells (both granulocytic and erythroid), and very few to no myeloblasts (<5%). The BM biopsy shows a markedly hypercellular marrow with marked myeloid hyperplasia and no evidence or dysplasia or increased blasts (<5%). Other cytologic clues to a diagnosis of CML include basophilia, monolobated "dwarf" megakaryocytes, pseudo-Gaucher cells, and sea blue histiocytes.

Clinical features of AP include development of new cytogenetic abnormalities other than t(9;22), duplication of t(9;22), progressive leukocytosis or thrombocytosis despite therapy, massive splenomegaly, and increases of basophils (>20%) or blasts (10–19%) in the blood or BM. BC represents transformation to an acute leukemia, in which blasts account for greater than 20% in the peripheral blood or BM [120].

Therapy of CML

Historical Overview

Prior to the discovery of targeted TKIs against the BCR-ABL1 fusion gene, CML was a fatal disease for patients without an allogeneic SCT. First-line therapy for CML consisted of hydroxyurea, interferon (IFN), and an allogeneic SCT. However, the discovery and success of TKIs for CML revolutionized the landscape of targeted therapy for cancer.

First-Line Therapy for CP CML

Imatinib (IM), a potent inhibitor of *BCR-ABL1* as well as other kinases such as *PDGF-R* and *KIT*, was the first TKI clinically tested in CML patients. After initial studies of IM in patients who failed prior interferon therapy demonstrated its clinical activity, including hematologic and cytogenetic response of more than 95% and 50%, respectively, IM 400 mg quickly became the standard front-line therapy for CML [122, 123]. Subsequently, IM was compared with IFN plus low-dose cytarabine in newly diagnosed CP CML patients (IRIS study), and demonstrated significant improvement in the freedom from progression and the rate of complete cytogenetic responses (CCyR) by 18 months (87% vs 34%) [124]. With 6-year follow-up on IM treated patients, the estimated rate of the freedom from progression to AP or BC was 93% with a long-term OS of 88% [125]. IM is very well tolerated with the most common side effects being nausea, vomiting, muscle cramping, peripheral edema, diarrhea, and cytopenias.

In an effort to increase cytogenetic and molecular responses, higher doses of IM have been explored (600 mg or 800 mg). Higher doses of IM have generally led to faster CCyRs and major molecular responses (MMR), but after 24 months the differences in CCyR, MMR, and progression-free survival become negligible [126]. Recent data suggest that initial treatment with IM 800 mg leads to deeper molecular responses than IM 400 mg and shows a trend toward improved PFS and OS, albeit with more toxicity [127]. The recommended dose of IM for patients with CP CML remains 400 mg/day.

Second-generation TKIs have been developed and demonstrated activity in patients failing upfront IM. In an effort to increase responses and improve outcomes, including reducing the TKI resistance rate, dasatinib (DAS) and nilotinib (NIL) were tested in upfront therapy of CP CML patients. Both agents are more potent inhibitors of BCR-ABL than IM, with DAS also having potent activity against *SRC*. The efficacy and safety of DAS 100 mg was compared with IM 400 mg among newly diagnosed CP CML patients in the DASISION trial. At 12 months, DAS led to higher rates of both CCyR (77% vs 66%) and MMR (46% vs 28%), and the responses were achieved faster on the DAS arm. Although not statistically significant, progression to AP or BC was also lower in the DAS arm (1.9% vs 3.5%) [128]. DAS was approved for the first-line treatment of CML in 2010. A recent update of the DASISION trial demonstrated that these higher responses on DAS were maintained at 5 years but there is no appreciable difference in OS between DAS and IM [129]. NIL 300 mg and 400 mg twice a day was also compared with IM 400 mg in a randomized phase 3 trial for newly diagnosed CML patients. At 12 months, NIL demonstrated superior rates of CCyR (80% and 78% vs 65%) and MMR (44% and 43% vs 22%) as well as a statistically significant decrease in progression to AP and BC (<1% in both NIL doses vs 4%) when compared to IM. These results persisted at 4 years [130, 131]. NIL was also approved for first-line treatment of CML in 2010 at a dose of 300 mg twice daily.

Upon diagnosis of CML, the decision to begin with IM, DAS, or NIL is controversial and depends upon many factors, including age, side effect profile (DAS is associated with pleural effusions and pulmonary arterial hypertension, whereas NIL is associated with hyperglycemia, pancreatitis, and vascular events), cost, risk score, and phase of CML. In general, DAS and NIL lead to earlier and deeper responses than IM; however, it is unclear if this translates to an overall improved outcome and prolonged OS. Given the deeper responses seen with DAS and NIL, it would be reasonable, however, to begin with the more potent agents in younger patients in order to improve the possibility of long-term DFS. There is emerging evidence that approximately 30–40% of patients who receive a deep stable complete molecular response (CMR) on TKI therapy may be able to safely discontinue TKI therapy with long-term DFS [132].Future studies are ongoing to better predict which patients are more likely to remain in CMR after treatment discontinuation. On the other hand, given the long-term safety and efficacy data of IM, it is reasonable to begin with this agent in all ages, especially in an older patient population, in which treatment discontinuation may not be the ultimate goal.

Monitoring Response to TKI Therapy

One of the key aspects in managing patients with CML is to appropriately monitor responses while on TKI therapy. Criteria have been developed in order to determine optimal or suboptimal responses to therapy (Table 29.6). The goal of therapy for CML is to achieve a complete hematologic response (CHR) within 3 months, a CCyR within 12 months, and an MMR within 18 months. BCR-ABL FISH and PCR (via peripheral blood) should be checked at 3-month intervals after beginning therapy. Once a CCyR is achieved, PCR can then be followed at 3–6-month intervals in order to ensure continued optimal responses are achieved. Patients who are not achieving appropriate milestones, or patients with rising BCR-ABL1 PCR/FISH levels should be switched to an alternative TKI and tested for BCR-ABL mutations or additional genetic abnormalities. Recent studies suggest that early molecular response (BCR-ABL PCR ≤10% at 3 months) is an effective prognostic indicator for short-term and long-term success [134]. Patients who do not achieve this early molecular response should be considered to switch therapy to an alternative TKI.

Second-Line Therapy for CML

Although the response rates are high for IM in the front-line setting for CML, as many as 40% of patients will eventually fail IM therapy due to intolerance or resistance [135]. Causes of resistance can be subdivided into primary versus secondary causes. Primary resistance is due to the failure to meet optimal responses to IM over specified time periods (Table 29.6). Secondary resistance occurs after initially achieving a response to IM and then relapsing. The most common cause for secondary resistance is the development of mutations in the kinase domain of the ABL1 gene. Patients with primary or secondary resistance should first be questioned about their

Table 29.6 CML treatment milestone recommendations [133].

Time	Response	Treatment recommendations
3 months	No hematologic response BCR-ABL PCR >10%	Switch to alternate TKI Switch to alternate TKI
6 months	No CHR[1] No cytogenetic response[2]	Switch to alternate TKI Switch to alternate TKI
12 months	< Partial cytogenetic response[3]	Switch to alternate TKI
18 months	< CCyR[4]	Switch to alternate TKI

[1] CHR is defined as white blood cells <10,000/mm^3, basophils <5%, no myelocytes, promyelocytes, or myeloblasts on differential, platelets <450/mm^3.
[2] No cytogenetic response is defined as Philadelphia chromosome FISH or cytogenetics >95%.
[3] Less than partial cytogenetic response is defined as Philadelphia chromosome FISH or cytogenetics >35%.
[4] CCyR is defined as FISH or cytogenetics 0% BCR-ABL1.
CCyR, complete cytogenetic response; CHR, complete hematologic response; FISH, fluorescent *in situ* hybridization; PCR, polymerase chain reaction; TKI, tyrosine kinase inhibitor.

compliance. After eliminating compliance as a potential cause, patients with resistance should then receive a *BCR-ABL1* mutational analysis, in order to detect specific mutations and to guide further therapy.

NIL and DAS can result in CCyR in approximately 50% of patients in CP who failed IM, and the responses are durable with approximately 80% of patients maintaining response at 2 years [135]. Most recently, bosutinib (BOS), a *BCR-ABL1* and *SRC* kinase inhibitor, was approved for treatment of CML patients failing prior TKI therapy. The most common side effects of BOS include diarrhea, rash, and vomiting [136]. Certain mutations confer resistance to multiple TKIs, and therefore the mutational analysis should be used as a guide for switching therapy in the second-line setting. The second-generation TKIs (DAS, NIL, or BOS) are not active against the T315I mutation. A third-generation TKI, ponatinib, was approved for the treatment of CML in patients with resistance or intolerance to prior therapy. It is the only TKI to demonstrate durable activity in patients with T315I mutations (70% major cytogenetic response) [137]. Due to adverse events such as blood clots (arterial and venous) and narrowing of blood vessels in more than one-quarter of patients, its use is limited to patients with CML resistant to the other TKIs or those having T315I mutations. However, response to either of the second- or third-generation TKIs decreases after treatment failure with more than one TKI.

Finally, omacetaxine, a homoharringtonine analog, has demonstrated activity in patients who have failed two or more TKIs [138]. Given its novel mechanism of action as a protein synthesis inhibitor, omacetaxine is a viable option for patients who have developed multiple kinase mutations, including T315I mutations, and those who cannot tolerate ponatinib.

Advanced-Phase CML (AP/BC)

Patients who develop AP CML (blasts 10–30%) while on TKI therapy can be offered higher doses of second- and third-generation TKIs. Ponatinib can be used for patients with T315I mutations. However, responses in this setting tend to be short-lived, and an allogeneic SCT is recommended once patients achieve a second CP. Patients who progress to BC (>30% blasts) or who present with AP or BC at diagnosis have an extremely poor prognosis. Treatment options include the same TKI options as AP, or multiagent chemotherapy with or without a TKI [139]. Once a response is achieved, an allogeneic SCT is recommended to improve the possibility of long-term survival.

Allogeneic SCT in CML

Allogeneic SCT is the only known cure for CML, and was recommended to all CML patients, including those in CP, prior to the discovery of TKIs. Since the TKI era, allogeneic SCT rates have dropped dramatically for CML. Currently, allogeneic SCT is recommended for patients with high-risk disease (AP or BC), patients who are intolerant to or failed multiple TKIs, or patients with T315I mutations [140]. Allogeneic SCT yields the best outcomes when patients are transplanted in CP (as opposed to AP or BC). Therefore, patients presenting with AP or BC CML should be treated with TKI alone or in combination with chemotherapy prior to allogeneic SCT. Additionally, outcomes are better for patients transplanted in first CP when compared with second CP. Unfortunately, an increasing percentage of patients are transplanted in second CP and advanced phase in the TKI era, leading to worse overall outcomes post SCT [141].

Other Myeloproliferative Neoplasms

Epidemiology and Presentation

The three most common Ph-negative myeloproliferative neoplasms are polycythemia vera (PV), essential thrombocythemia (ET), and primary myelofibrosis (PMF). Signs of these MPNs include increases in peripheral blood measurements of various blood counts, splenomegaly, and marrow fibrosis. Disease transformation to AML is rare with PV or ET but may occur in up to 30% of patients with PMF. In general, patients with any of these disorders who receive cytotoxic chemotherapy appear to have higher AML transformation risk.

PV is a neoplasm of adults, with an incidence of 2.6 per 100,000 people per year and a median age at diagnosis of 60 years. Most commonly, patients present with asymptomatic hemoglobin elevation on routine blood work. Uncommonly, patients present with portal vein thrombosis (Budd–Chiari syndrome) [142] or a characteristic PV-associated pruritus and skin reddening after exposure to warm water (erythromelalgia). As a neoplastic process, the elevation of hemoglobin in PV occurs unrelated to erythropoietin (EPO) regulation and EPO levels should be low or low-normal. Among non-smokers, a hemoglobin of 18.5 g/dL in men or 16.5 g/dL in women fulfills a major criterion for PV in the current classification. The presence of an activating JAK2 mutation is the other major criterion for diagnosis. Either major criterion is not necessary if the patient has two of the following features: (i) appropriate histologic appearance on BM biopsy, (ii) low serum EPO level, or (iii) endogenous erythroid colony formation *in vitro*. Histologically, the BM for the cellular phase of PV shows not only increased erythroid cellularity, but panmyelosis, with an increase in myeloid cells and megakaryocytes [143].

ET presents with marked thrombocytosis (>450,000/µL), usually with the remaining blood counts being normal. It has an incidence of 0.3–1.0 per 100,000 persons per year with a female predominance and a median age of 67 years [144]. Patients can present with events related to hemorrhage and/or thrombosis, but most are asymptomatic and diagnosed after persistent thrombocytosis is seen on routine blood work. BM examination usually shows increased atypical megakaryocytes with normal to modestly increased cellularity.

Previously called chronic idiopathic myelofibrosis or agnogenic myeloid metaplasia, PMF has an incidence of 0.5–1.5 per 100,000 people a year [145]. Patients may be asymptomatic at initial diagnosis or have nonspecific constitutional symptoms, such as fevers, drenching night sweats, fatigue, or weight loss. Early satiety from splenomegaly may also be present. The majority of patients with PMF show abnormal peripheral counts with anemia and thrombocytosis being the most common abnormalities, often accompanied by leukocytosis.

Clinically, early stages of PMF's natural history may be difficult to discriminate from ET as the disease initially proceeds through a cellular phase with limited BM fibrosis. The presence of myeloid hyperplasia and large tight clusters of atypical megakaryocytes in the marrow usually differentiates cellular-phase PMF from ET. As the disease progresses, the marrow undergoes marked reticulin and eventually collagen fibrosis, likely related to cytokine release from megakaryocytes. Marrow fibrosis is often paired with the development of extramedullary hematopoiesis and progressive, often massive splenomegaly. Eventually, the disease progresses to an osteosclerotic phase, with marrow space being replaced by bone formation.

Mastocytosis is a heterogeneous group of diseases, often presenting with cutaneous symptoms such as pruritus or "Darier's sign," which is reddening and itching of the skin after stroking. In addition, in the case of systemic mastocytosis, symptoms may include fatigue, weight loss, diaphoresis, fever, gastrointestinal distress, or abdominal or musculoskeletal pain. Patients will also consistently have an elevated tryptase level. Histologically, mastocytosis is defined by multiple abnormal clusters of mast cells in any organ. Cutaneous lesions are seen as urticaria pigmentosa. Systemic mastocytosis may also present in association with another myeloid neoplasm, most often chronic myelomonocytic leukemia [146].

MPNs with abnormalities of *PDGFRA*, *PDGFRB*, and *FGFR1* are rare neoplasms that present with peripheral eosinophilia. *PDGFRA* rearrangements have a strong male predominance, while *PDGFRB* and *FGFR1* rearrangements occur with a lesser male predominance with a peak incidence of both in the 30s and 40s.

Pathogenesis and Genetics

A unifying biologic feature of all of the MPNs is their strong association with mutations that constitutively activate tyrosine kinase signal transduction. In CML, this occurs through the *BCR-ABL1* fusion while in PV, ET, and PMF it most often arises from a recurrent point mutation in *JAK2* (V617F). The *JAK2* gene encodes a tyrosine kinase that is essential for hematopoiesis. *JAK2* normally is activated by cytokines ligating to transmembrane receptors (e.g., erythropoietin). This causes conformational changes and dimerization of the receptor that aid *JAK2* docking and phosphorylation [147, 148]. Murine studies show that the *JAK2 V617F* mutation activates numerous signaling pathways, including *STAT5*, *STAT3*, *RAS/MAP* kinase, and *PI3* kinase/*AKT*. *JAK2 V617F* also confers hypersensitivity to erythropoietin [149].

Unlike CML, the *JAK2* mutation is not always seen in Ph-negative MPNs. While 95% of PV patients have the V617F activating *JAK2* point mutations, only 50% of ET and PMF patients carry this mutation [150]. Other mutations have been reported in each of these diseases and are thought to up-regulate signal transduction in a fashion similar to *JAK2 V617F*. Most commonly, frameshift mutations in calreticulin (*CALR*) can be found in *JAK2*-negative ET or PMF. Additionally, other activating *JAK2* mutations (e.g., exon 12) as well as rare mutations in c-MPL (thrombopoietin receptor), *SETBP1*, and *CSF3R* can be found in Ph-negative MPNs [151–156].

Mastocytosis commonly harbors activating *KIT* mutations, with the most common being *KIT D816V*. This particular mutation is unresponsive to several *KIT* tyrosine kinase inhibitors (e.g., imatinib). KIT mutations are not specific to mastocytosis, as they also occur in AML as well as numerous solid tumors, including gastrointestinal stromal tumors (GIST), melanoma, and gliomas.

Classification

The *JAK2* MPNs follow a progression from an early, cellular phase to a fibrotic marrow and eventually to an osteosclerotic marrow. A post-polycythemic or post-thrombocythemic myelofibrosis is difficult to distinguish from PMF, with only a previous history of either PV or ET suggesting a progression of that disease as opposed to a *bona fide* PMF case. However, this distinction is important, as PMF has a significantly higher transformation rate to AML [157].

Mastocytosis is classified into either isolated cutaneous mastocytosis or systemic mastocytosis. Most cases of systemic mastocytosis also contain a cutaneous component. In addition, based on numerous clinical criteria, systemic mastocytosis can be classified as indolent or aggressive. Aggressive systemic mastocytosis is identified by cytopenias, hepatomegaly with evidence of liver dysfunction, skeletal involvement, splenomegaly, or malabsorption due to gastrointestinal infiltrates [146]. In addition, identifying systemic mastocytosis in the presence of other hematologic malignancy is important.

Myeloid neoplasms with *PDGFRA*, *PDGFRB*, or *FGFR1* are classified by identifying an MPN along with evidence of the appropriate fusion gene.

Overlap MDS/MPN Neoplasms

Some neoplasms have overlapping MDS or MPN features that complicate assignment to one category. The four most common overlap syndromes are chronic myelomonocytic leukemia (CMML), juvenile myelomonocytic leukemia (JMML), atypical chronic myeloid leukemia (aCML), and chronic neutrophilic leukemia (CNL). CMML is defined as a clonal proliferation of myeloid cells, particularly monocytes and promonocytes. By definition, these cases are negative for *BCR–ABL1* or genetic events that define other disease entities. The presence of dysplasia is not always seen, and a presumptive diagnosis can be made if the patient has persistent peripheral blood monocytosis and an acquired genetic mutation is found, or if the monocytosis persists for 3 months without an underlying cause being found. CMML is subcategorized based on the percentage of blasts and monocytes into CMML-0 (<2% blasts in peripheral blood and <5% BM blasts), CMML-1 (2–4% blasts in peripheral blood and/or 5–9% BM blasts), or CMML-2 (5–19% blasts in peripheral blood, 10–19% BM blasts, and/or presence of Auer rods) [20]. JMML, as the name suggests, is a neoplasm found in infants and young children and has an incidence of 1.3 per 1,000,000 children per year with a 2:1 male predominance. Clinically, patients often present with vague symptoms or infection with leukocytosis, particularly peripheral monocytosis along with or without splenomegaly. Diagnostically this can be very challenging with a very large overlap of infectious causes that should be ruled out. The diagnosis can be made easier if evidence is found of a clonal chromosomal abnormality, of which monosomy 7 is the most prevalent. Finally, aCML is a rare MDS/MPN overlap disease that is genetically unrelated to CML, being negative for *BCR-ABL1*. These patients have a leukocytosis without monocytosis, and characteristically have dysplastic neutrophils in the peripheral blood. Over 80% of cases have cytogenetic abnormalities, with +8 and del(20q) being the most prevalent. aCML is now better defined molecularly as up to one-third of patients have *SETBP1* and/or *ETNK1* mutations. Driver mutations seen in other MPNs such as *BCR-ABL1*, *JAK2*, *CALR*, *MPL*, *KIT*, or *PDGFR* are typically absent in aCML [20]. As with aCML, CNL has also recently been defined molecularly, with a strong association with *CSF3R* mutations. Other diagnostic criteria for CNL include peripheral blood leukocytosis (WBC ≥25,000/μL) without a monocytosis, hypercellular BM, and not meeting other MPN criteria such as CML, PV, ET, or myelofibrosis [20].

Therapy of Myeloproliferative Neoplasms

Polycythemia Vera (PV)

In PV, the major therapeutic goals are to minimize symptoms of polycythemia by phlebotomy and to prevent long-term complications of the disease (Table 29.7). A landmark trial by the Polycythemia Vera Study Group (PVSG) randomized patients to phlebotomy alone, chlorambucil plus phlebotomy, or radioactive phosphate plus phlebotomy. The phlebotomy arm exhibited the longest OS as well as the lowest secondary malignancies. However, there were increased rates of thrombosis in the phlebotomy only arm during the first 3 years when compared to the other arms [158]. In order to determine the hematocrit (Hct) goal for patients undergoing phlebotomy for PV, an Italian collaborative group randomized patients to receive intensive phlebotomy (Hct <45%) or less intensive phlebotomy (Hct 45–50%). Patients assigned to the intensive phlebotomy arm had significantly decreased rates of thrombosis and cardiovascular deaths, thus establishing a standard Hct goal of <45% in patients with PV [159]. All patients with PV should also be treated with low-dose aspirin (100 mg/day), which has been shown to reduce the incidence of morbidity and mortality due to vascular events [160]. For patients at high risk of thrombosis (age >60 years or previous history of

Table 29.7 Treatment of myeloproliferative neoplasms (MPNs).

MPN disease	Symptoms and disease risk	Therapy options
Polycythemia vera (PV)	Low risk of vascular events [170]	Phlebotomy (goal Hct <45%) + low-dose aspirin Hydroxyurea ± IFN, or IFN alone
	High risk of vascular events [170]	Ruxolitinib as second-line
Essential thrombocythemia (ET)	Asymptomatic, <60 years without thrombosis, cardiovascular risk factors or JAK2 V617F mutation	Observation
	<60 years + symptoms of microvascular disease, or presence of cardiovascular risk factors, or JAK2 V617F mutation	Low-dose aspirin (twice-daily if continued symptoms with once-daily aspirin)
	History of thrombosis and <60 years	Hydroxyurea (second-line agent = IFN) Venous thrombosis = anticoagulation Arterial thrombosis = aspirin
	≥60 years	Hydroxyurea + aspirin
Myelofibrosis (MF)	Asymptomatic + low or intermediate-1 risk group[1]	Observation
	Symptomatic anemia	Androgen therapy, danazol, or thalidomide + prednisone
	Symptomatic splenomegaly	Ruxolitinib
	Intermediate-2 or high-risk	Consideration of allogeneic SCT or ruxolitinib, or investigational agents

[1] Risk factors (DIPSS) include age ≥65, hemoglobin <10 g/dL, leukocyte count >25,000/mm^3, circulating blasts >1%, constitutional symptoms, presence of unfavorable karyotype, platelet count <100/mm^3, and need for red blood cell transfusions.
Low-risk = 0 risk factors, intermediate-1 = 1 risk factor, intermediate-2 = 2–3 risk factors, high-risk = ≥4 risk factors.
DIPSS, Dynamic International Prognostic Scoring System; Hct, hematocrit; IFN, interferon; SCT, hematopoietic stem cell transplantation.

thrombosis), treatment should include cytoreductive therapy with hydroxyurea with or without interferon-α (IFN). A multicenter phase 2 study demonstrated high response rates (94.6%) in patients with PV treated with IFN [161]. The majority of patients with PV will have a *JAK2 V617F* mutation. Recently, ruxolitinib, a *JAK2* inhibitor, has been FDA approved for treatment of PV after failure to respond or tolerate hydroxyurea based on a phase 3 study [162]. When compared with best supportive care, ruxolitinib led to superior response rates and Hct control. Thrombotic complications are common in patients with PV, and when present, should be treated with standard anticoagulation therapy.

Essential Thrombocythemia (ET)

Most patients with ET achieve a relatively normal life expectancy and the disease follows an especially indolent course. The goal of treatment is to prevent complications from thrombocytosis, such as thrombosis and cardiovascular-related morbidities, as well as hemorrhagic events secondary to acquired von Willebrand disease. Low-dose aspirin therapy is recommended for younger patients (<60 years) with a history of thrombocytosis or the presence of additional cardiovascular disease or a *JAK2* V617F mutation. Otherwise, the majority of patients with ET can be observed without any treatment. As with PV, patients at high risk for thrombosis (age >60 years or previous history of thrombosis) should be managed with aspirin plus cytoreductive therapy (i.e., hydroxyurea). Anagrelide is also an option for patients with very high platelet counts [163].

Myelofibrosis (MF)

MF includes primary myelofibrosis (PMF) as well as PV and ET transforming to myelofibrosis, termed post-PV MF and post-ET MF, respectively. Approximately 5% of ET cases and 10–20% of PV cases transform to MF over 10–15 years [164]. MF has a much more aggressive course than PV and ET; therefore, more intensive therapies are recommended at diagnosis. The treatment of MF relies on appropriate risk stratification of patients based on specific risk factors into low, intermediate-1, intermediate-2, and high-risk categories (Table 29.7) [165]. Presently, the only known cure for MF is an allogeneic SCT, which is recommended in patients with intermediate/high-risk features. Other therapies are aimed at improving quality of life, decreasing symptoms, and decreasing progression of the disease. For patients who are not candidates for SCT, treatment options include androgens, corticosteroids, thalidomide, lenalidomide, and recent JAK2 inhibitors [163]. Almost all patients with MF have symptomatic splenomegaly. Splenectomy is a palliative option for patients with portal hypertension, splenic infarction, or splenic sequestration, or for symptomatic relief. Most recently, JAK2 inhibitors were developed as a therapeutic option for patients with MF, regardless of JAK2 mutation status. The COMFORT-1 study randomized patients with intermediate- or high-risk MF to ruxolitinib, a JAK2 inhibitor, or placebo. A significant reduction in spleen size and an associated improvement of symptoms were seen in the ruxolitinib arm when compared to placebo. Patients receiving ruxolitinib did develop more frequent cytopenias, however [166]. A second COMFORT-II trial randomized patients with MF to ruxolitinib or best available therapy with similar results seen with COMFORT-1 [167]. Based on these studies, ruxolitinib was FDA approved for treatment of intermediate- and high-risk MF, including PMF and post-PV and post-ET MF. Although ruxolitinib is extremely effective at reducing spleen size and associated symptoms, fibrosis and clinical disease still persist after treatment. With longer follow-up, however, ruxolitinib appears to improve OS in MF patients. Abrupt discontinuation of ruxolitinib can lead to exacerbation of symptoms and the dose should thus be tapered gradually in any patient who fails therapy or requires discontinuation [168].

Chronic Myelomonocytic Leukemia (CMML)

The management of CMML can be divided into patients who have a fusion gene with platelet derived growth factor receptor-β (*PDGFRB*) or not. Patients with a *PDGFRB* fusion gene (most commonly t(5;12)(q33;p13)) should be treated with imatinib, whereas patients without a *PDGFRB* fusion gene should be treated similarly to MDS, with hypomethylating agents as the preferred first-line agent [169]. Unfortunately, there is no uniform stratification criterion for CMML patients. An allogeneic SCT is an option for patients with high-risk disease (increased blast counts or adverse karyotype) or patients who fail first-line therapy. Unfortunately, there are limited data on effective therapies in patients with CMML, and primary management of CMML is thus controversial. Clinical trials are strongly recommended in this disease state, in order to learn more about the natural history of the disease, as well as to explore novel agents that may be most effective in treating symptoms of CMML and improving OS.

References

1 Cancer Genome Atlas Research Network, Ley TJ, Miller C, *et al.* Genomic and epigenomic landscapes of adult de novo acute myeloid leukemia. *N Engl J Med* 2013;368(22):2059–74.
2 Steensma DP, Bejar R, Jaiswal S, *et al.* Clonal hematopoiesis of indeterminate potential and its distinction from myelodysplastic syndromes. *Blood* 2015;126(1):9–16.
3 Jaiswal S, Fontanillas P, Flannick J, *et al.* Age-related clonal hematopoiesis associated with adverse outcomes. *N Engl J Med* 2014;371(26):2488–98.
4 Genovese G, Kahler AK, Handsaker RE, *et al.* Clonal hematopoiesis and blood-cancer risk inferred from blood DNA sequence. *N Engl J Med* 2014;371(26):2477–87.
5 Howlader N, Noone AM, Krapcho M, *et al.* (eds). SEER Cancer Statistics Review, 1975–2013, National Cancer Institute. Bethesda, MD, http://seer.cancer.gov/csr/1975_2013/, based on November 2015 SEER data submission, posted to the SEER web site, April 2016.
6 Ma X. Epidemiology of myelodysplastic syndromes. *Am J Med* 2012;125(7 Suppl):S2–5.

7 Bessler M, Wilson DB, Mason PJ. Dyskeratosis congenita. *FEBS Lett* 2010;584(17):3831–8.
8 Kee Y, D'Andrea AD. Molecular pathogenesis and clinical management of Fanconi anemia. *J Clin Invest* 2012;122(11):3799–806.
9 Owen CJ, Toze CL, Koochin A, *et al.* Five new pedigrees with inherited RUNX1 mutations causing familial platelet disorder with propensity to myeloid malignancy. *Blood* 2008;112(12):4639–45.
10 Hahn CN, Chong CE, Carmichael CL, *et al.* Heritable GATA2 mutations associated with familial myelodysplastic syndrome and acute myeloid leukemia. *Nat Genet* 2011;43(10):1012–7.
11 Pedersen-Bjergaard J, Andersen MK, Christiansen DH, Nerlov C. Genetic pathways in therapy-related myelodysplasia and acute myeloid leukemia. *Blood* 2002;99(6):1909–12.
12 Ebert BL, Pretz J, Bosco J, *et al.* Identification of RPS14 as a 5q- syndrome gene by RNA interference screen. *Nature* 2008;451(7176):335–9.
13 Bejar R, Stevenson K, Abdel-Wahab O, *et al.* Clinical effect of point mutations in myelodysplastic syndromes. *N Engl J Med* 2011;364(26):2496–506.
14 Papaemmanuil E, Gerstung M, Malcovati L, *et al.* Clinical and biological implications of driver mutations in myelodysplastic syndromes. *Blood* 2013;122(22):3616–27.
15 Haferlach T, Nagata Y, Grossmann V, *et al.* Landscape of genetic lesions in 944 patients with myelodysplastic syndromes. *Leukemia* 2014;28(2):241–7.
16 Figueroa ME, Skrabanek L, Li Y, *et al.* MDS and secondary AML display unique patterns and abundance of aberrant DNA methylation. *Blood* 2009;114(16):3448–58.
17 Yoshida K, Sanada M, Shiraishi Y, *et al.* Frequent pathway mutations of splicing machinery in myelodysplasia. *Nature* 2011;478(7367):64–9.
18 Visconte V, Makishima H, Maciejewski JP, Tiu RV. Emerging roles of the spliceosomal machinery in myelodysplastic syndromes and other hematological disorders. *Leukemia* 2012;26(12):2447–54.
19 Brunning RD, Orazi A, Germing U, *et al.* Myelodysplastic syndromes/neoplasms overview. In: *WHO Classification of Tumours of Haematopoietic and Lymphoid Tissue.* Lyon, France: IARC Press, 2008:88–93.
20 Arber DA, Orazi A, Hasserjian R, *et al.* The 2016 revision to the World Health Organization classification of myeloid neoplasms and acute leukemia. *Blood* 2016;127(20):2391–405.
21 List A, Kurtin S, Roe DJ, *et al.* Efficacy of lenalidomide in myelodysplastic syndromes. *N Engl J Med* 2005;352(6):549–57.
22 Patel JP, Gonen M, Figueroa ME, *et al.* Prognostic relevance of integrated genetic profiling in acute myeloid leukemia. *N Engl J Med* 2012;366(12):1079–89.
23 Greenberg P, Cox C, LeBeau MM, *et al.* International scoring system for evaluating prognosis in myelodysplastic syndromes. *Blood* 1997;89(6):2079–88.
24 Greenberg PL, Tuechler H, Schanz J, *et al.* Revised international prognostic scoring system for myelodysplastic syndromes. *Blood* 2012;120(12):2454–65.
25 Hellstrom-Lindberg E, Gulbrandsen N, Lindberg G, *et al.* A validated decision model for treating the anaemia of myelodysplastic syndromes with erythropoietin + granulocyte colony-stimulating factor: significant effects on quality of life. *Br J Haematol* 2003;120(6):1037–46.
26 Casadevall N, Durieux P, Dubois S, *et al.* Health, economic, and quality-of-life effects of erythropoietin and granulocyte colony-stimulating factor for the treatment of myelodysplastic syndromes: a randomized, controlled trial. *Blood* 2004;104(2):321–7.
27 Malcovati L. Impact of transfusion dependency and secondary iron overload on the survival of patients with myelodysplastic syndromes. *Leuk Res* 2007;31 Suppl 3:S2–6.
28 Greenberg PL, Attar E, Bennett JM, *et al.* NCCN Clinical Practice Guidelines in Oncology: myelodysplastic syndromes. *J Natl Compr Canc Netw* 2011;9(1):30–56.
29 Piga A, Galanello R, Forni GL, *et al.* Randomized phase II trial of deferasirox (Exjade, ICL670), a once-daily, orally-administered iron chelator, in comparison to deferoxamine in thalassemia patients with transfusional iron overload. *Haematologica* 2006;91(7):873–80.
30 Sloand EM, Wu CO, Greenberg P, Young N, Barrett J. Factors affecting response and survival in patients with myelodysplasia treated with immunosuppressive therapy. *J Clin Oncol* 2008; 26(15):2505–11.
31 Saunthararajah Y, Nakamura R, Nam JM, *et al.* HLA-DR15 (DR2) is overrepresented in myelodysplastic syndrome and aplastic anemia and predicts a response to immunosuppression in myelodysplastic syndrome. *Blood* 2002;100(5):1570–4.
32 Passweg JR, Giagounidis AA, Simcock M, *et al.* Immunosuppressive therapy for patients with myelodysplastic syndrome: a prospective randomized multicenter phase III trial comparing antithymocyte globulin plus cyclosporine with best supportive care – SAKK 33/99. *J Clin Oncol* 2011;29(3):303–9.
33 Castelli R, Cassin R, Cannavo A, Cugno M. Immunomodulatory drugs: new options for the treatment of myelodysplastic syndromes. *Clin Lymphoma Myeloma Leuk* 2013;13(1):1–7.
34 List A, Dewald G, Bennett J, *et al.* Lenalidomide in the myelodysplastic syndrome with chromosome 5q deletion. *N Engl J Med* 2006;355(14):1456–65.
35 Fenaux P, Giagounidis A, Selleslag D, *et al.* A randomized phase 3 study of lenalidomide versus placebo in RBC transfusion-dependent patients with Low-/Intermediate-1-risk myelodysplastic syndromes with del5q. *Blood* 2011;118(14):3765–76.
36 Raza A, Reeves JA, Feldman EJ, *et al.* Phase 2 study of lenalidomide in transfusion-dependent, low-risk, and intermediate-1 risk myelodysplastic syndromes with karyotypes other than deletion 5q. *Blood* 2008;111(1): 86–93.
37 Silverman LR, Demakos EP, Peterson BL, *et al.* Randomized controlled trial of azacitidine in patients with the myelodysplastic syndrome: a study of the cancer and leukemia group B. *J Clin Oncol* 2002;20(10):2429–40.
38 Fenaux P, Mufti GJ, Hellstrom-Lindberg E, *et al.* Efficacy of azacitidine compared with that of conventional care regimens in the treatment of higher-risk myelodysplastic syndromes: a randomised, open-label, phase III study. *Lancet Oncol* 2009;10(3):223–32.

39 Wijermans P, Lubbert M, Verhoef G, *et al.* Low-dose 5-aza-2'-deoxycytidine, a DNA hypomethylating agent, for the treatment of high-risk myelodysplastic syndrome: a multicenter phase II study in elderly patients. *J Clin Oncol* 2000;18(5):956–62.

40 Kantarjian H, Issa JP, Rosenfeld CS, *et al.* Decitabine improves patient outcomes in myelodysplastic syndromes: results of a phase III randomized study. *Cancer* 2006;106(8):1794–803.

41 Kantarjian H, Oki Y, Garcia-Manero G, *et al.* Results of a randomized study of 3 schedules of low-dose decitabine in higher-risk myelodysplastic syndrome and chronic myelomonocytic leukemia. *Blood* 2007;109(1):52–7.

42 de Witte T, Suciu S, Verhoef G, *et al.* Intensive chemotherapy followed by allogeneic or autologous stem cell transplantation for patients with myelodysplastic syndromes (MDSs) and acute myeloid leukemia following MDS. *Blood* 2001;98(8):2326–31.

43 Kantarjian H, Beran M, Cortes J, *et al.* Long-term follow-up results of the combination of topotecan and cytarabine and other intensive chemotherapy regimens in myelodysplastic syndrome. *Cancer* 2006;106(5):1099–109.

44 Damaj G, Duhamel A, Robin M, *et al.* Impact of azacitidine before allogeneic stem-cell transplantation for myelodysplastic syndromes: a study by the Societe Francaise de Greffe de Moelle et de Therapie-Cellulaire and the Groupe-Francophone des Myelodysplasies. *J Clin Oncol* 2012;30(36): 4533–40.

45 Appelbaum FR, Anderson J. Allogeneic bone marrow transplantation for myelodysplastic syndrome: outcomes analysis according to IPSS score. *Leukemia* 1998;12 Suppl 1:S25–9.

46 Martino R, Iacobelli S, Brand R, *et al.* Retrospective comparison of reduced-intensity conditioning and conventional high-dose conditioning for allogeneic hematopoietic stem cell transplantation using HLA-identical sibling donors in myelodysplastic syndromes. *Blood* 2006;108(3):836–46.

47 Cutler CS, Lee SJ, Greenberg P, *et al.* A decision analysis of allogeneic bone marrow transplantation for the myelodysplastic syndromes: delayed transplantation for low-risk myelodysplasia is associated with improved outcome. *Blood* 2004;104(2): 579–85.

48 Sierra J, Perez WS, Rozman C, *et al.* Bone marrow transplantation from HLA-identical siblings as treatment for myelodysplasia. *Blood* 2002;100(6):1997–2004.

49 Siegel RL, Miller KD, Jemal A. Cancer statistics, 2017. *CA Cancer J Clin* 2017;67(1):7–30.

50 Deschler B LM. Acute myeloid leukemia: epidemiology and etiology. *Cancer* 2006;107(6):2099–107.

51 Vardiman JW, Brunning RD, Arber DA, *et al.* Introduction and overview of the classification of myeloid neoplasms. *WHO Classification of Tumours of Haematopoietic and Lymphoid Tissues*. Lyon, France: IARC Press, 2008: 18–30.

52 Grimwade D, Hills RK, Moorman AV, *et al.* Refinement of cytogenetic classification in acute myeloid leukemia: determination of prognostic significance of rare recurring chromosomal abnormalities among 5876 younger adult patients treated in the United Kingdom Medical Research Council trials. *Blood* 2010;116(3):354–65.

53 Byrd JC, Mrozek K, Dodge RK, *et al.* Pretreatment cytogenetic abnormalities are predictive of induction success, cumulative incidence of relapse, and overall survival in adult patients with de novo acute myeloid leukemia: results from Cancer and Leukemia Group B (CALGB 8461). *Blood* 2002;100(13):4325–36.

54 Grimwade D, Walker H, Oliver F, *et al.* The importance of diagnostic cytogenetics on outcome in AML: analysis of 1,612 patients entered into the MRC AML 10 trial. The Medical Research Council Adult and Children's Leukaemia Working Parties. *Blood* 1998;92(7):2322–33.

55 Schlenk RF, Dohner K, Krauter J, *et al.* Mutations and treatment outcome in cytogenetically normal acute myeloid leukemia. *N Engl J Med* 2008;358(18):1909–18.

56 Pabst T, Mueller BU, Zhang P, *et al.* Dominant-negative mutations of CEBPA, encoding CCAAT/enhancer binding protein-alpha (C/EBPalpha), in acute myeloid leukemia. *Nat Genet* 2001;27(3):263–70.

57 Preudhomme C, Sagot C, Boissel N, *et al.* Favorable prognostic significance of CEBPA mutations in patients with de novo acute myeloid leukemia: a study from the Acute Leukemia French Association (ALFA). *Blood* 2002;100(8):2717–23.

58 Thiede C, Steudel C, Mohr B, *et al.* Analysis of FLT3-activating mutations in 979 patients with acute myelogenous leukemia: association with FAB subtypes and identification of subgroups with poor prognosis. *Blood* 2002;99(12): 4326–35.

59 Rombouts WJ, Blokland I, Löwenberg B, Ploemacher RE. Biological characteristics and prognosis of adult acute myeloid leukemia with internal tandem duplications in the Flt3 gene. *Leukemia* 2000;14(4):675–83.

60 Levis MJ, Perl AE, Dombret H, *et al.* Final Results of a Phase 2 Open-Label, Monotherapy Efficacy and Safety Study of Quizartinib (AC220) in Patients with FLT3-ITD Positive or Negative Relapsed/Refractory Acute Myeloid Leukemia After Second-Line Chemotherapy or Hematopoietic Stem Cell Transplantation. *ASH Annual Meeting Abstracts*. 2012;120(21):673.

61 Paschka P. Core binding factor acute myeloid leukemia. *Semin Oncol* 2008;35(4):410–7.

62 Bennett JM, Catovsky D, Daniel MT, *et al.* Proposals for the classification of the acute leukaemias. French-American-British (FAB) co-operative group. *Br J Haematol* 1976;33(4):451–8.

63 Craig FE, Foon KA. Flow cytometric immunophenotyping for hematologic neoplasms. *Blood* 2008;111(8):3941–67.

64 Jennings CD, Foon KA. Recent advances in flow cytometry: application to the diagnosis of hematologic malignancy. *Blood* 1997;90(8):2863–92.

65 Menell JS, Cesarman GM, Jacovina AT, *et al.* Annexin II and bleeding in acute promyelocytic leukemia. *N Engl J Med* 1999;340(13):994–1004.

66 Falanga A, Alessio MG, Donati MB, Barbui T. A new procoagulant in acute leukemia. *Blood* 1988;71(4):870–5.

67 Falanga A, Consonni R, Marchetti M, *et al.* Cancer procoagulant and tissue factor are differently modulated by all-trans-retinoic acid in acute promyelocytic leukemia cells. *Blood* 1998;92(1):143–51.

68 Dohner H, Estey EH, Amadori S, *et al.* Diagnosis and management of acute myeloid leukemia in adults: recommendations from an international expert panel, on behalf of the European LeukemiaNet. *Blood* 2010;115(3): 453–74.

69 Mrozek K, Marcucci G, Nicolet D, *et al.* Prognostic significance of the European LeukemiaNet standardized system for reporting cytogenetic and molecular alterations in adults with acute myeloid leukemia. *J Clin Oncol* 2012;30(36):4515–23.

70 Papaemmanuil E, Gerstung M, Bullinger L, *et al.* Genomic classification and prognosis in acute myeloid leukemia. *N Engl J Med* 2016;374(23):2209–21.

71 Yates J, Glidewell O, Wiernik P, *et al.* Cytosine arabinoside with daunorubicin or adriamycin for therapy of acute myelocytic leukemia: a CALGB study. *Blood* 1982;60(2):454–62.

72 Rai KR, Holland JF, Glidewell OJ, *et al.* Treatment of acute myelocytic leukemia: a study by cancer and leukemia group B. *Blood* 1981;58(6):1203–12.

73 Tefferi A, Letendre L. Going beyond 7 + 3 regimens in the treatment of adult acute myeloid leukemia. *J Clin Oncol* 2012;30(20):2425–8.

74 Fernandez HF, Sun Z, Yao X, *et al.* Anthracycline dose intensification in acute myeloid leukemia. *N Engl J Med* 2009;361(13):1249–59.

75 Lee JH, Joo YD, Kim H, *et al.* A randomized trial comparing standard versus high-dose daunorubicin induction in patients with acute myeloid leukemia. *Blood* 2011;118(14):3832–41.

76 Lowenberg B, Ossenkoppele GJ, van Putten W, *et al.* High-dose daunorubicin in older patients with acute myeloid leukemia. *N Engl J Med* 2009;361(13):1235–48.

77 Burnett AK, Russell NH, Hills RK, *et al.* A randomized comparison of daunorubicin 90 mg/m^2 vs 60 mg/m^2 in AML induction: results from the UK NCRI AML17 trial in 1206 patients. *Blood* 2015;125(25):3878–85.

78 Holowiecki J, Grosicki S, Giebel S, *et al.* Cladribine, but not fludarabine, added to daunorubicin and cytarabine during induction prolongs survival of patients with acute myeloid leukemia: a multicenter, randomized phase III study. *J Clin Oncol* 2012;30(20):2441–8.

79 Burnett AK, Russell NH, Hunter AE, *et al.* Clofarabine doubles the response rate in older patients with acute myeloid leukemia but does not improve survival. *Blood* 2013;122(8):1384–94.

80 Foran JM, Sun Z, Claxton JF, *et al.* North American leukemia, intergroup phase III randomized trial of single agent clofarabine as induction and post-remission therapy, and decitabine as maintenance therapy in newly-diagnosed AML in older adults (age > = 60years): A trial of the ECOG-ACRIN Cancer Research Group (E2906). *Blood (Abstract)* 2015;126:217.

81 Petersdorf SH, Kopecky KJ, Slovak M, *et al.* A phase 3 study of gemtuzumab ozogamicin during induction and postconsolidation therapy in younger patients with acute myeloid leukemia. *Blood* 2013;121(24):4854–60.

82 Rowe JM, Lowenberg B. Gemtuzumab ozogamicin in acute myeloid leukemia: a remarkable saga about an active drug. *Blood* 2013;121(24):4838–41.

83 Levis M. FLT3 mutations in acute myeloid leukemia: what is the best approach in 2013? *Hematology Am Soc Hematol Educ Program* 2013;2013:220–6.

84 Stone RM, Mandrekar S, Sanford BL, *et al.* The multi-kinase inhibitor midostaurin prolongs survival compared with placebo in combination with daunorubicin/cytarabine induction, high-dose cytarabine consolidation, and as maintenance therapy in newly diagnosed AML patients 18–60 with FLT3 mutations: An international prospective randomized controlled double-blind trial (CALGB 10603/ RATIFY [Alliance]). Blood (Abstract) 2015;126(6).

85 Stone RM, Mandrekar S, Sanford BL, *et al.* Midostaurin plus chemotherapy for AML with a FLT3 mutation. *N Engl J Med* 2017;377:454–64.

86 Rollig C, Serve H, Huttmann A, *et al.* Addition of sorafenib versus placebo to standard therapy in patients aged 60 years or younger with newly diagnosed acute myeloid leukaemia (SORAML): a multicentre, phase 2, randomised controlled trial. *Lancet Oncol* 2015;16(16):1691–9.

87 Cortes JE, Kantarjian H, Foran JM, *et al.* Phase I study of quizartinib administered daily to patients with relapsed or refractory acute myeloid leukemia irrespective of FMS-like tyrosine kinase 3-internal tandem duplication status. *J Clin Oncol* 2013;31(29):3681–7.

88 Mayer RJ, Davis RB, Schiffer CA, *et al.* Intensive postremission chemotherapy in adults with acute myeloid leukemia. Cancer and Leukemia Group B. *N Engl J Med* 1994;331(14):896–903.

89 Bloomfield CD, Lawrence D, Byrd JC, *et al.* Frequency of prolonged remission duration after high-dose cytarabine intensification in acute myeloid leukemia varies by cytogenetic subtype. *Cancer Res* 1998;58(18):4173–9.

90 Farag SS, Ruppert AS, Mrozek K, *et al.* Outcome of induction and postremission therapy in younger adults with acute myeloid leukemia with normal karyotype: a Cancer and Leukemia Group B study. *J Clin Oncol* 2005;23(3):482–93.

91 Burnett AK, Russell NH, Hills RK, *et al.* Optimization of chemotherapy for younger patients with acute myeloid leukemia: results of the medical research council AML15 trial. *J Clin Oncol* 2013;31(27):3360–8.

92 Gardin C, Turlure P, Fagot T, *et al.* Postremission treatment of elderly patients with acute myeloid leukemia in first complete remission after intensive induction chemotherapy: results of the multicenter randomized Acute Leukemia French Association (ALFA) 9803 trial. Blood2007;109(12):5129–35.

93 Luznik L, O'Donnell PV, Symons HJ, *et al.* HLA-haploidentical bone marrow transplantation for hematologic malignancies using nonmyeloablative conditioning and high-dose, posttransplantation cyclophosphamide. *Biol Blood Marrow Transplant* 2008;14(6):641–50.

94 Peffault de Latour R, Brunstein CG, Porcher R, *al.* Similar overall survival using sibling, unrelated donor, and cord blood grafts after reduced-intensity conditioning for older patients with acute myelogenous leukemia. *Biol Blood Marrow Transplant* 2013;19(9):1355–60.

95 Koreth J, Schlenk R, Kopecky KJ, *et al.* Allogeneic stem cell transplantation for acute myeloid leukemia in first complete remission: systematic review and meta-analysis of prospective clinical trials. *JAMA* 2009;301(22):2349–61.

96 Appelbaum FR. The current status of hematopoietic cell transplantation. *Annu Rev Med* 2003;54:491–512.

97 Fang M, Storer B, Estey E, *et al.* Outcome of patients with acute myeloid leukemia with monosomal karyotype who undergo hematopoietic cell transplantation. *Blood* 2011;118(6):1490–4.

98 Cornelissen JJ, Breems D, van Putten WL, *et al.* Comparative analysis of the value of allogeneic hematopoietic stem-cell transplantation in acute myeloid leukemia with monosomal karyotype versus other cytogenetic risk categories. *J Clin Oncol* 2012;30(17):2140–6.

99 Forman SJ, Rowe JM. The myth of the second remission of acute leukemia in the adult. *Blood* 2013;121(7):1077–82.

100 Wrzesien-Kus A, Robak T, Lech-Maranda E, *et al.* A multicenter, open, non-comparative, phase II study of the combination of cladribine (2-chlorodeoxyadenosine), cytarabine, and G-CSF as induction therapy in refractory acute myeloid leukemia – a report of the Polish Adult Leukemia Group (PALG). *Eur J Haematol* 2003;71(3): 155–62.

101 Becker PS, Kantarjian HM, Appelbaum FR, *et al.* Clofarabine with high dose cytarabine and granulocyte colony-stimulating factor (G-CSF) priming for relapsed and refractory acute myeloid leukaemia. *Br J Haematol* 2011;155(2):182–9.

102 Roboz G, Rosenblat T, Arellano M, *et al.* International randomized phase III study of elacytarabine versus investigator choice in patients with relapsed/refractory AML. *J Clin Oncol* 2014;32(18):1919–26.

103 Stein E, DiNardo CD, Pollyea DA, *et al.* Enasidenib in mutant-IDH2 relapsed or refractory AML. *Blood* 2017;130(6):722–31.

104 O'Donnell MR, Abboud CN, Altman J, *et al.* Acute myeloid leukemia. *J Natl Compr Canc Netw* 2012;10(8):984–1021.

105 Appelbaum FR, Gundacker H, Head DR, *et al.* Age and acute myeloid leukemia. *Blood* 2006;107(9):3481–5.

106 Juliusson G, Antunovic P, Derolf A, *et al.* Age and acute myeloid leukemia: real world data on decision to treat and outcomes from the Swedish Acute Leukemia Registry. *Blood* 2009;113(18):4179–87.

107 Champlin R. Reduced intensity allogeneic hematopoietic transplantation is an established standard of care for treatment of older patients with acute myeloid leukemia. *Best Pract Res Clin Haematol* 2013;26(3):297–300.

108 Burnett AK, Milligan D, Prentice AG, *et al.* A comparison of low-dose cytarabine and hydroxyurea with or without all-trans retinoic acid for acute myeloid leukemia and high-risk myelodysplastic syndrome in patients not considered fit for intensive treatment. *Cancer* 2007;109(6):1114–24.

109 Dombret H, Seymour JF, Butrym A, *et al.* International phase 3 study of azacitidine vs conventional care regimens in older patients with newly diagnosed AML with >30% blasts. *Blood* 2015;126(3):291–9.

110 Kantarjian HM, Thomas XG, Dmoszynska A, *et al.* Multicenter, randomized, open-label, phase III trial of decitabine versus patient choice, with physician advice, of either supportive care or low-dose cytarabine for the treatment of older patients with newly diagnosed acute myeloid leukemia. *J Clin Oncol* 2012;30(21):2670–7.

111 Blum W, Garzon R, Klisovic RB, *et al.* Clinical response and miR-29b predictive significance in older AML patients treated with a 10-day schedule of decitabine. *Proc Natl Acad Sci U S A* 2010;107(16):7473–8.

112 Lancet JE, Uy GL, Cortes JE, *et al.* Final results of a phase III randomized trial of CPX-351 versus 7 + 3 in older patients with newly diagnosed high risk (secondary) AML. *J Clin Oncol* 2016;34 (suppl; abstr 7000).

113 Sanz MA, Martin G, Gonzalez M, *et al.* Risk-adapted treatment of acute promyelocytic leukemia with all-trans-retinoic acid and anthracycline monochemotherapy: a multicenter study by the PETHEMA group. *Blood* 2004;103(4):1237–43.

114 Lo-Coco F, Avvisati G, Vignetti M, *et al.* Retinoic acid and arsenic trioxide for acute promyelocytic leukemia. *N Engl J Med* 2013;369(2):111–21.

115 Norsworthy KJ, Altman JK. Optimal treatment strategies for high-risk acute promyelocytic leukemia. *Curr Opin Hematol* 2016;23(2):127–36.

116 Tallman MS, Andersen JW, Schiffer CA, *et al.* Clinical description of 44 patients with acute promyelocytic leukemia who developed the retinoic acid syndrome. *Blood* 2000;95(1):90–5.

117 Ganzel C, Douer D, Tallman MS. Postconsolidation maintenance and monitoring in patients with acute promyelocytic leukemia. *J Natl Compr Canc Netw* 2013;11(12):1512–21.

118 Lo-Coco F, Cimino G, Breccia M, *et al.* Gemtuzumab ozogamicin (Mylotarg) as a single agent for molecularly relapsed acute promyelocytic leukemia. *Blood* 2004;104(7):1995–9.

119 Stam K, Heisterkamp N, Grosveld G, *et al.* Evidence of a new chimeric bcr/c-abl mRNA in patients with chronic myelocytic leukemia and the Philadelphia chromosome. *N Engl J Med* 1985;313(23):1429–33.

120 Vardiman JW, Melo JV, Baccarani M, Thiele J. Chronic myelogenous leukaemia, BCR-ABL1 positive. *WHO Classification of Tumours of Haematopoietic and Lymphoid Tissues*. Lyon, France: IARC Press, 2008: 32–7.

121 Jamieson CH, Ailles LE, Dylla SJ, *et al.* Granulocyte-macrophage progenitors as candidate leukemic stem cells in blast-crisis CML. *N Engl J Med* 2004;351(7):657–67.

122 Druker BJ, Sawyers CL, Kantarjian H, *et al.* Activity of a specific inhibitor of the BCR-ABL tyrosine kinase in the blast crisis of chronic myeloid leukemia and acute lymphoblastic leukemia with the Philadelphia chromosome. *N Engl J Med* 2001;344(14):1038–42.

123 Kantarjian H, Sawyers C, Hochhaus A, *et al.* Hematologic and cytogenetic responses to imatinib mesylate in chronic myelogenous leukemia. *N Engl J Med* 2002;346(9):645–52.

124 O'Brien SG, Guilhot F, Larson RA, *et al.* Imatinib compared with interferon and low-dose cytarabine for newly diagnosed chronic-phase chronic myeloid leukemia. *N Engl J Med* 2003;348(11):994–1004.

125 Hochhaus A, O'Brien SG, Guilhot F, *et al.* Six-year follow-up of patients receiving imatinib for the first-line treatment of chronic myeloid leukemia. *Leukemia* 2009;23(6):1054–61.

126 Cortes JE, Baccarani M, Guilhot F, *et al.* Phase III, randomized, open-label study of daily imatinib mesylate 400 mg versus 800 mg in patients with newly diagnosed, previously untreated

chronic myeloid leukemia in chronic phase using molecular end points: tyrosine kinase inhibitor optimization and selectivity study. *J Clin Oncol* 2010;28(3):424–30.

127 Deininger MW, Kopecky KJ, Radich JP, *et al.* Imatinib 800 mg daily induces deeper molecular responses than imatinib 400 mg daily: results of SWOG S0325, an intergroup randomized PHASE II trial in newly diagnosed chronic phase chronic myeloid leukaemia. *Br J Haematol* 2014;164(2):223–32.

128 Kantarjian H, Shah NP, Hochhaus A, *et al.* Dasatinib versus imatinib in newly diagnosed chronic-phase chronic myeloid leukemia. *N Engl J Med* 2010;362(24):2260–70.

129 Cortes JE, Saglio G, Kantarjian HM, *et al.* Final 5-Year Study Results of DASISION: The Dasatinib Versus Imatinib Study in Treatment-Naive Chronic Myeloid Leukemia Patients Trial. *J Clin Oncol* 2016;34(20):2333–40.

130 Saglio G, Kim DW, Issaragrisil S, *et al.* Nilotinib versus imatinib for newly diagnosed chronic myeloid leukemia. *N Engl J Med* 2010;362(24):2251–9.

131 Hughes TP, Saglio G, Kantarjian HM, *et al.* Early molecular response predicts outcomes in patients with chronic myeloid leukemia in chronic phase treated with frontline nilotinib or imatinib. *Blood* 2014;123(9):1353–60.

132 Mahon FX, Rea D, Guilhot J, *et al.* Discontinuation of imatinib in patients with chronic myeloid leukaemia who have maintained complete molecular remission for at least 2 years: the prospective, multicentre Stop Imatinib (STIM) trial. *Lancet Oncol* 2010;11(11):1029–35.

133 Baccarani M, Cortes J, Pane F, *et al.* Chronic myeloid leukemia: an update of concepts and management recommendations of European LeukemiaNet. *J Clin Oncol* 2009;27(35):6041–51.

134 Marin D, Ibrahim AR, Lucas C, *et al.* Assessment of BCR-ABL1 transcript levels at 3 months is the only requirement for predicting outcome for patients with chronic myeloid leukemia treated with tyrosine kinase inhibitors. *J Clin Oncol* 2012;30(3):232–8.

135 O'Brien S, Berman E, Moore JO, *et al.* NCCN Task Force report: tyrosine kinase inhibitor therapy selection in the management of patients with chronic myelogenous leukemia. *J Natl Compr Canc Netw* 2011;9 Suppl 2:S1–25.

136 Cortes JE, Kantarjian HM, Brummendorf TH, *et al.* Safety and efficacy of bosutinib (SKI-606) in chronic phase Philadelphia chromosome-positive chronic myeloid leukemia patients with resistance or intolerance to imatinib. *Blood* 2011;118(17):4567–76.

137 Cortes JE, Kantarjian H, Shah NP, *et al.* Ponatinib in refractory Philadelphia chromosome-positive leukemias. *N Engl J Med* 2012;367(22):2075–88.

138 Cortes J, Lipton JH, Rea D, *et al.* Phase 2 study of subcutaneous omacetaxine mepesuccinate after TKI failure in patients with chronic-phase CML with T315I mutation. *Blood* 2012;120(13):2573–80.

139 Deau B, Nicolini FE, Guilhot J, *et al.* The addition of daunorubicin to imatinib mesylate in combination with cytarabine improves the response rate and the survival of patients with myeloid blast crisis chronic myelogenous leukemia (AFR01 study). *Leuk Res* 2011;35(6):777–82.

140 Benyamini N, Rowe JM. Is there a role for allogeneic transplantation in chronic myeloid leukemia? *Expert Rev Hematol* 2013;6(6):759–65.

141 Bacher U, Klyuchnikov E, Zabelina T, *et al.* The changing scene of allogeneic stem cell transplantation for chronic myeloid leukemia – a report from the German Registry covering the period from 1998 to 2004. *Ann Hematol* 2009;88(12):1237–47.

142 Smalberg JH, Arends LR, Valla DC, *et al.* Myeloproliferative neoplasms in Budd-Chiari syndrome and portal vein thrombosis: a meta-analysis. *Blood* 2012;120(25):4921–8.

143 Tefferi A. Polycythemia vera and essential thrombocythemia: 2012 update on diagnosis, risk stratification, and management. *Am J Hematol* 2012;87(3):285–93.

144 Jensen MK, de Nully Brown P, Nielsen OJ, Hasselbalch HC. Incidence, clinical features and outcome of essential thrombocythaemia in a well defined geographical area. *Eur J Haematol* 2000;65(2):132–9.

145 Mesa RA, Silverstein MN, Jacobsen SJ, Wollan PC, Tefferi A. Population-based incidence and survival figures in essential thrombocythemia and agnogenic myeloid metaplasia: an Olmsted County Study, 1976–1995. *Am J Hematol* 1999;6(1):10–5.

146 Horny HP, Metcalfe DD, Bennett JM, *et al.* Mastocytosis. In: SH Swerdlow, E Campo, NL Harris, *et al.* (eds) *WHO Classification of Tumors of Hematopoietic and Lymphoid Tissues.* Lyon: IARC, 2008:54–63.

147 Richmond TD, Chohan M, Barber DL. Turning cells red: signal transduction mediated by erythropoietin. *Trends Cell Biol* 2005;15(3):146–55.

148 Quintás-Cardama A. The role of Janus kinase 2 (JAK2) in myeloproliferative neoplasms: Therapeutic implications. *Leukemia Res* 2013;37(4):465–72.

149 Zou H, Yan D, Mohi G. Differential biological activity of disease-associated JAK2 mutants. *FEBS Lett* 2011;585(7):1007–13.

150 Baxter EJ, Scott LM, Campbell PJ, *et al.* Acquired mutation of the tyrosine kinase JAK2 in human myeloproliferative disorders. *Lancet* 2005;365(9464):1054–61.

151 Nangalia J, Massie CE, Baxter EJ, *et al.* Somatic CALR mutations in myeloproliferative neoplasms with nonmutated JAK2. *N Engl J Med* 2013;369(25):2391–405.

152 Klampfl T, Gisslinger H, Harutyunyan AS, *et al.* Somatic mutations of calreticulin in myeloproliferative neoplasms. *N Engl J Med* 2013;369(25):2379–90.

153 Scott LM, Tong W, Levine RL, *et al.* JAK2 exon 12 mutations in polycythemia vera and idiopathic erythrocytosis. *N Engl J Med* 2007;356(5):459–68.

154 Pikman Y, Lee BH, Mercher T, *et al.* MPLW515L is a novel somatic activating mutation in myelofibrosis with myeloid metaplasia. *PLoS Med* 2006;3(7):e270.

155 Maxson JE, Gotlib J, Pollyea DA, *et al.* Oncogenic CSF3R mutations in chronic neutrophilic leukemia and atypical CML. *N Engl J Med* 2013;368(19):1781–90.

156 Dao KH, Tyner JW. What's different about atypical CML and chronic neutrophilic leukemia? *Hematology Am Soc Hematol Educ Program* 2015;2015:264–71.

157 Teffieri A. Primary myelofibrosis: 2013 update on diagnosis, risk-stratification, and management. *Am J Hematol* 2013;88(2):141–50.

158 Berk PD, Goldberg JD, Donovan PB, *et al.* Therapeutic recommendations in polycythemia vera based on

Polycythemia Vera Study Group protocols. *Semin Hematol* 1986;23(2):132–43.

159 Marchioli R, Finazzi G, Specchia G, *et al.* Cardiovascular events and intensity of treatment in polycythemia vera. *N Engl J Med* 2013;368(1):22–33.

160 Landolfi R, Marchioli R, Kutti J, *et al.* Efficacy and safety of low-dose aspirin in polycythemia vera. *N Engl J Med* 2004;350(2):114–24.

161 Kiladjian JJ, Cassinat B, Chevret S, *et al.* Pegylated interferon-alfa-2a induces complete hematologic and molecular responses with low toxicity in polycythemia vera. *Blood* 2008;112(8):3065–72.

162 Verstovsek S, Vannucchi AM, Griesshammer M, *et al.* Ruxolitinib versus best available therapy in patients with polycythemia vera: 80-week follow-up from the RESPONSE trial. *Haematologica* 2016;101(7):821–9.

163 Tefferi A. Polycythemia vera and essential thrombocythemia: 2013 update on diagnosis, risk-stratification, and management. *Am J Hematol* 2013;88(6):507–16.

164 Reilly JT, McMullin MF, Beer PA, *et al.* Guideline for the diagnosis and management of myelofibrosis. *Br J Haematol* 2012;158(4):453–71.

165 Gangat N, Caramazza D, Vaidya R, *et al.* DIPSS plus: a refined Dynamic International Prognostic Scoring System for primary myelofibrosis that incorporates prognostic information from karyotype, platelet count, and transfusion status. *J Clin Oncol* 2011;29(4):392–7.

166 Verstovsek S, Mesa RA, Gotlib J, *et al.* A double-blind, placebo-controlled trial of ruxolitinib for myelofibrosis. *N Engl J Med* 2012;366(9):799–807.

167 Harrison C, Kiladjian JJ, Al-Ali HK, *et al.* JAK inhibition with ruxolitinib versus best available therapy for myelofibrosis. *N Engl J Med* 2012;366(9):787–98.

168 Tefferi A, Pardanani A. Serious adverse events during ruxolitinib treatment discontinuation in patients with myelofibrosis. *Mayo Clin Proc* 2011;86(12):1188–91.

169 Galimberti S, Ferreri MI, Simi P, *et al.* Platelet-derived growth factor beta receptor (PDGFRB) gene is rearranged in a significant percentage of myelodysplastic syndromes with normal karyotype. *Br J Haematol* 2009;147(5): 763–6.

170 Hensley B, Geyer H, Mesa R. Polycythemia vera: current pharmacotherapy and future directions. *Expert Opin Pharmacother* 2013;14(5):609–17.

30

Lymphoid Leukemias in Adults

Nilanjan Ghosh[1], Jocelyn L. Wozney[2], and Michael R. Grunwald[1]

[1] *Levine Cancer Institute/Carolinas HealthCare System, Charlotte, North Carolina, USA*
[2] *Lancaster General Health, Lancaster, Pennsylvania, USA*

Acute Lymphoblastic Leukemia/ Lymphoma (ALL)

Incidence, Mortality, and Etiology

Acute lymphoblastic leukemia/lymphoma is an uncommon disease in adults. Approximately 6,000 new cases of ALL occur each year in the United States (US), but only 43% of these are diagnosed in adults. The disease has a bimodal age distribution, with peaks occurring between 2 and 4 years of age and again after age 50 [1–3]. Caucasians and Hispanics have higher incidence rates of ALL than other racial and ethnic groups [4]. Historically, higher incidence rates of childhood ALL have been reported in groups with higher socioeconomic status [5]; lower risk is associated with early immune stimulation (such as in infant daycare settings) [4]. However, associations of demographic characteristics, inherited predispositions, and environmental exposures with the development of ALL have not been studied as thoroughly in adults as in children. Approximately 1,400 deaths from ALL occur annually in the US, with 84% of these being among adults [1, 2, 6].

Decades of progress have resulted in the ability to cure approximately 90% of children diagnosed with ALL [3]. In contrast, the 5-year survival in standard-risk adult patients is approximately 40% [7]. The highly successful outcomes in pediatric ALL have laid the foundation for improvements in the treatment of adolescents and young adults (AYA) with this disease. Importantly, in the last three decades, improved survival has been noted for patients up to age 59, and progress has been most pronounced in the older adolescent age group (age 15–19) [8]. Factors contributing to the more favorable outcomes among children include the presence of robust support networks, greater tolerance of high-intensity therapy, the higher frequency of prognostically favorable cytogenetic and molecular abnormalities, and possibly differences in the biology driving leukemogenesis [9].

Diagnostic Evaluation

Most adults with ALL come to medical attention because of symptoms related to pancytopenia. However, the complete blood cell count can reveal leukocytosis or leukopenia, with anemia and thrombocytopenia. Presenting symptoms and signs can include fever, fatigue, bruising, bleeding, dyspnea, pallor, infections, or bone pain. Because central nervous system (CNS) involvement is relatively common in ALL, patients may present with neurologic symptoms including headaches, mental status changes, or cranial neuropathies. Patients with predominantly lymphomatous involvement may present with respiratory symptoms or superior vena cava syndrome due to a mediastinal mass [10–12].

ALL is a medical emergency, and an expeditious evaluation should be undertaken once the diagnosis is suspected. The peripheral blood smear should be examined to determine if circulating blasts are present. A bone marrow aspirate and biopsy is also required to confirm the diagnosis. The immunophenotype of the leukemic blasts, which establishes the proteins expressed on the surface of these cells, must be determined. The immunophenotype is typically ascertained using flow cytometry (and sometimes immunohistochemistry) to analyze the peripheral blood or bone marrow. Immunophenotyping distinguishes ALL from other entities in the differential diagnosis, including acute myeloid leukemia and the mature lymphoid leukemias. It also permits further classification of the disease into one of three broad groups based on lineage and the stage of maturation arrest: precursor B-ALL, mature B-ALL, and T-ALL [13–15]. Mature B-ALL is also known as Burkitt leukemia/ lymphoma and has clinical, pathologic, and prognostic features distinct from precursor B- and T-ALL.

Some patients with ALL present with predominantly lymphomatous involvement, with a mediastinal mass or bulky lymphadenopathy and a paucity of circulating blasts. In these cases, immunohistochemistry or flow cytometry should be performed

The American Cancer Society's Oncology in Practice: Clinical Management, First Edition. Edited by The American Cancer Society.

Table 30.1 Prognostic factors in adult acute lymphoblastic leukemia. Adapted from [16–18].

Standard-risk	Age <35 years WBC <30 × 10^9/L for B-ALL WBC <100 × 10^9/L for T-ALL Hyperdiploidy (51–65 chromosomes) Minimal residual disease after induction: <0.01%
High-risk	Age >35 years WBC >30 × 10^9/L for B-ALL WBC >100 × 10^9/L for T-ALL t(9;22) (Philadelphia chromosome-positive) *MLL* rearrangements: t(4;11), t(9;11), t(11;19) t(8;14) (c-Myc translocation) Complex karyotype (5 or more abnormalities) Hypodiploidy (30–39 chromosomes) Minimal residual disease after induction: >0.01%

B-ALL, B-cell acute lymphocytic leukemia; T-ALL, T-cell acute lymphocytic leukemia; WBC, white blood cells.

on a biopsy specimen to further classify the immunophenotype. Lymphoblastic leukemia and lymphoblastic lymphoma are terms used to describe the same disease with different clinical presentations. Patients with predominantly lymphomatous involvement are classified as having lymphoblastic lymphoma, while patients with circulating blasts (with or without a mass lesion) are classified as having lymphoblastic leukemia [14].

Relevant prognostic factors for adult ALL are summarized in Table 30.1. Cytogenetic and molecular studies are important components of the diagnostic evaluation, serving to characterize the disease, risk-stratify patients, and identify potential therapeutic targets. The most commonly identified cytogenetic abnormality in adult ALL is the t(9;22) translocation (also known as the Philadelphia chromosome). It is found in approximately 25–30% of adults with precursor B-ALL. This translocation gives rise to the BCR-ABL fusion protein, a constitutively activated tyrosine kinase that results in dysregulated cell proliferation. The presence of the Philadelphia chromosome is relevant to treatment, since inhibition of BCR-ABL signaling can be achieved with tyrosine kinase inhibitors (TKIs). Historically, the Philadelphia chromosome has been viewed as a negative prognostic factor, but the incorporation of TKIs into multiagent chemotherapy regimens for ALL has led to improved outcomes for this group of patients. Other cytogenetic abnormalities that have been well-characterized in pediatric ALL, such as hyperdiploidy and the *TEL-AML1* translocation (t(12;21)), are less common in adults. Differences in the incidence of these favorable-risk cytogenetic abnormalities may partially account for the disparity in outcomes between pediatric and adult ALL patients [16, 17, 19, 20].

Treatment

The pretreatment evaluation for a newly diagnosed patient with ALL should include a thorough history and physical examination. Because involvement of the mediastinum and testis is common in T-ALL, patients with this subtype should undergo testicular examination as well as a computed tomography (CT) scan of the chest. Since disseminated intravascular coagulation (DIC) may exist at presentation or develop during treatment, a coagulation profile that includes the fibrinogen level should be obtained. Monitoring for tumor lysis syndrome is also essential, with attention to the uric acid, lactate dehydrogenase, potassium, phosphate, calcium, and creatinine levels. Since anthracyclines comprise an integral component of the commonly used chemotherapy regimens for ALL, cardiac function should be assessed, typically with an echocardiogram. Human leukocyte antigen (HLA) typing should be performed in patients who do not have a major contraindication to future allogeneic hematopoietic stem cell transplantation (SCT) [12, 13, 15].

Because CNS disease is present in approximately 5% of newly diagnosed patients, assessment of the cerebrospinal fluid for the presence of leukemic cells is mandatory. The presence of neurologic symptoms heightens the suspicion of CNS involvement, but most patients with this complication are asymptomatic. If CNS leukemia is present, then additional treatment with cranial irradiation, intrathecal chemotherapy, and/or administration of systemic high-dose methotrexate or cytarabine is necessary. Most patients with CNS disease are treated with a combination of these strategies. Even in patients without CNS involvement, prophylaxis with drugs that cross the blood–brain barrier is an important part of any ALL treatment regimen [10, 12, 15, 21].

The multiagent chemotherapy regimens employed for the treatment of ALL are among the most complex and intensive in all of oncology. Most experts recommend that patients receive treatment in specialized oncology centers with experience in treating this relatively rare disease. In general, the selection of the optimal treatment regimen for an individual patient depends heavily on age, the presence or absence of the Philadelphia chromosome, and institutional preference. Induction therapy is designed to eradicate the bulk of disease and to deliver CNS prophylaxis. One commonly used regimen in older adults (known as "hyperCVAD") utilizes hyperfractionated dosing of cyclophosphamide, vincristine, doxorubicin, and dexamethasone, alternating with doses of methotrexate and cytarabine that are sufficient to cross the blood–brain barrier. For patients whose leukemic blasts express CD20, the anti-CD20 monoclonal antibody rituximab is incorporated into this regimen. The AYA population is often treated with pediatric-inspired chemotherapy regimens that build upon the same drugs used in the hyperCVAD regimen but that also incorporate L-asparaginase, higher cumulative doses of vincristine and corticosteroids, and more intense CNS prophylaxis. L-asparaginase is usually avoided in older adults, who often have difficulty tolerating this drug. In patients with substantial comorbidities or impaired organ function, the intense chemotherapy regimens typically used in the treatment of ALL are not well tolerated. Unfortunately, there are few clinical trial data to guide management of these patients. Individualized modifications of the standard multiagent chemotherapy regimens are often necessary for these patients [12, 13, 15, 22–26].

In Philadelphia chromosome-positive (Ph+) ALL, it has become standard of care to combine chemotherapy with a TKI targeting BCR-ABL. Multiple clinical trials have shown improved remission rates with this strategy. TKIs have also been used as single agents as upfront therapy in the elderly and unfit population and as therapy in the relapsed/refractory population. None of the TKIs has been proven superior and the selection of the optimal agent must be based on patient-specific factors, side effect profiles, and ABL kinase domain mutational status (if used in the setting of relapsed/refractory disease) [12, 13, 15, 27–32]. While imatinib has the largest amount of long-term data of the TKIs, dasatinib is often chosen due to its CNS penetration as well as robust clinical trial data demonstrating the efficacy of this agent. Ponatinib is the only approved agent with activity against the BCR-ABL T315I mutation and is frequently used in the setting of relapsed/refractory Ph + ALL. TKIs are now often used as post-consolidation and post-transplant maintenance therapy in Ph + ALL [33–35].

After the bulk of disease is cleared with induction, patients then proceed on to the consolidation and delayed intensification phases of treatment. A 2- to 3-year period of maintenance chemotherapy follows, usually involving oral chemotherapy with 6-mercaptopurine punctuated with periodic doses of methotrexate, vincristine, and corticosteroids. Fit patients who are deemed high-risk are often directed to allogeneic SCT after induction, if remission has been achieved [12, 13, 15].

Approximately 90% of adults with ALL will achieve a complete clinical remission with induction chemotherapy [24, 25]. However, a large number of these patients will ultimately relapse. One of the potential explanations for this is the persistence of minimal residual disease (MRD), defined as the persistence of leukemic blasts below the threshold for morphologic detection. Sensitive techniques have been developed to assess for MRD. Flow cytometry and polymerase chain reaction (PCR) assays are used most frequently and are well validated as sensitive techniques. Several studies in both adults and children have shown that the presence of MRD at the end of induction therapy has prognostic value and is associated with a higher risk of relapse [18, 36].

Relapse is common in adults with ALL, and patients with relapsed disease have a poor prognosis [37]. Treatment options include the nucleoside analogs clofarabine and nelarabine (which has been shown to have efficacy in T-cell ALL), liposomal vincristine, or a modified multiagent chemotherapy regimen. Blinatumomab is a bispecific antibody that is now approved by the US Food and Drug Administration (FDA) for the treatment of relapsed/refractory pre-B-cell ALL. This agent engages T cells via its anti-CD3 arm and directs the targeting of B cells via its anti-CD19 arm, thereby juxtaposing the two cells and promoting T-cell mediated cytotoxicity [38–40]. Trials have not only shown promising efficacy for blinatumomab in the relapsed/refractory setting, but it has also been demonstrated that blinatumomab can eradicate MRD and prolong relapse-free survival in B-ALL patients [41, 42].

Inotuzumab ozogamicin, which is an anti-CD22 monoclonal antibody conjugated to the potent toxin calicheamicin, has induced remissions in relapsed ALL patients and has been demonstrated to have a progression-free survival (PFS) benefit and overall survival (OS) benefit compared to standard chemotherapy [43, 44]. Veno-occlusive disease of the liver is a major complication that can occur with use of inotuzumab ozogamicin. This agent is now approved in the US for adults with relapsed or refractory B-cell precursor ALL.

Moreover, chimeric antigen receptor T cells (CAR-T cells) targeting CD19 are showing great promise in pre-B-cell ALL [45–50]. The CAR-T therapy tisagenlecleucel was recently approved by the FDA for patients 25 years and younger with B-cell precursor ALL that is refractory or in second or later relapse. CAR-T cells targeting CD22 are also under development [51]. Cytokine release syndrome has been a common toxicity in patients receiving CAR-T cell therapy on clinical trials. Finally, because *NOTCH* mutations are common in patients with T-ALL, agents targeting this pathway are under evaluation [52].

Patients with Ph + ALL should undergo ABL kinase domain mutation testing to assess for the emergence of mutations that confer drug resistance. Switching to an alternate TKI may prove effective in such patients. Patients with relapsed disease who achieve remission should be considered for allogeneic SCT [12, 28, 29, 53–55].

Supportive Care

Patients with ALL require intensive supportive care. Given the complexity of the chemotherapy regimens, the lengthy treatment course, and the inherent immunosuppression associated with a lymphoid cancer, these patients are at risk of a multitude of complications both as a consequence of the disease itself as well as its treatment. During therapy, patients require aggressive transfusion support along with monitoring and prophylaxis for complications such as tumor lysis syndrome and DIC. Such complications are common during induction therapy. Patients are also at risk for chemotherapy-derived toxicity. L-asparaginase is associated with a myriad of side effects, including hypersensitivity reactions, pancreatitis, liver dysfunction, thrombosis, and hemorrhage. ALL patients must also be monitored for steroid-induced hyperglycemia and treated with insulin if this is identified. Finally, infection remains a major cause of morbidity and mortality in patients with ALL. Prophylaxis against the herpesviruses, *Pneumocystis jirovecii*, candida species, and the invasive molds is strongly recommended. During periods of neutropenia, antibacterial prophylaxis is also necessary [10, 13, 15].

Follow-Up and Survivorship

Periodic assessment with history, physical examination, blood counts and, if indicated, bone marrow biopsy is recommended after completing therapy. Patients with Ph + ALL often continue on prolonged therapy with TKIs and need to be monitored closely for adverse effects from treatment. Late effects of chemotherapy for ALL include avascular necrosis, heart failure, secondary malignancies, and neuropathy. Patients undergoing allogeneic SCT may develop infertility, thyroid dysfunction, chronic fatigue, and secondary cancers.

Chronic Lymphocytic Leukemia (CLL)

Incidence, Mortality, and Etiology

Chronic lymphocytic leukemia accounts for approximately 32% of all leukemia cases. In the US, the estimated number of new cases in 2017 is 20,110, and about 4,660 deaths occur annually in the US from CLL [1]. It is primarily a disease of older persons, and the median age at diagnosis is 71 years. The disease has a male predominance and in the US is most common in Caucasians and least common among Asian Americans/Pacific Islanders and American Indians/Alaska Natives for reasons that are unknown [56].

Family history is an important risk factor and approximately 8–10% of newly diagnosed patients have an afflicted family member [57, 58]. Many other putative risk factors have been investigated. Sun exposure and atopy have been inversely associated with CLL. Hepatitis C seropositivity and farming exposure have been associated with a higher incidence of CLL [59], with the exception of agent orange. The Institute of Medicine issued a report "Veterans and Agent Orange: Update 2002," which concluded that there was sufficient evidence of an association between herbicides used in Vietnam and CLL.

The diagnosis of CLL may be preceded by a premalignant, asymptomatic condition called monoclonal B-cell lymphocytosis (MBL). The link between MBL and CLL is analogous to the relationship between monoclonal gammopathy of undetermined significance (MGUS) and multiple myeloma. MBL is characterized by fewer than 5×10^9/L circulating monoclonal B cells and the absence of lymphadenopathy, organomegaly, cytopenias, and disease-related symptoms [60–62]. Longitudinal studies have suggested that patients with MBL that is detected during a clinical evaluation of lymphocytosis have an approximate rate of progression to CLL of 1–2% per year. Importantly, not all patients with MBL will progress to CLL. Guidelines for follow-up of patients with MBL do not exist, but most experts recommend annual clinical evaluations and blood count monitoring [63–65].

Diagnostic Evaluation

CLL is a heterogeneous disease with a variable clinical presentation. Many patients are asymptomatic at the time of diagnosis, having come to medical attention after routine laboratory studies showed an unexpected elevation in the white blood cell count. In symptomatic patients, the most common clinical features are fatigue, weight loss, and lymphadenopathy. Patients may report other "B" symptoms such as fevers and night sweats, which are typical of CLL and other lymphoproliferative disorders. In more advanced stages of disease, splenomegaly is common [66, 67]. Impaired immunity is a hallmark of CLL, due to both quantitative and qualitative defects in leukocyte function. This is often manifested by recurrent or severe infections, autoimmune phenomena, and hypogammaglobulinemia [68].

The diagnosis of CLL is usually first suspected when laboratory studies demonstrate an absolute lymphocytosis. According to the World Health Organization (WHO) Classification of Lymphoid Neoplasms, in order to diagnose CLL, a patient must have more than 5×10^9/L circulating monoclonal B cells that express cell surface markers such as CD5, CD19, and CD23, along with low levels of CD20 and membrane immunoglobulin. Clonality must be established by showing that the abnormal B cells are restricted to expression of either kappa or lambda light chains. The diagnostic criteria also allow for a diagnosis of CLL in the setting of lower lymphocyte counts, provided that there is evidence of CLL in the bone marrow and disease-related symptoms or cytopenias not caused by an autoimmune process. A similar disease entity, SLL (small lymphocytic lymphoma), is essentially the tissue equivalent of CLL. Although the WHO Classification system distinguishes between the clinical presentations of CLL and SLL, the malignant cells in each disorder are identical pathologically and immunophenotypically. Except for rare cases of localized SLL, the prognosis for these two entities is quite similar and they are managed in a similar fashion. The diagnostic criteria for MBL, CLL, and SLL are summarized in Table 30.2 [60–62].

An important first step in the evaluation of a patient with suspected CLL involves a careful examination of the peripheral blood smear. The monoclonal B cells of CLL are similar in appearance to small, mature lymphocytes with scant cytoplasm, absent nucleoli, and densely packed chromatin. Classically, the peripheral blood smear will also show "smudge cells," which are larger cells that appear flattened or smeared. Flow cytometry of the peripheral blood can be sufficient to confirm the diagnosis and is helpful in ruling out other disorders that can present in a similar fashion. The differential diagnosis includes lymphocytosis secondary to infection (such as infectious mononucleosis), mantle cell lymphoma, marginal zone lymphoma, lymphoplasmacytic lymphoma (also known as Waldenstrom macroglobulinemia), hairy cell leukemia, prolymphocytic leukemia, and follicular lymphoma. A bone marrow biopsy is not required to establish a diagnosis of CLL [60, 62]. However, examination of the bone marrow can be quite helpful in determining the karyotype abnormalities associated with CLL and determining the etiology of anemia and thrombocytopenia in CLL.

Once the diagnosis of CLL has been established, additional studies may be useful in interpreting the disease burden and predicting prognosis. The disease burden is best assessed using the Rai or Binet staging systems (summarized in Table 30.3), or a combination of the two. Each system has limitations, but both have been well validated and are simple to use, relying only on the physical examination and routine laboratory studies [68, 69]. Critics of the Rai and Binet staging systems argue that most patients are diagnosed with low-risk, early-stage disease, where there is the greatest variability in outcomes [70]. Therefore, considerable attention has been paid to identifying other prognostic factors that might better predict the clinical course of an individual patient.

Table 30.2 Diagnostic criteria for MBL, SLL, and CLL. Adapted from [60–62].

Monoclonal B-cell lymphocytosis (MBL)	**Small lymphocytic lymphoma (SLL)**	**Chronic lymphocytic leukemia (CLL)**
Less than 5×10^9/L clonal B lymphocytes in circulation, *and* Absence of disease-related symptoms, lymphadenopathy, organomegaly, cytopenias	Less than 5×10^9/L clonal B lymphocytes in circulation, *and* Presence of disease-related symptoms, lymphadenopathy, or organomegaly	At least 5×10^9/L clonal B lymphocytes in circulation, *or* Presence of disease-related symptoms, lymphadenopathy, organomegaly, and/or cytopenias, *and* Less than 5×10^9/L clonal B lymphocytes in circulation

Table 30.3 Rai and Binet staging systems for CLL. Adapted from [68, 69].

Rai system for staging CLL

Stage	Description	Risk status
0	Lymphocytosis	Low
I	Lymphocytosis and lymphadenopathy	Intermediate
II	Lymphocytosis and/or lymphadenopathy with hepato/splenomegaly	Intermediate
III	Stage 0, I, or II and hemoglobin <11 g/dL or hematocrit <33%[1]	High
IV	Stage 0, I, or II and platelets <100,000/μL[1]	High

Binet system for staging CLL

Stage	Description
A	Hemoglobin ≥10 g/dL and platelets ≥100,000/mm^3 and <3 enlarged areas[2]
B	Hemoglobin ≥10 g/dL and platelets ≥100,000/mm^3 and >3 enlarged areas[2]
C	Hemoglobin <10 g/dL and/or platelets ≤100,000/mm^3 and any number of enlarged areas[2]

[1] Cytopenias not immune-mediated.
[2] Cytopenias not immune-mediated; areas of involvement considered for staging include head and neck, axillae, groin, spleen, and liver.

Over 35 different prognostic markers for CLL have been reported in the literature. Table 30.4 summarizes the most common and clinically useful tests utilized in practice [62, 71–82]. Besides clinical staging, the lymphocyte doubling time (LDT) is one of the earliest identified prognostic factors in CLL. Having an LDT of 12 months or less was found to correlate with a shorter progression-free and overall survival [73]. One of the most important prognostic factors in CLL is the presence of an unmutated immunoglobulin heavy chain variable (IgVH) region in the genome of the malignant lymphocytes. Multiple studies have shown that this correlates with poorer responses to therapy, shorter remissions, and inferior survival [76]. Presumably, this denotes a more primitive, and perhaps treatment-resistant, B-cell clone. Conversely, patients with a mutated IgVH have improved outcomes [77–79].

Table 30.4 Prognostic factors in CLL.

Genetic factors	Risk of poor prognosis
Deletion 17p	Very high
TP53 mutation	Very high
Complex karyotype	Very high
SF3B1 mutation	High
NOTCH1 mutation	High
Unmutated *IGHV*	High
Trisomy 12	High
Deletion 11 q	High
Deletion 13q	Low

Acquired chromosomal abnormalities, which can be assessed using interphase fluorescence *in situ* hybridization (FISH), represent another set of important prognostic factors for CLL. The most commonly encountered cytogenetic abnormality is deletion of chromosome 13q14, which appears to predict better outcomes. In contrast, partial deletions of chromosomes 17p (where the p53 gene resides) and 11q have been associated with inferior outcomes [80, 81]. Clonal evolution, defined as the acquisition of new cytogenetic abnormalities from a baseline analysis, has been observed in CLL and may be an independently negative predictor of survival [82]. Complex karyotype is a strong predictor of inferior outcomes in CLL [83–85]. CD49d is an independent prognostic factor in CLL [86]. It should be noted that none of these prognostic factors serves as an indicator to initiate treatment. Rather, they enable a clinician to better predict the prognosis for an individual patient, to understand the rate at which an individual's disease might progress, and to estimate the likelihood of response to treatment [62, 71].

Treatment

When evaluating a patient who is newly diagnosed with CLL, one of the first questions that must be addressed is whether the patient requires immediate therapy. Not all patients with CLL require treatment at the time of diagnosis. Many patients are diagnosed with early-stage disease, are asymptomatic, and can be safely monitored for months or even years without treatment. CLL cannot be cured with conventional chemotherapy alone and clinical trials assessing the benefit of immediate versus deferred treatment for early-stage CLL have failed to show a benefit for an aggressive approach [87]. Furthermore, while these instances are rare, spontaneous regression of CLL has been reported [88]. Patients who do not require therapy at the time of initial diagnosis should undergo careful monitoring for disease progression and/or complications.

Expert guidelines have been adopted to guide clinicians regarding the optimal timing of initial therapy. At least one of the following criteria indicative of progressive disease should be met: progressive bone marrow failure (worsening anemia or thrombocytopenia); massive or progressive splenomegaly; massive or progressive lymphadenopathy; autoimmune cytopenias that have not responded to standard therapies; and/or disease-related constitutional symptoms (significant fatigue, fevers or night sweats, weight loss of more than 10% body weight in 6 months). Rapidly progressive lymphocytosis, with an LDT of less than 6 months, may serve as another reason for starting treatment, particularly if there are other signs of worsening disease [62]. Of note, there is no threshold absolute lymphocyte count that serves as an indicator of when treatment is needed. Symptoms associated with aggregation of white blood cells in the microvasculature, as in the acute leukemias, occur only in very rare instances in CLL.

Once a decision has been made to initiate therapy, the clinician must take into account various patient factors to guide the selection of specific treatment. These include, but are not limited to, age, performance status, medical comorbidities, and organ dysfunction, along with disease-specific factors such as FISH and IgVH mutation results. Generally, in additional to the physical examination and routine laboratory studies, the pretreatment evaluation for a patient with CLL should include testing for HIV and hepatitis B and C, measurement of serum immunoglobulin levels and lactate dehydrogenase (LDH), a direct antiglobulin test, and imaging. It is also important to perform interphase FISH to assess for chromosomal abnormalities, along with testing to determine the IgVH mutational status [62].

Chemoimmunotherapy

A number of drugs and combination therapies are FDA approved for the treatment of CLL. Many treatment guidelines suggest regimens containing the purine analog fludarabine for first-line treatment in non-frail patients. Fludarabine is often combined with the alkylating agent cyclophosphamide and the anti-CD20 monoclonal antibody rituximab, forming the commonly used FCR regimen [89]. A large randomized clinical trial investigating chemoimmunotherapy with FCR achieved response rates of 90% in previously untreated patients, versus 80% with chemotherapy using FC alone. Survival was longer in the FCR arm [90]. However, fludarabine has been associated with significant toxicities including autoimmune hemolytic anemia and prolonged cytopenias [91–94.]

The alkylating agents chlorambucil and bendamustine have been extensively studied in CLL. Bendamustine was approved by the FDA on the basis of a phase 3 trial that showed improved response rates and PFS compared to chlorambucil [95, 96]. The most common side effects observed with bendamustine are myelosuppression, rash, and hypersensitivity reactions. Bendamustine is commonly combined with rituximab (BR) for the treatment of CLL. A randomized comparison of FCR versus BR showed improved PFS with FCR in patients. However, severe neutropenia and infections were more frequently observed with FCR and were more pronounced in patients >65 years [97]. No difference in overall survival has been reported with a median follow-up of 3 years. Treatment with FCR has led to very long remissions in patients who have IgVH mutated disease [98–100]. A humanized CD20 antibody, obinutuzumab, in combination with chlorambucil was recently approved by the FDA to treat patients with previously untreated CLL [101]. Obinituzumab monotherapy also has excellent responses in newly diagnosed CLL [102].

Small Molecule Inhibitors

The identification of the B-cell receptor pathway (BCR) and BCL-2 in the pathogenesis of CLL has led to development of small molecule inhibitors (SMI) which are highly effective agents in the treatment of CLL. Ibrutinib was the first in class irreversible inhibitor of Bruton's tyrosine kinase (BTK), an essential component of the BCR pathway involved in survival of CLL cells. Ibrutinib has been approved by the FDA in newly diagnosed CLL and relapsed/refractory CLL based on randomized comparisons with chlorambucil (newly diagnosed) and ofatumumab (relapsed/refractory) disease [103, 104]. Ibrutinib showed superiority in overall response rates, PFS, and OS in these studies. Impressively, ibrutinib has a high response rate and leads to durable remissions in deletion 17p CLL [105]. Although ibrutinib is a BTK inhibitor, it can have some off-target effects due to inhibition of other kinases such as interleukin-2-inducible T-cell kinase (ITK) and tyrosine-protein kinase (TEC). Ibrutinib affects collagen and von Willebrand factor-dependent platelet function and has been associated with bleeding complications, especially in patients who are on anticoagulation [106]. Ibrutinib is also associated with atrial fibrillation [107]. Patients who are on ibrutinib need monitoring for bleeding, infections, and atrial fibrillation. Second-generation BTK inhibitors such as acalabrutinib have more selective BTK inhibition, and bleeding events or atrial fibrillation have not been observed with this agent [108].

Idelalisib is a phosphatidylinositol 3-kinase delta (PI3Kδ) inhibitor and has significant clinical activity in relapsed and refractory CLL. However, it is associated with immune-mediated adverse effects such as hepatitis, colitis, and pneumonitis [109]. Therefore, patients need to be monitored closely. It is approved by the FDA for the treatment of patients with relapsed CLL, in combination with rituximab. TGR 1202 is a next-generation PI3Kδ inhibitor which retains potent efficacy against CLL but has a much improved adverse event profile [110].

Venetoclax is an inhibitor of the antiapoptotic protein BCL-2 and works via a p53 and BCR-independent mechanism. Venetoclax has potent anti-CLL activity and retains remarkable activity in deletion 17p CLL [111]. It has also demonstrated activity after failure of ibrutinib or idelalisib [112]. Clinically significant tumor lysis syndrome was seen in early studies which led to establishment of a stepwise weekly ramp-up with risk-based prophylaxis to mitigate against tumor lysis syndrome. Venetoclax is approved by the FDA for treatment of relapsed deletion 17p CLL.

Ofatumumab, a monoclonal antibody that targets a different epitope on the CD20 molecule, is also approved for the treatment of relapsed CLL [89, 113]. The benefits of autologous SCT for patients with CLL have been investigated in prospective randomized trials. Autologous SCT has been shown to prolong disease-free survival, but not OS [114–116]. Allogeneic SCT is the only potentially curative treatment for CLL. Candidates for allogeneic SCT are those with high-risk disease. Because of the high rate of treatment-related morbidity and mortality associated with myeloablative transplant regimens, nonmyeloablative or reduced-intensity transplants have emerged as the preferred options. However, there remains considerable debate regarding the selection of patients, ideal timing, and optimal transplantation regimen for CLL [114]. Moreover, with the emergence of multiple oral treatment options with favorable toxicity profiles, the attainment of cure may not be a necessary goal in the majority of patients. In addition, the activity of genetically modified chimeric antigen receptor (CAR) T cells has presented the opportunity to harness the immune system to kill CLL cells without the need of an allogeneic graft-versus-leukemia effect. Treatment of relapsed and refractory high-risk CLL with anti-CD19 CAR modified T cells has resulted in sustained remissions [117, 118].

Response to therapy is assessed by the international working group CLL response criteria [119]. The criteria are summarized in Table 30.5. More recently, PR with lymphocytosis (PR-L) has been defined as partial remission with prolonged lymphocytosis with <50% decline in lymphocyte count. This is commonly seen in patients who are treated with ibrutinib. Multicolor flow cytometry or PCR can be used to test for MRD in CLL.

Table 30.5 iwCLL response criteria.

CR	LN ≤1.5 cm, absence of B symptoms, hepatomegaly or splenomegaly, absence of clonal lymphocytes in peripheral blood
PR	≥50% decrease in lymphocyte count, ≥50% decrease in LN size
SD	Absence of PD and failure to achieve at least a PR
PD	≥50% increase in lymphocyte count, ≥50% increase in LN size

iwCLL, International Workshop on CLL; CR, complete remission; LN, lymph nodes; PD, progressive disease; PR, partial remission; SD, stable disease.

Achieving BM MRD-negative complete remission (CR) is associated with superior PFS and overall survival; MRD status is the single best post-treatment predictor of long-term outcomes after chemoimmunotherapy regimens such as FCR.

Supportive Care

Supportive care is an integral part of the management of patients with CLL. A wide range of complications can arise during the course of treatment, including infections, autoimmune phenomena, and Richter transformation.

Patients with CLL suffer from both quantitative and qualitative deficits in immune function, involving not only the lymphoid lineage but also natural killer (NK) cells, neutrophils, monocytes, and macrophages. It is important to note that the risk of infection is not limited to patients undergoing active treatment; rather, untreated patients are also at an increased risk of infection from both common and opportunistic pathogens [120]. Because infection is a common cause of death in patients with CLL, specific guidelines have been assembled to guide decision-making about antimicrobial prophylaxis and monitoring for patients. This is particularly relevant for patients receiving therapy with the purine analogs or alemtuzumab. These agents are quite immunosuppressive and have been associated with *Pneumocystis jirovecii* pneumonia and cytomegalovirus (CMV) reactivation. Patients treated with alemtuzumab must be monitored for CMV reactivation during treatment and for 2 months beyond the conclusion of therapy [89, 121].

Almost two-thirds of patients with CLL will develop hypogammaglobulinemia during the course of their disease. Patients with hypogammaglobulinemia and recurrent bacterial infections should be considered for treatment with prophylactic intravenous immunoglobulin treatments on a regular basis. It is recommended that patients receive the influenza vaccination yearly and the pneumococcal vaccination every 5 years. All live virus vaccines, including the herpes zoster vaccine, should be avoided [89, 120, 121].

Patients with CLL are also at risk for a variety of autoimmune complications. Hematological autoimmunity, manifesting as autoimmune hemolytic anemia or immune thrombocytopenia, is most common. In the evaluation of a CLL patient with anemia or thrombocytopenia, it is important to distinguish between disease-related bone marrow failure and autoimmunity. Examination of the bone marrow can be quite helpful in making this distinction. When autoimmune hemolytic anemia, pure red cell aplasia or immune thrombocytopenia is suspected, standard immunosuppressive treatments such as corticosteroids, intravenous immunoglobulin, cyclosporine, or rituximab should be instituted. Immune-mediated cytopenias are not an immediate indication for the institution of chemo- or immunotherapy for CLL, unless they cannot be controlled with standard immunosuppressive therapies [62, 89, 122]. Other manifestations of autoimmunity have been associated with CLL, including acquired angioedema, paraneoplastic pemphigus, thyroiditis, vasculitis, polyneuropathy, glomerulonephritis, rheumatoid arthritis, and inflammatory bowel disease. As is the case with the immune-mediated cytopenias, treatment should first be directed at the underlying autoimmune disorder. If the autoimmune condition cannot be controlled with standard therapy, then it is reasonable to initiate treatment directed at CLL [89, 120, 122].

With effective therapies, patients with CLL are at risk for tumor lysis syndrome, which is caused by the sudden release of intracellular contents. Precautions, including aggressive intravenous hydration and administration of allopurinol, should be taken to prevent the complications associated with this syndrome. Patients with bulky disease and/or a high white blood cell count are at the highest risk for tumor lysis syndrome [89, 123].

Richter transformation/syndrome, which is the transformation of CLL into aggressive diffuse large B-cell lymphoma (90%) or Hodgkin lymphoma, occurs at a rate of 0.5–1% per year. Patients with bulky disease, deletion 17p or *NOTCH1* mutations and those without deletion 13q CLL are at a higher risk of developing Richter transformation. Patients usually present with systemic "B" symptoms such as fever, weight loss, and night sweats in conjunction with rapidly enlarging lymphadenopathy. Laboratory studies often show an elevated LDH level. Positron emission tomography (PET) scan can be helpful in making the diagnosis, since affected sites are usually markedly fluorodeoxyglucose (FDG)-avid. Biopsy is necessary for confirming the diagnosis of Richter syndrome. Treatment with aggressive multidrug chemotherapy regimens (such as RCHOP) is often required to achieve a treatment response, but durable remissions are uncommon and the prognosis is poor. Patients who respond to chemotherapy should be considered for allogeneic transplant or clinical trials [124].

Prolymphocytic Leukemia (PLL)

B- and T-prolymphocytic leukemia are rare, mature lymphoid leukemias that typically affect older adults. These entities can be distinguished from CLL morphologically and immunophenotypically. On the peripheral blood smear, prolymphocytes appear as medium-sized cells with a high nuclear-to-cytoplasmic ratio and prominent nucleoli. The diagnosis is confirmed with flow cytometry of the peripheral blood, through which the subtype of PLL can also be established. The presentation of B-PLL is quite similar to CLL. *De novo* B-PLL is extremely rare, but the disease can evolve from CLL as a consequence of transformation. The treatment approaches in B-PLL and CLL are the same. In contrast, T-PLL is more common than B-PLL and comprises approximately 2% of all mature lymphoid malignancies. T-PLL typically presents with lymphocytosis, lymphadenopathy, and hepatosplenomegaly, and patients may also have a rash due to leukemic infiltration of the skin. The use of alemtuzumab has led to improved outcomes in

T-PLL and this agent should be included in the treatment of patients with this disease [89, 125, 126].

Hairy Cell Leukemia (HCL)

Hairy cell leukemia is a mature B-cell neoplasm that accounts for approximately 2% of all lymphoid leukemias, with approximately 1,100 patients diagnosed annually in the US [1, 127]. Most patients present with pancytopenia and splenomegaly. The peripheral blood smear characteristically shows small leukemic cells with abundant cytoplasm and prominent hair-like cytoplasmic projections. In the past, the diagnosis of HCL was confirmed by showing positive staining for tartrate-resistant acid phosphatase. However, in the modern era, the diagnosis is typically established through immunophenotyping. HCL characteristically expresses CD20, CD25, CD103, and CD11c. The disease tends to behave in an indolent fashion, and patients may be observed until symptoms develop that merit treatment. First-line treatment should utilize one of the purine analogs, pentostatin or cladribine. Complete response rates exceed 80% with these drugs and most patients exhibit durable remissions [89, 128]. Rituximab has also been used in the treatment of HCL, typically in the setting of relapsed or minimal residual disease [129–131]. Investigators have reported that the presence of BRAF V600E mutations is a universal finding in HCL. Vemurafenib is an oral BRAF inhibitor which is highly effective in relapsed hairy cell leukemia [132].

References

1 Siegel RL, Miller KD, Jemal A. Cancer statistics, 2017. *CA Cancer J Clin* 2017;67(1):7–30.
2 SEER Cancer Stat Facts: Acute Lymphocytic Leukemia. National Cancer Institute. Bethesda, MD. Available from http://seer.cancer.gov/statfacts/html/alyl.html (accessed 13 January, 2017).
3 Ward E, DeSantis C, Robbins A, Kohler B, Jemal A. Childhood and adolescent cancer statistics, 2014. *CA Cancer J Clin* 2014;64(2):83–103.
4 Rudant J, Lightfoot T, Urayama KY, *et al.* Childhood acute lymphoblastic leukemia and indicators of early immune stimulation: a childhood leukemia international consortium study. *Am J Epidemiol* 2015;181(8):549–62.
5 Greenberg RS, Shuster JL. Epidemiology of cancer in children. *Epidemiol Rev* 1985;7:22–48.
6 American Cancer Society. *Cancer Facts & Figures 2016.* Atlanta, GA: American Cancer Society, 2016.
7 Goldstone AH, Richards SM, Lazarus HM, *et al.* In adults with standard-risk acute lymphoblastic leukemia, the greatest benefit is achieved from a matched sibling allogeneic transplantation in first complete remission, and an autologous transplantation is less effective than conventional consolidation/maintenance chemotherapy in all patients: final results of the International ALL Trial (MRC UKALL XII/ ECOG E2993). *Blood* 2008;111:1827–33.
8 Pulte D, Gondos A, Brenner H. Improvement in survival in younger patients with acute lymphoblastic leukemia from the 1980s to the early 21st century. *Blood* 2009;7:1408–11.
9 Schiffer CA. A perspective on the treatment of acute lymphoblastic leukemia in adults. In: AS Advani, HM Lazarus (eds) *Adult Acute Lymphocytic Leukemia: Biology and Treatment.* New York: Springer, 2010: 1–5.
10 Bassan R, Gatta G, Tondini C, *et al.* Adult acute lymphoblastic leukemia. *Crit Rev Oncol Hematol* 2004;50:223–61.
11 Faderl S, O'Brien S, Pui C, *et al.* Adult acute lymphoblastic leukemia: concepts and strategies. *Cancer* 2010;116:1165–76.
12 Narayanan S, Shami PJ. Treatment of acute lymphoblastic leukemia in adults. *Crit Rev Oncol Hematol* 2012;81:94–102.
13 Fielding AK. Current therapeutic strategies in adult acute lymphoblastic leukemia. *Hematol Oncol Clin North Am* 2011;25:1255–79.
14 Borowitz MJ, Chan JKC. Precursor lymphoid neoplasms. In: SH Swerdlow, E Campo, NL Harris, *et al.* (eds) *WHO Classification of tumors of Hematopoietic and Lymphoid Tissues.* Lyon: IARC Press, 2008:167–78.
15 Alvarnas JC, Brown PA, Aoun P, *et al.* Acute lymphoblastic leukemia. *J Natl Compr Canc Netw* 2012;10:858–914.
16 Rowe JM, Buck G, Burnett AK, *et al.* Induction therapy for adults with acute lymphoblastic leukemia: results of more than 1500 patients from the international ALL trial: MRC UKALL XII/ECOG E2993. *Blood* 2005;106:3760–7.
17 Moorman AV, Harrison CJ, Buck GAN, *et al.* Karyotype is an independent prognostic factor in adult acute lymphoblastic leukemia (ALL): analysis of cytogenetic data from patients treated on the Medical Research Council (MRC) UKALLXII/ Eastern Cooperative Oncology Group (ECOG) 2993 trial. *Blood* 2007;109:3189–97.
18 Patel B, Rai L, Buck G, *et al.* Minimal residual disease is a significant predictor of treatment failure in non T-lineage adult acute lymphoblastic leukemia: final results of the international trial UKALL XII/ECOG2993. *Br J Haematol* 2010;148:80–9.
19 Armstrong S, Look AT. Molecular genetics of acute lymphoblastic leukemia. *J Clin Oncol* 2005;23:6306–15.
20 Moorman AV, Harrison CJ. Cytogenetics. In: AS Advani, HM Lazarus (eds) *Adult Acute Lymphocytic Leukemia: Biology and Treatment.* New York: Springer, 2010:61–75.
21 Lazarus HM, Richards SM, Chopra R, *et al.* Central nervous system involvement in adult acute lymphoblastic leukemia at diagnosis: results from the international ALL trial MRC UKALL XII/ECOG E2993. *Blood* 2006;108:465–72.
22 Larson RA, Dodge RK, Burns CP, *et al.* A five-drug remission induction regimen with intensive consolidation for adults with acute lymphocytic leukemia: cancer and leukemia group B study 8811. *Blood* 1995;85:2025–37.
23 Schrappe M, Reiter A, Zimmerman M, *et al.* Long-term results of four consecutive trials in childhood ALL performed by the ALL-BFM study group from 1981 to 1995. *Berlin-Frankfurt-Munster. Leukemia* 2000;14:2205–22.
24 Kantarjian HM, O'Brien S, Smith TL, *et al.* Results of treatment with hyper-CVAD, a dose-intensive regimen, in adult acute lymphocytic leukemia. *J Clin Oncol* 2000;18:547–61.

25 Rowe JM, Buck G, Burnett AK, *et al.* Induction therapy for adults with acute lymphoblastic leukemia: results of more than 1500 patients from the international ALL trial: MRC UKALL XII/ECOG E2993. *Blood* 2005;106:3760–7.

26 Stock W, La M, Sanford B, *et al.* What determines the outcomes for adolescents and young adults with acute lymphoblastic leukemia treated on cooperative group protocols? A comparison of Children's Cancer Group and Cancer and Leukemia Group B studies. *Blood* 2008;112:1646–54.

27 Thomas DA, Faderl S, Cortes J, *et al.* Treatment of Philadelphia chromosome-positive acute lymphocytic leukemia with hyperCVAD and imatinib mesylate. *Blood* 2004;103:4396–407.

28 Ottmann O, Dombret H, Martinelli G, *et al.* Dasatinib induces rapid hematologic and cytogenetic responses in adult patients with Philadelphia chromosome positive acute lymphoblastic leukemia with resistance or intolerance to imatinib: interim results of a phase 2 study. *Blood* 2007;110:2309–15.

29 Ottmann OG, Pfeifer H. Management of Philadelphia chromosome-positive acute lymphoblastic leukemia. *Hematology Am Soc Hematol Educ Program* 2009;1:371–81.

30 Ravandi F, O'Brien S, Thomas D, *et al.* First report of phase 2 study of dasatinib with hyper-CVAD for the frontline treatment of patients with Philadelphia chromosome-positive (Ph+) acute lymphoblastic leukemia. *Blood* 2010;116:2070–7.

31 Jabbour E, Kantarjian H, Ravandi F, *et al.* Combination of hyper-CVAD with ponatinib as first-line therapy for patients with Philadelphia chromosome-positive acute lymphoblastic leukaemia: a single-centre, phase 2 study. *Lancet Oncol* 2015;16(15):1547–55.

32 Cortes JE, Kim DW, Pinilla-Ibarz J, et al. A phase 2 trial of ponatinib in Philadelphia chromosome–positive leukemias. *N Engl J Med* 2013;369(19):1783–96.

33 Fielding AK, Rowe JM, Buck G, *et al.* UKALLXII/ECOG2993: addition of imatinib to a standard treatment regimen enhances long-term outcomes in Philadelphia positive acute lymphoblastic leukemia. *Blood* 2014;123(6):843–50.

34 Carpenter PA, Snyder DS, Flowers ME, *et al.* Prophylactic administration of imatinib after hematopoietic cell transplantation for high-risk Philadelphia chromosome–positive leukemia. *Blood* 2007;109(7):2791–3.

35 Ravandi F, O'Brien S, Thomas D, *et al.* First report of phase 2 study of dasatinib with hyper-CVAD for the frontline treatment of patients with Philadelphia chromosome–positive (Ph+) acute lymphoblastic leukemia. *Blood* 2010;116(12):2070–7.

36 Bruggemann M, Gokbuget N, Kneba M. Acute lymphoblastic leukemia: monitoring minimal residual disease as a therapeutic principle. *Semin Oncol* 2012;39:47–57.

37 Kantarjian HM, Thomas D, Ravandi F, *et al.* Defining the course and prognosis of adults with acute lymphocytic leukemia in first salvage after induction failure or short first remission duration. *Cancer* 2010;116:5568–74.

38 Topp MS, Gökbuget N, Zugmaier G, *et al.* Phase II trial of the anti-CD19 bispecific T cell-engager blinatumomab shows hematologic and molecular remissions in patients with relapsed or refractory B-precursor acute lymphoblastic leukemia. *J Clin Oncol* 2014;32(36):4134–40.

39 Topp MS, Gökbuget N, Stein AS, *et al.* Safety and activity of blinatumomab for adult patients with relapsed or refractory B-precursor acute lymphoblastic leukaemia: a multicentre, single-arm, phase 2 study. *Lancet Oncol* 2015;16(1):57–66.

40 Topp MS, Stein A, Gökbuget N, *et al.* Blinatumomab improved overall survival in patients with relapsed or refractory Philadelphia negative B-cell precursor acute lymphoblastic leukemia in a randomized, open-label phase 3 study (TOWER). Haematologica 2016;101: 24–5).

41 Topp MS, Gokbuget N, Zugmaier G, *et al.* Long-term follow-up of hematologic relapse-free survival in a phase 2 study of blinatumomab in patients with MRD in B-lineage ALL. *Blood* 2012;120:5185–7.

42 Goekbuget N, Dombret H, Bonifacio M, *et al.* BLAST: a confirmatory, single-arm, phase 2 study of blinatumomab, a bispecific T-cell engager (BiTE®) antibody construct, in patients with minimal residual disease B-precursor acute lymphoblastic leukemia (ALL). *Blood* 2014;124(21):379.

43 Kantarjian H, Thomas D, Jorgensen J, *et al.* Inotuzumab ozogamicin, an anti-CD22-calecheamicin conjugate, for refractory and relapsed acute lymphocytic leukemia: a phase 2 study. *Lancet Oncol* 2012;13:403–11.

44 Kantarjian HM, DeAngelo DJ, Stelljes M, *et al.* Inotuzumab ozogamicin versus standard therapy for acute lymphoblastic leukemia. *N Engl J Med* 2016;375(8):740–53.

45 Brentjens RJ, Davila ML, Riviere I, *et al.* CD19-targeted T cells rapidly induce molecular remissions in adults with chemotherapy-refractory acute lymphoblastic leukemia. *Sci Trans Med* 2013;5(177):177ra38.

46 Grupp SA, Kalos M, Barrett D, *et al.* Chimeric antigen receptor–modified T cells for acute lymphoid leukemia. *N Engl J Med* 2013;368(16):1509–18.

47 Maude S, Frey N, Shaw P, *et al.* Sustained remissions with chimeric antigen receptor T cells for leukemia. *N Engl J Med* 2014;371:1507–17.

48 Brudno JN, Somerville RP, Shi V, *et al.* Allogeneic T cells that express an anti-CD19 chimeric antigen receptor induce remissions of B-cell malignancies that progress after allogeneic hematopoietic stem-cell transplantation without causing graft-versus-host disease. *J Clin Oncol* 2016;34(10):1112–21.

49 Park JH, Riviere I, Wang X, *et al.* Impact of disease burden on long-term outcome of 19-28z CAR modified T cells in adult patients with relapsed B-ALL. J Clin Oncol 2016;34(Suppl.).

50 Frey NV, Shaw PA, Hexner EO, *et al.* Optimizing chimeric antigen receptor (CAR) T cell therapy for adult patients with relapsed or refractory (r/r) acute lymphoblastic leukemia (ALL). *J Clin Oncol* 2016;34(15 suppl):7002.

51 Haso W, Lee DW, Shah NN, *et al.* Anti-CD22–chimeric antigen receptors targeting B-cell precursor acute lymphoblastic leukemia. *Blood* 2013;121(7):1165–74.

52 Douer D. What is the impact, present and future, or novel targeted agents in acute lymphoblastic leukemia? *Best Pract Res Clin Haematol* 2012;25:453–64.

53 DeAngelo DJ, Yu D, Johnson JL, *et al.* Nelarabine induces complete remissions in adults with relapsed or refractory T-lineage acute lymphoblastic leukemia or lymphoblastic lymphoma: Cancer and Leukemia Group B study 19801. *Blood* 2007;109:5136–42

54 O'Brien S, Schiller G, Lister J, *et al.* High-dose vincristine sulfate liposome injection for advanced, relapsed, and refractory adult Philadelphia chromosome-negative acute lymphoblastic leukemia. *J Clin Oncol* 2013;31:676–83.
55 Koller CA, Kantarjian D, Thomas D, *et al.* The hyper-CVAD regimen improves outcome in relapsed acute lymphoblastic leukemia. *Leukemia* 1997;11:2039–44.
56 SEER Cancer Stat Facts: Chronic Lymphocytic Leukemia. National Cancer Institute. Bethesda, MD. Available from: http://seer.cancer.gov/statfacts/html/clyl.html (accessed 14 January, 2017).
57 Lanasa M. Novel insights into the biology of CLL. Hematology Am Soc Hematol Educ Program 2010;70–6.
58 Linet M, Schubauer-Berigan M, Weisenburger D, *et al.* Chronic lymphocytic leukemia: an overview of etiology in light of recent developments in classification and pathogenesis. *Br J Haematol* 2007;139:672–86.
59 Slager SL, Benavente Y, Blair A, *et al.* Medical history, lifestyle, family history, and occupational risk factors for chronic lymphocytic leukemia/small lymphocytic lymphoma: the InterLymph Non-Hodgkin Lymphoma Subtypes Project. *J Natl Cancer Inst Monogr* 2014;2014(48):41–51.
60 Muller-Hermelink HK, Montserrat E, Catovsky D, *et al.* Chronic lymphocytic leukemia/small lymphocytic lymphoma. In: SH Swerdlow, E Campo, NL Harris, *et al.* (eds) *WHO Classification of Tumors of Hematopoietic and Lymphoid Tissues.* Lyon: IARC Press, 2008:180–2.
61 Campo E, Swerdlow SH, Harris NL, *et al.* The 2008 WHO classification of lymphoid neoplasms and beyond: evolving concepts and practical applications. *Blood* 2011;117:5019–32.
62 Hallek M, Cheson BD, Catovsky D, *et al.* Guidelines for the diagnosis and treatment of chronic lymphocytic leukemia: a report from the International Workshop on Chronic Lymphocytic Leukemia updating the National Cancer Institute-Working Group 1996 guidelines. *Blood* 2008;111:5446–56.
63 Molica S, Mauro FR, Molica M, *et al.* Monoclonal B-cell lymphocytosis: a reappraisal of its clinical applications. *Leuk Lymphoma* 2012;53:1660–5.
64 Rawstron AC, Bennett FL, O'Connor SJM, *et al.* Monoclonal B-cell lymphocytosis and chronic lymphocytic leukemia. *N Engl J Med* 2008;359:575–83.
65 Landgren O, Albitar M, Ma W, *et al.* B-cell clones as early markers for chronic lymphocytic leukemia. *N Engl J Med* 2009;360:659–67.
66 Rozman C, Montserrat E. Chronic lymphocytic leukemia. *N Engl J Med* 1995;333:1052–7.
67 Ghia P, Ferreri AJM, Caligaris-Cappio F. Chronic lymphocytic leukemia. *Crit Rev Oncol Hematol* 2007;64:234–46.
68 Rai KR, Sawitsky A, Cronkite EP, *et al.* Clinical staging of chronic lymphocytic leukemia. *Blood* 1975;46:219–34.
69 Binet JL, Auquier A, Dighiero G, *et al.* A new prognostic classification of chronic lymphocytic leukemia derived from a multivariate survival analysis. *Cancer* 1981; 48:198–206.
70 Shanafelt TD. Predicting clinical outcome in CLL: how and why. Hematology Am Soc Hematol Educ Program 2009:421–9.
71 Furman RR. Prognostic markers and stratification of chronic lymphocytic leukemia. Hematology Am Soc Hematol Educ Program 2010: 77–81.
72 Lipshutz MD, Mir R, Rai KR, *et al.* Bone marrow biopsy and clinical staging in chronic lymphocytic leukemia. *Cancer* 1980;46:1422–7.
73 Montserrat E, Sanchez-Bisono J, Vinolas N, *et al.* Lymphocyte doubling time in chronic lymphocytic leukemia: analysis of its prognostic significance. *Br J Haematol* 1986;62:567–75.
74 Ibrahim S, Keating M, Do KA, *et al.* CD38 expression as an important prognostic factor in B-cell chronic lymphocytic leukemia. *Blood* 2001;98:181–6.
75 Rassenti LZ, Huynh L, Toy TL, *et al.* ZAP-70 compared with immunoglobulin heavy-chain gene mutation status as a predictor of disease progression in chronic lymphocytic leukemia. *N Engl J Med* 2004;351:893–901.
76 Kharfan-Dabaja MA, Chavez JC, Khorfan KA, *et al.* Clinical and therapeutic implications of the mutational status of IgVH in patients with chronic lymphocytic leukemia. *Cancer* 2008; 113: 897–906.
77 Damle RN, Wasil T, Fais F, *et al.* IgV gene mutation status and CD38 expression as novel prognostic indicators in chronic lymphocytic leukemia. *Blood* 1999;94:1840–7.
78 Hamblin TJ, Davis Z, Gardiner A, *et al.* Unmutated IgVH genes are associated with a more aggressive form of chronic lymphocytic leukemia. *Blood* 1999;94:1848–54.
79 Gladstone DE, Blackford A, Cho E, *et al.* The importance of IGHV mutational status in del(11q) and del(17p) chronic lymphocytic leukemia. *Clin Lymphoma Myeloma Leuk* 2012;12:132–7.
80 Dohner H, Stilgenbauer S, Benner A, *et al.* Genomic aberrations and survival in chronic lymphocytic leukemia. *N Engl J Med* 2000;343:1910–6.
81 Chiorazzi, N. Implications of new prognostic markers in chronic lymphocytic leukemia. Hematology Am Soc Hematol Educ Program 2012:76–87.
82 Janssens A, Van Roy N, Poppe B, *et al.* High-risk clonal evolution in chronic B-lymphocytic leukemia: single-center interphase fluorescence in situ hybridization study and review of the literature. *Eur J Haematol* 2012;89:72–80.
83 Thompson PA, O'Brien SM, Wierda WG, *et al.* Complex karyotype is a stronger predictor than del (17p) for an inferior outcome in relapsed or refractory chronic lymphocytic leukemia patients treated with ibrutinib-based regimens. *Cancer* 2015;121(20):3612–21.
84 Jaglowski SM, Ruppert AS, Heerema NA, *et al.* Complex karyotype predicts for inferior outcomes following reduced-intensity conditioning allogeneic transplant for chronic lymphocytic leukaemia. *Br J Haematol* 2012;159(1):82–7.
85 Le Bris Y, Struski S, Guièze R, *et al.* Major prognostic value of complex karyotype in addition to TP53 and IGHV mutational status in first-line chronic lymphocytic leukemia. Hematol Oncol 2016 Sep 28. doi: 10.1002/hon.2349. [Epub ahead of print]
86 Dal Bo M, Bulian P, Bomben R, *et al.* CD49d prevails over the novel recurrent mutations as independent prognosticator of overall survival in chronic lymphocytic leukemia. *Leukemia* 2016; 30(10):2011–8.

87 CLL trialists' Collaborative Group. Chemotherapeutic options in chronic lymphocytic leukemia: A meta-analysis of the randomized trials. *J Natl Cancer Inst* 1999;91:861–8.

88 Del Guidice I, Chiaretti S, Tavolaro S, *et al.* Spontaneous regression of chronic lymphocytic leukemia: clinical and biologic features of 9 cases. *Blood* 2009;114:638–46.

89 Zelenetz AD, Abramson JS, Advani RH, *et al.* Non-Hodgkin's lymphomas. *J Natl Compr Canc Netw* 2011;9:484–560.

90 Hallek M, Fischer K, Fingerle-Rowson G, *et al.* Addition of rituximab to fludarabine and cyclophosphamide in patients with chronic lymphocytic leukemia: a randomized, open-label, phase 3 trial. *Lancet* 2010;376:1164–74.

91 Weiss RB, Freiman J, Kweder SL, *et al.* Hemolytic anemia after fludarabine therapy for chronic lymphocytic leukemia. *J Clin Oncol* 1998;16:1885–9.

92 Borthakur G, O'Brien S, Wierda WG, *et al.* Immune anemias in patients with chronic lymphocytic leukemia treated with fludarabine, cyclophosphamide, and rituximab – incidence and predictors. *Br J Haematol* 2007;136:800–5.

93 Gill S, Carney D, Ritchie D, *et al.* The frequency, manifestations, and duration of prolonged cytopenias after first-line fludarabine combination chemotherapy. *Ann Oncol* 2010;21:331–4.

94 Kay NE, Geyer SM, Call TG, *et al.* Combination chemoimmunotherapy with pentostatin, cyclophosphamide, and rituximab shows significant clinical activity with low accompanying toxicity in previously untreated B chronic lymphocytic leukemia. *Blood* 2007;109:405–11.

95 Knauf WU, Lissichkov T, Aldaoud A, *et al.* Phase III randomized study of bendamustine compared with chlorambucil in previously untreated patients with chronic lymphocytic leukemia. *J Clin Oncol* 2009;27:4378–84.

96 Knauf WU, Lissitchkov T, Aldaoud A, *et al.* Bendamustine compared with chlorambucil in previously untreated patients with chronic lymphocytic leukemia: updated results of a randomized phase III trial. *Br J Haematol* 2012;159:67–77.

97 Eichhorst B, Fink AM, Bahlo J, *et al.* First-line chemoimmunotherapy with bendamustine and rituximab versus fludarabine, cyclophosphamide, and rituximab in patients with advanced chronic lymphocytic leukaemia (CLL10): an international, open-label, randomised, phase 3, non-inferiority trial. *Lancet Oncol* 2016;17(7):928–42.

98 Thompson PA, Tam CS, O'Brien SM, *et al.* Fludarabine, cyclophosphamide, and rituximab treatment achieves long-term disease-free survival in IGHV-mutated chronic lymphocytic leukemia. *Blood* 2016;127(3):303–9.

99 Fischer K, Bahlo J, Fink AM, *et al.* Long term remissions after FCR chemoimmunotherapy in previously untreated patients with CLL: updated results of the CLL8 trial. *Blood* 2015;127(2):208–15.

100 Rossi D, Terzi-di-Bergamo L, De Paoli L, *et al.* Molecular prediction of durable remission after first-line fludarabine-cyclophosphamide-rituximab in chronic lymphocytic leukemia. *Blood* 2015;126(16):1921–4.

101 Goede V, Fischer K, Busch R, *et al.* Obinutuzumab plus chlorambucil in patients with CLL and coexisting conditions. *N Engl J Med* 2014;370:1101–10.

102 Byrd JC, Flynn JM, Kipps TJ, *et al.* Randomized phase 2 study of obinutuzumab monotherapy in symptomatic, previously untreated chronic lymphocytic leukemia. *Blood* 2016;127(1):79–86.

103 Burger JA, Tedeschi A, Barr PM, *et al.* Ibrutinib as initial therapy for patients with chronic lymphocytic leukemia. *N Engl J Med* 2015;373(25):2425–37.

104 Byrd JC, Brown JR, O'Brien S, *et al.* Ibrutinib versus ofatumumab in previously treated chronic lymphoid leukemia. *N Engl J Med* 2014;371:213–23.

105 O'Brien S, Jones JA, Coutre SE, *et al.* Ibrutinib for patients with relapsed or refractory chronic lymphocytic leukaemia with 17p deletion (RESONATE-17): a phase 2, open-label, multicentre study. *Lancet Oncol* 2016;17(10):1409–18.

106 Levade M, David E, Garcia C, *et al.* Ibrutinib treatment affects collagen and von Willebrand factor-dependent platelet functions. *Blood* 2014;124(26):3991–5.

107 McMullen JR, Boey EJ, Ooi JY, *et al.* Ibrutinib increases the risk of atrial fibrillation, potentially through inhibition of cardiac PI3K-Akt signaling. *Blood* 2014;124(25):3829–30.

108 Byrd JC, Harrington B, O'Brien S, *et al.* Acalabrutinib (ACP-196) in relapsed chronic lymphocytic leukemia. *N Engl J Med* 2016;374(4):323–32.

109 Furman RR, Sharman JP, Coutre SE, *et al.* Idelalisib and rituximab in relapsed chronic lymphocytic leukemia. *N Engl J Med* 2014;370(11):997–1007.

110 Burris HA, Patel MR, Brander DM, *et al.* TGR-1202, a novel once daily PI3Kδ inhibitor, demonstrates clinical activity with a favorable safety profile, lacking hepatotoxicity, in patients with chronic lymphocytic leukemia and B-cell lymphoma. *Blood* 2014;124(21):1984.

111 Stilgenbauer S, Eichhorst B, Schetelig J, *et al.* Venetoclax in relapsed or refractory chronic lymphocytic leukaemia with 17p deletion: a multicentre, open-label, phase 2 study. *Lancet Oncol* 2016;17(6):768–78.

112 Jones J, Mato AR, Coutre S, *et al.* Preliminary results of a phase 2, open-label study of venetoclax (ABT-199/GDC-0199) monotherapy in patients with chronic lymphocytic leukemia relapsed after or refractory to ibrutinib or idelalisib therapy. *Blood* 2015;126(23):715.

113 Wierda WG, Kipps TJ, Mayer J, *et al.* Ofatumumab as single-agent CD20 immunotherapy in fludarabine-refractory chronic lymphocytic leukemia. *J Clin Oncol* 2010;28:1749–55.

114 Gladstone DE, Fuchs E. Hematopoietic stem cell transplantation for chronic lymphocytic leukemia. *Curr Opin Oncol* 2012;24:176–81.

115 Michallet M, Dreger P, Sutton L, *et al.* Autologous hematopoietic stem cell transplantation in chronic lymphocytic leukemia: results of European intergroup randomized trial comparing autografting versus observation. *Blood* 2011;117:1516–21.

116 Sutton L, Chevret S, Tournilhac O, *et al.* Autologous stem cell transplantation as a first-line treatment strategy for chronic lymphocytic leukemia: a multicenter, randomized, controlled trial from the SFGM-TC and GFLLC. *Blood* 2011;117:6109–19.

117 Porter DL, Levine BL, Bunin N, *et al.* A phase 1 trial of donor lymphocyte infusions expanded and activated ex vivo via CD3/CD28 costimulation. *Blood* 2006;107(4):1325–31.

118 Porter DL, Hwang WT, Frey NV, *et al.* Chimeric antigen receptor T cells persist and induce sustained remissions in relapsed refractory chronic lymphocytic leukemia. *Sci Trans Med* 2015;7(303):303ra139–.

119 Hallek M, Cheson BD, Catovsky D, *et al.* Guidelines for the diagnosis and treatment of chronic lymphocytic leukemia: a report from the International Workshop on Chronic Lymphocytic Leukemia updating the National Cancer Institute–Working Group 1996 guidelines. *Blood* 2008;111(12):5446–56.

120 Dearden C. Disease-specific complications of chronic lymphocytic leukemia. Hematology Am Soc Hematol Educ Program 2008;450–6.

121 Morrison VA. Management of infectious complications in patients with chronic lymphocytic leukemia. Hematology Am Soc Hematol Educ Program 2007:332–8.

122 Hamblin TJ. Autoimmune complications of chronic lymphocytic leukemia. *Semin Oncol* 2006;33:230–9.

123 Cheson BD. Etiology and management of tumor lysis syndrome in patients with chronic lymphocytic leukemia. *Clinical Advances in Hematology & Oncology* 2009; 7: 263–271.

124 Tsimberidou AM, Keating MJ. Richter syndrome: biology, incidence, and therapeutic strategies. *Cancer* 2005;103:216–28.

125 Dearden CE. T cell prolymphocytic leukemia. *Clin Lymphoma Myeloma* 2009;9 Suppl 3:S239–43.

126 Dearden C. How I treat prolymphocytic leukemia. *Blood* 2012;120:538–51.

127 Teras LR, DeSantis CE, Cerhan JR, *et al.* 2016 US lymphoid malignancy statistics by World Health Organization subtypes. *CA Cancer J Clin* 2016;66(6):443–59.

128 Naik RR, Saven A. My treatment approach to hairy cell leukemia. *Mayo Clin Proc* 2012;87:67–76.

129 Ravandi F, Jorgensen JL, O'Brien SM, *et al.* Eradication of minimal residual disease in hairy cell leukemia. *Blood* 2006; 107: 4658–62.

130 Cervetti G, Galimberti S, Andreazzoli F, *et al.* Rituximab as treatment for minimal residual disease in hairy cell leukemia. *Eur J Hematol* 2004;73:412–7.

131 Nieva J, Bethel K, Saven A. Phase 2 study of rituximab in the treatment of cladribine-failed patients with hairy cell leukemia. *Blood* 2003;102:810–3.

132 Tiacci E, Park JH, De Carolis L, *et al.* Targeting mutant BRAF in relapsed or refractory hairy-cell leukemia. *N Engl J Med* 2015;373(18):1733–47.

31

Hodgkin Lymphoma in Adults

Satish Shanbhag and Richard Ambinder

Johns Hopkins University School of Medicine, Baltimore, Maryland, USA

Introduction

Hodgkin disease was first described in an autopsy case series of patients with lymphadenopathy and splenic enlargement by the English pathologist Thomas Hodgkin in 1832 [1]. Huge strides have been made in diagnosis, subclassification, staging, and treatment since that time – Hodgkin lymphoma (HL) is one of the few types of cancer that is often curable even when it presents at an advanced stage. The term "disease" was used as there was no clear understanding as to whether the entity described was a malignancy or not. Since the late 1990s the term "lymphoma" rather than "disease" is gaining favor as the character of the entity is no longer in doubt [2]. HL is unique among cancers in that only a small minority of cells in the tumor mass are of the malignant clone. The remainder are reactive or inflammatory cells. The malignant cells are recognized as multinucleate giant cells, referred to as Reed–Sternberg cells, or as mononuclear large cells, often referred to as Hodgkin cells. Although for many years the origins of the Reed–Sternberg and Hodgkin cells were obscure, it is now accepted that they are of B-lymphocyte lineage as indicated by the presence of rearranged immunoglobulin genes. Despite the presence of rearranged immunoglobulin genes, the tumor cells do not express immunoglobulin. In some instances, this is because the immunoglobulin gene rearrangements led to nonsense mutations that could not be expressed. In other instances, particular transcription factors are absent [3, 4].

Classification of Hodgkin Lymphoma

Hodgkin lymphoma is subdivided into classic Hodgkin lymphoma (cHL) and lymphocyte predominant (LPHL) types on the basis of morphology and histopathology. Over 90% of HL cases are cHL, and cHL is the major focus of this chapter [5, 6]. The clinical differences between cHL and LPHL are substantive with cHL behaving as a more aggressive neoplasm while LPHL is often quite indolent. The two types of Hodgkin lymphoma also differ in terms of patterns of spread, and probability and time course of recurrence.

Pathologic characteristics are used to further subclassify cHL. Fibrosis, the inflammatory infiltrate, the abundance of malignant cells, and the morphology of the malignant cells are used to subclassify cHL into nodular sclerosis, mixed cellularity, and other less common subtypes. The malignant Hodgkin Reed–Sternberg cell in cHL is usually positive for CD15 and CD30 and negative for CD45, while CD20 expression is variable.

Nodular sclerosis cHL (NSHL) is the most common form in the developed world, accounting for about 75% of cHL and characterized by neoplastic cells in an inflammatory background of band-forming sclerosis. NSHL is more common in girls and women than in men, and is more common in young adult populations than in childhood or older adult populations. Characteristic presentations are in the mediastinum, supraclavicular, and cervical nodes. Mixed cellularity is the second most common subtype of cHL. It is more common in boys and men than in women, and is more common in very young and older adult populations. It is also more common in immunocompromised populations such as those with HIV infection or those with a history of organ transplantation. Lymphocyte-rich and lymphocyte-depleted subtypes are much less common, accounting together for about 5% of total cases of cHL [6].

Nodular lymphocyte predominant HL (LPHL) differs from cHL and comprises a small percentage (about 5%) of total diagnoses of HL. LPHL is invariably negative for Epstein–Barr virus-encoded RNA (EBER), with a nodular pattern of growth and popcorn-like lymphocytic–histiocytic malignant cells without much fibrosis. The malignant cells in LPHL are CD15 and CD30 negative and express CD20 and CD45. The malignancy is also more indolent in its behavior. B symptoms (fevers, night sweats, weight loss) are less common than in cHL.

In addition to subtyping, grading systems have been developed to risk stratify cHL, but are not widely used. The British grading system for NSHL attempted to categorize patients based on the abundance (or lack) of malignant Hodgkin Reed–Sternberg cells within the reactive infiltrate, with higher relative

The American Cancer Society's Oncology in Practice: Clinical Management, First Edition. Edited by The American Cancer Society.

numbers of malignant cells predicting a worse outcome [7]. The British grading did not stand the test of time, losing relevance with modern therapies, therefore the German Hodgkin Lymphoma Study Group (GHSG) developed a new grading system based on three histopathologic criteria – eosinophilia, lymphocyte depletion, and atypia of the Hodgkin Reed–Sternberg cells; these three together were a significant indicator of prognosis in intermediate and advanced stages of nodular sclerosis cHL [8].

Incidence and Mortality

Approximately 8,260 new cases of HL (4,650 in males and 3,610 in females) are diagnosed each year, and approximately 1,070 (630 in males and 440 in females) deaths from these cancers occur annually in the United States (US) [9]. The incidence rate of HL, based on cases diagnosed in 2009–2013, was approximately 2.6 per 100,000 persons per year. During the same time period, the death rate was 0.4 per 100,000 persons per year. The lifetime risk of HL is approximately 0.2%. The median age at diagnosis is 39 years, and the highest incidence rates are among individuals aged 20–34 years. However, approximately 17.8% of new diagnoses and 51.6% of deaths are among individuals aged 65 years and older [10] (Figure 31.1).

Etiology and Prevention

The etiology of HL is poorly understood. Recognized cofactors include Epstein–Barr virus (EBV), genetics, and immunodeficiency. Most adults and many children are infected by EBV but EBV is rarely detected in cancers. EBV is present in the tumor cells of cHL in some patients as evidenced by the ability to detect viral RNA and viral proteins in those cells. These cases are referred to as EBV-associated. Only a minority of patients with cHL in North America and Western Europe have EBV-associated cHL. The viral association is present in a substantially higher percentage of tumors from patients in developing nations and in patients with immunodeficiencies [11]. Symptomatic EBV infection (acute infectious mononucleosis) is associated with an increased risk of EBV-associated cHL but not EBV-negative cHL. The importance of genetics for cHL was first recognized in family studies. More recently, genome-wide association studies (GWAS) have identified several links with cHL and in some instances with EBV association as a function of genetic makeup. Several loci associated with cHL have been identified in the major histocompatibility complex region [12]. There is an association between cHL and immunosuppression (in patients with HIV or following organ transplantation). In these populations, cHL is almost always EBV-associated and usually of the mixed cellularity subtype. There are no established prevention strategies.

Clinical Presentation

The most common presentation of cHL is a young person with enlarging lymph nodes in the neck and chest regions. Not as well known is the rise in incidence rates in the elderly population during their sixth and seventh decades of life leading to a bimodal age distribution curve [13]. A majority of the data collected in treating patients on clinical trials with Hodgkin lymphoma has been in younger patients. Patients with cHL may present with fevers, night sweats, and unintentional weight loss. These constitutional symptoms are referred to as "B symptoms" and are included in tumor staging (see next section). Because malignancy is so rare in this age group (the highest incidence is in 20- to 34-year-olds), imaging studies are often delayed and it is not uncommon for diagnoses to be made many months after the onset of symptoms. Lymphadenopathy, wheezing, or shortness of breath is attributed to presumed upper respiratory infection and patients have often been treated with a series of antibiotics before a diagnosis is established.

The diagnosis can only be established by biopsy. Excisional biopsy is preferred so as to allow assessment of the characteristic tumor cells and of the surrounding infiltrate. Fine-needle aspirates or core biopsy will in some cases show tumor cells, but the small specimen size often precludes assessment of the infiltrate and architecture of the lymph node. Fine-needle aspirates and core biopsy may also miss the tumor cells. A common error is to assume a negative needle biopsy rules out cHL.

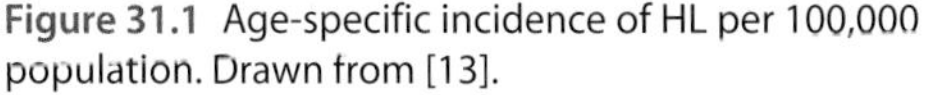

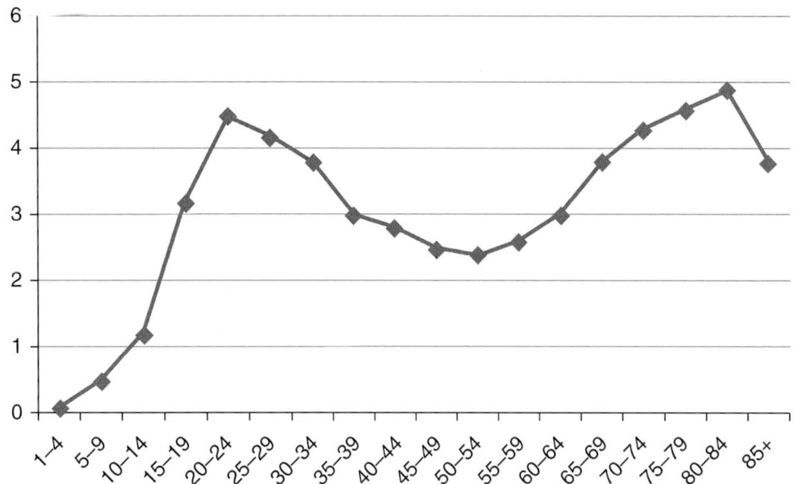

Figure 31.1 Age-specific incidence of HL per 100,000 population. Drawn from [13].

Staging Hodgkin Lymphoma

Staging HL has been in accord with the Ann Arbor staging system developed in the 1970s (Table 31.1) [14]. Ann Arbor staging relied heavily on laparotomy with splenectomy and multiple biopsies of liver and lymph nodes to determine the extent of disease [15–17]. With improvements in imaging, computed tomography (CT) and 2-[^{18}F]fluoro-2-deoxy-d-glucose positron emission tomography (PET/CT) have replaced staging laparotomy (Figure 31.2). Bone marrow biopsy has also been routine for decades, although its role is increasingly being questioned. In a retrospective study of 454 patients with cHL, no patient with bone marrow involvement was assessed as having limited-stage disease by PET-CT. Although a few patients with stage III disease by PET-CT were up-staged to IV by a bone marrow biopsy, none of the 454 patients would have been allocated to another treatment on the basis of marrow involvement [18].

Prognosis in Hodgkin Lymphoma

As in other malignancies, mortality correlates with stage at presentation. Early-stage cHL is usually curable, with cure rates of 85–95% with stage I–II disease [19]. However, even in patients presenting with stage II disease there are those who do poorly. Various groups have made efforts to subclassify these high-risk patients separately; there is no consensus on how exactly to define this "high-risk" group, but characteristics of this patient population include systemic B symptoms, bulky disease (>10 cm at presentation), older age, greater number of involved nodal sites, elevated erythrocyte sedimentation rate (ESR) at diagnosis, etc. [20].

Patients with advanced-stage disease at presentation (stage IIB–IV) have lower long-term survival rates, but a large proportion (80–90% for stage IIIA–IVA) are curable with current therapies. Patients with stage IVB disease at presentation have 10-year survival rates of about 60%. Figure 31.3 shows survival by stage in HL [19].

Patients with advanced cHL may be risk stratified according to the International Prognostic Score (IPS). The IPS uses seven factors: gender, hemoglobin, serum albumin, age, stage, and leukocyte parameters. Those with 0–2 risk factors have long-term freedom from disease progression of about 80% while those with 3 or more risk factors have a significantly lower freedom from progression of about 60% [21].

A European study of patients with either early-stage disease with adverse prognostic factors or advanced-stage cHL used interim PET imaging (done after 2 months of chemotherapy) to risk stratify patients. Those with positive interim PET scans had a poor outcome of 12.8% progression-free survival at the 2-year mark, whereas those with complete response on the interim PET scan seemed to do very well with 95% progression-free survival [22]. Interim PET also supersedes the IPS in prognostication; treatment outcomes were similar for patients with positive interim PET scans irrespective of their IPS scores at diagnosis, and patients with negative interim PET scans had excellent outcomes. Thus interim PET is increasingly used to risk stratify patients.

Table 31.1 Staging Hodgkin lymphoma – Cotswold modification of Ann Arbor staging. Adapted from [14].

Stage	Symptoms/other classifiers
I) Involvement of a single lymph node region II) Involvement of two or more lymph node regions or lymph node structures on the same side of the diaphragm III) Involvement of lymph node regions or lymphoid structures on both sides of the diaphragm IV) Extensive extranodal disease (lung, liver, bone, bone marrow)	• B – fevers, night sweats, – >10% weight loss over 6 months • A – no systemic symptoms – e – local extension – x – bulky – s – splenic involvement

Treatment of Hodgkin Lymphoma

The treatment of HL has improved substantially in the last 50 years. SEER data for the period 1975–2008 from the US attest to the decline in mortality rates related to HL to about a third of the rates in the 1970s, while incidence rates have been stable to rising [23]. Radiation therapy was a mainstay of treatment in the early twentieth century, but it was only in the 1960s that Henry Kaplan at Stanford University established the doses and fields required to treat patients with both limited and advanced-stage HL [24–26]. Aggressive staging procedures including laparotomy with liver and lymph node biopsies and diagnostic splenectomy were employed to define the extent of disease. Because, in almost all cases, HL progresses from nodal site to contiguous nodal site, fields involved by tumor and adjacent fields could be irradiated allowing cure of many patients with early, and in some cases, advanced-stage disease. Regardless, radiotherapy alone cured only a small minority of patients even with limited HL. For patients with advanced-stage disease, mantle field radiation (covering neck, axillae, mediastinum, and hilar regions) along with an inverted Y field to treat the abdomen and spleen together formed what was called "total nodal irradiation" – effective in controlling the cancer in a small percentage of patients with advanced-stage HL. However extensive radiation is associated with many long-term toxicities, elaborated further under "Survivorship."

Cytotoxic drugs were also effective in achieving tumor response in cHL but patients invariably relapsed until the drugs were used in combination [27]. Devita *et al.* at the National Cancer Institute published one of the first few trials looking at combination chemotherapy in HL: 43 patients with advanced-stage newly diagnosed Hodgkin lymphoma were treated with a combination of vincristine, nitrogen mustard (or cyclophosphamide), procarbazine, and prednisone (MOPP), given in cyclical fashion for 6 months [28]. The MOPP chemotherapy regimen was the first potent systemic treatment for advanced Hodgkin lymphoma, achieving complete remission rates of 81% of the 43 patients on trial, an astounding result for those times; but accompanying this

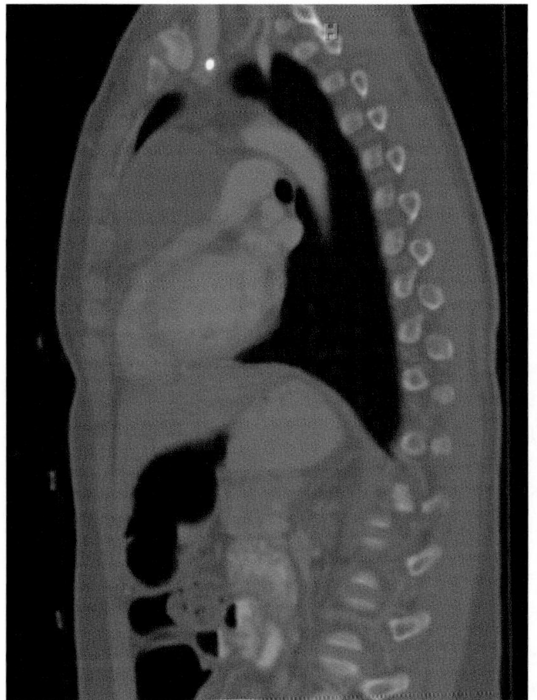
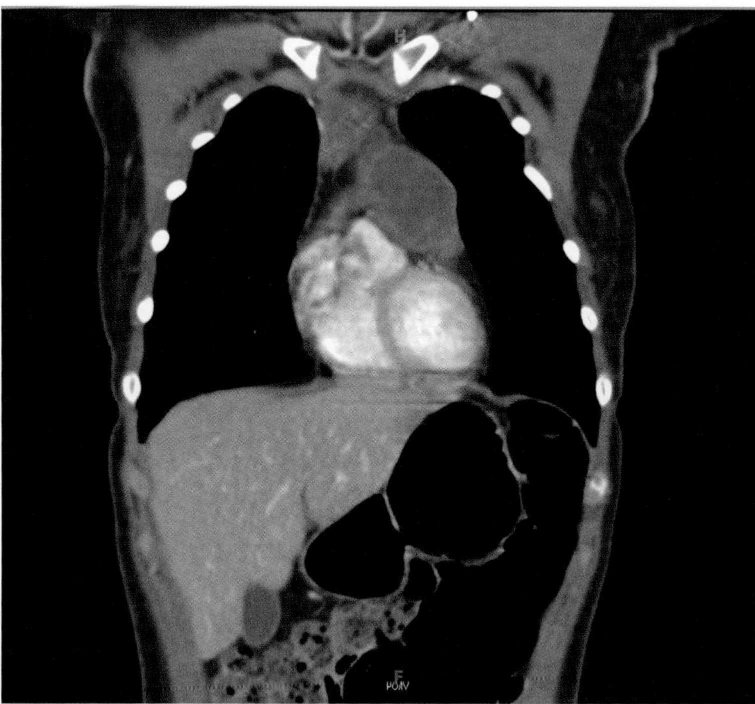
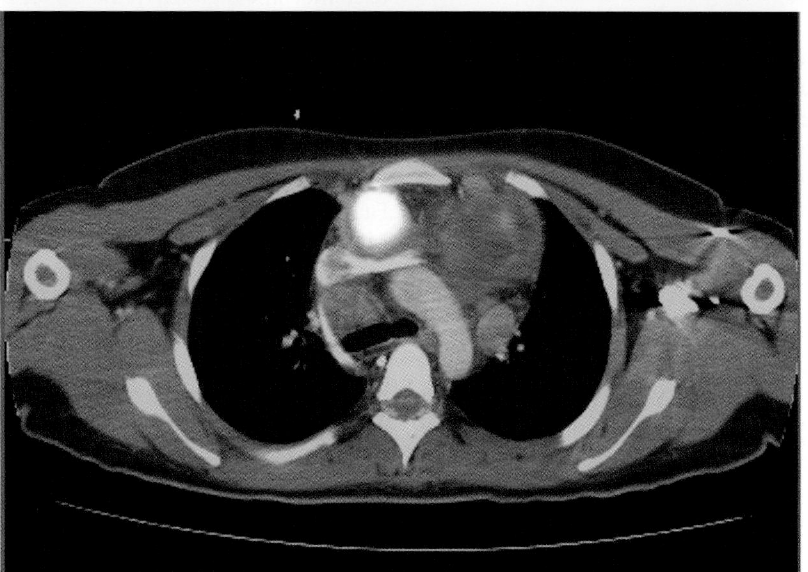

Figure 31.2 CT and fused PET-CT of a 18-year-old female with bulky mediastinal presentation of Hodgkin lymphoma (sagittal, coronal, and transverse views).

success, a large percentage of survivors had long-term bone marrow toxicity and sterility induced by the MOPP regimen.

The Italian Istituto Nazionale Tumori under Gianni Bonadonna developed a combination regimen ABVD (Adriamycin, i.e., doxorubicin, bleomycin, vinblastine, and dacarbazine) based on non-overlapping chemosensitivity profiles with MOPP. A randomized trial showed that 6 cycles of either MOPP or ABVD yielded similar complete remission rates in advanced HL [29, 30]. Due to a better toxicity profile ABVD has become the *de facto* standard as combination chemotherapy for HL. Important toxicities of the ABVD regimen include pulmonary toxicity associated with bleomycin, doxorubicin cardiomyopathy, and neuropathy associated with vinblastine.

Early-Stage cHL with Favorable Prognostic Factors

Patients with early-stage cHL with favorable prognostic features have an excellent prognosis and the goals of clinical trials have been to de-escalate intensity of therapy to minimize chemotherapy- and radiotherapy-associated toxicities. From the early days, radiotherapy was found to be curative in a significant percentage of patients with early-stage cHL, but with significant cardiopulmonary toxicities and increased incidence of breast cancer in females. The goal of combined modality therapy (incorporating chemotherapy with radiation therapy) has been to minimize doses of radiotherapy and substitute with combination chemotherapy while also improving remission rates.

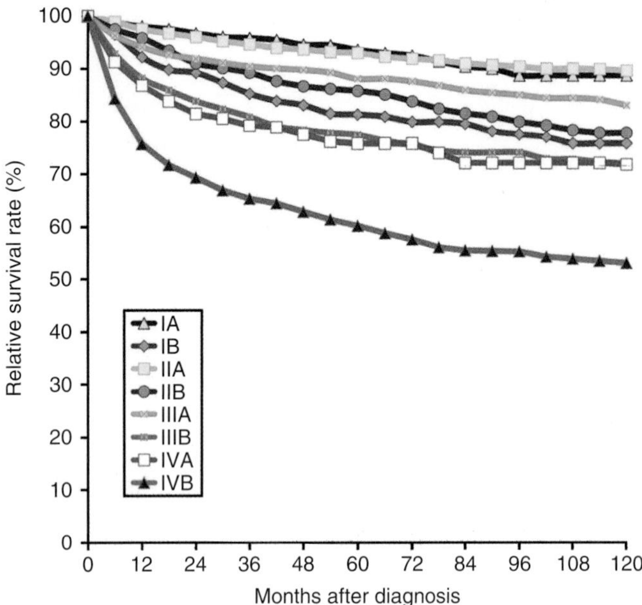

Figure 31.3 Relative survival rates (%) by stage and B symptoms, ages 15+ [19]. SEER long-term survival data for 1988–2001 show significant long-term survivors even in patients with advanced HL.

Early trials of combined modality therapy used the MOPP regimen [31, 32] and clearly demonstrated benefit to the addition of combination chemotherapy. A 1,500-patient European trial compared 3 cycles of MOPP combined with doxorubicin, bleomycin, and vinblastine (ABV) plus involved-field radiotherapy versus subtotal nodal radiotherapy alone; the 5-year event-free survival rate was significantly higher for the combined modality arm at 98% versus 74%. This also translated into improved 10-year overall survival rates, definitively establishing combination therapy as standard of care [33].

A GHSG trial looked into the possibility of further treatment de-escalation in patients with early-stage cHL, comparing four treatment groups of a combination chemotherapy regimen of two different intensities followed by involved-field radiation therapy at two different dose levels [34]: 1370 patients with newly diagnosed early-stage cHL with a favorable prognosis were randomized to receive either 2 or 4 cycles of ABVD followed by 20 or 30 Gray (Gy) of radiation therapy. There did not seem to be a significant difference between any of the groups in terms of freedom from treatment failure or survival, making a case for using the least toxic regimen – 2 cycles of ABVD followed by 20 Gy of involved-field radiation [34].

Trials looking at the necessity of radiotherapy in early-stage favorable risk cHL have not been optimal, using older radiotherapy techniques with extended fields rather than modern involved-field radiotherapy [35]. The general rule of thumb seems to be that skipping radiation results in short-term loss of benefit but might be beneficial by sparing patients long-term toxicities. However, there remains considerable controversy as to the best strategies to optimize outcomes as chemotherapy and radiation therapy both continue to improve. Discussions about optimal therapy in this group of patients with an overall excellent prognosis should be individualized keeping in mind the patient's age, sex, and comorbidities.

Early-Stage cHL with Unfavorable Prognostic Factors

Combined modality therapy is commonly used in this subgroup of patients, although the choice of combination chemotherapy is not clear. As in early-stage favorable risk HL, MOPP was one of the first regimens to be studied. The H8-U trial compared 6 cycles of MOPP-ABV plus involved-field radiotherapy, 4 cycles of MOPP-ABV plus involved-field radiotherapy, and 4 cycles of MOPP-ABV plus subtotal nodal radiotherapy with similar estimated 5-year event-free survival rates in all three treatment groups [33].

The GHSG has tried to improve upon results with ABVD with a more intense regimen termed escalated BEACOPP (bleomycin, etoposide, doxorubicin, cyclophosphamide, vincristine, procarbazine, and prednisone). Despite being a more "potent" regimen it is fraught with significant marrow toxicity and has not shown significant overall survival benefit in this patient population, although it resulted in better progression-free survival [36].

Advanced-Stage cHL

The mainstay of treatment for advanced-stage cHL (stage III–IV) is combination chemotherapy. ABVD is the most commonly used first-line regimen in the US for patients in this group. One of the early definitive trials (published in 1992) to establish ABVD as the first-line regimen of choice was conducted by George Canellos comparing the then-established standard of 6–8 cycles MOPP with MOPP alternating with ABVD for 12 cycles, and ABVD alone for 6–8 cycles. Response rates were significantly better with the anthracycline-containing regimens. Failure-free survival and overall survival at 5 years (66% for MOPP, 73% for ABVD, and 75% for MOPP-ABVD, $P = 0.28$) were similar for all three regimens, but the ABVD arm had fewer treatment treatment-related toxicities [37].

ABVD was compared to mechlorethamine, vincristine, procarbazine, prednisone, doxorubicin, bleomycin, and vinblastine (MOPP-ABV) in a randomized trial of 856 patients with advanced HL. The rates of complete remission (76% vs 80%, $P = 0.16$), failure-free survival at 5 years (63% vs 66%, $P = 0.42$), and overall survival at 5 years (82% vs 81%, $P = 0.82$) were essentially the same. However toxicities were less with ABVD; the MOPP-ABV arm had much higher acute pulmonary and hematologic toxicity, treatment-related deaths, and secondary (especially hematological) malignancies [38]. Therefore, the addition of MOPP to ABVD did not improve outcomes but increased toxicity.

The strongest rationale for challenging ABVD as standard of care was the GHSG conducted HD9 trial comparing three chemotherapy regimens: 8 cycles of cyclophosphamide, vincristine, procarbazine, and prednisone (COPP) alternating with doxorubicin, bleomycin, vinblastine, and dacarbazine (ABVD); 8 cycles of BEACOPP; or 8 cycles of escalated BEACOPP. "Escalating" the BEACOPP regimen involves titrating doses of etoposide, doxorubicin, and cyclophosphamide based on hematological toxicities from the prior cycle of chemotherapy. The 10-year freedom from treatment failure was 64%, 70%, and 82% with overall survival rates of 75%, 80%, and 86% for patients treated with COPP/ABVD, BEACOPP baseline, and BEACOPP escalated respectively ($P<0.001$) [39].

The Italians compared ABVD versus escalated BEACOPP with a plan for high-dose salvage therapy in patients who relapsed after their first-line regimen. The 7-year rate of freedom from first progression was 85% among patients who had received BEACOPP and 73% among those who had received initial treatment with ABVD ($P = 0.004$). After completion of the overall planned first-line and salvage therapy, the 7-year rate of overall survival (a secondary endpoint) was 89% and 84%, respectively, indicating no significant difference between the arms ($P = 0.39$). As would be expected, severe adverse events were more common in the BEACOPP arm [40]. Thus ABVD is a better-tolerated regimen for first-line therapy, and with the use of salvage therapy yields similar long-term overall survival.

Since the interim PET scan is highly predictive of long-term outcomes, the focus in first-line treatment for advanced cHL has shifted towards risk stratifying patients and modifying the intensity of chemotherapy based on their prognosis. The RATHL (Risk Adapted Therapy in Hodgkin Lymphoma) study enrolled 1,200 patients with advanced cHL, all of whom received 2 cycles of ABVD followed by an interim PET-CT scan. Eighty-four percent of patients had a negative scan: in these patients who had a very good long-term prognosis, no difference in 3-year progression-free survival (85%) or overall survival was found by omitting bleomycin from the last 4 cycles of chemotherapy. Patients on the AVD (without bleomycin) arm had lower rates of febrile neutropenia and lung toxicity. In contrast, the 16% of patients who had a positive interim PET scan were switched from ABVD to BEACOPP-based regimens: even these poor-risk patients had an excellent 3-year progression-free survival of 67%, much higher than the expected 15% if ABVD were continued. This strategy is very attractive for sparing patients with good risk features from toxicities of treatment, while only those with poor-risk advanced cHL who would likely benefit from more aggressive chemotherapy would be treated with intensive regimens [41].

Stanford V is a 12-week intense multiagent chemotherapy (doxorubicin, vinblastine, mechlorethamine, vincristine, bleomycin, etoposide, and prednisone) regimen combined with radiation therapy to bulky nodal sites. It has the advantage of being half as long as 6 cycles of ABVD and uses lower cumulative doses of anthracycline and bleomycin which may be associated with less cardiopulmonary toxicity. However, several trials have not shown improved outcomes when Stanford V was compared to ABVD in advanced stage HL [42, 43].

The addition of radiation may have a role in patients with advanced HL who have bulky nodal disease with a diameter of >10 cm but is unlikely to benefit patients who are in a complete response at the completion of their therapy.

Relapsed/Refractory cHL

Primary refractory advanced-stage cHL is a not-so-rare entity, occurring in about 15% of patients treated with ABVD chemotherapy despite addition of local radiotherapy [40]. As HL, particularly nodular sclerosis, is often associated with scarring, a residual mass commonly persists on CT imaging at completion of therapy. A growing or highly FDG-avid mass on PET-CT at completion of therapy should raise suspicion for residual or progressive disease. Thymic rebound, sarcoidosis, and other inflammatory lesions may also be FDG avid. Therefore, biopsy confirmation is important before embarking upon salvage. In patients who relapse after completion of chemotherapy (i.e., after going into a temporary remission), those who relapse over a year after completing therapy tend to do better overall than those who suffer an early relapse: generally the shorter the time to relapse, the worse is the overall prognosis [44].

The GHSG conducted a clinical trial to compare salvage chemotherapy alone with chemotherapy followed by high-dose therapy with autologous stem cell transplantation (SCT) in 161 patients with relapsed cHL. Patients were randomly assigned 2 cycles of Dexa-BEAM (dexamethasone and carmustine, etoposide, cytarabine, and melphalan) and either 2 further courses of Dexa-BEAM or high-dose BEAM and transplantation of hematopoietic stem cells. Of those patients with chemosensitive disease (complete or partial responders to 2 cycles of DEXA-BEAM), freedom from treatment failure at 3 years was significantly better for patients given BEAM-SCT (55%) than for those on Dexa-BEAM (34%; $P = 0.019$). This benefit persisted in both patients with early and late relapse. Overall survival did not differ, however [45]. Other consolidative approaches have included high-dose cyclophosphamide, rituximab, and a cancer vaccine for relapsed cHL [46].

A recent advance involves immunotherapeutic targeting of the CD30-positive cells (CD30 is characteristic of Hodgkin Reed–Sternberg cells). Brentuximab vedotin is a CD30-specific monoclonal antibody with an antitubulin agent, monomethyl auristatin E (MMAE), attached by an enzyme-cleavable linker. MMAE is released following endocytosis when the antibody–drug conjugate (ADC) reaches the lysosome. Prior attempts to target CD30 with naked antibody had been much less successful, but the ADC dramatically increased the efficacy of the targeted approach [47].

In a pivotal Phase 2 study in patients with relapsed/refractory cHL (75% of whom had failed high-dose therapy with autologous SCT) overall response rates of 75% were seen with complete responses in 34% of patients. Median progression-free survival was 5.6 months, and those getting complete remissions had median duration of response of 20.5 months. Brentuximab is well tolerated with major toxicities being peripheral neuropathy and cytopenias [48]. Five-year end-of-study results showed that a small proportion of patients who get a complete response may have durable remissions without any further therapy, but the majority required salvage treatment or consolidation [49]. Brentuximab is a well-tolerated option for consolidation of high-risk patients after autologous SCT, those who relapse after high-dose therapy, and those who may not be good candidates for traditional cytotoxic therapy, such as elderly patients with relapsed disease [50]. Brentuximab is actively being studied in clinical trials as a part of upfront therapy.

Immunotherapy has shown great promise in the treatment of cHL, in part due to the high expression of programmed death 1 (PD-1) ligands on Reed–Sternberg cells. The PD-1 inhibitor nivolumab showed impressive clinical activity in heavily pretreated patients with relapsed cHL with an 87% response rate; thereby several immunotherapeutic drugs are being studied in this patient population [51].

Allogeneic stem cell transplantation is potentially curative in relapsed cHL. However, the approach has been limited by the availability of donors, by acute toxicities associated with preparative regimens, and by mortality associated with graft-versus-host disease [52, 53]. Nonetheless a consensus has emerged that there is a graft-versus-lymphoma effect in HL [54].

With the advent of a new approach to graft-versus-host disease prophylaxis involving post-transplantation cyclophosphamide, it has been possible to use reduced-intensity conditioning with matched or related haploidentical donors [55]. An international retrospective analysis compared the outcome of nonmyeloablative allogeneic (SCT) for patients with relapsed or refractory HL based on donor cell source. Ninety heavily pretreated patients with HL underwent reduced-intensity conditioning followed by allogeneic SCT from HLA-matched related ($n = 38$), unrelated ($n = 24$), or HLA-haploidentical related ($n = 28$) donors. In this study the HLA-haploidentical group received post-transplant cyclophosphamide prophylaxis. Two-year overall survival (OS) and progression-free survival (PFS) were 53%and 23% (HLA-matched related), 58% and 29% (unrelated), and 58% and 51% (HLA-haploidentical related), respectively. The risks of relapse were lower in the HLA-haploidentical recipients compared to the other two groups and neither acute nor chronic graft-versus-disease rates were increased.

Considerations in Treatment of Nodular LP Hodgkin Lymphoma

Treatment of LPHL is conceptually very different from cHL. In most cases LPHL is an indolent disease with many characteristics of a low-grade non-Hodgkin B-cell lymphoma (similar to follicular lymphoma or marginal zone lymphoma). As in other low-grade lymphomas, observation alone is adequate in some situations [56]. For limited stage IA/IIA presentation, there are no randomized data comparing treatment approaches but definitive radiotherapy is the norm without any proven benefit from the addition of cytotoxic chemotherapy [57, 58]. Advanced stage (III/IV) LPHL tends to behave worse, causing B symptoms, and relapses over an extended period of time. In the largest study evaluating advanced LPHL, a multicenter retrospective analysis reported that virtually all patients responded to first-line chemotherapy but about 38% of stage III and 76% of patients with stage IV disease relapsed over an 8-year period post completion of chemotherapy [59]. Rituximab is a monoclonal antibody targeting CD20 which has revolutionized treatment of CD20-positive non-Hodgkin lymphomas. Several small trials have reported very encouraging results using rituximab alone in treating patients with LPHL [60, 61]. Response rates of over 90% have been observed using this "gentler" immunotherapeutic in patients with LPHL who are treatment naïve and those who have relapsed/refractory disease after prior chemotherapy or radiotherapy. Although not validated in prospective clinical trials in this rare entity of advanced-stage LPHL, we follow the National Comprehensive Cancer Network (NCCN) consensus guidelines in treating this disease with rituximab-based combination chemotherapy (a strategy with extensive data in patients with both low-grade and aggressive non-Hodgkin lymphoma) when symptomatology dictates the need for therapy [20].

Survivorship

The dictum *primum non nocere* is important when we consider that most patients are cured and go on to live long lives [19]. The young age of patients with HL compared with other cancers makes the issue of long-term toxicities related to therapy even more important. While 20-year actuarial survival estimates improved from 65% to 87% from the 1960s to 1980s, so did the incidence of malignancies in those survivors [62]. Most of the published data on long-term toxicities have looked at patients treated with older chemotherapeutic regimens (MOPP) and more aggressive/extensive radiation (total nodal radiation, mantle radiation) than would be considered standard today, but are important as a general guide to mechanisms of side effects. Since a large portion of survivors of HL were treated using older modalities of therapy, revisiting some of these toxicities is important, especially for newly minted oncologists and other doctors who may not have experience with them. Some of the important long-term complications of HL therapy are listed in Table 31.2.

In a Dutch study published in 2003 looking at 1,261 patients treated for HL (all stages), 291 had died: HL accounted for 54.5% of all deaths, while second malignancies formed the next most numerous group accounting for 21.7%; cardiovascular disease accounted for 9.4% of all deaths. Death from second malignancies, especially solid tumors, occurred at an increased rate with a relative risk of about 6.6 times the general population [62]. Therapy-related acute myeloid leukemia (AML) and myelodysplastic syndrome (MDS) were responsible for 4.5% of deaths while gastrointestinal and lung malignancies accounted for 4.7% and 4.3% respectively.

Patients treated initially with chemotherapy have an increased excess absolute risk (EAR) for AML compared with those treated with radiotherapy alone (11.3 vs 5.4, $P<0.001$) [63]. As would be expected, the EAR of AML declined significantly after 1984 (7.0 to 4.2 and 16.4 to 9.9 in the <35 and ≥35 age groups, respectively) related to replacement of MOPP by ABVD. Risk for AML/MDS is highest in the first 10 years and subsequently declines close to baseline population risk [63, 64].

The risk of breast cancer secondary to radiotherapy is particularly high in those who received radiation as young women (i.e., <30 years of age). The risk remains high for decades after completion of radiotherapy. In a study of 111 women who received mantle irradiation, the relative risk of breast carcinoma was 56 (confidence interval (CI), 23.3–107) for those 19 years or younger at the time of treatment, 7.0 (CI, 2.3–16.4) for those aged 20–29 years, and 0.9 (CI, 0–5.3) for those 30 years and older [65]. Other studies have reproduced similar results

Table 31.2 Important long-term complications of HL therapy.

Myelodysplasia and acute myeloid leukemia
Bleomycin-induced lung injury
Anthracycline cardiotoxicity
Radiation pneumonitis
Premature coronary atherosclerosis
Infertility
Breast cancer and lung cancer

confirming that breast tissue is likely highly susceptible to ionizing radiation in younger patients, necessitating long-term surveillance [66]. With newer radiation techniques and lower dose delivery to surrounding tissue, the rates of breast cancer are hypothesized to be lower than in the past. Screening MRI may be useful as an adjunct to routine mammography for women with an approximately 20–25% or greater lifetime risk of breast cancer, including women who were treated with mediastinal radiation for HL [67].

Patients with HL are susceptible to nonischemic cardiovascular disease from anthracyclines (involving oxidative stress and apoptosis) which form the backbone of virtually all modern chemotherapeutic regimens for HL. This is usually dose dependent and a major problem once cumulative doses of doxorubicin exceed 400 mg/m^2 [68]. Older adults, those who are receiving additional radiotherapy to the tissues surrounding the heart, and those with cardiomyopathy preceding diagnosis of HL are more susceptible to cardiotoxicity, which can sometimes occur at much lower cumulative doses. While one can be vigilant about checking cardiac function during chemo- or radiotherapy, there is also associated long-term cardiovascular risk associated with combined modality therapy. Long-term survivors are at risk for premature atherosclerosis of the coronary arteries, valvular dysfunction, and congestive heart failure from cumulative toxicities of chemotherapy with radiation [69].

Pulmonary toxicities can arise both acutely and subacutely during therapy (bleomycin- and radiation-induced pneumonitis) and when undiagnosed/untreated can cause havoc to a patient's pulmonary diffusion capacity leading to chronic respiratory impairment. Once patients are exposed to bleomycin they are indefinitely forewarned against exposure to high concentrations of oxygen for fear of worsening bleomycin-induced lung damage.

MOPP and BEACOPP (containing drugs such as nitrogen mustard and procarbazine) are much worse for gonadal function and recovery of fertility post chemotherapy than ABVD. Younger age during institution of chemotherapy also predicts for a greater chance of recovery of ovarian function upon completion [70]. In a Life Situation Questionnaire sent to 1,700 women who had been treated for HL, the cumulative risk of premature ovarian failure (POF) after such chemotherapy was 60% (95% CI, 41– 79%) but only 3% (95% CI, 1– 7%) after ABVD chemotherapy. Also, the risk of POF was found to show positive linear relationships for chemotherapy dose and age at treatment [71]. In patients with relapsed disease receiving salvage chemotherapy/high-dose therapy, preservation of ovarian function and fertility is unlikely. Sperm banking, embryo cryopreservation, and oocyte freezing are all being used to provide fertility preservation options for patients with Hodgkin lymphoma before initiation of therapy.

References

1 Hodgkin T. On some Morbid Appearances of the Absorbent Glands and Spleen. *Med Chir Trans* 1832;17:68–114.

2 Jaffe ES HN, Stein H, Vardiman JW. Pathology and Genetics of Tumours of Haematopoietic and Lymphoid Tissues. *WHO/IARC Classification of Tumours*. Lyon: IARC, 2001.

3 Küppers R, Rajewsky K, Zhao M, *et al.* Hodgkin disease: Hodgkin and Reed-Sternberg cells picked from histological sections show clonal immunoglobulin gene rearrangements and appear to be derived from B cells at various stages of development. *Proc Natl Acad Sci U S A* 1994;91(23):10962–6.

4 Foss H-D, Reusch R, Demel G, *et al.* Frequent expression of the B-cell–specific activator protein in Reed-Sternberg cells of classical Hodgkin's Disease provides further evidence for its B-cell origin. *Blood* 1999;94(9):3108–13.

5 Swerdlow SH, Campo E, Harris NL, *et al. WHO Classification of Tumours of Haematopoietic and Lymphoid Tissues*, 4th edn. Lyon: IARC.

6 Harris NL, Jaffe ES, Stein H, *et al.* A revised European-American classification of lymphoid neoplasms: a proposal from the International Lymphoma Study Group. *Blood* 1994;84(5):1361–92.

7 bMacLennan KA, Bennett MH, Tu A, *et al.* Relationship of histopathologic features to survival and relapse in nodular sclerosing Hodgkin's disease. A study of 1659 patients. *Cancer* 1989;64(8):1686–93.

8 von Wasielewski S, Franklin J, Fischer R, *et al.* Nodular sclerosing Hodgkin disease: new grading predicts prognosis in intermediate and advanced stages. *Blood* 2003;101(10):4063–9.

9 Siegel RL, Miller KD, Jemal A. Cancer statistics, 2017. *CA Cancer J Clin* 2017;67(1):7–30.

10 Howlader N, Noone AM, Krapcho M, *et al.* (eds). SEER Cancer Statistics Review, 1975-2013 Bethesda MD: National Cancer Institute. http://seer.cancer.gov/csr/1975_2013/, based on November 2015 SEER data submission, posted to the SEER web site, April 2016.

11 Siebert JD, Ambinder RF, Napoli VM, *et al.* Human immunodeficiency virus-associated Hodgkin's disease contains latent, not replicative, *Epstein-Barr virus. Hum Pathol* 1995;26(11):1191–5.

12 Urayama KY, Jarrett RF, Hjalgrim H, *et al.* Genome-wide association study of classical Hodgkin lymphoma and Epstein-Barr virus status-defined subgroups. *J Natl Cancer Inst* 2012;104(3):240–53.

13 Fast Stats: An interactive tool for access to SEER cancer statistics. Surveillance Research Program, National Cancer Institute. https://seer.cancer.gov/faststats (accessed 13 January 2017).

14 Lister TA, Crowther D, Sutcliffe SB, *et al.* Report of a committee convened to discuss the evaluation and staging of patients with Hodgkin's disease: Cotswolds meeting. *J Clin Oncol* 1989;7(11):1630–6.

15 Carbone PP, Kaplan HS, Musshoff K, Smithers DW, Tubiana M. Report of the Committee on Hodgkin's Disease Staging Classification. *Cancer Res* 1971;31(11):1860–1.

16 Rosenberg SA, Boiron M, DeVita VT, Jr., *et al.* Report of the Committee on Hodgkin's Disease Staging Procedures. *Cancer Res* 1971;31(11):1862-–3.

17 Rosenberg SA. A critique of the value of laparotomy and splenectomy in the evaluation of patients with Hodgkin's disease. *Cancer Res*1971;31(11):1737–40.

18 El-Galaly TC, d'Amore F, Mylam KJ, *et al.* Routine bone marrow biopsy has little or no therapeutic consequence for positron emission tomography/computed tomography-staged treatment-naive patients with Hodgkin lymphoma. *J Clin Oncol* 2012;30(36):4508–14.

19 Christina Clarke COM, and Sally Glaser. SEER Survival Monograph: Cancer Survival Among Adults: U. S. SEER Program, 1988-2001. Bethesda MD: SEER, 2007. Available from: http://seer.cancer.gov/publications/survival/surv_hodgkin.pdf (accessed 20 September 2017).

20 Hoppe RT, Advani RH, Ai WZ, *et al.* Hodgkin lymphoma, version 2.2012 featured updates to the NCCN guidelines. *J Natl Compr Canc Netw* 2012;10(5):589–97.

21 Hasenclever D, Diehl V. A prognostic score for advanced Hodgkin's disease. International Prognostic Factors Project on Advanced Hodgkin's Disease. *N Engl J Med* 1998;339(21):1506–14.

22 Gallamini A, Hutchings M, Rigacci L, *et al.* Early interim 2-[18F]fluoro-2-deoxy-D-glucose positron emission tomography is prognostically superior to international prognostic score in advanced-stage Hodgkin's lymphoma: a report from a joint Italian-Danish study. *J Clin Oncol* 2007;25(24):3746–52.

23 Seer Cancer Statistics Review 1975-2008. Available from: http://seer.cancer.gov/csr/1975_2008/ (accessed 27 October 2017).

24 Kaplan HS, Rosenberg SA. Extended-field radical radiotherapy in advanced Hodgkin's disease: short-term results of 2 randomized clinical trials. *Cancer Res* 1966;26(6):1268–76.

25 Kaplan HS. Long-term results of palliative and radical radiotherapy of Hodgkin's disease. *Cancer Res* 1966;26(6):1250–3.

26 Kaplan HS. Evidence for a tumoricidal dose level in the radiotherapy of Hodgkin's disease. *Cancer Res* 1966;26(6):1221–4.

27 DeVita VT, Jr. A selective history of the therapy of Hodgkin's disease. *Br J Haematol* 2003;122(5):718–27.

28 Devita VT, Jr., Serpick AA, Carbone PP. Combination chemotherapy in the treatment of advanced Hodgkin's disease. *Ann Intern Med*1970;73(6):881–95.

29 Bonadonna G, Zucali R, Monfardini S, De Lena M, Uslenghi C. Combination chemotherapy of Hodgkin's disease with adriamycin, bleomycin, vinblastine, and imidazole carboxamide versus MOPP. *Cancer* 1975;36(1):252–9.

30 Bonadonna G, Valagussa P, Santoro A. Alternating non-cross-resistant combination chemotherapy or MOPP in stage IV Hodgkin's disease. A report of 8-year results. *Ann Intern Med* 1986;104(6):739–46.

31 Longo DL, Glatstein E, Duffey PL, *et al.* Radiation therapy versus combination chemotherapy in the treatment of early-stage Hodgkin's disease: seven-year results of a prospective randomized trial. *J Clin Oncol* 1991;9(6):906–17.

32 Nissen NI, Nordentoft AM. Radiotherapy versus combined modality treatment of stage I and II Hodgkin's disease. *Cancer Treat Rep* 1982;66(4):799–803.

33 Ferme C, Eghbali H, Meerwaldt JH, *et al.* Chemotherapy plus involved-field radiation in early-stage Hodgkin's disease. *N Engl J Med* 2007;357(19):1916–27.

34 Engert A, Plutschow A, Eich HT, *et al.* Reduced treatment intensity in patients with early-stage Hodgkin's lymphoma. *N Engl J Med* 2010;363(7):640–52.

35 Meyer RM, Gospodarowicz MK, Connors JM, *et al.* ABVD alone versus radiation-based therapy in limited-stage Hodgkin's lymphoma. *N Engl J Med* 2012;366(5):399–408.

36 von Tresckow B, Plutschow A, Fuchs M, *et al.* Dose-intensification in early unfavorable Hodgkin's lymphoma: final analysis of the German hodgkin study group HD14 trial. *J Clin Oncol* 2012;30(9):907–13.

37 Canellos GP, Anderson JR, Propert KJ, *et al.* Chemotherapy of advanced Hodgkin's disease with MOPP, ABVD, or MOPP alternating with ABVD. *N Engl J Med* 1992;327(21):1478–84.

38 Duggan DB, Petroni GR, Johnson JL, *et al.* Randomized comparison of ABVD and MOPP/ABV hybrid for the treatment of advanced Hodgkin's disease: report of an intergroup trial. *J Clin Oncol* 2003;21(4):607–14.

39 Engert A, Diehl V, Franklin J, *et al.* Escalated-dose BEACOPP in the treatment of patients with advanced-stage Hodgkin's lymphoma: 10 years of follow-up of the GHSG HD9 study. *J Clin Oncol* 2009;27(27):4548–54.

40 Viviani S, Zinzani PL, Rambaldi A, *et al.* ABVD versus BEACOPP for Hodgkin's lymphoma when high-dose salvage is planned. *N Engl J Med* 2011;365(3):203–12.

41 Johnson P, Federico M, Kirkwood A, *et al.* Adapted treatment guided by interim PET-CT scan in advanced Hodgkin's lymphoma. *N Engl J Med* 2016;374(25):2419–29.

42 Gordon LI, Hong F, Fisher RI, *et al.* Randomized phase III trial of ABVD versus Stanford V with or without radiation therapy in locally extensive and advanced-stage Hodgkin lymphoma: an intergroup study coordinated by the Eastern Cooperative Oncology Group (E2496). *J Clin Oncol* 2013;31(6):684–91.

43 Hoskin PJ, Lowry L, Horwich A, *et al.* Randomized comparison of the stanford V regimen and ABVD in the treatment of advanced Hodgkin's Lymphoma: United Kingdom National Cancer Research Institute Lymphoma Group Study ISRCTN 64141244. *J Clin Oncol* 2009;27(32):5390–6.

44 Lohri A, Barnett M, Fairey RN, *et al.* Outcome of treatment of first relapse of Hodgkin's disease after primary chemotherapy: identification of risk factors from the British Columbia experience 1970 to 1988. *Blood* 1991;77(10):2292–8.

45 Schmitz N, Pfistner B, Sextro M, *et al.* Aggressive conventional chemotherapy compared with high-dose chemotherapy with autologous haemopoietic stem-cell transplantation for relapsed chemosensitive Hodgkin's disease: a randomised trial. *Lancet* 2002;359(9323):2065–71.

46 Yvette L. Kasamon RJJ, Hyam I, *et al.* *High-Dose Cyclophosphamide (Cy), Rituximab, and a Cancer Vaccine for Relapsed Classical Hodgkin's Lymphoma (cHL).* Orlando, FL: American Society of Hematology, 2010:Abstract 3954.

47 Younes A, Bartlett NL, Leonard JP, *et al.* Brentuximab vedotin (SGN-35) for relapsed CD30-positive lymphomas. *N Engl J Med* 2010;363(19):1812–21.

48 Younes A, Gopal AK, Smith SE, *et al.* Results of a pivotal phase II study of brentuximab vedotin for patients with relapsed or refractory Hodgkin's lymphoma. *J Clin Oncol* 2012;30(18):2183–9.

49 Chen R, Gopal AK, Smith SE, *et al.* Five-year survival and durability results of brentuximab vedotin in patients with relapsed or refractory Hodgkin lymphoma. *Blood* 2016;128(12):1562–6.

50 Moskowitz CH, Nademanee A, Masszi T, *et al.* Brentuximab vedotin as consolidation therapy after autologous stem-cell transplantation in patients with Hodgkin's lymphoma at risk of relapse or progression (AETHERA): a randomised, double-blind, placebo-controlled, phase 3 trial. *Lancet* 2015;385(9980):1853–62.

51 Ansell SM, Lesokhin AM, Borrello I, *et al.* PD-1 blockade with nivolumab in relapsed or refractory Hodgkin's lymphoma. *N Engl J Med* 2015;372(4):311–9.

52 Thomson KJ, Peggs KS, Smith P, *et al.* Superiority of reduced-intensity allogeneic transplantation over conventional treatment for relapse of Hodgkin's lymphoma following autologous stem cell transplantation. *Bone Marrow Transplant* 2008;41(9):765–70.

53 Sureda A, Robinson S, Canals C, *et al.* Reduced-intensity conditioning compared with conventional allogeneic stem-cell transplantation in relapsed or refractory Hodgkin's lymphoma: an analysis from the Lymphoma Working Party of the European Group for Blood and Marrow Transplantation. *J Clin Oncol* 2008;26(3):455–62.

54 Sureda A, Canals C, Arranz R, *et al.* Allogeneic stem cell transplantation after reduced intensity conditioning in patients with relapsed or refractory Hodgkin's lymphoma. Results of the HDR-ALLO study - a prospective clinical trial by the Grupo Espanol de Linfomas/Trasplante de Medula Osea (GEL/TAMO) and the Lymphoma Working Party of the European Group for Blood and Marrow Transplantation. *Haematologica* 2012;97(2):310–7.

55 Burroughs LM, O'Donnell PV, Sandmaier BM, *et al.* Comparison of outcomes of HLA-matched related, unrelated, or HLA-haploidentical related hematopoietic cell transplantation following nonmyeloablative conditioning for relapsed or refractory Hodgkin lymphoma. *Biol Blood Marrow Transplant* 2008;14(11):1279–87.

56 Mauz-Korholz C, Gorde-Grosjean S, *et al.* Resection alone in 58 children with limited stage, lymphocyte-predominant Hodgkin lymphoma-experience from the European network group on pediatric Hodgkin lymphoma. *Cancer* 2007;110(1):179–85.

57 Wirth A, Yuen K, Barton M, *et al.* Long-term outcome after radiotherapy alone for lymphocyte-predominant Hodgkin lymphoma: a retrospective multicenter study of the Australasian Radiation Oncology Lymphoma Group. *Cancer* 2005;104(6):1221–9.

58 Canellos GP, Mauch P. What is the appropriate systemic chemotherapy for lymphocyte-predominant Hodgkin's lymphoma? *J Clin Oncol* 2010;28(1):e8.

59 Diehl V, Sextro M, Franklin J, *et al.* Clinical presentation, course, and prognostic factors in lymphocyte-predominant Hodgkin's disease and lymphocyte-rich classical Hodgkin's disease: report from the European Task Force on Lymphoma Project on Lymphocyte-Predominant Hodgkin's Disease. *J Clin Oncol*1999;17(3):776–83.

60 Schulz H, Rehwald U, Morschhauser F, *et al.* Rituximab in relapsed lymphocyte-predominant Hodgkin lymphoma: long-term results of a phase 2 trial by the German Hodgkin Lymphoma Study Group (GHSG). *Blood* 2008;111(1):109–11.

61 Eichenauer DA, Fuchs M, Pluetschow A, *et al.* Phase 2 study of rituximab in newly diagnosed stage IA nodular lymphocyte-predominant Hodgkin lymphoma: a report from the German Hodgkin Study Group. *Blood* 2011;118(16):4363–5.

62 Aleman BM, van den Belt-Dusebout AW, Klokman WJ, *et al.* Long-term cause-specific mortality of patients treated for Hodgkin's disease. *J Clin Oncol* 2003;21(18):3431–9.

63 Schonfeld SJ, Gilbert ES, Dores GM, *et al.* Acute myeloid leukemia following Hodgkin lymphoma: a population-based study of 35,511 patients. *J Natl Cancer Inst.* 2006;98(3):215–8.

64 Swerdlow AJ, Douglas AJ, Hudson GV, *et al.* Risk of second primary cancers after Hodgkin's disease by type of treatment: analysis of 2846 patients in the British National Lymphoma Investigation. *BMJ* 1992;304(6835):1137–43.

65 Aisenberg AC, Finkelstein DM, Doppke KP, *et al.* High risk of breast carcinoma after irradiation of young women with Hodgkin's disease. *Cancer* 1997;79(6):1203–10.

66 Hancock SL, Tucker MA, Hoppe RT. Breast cancer after treatment of Hodgkin's disease. *J Natl Cancer Inst* 1993;85(1):25–31.

67 Saslow D, Boetes C, Burke W, *et al.* American Cancer Society guidelines for breast screening with MRI as an adjunct to mammography. *CA Cancer J Clin* 2007;57(2):75–89.

68 Monsuez JJ, Charniot JC, Vignat N, Artigou JY. Cardiac side-effects of cancer chemotherapy. *Int J Cardiol* 2010;144(1):3–15.

69 Aleman BM, van den Belt-Dusebout AW, De Bruin ML, *et al.* Late cardiotoxicity after treatment for Hodgkin lymphoma. *Blood* 2007;109(5):1878–86.

70 van der Kaaij MAE, van Echten-Arends J, Simons AHM, Kluin-Nelemans HC. Fertility preservation after chemotherapy for Hodgkin lymphoma. *Hematol Oncol* 2010;28(4):168–79.

71 van der Kaaij MAE, Heutte N, Meijnders P, *et al.* Premature ovarian failure and fertility in long-term survivors of Hodgkin's lymphoma: A European Organisation for Research and Treatment of Cancer Lymphoma Group and Groupe d'Étude des Lymphomes de l'Adulte Cohort Study. *J Clin Oncol* 2012;30(3):291–9.

32

Non-Hodgkin Lymphoma in Adults

Loretta J. Nastoupil[1], Jean L. Koff[2], Leon Bernal-Mizrachi[2], and Christopher R. Flowers[2]

[1] MD Anderson Cancer Center, Houston, Texas, USA
[2] Winship Cancer Institute, Emory University, Atlanta, Georgia, USA

Introduction

Lymphoid malignancies are a complex and heterogeneous group of cancers. The lymphomas constitute a cluster of cancers of the lymphatic system that occur when B or T lymphocytes undergo malignant transformation. The heterogeneity seen in this collection of cancers reflects the complexity of the normal hematopoietic and immune systems. These diseases include Hodgkin's disease (now termed Hodgkin lymphoma (HL)) and the non-Hodgkin lymphomas (NHL); the latter are the subject of this chapter, whereas the former is addressed by Chapter 31.

In the United States (US) approximately 40,080 men and 32,160 women are diagnosed with NHL each year, and an estimated 11,450 men and 8,690 women die from NHL annually [1]. Incidence rates for NHL increased by an average of 3.6% per year between 1975 and 1991, then increased by an average of 0.7% annually from 1991 through 2009, and most recently decreased by an average of 1.5% annually from 2009 through 2013 [2].

The etiology of the great majority of lymphomas remains unknown. Thus, the lack of effective prevention strategies for lymphoma has made the development of novel therapies and improved management strategies clinical priorities. Risk factors identified for some NHL types are discussed later in this chapter in the sections addressing those types.

NHL Classification System

NHL is comprised of many biologically distinct subtypes that can be distinguished using the World Health Organization (WHO) classification system introduced in 2001 [3]. This classification provides a foundation for understanding the biological and clinical variability among lymphomas and over time has been adopted broadly by hematopathologists, clinicians, and investigators. In addition, the WHO synthesizes clinical, cytogenetic, and immunophenotypic features into diagnostic categories, emphasizing that many lymphomas are clinicopathologic entities. Approximately 136,960 new lymphoid neoplasms are diagnosed annually in the US, among which 72,240 are NHL [1, 4]. Collectively, lymphoid neoplasms are the fourth most common cancer and the sixth leading cause of cancer death in the US. However, incidence and survival vary greatly by race, gender, and subtype. For instance, while it is well known that the incidence of lymphoma is lower in Black Americans (as well as Asian Americans/Pacific Islanders and American Indians/Alaska Natives) relative to White Americans [5], Black patients in the US with several lymphoid cancers present at a younger age, at a more advanced stage, and have inferior survival [5–14].

In 2008, the Fourth Edition of the *WHO Classification of Tumours of Haematopoietic and Lymphoid Tissues* was published, building upon the 2001 edition (Table 32.1) [3, 15]. This revision refined some categories of lymphoma subtypes and defined new clinical and pathological entities. These modifications highlight the growing appreciation over the last decade of the heterogeneity across the NHLs and the overlap between disease states. One such example is the overlap between primary mediastinal large B-cell lymphoma (PMBL) and nodular sclerosis classical HL involving the mediastinum. Lymphomas that occur with these overlapping features, formerly called "gray zone" lymphomas, are now known to have similar gene expression profiles to both PMBL and classical HL [16, 17]. In the 2008 WHO classification system, a provisional category was created for these B-cell neoplasms with features intermediate between diffuse large B-cell lymphoma (DLBCL) and classical HL [18]. A similar provisional category was established for an entity termed "B-cell lymphoma, unclassifiable, with features intermediate between DLBCL and Burkitt lymphoma (BL)." Although creating overlapping diagnostic categories may seem to disregard the increased specificity sought by contemporary pathological classification, this approach provides a consistent definition

The American Cancer Society's Oncology in Practice: Clinical Management, First Edition. Edited by The American Cancer Society.

Table 32.1 Simplified World Health Organization classification of the most common lymphoid malignancies [15].

Mature B-cell neoplasms	*Mature T-cell and NK-cell neoplasms*
Diffuse large B-cell lymphoma (DLBCL), NOS	Peripheral T-cell lymphoma, NOS
T-cell/histiocyte rich large B-cell lymphoma	Angioimmunoblastic T-cell lymphoma
Primary DLBCL of the CNS	Anaplastic large cell lymphoma, ALK-positive
Primary cutaneous DLBCL, leg type	Anaplastic large cell lymphoma, ALK-negative
EBV-positive DLBCL of the elderly	Aggressive NK-cell leukemia
DLBCL associated with chronic inflammation	Adult T-cell leukemia/lymphoma
Lymphomatoid granulomatosis	Extranodal NK/T-cell lymphoma, nasal type
Primary mediastinal (thymic) large B-cell lymphoma	Enteropathy-associated T-cell lymphoma
Intravascular large B-cell lymphoma	Hepatosplenic T-cell lymphoma
ALK-positive large B-cell lymphoma	Subcutaneous panniculitis-like T-cell lymphoma
Primary effusion lymphoma	T-cell prolymphocytic leukemia
B-cell lymphoma, unclassifiable, with features intermediate between diffuse large B-cell lymphoma and classical Hodgkin lymphoma	T-cell large granular lymphocytic leukemia
B-cell lymphoma, unclassifiable, with features intermediate between diffuse large B-cell lymphoma and Burkitt lymphoma	Mycosis fungoides
Burkitt lymphoma	Sézary syndrome
Plasmablastic lymphoma	Primary cutaneous CD30+ T-cell lymphoproliferative disorders
Follicular lymphoma	Lymphomatoid papulosis
Primary cutaneous follicle centre lymphoma	Primary cutaneous anaplastic large cell lymphoma
Mantle cell lymphoma	Primary cutaneous $\gamma\delta$ T-cell lymphoma
Hairy cell leukemia	Primary cutaneous CD8+ aggressive epidermotropic cytotoxic T-cell lymphoma
Splenic lymphoma/leukemia, unclassifiable	Primary cutaneous CD4+ small/medium T-cell lymphoma
Marginal zone lymphomas	
Splenic marginal zone lymphoma	
Extranodal marginal zone lymphoma of mucosa-associated lymphoid tissue (MALT lymphoma)	
Nodal marginal zone lymphoma	
Lymphoplasmacytic lymphoma/Waldenström macroglobulinemia	
Multiple myeloma/solitary plasmacytoma of bone	
Chronic lymphocytic leukemia/small lymphocytic lymphoma	
Post-transplant lymphoproliferative disorders (PTLD)	
Early lesions	
Plasmacytic hyperplasia	
Infectious mononucleosis-like PTLD	
Polymorphic PTLD	
Monomorphic PTLD (B- and T/NK-cell types)	
Classical Hodgkin lymphoma type PTLD	

ALK, anaplastic lymphoma kinase; CNS, central nervous system; EBV, Epstein–Barr virus; NOS, not otherwise specified.

for such cases so that consensus treatment algorithms may be applied to these diagnostically challenging cases. As more specific and advanced analytic techniques and strategies for establishing a pathological diagnosis are being employed, the classifications of malignant lymphomas have been continually updated and improved and in 2016 have been subject to additional modifications with significant clinical and biologic implications. This resulted in revisions in the WHO classification system that present new and clearer guidelines that define discrete lymphoma subgroups with distinct diagnostic approaches, clinical expectations, and therapeutic strategies [19].

NHL Biology and Lymphomagenesis

Normal B-Cell Development

B-cell NHLs are a heterogeneous group of malignant lymphoid tumors, with each subtype phenotypically resembling the normal B lymphocyte at a particular stage of maturation. Thus, an understanding of physiologic B-cell development and the generation of a diverse immunoglobulin repertoire lends insight into many of the mechanisms underlying lymphomagenesis. A brief review is provided here.

B-cell development begins in the bone marrow, where B-cell progenitors progress through a series of steps eventually resulting in the production of immunoglobulin (Ig). During this process, B cells remodel DNA within the Ig loci in order to generate secondary Ig isotypes [20]. Ultimately, this process results in expression of IgM on the cell surface of antigen-naïve B cells. In addition to binding antigen as part of the immune response, surface IgM is noncovalently coupled to CD79a and CD79b subunits to form the B-cell receptor, which allows the maturing cells to transduce survival signals throughout their development. In the bone marrow, a large proportion of B cells undergo apoptosis if they fail to produce surface IgM, or if their IgM binds self-antigen.

Next, those mature B cells that survive the first round of selection leave the bone marrow and are exposed to antigen in secondary lymphoid tissues (e.g., lymph nodes and spleen). Following antigen exposure, these cells continue to one of three fates: a small percentage enter into a state of anergy, some undergo plasmacytic differentiation in the peripheral blood, but the majority migrate to the germinal center. Here, B cells proliferate in primary lymphoid follicles and undergo further modification of the Ig gene via somatic hypermutation and class switch recombination (CSR). Somatic hypermutation introduces point mutations, small deletions, and insertions into the variable region to increase an antibody's affinity for antigen. Those few B cells with antibodies exhibiting high antigen affinity receive survival signaling through the Ig receptor; however, most will die. Through CSR, exons in the constant region of the Ig heavy chain are replaced by a recombination/deletion process, thus facilitating the production of secondary Ig isotypes: IgG, IgA, or IgE [21]. Once B cells exit the germinal center, they differentiate either into plasmablasts, which ultimately develop into plasma cells, or into memory B cells.

Genetic Lesions and Mechanisms of Genomic Damage

During the process of differentiation, naïve B cells undergo massive clonal expansion and mutagenesis. The germinal center reaction requires major changes in gene expression, mediated in part by transcription factors, histone-modifying enzymes, and methylation changes in the CpG dinucleotides. Some genetic instability is inherent to the physiologic processes responsible for producing antibody diversity, as the involved enzymes introduce DNA double-strand breaks and point mutations to the Ig gene. B cells are thus particularly predisposed to acquire chromosomal translocations and other oncogenic mutations when these processes go awry, providing footing for malignant transformation to lymphoma.

Balanced translocations leading to activated oncogenes are common events in many lymphoma subtypes, with characteristic lesions of each subtype arising during specific phases of B-cell differentiation. Often, the promoter of constitutively expressed Ig on chromosome 14 serves as a translocation partner. For instance, in follicular lymphoma (FL), t(14,18) leads to overexpression of BCL2, an anti-apoptotic protein that promotes cell survival even in the harshly pro-death environment of the germinal center [22]. Similarly, constitutive expression of cyclin D1 in mantle cell lymphoma (MCL) results from t(11,14) and promotes cellular proliferation [23].

The machinery involved in somatic hypermutation offers ample opportunity for gaining genetic lesions. For example, t(8,14) observed in endemic Burkitt lymphoma (BL) is thought to occur during somatic hypermutation, since the *MYC* gene is often joined to an Ig locus whose V region exon is rearranged and somatically mutated [24].

DNA breaks also occur in CSR, signifying yet another process that may yield translocations if disrupted. CSR is implicated in many translocations found in multiple myeloma, as well as in the t(8,14) seen in *sporadic* BL, in which translocation breakpoints involve the Ig heavy chain switch locus [24]. Furthermore, defects in CSR are seen in activated B cell-like (ABC) DLBCL but not in the germinal center B cell-like (GCB) subset [25]. It is possible that this difference in CSR may contribute to the distinct mutations described in each subtype (e.g., in *MYOM2*, *CD79*, and *MYD88* in ABC, and in *MLL2*, *BCL2*, and *CREBBP* in GCB) [26].

While balanced translocations may be initiating pathogenic events, unbalanced chromosomal gains and losses likely represent cooperating contributors to malignant transformation and cancer cell survival advantage. For instance, deletions and mutations of the gene coding for the tumor suppressor p53 have been described in FL, MCL, BL, and chronic lymphocytic leukemia/small lymphocytic lymphoma (CLL/SLL) [27]. Similarly, deletion of 6q portends poor prognosis in FL [28]. More recent studies also suggest that dysregulated epigenetic mechanisms contribute to lymphomagenesis; an overview and examples of these mechanisms are provided in the following paragraphs.

Epigenetic Changes

Histone Modification

Transcriptional access to DNA is controlled by histones, proteins that may undergo modification by many different enzymes (often by methylation or acetylation). Certain histone modifications are linked to actively transcribed chromatin, while others are linked to repressed chromatin. Thus, structural alteration of histone-modifying enzymes can significantly impact transcriptional output, and recurrent examples of such alterations have been revealed by cancer genomics studies [29]. In lymphoma, the exact oncogenic advantage conferred by altering these enzymes remains largely unknown, but instances of both oncogenes and tumor suppressors have been described.

DNA Methylation

DNA methylation patterning represents another determinant factor in transcriptional control that, when perturbed, may contribute to malignant transformation. In general, hypermethylation of regulatory sequences is associated with gene silencing, while hypomethylation is associated with expression. Studies that identified changes in methylation of DNA repair genes such as *MGMT* highlighted the possibility that abnormalities among lymphomas could be expected [30]. Furthermore, distinct methylation patterns have been identified among CLL/SLL, FL, MCL, GCB DLBCL, and ABC DLBCL, suggesting that epigenetic programming may contribute to the phenotype of these tumors [31]. Although many advances have been made in this field, more work needs to be done to further elucidate the role of aberrant DNA methylation in lymphoma development.

MicroRNAs

MicroRNAs (miRNAs) are small, noncoding RNAs that target specific genes for down-regulation by decreasing their mRNA levels. miRNAs are involved in regulating differentiation and CSR in normal B cells, and may play a role in lymphoma pathogenesis [32, 33]. The causative role of miRNAs in lymphomagenesis was first inferred by identifying a frequent loss of microRNAs miR-15a and miR-16-1 in CLL/SLL [34]. Suspected targets of miR-15a and miR-16-1 include BCL2 and regulators of the cell cycle, indicating that they may act as tumor suppressors. In fact, many hypothesize that up-regulated miRNAs may repress tumor suppressor genes, while down-regulation of other miRNAs may induce expression of oncogenes. Studies have also found occasional deletion of the miRNA recognition sequences in the untranslated region of the gene encoding cyclin D1, uncovering an alternative pathway to its constitutive expression in MCL [35].

Affected Signaling Pathways

Genetic lesions resulting in oncogenic gain of function or suppression of negative regulators allow lymphomas to hijack normal B-cell signaling pathways that potentiate their own survival and proliferation. Fundamental examples of these expropriated networks and their downstream effects are explored in the following paragraphs.

Enhancing Growth and Proliferation

As a proto-oncogene implicated in many different cancers, *MYC* encodes for a transcription factor involved in multiple cellular functions, including cell cycle regulation, growth, metabolism, adhesion, and differentiation. It induces proliferation by up-regulating genes involved in cell cycle control and down-regulating genes responsible for growth arrest [36]. Induction of cell immortalization has also been attributed to c-*MYC*. Normally, c-*MYC* is subject to tight transcriptional and post-transcriptional control, which stands to reason given its broad range of biologic activity. When c-*MYC*'s regulatory network is circumvented by translocation, constitutive expression results in a decidedly oncogenic effect [37]. Translocations involving the Ig and *c-MYC* genes are associated with aggressive clinical behavior and are present in virtually all BL, as well as in some DLBCL and even FL. Interestingly, t(8,14) appears to be a driving mutation in BL, but may represent a secondary event in other lymphomas.

Escaping Apoptosis

Apoptosis avoidance is a hallmark of malignant transformation, but it is especially vital in the context of the germinal center, where B cells are poised for apoptosis unless rescued by positive selection. Many lymphoma subtypes utilize the anti-apoptotic nuclear factor-κB (NF-κB) pathway as a strategic cornerstone in their evasion of cell death [38]. Controlled activity of NF-κB transcription factors is a key player in physiologic lymphocyte maturation, proliferation, and survival, and is required for the normal immune response [39]. Dysregulation of this pathway can result from a variety of mechanisms, many of which appear to be specific to certain lymphoma subtypes. In fact, the two main subsets of DLBCL (GCB and ABC) may also be characterized by distinct mechanisms of NF-κB activation, often by mutations in upstream regulators [40–42]. In other DLBCL, translocations and truncations of the NF-κB2 gene result in constitutive pathway activity.

Still other mechanisms of NF-κB activation may be found in mucosa-associated lymphoid tissue (MALT) lymphomas. In 30–50% of this subtype, t(11,18) leads to formation of the fusion protein AP12/MLT1, which activates the NF-κB pathway even though neither AP12 nor MLT1 does so on its own. Less frequently, t(1,14) results in constitutive expression of BCL10, a protein necessary for NF-κB activation downstream of receptor signaling.

The anti-apoptotic protein BCL2 is up-regulated by NF-κB signaling, but overexpression may be induced by other processes as well. Translocation of the *BCL2* gene with Ig loci represents the characterizing genetic lesion in FL and is also found in ~25% DLBCL (nearly all of which are GCB) [43]. In other lymphomas, *BCL2* may be amplified or transcriptionally up-regulated by mechanisms that remain unclear.

Blocking Differentiation

Rather than promoting proliferation or inhibiting apoptosis, some genetic aberrations in lymphoma appear to "trap" the cell in a particular stage of development. Mutation of *BCL6* is a prime example of such a lesion. Since BCL6 represses genes involved in B-cell activation and terminal differentiation during the normal germinal center reaction, dysregulated BCL6 acts to prevent plasmacytic development [44]. Furthermore, BCL6 facilitates somatic hypermutation by dampening the DNA damage response, thus potentially exposing the cell to increased acquisition of genetic lesions. Translocations coupling constitutively active promoters to the 5′ region of *BCL6* are found in ~40% of DLBCL and in 5–10% of FL.

Cells of Origin?

As mentioned previously, B-cell NHL is categorized into several subtypes, each bearing resemblance to a normal B-cell counterpart at a specific phase of differentiation. Subtypes are distinguished from each other based on histologic characteristics, flow cytometry patterns measured by cluster of differentiation (CD) markers, presence or absence of mutations in the Ig V region (indicating whether or not somatic hypermutation has occurred), and gene expression profiling (see Table 32.2).

Normal T-Cell Development

Ten to 15% of NHL derive from T- and natural killer (NK) cell precursors, although the biology of T-cell lymphomagenesis is less well understood than that of B-cell NHL. While some T-cell NHL resemble normal lymphocytes at a distinct developmental stage (especially when gene expression profiling is considered), determining the cellular origin of many subtypes remains difficult. This is in sharp contrast to B-cell lymphoma, in which each subtype corresponds with a normal cellular phenotype [45]. Interestingly, normal T-cell maturation mirrors that of B cells in many ways: lymphoid cells progress through a series of coordinated developmental steps, undergoing positive and negative selection in the thymus so that mature cells ultimately express a functional antigen-receptor gene – in this case, the T cell receptor (TCR). Unlike T cells, NK cells do not require the thymus for

Table 32.2 Cell of origin and characteristic genetic lesions of B-cell lymphomas.

	Cell of origin	Lymphoma subtype	Characteristic genetic lesions
Pre-germinal center	Naïve mature B cell	Mantle cell lymphoma	Cyclin D1 overexpression via t(11,14) (>95%)
	Antigen-exposed B cell	Mantle cell lymphoma	Cyclin D1 overexpression
		CLL/SLL	
Germinal center	Centroblast	Burkitt lymphoma	c-*MYC* overexpression via t(8,14)
		GCB DLBCL	BCL6 overexpression via multiple mechanisms (50%)
	Centrocyte	Follicular lymphoma	BCL2 overexpression via t(14,18) (>80%)
	Marginal zone B cell	Marginal zone lymphoma (e.g., MALT lymphoma)	BCL10 overexpression AP12-MALT1 fusion protein via t(11,18) in 60% MALT lymphoma
Post-germinal center	Memory B cell	CLL/SLL	
		Hairy cell lymphoma	BRAF mutation
	Plasmablast	ABC DLBCL	Chronic active BCR signaling via multiple mechanisms
	Plasma cell	Multiple myeloma	

Source: Shaffer AL, Young RM, Staudt LM. Pathogenesis of human B cell lymphomas. Annu Rev Immunol 2012;30:565–610.
ABC DLBCL, activated B cell-like diffuse large B-cell lymphoma; CLL/SLL, chronic lymphocytic leukemia/small lymphocytic lymphoma; GCB DLBCL, germinal center B cell-like diffuse large B-cell lymphoma; MALT, mucosa-associated lymphoid tissue.

development and lack a unique antigen receptor. Instead, they mature primarily in the bone marrow before migrating to the periphery [46].

Cells of Origin?

Although cell of origin is often difficult to pinpoint, the majority of T-cell lymphomas appear to be post-thymic in origin. Interestingly, NK cells share many phenotypic and functional traits with γ/δ T cells, despite their apparently disparate developmental paths. When distinction between the two cell types is unclear, the term "NK/T" cell NHL is utilized [47].

Genetic Lesions and Mechanisms of Genomic Damage

Unlike in B-cell lymphoma, most T-cell NHL subtypes have not been associated with specific genetic or biologic changes. Moreover, the balanced translocations that often characterize B-cell NHL subtypes are uncommon in T-cell lymphomas. One important exception is the anaplastic lymphoma kinase (*ALK*) translocation found in a subset of anaplastic large cell lymphoma (ALCL). The *ALK* locus may be juxtaposed with a variety of partners, each resulting in an oncogenic hybrid protein. The most common fusion, t(2,5), links the promoter of nucleophosmin to the catalytic *ALK* domain, generating a constitutively active tyrosine kinase implicated in malignant transformation and activation of anti-apoptotic pathways. Notably, ALK-positive ALCLs carry a more favorable prognosis than their ALK-negative counterparts [48].

Given the difficulty in defining a genetic basis for most T-cell lymphomas, recent research efforts have employed gene expression profiling (GEP) to attempt to identify phenotypic differences in these tumors. For instance, GEP studies have demonstrated that hepatosplenic T-cell lymphomas may be completely segregated from other T-cell NHL, highlighting the distinct clinicopathological characteristics of this subtype. Supervised analysis has also allowed investigators to differentiate between αβ and γδ T-cell lymphomas [49]. Interestingly, although *TP53* mutations themselves are uncommon in T-cell NHL, next-generation whole-genome sequencing has demonstrated recurrent rearrangements of p53-related genes in peripheral T-cell lymphoma (PTCL). One such rearrangement encodes a truncated p63 protein known to be oncogenic and to inhibit p53 in a dominant negative fashion, thus positing an alternative genetic mechanism for silencing the p53 tumor suppressor effect [50].

Clearly, our current understanding of T-cell lymphomagenesis leaves much to be desired. Continuing research is necessary for further elucidation of the molecular mechanisms underlying pathogenesis in this enigmatic group of malignancies.

General Management Principles

Diagnostic Workup

At present, there is no single marker that can be used as the gold standard for the diagnosis of NHL, and therefore a combination of assessments and techniques is used. Patterns of presentation for NHL can be quite varied. Patients with NHL subtypes commonly present with nontender lymphadenopathy and may present with constitutional symptoms (B symptoms) such as fever, night sweats, weight loss, and fatigue. On occasion, patients may have symptoms related to enlarged lymph nodes, the most concerning of which arise when a bulky mediastinal mass produces stridor or superior vena cava (SVC) syndrome, which are oncologic emergencies. Other symptoms may stem from cytopenias that result from bone marrow compromise. Central nervous system involvement at presentation is uncommon. A careful history and physical examination are important in the initial workup with particular attention paid to nodal areas, the size of the liver and spleen, presence of B symptoms, and assessment of performance status.

An excisional or incisional lymph node biopsy is recommended in order to provide adequate tissue for assessment of nodal architecture and establish the diagnosis of NHL. It is also important to consider that the most accessible lymph node may not be the most informative or representative one. Communication of the treating physician with the pathologist and surgeon may be advisable if treatment decisions may be impacted by distinguishing between an indolent lymphoma and a transformed lymphoma, as well as to ensure that unfixed material is saved for appropriate ancillary tests.

Once the diagnosis of NHL has been established, patients should undergo additional testing to determine stage, prognostic risk factors, and general evaluation of accompanying medical conditions. Laboratory studies should include a complete blood count (CBC), comprehensive metabolic panel, and lactate dehydrogenase (LDH). Depending on the subtype of NHL, evaluation of human immunodeficiency virus (HIV), human T-lymphotropic virus type 1 (HTLV-1), hepatitis B serologies, or testing for other infectious agents may be appropriate.

A bone marrow biopsy is recommended as part of the staging workup in most situations. However, imaging modalities at diagnosis are somewhat controversial. All patients should receive dedicated imaging of the neck, chest, and abdomen/pelvis by computed tomography (CT) with IV and oral contrast as clinically indicated. In the US, integrated positron emission tomography (PET) fused with CT (PET-CT) is commonly utilized instead of dedicated CT scans. However, further studies are needed to support this practice. Pretreatment PET is now recommended for DLBCL and HL and can be considered for other NHL subtypes according to national guidelines [51].

Staging is performed according to the Lugano classification [52]. Stage I indicates that the lymphoma is located in a single region, usually one lymph node and the surrounding area. Stage II denotes lymphoma located in two separate regions, an affected lymph node or organ and a second affected area, all confined to one side of the diaphragm. The modifier "E" is added if extranodal extension is present in early-stage disease. Stage III denotes lymphoma identified on both sides of the diaphragm, including one organ or area near the lymph nodes, or the spleen. Stage IV indicates diffuse or disseminated involvement of one or more extralymphatic organs, including but not limited to any involvement of the liver, bone marrow, or lungs.

Factors that have been shown to predict survival in patients with NHL include degree of tumor burden, host factors such as age, B symptoms, hemoglobin, and performance status, and response to therapy. The International Prognostic Index (IPI) was devised to predict prognosis in aggressive lymphomas and consists of five variables: age, performance status, stage, extranodal involvement, and serum LDH level [53]. For indolent lymphomas, the Follicular Lymphoma IPI (FLIPI) uses five parameters: age, stage, LDH, hemoglobin, and number of nodal sites [53]. Table 32.3 shows the expected outcomes for patients with aggressive NHL stratified by IPI category from the original publication of this prognostic model [53]. Of course, counseling individual patients regarding prognosis requires interpreting prognostic indices as general guidelines in addition to incorporating other disease- and patient-specific risk factors.

Assessment of Treatment Response

Radiological tests should be performed midterm and after completion of chemotherapy, because patients with insufficient or no response should be evaluated for early salvage regimens. A growing body of data suggests that PET-CT may be an effective means to evaluate response quality for certain aggressive NHL subtypes, but this approach remains investigational [54].

Management Strategies by Subtype

Since the NHL comprise >60 distinct entities, each with its own clinical features, prognosis, treatment strategies, and outcomes, detailed discussion of the nuances of management for all entities is beyond the scope of this text. Individualized discussion of particular rare clinical entities is available in several reviews. The level of detail in the discussion of each entity here corresponds roughly to its relative frequency in the population.

Mature B-Cell Neoplasms

The indolent NHLs represent approximately one-third of all malignant lymphomas, and most are of B-cell origin. FL is the most common indolent lymphoma subtype; others include CLL/SLL, and marginal zone B-cell lymphomas (MZL). The clinical behavior of mantle cell lymphoma is commonly debated. It is listed here among the indolent NHLs of mature B-cell origin, but this entity can behave aggressively.

Follicular Lymphoma

Epidemiology

FL is the second most commonly occurring lymphoma in the western world after DLBCL, and accounts for ~22% of B-cell lymphomas [55]. FL is more common in Caucasians than in Black or Asian Americans. Unlike other NHL subtypes, the incidence rates in men and women are similar. FL usually affects adults, with a median age in the sixth decade [55].

Clinical Presentation

Patients typically present with superficial lymph nodes, which in many cases have remained unnoticed. In contrast to other B-cell lymphomas, B symptoms (i.e., fever (>38 °C), drenching night sweats, and weight loss (≥10% body weight over 6 months)) and altered performance status are rare in patients presenting with FL. Although lymph nodes are the main site of presentation, involvement of the peripheral blood and bone marrow is common, and two-thirds of patients have advanced disease at presentation. On rare occasions, the disease may present in other organs such as the gastrointestinal tract and the testis [22, 55, 56].

Although FL is initially an indolent disease that is sensitive to a variety of immunotherapy and chemotherapy agents, this subtype exhibits a continuous pattern of relapses with decreasing sensitivity to treatment [56–58]. The median survival of patients with FL has conventionally been reported as ~8–10 years, but modern series suggest a much longer natural history [58]. Histological grade 1 and 2 FL are usually indolent and incurable unless they are localized, while grade 3 cases often follow a more aggressive clinical course but can be further divided into FL grade 3a and FL grade 3b (now classified as DLBCL), each

Table 32.3 Available prognostic indices for common B-cell lymphoma subtypes.

International Prognostic Index (IPI) [133]

Risk factor	Points
Age >60 years	1
Stage III or IV disease	1
Elevated serum LDH	1
ECOG performance status of ≥2	1
≥2 extranodal sites	1

Risk category	Points	Expected 5-year survival
Low risk	0–1	73%
Low-intermediate risk	2	51%
High-intermediate risk	3	43%
High risk	4–5	26%

Follicular Lymphoma International Prognostic Index (FLIPI) [71]

Risk factor	Points
Age >60 years	1
Stage III or IV disease	1
>4 lymph node groups involved	1
Serum hemoglobin <12 g/dL	1
Elevated serum LDH	1

Risk category	Points	Expected 5-year survival	Expected 10-year survival
Low risk	0–1	91%	71%
Intermediate risk	2	78%	51%
High risk	3–5	53%	36%

Mantle Cell Lymphoma International Prognostic Index (MIPI) [171]

Risk factor	Points
Age <50 years ECOG performance status of 0–1 LDH <0.67 × upper limit of normal WBC of <6,700 cells/μL	0
Age 50–59 LDH 0.67–0.99 × upper limit of normal WBC 6,700–9,999 cells/μL	1
Age 60–69 ECOG performance status of 2–4 LDH 1–1.49 × upper limit of normal WBC 10,000–14,000 cells/μL	2
Age ≥70 years LDH 1.5 × upper limit of normal WBC ≥15,000 cells/μL	3

Risk category	Points	Median expected survival
Low risk	0–3	Not reached
Intermediate risk	4–5	51 months
High risk	6–11	29 months

ECOG, Eastern Cooperative Oncology Group; LDH, lactic dehydrogenase; WBC, white blood cells.

with its own prognosis [22, 59]. Histological transformation into a high-grade lymphoma is observed in ~3% of patients per year and is associated with a progressive clinical course, poor response to treatment, and shorter survival; median survival is presently estimated at ~18 months [22, 56, 57].

First-Line Treatment

Over the past several years, the treatment paradigm for patients with FL has undergone significant changes, with the development of effective new agents that are now used in the front-line, maintenance, and relapse settings. Although these new therapies have led to improvements in patient outcomes, numerous questions remain regarding their optimal use. Treatment options depend on stage and degree of tumor burden. FL usually is considered an incurable disease, and the most common goal of therapy is to extend the lives of patients and obtain adequate disease control to maintain a good quality of life. Other considerations when deciding on management strategies include investigating options for available clinical trials that may address unanswered questions or provide access to novel therapeutics.

Depending on stage of disease and presenting characteristics, there are numerous available options for the initial management of FL. These include observation (i.e., watchful waiting), radiation alone, single-agent chemotherapy, single-agent rituximab, and rituximab–chemotherapy combinations (i.e., immunochemotherapy) [56, 57, 60, 61]. Stage I/II FL is often managed with radiation therapy, based on observational studies indicating long-term disease-free survival for select patients [60]. However, emerging data on practice patterns from a large cohort study in the US suggest that other management strategies for patients with localized disease may produce outcomes similar to those achieved with radiation [60].

Stage I–Contiguous Stage II Radiotherapy has also been suggested as an alternative to the "watch and wait strategy" in the rare cases of patients with low-stage, low-tumor-burden FL; however, findings are currently inconclusive. To date there have been no prospective randomized trials comparing these approaches and so conclusions must be drawn from retrospective analyses or observational studies. Several observational studies have demonstrated that patients with early-stage disease treated with radiotherapy have 10-year overall survival (OS) rates of 60–80%, with 10-year relapse-free survival rates of 45–60%, and median survival of approximately 15–20 years [56, 58]. In fact, a subset of patients with limited-stage FL may be cured with radiotherapy alone [22, 56, 60, 62]. Patients with stage I/II FL with high tumor burden should be treated with systemic therapy similarly to those with stage II noncontiguous, stage III, and stage IV FL [51, 56].

Stage II Noncontiguous, Stage III, and Stage IV Patients with FL and a low tumor burden have a median OS of around 12–15 years [56, 58]. Watchful waiting until treatment is indicated (e.g., due to bulky disease or systemic symptoms) has been the standard of care for many patients, with a period of 2–3 years usually passing before initiation of chemotherapy. Continual monitoring is an integral part of a watchful waiting strategy.

Rituximab Monotherapy Rituximab, a monoclonal antibody that targets the CD20 antigen found on B cells, has been in clinical use since it was initially approved in 1997 for patients with relapsed FL. Rituximab is thought to induce lymphoma cell lysis through complement-mediated cytolysis, antibody-dependent cell cytotoxicity, and induction of apoptosis, and acts synergistically with chemotherapy [63–65]. Other than infusion-related toxicities, it is generally well tolerated [53]. A prospective study addressing the role of rituximab monotherapy for patients with previously untreated, advanced-stage, asymptomatic grade 1 FL demonstrated an overall response rate (ORR) of 72%, with a 36% complete response and median time to progression of 2.2 years. Furthermore, two large trials looking at patients with non-bulky FL demonstrated that initial treatment with rituximab significantly delayed the need for new therapy compared to watchful waiting [66, 67]. Thus, rituximab may be considered as an option for low-tumor-burden FL as a brief course with or without ongoing maintenance. However, rituximab monotherapy is not yet recommended broadly, given that it may be safely used at progression and there is no indication that early initiation of therapy improves OS [56, 62, 65, 68, 69].

Rituximab Plus Chemotherapy In general, indications for more aggressive treatment include a high-risk FLIPI score or presence of any of the criteria outlined by the French Groupe d'Etude des Lymphomes Folliculaire (GELF), which include bulky tumors, systemic symptoms, poor performance status, and serum LDH and β2-microglobulin levels above normal limits [70, 71]. However, the optimal treatment approach for patients with advanced stages of FL remains undefined because of the low cure rates with current therapeutic options and the ability to use therapies sequentially. In previously untreated symptomatic patients with FL, standard induction treatment options include bendamustine (B) or combination chemotherapy regimens such as cyclophosphamide, doxorubicin, vincristine, and prednisone (CHOP), cyclophosphamide, vincristine, and prednisone (CVP), or a fludarabine-containing regimen such as fludarabine, mitoxantrone, and dexamethasone or fludarabine and mitoxantrone (FM). Chemotherapy is not indicated alone, as trials that have compared chemotherapy alone with chemotherapy plus rituximab have shown unequivocally that rituximab improves patient outcomes [56, 57]. At present, there is no consensus on the initial choice of chemotherapy to be used in combination with rituximab. Although several studies have compared regimens such as R-CHOP, R-CVP, and R-FM, to date the data have not been sufficiently compelling to lead to firm recommendations.

Regarding stage III/IV disease, the Primary Rituximab and Maintenance (PRIMA) trial reported that R-CHOP produces both higher response rates and longer progression-free survival (PFS) than does R-CVP, with comparable tolerability [56, 57, 62, 65]. Rummel and colleagues investigated a regimen of bendamustine plus rituximab (BR) versus R-CHOP for indolent lymphomas, with favorable outcomes. At a median follow-up of 45 months, results indicated a significant prolongation of PFS with BR, which was independent of FLIPI score in the FL subgroup [72]. In addition, BR was associated with less hematologic toxicity and no alopecia greater than grade 1. No significant difference in OS was reported between groups, although the authors suggest that interpretation of OS may be confounded by the fact that some patients treated with R-CHOP received BR as a salvage treatment. For older or infirm patients unable to tolerate standard therapy, radioimmunotherapy, rituximab monotherapy, single-agent alkylators with or without rituximab, or BR are good options given their tolerability.

Maintenance Therapy Rituximab has shown remarkable efficacy in prolonging the duration of remission achieved with induction therapy, as confirmed by a meta-analysis of randomized trials. Similarly, results from the PRIMA trial showed significant improvements in PFS with rituximab maintenance versus observation following first-line induction with a variety of immunochemotherapy regimens [73].

Radioimmunotherapy (RIT) represents another post-chemotherapy treatment strategy under investigation. An international phase 3 trial reported on the efficacy and safety of consolidation with yttrium-90 (^{90}Y)-ibritumomab tiuxetan in patients with advanced-stage FL in first remission. ^{90}Y-ibritumomab tiuxetan consolidation significantly prolonged median PFS, with a complete response rate of 87% [74]. The most common toxicity with ^{90}Y-ibritumomab tiuxetan was hematologic. However, only 31 patients received rituximab-based induction therapy, raising the question of the effectiveness of RIT consolidation after rituximab–chemotherapy induction.

Subsequent Treatment for Relapsed FL Despite the substantial improvements in PFS with front-line chemoimmunotherapy and maintenance regimens, almost all patients with FL eventually relapse. Nearly all chemoimmunotherapy regimens that are used in the front-line setting can also be used at relapse. Autologous stem cell transplantation may provide benefits for select patients with relapsed FL [62, 75].Therefore, approaches aimed at treating relapsed disease are the focus of numerous studies. All regimens discussed as first-line therapy have been utilized in patients with relapsed FL. Allogeneic stem cell transplantation is the only approach that has been demonstrated to cure patients with relapsed FL [62]. Three agents are now approved for patients with relapsed FL: idelalisib, bendamustine, and the combination of bendamustine and obinutuzumab [76–78]. Bendamustine is now more commonly used in the front-line setting, and its role in the relapsed setting alone or in combination with an anti-CD20 antibody remains unclear. Other oral targeted agents are also being explored as single agents and in combination therapies, which likely will change the therapeutic options for relapsed patients in the future.

Allogeneic Stem Cell Transplant

Myeloablative allogeneic stem cell transplantation (SCT) is associated with a treatment-related mortality rate of approximately 30%. Given this high mortality rate, myeloablative allogeneic SCT is reserved for young, highly motivated patients with relapsed or resistant follicular lymphoma. In contrast, nonmyeloablative or reduced-intensity conditioning (RIC) regimens are associated with lower transplant-related mortality. Nonmyeloablative conditioning regimens may be preferred for patients who have attained a second complete remission but are not ideal candidates for conventional myeloablative SCT. In addition, patients who relapse after autologous SCT may be considered for nonmyeloablative allogeneic SCT. As suggested by several single-center studies [79] and registry analysis [80], long-term disease control can be achieved in 40–75% of transplanted patients using an RIC approach.

Chronic Lymphocytic Leukemia/Small Lymphocytic Lymphoma

According to the WHO classification, chronic lymphocytic leukemia (CLL) and small lymphocytic lymphoma (SLL) represent two different stages of the same disease, each characterized by the accumulation of functionally incompetent lymphocytes. With identical pathologic and immunophenotypic features, the distinction between the two is based on clinical presentation: in CLL, malignant cells appear primarily in the peripheral blood and bone marrow, while SLL presents in the lymph nodes [19]. Further discussion of the management of this disease may be found in Chapter 30.

Marginal Zone Lymphomas

MZLs represent a group of lymphomas that originate from memory B lymphocytes normally present in the "marginal zone" of secondary lymphoid follicles. The most recent lymphoma classification identifies three subtypes of MZLs: extranodal MZL of mucosa-associated lymphoid tissue (MALT), splenic MZL (SMZL), and nodal MZL (NMZL). Most cases occur in adults, with a median age of 60 years and a slight female predominance. MALT lymphoma differs from SMZL and NMZL in that it arises in organs (i.e., stomach, lungs, salivary glands, lacrimal glands, skin, thyroid) that normally lack lymphoid tissue but have accumulated B cells in response to chronic infections or autoimmune diseases. The list of infectious species associated with MALT lymphoma includes *Helicobacter pylori*, *H. heilmannii*, hepatitis C virus, *Campylobacter jejuni*, *Borrelia burgdorferi*, and *Chlamydia psittaci*. A very high prevalence (up to 90% of cases) of *H. pylori* infection has been reported with gastric MALT lymphoma. There is compelling evidence that gastric MALT arises from *H. pylori*-stimulated, autoreactive B cells [81].

The clinical aspects and presenting symptoms of extranodal MZL are generally related to location of primary involvement. The stomach is the most common site of localization, often with multifocal involvement. Patients often present with signs and symptoms suggestive of peptic ulcer disease, including epigastric discomfort, nausea, and dyspepsia. Anemia, weight loss, and gastrointestinal bleeding can be seen in patients with more advanced disease. MALT lymphomas most commonly present as localized disease (Lugano stage IE), and bone marrow and peripheral lymph node involvement are uncommon. Advanced disease at diagnosis appears to be more common in MALT lymphomas that arise outside of the gastrointestinal tract. Other presentation sites include the salivary glands, ocular adnexa, thyroid, lungs, skin, breast, liver, and other gastrointestinal sites.

Gastric Marginal Zone Lymphomas

Antibiotic eradication of *H. pylori* results in regression of MALT lymphoma in approximately half of treated patients [82, 83].

The most common approach to eradication is triple therapy with a proton pump inhibitor, amoxicillin, and clarithromycin. Follow-up endoscopy 2 3 months after triple therapy is recommended to document *H. pylori* eradication. For patients who remain positive for *H. pylori*, a second-line anti-Helicobacter regimen is recommended. More extensive disease is less likely to respond to antibiotic therapy. Lack of response has also been correlated with presence of t(11;18). The role of additional chemotherapy after antibiotics was reported in a randomized study comparing chlorambucil versus observation after *H. pylori* treatment; in this study, chlorambucil did not increase the survival rates [84].

For patients with early-stage MALT lymphoma of the stomach without evidence of *H. pylori* infection, those with persistent lymphoma after attempted eradication, and for localized nongastric presentations, involved-field radiotherapy (25–35 Gy) has been associated with excellent disease control [85]. Surgery has also been a therapeutic option for localized disease. However, gastric MALT lymphoma is often multifocal, and adequate gastrectomy can severely impact patients' quality of life. Additionally, residual disease at the margins may require additional radiation and/or chemotherapy.

A randomized study of patients with nongastric and gastric MALT lymphomas failing antibiotic therapy suggested that the combination of chlorambucil plus rituximab resulted in superior event-free survival compared to chlorambucil alone [86]. Furthermore, a fludarabine-containing front-line regimen has demonstrated activity in nongastric MALT lymphoma [87]. Extrapolation from the data in FL has also been applied in this setting, with observation, single-agent rituximab, and rituximab in combination with chemotherapy posited as additional management strategies depending on goals of therapy.

Nongastric Marginal Zone Lymphomas

A strong rationale for antibiotic treatment of localized lesions in nongastric MALT lymphoma is supported by the finding that *C. psittaci* has a potential pathogenic role in the development of MALT lymphoma of the ocular adnexa. A prospective phase 2 study showed lymphoma regression in more than 60% of patients with MALT lymphoma of the ocular adnexa after doxycycline treatment [88]. Lymphoma regression was even observed in some lymphomas with no evidence of *C. psittaci* and/or failed eradication of *C. psittaci* infection.

Nodal Marginal Zone Lymphomas

The majority of patients with NMZL present with disseminated peripheral and/or abdominal nodal involvement. Bone marrow involvement occurs in less than half of patients, and peripheral blood involvement is rare. A serum monoclonal protein is detected in about 10% of patients. Interestingly, hepatitis C virus infection has been reported to be associated with NMZL. There is no current treatment consensus for NMZLs, but many patients are managed according to guidelines established for FL. In limited-stage disease, surgery and/or radiotherapy may be appropriate. In advanced-stage disease, chemoimmunotherapy is an option. In patients with hepatitis C virus-associated chronic hepatitis and no indication for immediate chemotherapy, antiviral treatment with pegylated interferon and ribavirin is recommended.

Splenic Marginal Zone Lymphomas

Splenic marginal zone lymphoma (SMZL) is a B-cell NHL consisting predominantly of small cells involving the white pulp follicles of the spleen, but it may also involve the splenic hilar lymph nodes, bone marrow, and peripheral blood. Most SMZL patients present with splenomegaly and abnormal blood cell counts, including anemia and/or thrombocytopenia (usually due to splenic sequestration rather than bone marrow infiltration) with lymphocytosis; patients commonly are asymptomatic. SMZL can be associated with autoimmune phenomena, including autoimmune hemolytic anemia or autoimmune thrombocytopenia. A subset of patients (10–40%) may also have a monoclonal paraprotein.

Treatment is required only in symptomatic patients (e.g., with symptomatic splenomegaly or cytopenias secondary to hypersplenism). Approximately one-third of patients with SMZL will never require therapy. Options for front-line therapy include: splenectomy, single-agent rituximab, and chemoimmunotherapy approaches similar to other forms of indolent B-cell NHL. Chemotherapy may be proposed to patients with contraindications to surgery, elderly patients, or those who have progression after surgery. Regimens are based on alkylating agents (i.e., chlorambucil or cyclophosphamide), fludarabine, or rituximab as a single agent or in combination with chemotherapy. Splenic irradiation represents an additional alternative.

Mantle Cell Lymphoma (MCL)

MCL comprises 5–7% of all non-Hodgkin lymphoma and is characterized by overexpression of cyclin D1, a cell cycle regulator that promotes proliferation, typically resulting from t(11,14). Commonly, patients present in their late 60s with advanced-stage disease and extranodal involvement [89–91], particularly in the gastrointestinal tract where involvement may be subtly detected on biopsy [92, 93] or extensively, as in the case of multiple lymphomatous polyposis [93–96]. Two studies independently estimated that >80% of patients with MCL have gastrointestinal tract involvement [92, 93]. MCL is thought to exhibit both aggressive and indolent phenotypes, but identifying patients with indolent disease remains difficult. Several research groups have defined indolence as stable disease without the need for treatment over a variable period of time [97–99].

First-Line Treatment

MCL remains a therapeutic challenge, as it is incurable with conventional chemotherapeutic approaches. Some clinical series and trials suggest that outcomes are improved with intensive induction regimens containing cytarabine (Ara-C) [100] and/or the use of high-dose therapy (HDT) and autologous stem cell transplantation (SCT) once patients achieve remission [101–105]. Given the demographics of this patient population, additional strategies such as maintenance have been explored for elderly patients not eligible for intensive consolidation, in an attempt to improve the duration of remission after induction [106]. There is no current consensus on the optimal initial management strategies for patients with untreated MCL in the US. Rummel and colleagues investigated a regimen of bendamustine plus rituximab (BR) versus R-CHOP for MCL, demonstrating a significantly longer PFS with BR [72]. Other authors have demonstrated a benefit for rituximab maintenance following chemoimmunotherapy which may be a useful approach for older individuals with MCL [107].

Relapsed MCL: A Signaling Approach

An exciting area of clinical research activity in MCL involves targeting the BCR signaling pathway. Activation of BCR engages the prosurvival nuclear factor kappa B (NF-κB) pathway [108]. Bortezomib, a proteasome inhibitor that inhibits NF-κB, received US Food and Drug Administration (FDA) approval for use in relapsed MCL based on results of a phase 2 multicenter trial that showed an ORR of 32% and 8% CR [109, 110]. Interestingly, in patients who achieved CR, median response duration and time to progression were not reached after a median follow-up of 26.4 months, with median OS of 36.0 months.

Ibrutinib is an orally available, highly selective, irreversible inhibitor of BTK that provides more direct targeting of BCR signaling pathway upstream. Early clinical studies involving ibrutinib demonstrated activity in several B-cell malignancies [111–113]. A phase 2 international study investigated the efficacy and safety of ibrutinib in patients with relapsed or refractory MCL [114]. With a median follow-up of ~15 months, the ORR in patients who received ibrutinib was 68%, with 21% achieving CR and 47% achieving PR. Importantly, response did not vary according to baseline characteristics or prior therapy, and responses improved over time with continued therapy. The estimated median PFS among treated patients was 13.9 months, and the median OS was not reached.

Mechanistic target of rapamycin (mTOR) kinase is a key downstream component of the PI3K/AKT pathway. Temsirolimus, a specific inhibitor of mTOR kinase, was associated with significant improvement in PFS (4.8 months vs 1.9 months, respectively) and ORR (22% vs 2%, respectively) in comparison to standard chemotherapeutic single agents in an open-label, randomized phase 3 study of patients with relapsed or refractory MCL [115]. However, median OS was not significantly different for the temsirolimus group and the investigator's choice group. Based on this study, temsirolimus is approved for relapsed MCL in Europe.

Although the precise mechanisms of action of lenalidomide, an analog of thalidomide, are unknown, its efficacy has been attributed to targeting the tumor microenvironment by enhancing the proliferative and functional capacity of T cells and increasing natural killer cell mediated antibody-dependent cell cytotoxicity [116–119]. Preliminary results of a multicenter phase 2 study investigating single-agent lenalidomide in MCL patients who had relapsed after or were refractory to bortezomib therapy led to FDA approval of lenalidomide for this patient population [120]. ORR was 28% (CR or CR unconfirmed 8%), median duration of response was 16.6 months, median PFS was 4 months, and median OS was 19 months. While these promising agents provide the foundation for constructing treatment strategies for MCL that avoid or limit the use of chemotherapy, additional studies are needed to determine the best ways to utilize and sequence these therapies.

Allogeneic Stem Cell Transplant

Evidence for graft-versus-lymphoma (GVL) effect in MCL is sparse, but long-term disease control seen after autologous SCT failure suggests that there is an important role for allogeneic SCT in MCL. The nonrelapse mortality for allogeneic SCT in MCL is higher than that reported for FL and CLL, even if RIC is applied [121]. This observation may be due to the more aggressive nature of mantle cell lymphoma. Single centers have reported long-term disease control rates of approximately 50% [121, 122] with allogeneic transplant.

Aggressive Lymphomas

Burkitt Lymphoma

Burkitt lymphoma (BL) is a highly aggressive NHL that often presents in extranodal sites or similarly to acute leukemia. The hallmark of this disease is the overexpression of c-*MYC*, most commonly resulting from t(8;14). Three different clinical variants of BL have been described: endemic (most commonly seen involving the jaw of children aged 4–7 years in equatorial Africa), sporadic (1– 2% of adult NHLs), and immunodeficiency BL (in HIV-infected patients). Symptoms at presentation may include abdominal pain, gastrointestinal bleeding, bowel obstruction, nausea, and vomiting. Bone marrow and central nervous system (CNS) involvement is reported in 30–38% of pediatric cases and 13–17% of adults, respectively [19].

BL is one of the few cancers that is routinely cured when diagnosed and treated appropriately. However, the diagnosis can be confounded by the overlapping morphology, immunophenotype, and t(8;14) translocations shared with diffuse large B cell lymphoma (DLBCL). Importantly, BL patients invariably relapse or progress when standard regimens for DLBCL are given. However, with high-intensity, brief-duration regimens, 65–100% of adults achieve CR, with 47–86% of patients maintaining these remissions at least 1 year following therapy[123–126]. Patients with BL can be successfully treated with cyclophosphamide, vincristine, doxorubicin, high-dose methotrexate/ifosfamide, etoposide, high-dose cytarabine (CODOX-M/IVAC), modified fractionated cyclophosphamide, vincristine, doxorubicin, and dexamethasone alternating with methotrexate and cytarabine (hyper-CVAD/MTX-Ara-C), and Cancer and Leukemia Group B (CALGB) 9251. Comparison of these treatment regimens is difficult in adult BL because of differences in pathology, staging, and patient populations across trials. Examining the genetic basis for the unique biological and clinical characteristics of BL [127] can aid in understanding why BL responds well to multiagent chemotherapy whereas most other cancers do not.

Diffuse Large B-Cell Lymphoma

Epidemiology

DLBCL is the most commonly occurring form of non-Hodgkin lymphoma (NHL) in the western world, encompassing approximately one-third of all lymphomas in adults. DLBCL represents a significant clinical problem in that it is a highly curable disease, but one that is universally fatal if untreated or improperly treated [128]. Untreated DLBCL patients have an expected survival of <1 year [59], whereas with modern therapy more than 50% of patients are alive and disease-free at 5 years [129–131]. Despite the high cure rates in this disease, outcomes remain heterogeneous. The median age at diagnosis for DLBCL is in the seventh decade, with patients commonly presenting with a rapidly enlarging, painless lymph node. However, in up to 40% of patients, the first site involved is extranodal. Approximately

15% of patients present with bone marrow involvement, about one-third have B symptoms (fever, night sweats, and weight loss), nearly half have stage III/IV disease, and more than half have an elevated serum LDH at diagnosis [132]. Patients diagnosed with DLBCL need to undergo full staging workup, which will help determine the treatment schedule and aid in predicting the expected likelihood of survival.

The IPI remains the primary clinical tool used to predict outcome for patients with DLBCL [133], and allows for patients to be stratified into four discrete groups: low risk, low intermediate risk, high intermediate risk, and high risk, with a 5-year OS ranging from 26% to 73%. For patients with IPI scores of 0–1, 2, 3, 4–5 points, the 5-year OS is 73%, 51%, 43%, and 26%, respectively. However, the IPI was developed prior to the era of rituximab. The revised IPI published by Sehn and colleagues defines three separate outcome categories [134]. Among patients treated with rituximab-containing regimens, those with zero risk factors had a >90% chance of 4-year PFS, those with 1–2 risk factors had ~80% expected PFS, and those with ≥3 risk factors had ~50% PFS. However, this system was not prospectively developed and has not been prospectively evaluated, so the original IPI method remains the best validated prognostic approach.

Pathophysiology

Growing knowledge of DLBCL biology has led to the understanding that DLBCL is composed of biologically distinct pathophysiologic entities, as initially described by Alizadeh, Staudt, and colleagues [135]. The subgrouping of DLBCL tumors with distinct gene expression patterns has been defined using hierarchical clustering and identifies signatures that have been associated with differences in cell of origin. One subtype clustered with normal germinal center B cells (GCB) and the other with activated B cells (ABC) [43]. The Lymphoma/Leukemia Molecular Profiling Project reported approximately 60% GCB and 40% non-GCB in 240 newly diagnosed DLBCL patient biopsy samples examined by gene expression [43, 136]. Importantly, patients with ABC DLBCL have a poorer prognosis than their GCB counterparts, an observation that has held up in the era of rituximab [137]. Because gene expression profiling is not yet readily applied in clinical practice, immunohistochemistry (IHC) algorithms have been developed and validated for classifying DLBCL into ABC and GCB subtypes, but it remains to be seen whether such algorithms will be incorporated outside the research setting [14–16].

First-Line Treatment

Limited Stage: Stage I/Contiguous Stage II Approximately one-third of DLBCL patients present with limited-stage disease, which includes Lugano stage I and non-bulky stage II disease and can be more clearly defined as disease contained within one irradiation field. Those patients presenting with bulky stage II disease (e.g., mass >10 cm) have similar outcomes as stage III and IV disease and should be treated as advanced-stage disease [13]. Most patients with non-bulky, limited-stage DLBCL are treated with combined modality therapy consisting of systemic chemotherapy (i.e., 2–4 cycles of CHOP) with rituximab, followed by locoregional radiation therapy. There have been several trials comparing chemotherapy followed by radiation therapy versus chemotherapy alone for patients with limited-stage lymphoma, with variable results [138–141], but all these trials were performed in the period prior to routine rituximab use, which allows for a continued debate as to the most appropriate treatment for patients with limited-stage disease. In addition, there are no definitive, randomized controlled trials in the era of rituximab comparing chemoimmunotherapy with or without radiation therapy [142].

Stage II Noncontiguous, Stage III and Stage IV For the majority of patients, DLBCL is a systemic disease at the time of diagnosis. Although the standard chemotherapy regimen has not significantly changed over the past three decades, the incorporation of monoclonal antibody therapy into the standard treatment program represents an improvement in OS for the majority of patients with DLBCL. CHOP was known to cure approximately 30% of patients with advanced stages of intermediate-grade or high-grade NHL [143, 144]. Then, in 2002, a randomized trial comparing CHOP and R-CHOP demonstrated that R-CHOP improved 2-year OS from 57% to 70% [145]. Follow-up data from this and other randomized trials confirmed the benefits of R-CHOP for 6 cycles, demonstrating cure in ~60% of patients and establishing the regimen as the standard of care in DLBCL [129–131, 146–148].

Second-Line Therapy

A number of standard regimens exist for salvage lymphoma therapy, including ICE (ifosfamide, carboplatin, etoposide), ESHAP (etoposide, methyl prednisolone, high-dose cytarabine, cisplatin), DHAP (dexamethasone, cisplatin, cytarabine), and GDP (dexamethasone, cisplatin, gemcitabine), with varying response rates. The choice of salvage therapy is still debated, although it is clear that the addition of rituximab to these re-induction regimens yields superior results compared to the same regimen without rituximab [149, 150]. The choice of salvage chemotherapy after R-CHOP failures was addressed by a prospective multicenter phase III study, the COllaborative trial in Relapsed Aggressive Lymphoma (CORAL) [151]. DLBCL patients in first relapse or who were refractory after first-line therapy were randomly assigned to salvage therapy with R-ICE or R-DHAP. After three courses of therapy, DLBCL patients who responded were treated with HDT and autologous SCT. The response rates for R-ICE and R-DHAP were identical, suggesting that either regimen can be used for salvage therapy. However, an analysis of the 396 patients enrolled on the trial also showed much poorer outcomes for patients who had: (i) second-line IPI score of 2/3 versus 0/1 (3-year event-free survival 18% vs 40%, respectively), (ii) relapse <12 months after completion of first-line therapy (20% vs 45%, respectively) or (iii) prior rituximab exposure in the front-line setting (21% vs 47%, respectively), regardless of their type of salvage therapy. Moreover, patients who relapsed early following upfront R-chemotherapy had a very poor prognosis with a 3-year PFS of 23%, which remained poor even when consolidated with HDT and autologous SCT (3-year PFS of 39%) [151].

Despite our understanding of the heterogeneity of DLBCL and an increasing number of treatment combinations and experimental agents, most clinicians continue to treat DLBCL with a single management strategy at initial presentation and at relapse. Novel approaches to managing patients with relapsed DLBCL are needed [62, 152]. Nevertheless, autologous transplantation remains a preferred option for relapsed patients with DLBCL who demonstrate evidence of chemosensitive disease.

Allogeneic Transplant for Diffuse Large B-Cell Lymphoma The optimal management of autologous SCT recipients experiencing DLBCL relapse is unknown. A third chemotherapy regimen may be administered in an attempt to attain another response. Patients with chemotherapy-sensitive disease may be candidates for an allogeneic SCT, preferably in the context of a clinical trial. In most centers in the US, patients are considered eligible for nonmyeloablative allogeneic SCT only if they are <65 years of age, with normal cardiac, liver, and renal function, and good performance status (Eastern Cooperative Oncology Group (ECOG) performance status 0 or 1). Eligibility for conventional myeloablative transplantation is typically restricted to patients younger than 55 years of age. There have been several studies reporting on the use of RIC allogeneic SCT for patients with DLCBL who have failed an autologous SCT [153, 154]. Although the nonrelapse mortality was <30% in most of these studies, the 3-year PFS rates were less than <40%, suggesting that the graft-versus-lymphoma effect for DLBCL may not be as strong as it is for FL or CLL.

Mature T-Cell Neoplasms

Peripheral T-Cell Lymphoma

PTCL is a heterogeneous group of NHLs characterized by poor treatment outcome with conventional chemotherapy. Despite great strides in the management of B-cell NHL, peripheral T-cell lymphoma (PTCL) remains a therapeutic challenge. Anthracycline-based chemotherapy remains the standard treatment for patients with PTCL. There are well-established favorable outcomes for patients with ALK-positive anaplastic large cell lymphomas (ALCL) [155] with CHOP, but such regimens have failed to induce sustained remissions for most patients. The International Peripheral T-cell Lymphoma Clinical and Pathologic Review Project retrospectively demonstrated no difference in OS comparing patients who did or did not receive an anthracycline [156]. Prior studies have established worse outcome for PTCL compared to aggressive B-cell NHL treated with anthracycline-based chemotherapy, in terms of response, relapse, and OS rates [157–159]. In a meta-analysis, the CR rate achieved with anthracycline-based regimens ranged from 36% in enteropathy-type T-cell lymphoma (ETTL) to 66% in ALCL [160]. Five-year OS across PTCL subtypes also ranged widely from 20% in ETTL to 57% in ALCL. ALCL patients had a markedly better 5-year OS than other PTCL patients (57% vs 37%, $P<0.001$).

Among patients who relapse, the median OS was only 5.5 months in a series of 153 patients (including 11 with ALK-positive anaplastic large cell lymphoma). This was only marginally improved to 6.5 months if a patient received chemotherapy at the time of relapse, an indication of the poor response to currently available therapy options [161]. Given the poor prognosis for most patients, patients with PTCL should be encouraged to enroll on prospective clinical trials at diagnosis and at relapse.

Follow-Up

There are few well-designed controlled trials that aid in determining the best approaches for surveillance in patients with NHL [162]. Although the routine use of surveillance imaging traditionally has been a common component of patient care, observational and modeling studies suggest that this approach to secondary screening provides limited benefits for detecting asymptomatic disease in a manner that improves overall survival [162–165]. The majority of patients with relapsed NHL present clinical signs or symptoms between imaging studies or at the same time as a scheduled imaging examination which prompts further evaluation. Ten percent or fewer patients experience relapse detected on a routine scan while being otherwise asymptomatic [165].

Because surveillance imaging is costly, might expose patients to minimal risks of radiation-related secondary cancers, and can produce false-positive findings leading to unnecessary biopsies, current recommendations suggest avoiding their routine use in asymptomatic NHL patients determined to be in complete remission. No prospective study has shown a significant improvement in survival for NHL patients who have relapse discovered on a routine scan versus those who present with clinical symptoms. Current national and international guidelines recommend that a medical history is taken and a physical examination is conducted every 3–6 months for 2–5 years, and subsequently once a year unless clinically indicated [166–169]. While many guidelines continue to recommend radiological examinations every 6 months for 2 years and annually thereafter, this approach is changing based on the findings previously discussed [162, 169]. While the identification of other late effects such as hypothyroidism, sexual dysfunction, cardiovascular disease, and secondary malignancies has been better articulated for survivors of Hodgkin lymphoma [170] these same risks of late effects are present for NHL survivors. Other surveillance strategies also are needed to detect these late effects and identify risk factors for them [170]. These interventions should be pursued for NHL patients who often are long-term survivors with indolent NHL or following cure of an aggressive NHL.

References

1 Siegel RL, Miller KD, Jemal A. Cancer statistics, 2017. *CA Cancer J Clin* 2017;67(1):7–30.

2 Howlader N, Noone AM, Krapcho M, *et al.* (eds). SEER Cancer Statistics Review, 1975-2013, National Cancer Institute. Bethesda, MD, http://seer.cancer.gov/csr/1975_2013/, based on November 2015 SEER data submission, posted to the SEER web site, April 2016.

3 Jaffe ES, Harris NL, Stein H, *et al. World Health Organization Classification of Tumours.* Pathology and Genetics of Tumours of Hematopoietic and Lymphoid Tissues. Lyon: IARC Press, 2001.

4 Teras LR, DeSantis CE, Cerhan JR, *et al.* 2016 US lymphoid malignancy statistics by World Health Organization subtypes. *CA Cancer J Clin* 2016;66(6):443–59
5 Flowers CR, Glover R, Lonial S, Brawley OW. Racial differences in the incidence and outcomes for patients with hematological malignancies. *Curr Probl Cancer* 2007;31(3):182–201.
6 Abouyabis AN, Shenoy PJ, Lechowicz MJ, Flowers CR. Incidence and outcomes of the peripheral T-cell lymphoma subtypes in the United States. *Leuk Lymphoma* 2008;49(11):2099–107.
7 Berry J, Bumpers K, Ogunlade V, *et al.* Examining racial disparities in colorectal cancer care. *J Psychosoc Oncol* 2009;27(1):59–83.
8 Imam MH, Shenoy PJ, Flowers CR, Phillips A, Lechowicz MJ. Incidence and survival patterns of cutaneous T-cell lymphomas in the United States. *Leuk Lymphoma* 2013;54(4):752–9
9 Nabhan C, Byrtek M, Taylor MD, *et al.* Racial differences in presentation and management of follicular non-Hodgkin lymphoma in the United States: report from the National LymphoCare Study. *Cancer* 2012;118(19):4842–50.
10 Shenoy PJ, Maggioncalda A, Malik N, Flowers CR. Incidence patterns and outcomes for hodgkin lymphoma patients in the United States. *Adv Hematol* 2011;2011:725219.
11 Shenoy PJ, Borate U, Bumpers K, *et al.* Examining the Racial Disparities In Presentation and Treatment for Patients with Diffuse Large B-Cell Lymphoma (DLBCL). *ASH Annual Meeting Abstracts.* 2010;116:1521.
12 Shenoy PJ, Bumpers K, King N, *et al.* Black/White Differences in the Treatment and Outcomes of Diffuse Large B Cell Lymphoma: A Matched Cohort Analysis. *ASH Annual Meeting Abstracts.* 2009;114(22):1392.
13 Shenoy PJ, Malik N, Nooka A, *et al.* Racial differences in the presentation and outcomes of diffuse large B-cell lymphoma in the United States. *Cancer* 2011;117(11):2530–40.
14 Shenoy PJ, Malik N, Sinha R, *et al.* Racial differences in the presentation and outcomes of chronic lymphocytic leukemia and variants in the United States. *Clin Lymphoma Myeloma Leuk* 2011;11(6):498–506.
15 Jaffe ES, Harris NL, Stein H, Isaacson PG. Classification of lymphoid neoplasms: the microscope as a tool for disease discovery. *Blood* 2008;112(12):4384–99.
16 Rosenwald A, Wright G, Leroy K, *et al.* Molecular diagnosis of primary mediastinal B cell lymphoma identifies a clinically favorable subgroup of diffuse large B cell lymphoma related to Hodgkin lymphoma. *J Exp Med* 2003;198(6):851–62.
17 Savage KJ, Monti S, Kutok JL, *et al.* The molecular signature of mediastinal large B-cell lymphoma differs from that of other diffuse large B-cell lymphomas and shares features with classical Hodgkin lymphoma. *Blood* 2003;102(12):3871–9.
18 Traverse-Glehen A, Pittaluga S, Gaulard P, *et al.* Mediastinal gray zone lymphoma: the missing link between classic Hodgkin's lymphoma and mediastinal large B-cell lymphoma. *Am J Surg Pathol* 2005;29(11):1411–21.
19 Swerdlow SH, Campo E, Pileri SA, *et al.* The 2016 revision of the World Health Organization classification of lymphoid neoplasms. *Blood* 2016;127(20):2375–90.
20 Taccioli GE, Rathbun G, Oltz E, *et al.* Impairment of V(D)J recombination in double-strand break repair mutants. *Science* 1993;260(5105):207–10.
21 Li Z, Woo CJ, Iglesias-Ussel MD, Ronai D, Scharff MD. The generation of antibody diversity through somatic hypermutation and class switch recombination. *Genes Dev* 2004;18(1):1–11.
22 Kridel R, Sehn LH, Gascoyne RD. Pathogenesis of follicular lymphoma. *J Clin Invest* 2012;122(10):3424–31.
23 Pérez-Galán P, Dreyling M, Wiestner A. Mantle cell lymphoma: biology, pathogenesis, and the molecular basis of treatment in the genomic era. *Blood* 2011;117(1):26–38.
24 Shaffer AL, Rosenwald A, Staudt LM. Decision making in the immune system: Lymphoid Malignancies: the dark side of B-cell differentiation. *Nat Rev Immunol* 2002;2(12):920.
25 Lenz G, Nagel I, Siebert R, *et al.* Aberrant immunoglobulin class switch recombination and switch translocations in activated B cell–like diffuse large B cell lymphoma. *J Exp Med* 2007;204(3):633–43.
26 Pasqualucci L, Trifonov V, Fabbri G, *et al.* Analysis of the coding genome of diffuse large B-cell lymphoma. *Nat Genet* 2011;43(9):830–7.
27 Xu-Monette ZY, Medeiros LJ, Li Y, *et al.* Dysfunction of the TP53 tumor suppressor gene in lymphoid malignancies. *Blood* 2012;119(16):3668–83.
28 Offit K, Wong G, Filippa D, Tao Y, Chaganti R. Cytogenetic analysis of 434 consecutively ascertained specimens of non-Hodgkin's lymphoma: clinical correlations. *Blood* 1991;77(7):1508–15.
29 Ping C, Allis CD, Wang GG. Covalent histone modifications – miswritten, misinterpreted and mis-erased in human cancers. *Nat Rev Cancer* 2010;10(7):457–69.
30 Esteller M, Gaidano G, Goodman SN, *et al.* Hypermethylation of the DNA repair gene O6-methylguanine DNA methyltransferase and survival of patients with diffuse large B-cell lymphoma. *J Natl Cancer Inst* 2002;94(1):26–32.
31 Shaknovich R, Melnick A. Epigenetics and B-cell lymphoma. *Curr Opin Hematol* 2011;18(4):293–9.
32 Ventura A, Young AG, Winslow MM, *et al.* Targeted deletion reveals essential and overlapping functions of the miR-17 ~ 92 family of miRNA clusters. *Cell* 2008;132(5):875–86.
33 Malumbres R, Sarosiek KA, Cubedo E, *et al.* Differentiation stage–specific expression of microRNAs in B lymphocytes and diffuse large B-cell lymphomas. *Blood* 2009;113(16):3754–64.
34 Klein U, Lia M, Crespo M, *et al.* The DLEU2/miR-15a/16-1 cluster controls B cell proliferation and its deletion leads to chronic lymphocytic leukemia. *Cancer Cell* 2010;17(1):28–40.
35 Di Lisio L, Martinez N, Montes-Moreno S, *et al.* The role of miRNAs in the pathogenesis and diagnosis of B-cell lymphomas. *Blood* 2012;120(9):1782–90.
36 Sánchez-Beato M, Sánchez-Aguilera A, Piris MA. Cell cycle deregulation in B-cell lymphomas. *Blood* 2003;101(4):1220–35.
37 Klapproth K, Wirth T. Advances in the understanding of MYC-induced lymphomagenesis. *Br J Haematol* 2010;149(4): 484–97.
38 Staudt LM. Oncogenic activation of NF-κB. *Cold Spring Harb Perspect Biol* 2010;2(6):a000109.
39 Jost PJ, Ruland J. Aberrant NF-κB signaling in lymphoma: mechanisms, consequences, and therapeutic implications. *Blood* 2007;109(7):2700–7.

40 Compagno M, Lim WK, Grunn A, *et al.* Mutations of multiple genes cause deregulation of NF-κB in diffuse large B-cell lymphoma. *Nature* 2009;459(7247):717–21.

41 Zhang J, Grubor V, Love CL, *et al.* Genetic heterogeneity of diffuse large B-cell lymphoma. *Proc Natl Acad Sci U S A* 2013;110(4):1398–403.

42 Lenz G, Davis RE, Ngo VN, *et al.* Oncogenic CARD11 mutations in human diffuse large B cell lymphoma. *Science* 2008;319(5870):1676–9.

43 Rosenwald A, Wright G, Chan WC, *et al.* The use of molecular profiling to predict survival after chemotherapy for diffuse large-B-cell lymphoma. *N Engl J Med* 2002;346(25):1937–47.

44 Basso K, Dalla-Favera R. Chapter 7. BCL6: Master regulator of the germinal center reaction and key oncogene in B cell lymphomagenesis. In: WA Frederick (ed.) *Advances in Immunology*. Volume 105. Academic Press, 2010:193–210.

45 Costello R, Sanchez C, Le Treut T, *et al.* Peripheral T-cell lymphoma gene expression profiling and potential therapeutic exploitations. *Br J Haematol* 2010;150(1):21–7.

46 Sun JC, Lanier LL. NK cell development, homeostasis and function: parallels with CD8+ T cells. *Nat Rev Immunol* 2011;11(10):645–57.

47 Shankland KR, Armitage JO, Hancock BW. Non-Hodgkin lymphoma. *Lancet* 380(9844):848–57.

48 Ferreri AJM, Govi S, Pileri SA, Savage KJ. Anaplastic large cell lymphoma, *ALK-positive. Crit Rev Oncol Hematol* 2012;83(2):293–302.

49 Miyazaki K, Yamaguchi M, Imai H, *et al.* Gene expression profiling of peripheral T-cell lymphoma including γδ T-cell lymphoma. *Blood* 2009;113(5):1071–4.

50 Vasmatzis G, Johnson SH, Knudson RA, *et al.* Genome-wide analysis reveals recurrent structural abnormalities of TP63 and other p53-related genes in peripheral T-cell lymphomas. *Blood* 2012;120(11):2280–9.

51 National Comprehensive Cancer Network (NCCN) Clinical Practice Guidelines in Oncology B cell Non-Hodgkin's Lymphoma, version 5.2017. http://wwwnccnorg/professionals/physician_gls/pdf/nhlpdf (accessed 22 October, 2017).

52 Cheson BD, Fisher RI, Barrington SF, *et al.* Recommendations for Initial Evaluation, Staging, and Response Assessment of Hodgkin and Non-Hodgkin Lymphoma: The Lugano Classification. *J Clin Oncol* 2014;32(27):3059–67.

53 Le Gouill S, Milpied N, Buzyn A, *et al.* Graft-versus-lymphoma effect for aggressive T-cell lymphomas in adults: a study by the Societe Francaise de Greffe de Moelle et de Therapie Cellulaire. *J Clin Oncol* 2008;26(14):2264–71.

54 Trotman J, Fournier M, Lamy T, *et al.* Positron emission tomography-computed tomography (PET-CT) after induction therapy is highly predictive of patient outcome in follicular lymphoma: analysis of PET-CT in a subset of PRIMA trial participants. *J Clin Oncol* 2011;29(23):3194–200.

55 Linet MS, Vajdic CM, Morton LM, *et al.* Medical history, lifestyle, family history, and occupational risk factors for follicular lymphoma: the InterLymph Non-Hodgkin Lymphoma Subtypes Project. *J Natl Cancer Inst Monogr* 2014;2014(48):26–40.

56 Chen Q, Ayer T, Nastoupil LJ, *et al.* Initial management strategies for follicular lymphoma. *Int J Hematol Oncol* 2012;1(1):35–45.

57 Nastoupil LJ, Sinha R, Byrtek M, *et al.* Comparison of the effectiveness of frontline chemoimmunotherapy regimens for follicular lymphoma used in the United States. *Leuk Lymphoma* 2015;56(5):1295–302.

58 Tan D, Horning SJ, Hoppe RT, *et al.* Improvements in observed and relative survival in follicular grade 1–2 lymphoma during 4 decades: the Stanford University experience. *Blood* 2013;122(6):981–7.

59 Flowers CR, Sinha R, Vose JM. Improving outcomes for patients with diffuse large B-cell lymphoma. *CA Cancer J Clin* 2010;60(6):393–408.

60 Friedberg JW, Byrtek M, Link BK, *et al.* Effectiveness of first-line management strategies for stage I follicular lymphoma: analysis of the National LymphoCare Study. *J Clin Oncol* 2012;30(27):3368–75.

61 Nastoupil LJ, Sinha R, Byrtek M, *et al.* The use and effectiveness of rituximab maintenance in patients with follicular lymphoma diagnosed between 2004 and 2007 in the United States. *Cancer* 2014;120(12):1830–7.

62 Flowers CR, Armitage JO. A decade of progress in lymphoma: advances and continuing challenges. *Clin Lymphoma Myeloma Leuk* 2010;10(6):414–23.

63 Cartron G, Watier H, Golay J, Solal-Celigny P. From the bench to the bedside: ways to improve rituximab efficacy. *Blood* 2004;104(9):2635–42.

64 Cragg MS, Bayne MC, Illidge TM, *et al.* Apparent modulation of CD20 by rituximab: an alternative explanation. *Blood* 2004;103(10):3989–90; author reply 90–1.

65 Flowers CR. Improving our use and understanding of antibodies in B-cell lymphomas. *Oncology (Williston Park)* 2010;24(2):176–7.

66 Ardeshna KM, Qian W, Smith P, *et al.* Rituximab versus a watch-and-wait approach in patients with advanced-stage, asymptomatic, non-bulky follicular lymphoma: an open-label randomised phase 3 trial. *Lancet Oncol* 2014;15(4):424–35.

67 Kahl BS, Hong F, Williams ME, *et al.* Rituximab extended schedule or re-treatment trial for low-tumor burden follicular lymphoma: Eastern Cooperative Oncology Group Protocol E4402. *J Clin Oncol* 2014;32(28):3096–102.

68 Kahl B. Is there a role for "watch and wait" in follicular lymphoma in the rituximab era? *Hematology Am Soc Hematol Educ Program* 2012;2012:433–8.

69 Solal-Celigny P, Bellei M, Marcheselli L, *et al.* Watchful waiting in low-tumor burden follicular lymphoma in the rituximab era: results of an F2-study database. *J Clin Oncol* 2012;30(31):3848–53.

70 Nooka AK, Nabhan C, Zhou X, *et al.* Examination of the follicular lymphoma international prognostic index (FLIPI) in the National LymphoCare study (NLCS): a prospective US patient cohort treated predominantly in community practices. *Ann Oncol* 2013;24(2):441–8.

71 Solal-Celigny P, Roy P, Colombat P, *et al.* Follicular lymphoma international prognostic index. *Blood* 2004;104(5):1258–65.

72 Rummel MJ, Niederle N, Maschmeyer G, *et al.* Bendamustine plus rituximab versus CHOP plus rituximab as first-line treatment for patients with indolent and mantle-cell lymphomas: an open-label, multicentre, randomised, phase 3 non-inferiority trial. *Lancet* 2013;381(9873):1203–10.

73 Salles G, Seymour JF, Offner F, *et al.* Rituximab maintenance for 2 years in patients with high tumour burden follicular lymphoma responding to rituximab plus chemotherapy (PRIMA): a phase 3, randomised controlled trial. *Lancet* 2011;377(9759):42–51.

74 Morschhauser F, Radford J, Van Hoof A, *et al.* 90Yttrium-ibritumomab tiuxetan consolidation of first remission in advanced-stage follicular non-Hodgkin lymphoma: updated results after a median follow-up of 7.3 years from the International, Randomized, Phase III First-LineIndolent trial. *J Clin Oncol* 2013;31(16):1977–83.

75 Brice P, Simon D, Bouabdallah R, *et al.* High-dose therapy with autologous stem-cell transplantation (ASCT) after first progression prolonged survival of follicular lymphoma patients included in the prospective GELF 86 protocol. *Ann Oncol* 2000;11(12):1585–90.

76 Gopal AK, Kahl BS, de Vos S, *et al.* PI3Kdelta inhibition by idelalisib in patients with relapsed indolent lymphoma. *N Engl J Med* 2014;370(11):1008–18.

77 Kahl BS, Bartlett NL, Leonard JP, *et al.* Bendamustine is effective therapy in patients with rituximab-refractory, indolent B-cell non-Hodgkin lymphoma: results from a Multicenter Study. *Cancer* 2010;116(1):106–14.

78 Sehn LH, Chua N, Mayer J, *et al.* Obinutuzumab plus bendamustine versus bendamustine monotherapy in patients with rituximab-refractory indolent non-Hodgkin lymphoma (GADOLIN): a randomised, controlled, open-label, multicentre, phase 3 trial. *Lancet Oncol* 2016;17(8):1081–93.

79 Thomson KJ, Morris EC, Bloor A, *et al.* Favorable long-term survival after reduced-intensity allogeneic transplantation for multiple-relapse aggressive non-Hodgkin's lymphoma. *J Clin Oncol* 2009;27(3):426–32.

80 Delgado J, Canals C, Attal M, *et al.* The role of in vivo T-cell depletion on reduced-intensity conditioning allogeneic stem cell transplantation from HLA-identical siblings in patients with follicular lymphoma. *Leukemia* 2011;25(3):551–5.

81 Raderer M, Kiesewetter B, Ferreri AJ. Clinicopathologic characteristics and treatment of marginal zone lymphoma of mucosa-associated lymphoid tissue (MALT lymphoma). *CA Cancer J Clin* 2015;66(2):152–71.

82 Malfertheiner P, Megraud F, O'Morain C, *et al.* Current concepts in the management of Helicobacter pylori infection: the Maastricht III Consensus Report. *Gut* 2007;56(6):772–81.

83 Chey WD, Wong BC, Practice Parameters Committee of the American College of Gastroenterology. American College of Gastroenterology guideline on the management of Helicobacter pylori infection. *Am J Gastroenterol* 2007;102(8):1808–25.

84 Hancock BW, Qian W, Linch D, *et al.* Chlorambucil versus observation after anti-Helicobacter therapy in gastric MALT lymphomas: results of the international randomised LY03 trial. *Br J Haematol* 2009;144(3):367–75.

85 Koch P, Probst A, Berdel WE, *et al.* Treatment results in localized primary gastric lymphoma: data of patients registered within the German multicenter study (GIT NHL 02/96). *J Clin Oncol* 2005;23(28):7050–9.

86 Zucca E, Conconi A, Martinelli G, et al. Chlorambucil plus rituximab produces better eventfree survival in comparison with chlorambucil alone in the treatment of MALT lymphoma: 5-year analysis of the 2-arms part of the IELSG-19 randomized study [abstract]. Blood (ASH Annual Meeting Abstracts) 2010;116:432. 2010.

87 Zinzani PL, Stefoni V, Musuraca G, *et al.* Fludarabine-containing chemotherapy as frontline treatment of nongastrointestinal mucosa-associated lymphoid tissue lymphoma. *Cancer* 2004;100(10):2190–4.

88 Ferreri AJ, Govi S, Pasini E, *et al.* Chlamydophila psittaci eradication with doxycycline as first-line targeted therapy for ocular adnexae lymphoma: final results of an international phase II trial. *J Clin Oncol* 2012;30(24):2988–94.

89 Zhou Y, Wang H, Fang W, *et al.* Incidence trends of mantle cell lymphoma in the United States between 1992 and 2004. *Cancer* 2008;113(4):791–8.

90 Ambinder AJ, Shenoy PJ, Nastoupil LJ, Flowers CR. Using primary site as a predictor of survival in mantle cell lymphoma. *Cancer* 2013;119(8):1570–7.

91 A clinical evaluation of the International Lymphoma Study Group classification of non-Hodgkin's lymphoma. The Non-Hodgkin's Lymphoma Classification Project. *Blood* 1997;89(11):3909–18.

92 Romaguera JE, Medeiros LJ, Hagemeister FB, *et al.* Frequency of gastrointestinal involvement and its clinical significance in mantle cell lymphoma. *Cancer* 2003;97(3):586–91.

93 Salar A, Juanpere N, Bellosillo B, *et al.* Gastrointestinal involvement in mantle cell lymphoma: a prospective clinic, endoscopic, and pathologic study. *Am J Surg Pathol* 2006;30(10):1274–80.

94 Isaacson PG, Spencer J, Wright DH. Classifying primary gut lymphomas. *Lancet* 1988;2(8620):1148–9.

95 Lavergne A, Brouland JP, Launay E, *et al.* Multiple lymphomatous polyposis of the gastrointestinal tract. An extensive histopathologic and immunohistochemical study of 12 cases. *Cancer* 1994;74(11):3042–50.

96 Fraga M, Lloret E, Sanchez-Verde L, Orradre JL, Campo E, Bosch F, et al. Mucosal mantle cell (centrocytic) lymphomas. *Histopathology.* 1995;26(5):413–22.

97 Martin P, Chadburn A, Christos P, *et al.* Outcome of deferred initial therapy in mantle-cell lymphoma. *J Clin Oncol* 2009;27(8):1209–13.

98 Fernandez V, Salamero O, Espinet B, *et al.* Genomic and gene expression profiling defines indolent forms of mantle cell lymphoma. *Cancer Res* 2010;70(4):1408–18.

99 Nygren L, Baumgartner Wennerholm S, *et al.* Prognostic role of SOX11 in a population-based cohort of mantle cell lymphoma. *Blood* 2012;119(18):4215–23.

100 Romaguera JE, Fayad LE, Feng L, *et al.* Ten-year follow-up after intense chemoimmunotherapy with Rituximab-HyperCVAD alternating with Rituximab-high dose methotrexate/cytarabine (R-MA) and without stem cell transplantation in patients with untreated aggressive mantle cell lymphoma. *Br J Haematol* 2010;150(2):200–8.

101 Dreyling M, Lenz G, Hoster E, *et al.* Early consolidation by myeloablative radiochemotherapy followed by autologous stem cell transplantation in first remission significantly prolongs progression-free survival in mantle-cell lymphoma: results of a prospective randomized trial of the European MCL Network. *Blood* 2005;105(7):2677–84.

102 Delarue R, Haioun C, Ribrag V, *et al.* CHOP and DHAP plus rituximab followed by autologous stem cell transplantation in mantle cell lymphoma: a phase 2 study from the Groupe d'Etude des Lymphomes de l'Adulte. *Blood* 2013;121(1):48–53.

103 Damon LE, Johnson JL, Niedzwiecki D, *et al.* Immunochemotherapy and autologous stem-cell transplantation for untreated patients with mantle-cell lymphoma: CALGB 59909. *J Clin Oncol* 2009;27(36):6101–8.

104 Geisler CH, Kolstad A, Laurell A, *et al.* Long-term progression-free survival of mantle cell lymphoma after intensive front-line immunochemotherapy with in vivo-purged stem cell rescue: a nonrandomized phase 2 multicenter study by the Nordic Lymphoma Group. *Blood* 2008;112(7):2687–93.

105 Weisenburger DD, Vose JM, Greiner TC, *et al.* Mantle cell lymphoma. A clinicopathologic study of 68 cases from the Nebraska Lymphoma Study Group. *Am J Hematol* 2000;64(3):190–6.

106 Kluin-Nelemans HC, Hoster E, Hermine O, *et al.* Treatment of older patients with mantle-cell lymphoma. *N Engl J Med* 2012;367(6):520–31.

107 Forstpointner R, Unterhalt M, Dreyling M, *et al.* Maintenance therapy with rituximab leads to a significant prolongation of response duration after salvage therapy with a combination of rituximab, fludarabine, cyclophosphamide, and mitoxantrone (R-FCM) in patients with recurring and refractory follicular and mantle cell lymphomas: Results of a prospective randomized study of the German Low Grade Lymphoma Study Group (GLSG). *Blood* 2006;108(13):4003–8.

108 Lim KH, Yang Y, Staudt LM. Pathogenetic importance and therapeutic implications of NF-kappaB in lymphoid malignancies. *Immunol Rev* 2012;246(1):359–78.

109 Fisher RI, Bernstein SH, Kahl BS, *et al.* Multicenter phase II study of bortezomib in patients with relapsed or refractory mantle cell lymphoma. *J Clin Oncol* 2006;24(30):4867–74.

110 Goy A, Bernstein SH, Kahl BS, *et al.* Bortezomib in patients with relapsed or refractory mantle cell lymphoma: updated time-to-event analyses of the multicenter phase 2 PINNACLE study. *Ann Oncol* 2009;20(3):520–5.

111 Advani RH, Buggy JJ, Sharman JP, *et al.* Bruton tyrosine kinase inhibitor ibrutinib (PCI-32765) has significant activity in patients with relapsed/refractory B-cell malignancies. *J Clin Oncol* 2013;31(1):88–94.

112 Herman SE, Gordon AL, Hertlein E, *et al.* Bruton tyrosine kinase represents a promising therapeutic target for treatment of chronic lymphocytic leukemia and is effectively targeted by PCI-32765. *Blood* 2011;117(23):6287–96.

113 Byrd JC, Furman RR, Coutre SE, *et al.* Targeting BTK with ibrutinib in relapsed chronic lymphocytic leukemia. *N Engl J Med* 2013;369(1):32–42.

114 Wang ML, Rule S, Martin P, *et al.* Targeting BTK with ibrutinib in relapsed or refractory mantle-cell lymphoma. *N Engl J Med* 2013;369(6):507–16.

115 Hess G, Herbrecht R, Romaguera J, *et al.* Phase III study to evaluate temsirolimus compared with investigator's choice therapy for the treatment of relapsed or refractory mantle cell lymphoma. *J Clin Oncol* 2009;27(23):3822–9.

116 Chanan-Khan AA, Chitta K, Ersing N, *et al.* Biological effects and clinical significance of lenalidomide-induced tumour flare reaction in patients with chronic lymphocytic leukaemia: in vivo evidence of immune activation and antitumour response. *Br J Haematol* 2011;155(4):457–67.

117 Chang DH, Liu N, Klimek V, *et al.* Enhancement of ligand-dependent activation of human natural killer T cells by lenalidomide: therapeutic implications. *Blood* 2006;108(2):618–21.

118 Wu L, Adams M, Carter T, *et al.* Lenalidomide enhances natural killer cell and monocyte-mediated antibody-dependent cellular cytotoxicity of rituximab-treated CD20+ tumor cells. *Clin Cancer Res* 2008;14(14):4650–7.

119 Ramsay AG, Clear AJ, Kelly G, *et al.* Follicular lymphoma cells induce T-cell immunologic synapse dysfunction that can be repaired with lenalidomide: implications for the tumor microenvironment and immunotherapy. *Blood* 2009;114(21):4713–20.

120 Goy A, Sinha R, Williams ME, *et al.* Phase II multicenter study of single-agent lenalidomide in subjects with mantle cell lymphoma who relapsed or progressed after or were refractory to bortezomib: The MCL-001 "EMERGE" Study. Blood (ASH Annual Meeting Abstracts) 2012;120:Abstract 905.

121 Dreger P, Dohner H, Ritgen M, *et al.* Allogeneic stem cell transplantation provides durable disease control in poor-risk chronic lymphocytic leukemia: long-term clinical and MRD results of the German CLL Study Group CLL3X trial. *Blood* 2010;116(14):2438–47.

122 Tam CS, Bassett R, Ledesma C, *et al.* Mature results of the M. D. Anderson Cancer Center risk-adapted transplantation strategy in mantle cell lymphoma. *Blood* 2009;113(18):4144–52.

123 Magrath I, Adde M, Shad A, *et al.* Adults and children with small non-cleaved-cell lymphoma have a similar excellent outcome when treated with the same chemotherapy regimen. *J Clin Oncol* 1996;14(3):925–34.

124 McMaster ML, Greer JP, Greco FA, *et al.* Effective treatment of small-noncleaved-cell lymphoma with high-intensity, brief-duration chemotherapy. *J Clin Oncol* 1991;9(6):941–6.

125 Mead GM, Sydes MR, Walewski J, *et al.* An international evaluation of CODOX-M and CODOX-M alternating with IVAC in adult Burkitt's lymphoma: results of United Kingdom Lymphoma Group LY06 study. *Ann Oncol* 2002;13(8):1264–74.

126 Thomas DA, Cortes J, O'Brien S, *et al.* Hyper-CVAD program in Burkitt's-type adult acute lymphoblastic leukemia. *J Clin Oncol* 1999;17(8):2461–70.

127 Love C, Sun Z, Jima D, *et al.* The genetic landscape of mutations in Burkitt lymphoma. *Nat Genet* 2012;44(12):1321–5.

128 Sinha R, Nastoupil LJ, Flowers C. Treatment strategies for patients with diffuse large B-cell lymphoma: Past, present, and future. *Blood Lymphat Cancer* 2012;2012(2):87–98.

129 Coiffier B, Thieblemont C, Van Den Neste E, *et al.* Long-term outcome of patients in the LNH-98.5 trial, the first randomized study comparing rituximab-CHOP to standard CHOP chemotherapy in DLBCL patients: a study by the Groupe d'Etudes des Lymphomes de l'Adulte. *Blood* 2010;116(12):2040–5.

130 Feugier P, Van Hoof A, Sebban C, *et al.* Long-term results of the R-CHOP study in the treatment of elderly patients with diffuse large B-cell lymphoma: a study by the Groupe d'Etude des Lymphomes de l'Adulte. *J Clin Oncol* 2005;23(18):4117–26.

131 Pfreundschuh M, Kuhnt E, Trumper L, *et al.* CHOP-like chemotherapy with or without rituximab in young patients with good-prognosis diffuse large-B-cell lymphoma: 6-year results of an open-label randomised study of the MabThera International Trial (MInT) Group. *Lancet Oncol* 2011;12(11):1013–22.

132 Friedberg JW, Fisher RI. Diffuse large B-cell lymphoma. *Hematol Oncol Clin North Am* 2008;22(5):941–52, ix.

133 A predictive model for aggressive non-Hodgkin's lymphoma. The International Non-Hodgkin's Lymphoma Prognostic Factors Project. *N Engl J Med* 1993;329(14):987–94.

134 Sehn LH, Berry B, Chhanabhai M, *et al.* The revised International Prognostic Index (R-IPI) is a better predictor of outcome than the standard IPI for patients with diffuse large B-cell lymphoma treated with R-CHOP. *Blood* 2007;109(5):1857–61.

135 Alizadeh AA, Eisen MB, Davis RE, *et al.* Distinct types of diffuse large B-cell lymphoma identified by gene expression profiling. *Nature* 2000;403(6769):503–11.

136 Fu K, Weisenburger DD, Choi WW, *et al.* Addition of rituximab to standard chemotherapy improves the survival of both the germinal center B-cell-like and non-germinal center B-cell-like subtypes of diffuse large B-cell lymphoma. *J Clin Oncol* 2008;26(28):4587–94.

137 Read JA, Koff JL, Nastoupil LJ, *et al.* Evaluating cell-of-origin subtype methods for predicting diffuse large B-cell lymphoma survival: a meta-analysis of gene expression profiling and immunohistochemistry algorithms. *Clin Lymphoma Myeloma Leuk* 2014;14(6):460–7 e2.

138 Miller TP, Dahlberg S, Cassady JR, *et al.* Chemotherapy alone compared with chemotherapy plus radiotherapy for localized intermediate- and high-grade non-Hodgkin's lymphoma. *N Engl J Med* 1998;339(1):21–6.

139 Reyes F, Lepage E, Ganem G, *et al.* ACVBP versus CHOP plus radiotherapy for localized aggressive lymphoma. *N Engl J Med* 2005;352(12):1197–205.

140 Horning SJ, Weller E, Kim K, *et al.* Chemotherapy with or without radiotherapy in limited-stage diffuse aggressive non-Hodgkin's lymphoma: Eastern Cooperative Oncology Group study 1484. *J Clin Oncol* 2004;22(15):3032–8.

141 Bonnet C, Fillet G, Mounier N, *et al.* CHOP alone compared with CHOP plus radiotherapy for localized aggressive lymphoma in elderly patients: a study by the Groupe d'Etude des Lymphomes de l'Adulte. *J Clin Oncol* 2007;25(7):787–92.

142 Persky DO, Unger JM, Spier CM, *et al.* Phase II study of rituximab plus three cycles of CHOP and involved-field radiotherapy for patients with limited-stage aggressive B-cell lymphoma: Southwest Oncology Group study 0014. *J Clin Oncol* 2008;26(14):2258–63.

143 Fisher RI, Gaynor ER, Dahlberg S, *et al.* Comparison of a standard regimen (CHOP) with three intensive chemotherapy regimens for advanced non-Hodgkin's lymphoma. *N Engl J Med* 1993;328(14):1002–6.

144 McKelvey EM, Gottlieb JA, Wilson HE, *et al.* Hydroxyldaunomycin (Adriamycin) combination chemotherapy in malignant lymphoma. *Cancer* 1976;38(4):1484–93.

145 Coiffier B, Lepage E, Briere J, *et al.* CHOP chemotherapy plus rituximab compared with CHOP alone in elderly patients with diffuse large-B-cell lymphoma. *N Engl J Med* 2002;346(4):235–42.

146 Coiffier B, Feugier P, Mounier N, *et al.* Long-term results of the GELA study comparing R-CHOP and CHOP chemotherapy in older patients with diffuse large B-cell lymphoma show good survival in poor-risk patientsthe Groupe d'Etude des Lymphomes de l'Adulte. J Clin Oncol ASCO Annual Meeting Proceedings Part I. 2007;25(18S):Abstract#8009.

147 Pfreundschuh MG, Trumper L, Ma D, *et al.* Randomized intergroup trial of first line treatment for patients < =60 years with diffuse large B-cell non-Hodgkin's lymphoma (DLBCL) with a CHOP-like regimen with or without the anti-CD20 antibody rituximab – early stopping after the first interim analysis. Proc Am Soc Clin Oncol 2004:Abstract #6500

148 Habermann TM, Weller EA, Morrison VA, *et al.* Rituximab-CHOP versus CHOP alone or with maintenance rituximab in older patients with diffuse large B-cell lymphoma. *J Clin Oncol* 2006;24(19):3121–7.

149 Fenske TS, Hari PN, Carreras J, *et al.* Impact of pre-transplant rituximab on survival after autologous hematopoietic stem cell transplantation for diffuse large B cell lymphoma. *Biol Blood Marrow Transplant* 2009;15(11):1455–64.

150 Kewalramani T, Zelenetz AD, Nimer SD, *et al.* Rituximab and ICE as second-line therapy before autologous stem cell transplantation for relapsed or primary refractory diffuse large B-cell lymphoma. *Blood* 2004;103(10):3684–8.

151 Gisselbrecht C, Glass B, Mounier N. R-ICE versus R-DHAP in relapsed patients with CD20 diffuse large B cell lymphoma (DLBCL) followed by an autologous transplantation: CORAL study. J Clin Oncol 2009;27(Abstract 8509).

152 Lonial S, Arellano M, Hutcherson D, *et al.* Results of a clinical phase I dose-escalation study of cytarabine in combination with fixed-dose vinorelbine, paclitaxel, etoposide and cisplatin for the treatment of relapsed/refractory lymphoma. *Leuk Lymphoma* 2006;47(10):2155–62.

153 Sirvent A, Dhedin N, Michallet M, *et al.* Low nonrelapse mortality and prolonged long-term survival after reduced-intensity allogeneic stem cell transplantation for relapsed or refractory diffuse large B cell lymphoma: report of the Societe Francaise de Greffe de Moelle et de Therapie Cellulaire. *Biol Blood Marrow Transplant* 2010;16(1):78–85.

154 Rezvani AR, Norasetthada L, Gooley T, *et al.* Non-myeloablative allogeneic haematopoietic cell transplantation for relapsed diffuse large B-cell lymphoma: a multicentre experience. *Br J Haematol* 2008;143(3):395–403.

155 Savage KJ. Prognosis and Primary Therapy in Peripheral T-cell Lymphomas. Hematology Am Soc Hematol Educ Program 2008:280–8.

156 Vose JM, Armitage J, Weisenburger D. International Peripheral T-Cell and Natural Killer/T-Cell Lymphoma

Study: Pathology Findings and Clinical Outcomes. *J Clin Oncol* 2008;26(25):4124–30.

157 Cheung MM, Chan JK, Lau WH, *et al.* Primary non-Hodgkin's lymphoma of the nose and nasopharynx: clinical features, tumor immunophenotype, and treatment outcome in 113 patients. *J Clin Oncol* 1998;16(1):70–7.

158 Coiffier B, Brousse N, Peuchmaur M, *et al.* Peripheral T-cell lymphomas have a worse prognosis than B-cell lymphomas: a prospective study of 361 immunophenotyped patients treated with the LNH-84 regimen. The GELA (Groupe d'Etude des Lymphomes Agressives). *Ann Oncol* 1990;1(1):45–50.

159 Gisselbrecht C, Gaulard P, Lepage E, *et al.* Prognostic significance of T-cell phenotype in aggressive non-Hodgkin's lymphomas. Groupe d'Etudes des Lymphomes de l'Adulte (GELA). *Blood* 1998;92(1):76–82.

160 Abouyabis AN, Shenoy PJ, Sinha R, Flowers CR, Lechowicz MJ. A systematic review and meta-analysis of front-line anthracycline-based chemotherapy regimens for peripheral T-cell lymphoma. *ISRN Hematol* 2011;2011:623924.

161 Mak V, Hamm J, Chhanabhai M, *et al.* Survival of patients with peripheral T-cell lymphoma after first relapse or progression: spectrum of disease and rare long-term survivors. *J Clin Oncol* 2013;31(16):1970–6.

162 Cohen JB, Flowers CR. Optimal disease surveillance strategies in non-Hodgkin lymphoma. *ASH Education Program Book* 2014;2014(1):481–7.

163 Brenner DJ, Hall EJ. Computed tomography – an increasing source of radiation exposure. *N Engl J Med* 2007;357(22):2277–84.

164 Shenoy P, Sinha R, Tumeh JW, Lechowicz MJ, Flowers CR. Surveillance computed tomography scans for patients with lymphoma: is the risk worth the benefits? *Clin Lymphoma Myeloma Leuk* 2010;10(4):270–7.

165 Thompson CA, Ghesquieres H, Maurer MJ, *et al.* Utility of routine post-therapy surveillance imaging in diffuse large B-cell lymphoma. *J Clin Oncol* 2014;32(31):3506–12.

166 Dreyling M. Newly diagnosed and relapsed follicular lymphoma: ESMO Clinical Practice Guidelines for diagnosis, treatment and follow-up. *Ann Oncol* 2010;21 Suppl 5:v181–3.

167 Tilly H, Dreyling M. Diffuse large B-cell non-Hodgkin's lymphoma: ESMO Clinical Practice Guidelines for diagnosis, treatment and follow-up. *Ann Oncol* 2010;21 Suppl 5:v172–4.

168 Ng A, Constine L, Advani R, *et al.* ACR Appropriateness Criteria (R): Follow-Up of Hodgkin's Lymphoma. *Curr Prob Cancer* 2010;34(3):211–27.

169 Cheson BD, Fisher RI, Barrington SF, *et al.* Recommendations for initial evaluation, staging, and response assessment of Hodgkin and non-Hodgkin lymphoma: the Lugano classification. *J Clin Oncol* 2014;32(27):3059–68.

170 Ng AK. Current survivorship recommendations for patients with Hodgkin lymphoma: focus on late effects. *ASH Education Program Book* 2014;2014(1):488–94.

171 Hoster E, Dreyling M, Klapper W, *et al.* A new prognostic index (MIPI) for patients with advanced-stage mantle cell lymphoma. *Blood* 2008;111(2):558–65.

33

Multiple Myeloma

Giada Bianchi and Kenneth C. Anderson

Dana Farber Cancer Institute, Boston, Massachusetts, USA

Incidence and Mortality

Multiple myeloma (MM) represents 1.8% of all newly diagnosed cancer in the United States (US), with 30,280 new cases and 12,590 deaths estimated for the year 2017 [1]. Median age at diagnosis is 69 years, and the age-adjusted incidence rate is 6.5 per 100,000 men and women per year with a male predominance (8.2 vs 5.2 per 100,000 per year for men and women, respectively). Incidence and mortality rates among Blacks are approximately twice those of Whites; in contrast, incidence and mortality rates are lower for Asians/Pacific Islanders and American Indians/Alaska Natives. Median age of death is 75 years, with age-adjusted death rates of 4.2 and 2.7 per 100,000 persons per year for men and women, respectively [2].

Risk Factors and Prevention

Although several risk factors for MM have been identified, the exact etiopathogenic mechanism of the disease is largely unknown.

Environmental and occupational exposures: Nuclear radiation and petroleum products exposures are the only recognized environmental risk factors. However, a higher than expected incidence in farmers and wood and leather manufacturers raises the suspicion for other unidentified environmental exposures.

Prior B-cell neoplasia: The occurrence of B-cell neoplasia, including MM and its precursors, monoclonal gammopathy of undetermined significance (MGUS) and smoldering MM (SMM), in family clusters was first recognized over 50 years ago.

Family history: Recent epidemiologic studies have reported an increased incidence of MM in first-degree relatives of patients with MGUS or MM, further suggesting a genetic predisposition. Nonparametric and parametric linkage analysis in familial cases of MM and/or MGUS identified the loci 1q and 4q as the regions of interest for genetic mutations [3]. The hyperphosphorylated form of Paratarg-7 (P-7), a protein of unknown function, is inherited as an autosomal dominant trait in familial cases of MM and MGUS, suggesting a potential pathogenic role [4].

Other cancers: Approximately 10% of MM patients are diagnosed with another primary neoplasm, most commonly a solid tumor, although a higher than expected incidence of acute myeloid leukemia and myelodysplastic syndrome has been noted in patients with immunoglobulin (Ig) A and IgG MGUS [5].

Etiopathogenesis

MM is believed to be a cancer of long-lived plasma cells (PCs) [6]. These long-lived PCs home to and survive in the bone marrow (BM) niche rather than undergo apoptosis after a few days of intense Ig production as short-lived PCs. Long-lived PCs produce low-titer, high-affinity antibodies for months to years, thus contributing to immunological memory [7]. B cells differentiate into long-lived PCs after encountering a specific antigen and maturing in the germinal center (GC). In a T-helper mediated process, naïve B lymphocytes undergo proliferation and Ig class switching, as well as rearrangement and somatic mutation of the V(D)J sequence within the GC to give rise to either memory B cells or PCs [8]. Gene sequence analysis of the Ig variable region (VH) of MM cells (MMCs) showed a common, monoclonal, mutated sequence, thus confirming their post-GC origin [9]. Interestingly, no subclones were identified based on IgVH in primary MMCs, arguing against continued hypermutation [10]. Indeed, based on antigenic profile analysis, the early genetic mutations in MM occur at the pre-B cell stage, while the crucial oncogenic process appears to take place after terminal differentiation into antibody-secreting PCs [11]. Two recent studies showed MM to be (almost) inevitably preceded by MGUS, a premalignant, common condition with a 1% per year, life-long risk of progression to MM or other B-cell malignancies [12, 13]. The molecular bases underlying the malignant evolution of MGUS have not yet been delineated [14]. However, on the base of retrospective epidemiologic studies, non-IgG Ig

The American Cancer Society's Oncology in Practice: Clinical Management, First Edition. Edited by The American Cancer Society.

subtype, elevated monoclonal (M) protein, and abnormal serum free light chain (FLC) ratio have been identified as risk factors for progression of MGUS to MM or lymphoproliferative syndrome [15]. A risk progression model based on the proportion of malignant PCs detected via multiparametric flow cytometry within the pool of BM PCs has also recently been developed. Combined with DNA aneuploidy in the malignant clone, a 95% preponderance of malignant PCs predicted a risk of evolution to active MM of almost 50% at 5 years, compared to 10% and 2% risk when one or none of the two risk factors was detected, respectively [16].

Histopathology and Molecular Pathology

MM histological diagnosis is based on the presence of an excess of monotypic malignant PCs in the BM. Extramedullary localization of MMCs occurs in solitary plasmacytoma and/or in advanced, aggressive disease when malignant cells can be detected in the peripheral blood (plasma cell leukemia), pleural or pericardial fluid, skin, and/or parenchymal tissues. On microscopy, MMCs appear large, round or oval-shaped with an eccentric nucleus and coarsely clumped chromatin, along with abundant basophilic cytoplasm (Figure 33.1). A perinuclear clear area is usually visible

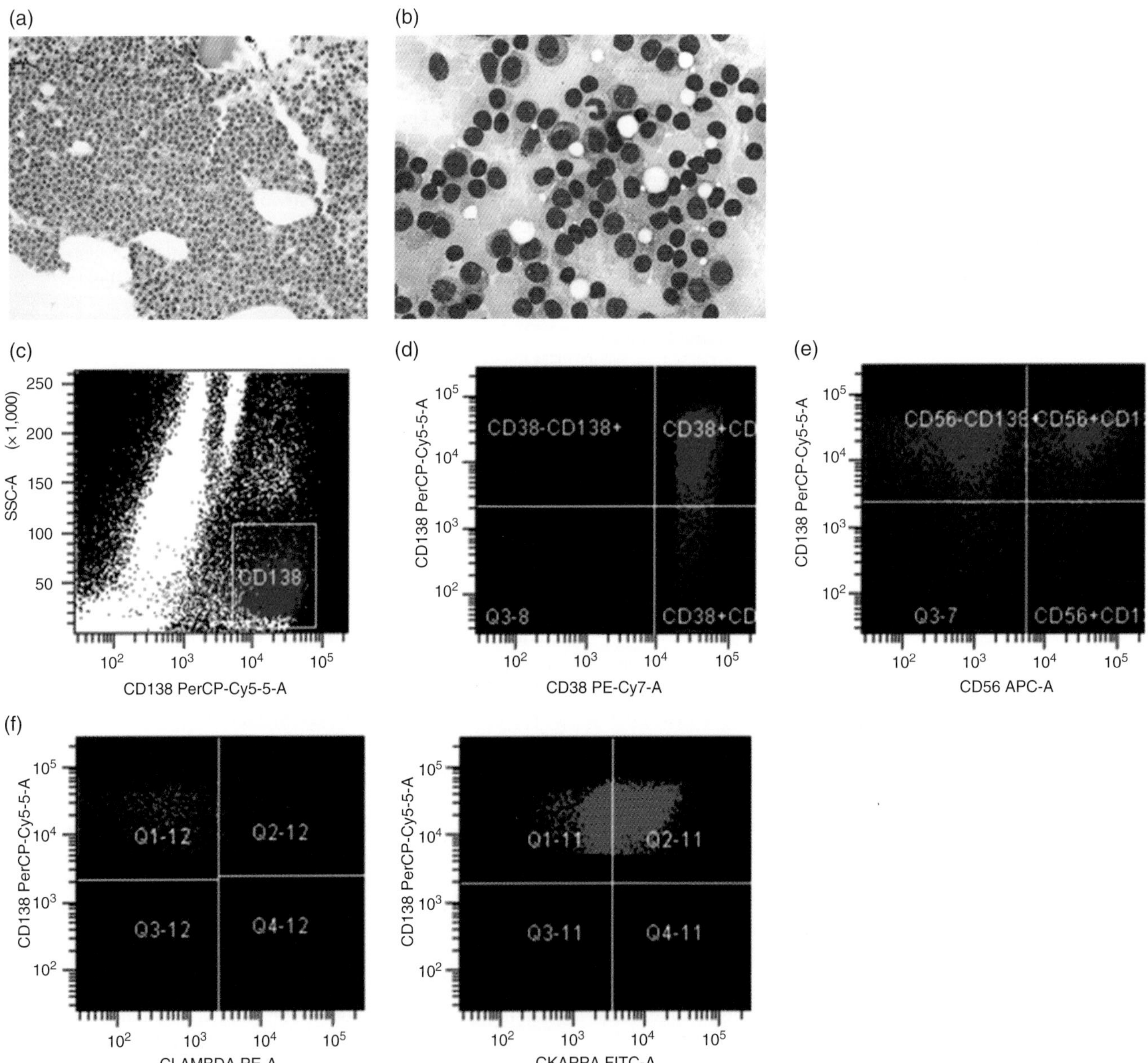

Figure 33.1 Diagnostic features of MM. A sheet of malignant plasma cells (PCs) is visible at 40× magnification on hematoxylin–eosin stain of a bone marrow biopsy (a); (b) shows a higher magnification (100×) view of the malignant MMCs on Wright–Giemsa stain on the bone marrow aspirate. Immunohistochemistry staining for κ light chain confirmed the monoclonality of the PC infiltrate. (c) shows a population briskly positive for CD138 (x axis) which is largely CD38 positive (panel d) and with aberrant expression of CD56 in a subset of cells (panel e). Panel (f) shows the monoclonality of the CD138 positive cells: they are negative for λ (first panel) but positive for κ (second panel) light chain.

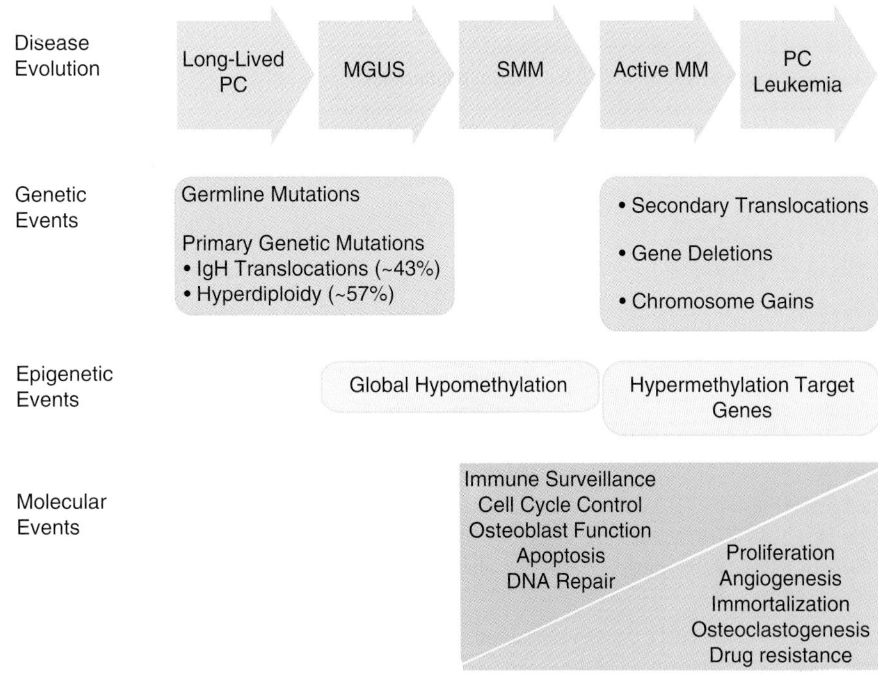

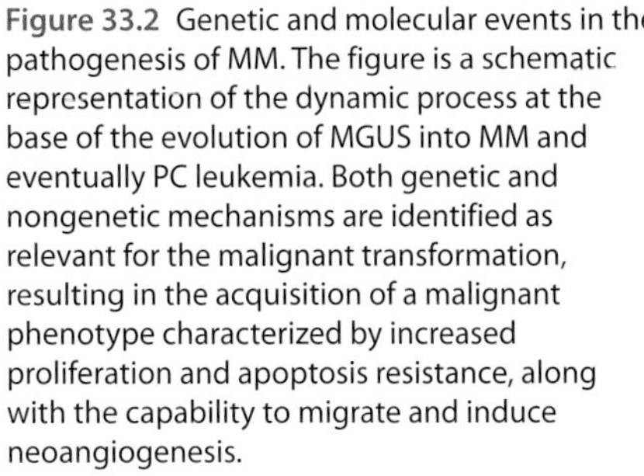
Figure 33.2 Genetic and molecular events in the pathogenesis of MM. The figure is a schematic representation of the dynamic process at the base of the evolution of MGUS into MM and eventually PC leukemia. Both genetic and nongenetic mechanisms are identified as relevant for the malignant transformation, resulting in the acquisition of a malignant phenotype characterized by increased proliferation and apoptosis resistance, along with the capability to migrate and induce neoangiogenesis.

corresponding to the Golgi apparatus. Binucleate or multinucleate cells, mitosis, and prominent nucleoli are often detected. Under electron microscopy, MMCs show a large amount of endoplasmic reticulum, reflecting the Ig production. Immunophenotypically, MMCs strongly express CD138 (syndecan-1) and a monotypic light chain (either κ or λ). In contrast to PCs, MMCs typically lack expression of CD19, CD27, and CD45, and aberrantly express CD56, CD28, and CD38. These differences provide the basis for use of multiparametric flow cytometry to detect minimal residual disease and/or to monitor disease [17, 18].

Genetically, MM is a heterogeneous disease. About 50–60% of cases are hyperdiploid with trisomies in odd chromosomes (3, 5, 7, 9, 11, 15, 19, and 21). The initial genetic event in the non-hyperdiploid tumors is typically a translocation between the IgH locus on chromosome 14q32 and one of the following oncogenes: fibroblast growth factor receptor 3 (*FGFR3*); multiple myeloma SET domain (*MMSET*); cyclin D1 and D3; *MAF*; and *MAFB*. Secondary genetic events involve activating mutations in pathways involved in proliferation, immortalization, and apoptosis resistance such as *MYC*, *K-RAS* and *N-RAS*, *BRAF*, *PI3K*, and *AKT*, and/or deletion of oncosuppressors such as *TP53* (del 17p). Recently, genetic or nongenetic disruption of key regulators of PC differentiation, XBP1, Blimp-1, and IRF-4, has proved crucial for MM pathogenesis [19, 20]. While epigenetic changes in MM have been less well characterized, generalized gene hypomethylation is associated with the transition between MGUS and MM, whereas hypermethylation of specific, target genes correlates with progression of MM into PC leukemia (Figure 33.2) [21].

Clinical Presentation

The most common presenting symptoms of MM are fatigue and bone pain. Aberrant proliferation of MMCs in the BM with impairment of normal hematopoiesis, excess production of monoclonal Ig or FLC, and perturbation of the homeostatic cytokine milieu in the BM underlie the clinical presentation of MM. Active MM is typically suspected when hypercalcemia (C), acute kidney injury (AKI, R), anemia (A), and/or osteolytic lesions or pathologic fractures (B) are detected (Table 33.1). These four presenting signs constitute the CRAB criteria. Increased osteoclastic activity and proliferation, along with impairment of osteoblastogenesis, is the cause of hypercalcemia and bone disease in MM. Via both autocrine and paracrine mechanisms, MMCs cause an imbalance favoring osteoclast- versus osteoblast-activating cytokines in the BM milieu, resulting in unopposed bone destruction [23]. A bone survey to include long bones and skull is typically specific, but not very sensitive, to detect MM-related disease. Given the lytic nature of MM lesions, bone scan and/or alkaline phosphatase are generally normal. For selected patients with unexplained bone pain and negative bone survey, PET-CT and MRI are highly sensitive for the detection of radiographically occult lytic lesions [24, 25]. PET-CT has also been shown to be a sensitive tool to assess for early treatment response and/or disease relapse after autologous hematopoietic stem cell transplant (SCT) [26].

AKI is present in approximately 50% of newly diagnosed MM patients and can result from several pathogenic mechanisms: full or fragment Ig deposition in the renal tubules or glomeruli causes cast nephropathy or light chain deposition disease; deposition of the heavy chain component of Ig, as in heavy chain disease; infiltration of kidney parenchyma by either MMCs or amyloidogenic light chain with nephrotic syndrome; as well as hypercalcemia and associated arteriolar vasoconstriction and prerenal state due to brisk polyuria. Depending on the etiology of AKI, Bence Jones (light chain) proteinuria (cast nephropathy), nephrotic-range proteinuria with prevalent albuminuria (immunoglobulin light chain AL amyloidosis), or bland sediment (hypercalcemia, hyperuricemia) is detected [27]. Early decline in FLC has been associated

Table 33.1 The most common presenting symptoms/signs in MM patients with their related diagnostic findings and underlying pathogenic mechanisms.

Signs and symptoms	Diagnostic findings	Pathogenic mechanisms
Bone/back pain, cord compression, cauda equina	Lytic lesions, pathologic fractures, severe osteopenia	Myelophthisis, increased osteoclastogenesis, osteoblast inhibition, solitary plasmacytoma
Fatigue, malaise	Anemia	Myelophthisis, decreased EPO, hemolysis
	Renal failure	Light chain deposition, cast nephropathy, hypercalcemia-induced vasoconstriction, amyloidosis, urate nephropathy
	Hypercalcemia	Bone reabsorption secondary to myelophthisis and cytokine release
	Hepatitis, liver failure	Amyloid infiltration, MM cell infiltration
Recurrent infections	Hypogammaglobulinemia, leukopenia	Myelophthisis
Neurologic symptoms	Polyradiculopathy, ischemic strokes, altered mental status	Amyloid deposition, cryoglobulinemia type I, hyperviscosity, hypercalcemia, uremia
Respiratory distress	Infiltrative cardiomyopathy, arrhythmias, pleural effusions, pulmonary edema	Cardiac or pulmonary amyloid, plasmacytoma, malignant pleural effusions, hyperviscosity
Purpura, petechiae, bleeding, acrocyanosis	Cryoglobulinemia type I, thrombocytopenia, hyperviscosity	M spike deposition, myelophthisis, hyperviscosity

Source: Bianchi G, Ghobrial I. Does my patient with a serum monoclonal spike have multiple myeloma? Hematol Oncol Clin North Am 2012;26(2):383–93 [22]. Reproduced with permission of Elsevier.
EPO, erythropoietin; M, monoclonal.

Table 33.2 Myeloma-defining events (MDE). According to the revised criteria for MM diagnosis, the presence of MDE in a patient with more than 10%, clonal BM PC and/or biopsy-proven nonosseous plasmacytoma defines active MM. The table lists ROTI and biomarkers which are now considered as MDE according to the revised diagnostic criteria.

ROTI	Biomarkers
Revised CRAB criteria: • *C* (hyper*c*alcemia): total serum calcium >1 mg/dL higher than the ULN or >11 mg/dL • *R*enal insufficiency: estimated GFR <40 mL/min/m^2 or serum creatinine >2 mg/dL secondary to cast nephropathy • *A*nemia: hemoglobin >2 g/dL below the LLN or hemoglobin <10 g/dL • *B*one lesions: one or more osteolytic lesions on skeletal radiography, CT, or PET-CT	• Clonal BM PC infiltrate ≥60% • Ratio of involved:uninvolved sFLC ≥100 • >1 focal lesions of at least 5 mm diameter on MRI studies

BM, bone marrow; GFR, glomerular filtration rate; LLN, lower limit of normal; MRI, magnetic resonance imaging; PC, plasma cell; PET-CT, positron emission tomography–computed tomography; ROTI, related organ or tissue impairment; sFLC, serum free light chain; ULN, upper limit of normal.

with recovery of renal function in patients presenting with myeloma kidney. In this setting, early commencement of cytoreductive chemotherapy with bortezomib is essential. Supplemental removal of FLC via either plasma exchange or high cut-off hemodialysis may be considered, although conclusive data are lacking [28]. It is worth noting that the only form of renal failure which is diagnostic of active MM is cast nephropathy [29].

The etiology of anemia is multifactorial: direct impairment of hematopoiesis by MMCs; cytokine-induced suppression of erythropoiesis with features typical of anemia of chronic disease; and erythropoietin (EPO) deficiency.

Previously, peripheral neuropathy, AL amyloidosis, hyperviscosity syndrome, and recurrent infections were also considered related organ or tissue impairment (ROTI) and thus diagnostic of active MM. However, the revised diagnostic criteria for active MM no longer include these signs and syndromes, as their occurrence in the absence of CRAB criteria or biomarkers of active MM (Table 33.2, myeloma-defining events or MDE) is rare [29]. Peripheral neuropathy in the context of active MM is related to direct axonal degeneration, with or without amyloid protein deposition, as well as to demyelination related to paraneoplastic antimyelin autoantibody production [30].

AL amyloidosis is typically diagnosed on periumbilical fat aspirate. Amyloidogenic protein causes the pathognomonic "apple-green" pattern of polarized light birefringence upon Congo red staining. The clinical presentation of AL amyloidosis depends on the pattern of organ involvement, most frequently: myocardium, presenting with heart failure secondary to restrictive or dilated cardiomyopathy; liver, with hepatic failure; gastrointestinal tract, manifesting as diarrhea or gastrointestinal bleed; nephrotic syndrome in the case of kidney involvement; and peripheral neuropathy related to nerve injury. AL amyloidosis is a true, distinct clinical entity from MM and only a minority of patients diagnosed with AL amyloidosis carry a concurrent diagnosis of MM or will transform into active MM. However, diagnostic criteria are poorly defined and variable thresholds of BM involvement have been used to distinguish primary AL amyloidosis versus AL amyloidosis secondary to MM. A recent, retrospective study from the Mayo Clinic showed that the prognosis of patients with AL amyloidosis and more than 10% clonal BM PC involvement was similar to patients with AL amyloidosis in the context of active MM (based on CRAB criteria) [31].

Hyperviscosity syndrome typically manifests with cerebrovascular events, ocular signs, respiratory distress, and tendency to bleed. In MM, it occurs most often in patients with elevated paraprotein of IgM subtype (22% of cases with M spike over 5 g/dL), followed by IgA and IgG3, due to chemical–physical properties. In patients with IgG MM, hyperviscosity syndrome occurs with a frequency of one in 25 patients [32]. Prompt initiation of plasmapheresis and cytoreductive therapy usually results in rapid clinical improvement.

Immunoparesis with hypogammaglobulinemia and leukopenia can occur in MM and explains the propensity to recurrent infections. In case of frequent, life-threatening infections, intravenous (IV) Ig supplementation is recommended.

Diagnosis of Multiple Myeloma and Related Dyscrasias

When MM is suspected, evaluation should include complete blood cell count with differential, full chemistry including calcium and albumin, β2-microglobulin, lactate dehydrogenase (LDH), Ig fractions with serum protein electrophoresis (SPEP) and immunofixation (IF), serum FLC, 24-hour urinalysis with urine protein electrophoresis (UPEP) and IF, and bone survey. An M protein (or M spike) on SPEP and/or UPEP and IF and/or the presence of an abnormal FLC ratio is the laboratory hallmark of MM, with less than 1% of MM patients presenting with true, nonsecretory disease characterized by negative SPEP, UPEP, and FLC assay [33]. Confirmation of malignant PC infiltrate in the BM is indicated for diagnostic and prognostic purposes. Beyond morphologic review of the aspirate, immunohistochemistry, cytogenetics, and fluorescence *in situ* hybridization (FISH) should be ordered. Diagnostic criteria for MM were updated in 2014 to include patients whose disease was previously classified as SMM but whose biologic aggressiveness was more consistent with active MM [29]. Active MM is currently defined by the presence of a clonal, BM PC infiltrate of 10% or more or biopsy-proven osseous or extraosseous plasmacytoma plus one or more MDE which include: ROTI and biomarkers of malignancy (malignant PC accounting for 60% or more of BM cellularity; ratio of involved to uninvolved serum FLC exceeding 100; and/or two or more focal lesions on MRI measuring 5 mm or more) (Table 33.2). Active MM needs to be distinguished from other monoclonal gammopathies, in particular SMM and MGUS (Table 33.3). SMM is a precancerous condition with a risk of progression to active MM of 10% per year during the first 5 years, 3% per year in the following 5 years, and 1% per year thereafter, accounting for a cumulative likelihood of malignant evolution of 70% at 15 years. A risk stratification model based on BM involvement exceeding 10%, an M spike ≥3 g/dL, and an abnormal FLC ratio has been developed to aid in counseling and help with therapeutic decisions [34]. According to the revised diagnostic criteria, SMM is diagnosed in the presence of an M spike ≥3 g/dL, or urinary monoclonal protein ≥500 mg over 24 hours, and/or malignant PC infiltrate in the BM between 10 and 60%, in the absence of MDE as listed above. No treatment outside of clinical trials, with the exception of consideration for bisphosphonates, is recommended for SMM patients [24]. Routine ambulatory visits with laboratory analysis every 3–6 months and annual bone survey are indicated for early detection of malignant evolution [14]. Prompt interim evaluation is warranted in case of symptoms/signs suspicious of active disease including back pain, fatigue, and confusion. Ongoing trials are evaluating the effect of early treatment in high-risk SMM. While delayed progression to MM is anticipated and has been shown, it is critical to demonstrate that treatment has not selected a more malignant clone and that overall survival (OS) is also extended [35].

In order for MGUS to be diagnosed, three criteria must be simultaneously fulfilled: less than 10% MMC infiltrate on BM biopsy; an M spike measuring less than 3 g/dL; and absence of MDE. MGUS is typically incidentally diagnosed, being detected in 3–7% of persons over age 50 years and with incidence increasing with age [36]. As with SMM, MGUS does not require treatment, and close medical follow-up with routine bloodwork is recommended, albeit of controversial value [14, 37].

Solitary plasmacytoma is a variant of PC dyscrasia, characterized by a single area of malignant PC proliferation in the bone (osseous plasmacytoma) or in the soft tissue (extraosseous plasmacytoma), without systemic symptoms and/or BM involvement. It carries an approximately 10% risk of evolution to active MM within 3 years. Solitary plasmacytoma with minimal marrow involvement differs from true solitary plasmacytoma by the presence of less than 10% clonal BM PC involvement and carries a significantly higher likelihood of evolution to active MM (about 60% for the osseous and 20% for the extraosseous variant within 3 years) [29]. In a large series, the median time to evolution was 21 months, with a wide range spanning from 2 to 135 months, and occasionally late disease progression (time to progression over 15 years) [38]. Older age and osseous (rather than extraosseous) localization were the only predictive factors of progression to MM identified in multivariate analysis [39, 40]. The OS rate in the largest series is 70% at 5 years [38]. Solitary plasmacytoma represents 3–5% of cases of PC dyscrasia and does not require systemic therapy, but only local management, generally with surgery or radiation therapy. If ROTI or systemic symptoms are present, then the plasmacytoma represents an extramedullary localization of MM and may warrant systemic therapy. The rate of local disease control for osseous and extraosseous plasmacytoma has been reported at 90% [41, 42].

PC leukemia is defined by the presence of circulating PCs exceeding 2×10^9/L or 20% of leukocytes. It can either represent the leukemic transformation of MM, typically in advanced stages (secondary PC leukemia) or occur *de novo* (primary PC, 60% of cases).

Table 33.3 Novel diagnostic criteria of plasma cell dyscrasia as accepted by the International Myeloma Working Group (IMWG).

	M protein		BM		MDE[1]	Comments
MGUS	<3 g/dL	*and*	<10%	*and*	Absent	Diagnosis requires exclusion of other lymphoproliferative diseases
SMM	≥3 g/dL or abnormal sFLC or ≥500 mg in 24-hour urine collection	*and/or*	≥10% and <60%	*and*	Absent	AL amyloidosis must also be excluded for diagnosis of SMM
MM	Any concentration on SPEP/UPEP or abnormal sFLC	*and*	≥10% or plasmacytoma	*and*	Present	In nonsecretory MM: SPEP, UPEP, and FLC are normal
Solitary plasmacytoma	Absent[3]	*and*	Absent	*and*	Absent	Defined as a single site of clonal, PC proliferation in the bone (osseous) or soft tissue (extraosseous)
Solitary plasmacytoma with minimal BM involvement	Absent[3]	*and*	<10%	*and*	Absent	Defined as a single site of clonal, PC proliferation in the bone (osseous) or soft tissue (extraosseous)
PC leukemia[2]	Absent/present	*and*	Absent/present	*and*	Absent/present	Defined as peripheral blood circulating clonal PCs $>2\times10^9$/L or 20% of leukocytes
Primary AL amyloidosis	Absent/present	*and/or*	If present, median 7–10%	*and*	Absent	Defined by: • Amyloid-related syndrome/organ involvement • Positive Congo red stain in any tissue • Mass spectrometry/IEM confirmation of light chain amyloid • Presence of a PC dyscrasia on lab/pathologic specimens
POEMS[4]	Absent/present	*and/or*	Absent/present	*and*	Absent	Defined by: • Polyneuropathy • Diagnosis of PC dyscrasia by lab/pathologic specimens Plus one other major criterion: • Sclerotic bone lesions • Castleman disease • Elevated serum VEGF-A Plus one minor criterion: Organomegaly (hepato-, spleno-megaly, adenopathies) Sign of volume overload (edema, effusion, ascites) Endocrinopathy (adrenal, thyroid, parathyroid, pituitary, gonadal, pancreatic) Skin changes Papilledema Thrombocytosis/polycythemia

Source: Bianchi G, Ghobrial I. Does my patient with a serum monoclonal spike have multiple myeloma? Hematol Oncol Clin North Am 2012;26(2):383–93 [22]. Reproduced with permission of Elsevier.

[1] Please refer to Table 33.2 for the definition of MDE. Hyperviscosity, recurrent infections related to hypogammaglobulinemia, and amyloidosis are no longer included in the list of ROTI.

[2] PC leukemia is further classified into primary when occurring *de novo*, or secondary, when representing the leukemic phase of MM.

[3] A small M spike can be occasionally seen.

[4] Differential diagnosis must be excluded prior to diagnosing POEMS.

AL, immunoglobulin light chain; BM, bone marrow invasion by monoclonal malignant plasma cells; CRAB, hypercalcemia, renal failure, anemia, bone lesions; FLC, free light chain; IEM, immunoelectron microscopy; M, monoclonal; MM, multiple myeloma; MGUS, monoclonal gammopathy of undetermined significance; PC, plasma cell; POEMS, polyneuropathy, organomegaly, endocrinopathy, monoclonal gammopathy, and skin changes; ROTI: related organ or tissue impairment; SMM, smoldering multiple myeloma; SPEP, serum protein electrophoresis; UPEP, urine protein electrophoresis; VEGF-A, vascular endothelial growth factor A.

The diagnosis of AL amyloidosis requires the concomitant presence of an amyloid-related organ involvement as detailed above; positive Congo red stain in any tissue, including fat aspirate, bone marrow biopsy, or organ biopsy; and finally the laboratory or pathologic evidence of PC dyscrasia (M spike in serum or urine, abnormal free light-chain ratio, or clonal BM PC) [29]. Mass spectrometry-based or immunoelectron microscopy is indicated to confirm the light-chain nature of amyloid if there is clinical suspicion of an alternative subtypes (transthyretin (ATTR) or serum amyloid A (SAA) amyloid).

Finally, POEMS (polyneuropathy, organomegaly, endocrinopathy, monoclonal gammopathy, and skin changes) syndrome is diagnosed in the presence of polyneuropathy, a PC dyscrasia, typically λ-restricted, and any one of three major and six minor criteria as listed in Table 33.3 [43].

Staging

The Durie–Salmon staging system was developed in the mid 1970s to provide surrogate laboratory values for tumor mass. Three stages were identified based on level of hemoglobin, serum calcium, M spike, and extent of bone disease, while kidney function would further stratify each stage into A and B (creatinine less than or exceeding 2 mg/dL, respectively). In the era of standard cytotoxic chemotherapy, OS correlated with Durie–Salmon staging; however, this system lost its prognostic utility with the introduction of novel agents [44]. The International Staging System (ISS) now stratifies MM patients into three groups based upon serum albumin and β2-microglobulin. Patients with stage I disease have an overall survival of 62 months compared to 44 and 29 in stage II and III, respectively [45]. This staging system has preserved its prognostic value in the era of targeted therapies, and is the most widely used (Table 33.4). Karyotype and FISH also provide helpful prognostic stratification and have been used to guide therapeutic decisions [46]. A number of genomic abnormalities, such as deletion of chromosome 13 or 13q, translocation t(4;14) and t(14;16), deletion(17p), and gain of long arm of chromosome 1 at locus 21 (1q21+) or loss of its short arm deletion(1p) have been investigated as predictive factors of response to therapy as well as prognostic factors [47]. The most recent consensus of the International Myeloma Working Group (IMWG) recognizes t(4;14), t(14;16), t(14;20), deletion(17/17p) and nonhyperdiploid karyotype as clearly adverse cytogenetics in newly diagnosed MM [48]. Together with ISS stage II and III, these cytogenetics identify high-risk, newly diagnosed MM and are key in informing therapeutic choices [49]. Gain(1q) and/or del(1p) have been recently recognized as poor-risk cytogenetics while the combination of three or more adverse cytogenetics identifies a MM patient population with ultra-high-risk disease, characterized by an OS less than 2 years [48, 50].

Treatment

The natural history of MM has been profoundly impacted by three therapeutic interventions: the introduction of melphalan and corticosteroid in the 1950s and 1960s; autologous SCT, pioneered in the 1980s; and the clinical use of the proteasome inhibitor (PI) bortezomib and the immunomodulatory drugs (IMiDs) thalidomide and lenalidomide in the late 1990s and early 2000s [51]. These treatments resulted in a stepwise improvement in OS from 1–2 years to the current 7–8 years, which is likely an underestimate of the effect of novel combination therapies as well as maintenance treatment [52].

Table 33.4 The Durie–Salmon staging system and the International Staging System for MM. Adapted from "A clinical staging system for multiple myeloma. Correlation of measured myeloma cell mass with presenting clinical features, response to treatment, and survival", BG Durie and SE Salmon, Cancer 1975 [44].

	Durie–Salmon[1]	ISS
Stage I	All of the following must be present: • Hemoglobin >10 g/dL • Serum calcium ≤12 mg/dL • Absence of bone disease or solitary plasmacytoma • M protein: <5 g/dL, if IgG, or <3 g/dL, if IgA, and/or Bence Jones proteinuria <4 g/24 hours	Serum β2-microglobulin <3.5 mg/dL *and* serum albumin ≥3.5 g/dL
Stage II	Meeting criteria for neither stage I nor III	Meeting criteria for neither stage I nor III
Stage III	One or more of the following must be present: • Hemoglobin <8.5 g/dL • Serum calcium >12 mg/dL • Extensive bone lesions • M protein: >7 g/dL, if IgG, >5 g/dL, if IgA, and/or Bence Jones proteinuria >12 g/24 hours	Serum β2-microglobulin ≥5.5 mg/dL

[1] Each stage is further subclassified into A or B depending on whether serum creatinine is <2 mg/dL (A) or ≥2 mg/dL (B).

More recently, the clinical use of monoclonal antibody against CD38 and signaling lymphocyte activation molecule family 7 (SLAMF7) in the context of IMiDs and PI-based regimens has proven extremely effective in newly diagnosed and relapsed/refractory MM. In a parallel fashion, ancillary care has also markedly improved, with better control of bone pain via pharmacologic, radiologic, or surgical means, as well as improved support of cytopenias and immunoparesis via growth factors, blood products, and IVIg. These advances in primary and supportive therapies have resulted in improved quality of life and reduced comorbidities.

The choice of treatment for newly diagnosed MM patients is based on whether or not they are eligible for autologous SCT (Table 33.5) [24].

Recently Approved Agents for Multiple Myeloma

A deeper understanding of the biology of MM and the role of the BM microenvironment in supporting proliferation, trafficking, and drug resistance has informed the design of novel therapies (Figure 33.3) [53]. Following the unexpected effectiveness of thalidomide in patients with refractory, relapsed MM, 15 treatments have been approved by the US Food and Drug Administration (FDA) for MM [54]. These novel agents proved effective in preclinical models of MM in the presence of stroma cells and cytokines such as interleukin 6 (IL-6), and similarly overcame the advantage of the BM niche in patients (Table 33.6).

Immunomodulatory Drugs (IMiDs)

Until its rediscovery as an anti-MM agent, thalidomide had been marketed as a potent antiemetic, particularly effective in hyperemesis gravidarum, and became tragically associated with its profound teratogenic effects (phocomelia). Its use in MM was based on the postulated antiangiogenic properties, although immunomodulation is a predominant effect of IMiDs [72]. The molecular base of effectiveness of IMiDs has been recently clarified with the identification of their target: the E3, ubiquitin ligase enzyme, cereblon (CRBN). Inhibition of this protein was shown to be responsible for thalidomide-induced phocomelia in animal models, as well as for IMiD-related antiproliferative and immunomodulatory activity [73, 74]. The combination of thalidomide with dexamethasone (dex) or with melphalan and prednisone (MPT) has been shown to be effective in randomized trials in newly diagnosed transplant candidates and those ineligible for transplant, respectively. Two derivative drugs of thalidomide, lenalidomide and pomalidomide, are also FDA approved for treatment of MM. Lenalidomide is an orally available agent with more potent immunomodulatory effects compared with thalidomide, and was approved as second-line therapy on the basis of two phase 3, randomized clinical trials in relapsed, refractory patients: compared to dex alone, the combination of lenalidomide and dex resulted in increased response rate (RR), progression-free survival (PFS), and OS [75]. Lenalidomide in combination with low-dose dex (Rd), as well as the triplet of lenalidomide/bortezomib/dex (RVd), achieved high extent and frequency of response as initial therapy in patients eligible for autologous SCT with manageable toxicities [61, 76]. However, grade 3 or higher peripheral neuropathy remains a concern in patients treated with intravenous bortezomib. RVd is an effective consolidation therapy post high-dose melphalan and autologous SCT. Moreover, lenalidomide maintenance can prolong the PFS and even OS post transplant, albeit with a small increased risk of secondary cancer [77, 78].

Pomalidomide was granted accelerated approval by the FDA in February 2013 for treatment of relapsed, refractory MM patients who have received at least two prior lines of therapy, including bortezomib and lenalidomide. Approval was based on the promising interim results of phase 1/2 studies and pending results of a phase 3, multicenter, randomized clinical trial in refractory, relapsed MM patients comparing bortezomib and dex to bortezomib plus dex plus pomalidomide [79–81]. Combination of pomalidomide with the oral PI ixazomib showed tolerable adverse events and promising effectiveness in a phase 1/2 trial in patients with lenalidomide and PI-refractory disease relapse [82].

Proteasome Inhibitors

The discovery of proteasome inhibitors as powerful anti-MM drugs has not only completely changed the prognosis of MM patients but also enhanced our understanding of MM molecular and cellular biology. The 26S proteasome is an ATP-dependent, multidomain proteolytic complex, which is ubiquitously expressed in eukaryotic cells and responsible for the bulk of short- and long-lived protein catabolism. Proteolysis is mediated by three proteasomal catalytic subunits: caspase-like ($\beta1$), trypsin-like ($\beta2$), and chymotryptic-like ($\beta5$) [83].

Initially developed as a research tool to study intracellular protein degradation, a potential market for PIs as pharmacologic treatment of cachexia was intuited [84]. Eventually the developmental interest moved to cancer and the first-in-class PI bortezomib, a boronate, reversible inhibitor of the chymotryptic-like activity of the proteasome, showed promising activity against a wide range of solid and hematologic malignancies in preclinical studies [85]. Despite the skepticism of the scientific community, bortezomib was remarkably well tolerated, with peripheral neuropathy and cyclic thrombocytopenia as common side effects [86]. MM was exquisitely sensitive to bortezomib, prompting rapid preclinical and clinical validation [87–89]. The molecular mechanisms underlying the sensitivity of MMCs to bortezomib and other PIs include their effects: (i) on the tumor cell (endoplasmic reticulum stress, cell cycle, NF-κB activation, heat shock protein response, apoptosis); (ii) on the tumor cell–host interaction (regulating binding of MMCs in the BM by regulating adhesion molecule expression); and (iii) in the microenvironment (transcription of cytokines mediating tumor cell growth, survival, and drug resistance, as well as triggering osteoclast apoptosis and osteoblastogenesis) [90, 91]. Bortezomib received accelerated FDA approval to treat relapsed, refractory disease in 2003, as second-line therapy in 2005, and as a first-line agent in 2008, and is now the backbone of the majority of upfront regimens in MM. Peripheral neuropathy emerged as a potentially severe side effect of bortezomib, and algorithms of schedule and dose reduction were developed for its management. Weekly rather than twice-weekly treatment and subcutaneous administration of bortezomib have markedly decreased the incidence of peripheral neuropathy without modifying the effectiveness of the treatment [92, 93]. Pre-existence of peripheral neuropathy is the only identified

Table 33.5 The results of phase 2/3 trials of the most commonly used induction regimens for transplant-eligible and transplant-ineligible patients.

Regimen	Setting	CR, %[1]	ORR[1]	PFS	OS	Side effects (%)	Reference trial
Transplant-eligible patients							
Bor/Dex	Phase 3 in NDMM	15 (≥VGPR)	79%	36 months (median)	81% at 3 years	Infection (10)	IFM 2005-01 [55]
Bor/Dox/Dex	Phase 2 and 3 in NDMM	21 (≥VGPR)	72%	35 months (median)[2]	61% at 5 years[2]	Infection (25), PN (15, grade ≥2), neutropenia (11, grade ≥3)	HOVON-65/GMMG-HD4 [56, 57]
Bor/Cy/Dex (CyBorD)	Phase 2 and 3 NDMM	22 (≥VGPR)	78%	100% at 1 year[2]	100% at 1 year[2]	Neutropenia (35, grade ≥3) and infections (22)	EVOLUTION, [57–59]
Bor/Thal/Dex (VTD)	Phase 3 NDMM	23	96%	60% at 3 years	90% at 3 years	Neuropathy (16, grade ≥3), infections (15), GI (13)	GIMEMA [60]
Bor/Len/Dex (VRD)	Phase 2 and 3 NDMM	16 (≥VGPR)	82%	43 months	~70% at 5 years	PN (23, grade ≥3), thrombocytopenia (18, grade ≥3), neutropenia (19, grade ≥3)	SWOG S0777 EVOLUTION [58, 61]
Len/Dex (Rd)	Phase 3	14 (≥VGPR)	70%	61% at 1 year	96% at 1 year	Neutropenia (20) and DVT (12)	[62]
Carf/Len/Dex (KRd)	Phase 3 RRMM	32	87%	26 months	73% at 2 years	Neutropenia (30), anemia (18), thrombocytopenia (17), cardiac failure (4), ischemic heart disease (3)	[63]
Dara/Len/Dex	Phase 3 RRMM	43	93%	63% risk reduction for PFS (P<0.0001)	N/A	Neutropenia (52, ≥grade 3), infections (28, ≥grade 3)	POLLUX (MMY3003) [64]
Dara/Bor/Dex	Phase 3 RRMM	19	83%	61% risk reduction for PFS (P<0.0001)	N/A	Infusion reaction (45), thrombocytopenia (59), PN (47), neutropenia (13)	CASTOR (MMY3004) [65]
Transplant-ineligible patients							
Bor/Mel/Pred (VMP)	Phase 3 NDMM	30 (≥VGPR)	81%	24 months	69% at 3 years	Cytopenias (40–50), herpes zoster reactivation (13), PN (44)	VISTA [66]
Mel/Pred/ Lena (MPR)	Phase 3 NDMM	33 (≥VGPR)	68–81	13–29 months	91% at 2 years	Neutropenia (60) and thrombocytopenia (30), second malignancies (7)	GIMEMA, MM-015 [67, 68]
Melphalan/ prednisone/ thalidomide (MPT)	Phase 3 NDMM	28 (≥VGPR)	57–76	13 months	40 months	Peripheral neuropathy (57%) and DVT (10%)	HOVON 49 [69]
Len/Dex (continuous)	Phase 3 NDMM	33(≥VGPR)	77	26 months	59% at 4 years	Grade 3 and 4, respectively: neutropenia (67 and 35), thrombocytopenia (35 and 11), anemia (24 and 3), infection (9 and 1)	[70]

[1] Clinical response was assessed by European Group for Blood and Marrow Transplantation criteria [71].
[2] Data from phase 2 study.
Bor, bortezomib; Carf, carfilzomib; CR, complete remission; Cy, cyclophosphamide; Dara, daratumumab; Dex, dexamethasone; Dox, doxorubicin; DVT, deep venous thrombosis; Len, lenalidomide; Mel, melphalan; NDMM, newly diagnosed multiple myeloma; ORR, overall response rate; OS, overall survival; PFS, progression-free survival; PN, peripheral neuropathy; RRMM, relapsed and/or refractory MM; Thal, thalidomide; VGPR, very good partial response.

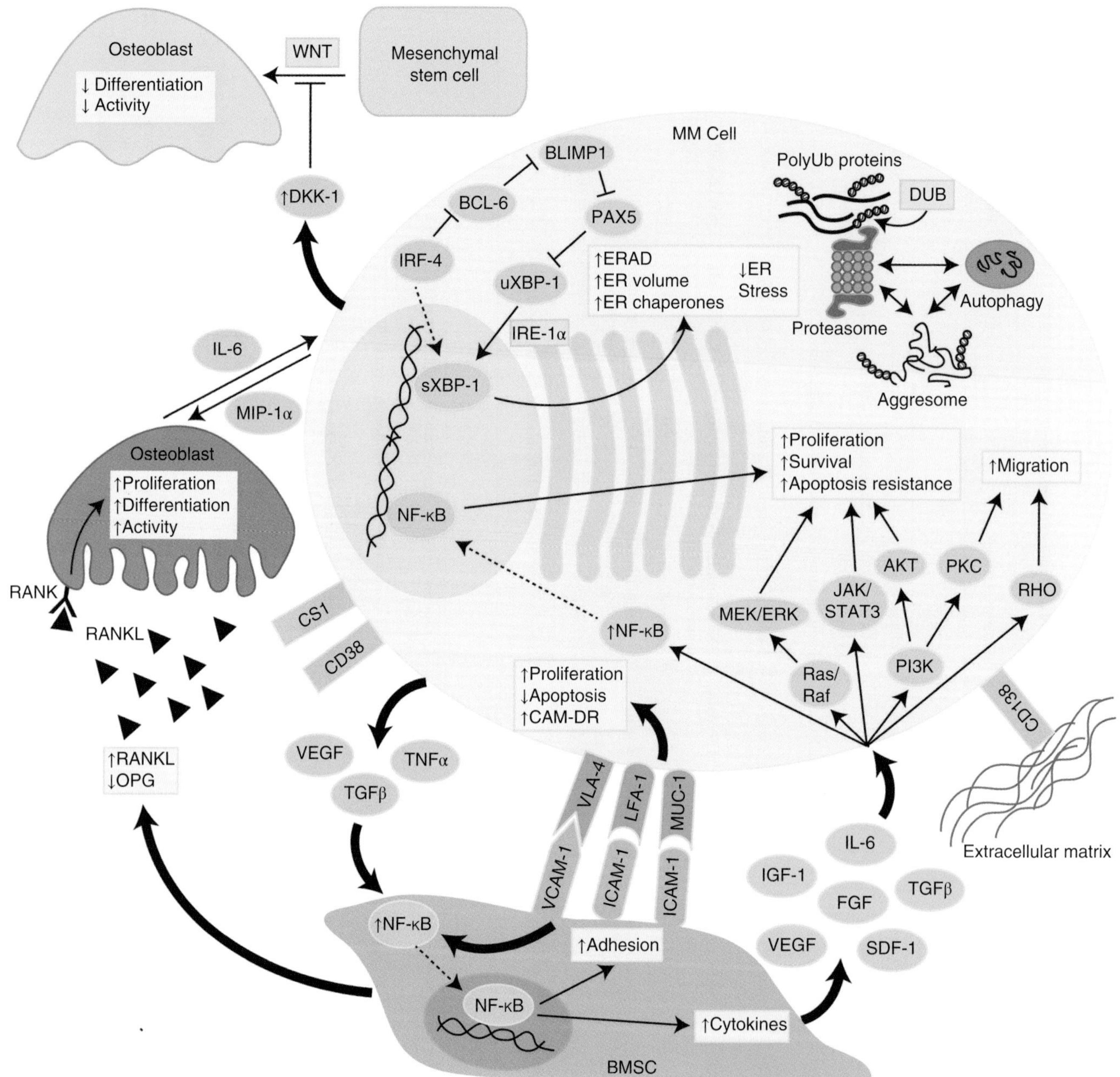

Figure 33.3 MM cells and microenvironment interaction. The cartoon is a representation of the maladaptive, bidirectional interaction between the malignant MMC and the BM niche with reciprocal activation of prosurvival, proliferative and antiapoptotic pathways in multiple myeloma cells (MMCs), osteoclasts and bone marrow stroma cells (BMSC). Abbreviations: AKT, serine/threonine kinase 1; BCL-6, interferon regulatory factor 4; BLIMP-1, B-lymphocyte-induced maturation protein 1; CAM-DR, cell adhesion mediated drug resistance; CS1, alias SLAM family member 7 (SLAMF7); DKK1, dickkopf WNT signaling pathway inhibitor 1; DUB, de-ubiquitinating enzyme; ERAD, endoplasmic reticulum associated degradation; FGF, fibroblast growth factor; ICAM1, intercellular adhesion molecule 1; IGF-1, insulin growth factor 1; IL-6, interleukin 6; IRE-1α, inositol-requiring enzyme-1α; IRF-4, interferon regulatory factor 4; JAK, Janus kinase; LFA-1, lymphocyte function-associated antigen 1; MEK/ERK, MAP (mitogen-activated protein kinase) kinase/ERK (extracellular regulated MAP kinase) kinase; MIP-1α, macrophage inflammatory protein 1-alpha; MUC-1, mucin 1; NF-κB, nuclear factor kappa B; OPG, osteoprotegerin; PAX5, paired box 5; PI3K, phosphatidylinositol-4,5-bisphosphate 3-kinase; PKC, protein kinase C; PolyUB, polyubiquitinated; RANK, receptor activator of nuclear factor-kappa B; RANKL, RANK ligand; RHO, rhodopsin; SDF-1, stromal cell-derived factor 1; STAT, signal transducer and activator of transcription protein; TGFβ, transforming growth factor beta; TNFα, tumor necrosis factor alpha; VCAM-1, vascular cell adhesion molecule 1; VEGF, vascular endothelial growth factor; VLA-4, very late antigen 4; WNT, wingless-type; X-BP1, X-box binding protein 1.

risk factor, while the molecular signature profile appears to suggest a different pattern of gene expression in patients who develop bortezomib-related neuropathy versus controls [94, 95]. Nevertheless, *de novo* or acquired resistance to bortezomib has prompted the development of second-generation PIs, characterized by higher potency, improved pharmacokinetics, or broader activity on all three catalytic subunits. Carfilzomib (PR-171) is an epoxyketone PI which irreversibly inhibits the chymotryptic-like activity of the proteasome [96]. Based upon activity in bortezomib-resistant MM, it received

Table 33.6 Important characteristics of FDA-approved, novel therapeutic agents in MM.

Name	Category	Molecular target	Predominant mechanisms of action	Route of administration	Notable side effects	Relevant PK	Increased risk of DVT	Pregnancy Category	FDA Approved Indication
Bortezomib (PS-341, Velcade)	PI	CT-L, C-L subunits of proteasome	PolyUb proteotoxicity NF-κB inhibition Caspase 8 and 9 cleavage UPR, HSR, and ROS induction BM niche-MM inhibition OC inhibition	IV, SQ	PN, thrombocytopenia (transient, cyclic)	Hepatic failure: dose reduction in moderate-severe Renal failure: no adjustment required	No	D[1]	First line (2008)
Carfilzomib (PR-171, Kyprolis)	PI	CT-L subunit of proteasome	PolyUb proteotoxicity Caspase 7, 8 and 9 cleavage UPR, HSR and ROS induction BM niche-MM inhibition	IV	Congestive heart failure, ischemic heart disease	Hepatic failure: N/A Renal failure: no dose adjustment required. Administer post HD in patients with ESRD	Yes Thromboprophylaxis required in combination with Dex or Len/Dex	D[1]	Third line (2012)
Ixazomib (MLN9708, Ninlaro)	PI	CT-L, C-L subunits of proteasome	PolyUb proteotoxicity NF-κB inhibition Caspase 8 and 9 cleavage UPR, HSR, and ROS induction BM niche-MM inhibition PIM1 down-regulation	PO	Rash, diarrhea, neutropenia, thrombocytopenia	Hepatic failure: dose reduction for moderate-severe Renal failure: dose reduction for stage 4 CKD and ESRDNon dialyzable	No	N/A. Teratogenic in rabbits and rats	Second line in combination with Rd (2015)
Thalidomide (Thalomid)	IMiD	CRBN	Proteasome-mediated degradation of IKZF1 and IKZF3	PO	PN, rash, constipation, somnolence	Hepatic failure: N/A Renal failure: no dose adjustment required	Yes Thromboprophylaxis required in combination with Dex[2]	X[1] (Teratogenic)	First line in combination with Dex (2006)
Lenalidomide (Revlimid)	IMiD	CRBN	Proteasome-mediated degradation of IKZF1 and IKZF3	PO	BLACK BOX WARNING for embryo-fetal toxicity, myelosuppression and venous and arterial thromboembolism Second primary malignancies[3]	Hepatic failure: N/A Renal failure: dose reduction for CKD stage ≥3 required Administer post dialysis on HD days	Yes Thromboprophylaxis required in combination with Dex[2]	X[1] (Teratogenic)	Second line in combination with Dex (2006)
Pomalidomide (Pomalyst)	IMiD	CRBN	Proteasome-mediated degradation of IKZF1 and IKZF3	PO	BLACK BOX WARNING for embryo-fetal toxicity and venous and arterial thromboembolism	Data not available for patients with moderate-severe hepatic or renal failure	Yes Thromboprophylaxis required in combination with Dex[2]	X[1] (Teratogenic)	Third line after Btz and IMiD (2013)
Panobinostat (LBH589, Farydak)	HDACi	HDAC class I, II, and IV	Reactivation of epigenetically silenced (deacetylated) oncosuppressors (p21,p27) Proteotoxicity secondary to blockade of aggresome formation	PO	BLACK BOX WARNING for potentially fatal cardiac ischemic events, arrhythmias and diarrhea	Hepatic failure: dose adjustment in mild and moderate. Use not recommended in severe Renal failure: no dose adjustment for stage 1–4 CKD. No data in ESRD	No	N/A Teratogenic in rats and rabbits	Third line in combination with VD after Btz and IMiDs-based regimens (2015)
Elotuzumab (Empliciti)	MoAb	SLAMF7	ADCC Increased NK function	IV	Infusion reaction Second primary malignancy, skin cancer Interference with IgG K M spike detection	Data not available for patients with moderate-severe hepatic failure Renal failure: no dose adjustment. Non dialyzable	No	N/A	Second line in combination with Rd (2015)
Daratumumab (Darzalex)	MoAb	CD38	ADCC CDC ADCP Direct cross-linking mediated cytotoxocity	IV	Infusion reactions Artifactual positive indirect Coombs test Interference with IgG K M spike detection	Data not available for patients with moderate-severe hepatic failure Renal failure: no dose adjustment	No	N/A	Third line after PI and IMiDs or in PI and IMiD-double refractory patients (2015)

[1] Category D: There is positive evidence of human fetal risk based on adverse reaction data from investigational or marketing experience or studies in humans, but potential benefits may warrant use of the drug in pregnant women despite potential risks. Category X: studies in animals or humans have demonstrated fetal abnormalities and/or there is positive evidence of human fetal risk based on adverse reaction data from investigational or marketing experience, and the risks involved in use of the drug in pregnant women clearly outweigh potential benefits. Dual contraception indicated.
[2] Increased risk of DVT was observed in combinatory regimens, particularly with high-dose dexamethasone.
[3] Increased risk of second primary malignancy was observed in patients receiving combination treatment with oral melphalan.
ADCC, antibody-dependent cell-mediated cytotoxicity; ADCP, antibody-dependent cellular phagocytosis; BM, bone marrow; Btz, bortezomib; CDC, complement-dependent cytotoxicity; CKD, chronic kidney disease; C-L, caspase-like; CRBN, cereblon; CT-L, chymotrypsin-like; DVT, deep venous thrombosis; ESRD, end-stage renal disease; HD, hemodialysis; HDAC, histone deacetylase; HDACi, histone deacetylase inhibitor; HSR, heat shock response; IKZF1, IKAROS family zinc finger 1; IKZF2, IKAROS family zinc finger 2; IMiD, immunomodulatory drug; IV, intravenous; MM, multiple myeloma. MoAb, monoclonal antibody; NF-κB, nuclear factor κB; OC, osteoclast; PI, proteasome inhibitors; PIM1, Pim-1 proto-oncogene, serine/threonine kinase; PK, pharmacokinetics; PN, peripheral neuropathy; PO, per os, by mouth; PolyUb, polyubiquitin; Rd, lenalidomide and low-dose dexamethasone; ROS, radical oxygen species; SLAMF7, SLAM family member 7; SQ, subcutaneous; UPR, unfolded protein response; VD, bortezomib and dexamethasone.

FDA approval in relapsed/refractory MM after at least two prior therapies, including an IMiD and bortezomib [97]. In a phase 3 trial in relapsed MM, the addition of carfilzomib to Rd (KRd) resulted in a significantly increased median PFS and overall response rate (ORR) [63]. However, ischemic cardiac disease and heart failure emerged as significant side effects in KRd-treated patients. As with bortezomib, carfilzomib at least partially overcomes the negative prognostic influence of adverse cytogenetics; importantly, it does not cause peripheral neuropathy, making it a valid alternative for patients unable to tolerate bortezomib [98]. Ixazomib is the first FDA-approved oral PI, based on interim results of a phase 3, randomized, double-blind study comparing ixazomib, lenalidomide, dex (IRd) versus Rd in relapsed and/or refractory MM (RRMM) patients. At the first interim analysis, the study met the primary endpoint of improved PFS in the study arm [99]. Importantly, IRd treatment seemed to overcome the negative impact of adverse cytogenetics, particularly del(17p). The most frequently observed, grade 3 and 4 side effect was thrombocytopenia. Ixazomib is further being evaluated in a phase 3 trial in newly diagnosed MM patients in combination with Rd as well as maintenance therapy post autologous SCT in patients with newly diagnosed MM.

Monoclonal Antibodies

Elotuzumab, targeting SLAMF7, and daratumumab, targeting CD38, are the first monoclonal antibodies (MoAb) to receive FDA approval in MM.

Elotuzumab is a humanized IgG1 antibody against SLAMF7 (also known as CS1), a protein highly expressed by MMCs whose function is still elusive. While no significant disease response was observed in patients treated with single-agent elotuzumab, the combination with Rd resulted in an 80–90% response rate in a phase 1/2 clinical trial [100]. Elotuzumab in combination with bortezomib also showed promising results even in bortezomib-resistant patients in a phase 1 study [101]. FDA approval was granted based on the results of a phase 3 trial of Rd ± elotuzumab in RRMM which showed prolongation of PFS and increased ORR [102]. Ongoing phase 3 studies are evaluating the addition of elotuzumab to Rd as first-line therapy as well as the incorporation of elotuzumab into RVd during induction, consolidation, and maintenance in newly diagnosed MM patients.

Daratumumab targets CD38, a transmembrane glycoprotein frequently expressed by MMCs and other hematologic malignancies. *In vitro*, it leads to antibody- and complement-dependent cytotoxicity (ADCC and CDC, respectively) and direct growth arrest in both MM cell lines and primary MMCs, providing the basis for its clinical development [103]. In contrast to elotuzumab, daratumumab proved effective as a single agent in heavily pretreated RRMM patients, with a partial response (PR) observed in 29–36% of patients across two distinct phase 2 studies [104, 105]. The side effect profile of daratumumab was favorable, with infusion reactions being the most frequently observed adverse event. Based on these results, the FDA granted approval for daratumumab as single-agent treatment in MM patients who have received three or more prior therapies, including an IMiD and PI, or who are double refractory to IMiD and PI. Interim results from phase 3, randomized control studies of daratumumab in combination with bortezomib and dex (DVd) and lenalidomide and dex (DRd) showed unprecedented ORR and time to progression [64,65]. Daratumumab appeared to be overall well tolerated with infusion reactions being the most frequent side effect. Clinical trials of daratumumab-based regimens are ongoing as front-line therapy in transplant-eligible and -ineligible patients.

Histone Deacetylase Inhibitors

The histone deacetylases (HDAC) are a family of enzymes characterized by distinct structure and target specificities that are involved in key cellular processes such as proliferation, survival, and migration by controlling epigenetic silencing of gene expression [106]. HDAC inhibitors (HDACi) have been preclinically validated as powerful anticancer drugs. In MM in particular, HDACi targeting HDAC6 were shown to disrupt aggresome formation and aggresome-mediated protein degradation, thus further accentuating proteotoxic stress in MM [90]. The combination of such HDACi with bortezomib proved synergistic *in vitro* and successfully overcame bortezomib resistance in preclinical models [107]. In a phase 3 trial, the combination of the class I/IIb HDACi vorinostat and bortezomib in RRMM achieved a significant ORR compared to the control arm, however PFS was only minimally improved (7.6 vs 6.8 months, respectively, $P = 0.01$), largely due to the severity and frequency of diarrhea, fatigue, and thrombocytopenia, leading to treatment discontinuation in a significant percentage of patients in the treatment arm [108]. Similarly, the combination of vorinostat with Rd proved effective but was poorly tolerated [109]. The clinical development of the pan-HDACi panobinostat showed a similarly narrow therapeutic index, however panobinostat was approved as third-line therapy in MM patients previously exposed to bortezomib and IMiDs based on a 4-month PFS prolongation and almost a doubling of near complete response (nCR) or better in the treatment arm compared to the control arm in a phase 3 trial [110]. Furthermore, adding panobinostat to VD led to a clinical response in about a third of patients with bortezomib-resistant disease and/or high-risk cytogenetics [111].

Front-Line Therapy for Non-Transplant Candidates

One of the major concerns for patients undergoing autologous SCT is the inability to collect an adequate amount of stem cells due to treatment-related damage of BM reserve. Predicated on this idea, the use of DNA alkylators as initial therapy in autologous SCT-eligible patients is discouraged. However, melphalan is an integral part of the first-line therapy for non-transplant candidates in combination with prednisone and novel agents. The VISTA trial first established the superiority of bortezomib/melphalan/prednisone (VMP) compared to MP, and was followed by several randomized clinical trials confirming the superiority of MPT and MPR compared to MP [66, 67, 112]. Cyclophosphamide, also an alkylator, in combination with bortezomib and dexamethasone (CyBorD), proved effective and well tolerated as first-line therapy [58]. Doublet therapy with either bortezomib or lenalidomide plus dex is a reasonable option as front-line therapy in non-transplant candidates with low-risk disease (low disease burden, early stage, high performance status, and absence of unfavorable cytogenetics).

Low-dose dex in combination with lenalidomide (Rd) showed improved OS and fewer side effects compared to lenalidomide/high-dose dex (RD), thus establishing Rd as the preferred regimen [62]. The randomized, phase 3, FIRST trial established continuous Rd as the standard of therapy in transplant-ineligible MM patients based on improvement in PFS and 4-year OS [113]. Of note, patients treated with continuous Rd had a lower incidence of neurologic and hematologic adverse events as well as second primary hematologic malignancies compared to patients receiving melphalan/prednisone/thalidomide (MPT). Continuous lenalidomide maintenance was already proven to be effective in transplant-ineligible patients based on PFS benefit. However, the observation that secondary cancers were more frequent in the lenalidomide arm compared to the control arm was of concern [67, 114]. A follow-up meta-analysis of randomized, controlled, phase 3 trials of newly diagnosed MM patients receiving lenalidomide showed that the combination of lenalidomide with oral melphalan was primarily associated with an increased risk for second primary cancer, particularly MDS, suggesting that this combination rather than lenalidomide per se is responsible for carcinogenesis [115].

The use of bortezomib and IMiDs may be limited by their availability (lenalidomide, for instance, is not readily available in several countries), costs, and side effects. In particular, both bortezomib and thalidomide can cause significant peripheral neuropathy, occasionally severe enough to prompt discontinuation of treatment. A modified RVd regimen (RVd lite) with reduced-dose lenalidomide and once-weekly subcutaneous bortezomib over a 35-day cycle is being evaluated in a phase 2 trial in elderly, transplant-ineligible patients and showing tolerable side effects and promising activity [116]. Overall, MP remains a valuable alternative as a front-line regimen in patients not eligible for transplant. The dosing of melphalan can be easily adjusted to achieve a mild degree of leukopenia/thrombocytopenia without causing profound BM suppression, making it a suitable drug also for elderly patients [117]. A recent pharmacoeconomic analysis of melphalan-based regimens suggests that VMP is more cost effective when compared to MP, MPT, and MPR without any detrimental effect on health outcomes [118].

Front-Line Therapy for Transplant Candidates

For younger patients with limited comorbidities, high-dose therapy followed by autologous SCT is the preferred treatment modality, since it provides more extended PFS and improved quality of life. However, the impact of early transplant on MM prognosis remains debatable, as improvement in OS was observed only in three out of five randomized clinical trials of autologous SCT in first remission versus at relapse [119–121]. The ongoing IFM/DFCI 2009 trial is exploring the benefit of autologous SCT in first remission versus autologous SCT in second remission in the context of RVD induction and consolidation and lenalidomide maintenance. Interim results suggest a 14 months PFS benefit in patients who received autologous SCT in first remission, however, OS at 4 years was not different between the groups [122].

In MM, tandem autologous SCT was found to benefit only those patients who did not achieve a VGPR after the first transplant [123]. Hypodiploid karyotype, t(4;14), t(14;16), del(17) or del(17p), and del(13) were associated with poor PFS and OS post autologous SCT, and are considered negative prognostic factors [124, 125]. Overall, the landscape of induction therapy for MM in transplant candidates has markedly improved. Highly effective front-line double, triple, and quadruple drug combinations incorporating novel agents have achieved unprecedented depth and ORR with VGPR or higher between 60 and 75% for the three drug regimens, thus largely overcoming the need for tandem autologous SCT. The EVOLUTION trial, a randomized, phase 2 study comparing bortezomib/dex plus either lenalidomide or cyclophosphamide versus the combination of all four drugs showed no substantial benefit in terms of PFS for the quadruple regimen [58]. Decreased treatment-related morbidity and mortality, as well as prolonged PFS and OS, have been noted with incorporation of combination novel agents as induction prior to, and consolidation post transplant, as well as in maintenance therapy. On the base of subset analysis and retrospective data, it appears that bortezomib can overcome the adverse prognosis of t(4;14) and del(13), while its effect on del(17) or del(17p) is still questionable [56, 126]. The recently approved oral PI ixazomib proved effective in MM patients with adverse cytogenetics, particularly del(17) [99].

Patients 65 years of age or younger with adequate renal, pulmonary, cardiac, and hepatic function have generally been considered eligible for autologous SCT [127]. However, the improved outcome with incorporation of novel agents into the transplant paradigm has now prompted studies to examine the role of transplantation in the era of novel therapies. These include RVD with or without early transplant, as well as MPR versus tandem transplantation therapy.

Initial therapy in transplant candidates should include combination novel therapies. In randomized trials, bortezomib or lenalidomide plus dex have been shown to be effective initial treatments. RVD, bortezomib/thalidomide/dex (VTD), or CyBorD achieve higher overall and extent of response than two drug combinations [24]. Inclusion of bortezomib in upfront therapy is recommended for patients with adverse cytogenetics, in particular t(4;14) and possibly del(17), as well as in patients presenting with AKI since dose adjustment is not required and bortezomib typically achieves rapid reduction in paraprotein [46]. Thalidomide also does not require dose adjustment based on eGFR, while dose reduction in renal failure is required for lenalidomide. In patients with significant baseline peripheral neuropathy and low-risk disease, the omission of bortezomib may be considered, although subcutaneous rather than intravenous injection drastically reduces the incidence of this side effect. In patients with high-risk disease, bortezomib should be incorporated and if not tolerated due to PN, strong consideration should be given to substitute carfilzomib or ixazomib.

Response to therapy should be assessed after two cycles according to the uniform response criteria from the IMWG, and stem cell collection is usually pursued between cycles 4 and 6, especially to avoid prolonged therapy with lenalidomide, which may compromise stem cell collection [128]. The timing of high-dose therapy and stem cell reinfusion is a matter of debate with some advocating continuation of induction treatment to achieve the deepest degree of response and others supporting early autologous SCT in order to avoid drug resistance or complications [129]. For patients who achieve a prompt stringent complete remission (sCR), the dilemma about continuing pharmacologic therapy followed by maintenance versus proceeding to autologous SCT is also being studied in randomized trials, as described previously.

In terms of conditioning regimen, a randomized trial from the Intergroupe Francophone du Myelome (IFM) established high-dose (200 mg/m^2) melphalan as the preferred regimen and total body radiation is no longer used [130]. Of note, the use of combination targeted therapies, i.e., VTD or RVD (2–4 cycles) as consolidation post transplant can increase depth and duration of response, with a significant fraction of patients now achieving sCR, as assessed by either polymerase chain reaction or multicolor flow cytometric techniques.

Maintenance Therapy

Both IMiDs and bortezomib have proven to be highly effective and well tolerated. Maintenance therapy with either single-agent or combination therapy has therefore been tested in MM patients as a strategy to prolong PFS and possibly OS. In patients ineligible for autologous SCT, bortezomib plus thalidomide maintenance following quadruple regimen MPVT was superior to MPV with respect to response rate and PFS, but showed no survival advantage and higher incidence of neutropenia and cardiac events [131]. In a similar patient population, lenalidomide maintenance proved to have statistically significant superior PFS, but not OS, at 4-year follow-up. In this trial, newly diagnosed patients were randomized to MP versus MPR versus MPR followed by lenalidomide maintenance (MPR-R). The median PFS was comparable for MP and MPR (13 vs 14 months), while it was 31 months for patients who received MPR-R [67]. Despite the lack of prolonged OS at 4-year follow-up, the reported quality of life was significantly improved in patients receiving continuous treatment with lenalidomide, favoring the maintenance strategy [132].

The data regarding the role of maintenance with either thalidomide or lenalidomide are less controversial in the post autologous SCT setting, since use of these agents as maintenance until disease progression has improved PFS, quality of life, and OS [133]. Although a small, but statistically significant increase in the incidence of both hematologic and solid secondary malignancies in patients treated with lenalidomide has been observed in retrospective analysis, the benefits of maintenance are felt to outweigh this risk [114]. Although maintenance therapy with bortezomib is expected to be effective in prolonging PFS post autologous SCT, only one phase 3 trial has been performed to date. Unfortunately, the schema of treatment and randomization of this study does not allow any clear conclusion regarding the benefit of bortezomib maintenance per se. However, the trial clearly demonstrated that prolonged treatment with bortezomib is feasible and safe, although dose reduction is likely to be required for a proportion of patients [56].

Allogeneic Transplant

The use of allogeneic SCT in MM has been largely disappointing. Predicated on the prolonged PFS and decreased rate of relapse observed in MM patients post syngeneic transplantation compared to autologous SCT, the graft-versus-myeloma effect was hypothesized to improve outcome [134, 135]. Although some patients have enjoyed prolonged PFS and OS, a high (40%) treatment-related mortality was noted in early studies with myeloablative, allogeneic SCT. Indeed, strategies to decrease the incidence of graft-versus-host disease (GVHD) via T-cell depletion or nonmyeloablative conditioning regimens have been evaluated to exploit the graft-versus-myeloma effect while avoiding attendant toxicity [136]. Tandem autologous SCT has been compared to autologous SCT followed by nonmyeloablative, HLA-identical sibling allogeneic transplant, with a trend supporting improved OS in patients receiving allogeneic transplant [137]. In these studies induction chemotherapy prior to transplant did not incorporate novel agents, resulting in a very low degree of VGPR or CR prior to conditioning, suggesting potential improved outcome with current regimens. However, a more recent phase 3 trial with biological randomization evaluated tandem autologous SCT versus autologous SCT followed by nonmyeloablative, allogeneic HSCT [138]. This study showed no improvement in PFS or OS at 3-year follow-up for standard-risk patients, suggesting that the benefit of graft-versus-myeloma effect is offset by the increased treatment-related mortality. In high-risk patients, treatment-related mortality in the first year approached 40%, but thereafter the OS curve tended to plateau, suggesting the possibility of a significantly improved survival with longer follow-up. At the present time, allogeneic transplant should be performed in the context of a clinical trial directed to achieve high rate of response while avoiding treatment-related morbidity and mortality.

Treatment of Recurrent Disease and Investigational Agents

Biochemical recurrence in MM warrants treatment in high-risk MM patients, but can be followed clinically and with frequent laboratory analysis in low-risk patients to assess the pace of disease progression. Myeloma therapies used in first-line treatment can be re-used if significant time has elapsed from initial treatment or can be incorporated in new combinations. Indeed, the same induction regimen can be effective in patients with late recurrence, although acquired comorbidities, decreased BM reserve, and higher incidence of side effects generally limit therapeutic success. Eventually, MMCs acquire resistance to treatment, prompting need for protocols evaluating novel agents in an attempt to extend survival.

Immune-based therapies, small molecules targeting the ubiquitin-proteasome pathway including novel PIs, and therapies directed at newly identified molecular targets including histone deacetylase 6, Bruton's tyrosine kinase (BTK), and bromodomain 4 are under evaluation in MM [139].

The orally bioavailable HDAC6 specific inhibitor ricolinostat (ACY-1215) was developed predicated on its preclinical activity against MM via disruption of the aggresomal pathway and with the goal of improving therapeutic index [140]. Phase 1/2 studies of ricolinostat in combination with VD or Rd in RRMM showed clinical activity even against bortezomib- or lenalidomide-refractory MM in the context of a favorable side effect profile [141–143].

Informed by bench research on the function of the ubiquitin-proteasome system (UPS) and adaptive response to PI, small molecule inhibitors of deubiquitinating enzymes have been validated preclinically and are entering early clinical development [144].

Similarly, BTK and bromodomain 4 were hypothesized to be good targets in MM given their role in mediating osteoclastogenesis and chromatin modification, respectively. On the base of this preclinical research, BTK inhibitors and JQ1 inhibitor of bromodomain 4 are currently under evaluation in derived clinical trials in MM [145, 146]. Combination of the Bcl-2 inhibitor venetoclax (ABT-199) with bortezomib and dexamethasone has recently shown positive results in a phase 1b trial in bortezomib-naïve or bortezomib-sensitive (ORR 83% and 68%, respectively) RRMM patients, consistent with the response pattern observed during preclinical development [147–149]. Patients harboring a t(11;14) were shown to be particularly sensitive to this compounds and single agent venotoclax has been proven effective in RRMM with t(11;14) [150].

Finally, the clinical development of immunotherapies, from monoclonal antibodies to checkpoint inhibitors and chimeric antigen receptor (CAR)-T cells, has profoundly changed the therapeutic landscape for cancer patients, with staggering, sustained responses observed in relapsed, refractory solid and hematologic malignancies [151–153]. Particularly, checkpoint inhibitors alone or in combination have proven a powerful tool to unleash self, anti-cancer immunity and cause cancer regression [154, 155]. Preliminary results of single-agent anti-PD1 antibody in MM patients have been disappointing with only one patient out of 27 enrolled in a phase 1b trial of nivolumab achieving an objective response; however, its combination with Rd appears active in a phase 1 trial in RRMM [156, 157]. Preclinical data are more encouraging for PD-L1 antibody and the combination of PD-1 and PD-L1 antibodies as well as their combination with novel agents, particularly IMiDs and HDAC inhibitors, and their clinical development is ongoing [158].

Chimeric antigen receptor (CAR)-T cells expressing a chimeric T-cell receptor composed of an anti-BCMA single-chain variable fragment, a CD28 or 4-1BB domain, and a CD3-zeta T-cell activation domain are currently in a first-in-humans clinical trial [159]. Two heavily pretreated patients receiving the highest dose escalation level experienced a rapid and profound response to CAR-T with one patient achieving an sCR 2 months after CAR-T cell infusion [160]. Interestingly, the group of Carl June reported a single case of MM remission after infusion of CAR-T cells directed against CD19 [161]. The mechanisms of disease clearance are unclear as 99.5% of the patient's MM cells did not have CD19 surface expression. CAR-T cells directed against NY-ESO-1 also induced profound and sustained responses in heavily pretreated MM patients in a phase 1/2 trial [162]. Predicated on the activity of daratumumab and elotuzumab and preclinical data, CAR-T cells directed against CD38 and SLAMF-7 are in development.

Ancillary Therapy

Myeloma-related bone disease and complications are the major determinant of poor quality of life and decreased performance status in patients with MM. Around 80–90% of MM patients will develop MM-related bone disease, ranging from osteopenia to pathologic fractures. The monthly intravenous administration of the aminobisphosphonate pamidronate was shown to decrease skeletal-related events (pathologic fractures, cord compression, need for orthopedic surgery or radiotherapy) in a large, double-blind study enrolling patients with stage 3 Durie–Salmon MM presenting with at least one bone lesion [163]. Along with diminished complications, treatment with pamidronate improved symptoms related to bone disease, performance status, and overall quality of life. Pamidronate has been largely replaced by zoledronic acid, a related bisphosphonate with higher potency, allowing for shorter infusion time (15 minutes vs 4 hours), less nephrotoxicity, and use in patients with mild to moderate kidney failure. Recently, direct antitumoral activity of nitrogen-containing bisphosphonates (pamidronate and zoledronic acid) was reported in a preclinical model of MM and in a clinical trial in breast cancer [164, 165]. Predicated on these results, a phase 3, randomized, prospective clinical trial was launched in MM comparing zoledronic acid to an orally available bisphosphonate, clodronate. The trial revealed improved OS in patients receiving zoledronic acid, providing the first clinical evidence of its anti-MM activity [166]. The length of duration of bisphosphonate therapy is a matter of debate due to its efficacy on the one hand versus the potential for significant side effects on the other. In particular, osteonecrosis of the jaw has been reported with the more potent zoledronic acid compared to pamidronate or clodronate. Meticulous dental care with at least annual examination is required for patients receiving high-dose bisphosphonates. Currently, bisphosphonates should be commenced in all MM patients receiving therapy, especially if presenting with bone lesions. Their use should be considered in patients with SMM, particularly in the context of clinical trials. Therapy should be continued in the presence of active disease and discontinuation considered in patients with CR or VGPR [167]. Close monitoring of renal function is recommended and use of the RANKL inhibitor, denosumab, in place of bisphosphonates can be considered in patients with renal compromise [168].

Prophylactic anticoagulation is recommended in patients receiving the combination of thalidomide, lenalidomide, or pomalidomide plus dex, given the excess incidence of venous thromboembolism noted in clinical trials. Depending on the presence or absence of patient-related risk factors for venous stasis, aspirin, low molecular weight heparin, or warfarin are accepted forms of anticoagulation [169].

Prophylactic antiviral therapy is recommended in patients receiving bortezomib, given the high incidence of varicella zoster virus reactivation noted in the APEX trial [170].

Follow-Up and Survivorship

The paradigm of MM as a rapidly fatal disease is changing. The development of novel therapies, largely designed based on the growing fund of knowledge of the biology of MM, has prolonged OS from a median of 1–2 years to 7–8 years. Ancillary therapies and mitigation of side effects have significantly improved the quality of life of MM patients, who now often have a chronic disease with the potential for prolonged survival post therapy.

Genomic studies are ongoing to help personalize treatment. Given the pace of approval of therapies in MM over the past 10 years, there is a reasonable hope that MM will soon become a chronic disease in the majority of patients, with curative potential. In this context, health care providers should be cautious in selecting anti-MM therapy with high potential for life-long complications and/or high treatment-related mortality. A close relationship between patients, families, and health care providers is indispensable to appropriately care for patients with MM. Improvement in quality of life, rather than just prolongation of survival, is becoming an increasingly important and feasible goal of therapy.

References

1 Siegel RL, Miller KD, Jemal A. Cancer statistics, 2017. *CA Cancer J Clin* 2017;67(1):7–30.
2 Howlader N, Noone AM, Krapcho M, *et al.* (eds). SEER Cancer Statistics Review, 1975-2013, National Cancer Institute. Bethesda, MD, http://seer.cancer.gov/csr/1975_2013/, based on November 2015 SEER data submission, posted to the SEER web site, April 2016.
3 Greenberg AJ, Rajkumar SV, Vachon CM. Familial monoclonal gammopathy of undetermined significance and multiple myeloma: epidemiology, risk factors, and biological characteristics. *Blood* 2012;119(23):5359–66.
4 Grass S, Preuss KD, Thome S, *et al.* Paraproteins of familial MGUS/multiple myeloma target family-typical antigens: hyperphosphorylation of autoantigens is a consistent finding in familial and sporadic MGUS/MM. *Blood* 2011;118(3):635–7.
5 Mailankody S, Pfeiffer RM, Kristinsson SY, *et al.* Risk of acute myeloid leukemia and myelodysplastic syndromes after multiple myeloma and its precursor disease (MGUS). *Blood* 2011;118(15):4086–92.
6 Anderson KC, Carrasco RD. Pathogenesis of myeloma. *Ann Rev Pathol* 2011;6:249–74.
7 Hauser AE, Muehlinghaus G, Manz RA, *et al.* Long-lived plasma cells in immunity and inflammation. *Ann NY Acad Sci* 2003;987:266–9.
8 Shapiro-Shelef M, Calame K. Regulation of plasma-cell development. *Nat Rev Immunol* 2005;5(3):230–42.
9 Sahota SS, Leo R, Hamblin TJ, Stevenson FK. Myeloma VL and VH gene sequences reveal a complementary imprint of antigen selection in tumor cells. *Blood* 1997;89(1):219–26.
10 Bakkus MH, Heirman C, Van Riet I, Van Camp B, Thielemans K. Evidence that multiple myeloma Ig heavy chain VDJ genes contain somatic mutations but show no intraclonal variation. *Blood* 1992;80(9):2326–35.
11 Bergsagel PL, Chesi M, Nardini E, *et al.* Promiscuous translocations into immunoglobulin heavy chain switch regions in multiple myeloma. *Proc Natl Acad Sci U S A* 1996;93(24):13931–6.
12 Landgren O, Kyle RA, Pfeiffer RM, *et al.* Monoclonal gammopathy of undetermined significance (MGUS) consistently precedes multiple myeloma: a prospective study. *Blood* 2009;113(22):5412–7.
13 Weiss BM, Abadie J, Verma P, Howard RS, Kuehl WM. A monoclonal gammopathy precedes multiple myeloma in most patients. *Blood* 2009;113(22):5418–22.
14 Kyle RA, Durie BG, Rajkumar SV, *et al.* Monoclonal gammopathy of undetermined significance (MGUS) and smoldering (asymptomatic) multiple myeloma: IMWG consensus perspectives risk factors for progression and guidelines for monitoring and management. *Leukemia* 2010;24(6):1121–7.
15 Rajkumar SV, Kyle RA, Therneau TM, *et al.* Serum free light chain ratio is an independent risk factor for progression in monoclonal gammopathy of undetermined significance. *Blood* 2005;106(3):812–7.
16 Perez-Persona E, Vidriales MB, Mateo G, *et al.* New criteria to identify risk of progression in monoclonal gammopathy of uncertain significance and smoldering multiple myeloma based on multiparameter flow cytometry analysis of bone marrow plasma cells. *Blood* 2007;110(7):2586–92.
17 San Miguel JF, Almeida J, Mateo G, *et al.* Immunophenotypic evaluation of the plasma cell compartment in multiple myeloma: a tool for comparing the efficacy of different treatment strategies and predicting outcome. *Blood* 2002;99(5):1853–6.
18 Rawstron AC, Davies FE, DasGupta R, *et al.* Flow cytometric disease monitoring in multiple myeloma: the relationship between normal and neoplastic plasma cells predicts outcome after transplantation. *Blood* 2002;100(9):3095–100.
19 Carrasco DR, Sukhdeo K, Protopopova M, *et al.* The differentiation and stress response factor XBP-1 drives multiple myeloma pathogenesis. *Cancer Cell* 2007;11(4):349–60.
20 Shaffer AL, Emre NC, Lamy L, *et al.* IRF4 addiction in multiple myeloma. *Nature* 2008;454(7201):226–31.
21 Morgan GJ, Walker BA, Davies FE. The genetic architecture of multiple myeloma. *Nat Rev Cancer* 2012;12(5):335–48.
22 Bianchi G, Ghobrial I. Does my patient with a serum monoclonal spike have multiple myeloma? *Hematol Oncol Clin North Am* 2012;26(2):383–93.
23 Raje N, Roodman GD. Advances in the biology and treatment of bone disease in multiple myeloma. *Clin Cancer Res* 2011;17(6):1278–86.
24 Anderson KC, Alsina M, Bensinger W, *et al.* Multiple myeloma. *J Natl Compr Canc Netw* 2011;9(10):1146–83.
25 Mena E, Choyke P, Tan E, Landgren O, Kurdziel K. Molecular imaging in myeloma precursor disease. *Semin Hematol* 2011;48(1):22–31.
26 Zamagni E, Patriarca F, Nanni C, *et al.* Prognostic relevance of 18-F FDG PET/CT in newly diagnosed multiple myeloma patients treated with up-front autologous transplantation. *Blood* 2011;118(23):5989–95.
27 Nasr SH, Valeri AM, Sethi S, *et al.* Clinicopathologic correlations in multiple myeloma: a case series of 190 patients with kidney biopsies. *Am J Kidney Dis* 2012;59(6):786–94.
28 Hutchison CA, Blade J, Cockwell P, *et al.* Novel approaches for reducing free light chains in patients with myeloma kidney. *Nat Rev Nephrol* 2012;8(4):234–43.
29 Rajkumar SV, Dimopoulos MA, Palumbo A, *et al.* International Myeloma Working Group updated criteria for the diagnosis of multiple myeloma. *Lancet Oncol* 2014;15(12):e538–e48.

30 Ropper AH, Gorson KC. Neuropathies associated with paraproteinemia. *N Engl J Med* 1998;338(22):1601–7.
31 Kourelis TV, Kumar SK, Gertz MA, *et al.* Coexistent multiple myeloma or increased bone marrow plasma cells define equally high-risk populations in patients with immunoglobulin light chain amyloidosis. *J Clin Oncol* 2013;31(34):4319–24.
32 Lindsley H, Teller D, Noonan B, Peterson M, Mannik M. Hyperviscosity syndrome in multiple myeloma. A reversible, concentration-dependent aggregation of the myeloma protein. *Am J Med* 1973;54(5):682–8.
33 Lorsbach RB, Hsi ED, Dogan A, Fend F. Plasma cell myeloma and related neoplasms. *Am J Clin Pathol* 2011;136(2): 168–82.
34 Dispenzieri A, Kyle RA, Katzmann JA, *et al.* Immunoglobulin free light chain ratio is an independent risk factor for progression of smoldering (asymptomatic) multiple myeloma. *Blood* 2008;111(2):785–9.
35 Mateos MV, Hernandez MT, Giraldo P, *et al.* Lenalidomide plus dexamethasone for high-risk smoldering multiple myeloma. *N Engl J Med* 2013;369(5):438–47.
36 Kyle RA, Therneau TM, Rajkumar SV, *et al.* A long-term study of prognosis in monoclonal gammopathy of undetermined significance. *N Engl J Med* 2002;346(8):564–9.
37 Bianchi G, Kyle RA, Colby CL, *et al.* Impact of optimal follow-up of monoclonal gammopathy of undetermined significance on early diagnosis and prevention of myeloma-related complications. *Blood* 2010;116(12):2019–25; quiz 197.
38 Knobel D, Zouhair A, Tsang RW, *et al.* Prognostic factors in solitary plasmacytoma of the bone: a multicenter Rare Cancer Network study. *BMC Cancer* 2006;6:118.
39 Jawad MU, Scully SP. Skeletal Plasmacytoma: progression of disease and impact of local treatment; an analysis of SEER database. *J Hematol Oncol* 2009;2:41.
40 Ozsahin M, Tsang RW, Poortmans P, *et al.* Outcomes and patterns of failure in solitary plasmacytoma: a multicenter Rare Cancer Network study of 258 patients. *Int J Radiat Oncol Biol Phys* 2006;64(1):210–7.
41 Dimopoulos MA, Moulopoulos LA, Maniatis A, Alexanian R. Solitary plasmacytoma of bone and asymptomatic multiple myeloma. *Blood* 2000;96(6):2037–44.
42 Liebross RH, Ha CS, Cox JD, *et al.* Clinical course of solitary extramedullary plasmacytoma. *Radiother Oncol* 1999;52(3):245–9.
43 Dispenzieri A. POEMS syndrome: update on diagnosis, risk-stratification, and management. *Am J Hematol* 2015;90(10):951–62.
44 Durie BG, Salmon SE. A clinical staging system for multiple myeloma. Correlation of measured myeloma cell mass with presenting clinical features, response to treatment, and survival. *Cancer* 1975;36(3):842–54.
45 Greipp PR, San Miguel J, Durie BG, *et al.* International staging system for multiple myeloma. *J Clin Oncol* 2005;23(15):3412–20.
46 Kumar SK, Mikhael JR, Buadi FK, *et al.* Management of newly diagnosed symptomatic multiple myeloma: updated Mayo Stratification of Myeloma and Risk-Adapted Therapy (mSMART) consensus guidelines. *Mayo Clin Proc* 2009;84(12):1095–110.
47 Chng WJ, Dispenzieri A, Chim CS, *et al.* IMWG consensus on risk stratification in multiple myeloma. *Leukemia* 2014;28(2): 269–77.
48 Sonneveld P, Avet-Loiseau H, Lonial S, *et al.* Treatment of multiple myeloma with high-risk cytogenetics: a consensus of the International Myeloma Working Group. *Blood* 2016;127(24):2955–62.
49 Bianchi G, Richardson PG, Anderson KC. Best treatment strategies in high-risk multiple myeloma: navigating a gray area. *J Clin Oncol* 2014;32(20):2125–32.
50 Avet-Loiseau H. Ultra high-risk myeloma. *Hematology Am Soc Hematol Educ Program* 2010;2010:489–93.
51 Kyle RA, Rajkumar SV. Multiple myeloma. *Blood* 2008;111(6): 2962–72.
52 Kumar SK, Rajkumar SV, Dispenzieri A, *et al.* Improved survival in multiple myeloma and the impact of novel therapies. *Blood* 2008;111(5):2516–20.
53 Hideshima T, Mitsiades C, Tonon G, Richardson PG, Anderson KC. Understanding multiple myeloma pathogenesis in the bone marrow to identify new therapeutic targets. *Nat Rev Cancer* 2007;7(8):585–98.
54 Singhal S, Mehta J, Desikan R, *et al.* Antitumor activity of thalidomide in refractory multiple myeloma. *N Engl J Med* 1999;341(21):1565–71.
55 Harousseau JL, Attal M, Avet-Loiseau H, *et al.* Bortezomib plus dexamethasone is superior to vincristine plus doxorubicin plus dexamethasone as induction treatment prior to autologous stem-cell transplantation in newly diagnosed multiple myeloma: results of the IFM 2005-01 phase III trial. *J Clin Oncol* 2010;28(30):4621–9.
56 Sonneveld P, Schmidt-Wolf IG, van der Holt B, *et al.* Bortezomib induction and maintenance treatment in patients with newly diagnosed multiple myeloma: results of the randomized phase III HOVON-65/GMMG-HD4 trial. *J Clin Oncol* 2012;30(24):2946–55.
57 Mai EK, Bertsch U, Durig J, *et al.* Phase III trial of bortezomib, cyclophosphamide and dexamethasone (VCD) versus bortezomib, doxorubicin and dexamethasone (PAd) in newly diagnosed myeloma. *Leukemia* 2015;29(8):1721–9.
58 Kumar S, Flinn I, Richardson PG, *et al.* Randomized, multicenter, phase 2 study (EVOLUTION) of combinations of bortezomib, dexamethasone, cyclophosphamide, and lenalidomide in previously untreated multiple myeloma. *Blood* 2012;119(19):4375–82.
59 Reeder CB, Reece DE, Kukreti V, *et al.* Cyclophosphamide, bortezomib and dexamethasone induction for newly diagnosed multiple myeloma: high response rates in a phase II clinical trial. *Leukemia* 2009;23(7):1337–41.
60 Cavo M, Pantani L, Petrucci MT, *et al.* Bortezomib-thalidomide-dexamethasone is superior to thalidomide-dexamethasone as consolidation therapy after autologous hematopoietic stem cell transplantation in patients with newly diagnosed multiple myeloma. *Blood* 2012;120(1):9–19.
61 Durie BG, Hoering A, Adibi MH, *et al.* Bortezomib with lenalidomide and dexamethasone versus lenalidomide and dexamethasone alone in patients with newly diagnosed myeloma without intent for immediate autologous stem-cell transplant (SWOG S0777): a randomised, open-label, phase 3 trial. *Lancet* 2017;389(10068):519–27.

62 Rajkumar SV, Jacobus S, Callander NS, *et al.* Lenalidomide plus high-dose dexamethasone versus lenalidomide plus low-dose dexamethasone as initial therapy for newly diagnosed multiple myeloma: an open-label randomised controlled trial. *Lancet Oncol* 2010;11(1):29–37.

63 Stewart AK, Rajkumar SV, Dimopoulos MA, *et al.* Carfilzomib, lenalidomide, and dexamethasone for relapsed multiple myeloma. *N Engl J Med* 2015;372(2):142–52.

64 Dimopoulos M, Oriol A, Nahi H, *et al.* Daratumumab, lenalidomide, and dexamethasone for multiple myeloma. *N Engl J Med* 2016;375(14):1319–31.

65 Palumbo A, Chanan-Khan A, Weisel K, *et al.* Daratumumab, bortezomib, and dexamethasone for multiple myeloma. *N Engl J Med* 2016;375(8):754–66.

66 San Miguel JF, Schlag R, Khuageva NK, *et al.* Bortezomib plus melphalan and prednisone for initial treatment of multiple myeloma. *N Engl J Med* 2008;359(9):906–17.

67 Palumbo A, Hajek R, Delforge M, *et al.* Continuous lenalidomide treatment for newly diagnosed multiple myeloma. *N Engl J Med* 2012;366(19):1759–69.

68 Palumbo A, Falco P, Corradini P, *et al.* Melphalan, prednisone, and lenalidomide treatment for newly diagnosed myeloma: a report from the GIMEMA – Italian Multiple Myeloma Network. *J Clin Oncol* 2007;25(28):4459–65.

69 Wijermans P, Schaafsma M, Termorshuizen F, *et al.* Phase III study of the value of thalidomide added to melphalan plus prednisone in elderly patients with newly diagnosed multiple myeloma: the HOVON 49 Study. *J Clin Oncol* 2010;28(19):3160–6.

70 Palumbo A, Hajek R, Delforge M, *et al.* Continuous lenalidomide treatment for newly diagnosed multiple myeloma. *N Engl J Med* 2012;366(19):1759–69.

71 Blade J, Samson D, Reece D, *et al.* Criteria for evaluating disease response and progression in patients with multiple myeloma treated by high-dose therapy and haemopoietic stem cell transplantation. Myeloma Subcommittee of the EBMT. European Group for Blood and Marrow Transplant. *Br J Haematol* 1998;102(5):1115–23.

72 Raje N, Anderson K. Thalidomide – a revival story. *N Engl J Med* 1999;341(21):1606–9.

73 Lopez-Girona A, Mendy D, Ito T, *et al.* Cereblon is a direct protein target for immunomodulatory and antiproliferative activities of lenalidomide and pomalidomide. *Leukemia* 2012;26(11):2326–35.

74 Ito T, Ando H, Suzuki T, *et al.* Identification of a primary target of thalidomide teratogenicity. *Science* 2010;327(5971):1345–50.

75 Weber DM, Chen C, Niesvizky R, *et al.* Lenalidomide plus dexamethasone for relapsed multiple myeloma in North America. *N Engl J Med* 2007;357(21):2133–42.

76 Richardson PG, Weller E, Lonial S, *et al.* Lenalidomide, bortezomib, and dexamethasone combination therapy in patients with newly diagnosed multiple myeloma. *Blood* 2010;116(5):679–86.

77 Attal M, Lauwers-Cances V, Marit G, *et al.* Lenalidomide maintenance after stem-cell transplantation for multiple myeloma. *N Engl J Med* 2012;366(19):1782–91.

78 McCarthy PL, Owzar K, Hofmeister CC, *et al.* Lenalidomide after stem-cell transplantation for multiple myeloma. *N Engl J Med* 2012;366(19):1770–81.

79 Lacy MQ, Hayman SR, Gertz MA, *et al.* Pomalidomide (CC4047) plus low dose dexamethasone (Pom/dex) is active and well tolerated in lenalidomide refractory multiple myeloma (MM). *Leukemia* 2010;24(11):1934–9.

80 Leleu X, Attal M, Arnulf B, *et al.* Pomalidomide plus low-dose dexamethasone is active and well tolerated in bortezomib and lenalidomide-refractory multiple myeloma: Intergroupe Francophone du Myelome 2009-02. *Blood* 2013;121(11):1968–75.

81 clinicaltrials.gov.

82 Voorhees PM, Mulkey F, Hassoun H, *et al.* Alliance A061202. a Phase I/II study of pomalidomide, dexamethasone and ixazomib versus pomalidomide and dexamethasone for patients with multiple myeloma refractory to lenalidomide and proteasome inhibitor based therapy: Phase I results. *Blood* 2015;126:375.

83 Goldberg AL. Functions of the proteasome: the lysis at the end of the tunnel. *Science* 1995;268(5210):522–3.

84 Lee DH, Goldberg AL. Proteasome inhibitors: valuable new tools for cell biologists. *Trends Cell Biol* 1998;8(10):397–403.

85 Kisselev AF, Goldberg AL. Proteasome inhibitors: from research tools to drug candidates. *Chem Biol* 2001;8(8):739–58.

86 Adams J. The proteasome: a suitable antineoplastic target. *Nature reviews Cancer.* 2004 May;4(5):349–60.

87 Hideshima T, Richardson P, Chauhan D, *et al.* The proteasome inhibitor PS-341 inhibits growth, induces apoptosis, and overcomes drug resistance in human multiple myeloma cells. *Cancer Res* 2001;61(7):3071–6.

88 Orlowski RZ, Stinchcombe TE, Mitchell BS, *et al.* Phase I trial of the proteasome inhibitor PS-341 in patients with refractory hematologic malignancies. *J Clin Oncol* 2002;20(22):4420–7.

89 Richardson PG, Sonneveld P, Schuster MW, *et al.* Bortezomib or high-dose dexamethasone for relapsed multiple myeloma. *N Engl J Med* 2005;352(24):2487–98.

90 Bianchi G, Oliva L, Cascio P, *et al.* The proteasome load versus capacity balance determines apoptotic sensitivity of multiple myeloma cells to proteasome inhibition. *Blood* 2009;113(13):3040–9.

91 McConkey DJ, Zhu K. Mechanisms of proteasome inhibitor action and resistance in cancer. *Drug resistance updates: reviews and commentaries in antimicrobial and anticancer chemotherapy.* 2008;11(4-5):164–79.

92 Richardson PG, Sonneveld P, Schuster MW, *et al.* Reversibility of symptomatic peripheral neuropathy with bortezomib in the phase III APEX trial in relapsed multiple myeloma: impact of a dose-modification guideline. *Br J Haematol* 2009;144(6):895–903.

93 Moreau P, Pylypenko H, Grosicki S, *et al.* Subcutaneous versus intravenous administration of bortezomib in patients with relapsed multiple myeloma: a randomised, phase 3, non-inferiority study. *Lancet Oncol* 2011;12(5):431–40.

94 Richardson PG, Xie W, Mitsiades C, *et al.* Single-agent bortezomib in previously untreated multiple myeloma: efficacy, characterization of peripheral neuropathy, and molecular correlations with response and neuropathy. *J Clin Oncol* 2009;27(21):3518–25.

95 Dimopoulos MA, Mateos MV, Richardson PG, *et al.* Risk factors for, and reversibility of, peripheral neuropathy associated with bortezomib-melphalan-prednisone in newly diagnosed patients with multiple myeloma: subanalysis of the phase 3 VISTA study. *Eur J Haematol* 2011;86(1):23–31.

96 Kortuem KM, Stewart AK. Carfilzomib. *Blood* 2013;121(6): 893–7.

97 Siegel DS, Martin T, Wang M, *et al.* A phase 2 study of single-agent carfilzomib (PX-171-003-A1) in patients with relapsed and refractory multiple myeloma. *Blood* 2012;120(14):2817–25.

98 Jakubowiak AJ, Siegel DS, Martin T, *et al.* Treatment outcomes in patients with relapsed and refractory multiple myeloma and high-risk cytogenetics receiving single-agent carfilzomib in the PX-171-003-A1 study. *Leukemia* 2013;27(12):2351–6.

99 Moreau P, Masszi T, Grzasko N, *et al.* Ixazomib, an investigational oral proteasome inhibitor (PI), in combination with lenalidomide and dexamethasone (IRd), significantly extends progression-free survival (PFS) for patients (pts) with relapsed and/or refractory multiple myeloma (RRMM): The Phase 3 Tourmaline-MM1 Study (NCT01564537). *Blood* 2015;126:727.

100 Lonial S, Vij R, Harousseau JL, *et al.* Elotuzumab in combination with lenalidomide and low-dose dexamethasone in relapsed or refractory multiple myeloma. *J Clin Oncol* 2012;30(16):1953–9.

101 Jakubowiak AJ, Benson DM, Bensinger W, *et al.* Phase I trial of anti-CS1 monoclonal antibody elotuzumab in combination with bortezomib in the treatment of relapsed/refractory multiple myeloma. *J Clin Oncol* 2012;30(16):1960–5.

102 Lonial S, Dimopoulos M, Palumbo A, *et al.* Elotuzumab therapy for relapsed or refractory multiple myeloma. *N Engl J Med* 2015;373(7):621–31.

103 de Weers M, Tai YT, van der Veer MS, *et al.* Daratumumab, a novel therapeutic human CD38 monoclonal antibody, induces killing of multiple myeloma and other hematological tumors. *J Immunol* 2011;186(3):1840–8.

104 Lonial S, Weiss BM, Usmani SZ, *et al.* Daratumumab monotherapy in patients with treatment-refractory multiple myeloma (SIRIUS): an open-label, randomised, phase 2 trial. *Lancet* 2016;387(10027):1551–60.

105 Lokhorst HM, Plesner T, Laubach JP, *et al.* Targeting CD38 with daratumumab monotherapy in multiple myeloma. *N Engl J Med* 2015;373(13):1207–19.

106 D'Arcy P, Brnjic S, Olofsson MH, *et al.* Inhibition of proteasome deubiquitinating activity as a new cancer therapy. *Nat Med* 2011;17(12):1636–40.

107 Hideshima T, Bradner JE, Wong J, *et al.* Small-molecule inhibition of proteasome and aggresome function induces synergistic antitumor activity in multiple myeloma. *Proc Natl Acad Sci U S A* 2005;102(24):8567–72.

108 Dimopoulos M, Siegel DS, Lonial S, *et al.* Vorinostat or placebo in combination with bortezomib in patients with multiple myeloma (VANTAGE 088): a multicentre, randomised, double-blind study. *Lancet Oncol* 2013;14(11):1129–40.

109 Siegel DS, Richardson P, Dimopoulos M, *et al.* Vorinostat in combination with lenalidomide and dexamethasone in patients with relapsed or refractory multiple myeloma. *Blood Cancer J* 2014;4:e182.

110 San-Miguel JF, Hungria VT, Yoon SS, *et al.* Panobinostat plus bortezomib and dexamethasone versus placebo plus bortezomib and dexamethasone in patients with relapsed or relapsed and refractory multiple myeloma: a multicentre, randomised, double-blind phase 3 trial. *Lancet Oncol* 2014;15(11):1195–206.

111 Richardson PG, Schlossman RL, Alsina M, *et al.* PANORAMA 2: panobinostat in combination with bortezomib and dexamethasone in patients with relapsed and bortezomib-refractory myeloma. *Blood* 2013;122(14):2331–7.

112 Facon T, Mary JY, Hulin C, *et al.* Melphalan and prednisone plus thalidomide versus melphalan and prednisone alone or reduced-intensity autologous stem cell transplantation in elderly patients with multiple myeloma (IFM 99-06): a randomised trial. *Lancet* 2007;370(9594):1209–18.

113 Benboubker L, Dimopoulos MA, Dispenzieri A, *et al.* Lenalidomide and dexamethasone in transplant-ineligible patients with myeloma. *N Engl J Med* 2014;371(10):906–17.

114 Dimopoulos MA, Richardson PG, Brandenburg N, *et al.* A review of second primary malignancy in patients with relapsed or refractory multiple myeloma treated with lenalidomide. *Blood* 2012;119(12):2764–7.

115 Palumbo A, Bringhen S, Kumar SK, *et al.* Second primary malignancies with lenalidomide therapy for newly diagnosed myeloma: a meta-analysis of individual patient data. *Lancet Oncol* 2014;15(3).333–42.

116 O'Donnell EK, Laubach JP, Yee AJ, *et al.* A Phase II study of modified lenalidomide, bortezomib, and dexamethasone (RVD-lite) for transplant-ineligible patients with newly diagnosed multiple myeloma. *Blood* 2014;124:3454.

117 Palumbo A, Anderson K. Multiple myeloma. *N Engl J Med* 2011;364(11):1046–60.

118 Garrison LP, Jr, Wang ST, Huang H, *et al.* The cost-effectiveness of initial treatment of multiple myeloma in the U.S. with bortezomib plus melphalan and prednisone versus thalidomide plus melphalan and prednisone or lenalidomide plus melphalan and prednisone with continuous lenalidomide maintenance treatment. *Oncologist* 2013;18(1):27–36.

119 Attal M, Harousseau JL, Stoppa AM, *et al.* A prospective, randomized trial of autologous bone marrow transplantation and chemotherapy in multiple myeloma. Intergroupe Francais du Myelome. *N Engl J Med* 1996;335(2):91–7.

120 Barlogie B, Attal M, Crowley J, *et al.* Long-term follow-up of autotransplantation trials for multiple myeloma: update of protocols conducted by the intergroupe francophone du myelome, southwest oncology group, and university of arkansas for medical sciences. *J Clin Oncol* 2010;28(7):1209–14.

121 Cavo M, Rajkumar SV, Palumbo A, *et al.* International Myeloma Working Group consensus approach to the treatment of multiple myeloma patients who are candidates for autologous stem cell transplantation. *Blood* 2011;117(23):6063–73.

122 Attal M, Lauwers-Cances V, Hulin C, *et al.* Lenalidomide, Bortezomib and Dexamethasone with Transplantation for Multiple Myeloma. *NEJM* 2017;376:1311–1320.

123 Attal M, Harousseau JL, Facon T, *et al.* Single versus double autologous stem-cell transplantation for multiple myeloma. *N Engl J Med* 2003;349(26):2495–502.

124 Gertz MA, Lacy MQ, Dispenzieri A, *et al.* Clinical implications of t(11;14)(q13;q32), t(4;14)(p16.3;q32), and -17p13 in myeloma patients treated with high-dose therapy. *Blood* 2005;106(8): 2837–40.

125 Cavo M, Terragna C, Renzulli M, *et al.* Poor outcome with front-line autologous transplantation in t(4;14) multiple myeloma: low complete remission rate and short duration of remission. *J Clin Oncol* 2006;24(3):e4–5.

126 Avet-Loiseau H, Leleu X, Roussel M, *et al.* Bortezomib plus dexamethasone induction improves outcome of patients with t(4;14) myeloma but not outcome of patients with del(17p). *J Clin Oncol* 2010;28(30):4630–4.

127 Kumar SK, Dingli D, Lacy MQ, *et al.* Autologous stem cell transplantation in patients of 70 years and older with multiple myeloma: Results from a matched pair analysis. *Am J Hematol* 2008;83(8):614–7.

128 Durie BG, Harousseau JL, Miguel JS, *et al.* International uniform response criteria for multiple myeloma. *Leukemia* 2006;20(9):1467–73.

129 Stewart AK, Richardson PG, San-Miguel JF. How I treat multiple myeloma in younger patients. *Blood* 2009;114(27):5436–43.

130 Moreau P, Facon T, Attal M, *et al.* Comparison of 200 mg/m(2) melphalan and 8 Gy total body irradiation plus 140 mg/m^2 melphalan as conditioning regimens for peripheral blood stem cell transplantation in patients with newly diagnosed multiple myeloma: final analysis of the Intergroupe Francophone du Myelome 9502 randomized trial. *Blood* 2002;99(3):731–5.

131 Palumbo A, Bringhen S, Rossi D, *et al.* Bortezomib-melphalan-prednisone-thalidomide followed by maintenance with bortezomib-thalidomide compared with bortezomib-melphalan-prednisone for initial treatment of multiple myeloma: a randomized controlled trial. *J Clin Oncol* 2010;28(34):5101–9.

132 Dimopoulos MA, Delforge M, Hajek R, *et al.* Lenalidomide, melphalan, and prednisone, followed by lenalidomide maintenance, improves health-related quality of life in newly diagnosed multiple myeloma patients aged 65 years or older: results of a randomized phase III trial. *Haematologica* 2013;98(5):784–8.

133 Ludwig H, Durie BG, McCarthy P, *et al.* IMWG consensus on maintenance therapy in multiple myeloma. *Blood* 2012;119(13):3003–15.

134 Bashey A, Perez WS, Zhang MJ, *et al.* Comparison of twin and autologous transplants for multiple myeloma. *Biol Blood Marrow Transplant* 2008;14(10):1118–24.

135 Gahrton G, Svensson H, Bjorkstrand B, *et al.* Syngeneic transplantation in multiple myeloma – a case-matched comparison with autologous and allogeneic transplantation. European Group for Blood and Marrow Transplantation. *Bone Marrow Transplant* 1999;24(7):741–5.

136 Alyea E, Weller E, Schlossman R, *et al.* T-cell–depleted allogeneic bone marrow transplantation followed by donor lymphocyte infusion in patients with multiple myeloma: induction of graft-versus-myeloma effect. *Blood* 2001;98(4): 934–9.

137 Bruno B, Rotta M, Patriarca F, *et al.* A comparison of allografting with autografting for newly diagnosed myeloma. *N Engl J Med* 2007;356(11):1110–20.

138 Krishnan A, Pasquini MC, Logan B, *et al.* Autologous haemopoietic stem-cell transplantation followed by allogeneic or autologous haemopoietic stem-cell transplantation in patients with multiple myeloma (BMT CTN 0102): a phase 3 biological assignment trial. *Lancet Oncol* 2011;12(13): 1195–203.

139 Bianchi G, Richardson PG, Anderson KC. Promising therapies in multiple myeloma. *Blood* 2015;126:300–310.

140 Santo L, Hideshima T, Kung AL, *et al.* Preclinical activity, pharmacodynamic, and pharmacokinetic properties of a selective HDAC6 inhibitor, ACY-1215, in combination with bortezomib in multiple myeloma. *Blood* 2012;119(11): 2579–89.

141 Vogl DT, Raje N, Hari P, *et al.* Phase 1B results of ricolinostat (ACY-1215) combination therapy with bortezomib and dexamethasone in patients with relapsed or relapsed and refractory multiple myeloma (MM). *Blood* 2014;124:4764.

142 Hideshima T, Cottini F, Ohguchi H, *et al.* Rational combination treatment with histone deacetylase inhibitors and immunomodulatory drugs in multiple myeloma. *Blood Cancer J* 2015;5:e312.

143 Yee AJ, Voorhees PM, Bensinger W, *et al.* Ricolinostat (ACY-1215), a selective HDAC6 inhibitor, in combination with lenalidomide and dexamethasone: results of a Phase 1b trial in relapsed and relapsed refractory multiple myeloma. *Blood* 2014;124:4772.

144 Chauhan D, Tian Z, Nicholson B, *et al.* A small molecule inhibitor of ubiquitin-specific protease-7 induces apoptosis in multiple myeloma cells and overcomes bortezomib resistance. *Cancer Cell* 2012;22(3):345–58.

145 Tai YT, Chang BY, Kong SY, *et al.* Bruton tyrosine kinase inhibition is a novel therapeutic strategy targeting tumor in the bone marrow microenvironment in multiple myeloma. *Blood* 2012;120(9):1877–87.

146 Delmore JE, Issa GC, Lemieux ME, *et al.* BET bromodomain inhibition as a therapeutic strategy to target c-Myc. *Cell* 2011;146(6):904–17.

147 Touzeau C, Chanan-Khan A, Roberts A, *et al.* Phase 1b interim results: venetoclax (ABT-199/GDC-0199) in combination with bortezomib (BTZ) and dexamethasone (Dex) in relapsed/refractory (R/R) multiple myeloma (MM). *J Clin Oncol* 2015;33(15 suppl):8580.

148 Punnoose EA, Leverson JD, Peale F, *et al.* Expression profile of BCL-2, BCL-XL, and MCL-1 predicts pharmacological response to the BCL-2 selective antagonist venetoclax in multiple myeloma models. *Mol Cancer Ther* 2016;15(5):1132–44.

149 Matulis SM, Gupta VA, Nooka AK, *et al.* Dexamethasone treatment promotes Bcl-2 dependence in multiple myeloma resulting in sensitivity to venetoclax. *Leukemia* 2016;30(5):1086–93.

150 Kumar S, Kaufman JL, Gasparetto C, *et al.* Efficacy of venetoclax as targeted therapy for relapsed/refractory t(11;14) multiple myeloma. *Blood* 2017 Available at: https://doi.org/10.1182/blood-2017-06-788786 (accessed 19 Dec 2017).

151 Topalian SL, Hodi FS, Brahmer JR, *et al.* Safety, activity, and immune correlates of anti-PD-1 antibody in cancer. *N Engl J Med* 2012;366(26):2443–54.

152 Maude SL, Frey N, Shaw PA, *et al.* Chimeric antigen receptor T cells for sustained remissions in leukemia. *N Engl J Med* 2014;371(16):1507–17.

153 Ansell SM, Lesokhin AM, Borrello I, *et al.* PD-1 blockade with nivolumab in relapsed or refractory Hodgkin's lymphoma. *N Engl J Med* 2015;372(4):311–9.

154 Callahan MK, Postow MA, Wolchok JD. Targeting T cell co-receptors for cancer therapy. *Immunity* 2016;44(5):1069–78.

155 Sharma P, Allison JP. The future of immune checkpoint therapy. *Science* 2015;348(6230):56–61.

156 Lesokhin AM, Ansell SM, Armand P, *et al.* Nivolumab in patients with relapsed or refractory hematologic malignancy: preliminary results of a Phase Ib Study. *J Clin Oncol* 2016;34(23):2698–704.

157 San Miguel J, Mateos M, Shah J, *et al.* Pembrolizumab in combination with lenalidomide and low-dose dexamethasone for relapsed/refractory multiple myeloma (RRMM): Keynote-023. *Blood* 2015;126:505.

158 Gorgun G, Samur MK, Cowens KB, *et al.* Lenalidomide enhances immune checkpoint blockade induced immune response in multiple myeloma. *Clin Cancer Res* 2015;21(20):4607–18.

159 Carpenter RO, Evbuomwan MO, Pittaluga S, *et al.* B-cell maturation antigen is a promising target for adoptive T-cell therapy of multiple myeloma. *Clin Cancer Res* 2013;19(8): 2048–60.

160 Ali S, Shi V, Wang M, *et al.* Remissions of multiple myeloma during a first-in-humans clinical trial of T cells expressing an anti-B-cell maturation antigen chimeric antigen receptor. *Blood* 2015;126:LBA-1.

161 Garfall AL, Maus MV, Hwang WT, *et al.* Chimeric antigen receptor T cells against CD19 for multiple myeloma. *N Engl J Med* 2015;373(11):1040–7.

162 Rapoport AP, Stadtmauer EA, Binder-Scholl GK, *et al.* NY-ESO-1-specific TCR-engineered T cells mediate sustained antigen-specific antitumor effects in myeloma. *Nat Med* 2015;21(8):914–21.

163 Berenson JR, Lichtenstein A, Porter L, *et al.* Long-term pamidronate treatment of advanced multiple myeloma patients reduces skeletal events. Myeloma Aredia Study Group. *J Clin Oncol* 1998;16(2):593–602.

164 Guenther A, Gordon S, Tiemann M, *et al.* The bisphosphonate zoledronic acid has antimyeloma activity in vivo by inhibition of protein prenylation. *Int J Cancer* 2010;126(1): 239–46.

165 Gnant M, Mlineritsch B, Schippinger W, *et al.* Endocrine therapy plus zoledronic acid in premenopausal breast cancer. *N Engl J Med* 2009;360(7):679–91.

166 Morgan GJ, Davies FE, Gregory WM, *et al.* First-line treatment with zoledronic acid as compared with clodronic acid in multiple myeloma (MRC Myeloma IX): a randomised controlled trial. *Lancet* 2010;376(9757):1989–99.

167 Terpos E, Morgan G, Dimopoulos MA, *et al.* International Myeloma Working Group recommendations for the treatment of multiple myeloma-related bone disease. *J Clin Oncol* 2013;31(18):2347–57.

168 Henry DH, Costa L, Goldwasser F, *et al.* Randomized, double-blind study of denosumab versus zoledronic acid in the treatment of bone metastases in patients with advanced cancer (excluding breast and prostate cancer) or multiple myeloma. *J Clin Oncol* 2011;29(9):1125–32.

169 Palumbo A, Rajkumar SV, Dimopoulos MA, *et al.* Prevention of thalidomide- and lenalidomide-associated thrombosis in myeloma. *Leukemia* 2008;22(2):414–23.

170 Chanan-Khan A, Sonneveld P, Schuster MW, *et al.* Analysis of herpes zoster events among bortezomib-treated patients in the phase III APEX study. *J Clin Oncol* 2008;26(29):4784–90.

Section 9

Skin Cancer

34

Melanoma

Justin M. Ko[1], Alan C. Geller[2], and Susan M. Swetter[3]

[1] Stanford University Medical Center, Stanford, California, USA
[2] Harvard TH Chan School of Public Health; Massachusetts General Hospital, Boston, Massachusetts, USA
[3] Stanford University Medical Center and Cancer Institute; VA Palo Alto Health Care System, Stanford, California, USA

Incidence and Mortality

Melanoma incidence is rising faster than that of almost all other cancer in the United States (US), and in 2017 there were an estimated 87,110 new cases of invasive melanoma [1]. Annual incidence rate increases of 2–3% per year have been noted in many European countries. In Australia and New Zealand, the two countries with the greatest burden of melanoma incidence, rates have doubled nearly every 10 years. Melanoma incidence has increased steadily over the past 30 years, and since 2004, by 3% annually in Caucasians [2]. Bimodal increases are apparent, with incidence rates rising more than twofold among young women (ages 20–29) and increasing even more sharply among middle-aged and older men.

The increase in melanoma incidence has been attributed to many factors: primarily, increased intermittent ultraviolet radiation (UVR) exposure among fair-skinned populations, via travel to sunny locales and through past wartime service. Several alternative factors have been proposed to contribute to the dramatically increased melanoma incidence in developed countries over the past 70 years, including higher rates of skin biopsies and screening resulting in the detection of thinner, more indolent lesions, and changes in the histologic interpretation of early evolving lesions.

Approximately 9,730 individuals in the US [1] and 23,000 Europeans die from melanoma each year, comprising about 75% of the world's melanoma deaths [3]. In the US and elsewhere, mortality rates for most cancers are dropping, whereas mortality rates of melanoma have only recently stabilized or continue to rise slightly. From 1969 through 2008, mortality declined among men and women aged 20–44. However, the mortality rate among men over age 65, who comprise 36% of all deaths but only 20% of all cases, rose by more than 150% during the same period [2]. These US mortality patterns are evident in most developed countries.

Prognostic Factors

Tumor Thickness

Survival rates decline steadily as the tumor thickness and disease stage increase. Over 95% of individuals diagnosed with melanoma ≤1 mm in thickness (T1) can expect prolonged survival and even cure, while individuals with thicker, later stage lesions (>4 mm) are more likely to die from metastatic disease (5-year survival rates ranging from 50 to 75% depending on other staging parameters) [4]. While a 5-year period is typically used to measure survival, a 2012 study in Queensland found 96% 20-year survival for individuals diagnosed with thin melanoma (≤1 mm) [4].

Many developed countries such as Australia, the US, and Sweden have 5-year survival rates exceeding 90%. In contrast, a number of countries in Eastern Europe have 5-year survival rates of 60%, similar to what was seen in advanced countries nearly 50 years ago. Of the more than 20,000 deaths from melanoma in Europe in 2008, Central and Eastern Europe comprise 35.5% of the total, although they have the smallest population in the region [3].

Patient Age and Gender, and Location of the Primary

A number of clinical factors affect patient prognosis including age, gender, and anatomic location of the primary tumor. In general, men, older individuals, and those with melanoma on the head and neck tend to fare worse. A population-based study in France during 2004–2008 showed that male patients had thicker and more frequently ulcerated tumors. Anatomic location varied between genders, involving the trunk in 47% of male patients and the legs in 48% of female patients. Older patients had thicker and more advanced melanomas, more frequently on the head and neck [5].

The American Cancer Society's Oncology in Practice: Clinical Management, First Edition. Edited by The American Cancer Society.

Melanoma Subtype

There is increasing evidence that the nodular subtype of melanoma accounts for a disproportionate number of melanoma deaths. In an Australian study, the median thickness of nodular melanoma (NM) at diagnosis was 2.6 mm compared with 0.6 mm for superficial spreading melanoma (SSM). A third of patients who died from melanoma during the follow-up period had thick tumors (>4 mm), most of which were NM (61%). Nodular melanoma accounted for 14% of invasive melanoma, but was responsible for 43% of melanoma deaths [4]. By comparison, SSM comprised 56% of invasive melanoma and 30% of deaths. A retrospective population-based cohort study of SEER data from 1978 to 2007 similarly demonstrated that among melanomas of known subtype, SSM comprised 66% of incident melanomas and 46% of ultimately fatal melanomas; in contrast, NM comprised only 14% of incident melanomas but 37% of fatal cases [6].

Etiology, Risk Factors, and Prevention

Melanoma Risk Factors and Assessment Models

Established risk factors for melanoma are discussed in *The American Cancer Society's Oncology in Practice: Clinical Management*, Chapter 10, and include: (i) increased numbers of common/typical melanocytic nevi ("moles"), presence of clinically atypical/dysplastic nevi; (ii) fair-complexion phenotype, often seen in tandem with red hair, light eye color, and increased sun sensitivity; (iii) personal history of non-melanoma skin cancer (NMSC), including basal cell and squamous cell carcinomas; (iv) family history of melanoma; and (v) excessive sun exposure through either natural or artificial ultraviolet light. Several risk assessment models have been used to target individuals who are at high risk for melanoma [7], though there are no available models to identify those at highest risk of developing lethal melanoma. Preliminary components of such a model include targeting white middle-aged and older (>65 years) men and those without partners or significant others, who play an instrumental role in early detection through examination of the skin, prompting or arranging physician skin examinations, and assisting in treatment and diagnostic decisions. Thorough skin examination of high-risk areas such as the back and scalp is warranted given the disproportionate number of fatal melanomas in these locations.

One current risk assessment model has been derived from a large case-control study of 718 non-Hispanic White patients and 945 controls that provided data for primary care clinicians and patients alike [7]. This tool involves inspection of the back for suspect moles and asks two questions about complexion and history of sun exposure. Mild freckling and light complexion were risk factors for both men and women. In addition, >17 small moles and ≥2 large moles in men or ≥12 small moles on the backs of women were also significant risk factors. These data led to the Melanoma Risk Assessment Tool, which is available from the National Cancer Institute (http://www.cancer.gov/melanomarisktool/). The tool calculates absolute risk of melanoma over the next 5 years up to age 70.

Novel Risk Factors for Melanoma

Screening and educational efforts can be more readily targeted to those with more established and identifiable risk factors. While individuals with the following risk factors are not as numerous as those noted earlier, jointly they represent a growing burden of risk thus requiring innovative behavioral strategies.

MC1R

The contribution of melanocortin-1 receptor (*MC1R*) gene variants to the development of early-onset melanoma is unknown. In an Australian population-based, case-control family study, *MC1R* sequencing of 565 young (18–39 years) patients with invasive cutaneous melanoma, 409 unrelated controls, and 518 sibling controls demonstrated that some *MC1R* variants were important determinants of early-onset melanoma, with strong associations in men and those with no or few nevi or with high childhood sun exposure [8].

Childhood Cancer History

History of cancer in childhood is a risk factor for subsequent malignancy, including melanoma. An analysis of childhood cancer survivors for subsequent melanoma risk demonstrated a standardized incidence ratio (SIR) of 2.42 (1.77, 3.23) [9]. The childhood cancer cases were generally those in the radiation field [9, 10].

Organ Transplantation

Organ transplant recipients receive long-term immunosuppression to prevent graft rejection. While transplant populations are at far greater risk of squamous cell carcinomas, they also develop more melanomas compared to the general population [11]. The age-adjusted incidence rate of melanoma among renal transplantation recipients was 55.9 diagnoses per 100,000 population representing a 3.6 times greater risk in age-adjusted, standardized risk from the SEER population [12].

Parkinson Disease

A large systematic meta-analysis reviewed the association of Parkinson disease (PD) and melanoma and demonstrated increased relative risk (RR) of 1.56 (1.27, 1.91) [13]. A more recent publication showed a significant relationship in cases where PD preceded melanoma, with OR 3.61 (1.49, 8.77) Conversely, if melanoma preceded PD, the OR was reported as 1.07 (0.62, 1.84). Many limitations exist, thus there is a need for well-conducted prospective studies that can also attempt to develop biological plausibility for a PD and melanoma association.

Indoor Tanning/Artificial Sunlamps

Indoor tanning is thought to be the major contributor to the increasing incidence of cutaneous melanoma among young women. Increased risk of melanoma has been associated with increasing years, hours, and sessions of tanning behavior [14]. A 2011 review found that ever-users of sunbeds had a 41% increased melanoma risk compared with never-users [15]. When further subdivided, those who used sunbeds >10 times had a higher risk (OR 2.01: 1.22, 3.31), as did those with earlier age of first use [15]. Alarmingly, 76% of melanomas in fair-skinned participants were attributed to tanning bed use at young ages. A meta-analysis of 27 studies found an overall summary RR for melanoma of 1.20 (1.08, 1.34) for "ever use" of sunbeds compared to those without this exposure. The RR for this exposure was even higher among individuals <35 years of age – 1.87 (1.41, 2.48) [16].

Pathology

Molecular Pathology and Pathogenesis

Despite the explosion in understanding of the molecular mechanisms driving melanoma, the sequence of events in which normal melanocytes transform into melanoma cells, referred to as melanomagenesis, remains poorly understood. It likely involves a multistep process of genetic mutations that (i) alter cell proliferation, differentiation, and death, and (ii) impact susceptibility to the carcinogenic effects of UVR [17].

The traditional Clark model of the progression of melanoma emphasized the stepwise transformation of melanocytes to melanoma, from the formation of nevi to the subsequent development of dysplasia, hyperplasia, invasion, and metastasis. However, this stepwise progression from melanocyte to mole to melanoma is relatively uncommon. In fact, fewer than 20–30% of melanomas are believed to arise from precursor nevi, though a higher proportion may be associated with histologically dysplastic nevi [18, 19]. The fact that most cutaneous melanomas arise *de novo* from normal-appearing skin suggests alternative pathways that bypass the nevus as a biologic intermediate, or that melanoma derives from transformed melanocyte stem cells or de-differentiated mature melanocytes [20]. This concept is supported by recent data suggesting difference in survival for patients with nevus-associated melanoma versus *de novo* melanoma, which may be more biologically aggressive [21]. However, Shain *et al.* defined the succession of genetic alterations during melanoma progression, suggesting an intermediate category of melanocytic neoplasia that may be defined by the controversial category of dysplastic nevi [22]. This study also underscored UVR as a major factor in both the initiation and progression of melanoma.

Signaling Pathways in Melanoma

A number of cellular pathways have been identified in the development of melanoma. These span signal transduction to developmental and transcriptional pathways and cell cycle deregulation. Understanding of signaling events involved in melanomagenesis may allow for more nuanced differentiation of subsets of melanoma and define molecular signatures and subtypes associated with response and resistance to targeted therapy.

One growth factor pathway that has garnered considerable attention as related to melanoma is the *RAS–RAF–MAPK–ERK* signal transduction cascade. Oncogenic lesions introduce changes in the primary sequence of *RAS* so that the protein is constitutively active. Much of the attention surrounding this pathway in human melanoma focuses on the fact that, in virtually all cases, there is an alteration at some level in the *RAS* signaling cascade [23]. Specifically, *NRAS* and *BRAF* mutations occur in about 80% of the most common subtypes of melanoma.

Activating mutations in *BRAF* are found in approximately half of all melanomas, with the majority arising in intermittently sun-exposed skin, as compared with melanomas from chronically sun-exposed areas, acral, mucosal, and uveal melanomas, suggesting an inverse association with high levels of cumulative UV exposure [24, 25]. The most common *BRAF* mutation is the T1799A point mutation, *BRAF* V600E, which results in the protein taking on a constitutive active configuration. Since *BRAF* mutations are common in both benign and dysplastic nevi, it is likely that such mutations are not sufficient for malignant transformation of melanocytes [26]. However, the high frequency of these mutations suggests a role in the earliest stages of neoplasia. The etiologic factors resulting in the *BRAF* mutation remain unclear, specifically the role of UVR.

The c-KIT receptor tyrosine kinase has been shown to be amplified or mutated in a subset of melanomas, specifically those that develop on body sites with little to no UV exposure, such as acral and mucosal melanomas, or on chronically sun-damaged skin [27]. Activation of this tyrosine kinase results in the stimulation of the *MAPK* and *PI3K–AKT* pathways, producing both proliferative and survival advantages [28].

None of the oncogenes or tumor suppressor genes identified in melanoma are thought to be solely responsible for melanoma pathogenesis. For instance, *NRAS*, as mentioned above, activates Raf kinases in response to growth factor receptor activation and harbors activating mutations in 15–20% of melanomas [29]. The loss of the p16 tumor suppressor is a relatively frequent event in melanoma, and there is significant overlap with *BRAF* mutation [30]. *PTEN* mutations and deletion have been described in a minority of melanomas and appear to coincide with *BRAF* mutation.

Clinicopathologic Subtypes

Four major clinicopathologic subtypes of primary cutaneous melanoma have been identified: superficial spreading melanoma, nodular melanoma, lentigo maligna melanoma, and acral lentiginous melanoma (Table 34.1, Figures 34.1, 34.2, 34.3, 34.4, and 34.5). In addition, there are rare variants (accounting for <5% of melanomas) including: (i) desmoplastic/neurotropic melanoma, (ii) mucosal (lentiginous) melanoma [31], (iii) malignant blue nevus, (iv) melanoma arising in a giant/large congenital nevus, and (v) melanoma of soft parts (clear cell sarcoma). Distinction among the subtypes is based on histologic growth pattern, anatomic site, and degree of sun damage. The pattern of sun exposure varies between the types (chronic in lentigo maligna; intermittent in superficial spreading and nodular subtypes; and non-contributory in acral lentiginous and mucosal subtypes). Whether the melanoma subtype affects the overall prognosis remains controversial [17].

Desmoplastic melanoma is a relatively rare but important melanoma subtype, given its predilection for older-age individuals and clinical features similar to NMSC. It may occur in association with macular, lentigo maligna-type pigmentation, or it may present *de novo* as a firm, amelanotic nodule or scar. It occurs most often on sun-exposed areas of the head and neck,

Table 34.1 Summary of major melanoma subtypes.

Melanoma subtype	Clinical features and anatomic site	Histologic features	Contributory role of UV exposure	Molecular features
Superficial spreading	Nearly 70% of cutaneous melanoma. Most common on the trunk in men and legs in women. Flat to slightly raised lesion that commonly displays the ABCD warning signs	Radial *in situ* growth phase of atypical melanocytes arranged haphazardly at the dermoepidermal junction, prominent upward (pagetoid) migration	Intermittent, high-intensity exposure	*BRAF* mutations more common
Nodular	15–30% of cutaneous melanoma. Most commonly on the legs and trunk in men and women. Dark brown to black papule or nodule demonstrating rapid growth over weeks to months	No preceding radial growth phase, direct vertical extension of population of melanoma cells demonstrating proliferation and nuclear pleomorphism into the dermis	Intermittent, high-intensity exposure	*NRAS* mutations more common
Lentigo maligna	Typically located on the head, neck, and arms (chronically sun-damaged skin) of fair-skinned older individuals (average age 65 years). Slowly growing over years to decades. Large brown macule (*in situ* component) with development of raised blue-black nodules (invasive component)	Radial *in situ* growth at the dermoepidermal junction with little tendency for pagetoid scatter, background	Chronic exposure	*KIT* mutations more common
Acral lentiginous	Least common subtype in White persons, most common subtype in African American, Asian, and Hispanic persons. Occurs on the palms, on the soles, or beneath the nail plate. Often delayed diagnosis as can mimic subungual hematoma, subungual wart, or fungal infection of the nail	Radial *in situ* growth at the dermoepidermal junction with little tendency for pagetoid scatter	Non-contributory	*KIT*, *CDK4*, and *CDKN2A* mutations more common

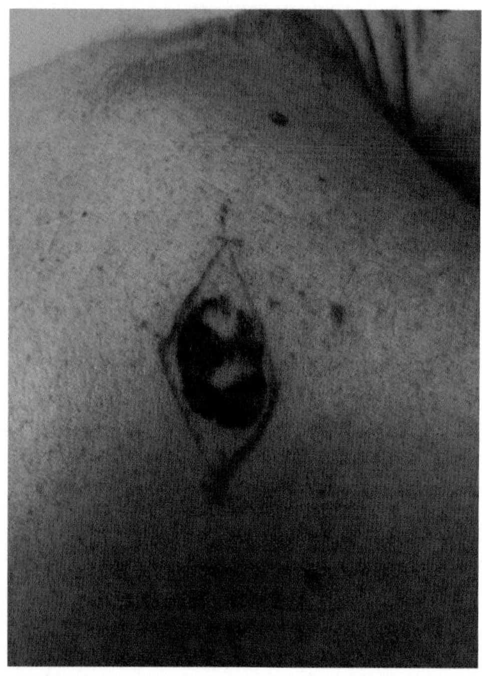

Figure 34.1 Superficial spreading melanoma on the right upper back of a middle-aged man.

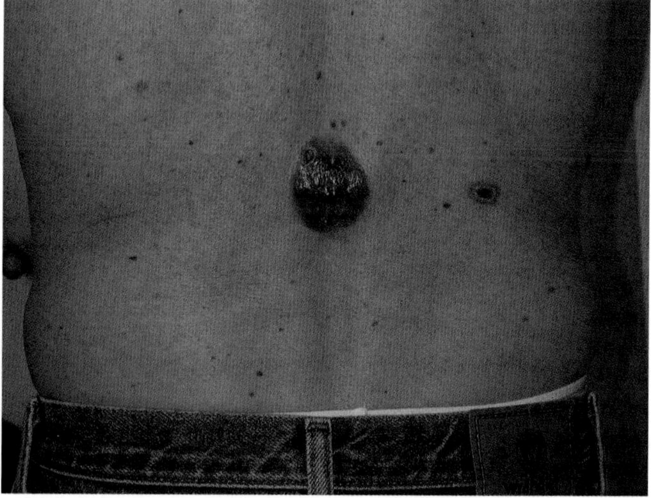

Figure 34.2 Nodular melanoma on the lower mid-back of a middle-aged man.

with a mean age of 60–65 years. Lack of pigmentation and clinical features more suggestive of keratinocytic skin cancer may result in delay in detection and thicker tumors at diagnosis. Desmoplastic melanoma frequently exhibits perineural extension and has a predilection for local recurrence.

Amelanotic melanoma is an uncommon clinical presentation (<5% of melanomas) and can be seen in any subtype. It is nonpigmented and clinically appears pink or flesh-colored, often mimicking basal cell or squamous cell carcinoma, dermatofibroma, or a ruptured hair follicle. Amelanotic melanoma occurs most commonly in the setting of the nodular or desmoplastic melanoma subtypes or melanoma metastasis to the skin, presumably because of the inability of these poorly differentiated cancer cells to synthesize melanin pigment (Figure 34.6).

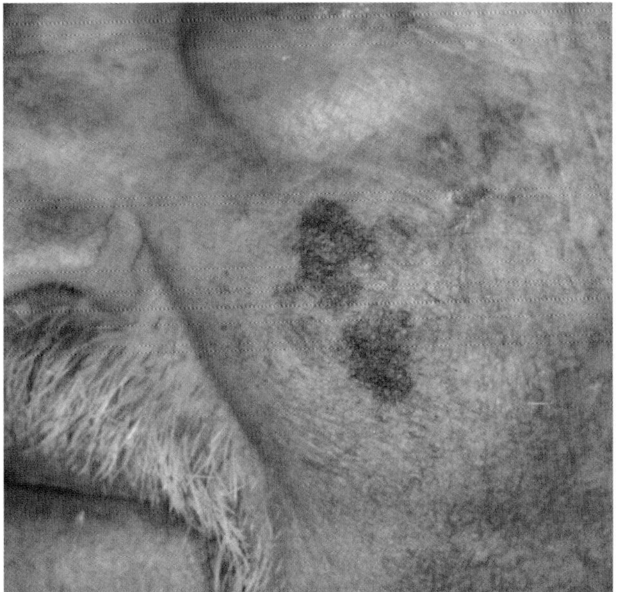

Figure 34.3 Lentigo maligna melanoma, left cheek.

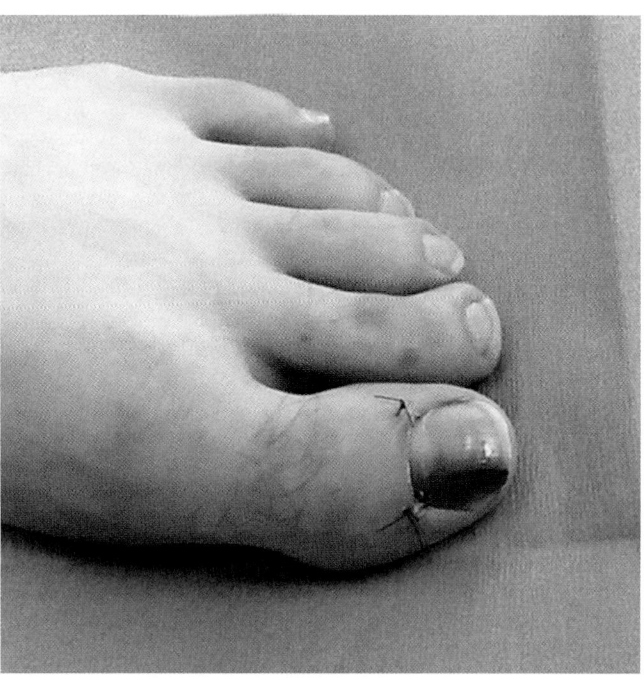

Figure 34.5 Subungual melanoma, left great toe.

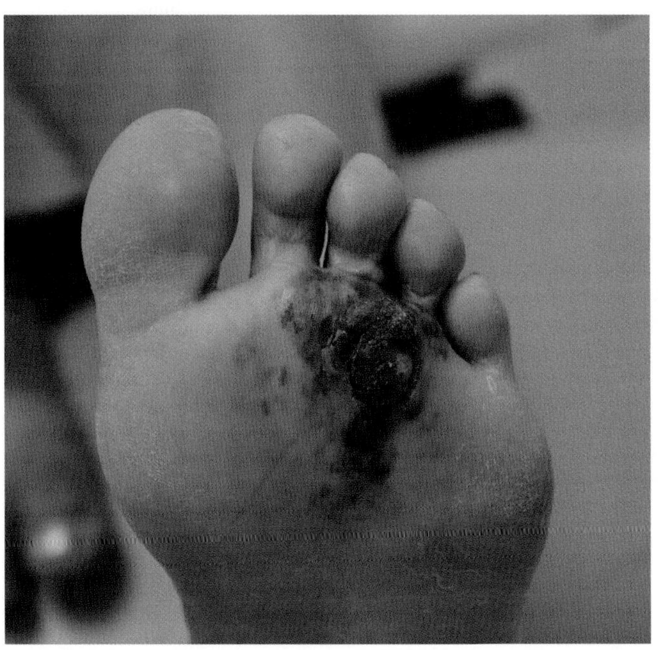

Figure 34.4 Acral lentiginous melanoma, sole of left foot.

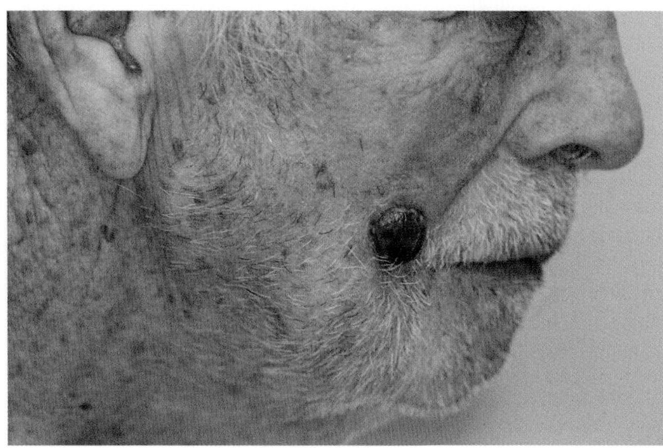

Figure 34.6 Amelanotic melanoma, right cheek.

Histopathologic Findings

With the exception of nodular melanoma, the growth patterns of the other clinicopathologic subtypes are characterized by a preceding *in situ* (radial growth) phase that lacks the biologic potential to metastasize and may last from months to years before dermal invasion occurs. Superficial spreading melanoma has an *in situ* (radial growth) phase characterized by increased numbers of atypical intraepithelial melanocytes arranged haphazardly at the dermoepidermal junction and demonstrates upward migration of cells through the epidermis (pagetoid spread). Lentigo maligna melanoma and acral lentiginous melanoma demonstrate predominant *in situ* growth at the dermoepidermal junction and little tendency for pagetoid spread.

Dermal invasion confers metastatic potential, although the greatest risk occurs in the setting of a vertical growth (tumorigenic) phase [32]. Immunohistochemical staining for lineage (S-100, homatropine methylbromide 45 (HMB-45), melan-A/Mart-1) or proliferation markers (proliferating cell nuclear antigen, Ki-67) may be helpful in some cases for histologic differentiation from histologic melanoma simulators such as melanocytic nevi, Spitz nevi, cellular blue nevus, clear cell sarcoma, or malignant peripheral nerve sheath tumor [33].

Diagnosis

Diagnosis of Cutaneous Melanoma

Melanoma can occur on any skin or mucosal surface, although a history of cutaneous melanoma does not appear to increase the risk of developing primary intraocular, oral, or other mucosal melanoma. Melanoma occurs most commonly on the trunk in White males and the lower legs in White females [34]. In African American, Hispanic, and Asian persons, the most common subtype of melanoma occurs on non-sun-exposed areas including plantar foot, subungual, palmar, and mucosal sites.

A total-body skin examination is critical when evaluating a patient at risk for melanoma, particularly those with increased mole count, presence of clinical atypical nevi, prior non-melanoma skin cancer, and/or strong family history of melanoma. Multiple studies have demonstrated that thinner melanomas are associated with physician detection during routine skin or physical examinations, compared with patient detection of melanoma when a lesion changes or becomes symptomatic [35].

From a clinical standpoint, a new or changing "mole" or other skin lesion is the most common warning sign for melanoma. Variation in color and/or an increase in diameter, height, or asymmetry of borders of a pigmented lesion are noted by the majority of patients with melanoma at the time of diagnosis. Symptoms such as bleeding, itching, ulceration, and pain in a pigmented lesion are less common but also warrant evaluation. Again, because the majority of cutaneous melanoma arise *de novo* and not in association with a precursor nevus, mass removal of melanocytic nevi is not warranted for melanoma prevention.

Clinician and patient education regarding the warning signs of early melanoma (particularly the superficial spreading subtype) has been enhanced through the use of the ABCDE clinical warning signs criteria [36] (Table 34.2). Lesions exhibiting these features should be evaluated for potential melanoma, although severely atypical/dysplastic nevi may be difficult to distinguish clinically. More recent use of the "ugly duckling" warning sign, in which skin examination is focused on recognition of a pigmented or clinically amelanotic lesion that simply looks different from the rest, may assist with detection of lesions that lack the classic ABCD criteria (e.g., nodular, amelanotic, or desmoplastic melanomas) [37].

Table 34.2 ABCDEs: clinical features of melanoma.

A	Asymmetry – the two halves of the lesion do not match each other
B	Border irregularity – may appear ragged, notched, or scalloped
C	Color variation – color is not uniform or lesion may be many colors displaying shades of tan, brown, or black. White, reddish, or blue-gray discoloration is of particular concern
D	Diameter – usually greater than 6 mm (roughly the diameter of a pencil eraser) although melanomas may be smaller in size; any growth in a nevus warrants an evaluation
E	Evolving lesion – changes in size or color; critical for nodular or amelanotic melanoma, which may not exhibit the ABCD criteria above

The standard for melanoma diagnosis is histopathologic examination of the suspicious skin lesion. An excisional biopsy with narrow margins (1–3 mm) of normal-appearing skin around the lesion is preferred when possible to provide accurate diagnosis and histologic microstaging. Acceptable excisional biopsy techniques include a punch biopsy around the visible pigmented lesion, saucerization shave (extending into the deep reticular dermis or subcutaneous fat), or fusiform excision [38, 39]. Superficial shave biopsies for suspicious pigmented lesions should be avoided because partial removal of the primary melanoma may compromise measurement of tumor thickness, which remains the most important histologic prognostic factor for cutaneous melanoma [40].

An important exception to this rule is the lentigo maligna subtype of melanoma *in situ*, in which the risk of misdiagnosis is high if partial biopsy specimens are taken. The best diagnostic biopsy technique in this case is often a broad shave biopsy that extends into at least the papillary dermis, which provides the opportunity to exclude microinvasive melanoma and allows for optimal histopathologic interpretation of the tumor [38, 39].

Staging

Tumor thickness, or Breslow depth, is the most important histologic determinant of prognosis and is measured vertically in millimeters from the top of the granular layer (or base of superficial ulceration) to the deepest point of tumor involvement. Importantly, the Eighth Edition of the *AJCC Cancer Staging Manual* records thickness to the nearest 0.1 mm, rather than the nearest 0.01 mm, due to the lack of precision in measurement beyond the 1/10th decimal point [41]. Increased tumor thickness confers a higher metastatic potential and a poorer prognosis [43]. The presence of ulceration microscopically, defined as a full-thickness epidermal defect overlying the melanoma, is the next most important histologic determinant of patient prognosis and, when present, up-stages both cutaneous and nodal disease [44].

Clark level has been used for more than 40 years and provides a measurement of tumor invasion anatomically. However, analysis of the worldwide American Joint Committee on Cancer/Union for International Cancer Control (AJCC/UICC) 2008 collaborative melanoma database demonstrated lower statistical correlation with melanoma survival when level of invasion was compared with thickness, mitotic rate, ulceration, age, sex, and site. As such, the Seventh Edition of the *AJCC Cancer Staging Manual* no longer included the Clark level in T1 melanomas (≤1 mm depth), except in cases when mitotic rate could be assessed [44]. The Eighth Edition of the *AJCC Cancer Staging Manual* excludes Clark level from staging, noting its lack of predictive value for survival, compared with other prognostic variables [41].

In contrast, cellular proliferation within the primary tumor, as reflected by the mitotic rate (measured per mm^2), emerged as an important predictor of survival [45]. Dermal mitotic rate $\geq 1/mm^2$ was used to up-stage T1a melanoma to T1b melanoma in the 2009 AJCC/UICC staging system [44]. However, tumor mitotic rate was removed as a staging criterion from the Eighth Edition of the *AJCC Cancer Staging Manual*, although histopathologic measurement of mitotic rate (#/mm^2) is recommended across all tumor thicknesses given its impact on prognosis [41].

The AJCC/UICC Melanoma Staging System recommends sentinel lymph node (SLN) – biopsy be performed as a staging procedure in patients for whom the information will have clinical relevance in planning subsequent treatment and follow-up. The procedure is currently recommended by the National Comprehensive Cancer Network (NCCN) for patients who have T2, T3, or T4 melanomas and clinically uninvolved regional lymph nodes (clinical stages IB and II), as well as for patients with T1 melanomas and secondary features associated with increased risk for nodal micrometastases, including ulceration, lymphovascular invasion, and elevated mitotic rate (proposed as ≥2/mm^2), especially when the primary melanoma is greater than 0.75 mm (now ≥0.8 mm, T1b) in thickness [44]. However, due to AJCC changes in the staging of T1a/b melanoma (effective January 2018), which recognize Breslow thickness ≥0.8 mm as the most reliable predictor of SLN positivity (regardless of histologic ulceration of dermal mitotic rate), current NCCN recommendations (www.nccn.org) utilize this tumor thickness as a threshold for SLNB consideration. Discussion of SLNB may also be appropriate in T1a melanoma (<0.8 mm without ulceration) when adverse histologic features are present, particularly in younger age patients [41, 42].

Treatment

Surgical Care

Excision of Cutaneous Melanoma

Wide local excision is the primary treatment for cutaneous melanoma (AJCC/UICC stages 0, I, and II). The goals of surgery are to achieve histopathologically clear margins and a low likelihood of local recurrence, including both true local recurrence at the margin (from inadequately excised primary melanoma) and metastatic local recurrence (i.e., satellites from intralymphatic spread of melanoma). Surgical margins of 5 mm were recommended for melanoma *in situ* by the National Institutes of Health (NIH) Consensus Development Conference on Diagnosis and Treatment of Early Melanoma in 1992, though this guideline was not based on prospectively controlled trials data [46]. In addition, certain melanoma *in situ* subtypes (e.g., lentigo maligna and acral lentiginous) often demonstrate subclinical extension and skip areas, making the use of histologically controlled margins through Mohs micrographic surgery or staged excision (e.g., "slow-Mohs") potentially more effective compared to conventional wide local excision [17, 47]. Mohs micrographic surgery is generally not recommended for treatment of invasive melanoma, though it has been successfully used in the management of thinner tumors. Studies have shown no increased local recurrence for Mohs surgery compared with historical controls, although much of the currently published data stem from thinner tumors with a lower risk of local recurrence and metastasis [48, 49].

Clinical margins of 1 cm are generally recommended for T1 melanoma [46, 50] and may be acceptable for tumors between 1.01 mm and 2.0 mm thickness (T2), although 2-cm margins are also deemed appropriate for T2 melanoma [51, 52]. Margins of 2 cm are recommended for cutaneous melanomas >2 mm (T3, T4) to prevent potential local recurrence in or around the scar site. In a recently concluded multicenter randomized controlled trial in nine European countries from 1994 to 2002, 936 patients with clinical stage IIA–IIC cutaneous melanoma >2 mm were randomized to wide excision with either 2- or 4-cm resection margins. With median follow-up of 6.7 years, the overall 5-year survival in both groups was 65%, suggesting that a 2-cm resection margin is sufficient and safe for patients with cutaneous melanoma thicker than 2 mm [53]. Both the NCCN and American Academy of Dermatology (AAD) melanoma practice guidelines recommend surgical margins of at least 1 cm and no greater than 2 cm for invasive melanoma, depending on tumor thickness [38, 39, 42].

Sentinel Lymph Node Biopsy

Pathologic staging of the regional nodes via sentinel lymph node biopsy (SLNB) allows a selective approach to identifying cutaneous melanoma patients with occult regional nodal metastasis, thereby up-staging the melanoma to AJCC/UICC stage III.

Preoperative lymphatic mapping (lymphoscintigraphy) and vital blue dye injection around the primary melanoma or biopsy scar at the time of wide local excision is performed to identify and remove the sentinel lymph node(s), which are then examined histopathologically for the presence of micrometastasis using both routine histology and immunohistochemistry. If present, a completion lymph node dissection (CLND) has traditionally been performed, though as yet no difference in overall survival (OS) has been observed for SLN-positive patients who underwent CLND compared to those who did not [54, 55]. Approximately 8–20% of CLND patients will have non-sentinel nodal metastases. Current NCCN guidelines recommend that CLND be discussed and offered in the setting of a positive SLNB, although active nodal basin surveillance, typically with ultrasound, is an alternative to CLND. However, CLND may be recommended in the setting of higher SLN tumor burden, greater number of positive SLNs, and/or adverse histologic features in the primary melanoma [42]. Surveillance regional nodal ultrasound is increasingly recognized for its role in monitoring the regional nodal basin in patients who are eligible for SLNB or CLND but do not undergo these procedures or in whom SLNB is technically not successful, although ultrasound is not considered a replacement for either SLNB or CLND at this point [56].

Sentinel node status (positive or negative) is widely regarded as the most important prognostic factor for recurrence and the most powerful predictor of survival in melanoma patients. Current NCCN and AAD clinical practice guidelines advocate pathologic staging of the regional lymph nodes with SLNB for cutaneous melanoma >1 mm depth and for thinner tumors with adverse features (e.g., ulceration, lymphovascular invasion, high mitotic rate) [39, 57]. A comprehensive systematic review of SLNB literature published from January 1990 through August 2011 was conducted by the American Society of Clinical Oncology and Society of Surgical Oncology and concurred with these recommendations [58]. As previously noted, NCCN guidelines stratify risk of SLN metastasis based on a Breslow depth cut-off point of 0.8mm (e.g. T1a/b), with recommendations to forego SLNB staging in patients with nonulcerated tumors 0.8 mm, unless other adverse histologic features are evident, for example lymphovascular invasion and/or very high mitotic index (particularly in younger age patients) [42].

While SLNB provides the most reliable and accurate means of staging appropriate patients with primary melanoma, its impact on overall survival has yet to be demonstrated. The final results of the first Multicenter Selective Lymphadenectomy Trial (MSLT-1), Florida Melanoma Trial, and Sunbelt Melanoma Trial have not shown a therapeutic benefit of SLNB in patients with cutaneous melanoma, although low rates of SLN positivity in these analyses limit their power to detect an overall survival difference [59]. Incorporation of novel molecular techniques may eventually aid in the selection of the most appropriate patients for SLNB and/or CLND.

Surgical Treatment of Metastatic Disease

Surgery may consist of excision of dermal recurrences or in-transit metastases, lymphadenectomy of nodal disease, and/or resection of visceral metastases. Distant metastases typically involve primarily the lung, liver, brain, gastrointestinal tract, and bone. Surgical treatment is generally offered for palliation of widespread metastases, although some data have suggested that metastasectomy of isolated visceral metastasis may result in improved survival for some patients with stage IV melanoma [60]. Candidates for operative intervention are generally those with isolated lung or brain metastases, although the role of metastasectomy for limited metastasis at other visceral sites has also been proposed. In rare cases, long-term survival may be achieved.

Medical Care

Adjuvant Systemic Therapy for Resected Melanoma

Numerous adjuvant therapies have been investigated for the treatment of cutaneous melanoma following surgical resection. High-dose interferon (IFN) alfa-2b and high-dose ipilimumab are currently approved by the US Food and Drug Administration (FDA) for adjuvant use in patients with melanoma at high risk for relapse (generally defined as resected stage III disease). Other immune checkpoint inhibitors, molecularly targeted agents (e.g., BRAF inhibitors), biologic response modifiers (e.g., granulocyte macrophage colony-stimulating factor (GM-CSF)), and various melanoma vaccines are currently being studied in the adjuvant setting for resected stage III and IV melanoma.

High-dose IFN alfa-2b was approved by the US Food and Drug Administration (FDA) in 1995 as an adjuvant therapy for resected primary tumors >4 mm in Breslow depth (AJCC stage IIB) and regional lymph node metastasis (stage III). High-dose pegylated IFN was FDA-approved as an adjuvant therapy for patients with resected stage III melanoma in 2011. Most trials of low-dose IFN have shown no benefit in disease-free survival (DFS) or OS rates, though a benefit in both DFS and OS was suggested in a study of low-dose IFN in resected stage III patients in a German Dermatologic Cooperative Oncology Group study [61]. A more recent analysis of adjuvant therapy with low-dose pegylated IFN (PEG-IFN) administered for 36 months versus low-dose IFN for 18 months in melanoma patients with macrometastastic nodes did not reveal differences in DFS, distant metastasis free survival (DMFS), or OS [62].

In the US, three prospective, multicenter, randomized, controlled trials were conducted to assess the effect of adjuvant high-dose IFN alfa-2b on relapse-free survival (RFS) and OS rates in patients with high-risk melanoma (primary tumors ≥4 mm depth and regional nodal disease) and have supported a consistent benefit in RFS but not OS [63].

A European Organisation for Research and Treatment of Cancer (EORTC) randomized, phase 3 trial of adjuvant high-dose pegylated interferon alfa-2b (PEG-IFN) in patients with resected stage III melanoma similarly showed no OS benefit but almost 12% improvement in RFS, though this was mostly limited to patients with microscopic lymph node involvement [64]. Long-term results of this trial at 7.6 years median follow-up demonstrated a slightly diminished impact on RFS, with a 7-year RFS rate of 39.1% in the PEG-IFN arm compared with 34.6% in the observation arm; however, no difference was observed in OS with longer follow-up. The subgroup of patients with ulcerated primary tumors and SLN metastasis have appeared to show the most consistent benefit from adjuvant treatment with PEG-IFN [65].

More recent systematic reviews and meta-analyses have demonstrated conflicting findings. A meta-analysis of 14 randomized controlled trials of IFN-alfa in varying doses (low, intermediate, and high) involving 8122 patients demonstrated significant improvement in DFS (hazard ratio (HR) for disease recurrence = 0.82; 95% confidence interval (CI) 0.77 to 0.87; P <0.001) and OS (HR for death = 0.89; 95% CI 0.83–0.96; P = 0.002), although the optimal IFN-alfa dose and treatment duration remain unclear [66]. However, an updated systematic review of seven trials comparing high-dose IFN-alfa with observation demonstrated benefit in only DFS (HR 0.77; 95% CI 0.6500.92; P = 0.004) and not OS (HR 0.93; 95% CI 0.78–1.12; P = 0.45) [67]. In any case, the potential benefits of high-dose IFN (whether administered for 1 year, or up to 5 years in the pegylated form), must be weighed against its substantial tolerability and toxicity issues, including the duration of therapy, commonly associated flu-like symptoms, and potential for significant adverse reactions.

Newer Adjuvant Immunotherapies/Regimens for Resected Stage III Melanoma

Ipilimumab, an immune checkpoint inhibitor of cytotoxic T-lymphocyte-associated antigen 4 (CTLA-4), was FDA approved in 2015 for adjuvant treatment of patients with cutaneous melanoma with pathologic involvement of regional lymph nodes (>1 mm) who have undergone CLND. Approval was based on results from the EORTC 18071 trial of 951 stage III patients that showed significantly increased RFS in the ipilimumab group compared with the placebo group at 1–3 years (46.5% vs 34.8% at 3 years) [68]. Patients in the ipilimumab group were 25% less likely to experience melanoma recurrence than those in the placebo group. However, the FDA-approved regimen for adjuvant ipilimumab is >3 times higher (10 mg/kg every 3 weeks for 4 doses then every 3 months for up to 3 years) and longer than that approved for patients with unresectable stage III and IV disease.

Improved RFS was again demonstrated at median follow-up of 5.3 years (HR 0.76; 95% CI 0.64–0.89; P = 0.0008) [69]. However for the first time, ipilimumab significantly reduced the risk of death – by 28% compared with placebo (11% absolute gain in OS at 5 years; HR 0.72; 95% CI 0.58–0.88; $P = 0.001$), and distant metastasis-free survival by 24% versus placebo (HR 0.76; 95% CI 0.64–0.92; $P = 0.002$), though rates of grade 3 or 4 immune-related adverse events (irAEs) remained high (41.6% vs 2.7%). Because irAEs are both dose and duration dependent, high-dose ipilimumab should be used with caution in the adjuvant setting. Results from a phase 3 cooperative group trial (ECOG E1609) assessing the use of low- versus high-dose ipilimumab compared with high-dose IFN in patients with resected stage IIIB and IV melanoma will help to establish the efficacy of low-dose ipilimumab in the adjuvant setting. Adjuvant trials utilizing anti-programmed-death receptors (PD-1 inhibitors) are underway with promising results [70].

Adjuvant biochemotherapy is also a consideration for resected stage III melanoma, based on results from a phase 3 SWOG S0008 trial utilizing a 9-week regimen consisting of cisplatin, vinblastine, dacarbazine, IL-2, and IFN, compared with the standard 52-week regimen of high-dose IFN alfa-2b in patients with resected stage III melanoma. Improved RFS survival was noted in biochemotherapy-treated patients compared with those on high-dose IFN (4.0 years vs 1.9 years, respectively, 95% CI 0.58–0.97), although median and 5-year OS rates did not significantly differ between the treatment groups [71]. However, substantial toxicity associated with the biochemotherapy regimen limits its use in clinical practice.

Melanoma Vaccines

Melanoma vaccines are a type of specific active immunotherapy based on melanoma cell expression of certain HLA- and tumor-associated antigens. Their appeal lies in lower toxicity (e.g., fatigue, myalgias, local inflammatory skin reactions) compared with other agents. Numerous melanoma-associated antigens have been identified, but it remains unclear which are the most important in eliciting the necessary cytotoxic and humoral responses to eradicate melanoma cells. In addition, HLA haplotype restriction (mainly to the A2 allele) limits the use of peptide vaccines in many patients. Most current trials for melanoma vaccines are for advanced disease (stages III and IV); trials aimed at prevention are not yet available. To date, no large, phase 3 randomized trial has demonstrated an OS advantage for vaccine-treated melanoma patients. However, a phase 3 trial of the glycoprotein peptide vaccine gp100:209-217(210M) in combination with high-dose interleukin-2 (IL-2) showed significant improvement in response rate and progression-free survival (PFS) compared with IL-2 alone and provided the first evidence of clinical benefit for vaccine strategies in patients with melanoma [72].

Systemic Treatment of Advanced Melanoma

Improved survival in patients with unresectable AJCC/UICC stage III and IV melanoma has been an elusive goal for the past several decades, with effective systemic therapies only recently becoming widely available. Following the FDA approval of IL-2 in 1998, a 13-year period elapsed with no new drugs approved for the treatment of advanced disease until ipilimumab and vemurafenib in 2011, heralding a new era of immunotherapy and molecularly targeted therapy for treatment of patients with advanced disease (Figure 34.7).

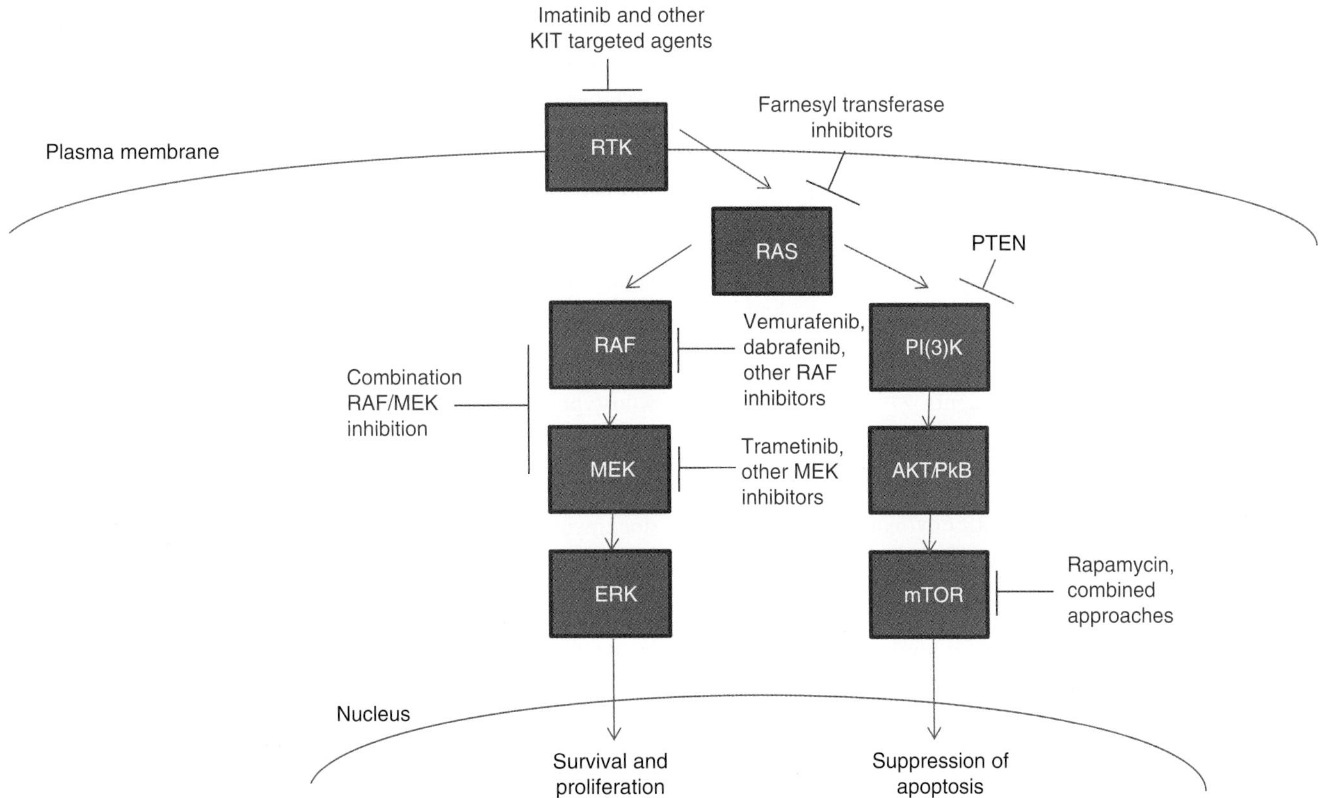

Figure 34.7 Schematic demonstrating therapeutic targets in the melanoma pathway. ERK, extracellular-signal-regulated kinase; MEK, MAPK/ERK kinase; mTOR, mechanistic target of rapamycin; PTEN, phosphatase and tensin homolog; RTK, receptor tyrosine kinase.

Chemotherapy

While no chemotherapeutic agent has demonstrated improved OS, chemotherapy may provide palliation for patients with unresectable melanoma. Dacarbazine (DTIC) was the first drug approved for the treatment of metastatic melanoma in 1975, with overall response rates ranging from 8 to 20%, although responses are typically partial, short-lived (4–6 months) and limited to skin, soft tissue, lymph node, and lung metastasis. The objective response rate (ORR) in a pooled analysis of 23 randomized controlled trials assessing the use of DTIC alone in 1,390 patients was 15.3%, the majority of which were partial (11.2%,) with complete response rates of only 4.2% [73]. In a phase 3 study of dacarbazine compared with its oral analog, temozolomide, the response rates were similar (12% vs 13%, respectively), although temozolomide has improved central nervous system penetration over DTIC [74]. To date, no combination chemotherapy or biochemotherapy regimen (incorporating IFN or IL-2 with combination chemotherapy) has demonstrated a survival advantage over single-agent DTIC, although combination regimens are associated with higher ORRs and longer PFS [75, 76]. Some data have demonstrated promising results for albumin-bound paclitaxel (*nab*-Paclitaxel) combined with carboplatin in chemotherapy-naïve patients with unresectable stage IV melanoma [77].

Immunomodulatory Agents

Interleukin-2 is a recombinant, T-cell-derived growth factor that was FDA approved in a high-dose bolus regimen in 1998 for the treatment of metastatic melanoma, due to the potential for durable complete responses in a small subset of patients. A pooled analysis of 270 patients treated with 600,000–720,000 units/kg administered every 8 hours for 5 days demonstrated an ORR of 16%, and complete response of 6%, mostly in patients with soft tissue and lung metastasis [78]. Forty-four percent of responders were long-term survivors beyond 5 years (range, >70 months to >150 months). Approximately 4% of responders will have durable remission after treatment [79]. However, treatment with high dose IL-2 requires hospitalization and intensive monitoring due to significant toxicities, including hypotension, fever, chills, vomiting, diarrhea, increased capillary permeability, cardiac arrhythmias, oliguria, and volume overload. Thus, treatment is often limited to specialized centers with experience in the management of this regimen and to younger patients with excellent performance status and organ function.

Immune Checkpoint Inhibitors

Ipilimumab is a monoclonal antibody against cytotoxic T-lymphocyte-associated antigen 4 (CTLA-4) which inhibits T-cell inactivation, allowing expansion of naturally developed melanoma-specific cytotoxic T cells. Ipilimumab was the first drug to demonstrate an OS advantage in stage IV melanoma and was FDA approved in 2011 for patients with unresectable stage III and IV melanoma. In the pivotal phase 3 trial, ipilimumab (given at 3 mg/kg every 3 weeks for 4 treatments) was shown to enhance the T-cell response in HLA-A2-positive patients and prolong OS in patients with metastatic melanoma compared with a glycoprotein 100 (gp 100) peptide vaccine (median OS 10.1 vs 6.4 months, respectively; HR for death 0.66; $P = 0.003$). Durable responses were observed for over 2 years in 9/15 (60%) of ipilimumab responders, suggesting a durable response benefit that has been demonstrated to be independent of HLA status [80]. Results of a phase 3 trial comparing DTIC plus ipilimumab (administered at 10 mg/kg) versus DTIC alone also demonstrated improved median OS in the ipilimumab-treated group (11.2 vs 9.1 months), with a consistent survival benefit noted at years 1, 2, and 3 or follow-up [81]. However, the use of both low- and high-dose ipilimumab is tempered by potential severe irAEs, primarily enterocolitis and hypophysitis, which require prompt initiation of high-dose corticosteroids and/or other immune response modifiers, as well as hormone replacement for pituitary axis alteration. Dermatitis, pruritus, and potential vitiligo may also be seen with ipilimumab therapy, emphasizing the importance of dermatologic consultation for management of associated skin conditions.

Enhanced antitumor activity with lower toxicity was demonstrated with human monoclonal antibodies against the programmed death-1 (PD-1) protein, a T-cell coinhibitory receptor, or its ligand, PD-L1. Objective responses, durable tumor regression, and prolonged stabilization of disease were initially observed in patients with a variety of advanced cancers, including non-small cell lung cancer, renal cell carcinoma, and melanoma following treatment with the anti-PD-L1 antibody BMS-936559, with reduced toxicity compared to ipilimumab. The PD-1 inhibitor pembrolizumab was FDA approved in 2014 for patients with advanced or unresectable stage III and IV melanoma and demonstrated efficacy in ipilimumab-refractory advanced melanoma [82]. An additional PD-1 inhibitor, nivolumab, was approved in 2015, and both PD-1 blockers are considered first-line monotherapy in patients with advanced melanoma [83].

Accelerated FDA approval of the PD-1 inhibitor pembrolizumab was granted in 2014 for patients with advanced or unresectable melanoma following progression on prior therapies, including ipilimumab and BRAF inhibitors [84]. Demonstration of superior survival and lower toxicity compared with ipilimumab in the phase 3 KEYNOTE-006 trial resulted in approval as first-line therapy in 2015.

Concurrent studies of the PD-1 inhibitor nivolumab showed similar durable tumor remission and long-term safety, with median OS of 16.8 months and 1- and 2-year survival rates of 62% and 43%, respectively, in patients with advanced, treatment-refractory melanoma [85]. In previously untreated BRAF wild-type melanoma patients, nivolumab was associated with significantly improved OS at 1 year compared with dacarbazine (72.9% vs 42.1%, respectively), with ORR of 40% versus 13.9%, respectively, resulting in FDA approval in 2015 [86]. Subsequent documented superior PFS over ipilimumab in the CheckMate 067 trial resulted in FDA approval of nivolumab as first-line monotherapy in metastatic melanoma.

The combination of CTLA-4 and PD-1 inhibitors showed even greater efficacy in patients with advanced melanoma but is associated with increased toxicity (grade 3 or 4 events) [87]. Combined nivolumab plus ipilimumab showed median PFS of 11.5 months compared with 2.9 months with ipilimumab and 6.9 months with nivolumab, and even higher responses in patients with tumors positive for the PD-1 ligand [88]. The nivolumab/ipilimumab combination was FDA approved in 2015 for previously untreated patients with BRAF V600 wild-type unresectable or metastatic melanoma [89]. Three-year OS analysis in the CheckMate 067 trial demonstrated superiority of combination therapy with nivolumab plus ipilimumab (58%) and nivolumab monotherapy (52%) over ipilimumab monotherapy (34%) [90]. Similar to BRAF/MEK inhibition, combination checkpoint blockade tends to work rapidly. However, significant immune-related adverse events occur on the dual regimen, making appropriate patient selection critical, along with careful monitoring during treatment, and prompt initiation of appropriate therapy for side effects.

In 2015, the FDA approved talimogene laherparepvec, commonly known as T-vec. This genetically modified, live-attenuated herpes simplex virus is programmed to replicate within tumors and produce the immune stimulatory protein GM-CSF. T-vec is indicated for the local treatment of unresectable cutaneous, subcutaneous, and nodal lesions in patients with melanoma recurrence after initial surgery but has demonstrated efficacy against visceral metastasis as well.

Approval of T-vec was based on the OPTiM randomized controlled trial in patients with unresectable regional or distant metastasis [91]. The durable response rate was significantly higher among patients who received talimogene laherparepvec compared with those given GM-CSF (16.3% vs 2.1%; odds ratio, 8.9; *P* <0.001). Overall response rate was also higher (26.4% vs 5.7%; *P* <0.001), with 32 (10.8%) patients demonstrating a complete response, although median OS was not statistically significant. Combination immunotherapies with T-vec and checkpoint inhibitors are now being studied for synergistic and/or abscopal immune responses [92].

BRAF and MEK Inhibitors

The mitogen-activated protein kinase (*MAPK*) signaling pathway (*RAS–RAF–MEK–ERK*) is constitutively activated in up to 80–90% of melanomas, with the most common mutations in either *NRAS* (15–30% of melanomas) or *BRAF* (50–66% of melanomas). Drugs that target this pathway, including multikinase inhibitors which decrease *BRAF* activity, have revolutionized treatment for patients with unresectable melanoma, although drug resistance is frequently encountered over time.

Vemurafenib is a selective small molecule inhibitor of some mutated forms of *BRAF* serine-threonine kinase, including *BRAF*-V600E and *BRAF*-V600K. In the pivotal phase 3 study, vemurafenib markedly improved PFS and OS compared with DTIC as a first-line agent in patients with advanced melanoma [93]. Vemurafenib-treated patients had a 74% reduction in the risk for disease progression or death compared with patients receiving DTIC (hazard ratio, 0.26; *P* <0.001). Mean PFS was 5.3 months in the vemurafenib group, compared with 1.6 months in the DTIC group. At 6 months, the estimated overall survival rate was 84% (95% CI, 78–89) in the vemurafenib group and 64% (95% CI, 56–73) in the DTIC group. Vemurafenib was FDA approved in 2011 for the treatment of unresectable or metastatic melanoma with the BRAF-V600 mutation. It is not indicated for patients whose tumors do not harbor the V600 mutation (i.e., wild-type BRAF melanoma).

Side effects from vemurafenib are mainly cutaneous in nature and include photosensitivity, alopecia, xerosis, follicular hyperkeratosis ("keratosis pilaris-like"), rash, and potential development of cutaneous squamous cell carcinoma (SCC), particularly the keratoacanthoma type. The keratinocyte proliferations observed with BRAF inhibition, ranging from benign papillomas to SCC, tend to appear early in the course of treatment and are believed to be related to paradoxical activation of the MAPK pathway. Recent reports of atypical melanocytic proliferations in patients on selective BRAF inhibitors, including new primary melanomas and dysplastic nevi, highlight the need for routine skin examination by a dermatologist in treated individuals [94].

Dabrafenib is another *BRAF* inhibitor that inhibits the mutant *BRAF* protein in melanomas with either the V600E or V600K genotype. A phase 3 study demonstrated high clinical response rates and improved PFS in *BRAF*(V600E) metastatic melanoma patients who received dabrafenib compared with DTIC [95]. Efficacy has also been demonstrated in *BRAF*-V600K patients and in those with brain metastasis. Dabrafenib appears similar to vemurafenib in terms of efficacy but is associated with less phototoxicity; it was FDA approved in May 2013 [96].

A phase 3 open-label trial assessing the use of an oral selective *MEK* inhibitor, trametinib, versus dacarbazine in 322 patients with metastatic melanoma (unresectable stage IIIC or IV) demonstrated improved rates of PFS and OS in patients with the *BRAF*-V600E or V600K mutation [97]. Rash, diarrhea, and peripheral edema were the most common toxic effects in the trametinib group, though secondary skin neoplasms, including cutaneous SCC, were not noted. Trametinib was FDA approved in May 2013 as a single agent, but is seldom used as monotherapy.

Two phase 3 trials (COMBI-v and coBRIM) demonstrated that combination *BRAF* and *MEK* inhibition is more efficacious than *BRAF* inhibitor monotherapy. Improved PFS resulted in FDA approval in 2014 for vemurafenib/dabrafenib as first-line therapy and for vemurafenib/cobimetinib in 2015. Combination therapy is considered standard of care for patients with high volume and/or rapidly progressing BRAF-mutant melanoma, and is also being investigated on the adjuvant therapy front [98].

Follow-Up/Survivorship

The key components to melanoma follow-up are careful physical examination (with attention to skin and lymph nodes) and review of systems. Patients should be educated in the performance of monthly skin self-examination for early detection of new primary melanoma as well as lymph node self-examinations.

Laboratory and Imaging Studies

Baseline and surveillance laboratory studies (e.g., lactate dehydrogenase (LDH) level, liver function tests, chemistry panel, CBC count), chest radiography (CXR), and other imaging studies (e.g., CT scanning, positron emission tomography (PET) scanning, bone scanning, magnetic resonance imaging (MRI)) are not typically beneficial for stage I/II (cutaneous) melanoma patients without signs or symptoms of metastasis [99–101].

A metastatic workup should be initiated if physical findings or symptoms suggest disease recurrence. Screening CT or PET-CT may be considered if the patient has documented nodal metastasis based on results from the SLNB, although the yield is low in this setting (0.5–3.7%) and positive findings tend to correlate with increased tumor thickness, ulceration of the primary tumor, and/or large tumor burden in the sentinel lymph node(s) [102]. A meta-analysis of 74 studies comprising over

10,000 melanoma patients demonstrated that ultrasonography was superior for detection of lymph node metastasis and PET-CT for detection of distant metastasis for both staging and surveillance in clinically appropriate patients [103].

Current NCCN guidelines recommend against surveillance laboratory or imaging studies for asymptomatic patients with stage IA, IB, and IIA melanoma (i.e., tumors ≤4 mm depth), unless clinically indicated for workup of signs or symptoms that suggest disease recurrence. Imaging studies (CT, PET-CT, or brain MRI) should be for confirmation of suspected metastasis or to delineate the extent of disease and may be considered to screen for recurrent/metastatic disease in asymptomatic patients with stage IIB–IV disease, although this latter recommendation remains optional. Routine laboratory or radiologic imaging in asymptomatic melanoma patients of any stage is not recommended after 3–5 years of follow-up [39, 42].

While abnormal laboratory test results are rarely the sole indicator of metastatic disease, serum LDH levels were incorporated into the AJCC melanoma staging in 2002 for the classification of stage IV (distant) disease, and they remain a key prognostic factor for this subgroup of patients. Elevated LDH levels are associated with worse survival in this subgroup, but routine testing is not recommended for patients with lower stage disease

Physical Examination

Cutaneous melanoma patients should be monitored regularly following diagnosis, particularly in the setting of tumors at increased risk of recurrence (e.g., >2 mm thickness, with ulceration, lymphovascular invasion, and/or high mitotic rate). While most metastases occur in the first 1–3 years after treatment of the primary tumor, skin examinations are recommended for life. An estimated 4–8% of patients with a history of melanoma develop a new primary melanoma, generally within the first 3–5 years following diagnosis. The risk of new primary melanoma is higher in the setting of increased nevus count; multiple clinical atypical/dysplastic nevi; family history of melanoma; fair skin/sun sensitivity; prior *in situ*, nodular, and lentigo maligna subtypes of melanoma; and male sex [104]. The frequency of dermatologic, surgical, and oncologic surveillance depends on individual patient risk for new primary melanoma as well as for recurrent disease.

Patient Education

Patients with a history of melanoma should be educated regarding sun-protective measures (including sun-protective clothing, hats, eyewear, and the use of sunscreen); skin self-examinations for new primary melanoma, which is particularly important in patients with numerous nevi (common or atypical) and/or a strong family history of melanoma; possible local recurrence within the melanoma scar; and screening of first-degree relatives for melanoma, particularly if they have a history of atypical moles. In addition, referral to a cancer genetics clinic for discussion of genetic testing for the *CDKN2A* (P16) mutation should be considered for individuals with 3 or more invasive melanomas (personal or in the same side of the family) or families with 3 or more "cancer events," including 2 invasive melanomas and 1 pancreatic cancer (or vice versa) [105]. However, a negative p16 mutation result does not preclude the need for ongoing dermatologic surveillance in patients with a history of melanoma.

Survivorship

As of 2012, an estimated one million Americans were living with a melanoma diagnosis, 21% of whom were under 50 years of age [106]. Delineating survivorship issues among melanoma survivors is vital to reducing the long-term social burden of this disease and improving quality of life. However, little survivorship research has been conducted to date among the growing population of melanoma survivors. Most melanoma survivors (74%) report fears of disease recurrence, and 33% report elevated levels of general distress and anxiety [107, 108]. In a recent analysis of 48 melanoma survivors of diverse ages, younger survivors expressed very specific concerns about insurability, career prospects, and family planning that differed from those reported by older survivors [109]. As melanoma becomes a more treatable disease in patients with advanced stages, attention to survivorship issues will be even more important.

References

1 Siegel RL, Miller KD, Jemal A. Cancer statistics, 2017. *CA Cancer J Clin* 2017;67(1):7–30.

2 Surveillance, Epidemiology, and End Results (SEER) Program Populations (1969-2011) (http://www.seer.cancer.gov/popdata), National Cancer Institute, DCCPS, Surveillance Research Program, Surveillance Systems Branch, released January 2013.

3 Forsea AM, Del Marmol V, de Vries E, Bailey EE, Geller AC. Melanoma incidence and mortality in Europe: new estimates, persistent disparities. *Br J Dermatol* 2012;167(5):1124–30.

4 Green AC, Baade P, Coory M, Aitken JF, Smithers M. Population-based 20-year survival among people diagnosed with thin melanomas in Queensland, *Australia. J Clin Oncol* 2012;30(13):1462–7.

5 Barbe C, Hibon E, Vitry F, Le Clainche A, Grange F. Clinical and pathological characteristics of melanoma: a population-based study in a French regional population. *J Eur Acad Dermatol Venereol.* 2012 Feb;26(2):159–64.

6 Shaikh WR, Xiong M, Weinstock MA. The contribution of nodular subtype to melanoma mortality in the United States, 1978 to 2007. *Arch Dermatol* 2012;148(1):30–6.

7 Fears TR, Guerry Dt, Pfeiffer RM, *et al.* Identifying individuals at high risk of melanoma: a practical predictor of absolute risk. *J Clin Oncol* 2006;24(22):3590–6.

8 Cust AE, Goumas C, Holland EA, *et al.* MC1R genotypes and risk of melanoma before age 40 years: a population-based case-control-family study. *Int J Cancer* 2012;131(3):E269–81.

9 Pappo AS, Armstrong GT, Liu W, *et al.* Melanoma as a subsequent neoplasm in adult survivors of childhood cancer: a report from the childhood cancer survivor study. *Pediatr Blood Cancer* 2013;60(3):461–6.

10 Watt TC, Inskip PD, Stratton K, *et al.* Radiation-related risk of basal cell carcinoma: a report from the Childhood Cancer Survivor Study. *J Natl Cancer Inst* 2012;104(16): 1240–50.

11 Brewer JD, Christenson LJ, Weaver AL, *et al.* Malignant melanoma in solid transplant recipients: collection of database cases and comparison with surveillance, epidemiology, and end results data for outcome analysis. *Arch Dermatol* 2011;147(7):790–6.

12 Hollenbeak CS, Todd MM, Billingsley EM, *et al.* Increased incidence of melanoma in renal transplantation recipients. *Cancer* 2005;104(9):1962–7.

13 Bajaj A, Driver JA, Schernhammer ES. Parkinson's disease and cancer risk: a systematic review and meta-analysis. *Cancer Causes Control* 2010;21(5):697–707.

14 Lazovich D, Vogel RI, Berwick M, *et al.* Indoor tanning and risk of melanoma: a case-control study in a highly exposed population. *Cancer Epidemiol Biomarkers Prev* 2010;19(6):1557–68.

15 Cust AE, Armstrong BK, Goumas C, *et al.* Sunbed use during adolescence and early adulthood is associated with increased risk of early-onset melanoma. *Int J Cancer* 2011;128(10):2425–35.

16 Boniol M, Autier P, Boyle P, Gandini S. Cutaneous melanoma attributable to sunbed use: systematic review and meta-analysis. *BMJ* 2012;345:e4757.

17 Swetter S. Cutaneous Melanoma. Medscape (serial online) 2013. Available from: http://emedicine.medscape.com/article/1100753-overview (accessed 2 October 2017).

18 Bevona C, Goggins W, Quinn T, Fullerton J, Tsao H. Cutaneous melanomas associated with nevi. *Arch Dermatol* 2003;139(12):1620–4; discussion 4.

19 Duman N, Erkin G, Gokoz O, *et al.* Nevus-associated versus de novo melanoma: do they have different characteristics and prognoses? *Dermatopathology* 2015;2(1):46–51.

20 Zabierowski SE, Herlyn M. Melanoma stem cells: the dark seed of melanoma. *J Clin Oncol* 2008;26(17):2890–4.

21 Cymerman RM, Shao Y, Wang K, *et al.* De novo vs nevus-associated melanomas: differences in associations with prognostic indicators and survival. J Natl Cancer Inst 2016;108(10).

22 Shain AH, Yeh I, Kovalyshyn I, *et al.* The genetic evolution of melanoma from precursor lesions. *N Engl J Med* 2015;373(20):1926–36.

23 Haluska FG, Tsao H, Wu H, *et al.* Genetic alterations in signaling pathways in melanoma. *Clin Cancer Res* 2006;12(7 Pt 2):2301 s–7 s.

24 Curtin JA, Fridlyand J, Kageshita T, *et al.* Distinct sets of genetic alterations in melanoma. *N Engl J Med* 2005;353(20):2135–47.

25 Hocker T, Tsao H. Ultraviolet radiation and melanoma: a systematic review and analysis of reported sequence variants. *Hum Mutat* 2007;28(6):578–88.

26 Saldanha G, Purnell D, Fletcher A, *et al.* High BRAF mutation frequency does not characterize all melanocytic tumor types. *Int J Cancer* 2004;111(5):705–10.

27 Curtin JA, Busam K, Pinkel D, Bastian BC. Somatic activation of KIT in distinct subtypes of melanoma. *J Clin Oncol* 2006;24(26):4340–6.

28 Webster JD, Kiupel M, Yuzbasiyan-Gurkan V. Evaluation of the kinase domain of c-KIT in canine cutaneous mast cell tumors. *BMC Cancer* 2006;6:85.

29 Padua RA, Barrass N, Currie GA. A novel transforming gene in a human malignant melanoma cell line. *Nature* 1984;311(5987):671–3.

30 Daniotti M, Oggionni M, Ranzani T, *et al.* BRAF alterations are associated with complex mutational profiles in malignant melanoma. *Oncogene* 2004;23(35):5968–77.

31 Rogers RS, 3rd, Gibson LE. Mucosal, genital, and unusual clinical variants of melanoma. *Mayo Clin Proc* 1997;72(4):362–6.

32 Guerry Dt, Synnestvedt M, Elder DE, Schultz D. Lessons from tumor progression: the invasive radial growth phase of melanoma is common, incapable of metastasis, and indolent. *J Invest Dermatol* 1993;100(3):342S–5S.

33 Ohsie SJ, Sarantopoulos GP, Cochran AJ, Binder SW. Immunohistochemical characteristics of melanoma. *J Cutan Pathol* 2008;35(5):433–44.

34 Pruthi DK, Guilfoyle R, Nugent Z, Wiseman MC, Demers AA. Incidence and anatomic presentation of cutaneous malignant melanoma in central Canada during a 50-year period: 1956 to 2005. *J Am Acad Dermatol* 2009;61(1):44–50.

35 Terushkin V, Halpern AC. Melanoma early detection. *Hematol Oncol Clin North Am* 2009;23(3):481–500, viii.

36 Abbasi NR, Shaw HM, Rigel DS, *et al.* Early diagnosis of cutaneous melanoma: revisiting the ABCD criteria. *JAMA* 2004;292(22):2771–6.

37 Gachon J, Beaulieu P, Sei JF, *et al.* First prospective study of the recognition process of melanoma in dermatological practice. *Arch Dermatol* 2005;141(4):434–8.

38 Bichakjian CK, Halpern AC, Johnson TM, *et al.* Guidelines of care for the management of primary cutaneous melanoma. American Academy of Dermatology. *J Am Acad Dermatol* 2011;65(5):1032–47.

39 Coit DG, Andtbacka R, Anker CJ, *et al.* Melanoma, Version 2.2013: Featured Updates to the NCCN Guidelines. *J Natl Compr Canc Netw* 2013;11(4):395–407.

40 Sober AJ, Balch CM. Method of biopsy and incidence of positive margins in primary melanoma. *Ann Surg Oncol* 2007;14(2):274-–5.

41 Gershenwald JE, Scolyer RA, Hess KR, *et al.* Melanoma of the skin. In: Amin M (ed.) *AJCC Cancer Staging Manual*, 8th edn. New York: Springer, 2017.

42 National Comprehensive Cancer Network Guidelines (Version 1.2018, 10/11/17 © National Comprehensive Cancer Network Inc. 2017.) Available at: https://www.nccn.org/professionals/physician_gls/recently_updated.aspx [accessed 18 December 2017].

43 Balch CM. Cutaneous melanoma: prognosis and treatment results worldwide. *Semin Surg Oncol* 1992;8(6): 400–14.

44 Edge SB, Byrd DR, Compton CC, *et al.* (eds). Melanoma of the skin. *AJCC Canter Staging Manual*, 7th edn. New York: Springer, 2009:325–40.

45 Francken AB, Shaw HM, Thompson JF, *et al.* The prognostic importance of tumor mitotic rate confirmed in 1317 patients with primary cutaneous melanoma and long follow-up. *Ann Surg Oncol* 2004;11(4):426–33.

46 National Institutes of Health Consensus Development Conference Statement on Diagnosis and Treatment of Early Melanoma, January 27–29, 1992. *Am J Dermatopathol* 1993;15(1):34–43; discussion 6–51.

47 Kunishige JH, Brodland DG, Zitelli JA. Surgical margins for melanoma in situ. *J Am Acad Dermatol* 2012;66(3):438–44.

48 Zitelli JA, Brown C, Hanusa BH. Mohs micrographic surgery for the treatment of primary cutaneous melanoma. *J Am Acad Dermatol* 1997;37(2 Pt 1):236–45.

49 Albertini JG, Elston DM, Libow LF, Smith SB, Farley MF. Mohs micrographic surgery for melanoma: a case series, a comparative study of immunostains, an informative case report, and a unique mapping technique. *Dermatol Surg* 2002;28(8):656–65.

50 Veronesi U, Cascinelli N. Narrow excision (1-cm margin). A safe procedure for thin cutaneous melanoma. *Arch Surg* 1991;126(4):438–41.

51 Veronesi U, Cascinelli N, Adamus J, *et al.* Thin stage I primary cutaneous malignant melanoma. Comparison of excision with margins of 1 or 3 cm. *N Engl J Med* 1988;318(18):1159–62.

52 Balch CM, Urist MM, Karakousis CP, *et al.* Efficacy of 2-cm surgical margins for intermediate-thickness melanomas (1 to 4 mm). Results of a multi-institutional randomized surgical trial. *Ann Surg* 1993;218(3):262–7; discussion 7–9.

53 Gillgren P, Drzewiecki KT, Niin M, *et al.* 2-cm versus 4-cm surgical excision margins for primary cutaneous melanoma thicker than 2 mm: a randomised, multicentre trial. *Lancet* 2011;378(9803):1635–42.

54 Leiter U, Stadler R, Mauch C, *et al.* Complete lymph node dissection versus no dissection in patients with sentinel lymph node biopsy positive melanoma (DeCOG-SLT): a multicentre, randomised, phase 3 trial. *Lancet Oncol* 2016;17(6):757–67.

55 Faires MB, Thompson JF, Cochhran AJ, *et al.* Completion dissection or observation for sentinel-node metastasis in melanoma. *NEJM* 2017;376(23):2211–2222.

56 Coit DG, Thompson JA, Algazi A, *et al.* NCCN Guidelines Insights: Melanoma, Version 3.2016. *J Natl Compr Canc Netw* 2016;14(8):945–58.

57 Balch CM, Gershenwald JE, Soong SJ, *et al.* Final version of 2009 AJCC melanoma staging and classification. *J Clin Oncol* 2009;27(36):6199–206.

58 Wong SL, Balch CM, Hurley P, *et al.* Sentinel lymph node biopsy for melanoma: American Society of Clinical Oncology and Society of Surgical Oncology joint clinical practice guideline. *J Clin Oncol* 2012;30(23):2912–8.

59 Morton DL, Thompson JF, Cochran AJ, *et al.* Sentinel-node biopsy or nodal observation in melanoma. *N Engl J Med* 2006;355(13):1307–17.

60 Howard JH, Thompson JF, Mozzillo N, *et al.* Metastasectomy for distant metastatic melanoma: analysis of data from the first Multicenter Selective Lymphadenectomy Trial (MSLT-I). *Ann Surg Oncol* 2012;19(8):2547–55.

61 Garbe C, Radny P, Linse R, *et al.* Adjuvant low-dose interferon {alpha}2a with or without dacarbazine compared with surgery alone: a prospective-randomized phase III DeCOG trial in melanoma patients with regional lymph node metastasis. *Ann Oncol* 2008;19(6):1195–201.

62 Grob JJ, Jouary T, Dreno B, *et al.* Adjuvant therapy with pegylated interferon alfa-2b (36 months) versus low-dose interferon alfa-2b (18 months) in melanoma patients without macrometastatic nodes: an open-label, randomised, phase 3 European Association for Dermato-Oncology (EADO) study. *Eur J Cancer* 2013;49(1):166–74.

63 Kirkwood JM, Manola J, Ibrahim J, *et al.* A pooled analysis of eastern cooperative oncology group and intergroup trials of adjuvant high-dose interferon for melanoma. *Clin Cancer Res* 2004;10(5):1670–7.

64 Eggermont AM, Suciu S, Santinami M, *et al.* Adjuvant therapy with pegylated interferon alfa-2b versus observation alone in resected stage III melanoma: final results of EORTC 18991, a randomised phase III trial. *Lancet* 2008;372(9633):117–26.

65 Eggermont AM, Suciu S, Testori A, *et al.* Long-term results of the randomized phase III trial EORTC 18991 of adjuvant therapy with pegylated interferon alfa-2b versus observation in resected stage III melanoma. *J Clin Oncol* 2012;30(31):3810–8.

66 Mocellin S, Pasquali S, Rossi CR, Nitti D. Interferon alpha adjuvant therapy in patients with high-risk melanoma: a systematic review and meta-analysis. *J Natl Cancer Inst* 2010;102(7):493–501.

67 Petrella T, Verma S, Spithoff K, Quirt I, McCready D, Melanoma Disease Site Group. Adjuvant interferon therapy for patients at high risk for recurrent melanoma: an updated systematic review and practice guideline. *Clin Oncol (R Coll Radiol)* 2012;24(6):413–23.

68 IEggermont AM, Chiarion-Sileni V, Grob JJ, *et al.* Adjuvant ipilimumab versus placebo after complete resection of high-risk stage III melanoma (EORTC 18071): a randomised, double-blind, phase 3 trial. *Lancet Oncol* 2015;16(5):522–30.

69 Eggermont AM, Chiarion-Sileni V, Grob JJ, *et al.* Prolonged Survival in Stage III Melanoma with Ipilimumab Adjuvant Therapy. *N Engl J Med* 2016;375(19):1845–55.

70 Weber J, Mandala M, Del Vecchio M, *et al.* Adjuvant Nivolumab versus Ipilimumab in Resected Stage III or IV Melanoma. *The New England journal of medicine* 2017;377:1824–35.

71 Flaherty LE, Othus M, Atkins MB, *et al.* Southwest Oncology Group S0008: a phase III trial of high-dose interferon Alfa-2b versus cisplatin, vinblastine, and dacarbazine, plus interleukin-2 and interferon in patients with high-risk melanoma – an intergroup study of cancer and leukemia Group B, Children's Oncology Group, Eastern Cooperative Oncology Group, and Southwest Oncology Group. *J Clin Oncol* 2014;32(33):3771–8.

72 Schwartzentruber DJ, Lawson DH, Richards JM, J Clin Oncol. gp100 peptide vaccine and interleukin-2 in patients with advanced melanoma. *N Engl J Med* 2011;364(22):2119–27.

73 Lui P, Cashin R, Machado M, *et al.* Treatments for metastatic melanoma: synthesis of evidence from randomized trials. *Cancer Treat Rev* 2007;33(8):665–80.

74 Middleton MR, Grob JJ, Aaronson N, *et al.* Randomized phase III study of temozolomide versus dacarbazine in the treatment of patients with advanced metastatic malignant melanoma. *J Clin Oncol* 2000;18(1):158–66.

75 Chapman PB, Einhorn LH, Meyers ML, *et al.* Phase III multicenter randomized trial of the Dartmouth regimen versus dacarbazine in patients with metastatic melanoma. *J Clin Oncol* 1999;17(9):2745–51.

76 Atkins MB, Hsu J, Lee S, *et al.* Phase III trial comparing concurrent biochemotherapy with cisplatin, vinblastine, dacarbazine, interleukin-2, and interferon alfa-2b with cisplatin, vinblastine, and dacarbazine alone in patients with metastatic malignant melanoma (E3695): a trial coordinated by the Eastern Cooperative Oncology Group. *J Clin Oncol* 2008;26(35):5748–54.

77 Hersh EM, O'Day SJ, Ribas A, *et al.* A phase 2 clinical trial of nab-paclitaxel in previously treated and chemotherapy-naive patients with metastatic melanoma. *Cancer* 2010;116(1):155–63.

78 Atkins MB, Lotze MT, Dutcher JP, *et al.* High-dose recombinant interleukin 2 therapy for patients with metastatic melanoma: analysis of 270 patients treated between 1985 and 1993. *J Clin Oncol* 1999;17(7):2105–16.

79 Atkins MB, Kunkel L, Sznol M, Rosenberg SA. High-dose recombinant interleukin-2 therapy in patients with metastatic melanoma: long-term survival update. *Cancer J Sci Am* 2000;6 Suppl 1:S11–4.

80 Hodi FS, O'Day SJ, McDermott DF, *et al.* Improved survival with ipilimumab in patients with metastatic melanoma. *N Engl J Med* 2010;363(8):711–23.

81 Robert C, Thomas L, Bondarenko I, *et al.* Ipilimumab plus dacarbazine for previously untreated metastatic melanoma. *N Engl J Med* 2011;364(26):2517–26.

82 Robert C, Ribas A, Wolchok JD, *et al.* Anti-programmed-death-receptor 1 treatment with pembrolizumab in ipilimumab-refractory advanced melanoma: a randomised dose-comparison cohort of a phase 1 trial. *Lancet* 2014;384(9948):1109–17.

83 Robert C, Schachter J, Long GV, *et al.* Pembrolizumab versus Ipilimumab in Advanced Melanoma. *N Engl J Med* 2015;372(26):2521–32.

84 Hamid O, Robert C, Daud A, *et al.* Safety and tumor responses with lambrolizumab (anti-PD-1) in melanoma. *N Engl J Med* 2013;369(2):134–44.

85 Topalian SL, Sznol M, McDermott DF, *et al.* Survival, durable tumor remission, and long-term safety in patients with advanced melanoma receiving nivolumab. *J Clin Oncol* 2014;32(10):1020–30.

86 Robert C, Long GV, Brady B, *et al.* Nivolumab in previously untreated melanoma without BRAF mutation. *N Engl J Med* 2015;372(4):320–30.

87 Wolchok JD, Kluger H, Callahan MK, *et al.* Nivolumab plus ipilimumab in advanced melanoma. *N Engl J Med* 2013;369(2):122–33.

88 Larkin J, Chiarion-Sileni V, Gonzalez R, *et al.* Combined nivolumab and ipilimumab or monotherapy in untreated melanoma. *N Engl J Med* 2015;373(1):23–34.

89 Postow MA, Chesney J, Pavlick AC, *et al.* Nivolumab and ipilimumab versus ipilimumab in untreated melanoma. *N Engl J Med* 2015;372(21):2006–17.

90 Wolchok JD, Chiarion-Sileni V, Gonzalez R, *et al.* Overall survival with combined nivolumab and ipilimumab in advanced melanoma. *N Eng J Med* 2017;377(14):1345–1356.

91 Andtbacka RH, Kaufman HL, Collichio F, *et al.* Talimogene laherparepvec improves durable response rate in patients with advanced melanoma. *J Clin Oncol* 2015;33(25):2780–8.

92 Ribas A, Dummer R, Puzanov I, *et al.* Oncolytic virotherapy promotes intrautmoral T cell infiltration and improves anti-PD-1 immunotherapy. *Cell* 2017;170:1109–1119.

93 Chapman PB, Hauschild A, Robert C, *et al.* Improved survival with vemurafenib in melanoma with BRAF V600E mutation. *N Engl J Med* 2011;364(26):2507–16.

94 Zimmer L, Hillen U, Livingstone E, *et al.* Atypical melanocytic proliferations and new primary melanomas in patients with advanced melanoma undergoing selective BRAF inhibition. *J Clin Oncol* 2012;30(19):2375–83.

95 Hauschild A, Grob JJ, Demidov LV, *et al.* Dabrafenib in BRAF-mutated metastatic melanoma: a multicentre, open-label, phase 3 randomised controlled trial. *Lancet* 2012;380(9839):358–65.

96 Menzies AM, Long GV, Murali R. Dabrafenib and its potential for the treatment of metastatic melanoma. *Drug Des Devel Ther* 2012;6:391–405.

97 Flaherty KT, Robert C, Hersey P, *et al.* Improved survival with MEK inhibition in BRAF-mutated melanoma. *N Engl J Med* 2012;367(2):107–14.

98 Long GV, Hauschild A, Santinami M, *et al.* The New England journal of medicine. *N Engl J Med* 2017;377:1813–23.

99 Wang TS, Johnson TM, Cascade PN, *et al.* Evaluation of staging chest radiographs and serum lactate dehydrogenase for localized melanoma. *J Am Acad Dermatol* 2004;51(3):399–405.

100 Hafner J, Schmid MH, Kempf W, *et al.* Baseline staging in cutaneous malignant melanoma. *Br J Dermatol* 2004;150(4):677–86.

101 Brown RE, Stromberg AJ, Hagendoorn LJ, *et al.* Surveillance after surgical treatment of melanoma: futility of routine chest radiography. *Surgery* 2010;148(4):711–6; discussion 6–7.

102 Miranda EP, Gertner M, Wall J, *et al.* Routine imaging of asymptomatic melanoma patients with metastasis to sentinel lymph nodes rarely identifies systemic disease. *Arch Surg* 2004;139(8):831–6; discussion 6–7.

103 Xing Y, Bronstein Y, Ross MI, *et al.* Contemporary diagnostic imaging modalities for the staging and surveillance of melanoma patients: a meta-analysis. *J Natl Cancer Inst* 2011;103(2):129–42.

104 Siskind V, Hughes MC, Palmer JM, *et al.* Nevi, family history, and fair skin increase the risk of second primary melanoma. *J Invest Dermatol* 2011;131(2):461–7.

105 Leachman SA, Carucci J, Kohlmann W, *et al.* Selection criteria for genetic assessment of patients with familial melanoma. *J Am Acad Dermatol* 2009;61(4):677 e1–14.

106 American Cancer Society. *Cancer Treatment & Survivorship: Facts & Figures 2012-2013*. Atlanta, GA: American Cancer Society, 2013.

107 Kasparian NA, McLoone JK, Butow PN. Psychological responses and coping strategies among patients with malignant melanoma: a systematic review of the literature. *Arch Dermatol* 2009;145(12):1415–27.

108 McLoone J, Menzies S, Meiser B, Mann GJ, Kasparian NA. Psycho-educational interventions for melanoma survivors: a systematic review. *Psychooncology* 2013;22(7): 1444–56

109 Oliveria SA, Shuk E, Hay JL, *et al.* Melanoma survivors: health behaviors, surveillance, psychosocial factors, and family concerns. *Psychooncology* 2013;22(1):106–16.

35

Non-Melanoma Skin Cancers

H. William Higgins, II[1] *and Martin A. Weinstock*[2]

[1] *Brown University School of Medicine, Providence, Rhode Island, USA*
[2] *VA Medical Center, Providence, Rhode Island, USA*

Introduction

Non-melanoma skin cancers (NMSC) vary in morbidity and mortality and affect all populations, from children to adults. NMSC encompass a variety of skin tumors, including basal and squamous cell carcinomas, keratoacanthomas, Merkel cell carcinoma, dermatofibrosarcoma protuberans, atypical fibroxanthomas, sebaceous carcinomas, and others. A more specific term, keratinocyte carcinoma (KC), is used to refer to only basal and squamous cell carcinomas of the skin (BCC, SCC). While ultraviolet (UV) light exposure has been shown to cause KC development, the link between sunlight and other NMSC is not as clear. This relationship is further discussed in *The American Cancer Society's Principles of Oncology: Prevention to Survivorship*, Chapter 10, "Sun Protection." This chapter will review the epidemiology, clinical characteristics, and treatment of NMSC.

Basal Cell Carcinoma (BCC)

Basal cell carcinomas are the most common form of skin cancer in the United States (US), Australia, and New Zealand, comprising approximately 75–80% of all KCs [1]. Because <0.1% of these lesions metastasize, they have low mortality. When they are fatal, it is usually because a large neglected lesion has invaded a vital structure [2–5]. However, these lesions can also grow to involve structures such as the nasal and ear cartilages, causing significant morbidity.

Incidence and Mortality

Epidemiologic data indicate that BCC incidence rates have risen between 20 and 80% over the last 30 years, making the morbidity associated with BCCs a growing public health concern [1]. The age-adjusted mortality rate for BCC has been estimated at 0.12 per 100,000. In general, men have higher rates of BCC than do women (1.5–2:1) [6].

Etiology and Risk Factors

Males and females are nearly equally affected (M:F ratio 0.92). The most common subtype is nodular BCC, followed by superficial BCC [6]. Genetic syndromes with a significant risk for developing BCCs include nevoid basal cell carcinoma syndrome (Gorlin syndrome), in which people develop hundreds of BCCs.

Individuals with fair skin are at highest risk, although BCCs can arise on darker skin with repeated and significant lifetime sun exposure [7]. The biggest risk factor is a prior history of BCC. Other common risk factors for development of BCC include: red hair, lentigines, melanocytic nevi, intermittent intense sun exposure, radiation therapy, extensive occupational sun exposure, and blistering sunburns as a child [1].

After diagnosis of one BCC, the risk of a second BCC is as high as 44% over the next 3 years, which represents a 10-fold increased risk compared to the general population [8]. Risk factors for development of a second BCC include older age, multiple tumors, and male gender [9].

Solid-organ transplantation increases the risk of KCs significantly, with the risk of BCCs estimated to be around 10 times the normal population. Risk factors for BCCs associated with solid-organ transplant include age at transplantation, fair skin, blistering sunburns as a child, type of immunosuppressive drug, and amount of cumulative sun exposure [10].

The occurrence of multiple BCCs is also associated with various genetic syndromes. In nevoid basal cell carcinoma syndrome, also known as Gorlin syndrome, affected individuals present with multiple abnormalities in various organ systems. In addition to developing multiple BCCs at a young age, they can develop odontogenic cysts of the jaw, palmar-plantar pits, bifid ribs, pectus excavatum, scoliosis, frontal bossing, coloboma, glaucoma, and medulloblastoma. This disorder is inherited in an autosomal dominant manner. In Bazex–Dupré–Christol syndrome, individuals develop follicular atrophoderma, hypotrichosis, hypohidrosis, and multiple BCCs. This disorder is

The American Cancer Society's Oncology in Practice: Clinical Management, First Edition. Edited by The American Cancer Society.

inherited in an X-linked dominant fashion. In Rombo syndrome, individuals develop atrophoderma vermiculatum, hypotrichosis, trichoepitheliomas, milia, cyanosis, acral erythema, and multiple BCCs. This disorder is inherited in an autosomal dominant manner [11].

Clinical Features (Figure 35.1)

BCCs can present with various clinical features, depending on the subtype of tumor. Because these clinical types have different histologic features and biologic behaviors, first-line treatment options can vary widely.

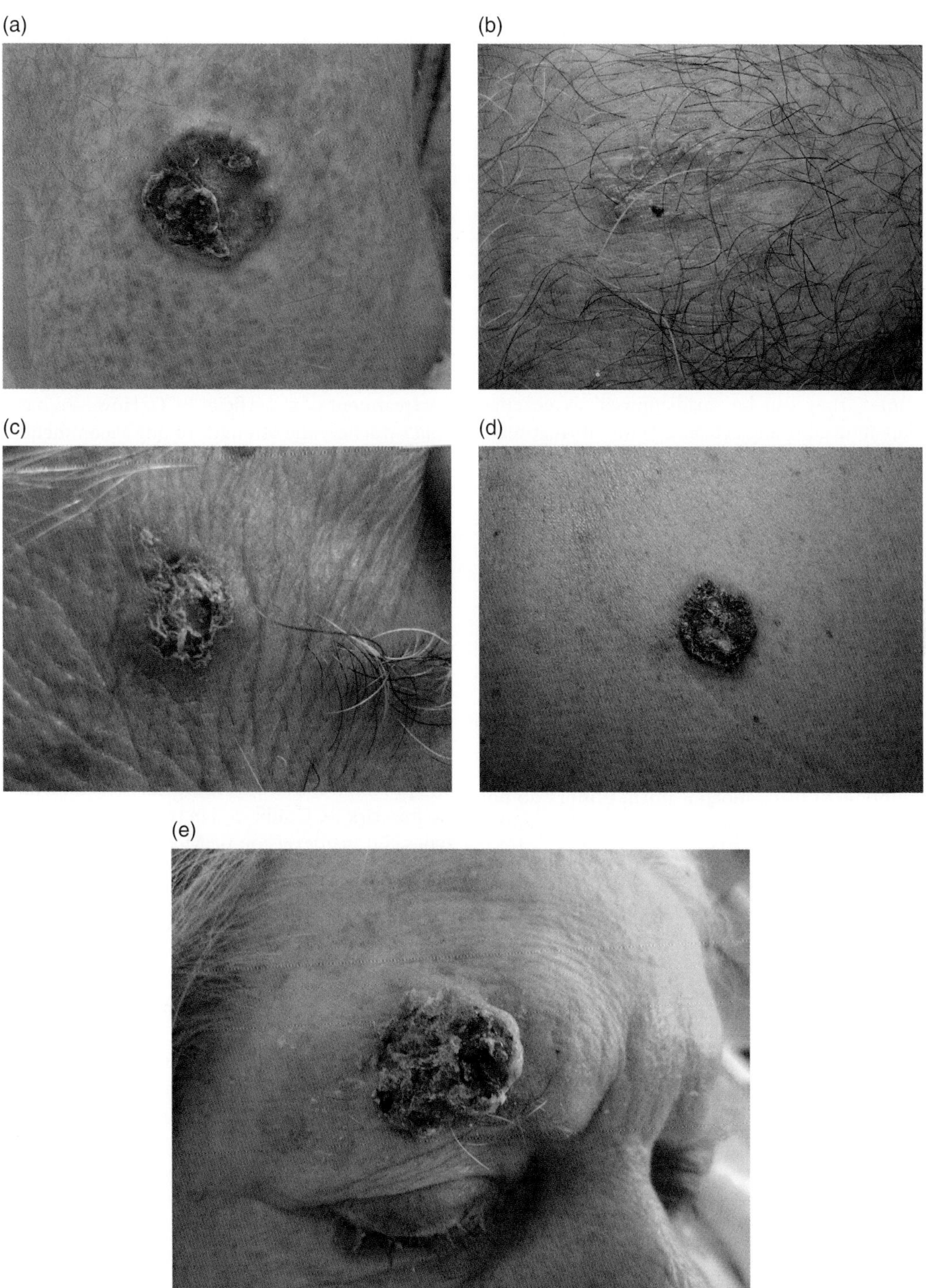

Figure 35.1 Clinical spectrum of basal cell carcinomas. (a) Nodular basal cell carcinoma. This lesion demonstrates classic features of basal cell carcinoma, including "rolled" borders, pearly pink color, central hemorrhagic crust, and prominent overlying telangiectasias. Hemorrhagic crusting is noted on the lesion secondary to trauma. (b) Superficial basal cell carcinoma. These lesions tend to be more subtle in appearance and present as an ill-defined, pink, flat papule or plaque. (c, d) Pigmented basal cell carcinoma. These well-defined pigmented plaques can often be confused with melanoma. (e) "Rodent ulcer." Longstanding basal cell carcinoma with central ulceration and crusting. A rolled border with prominent telangiectasias is present at the medial aspect of the tumor.

Low-Risk Subtypes: Nodular, Pigmented, Superficial

The *nodular* subtype is the most common type of BCC, accounting for up to 79% of all BCCs diagnosed [6]. Clinically, they present as waxy or pearly papules surrounding a small central depression. When the skin is stretched, the semi-translucent border is often accentuated. Centrally, the lesion can appear ulcerated or crusted. On closer examination, arborizing telangiectasias are often present throughout the lesion. As the tumor grows, central ulceration or crusting becomes more common, especially after minor trauma. The lesion will enlarge over time, with rare metastatic potential. Over time, nodular BCCs may develop central necrosis and ulceration with a clinical appearance aptly coined a "rodent ulcer."

The *pigmented* subtype is similar in appearance to other subtypes, with the addition of "floating" globules of brown or black pigment that can often be visualized within the lesion. They follow a similar clinical course as nodular BCCs.

The *superficial* subtype is the second most common form of BCC, comprising up to 15% of all BCCs diagnosed [6]. Clinically, these tumors present as pink to red patches or thin plaques. Telangiectasias are frequently present. Scale can sometimes be present. Oftentimes, they can be misdiagnosed as eczema, psoriasis, or solar-induced telangiectasias. Without treatment, this lesion can enlarge in size and may cause ulceration.

High-Risk Subtypes: Infiltrative, Micronodular, Morpheaform

The *infiltrative* BCC represents an aggressive tumor characterized by rapid infiltration of the upper and lower dermis by basaloid cells. Clinically, these lesions can resemble any of the aforementioned presentations of BCCs in this section.

Similarly, the *micronodular* subtype does not have distinctive clinical features, but acts in an aggressive manner of spread.

The *morpheaform* subtype presents as a scar-like plaque, and represents approximately 6% of all BCCs diagnosed [6]. Typically, these lesions occur on the head and neck. In contrast to the nodular subtype of BCC, morpheaform tumors do not characteristically show a rolled pearly border with central ulceration. In morpheaform tumors, telangiectasias can occasionally be present. They can be mistaken for a scar or other adnexal tumors of the head and neck. This subtype exhibits aggressive behavior.

Differential Diagnosis

The differential diagnosis for BCCs is broad and includes other types of NMSC. Oftentimes, it can be difficult to distinguish a small BCC from an actinic keratosis or a small SCC. An early BCC with a translucent border may also be confused with sebaceous hyperplasia, a benign lesion that commonly occurs on the face and like BCC may display a central depression. Ulcerated BCCs on the leg may be misdiagnosed as benign venous or arterial ulcers. Pigmented BCCs can resemble melanoma or nevi. Superficial BCCs can appear similar to a plaque of eczema or psoriasis.

Diagnosis

A skin biopsy is the gold standard for diagnosis of BCCs. Shave or punch biopsy may be utilized.

Pathology

On histopathology, nests of uniform, basaloid cells with peripheral palisading are seen. A loose, pink stroma typically surrounds each nest. Oftentimes, cleft-like retraction spaces can be identified. On molecular pathology, *TP53* mutations can be detected in each grouping of abnormal cells [6]. The percentage of BCCs with *TP53* mutations is not known.

On a molecular level, BCCs result from a defect in the sonic hedgehog signaling pathway, resulting in activation of tumor-promoting factors. *PTCH* is commonly mutated in those with BCCs, and new drug-based therapies targeting this pathway, such as vismodegib, have been developed.

Treatment

Various considerations are pertinent to choosing the optimal treatment, including tumor subtype, location, size of tumor, age and function of the patient, and patient preference.

Topical chemotherapeutic treatments can be effective for superficial BCCs. Both 5-fluorouracil (5-FU) and imiquimod are approved by the US Food and Drug Administration (FDA) for treatment of superficial BCC. However, based on the available evidence, the strength of any recommendations for these agents' use in primary treatment is weak. It is therefore recommended that their use be limited to patients who cannot undergo treatment with better-established therapies and ideally in small tumors in low-risk locations. Furthermore, the level of clearance is also highly influenced by patient compliance, as the patient is responsible for applying the medication [12]. Patients should also be aware that the course of topical treatment may take weeks or even months to complete. 5-FU is typically applied once or twice daily for 2–6 weeks and imiquimod is usually applied 5–7 days per week for 6–12 weeks.

Electrodesiccation and curettage is a commonly used treatment for low-risk subtypes of BCC, particularly on the trunk and proximal extremities. Surgical excision is also a good option for low-risk BCC subtypes in these locations. For high-risk subtypes, surgical excision or Mohs micrographic surgery (MMS) is typically the treatment of choice. MMS offers the highest cure rate for all BCC subtypes, but is only appropriate for tumors in locations where tissue conservation is of utmost importance such as the "mask areas" of face (eyelids, canthi, eyebrows, nose, chin, ears, preauricular cheek, and temple, and cutaneous/mucosal lips), the hands, feet, nail units, or genitals. Other factors such as underlying immunosuppression, tumor size, BCC subtype, recurrence after another treatment, and underlying genetic syndromes (e.g., basal cell nevus syndrome), would contribute to the decision to use MMS, but these details are beyond the scope of this chapter [13]. While MMS offers a high cure rate, its use should be guided by appropriate clinical indications in order to maintain cost-effective use of limited healthcare dollars.

Vismodegib and sonidegib are FDA-approved oral medications that act as antagonists to the smoothened receptor of the hedgehog signaling pathway. Abnormal signaling in this pathway has been implicated in the pathogenesis of BCCs. When the smoothened receptor is inhibited, transcription factors GLI1 and GLI2 remain inactive and are thus unable to promote abnormal growth of basaloid cells. These medications are only indicated for patients with multiple and/or advanced BCCs not amenable to surgery or radiation, such as those with nevoid basal cell carcinoma syndrome, BCCs that have relapsed after surgery, or metastatic BCC [14, 15].

Squamous Cell Carcinoma (SCC)

Squamous cell carcinomas are the second most common tumor of the skin, after BCC. Similar to BCC, UVR is an important cause of this tumor. In contrast to BCCs, SCCs have a higher overall risk of metastasis at 4% and may cause mortality in up to 1.5% [16].

Incidence and Mortality

In a systemic review of worldwide incidences of KCs, the incidence of SCC has been steadily increasing since 1960, with the rate of increase varying by geographic area. In Europe, Switzerland had the highest incidence with approximately 30/100,000 person years. In North America, SCC incidence rates vary by latitude. In Alberta, Canada, incidence rates were approximately 60/100,000 person years, compared to 290/100,000 person years in Arizona. Australia demonstrates the highest incidence rate of SCCs, with 386/100,000 person years for the continent, and specific areas, such as Queensland, showed rates as high as 1,035/100,000 [17].

Etiology and Risk Factors

Chronic, long-term UVR exposure is the primary risk factor for SCCs, as sun-exposed areas (face, scalp, neck, hands) are the most common locations for tumors. High-risk human papillomavirus subtypes may also have a role in transformation of actinic keratosis into SCCs, although this link has not been consistently demonstrated in clinical studies [18]. Genetic syndromes with a high risk of developing SCC include xeroderma pigmentosum and recessive dystrophic epidermolysis bullosa.

Risk factors for SCC include cumulative lifetime UVR exposure, prior occurrence of SCC, indoor tanning bed use, immunosuppression, older age, male gender, chronic nonhealing ulcerations, and fair skin [13].

After development of one SCC, the 3-year cumulative risk of subsequent SCC is 18%, or 10 times the incidence compared to the general population [8]. SCCs on genital skin are different clinically and epidemiologically; they are typically related to human papillomavirus infection (HPV) and are more likely than SCC arising in sun-exposed areas to result in metastasis or death.

SCCs are the most common type of NMSC to develop in the solid-organ transplant population, where squamous cell carcinoma *in situ* (SCCIS) and SCC of the lip are 65 and 20 times more likely to develop, respectively, compared to the general population. Up to 75% of these tumors occur on sun-exposed areas. The risk of SCC increases with time post transplant due to long-term use of immunosuppressive medications. These tumors are also more aggressive and have a higher risk of metastasis (0.5–5%) compared to SCCs in the nontransplant population. In the US, the risk of SCCs increases from 10 to 27% at 10 years post transplant to 40–60% at 20 years post transplant. In Australia, the risk is 80% at 20 years post transplant [19].

Several genetic syndromes related to increased photosensitivity can increase an individual's risk of developing SCCs. These photosensitivity syndromes include albinism, xeroderma pigmentosum, dyskeratosis congenita, Rothmund–Thomson syndrome, Bloom syndrome, and Werner syndrome. Other conditions with chronic scarring and remodeling of the dermis and epidermis can also lead to increased risk of SCC. These include dystrophic and junctional epidermolysis bullosa. SCCs may also develop as a result of BRAF inhibitor therapies used for treatment of malignant melanoma [20–22].

Clinical Features (Figure 35.2)

SCCs usually occur on sun-exposed areas such as the face, scalp, neck, forearms, dorsal hands, and lower legs. They can also occur on sites of chronic scars or ulceration. The clinical appearance usually ranges from erythematous to flesh-colored, plaque-like or papulonodular lesions that are often hyperkeratotic and, at times, exophytic. Overlying crusting, ulcerations, and erosions are secondary changes that can be observed. Eventually, the lesion may become fixed to deeper skin layers and can invade surrounding tissues. Tumors >2 cm are also most likely to metastasize to regional nodes, and are associated with a higher risk of local recurrence as well as mortality.

Actinic keratoses (AK), considered a precursor to SCC, appear as faint pink to red thin papules or plaques with rough scale. A hypertrophic variant exists, which can present with thicker scale. Over time, the lesion can transform into an SCCIS, also known as Bowen disease, which presents most commonly as a scaly pink or erythematous patch or plaque on sun-exposed skin. These lesions can evolve into an SCC, in which a firm, perhaps nodular, component can be palpated. The lesion can become ulcerated or can be hidden by a thick hyperkeratotic crust.

On the lip, SCC frequently develops first from actinic cheilitis, a precursor entity analogous to actinic keratosis but occurring on the mucosal epithelium of the lower lip. After repeated sunburns or cumulative sun exposure, the lip becomes persistently dry and scaly with progressive thickening and whitish

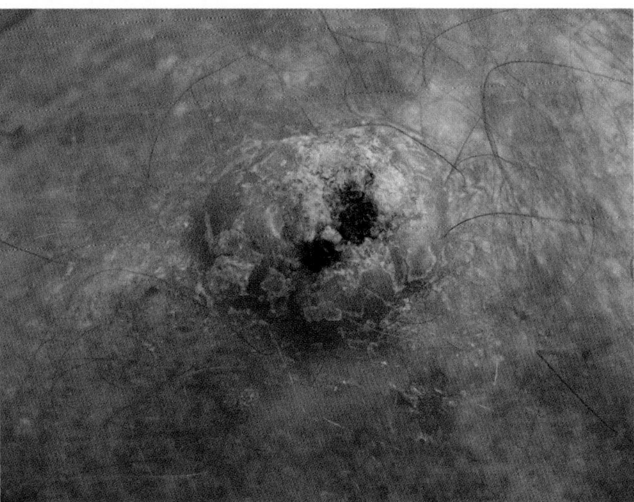

Figure 35.2 Squamous cell carcinoma: a pink, hyperkeratotic nodule. Crusting is present in this lesion.

discoloration of the lip at the border of the lip and skin. Over time, this thin plaque becomes more indurated and may eventually become a firm nodule that can ulcerate, signaling transformation into an SCC. A history of smoking is a strong risk factor for development of SCC of the lip. These lesions metastasize up to 10–15% of the time.

Differential Diagnosis

The differential diagnosis for SCC includes keratoacanthoma, granular cell tumor, infectious etiology, chronic ulceration, and seborrheic keratosis.

Diagnosis and Staging

Skin biopsy is the gold standard for diagnosis of this condition. Staging for non-melanoma cutaneous carcinomas of the head and neck (with the exception of Merkel cell carcinoma) according to the TNM (tumor, node, metastasis) system of the American Joint Committee on Cancer (AJCC) and the Union for International Cancer Control (UICC) is presented in Table 35.1. The Eighth Edition AJCC and UICC staging manuals limit application of this system to head and neck sites because non-melanoma cutaneous carcinomas of other anatomical regions are generally not staged. This represents a change from

Table 35.1 Head and neck cutaneous non-melanoma carcinoma staging, from the American Joint Committee on Cancer (AJCC) and the Union for International Cancer Control (UICC).

Definition of primary tumor (T)

T category	T criteria
TX	Primary tumor cannot be identified
Tis	Carcinoma *in situ*
T1	Tumor smaller than 2 cm in greatest dimension
T2	Tumor 2 cm or larger, but smaller than 4 cm in greatest dimension
T3	Tumor 4 cm or larger in maximum dimension or minor bone erosion or perineural invasion or deep invasion[1]
T4	Tumor with gross cortical bone/marrow, skull base invasion and/or skull base foramen invasion
T4a	Tumor with gross cortical bone/marrow invasion
T4b	Tumor with skull base invasion and/or skull base foramen involvement

[1]Deep invasion is defined as invasion beyond the subcutaneous fat or >6 mm (as measured from the granular layer of adjacent normal epidermis to the base of the tumor); perineural invasion for T3 classification is defined as tumor cells within the nerve sheath of a nerve lying deeper than the dermis or measuring 0.1 mm or larger in caliber, or presenting with clinical or radiographic involvement of named nerves without skull base invasion or transgression.

Definition of regional lymph node (N)

Clinical N (cN)

N category	N criteria
NX	Regional lymph nodes cannot be assessed
N0	No regional lymph node metastasis
N1	Metastasis in a single ipsilateral lymph node, 3 cm or smaller in greatest dimension and ENE(−)
N2	Metastasis in a single ipsilateral node larger than 3 cm but not larger than 6 cm in greatest dimension and ENE(−); *or* metastases in multiple ipsilateral lymph nodes, none larger than 6 cm in greatest dimension and ENE(−); *or* in bilateral or contralateral lymph nodes, none larger than 6 cm in greatest dimension and ENE(−)
N2a	Metastasis in a single ipsilateral node larger than 3 cm but not larger than 6 cm in greatest dimension and ENE(−)
N2b	Metastasis in multiple ipsilateral nodes, none larger than 6 cm in greatest dimension and ENE(−)
N2c	Metastasis in bilateral or contralateral lymph nodes, none larger than 6 cm in greatest dimension and ENE(−)
N3	Metastasis in a lymph node larger than 6 cm in greatest dimension and ENE(−); *or* metastasis in any node(s) and clinically overt ENE (ENE(+))
N3a	Metastasis in a lymph node larger than 6 cm in greatest dimension and ENE(−)
N3b	Metastasis in any node(s) and ENE(+)

Note: A designation of "U" or "L" may be used for any N category to indicate metastasis above the lower border of the cricoid (U) or below the lower border of the cricoid (L).
Similarly, clinical and pathological extranodal extension (ENE) should be recorded as ENE(−) or ENE(+).

Table 35.1 (Continued)

Pathological N (pN)

N category	N criteria
NX	Regional lymph nodes cannot be assessed
N0	No regional lymph node metastasis
N1	Metastasis in a single ipsilateral lymph node, 3 cm or smaller in greatest dimension and ENE(−)
N2	Metastasis in a single ipsilateral lymph node, 3 cm or smaller in greatest dimension and ENE(+); *or* larger than 3 cm but not larger than 6 cm in greatest dimension and ENE(−); *or* metastases in multiple ipsilateral lymph nodes, none larger than 6 cm in greatest dimension and ENE(−); *or* in bilateral or contralateral lymph nodes, none larger than 6 cm in greatest dimension, ENE(−)
N2a	Metastasis in single ipsilateral or contralateral node 3 cm or smaller in greatest dimension and ENE(+); *or* a single ipsilateral node larger than 3 cm but not larger than 6 cm in greatest dimension and ENE(−)
N2b	Metastasis in multiple ipsilateral nodes, none larger than 6 cm in greatest dimension and ENE(−)
N2c	Metastasis in bilateral or contralateral lymph nodes, none larger than 6 cm in greatest dimension and ENE(−)
N3	Metastasis in a lymph node larger than 6 cm in greatest dimension and ENE(−); *or* in a single ipsilateral node larger than 3 cm in greatest dimension and ENE(+); *or* multiple ipsilateral, contralateral, or bilateral nodes, any with ENE(+)
N3a	Metastasis in a lymph node larger than 6 cm in greatest dimension and ENE(−)
N3b	Metastasis in a single ipsilateral node larger than 3 cm in greatest dimension and ENE(+); *or* multiple ipsilateral, contralateral, or bilateral nodes, any with ENE(+)

Note: A designation of "U" or "L" may be used for any N category to indicate metastasis above the lower border of the cricoid (U) or below the lower border of the cricoid (L).
Similarly, clinical and pathological ENE should be recorded as ENE(−) or ENE(+).

Definition of distant metastasis (M)

M category	M criteria
M0	No distant metastasis
M1	Distant metastasis

AJCC prognostic stage groups

When T is...	And N is...	And M is...	Then the stage group is...
Tis	N0	M0	0
T1	N0	M0	I
T2	N0	M0	II
T3	N0	M0	III
T1	N1	M0	III
T2	N1	M0	III
T3	N1	M0	III
T1	N2	M0	IV
T2	N2	M0	IV
T3	N2	M0	IV
Any T	N3	M0	IV
T4	Any N	M0	IV
Any T	Any N	M1	IV

Source: Amin MB *et al.*, eds [23]. Used with permission of the American College of Surgeons, Chicago, Illinois. The original source for this information is the AJCC Cancer Staging Manual, Eighth Edition (2016), which is published by Springer Science + Business Media.

the Seventh Edition manual, in which non-melanoma cutaneous carcinomas were included regardless of anatomical region. The Eighth Edition can be used by clinicians to support patient care decisions starting in January 2017. However, until 1 January 2018, documentation of stage information in medical records should be based on the Seventh Edition.

There are no standard guidelines regarding referral for radiologic nodal staging or sentinel lymph node biopsy. Oftentimes, the presence of perineural invasion or evidence of in-transit metastasis will prompt surgeons to refer patients for additional radiographic staging, consideration of sentinel lymph node biopsy, or adjuvant radiotherapy if warranted [24–27].

Imaging studies should address the characteristics of the primary tumor, involved local structures, presence or absence of perineural invasion, lymph node involvement, and extranodal spread. Involvement of the extranodal locations correlates with a worse prognosis. Few studies have prospectively examined the impact of sentinel lymph node biopsy on overall patient survival.

Pathologic staging requires complete resection of the tumor. If lymph node involvement is suspected, a selective dissection of at least 10 nodes or a comprehensive dissection of 15 or more nodes is needed. Extranodal involvement should also be evaluated and assists with appropriate staging.

Pathology

In SCCIS, keratinocyte atypia is present throughout the entire depth of the epidermis but does not involve the underlying dermis. In SCC, there is invasion of these atypical keratinocytes into the dermis. Keratin pearls can also be seen throughout the tissue specimen. Poor cell differentiation, mitosis, intercellular bridging, pleomorphism, and spindle-shaped keratinocytes can also be seen in these tumors. Perineural invasion may be present in aggressive tumors. Molecular analysis of these tissue specimens can reveal a high frequency of *TP53* mutations and occasional *RAS* or *c-MYC* mutations [28–30].

Treatment

The primary treatment for invasive SCCs limited to the skin is surgical. In rare cases, tumors may metastasize to the lymph nodes, requiring further staging and workup. In these situations, systemic therapies such as chemotherapy may be used.

Mohs surgery is appropriate for lesions that fit the appropriate use criteria and is typically used for facial lesions in which cosmesis is a concern [13]. Topical 5-FU and imiquimod are also approved by the FDA for use in treating SCCIS. Other modalities, such as electrodesiccation and curettage, cryotherapy, 5-FU, imiquimod, and radiation, can also be used for SCCIS [31].

Radiation is another option for patients with SCC, especially for large lesions with perineural invasion or for those located in areas that would require extensive surgery and reconstruction. Radiation often provides a desirable cosmetic result, although effects of radiation dermatitis may be seen. Specific treatment recommendations for pattern and dose of radiation will depend on tumor characteristics (both clinical and histological), as well as tumor location. This therapy can also be considered for lesions that recur after surgery, and for those with histologically proven lymph node metastasis [32]. Contraindications to radiation include photosensitivity disorders such as xeroderma pigmentosum or albinism.

In addition to surgery and radiation, chemotherapy is an alternative treatment in patients with recurrent or advanced-stage lesions (stage III or IV). Because most tumors can be cured with surgery or radiation, few studies have compared the benefit of chemotherapy versus these more traditional methods for tumor removal.

Induction chemotherapy can be administered prior to surgery with the goal of decreasing total tumor burden before definitive treatment with surgery. This method can reduce the size of a large tumor making it more amenable to resection [33]. It is unclear whether this method improves survival. The regimens most commonly used for induction chemotherapy include 5-FU and cisplatin combinations.

Chemotherapy can also be used in combination with radiation for patients with unresectable disease or with comorbidities precluding use of surgery. This approach can improve survival compared to radiation alone, although this combined approach is associated with increased side effects [34–36]. Chemotherapy treatment regimens vary, but can include combinations of cisplatin, carboplatin, 5-FU, and paclitaxel.

Adjuvant chemotherapy is used postoperatively after surgical treatment of SCC. There are mixed data on the benefit of adjuvant therapy, with some studies suggesting a reduction in distant metastasis and other studies suggesting no additional benefit [37–40]. However, a survival benefit has not been definitively shown. Treatment regimens for adjuvant chemotherapy are similar to those of induction chemotherapy or chemotherapy combined with radiation [41].

In addition to use of traditional chemotherapy regimens, investigations into the use of epidermal growth factor blockers, monoclonal antibodies, and tyrosine kinase inhibitors have shown promise. Additional data are needed to definitively make a conclusion on the effectiveness of these therapies [37, 42, 43].

Keratoacanthoma (KAC)

Keratoacanthomas are considered by some to be a variant of SCC, although these two conditions do show histologic and clinical differences. The natural biologic course of KACs remains controversial, as some can regress spontaneously or after minor trauma, such as skin biopsy. Previously, KACs were thought to represent pseudomalignancies, given their frequent spontaneous regression. As such, they were not treated aggressively but were rather monitored for clearance. Currently, the view is that these tumors represent low-grade SCCs and should be treated surgically [44].

Incidence and Mortality

Because KACs are not reported to any central cancer registry, the true incidence and prevalence of this condition is unknown. Due to the low risk of metastasis associated with KACs, the mortality from this tumor is assumed to be minimal. However, no studies have directly investigated the mortality rates.

Etiology and Risk Factors

The prevalence of KACs in the population is unclear. Risk factors include immunosuppression, sunlight, and fair skin [45]. Reports of KACs developing after trauma suggest a role for skin injury in the pathogenesis of this disease. There is also a higher incidence of these tumors in warm climates [19]. KACs can also be associated with genetic syndromes, such as Muir–Torre syndrome and Ferguson Smith syndrome. Additionally, there are also reports of KACs resulting from BRAF inhibitor therapy for malignant melanoma [21].

Clinical Features

There are four recognized types of KACs: solitary (the most common type), and the relatively unusual variants – multiple, eruptive, and giant (keratoacanthoma centrifugum marginatum).

The *solitary* type (Figure 35.3) classically presents as a rapidly growing papule or nodule that enlarges over weeks. At presentation, it typically appears to be a firm red to skin-colored nodule with a central crater filled with keratinous debris of ulcerative crust. The nodule is well demarcated, and appears smoother and shiny. Telangiectasias may be present. This type of KAC often appears on sun-exposed areas, such as the hands, arms, and face. Lesions of the dorsal hands are common in men, whereas lesions on the lower legs are common in women.

The *multiple* type is similar to the solitary type, except that multiple tumors can be seen at once. This type of KAC is also known as the Ferguson Smith variant, in which multiple self-healing KACs form over the body. This condition can be traced back to its original description among Scottish families. Starting in the late teens or mid-20s, patients start to develop eruptive crops of KACs which appear clinically similar to solitary KACs. Lesions can grow over several weeks, but eventually involute within a few months. However, they do leave crateriform scarring after healing. As such, treatment with shave removal or cryotherapy may be warranted to reduce the appearance of scarring. Oral retinoids may also be useful in preventing the onset of new lesions.

The *eruptive* type of KAC is also known as the Grzybowski variant. This is a rare condition in which patients have no family history of a similar condition. Typically, patients present between 40 and 60 years of age and are in good general health without history of immunosuppression. Thousands of KACs may develop at the same time anywhere on the body, although they typically spare the palms and soles. Lesions can also appear in mucosal membrane areas, such as the mouth or larynx. Patients may complain of severe pruritus or facial disfigurement from scarring. Despite the sheer volume of KACs present, no reports of metastasis or increased risk of internal malignancy have been reported.

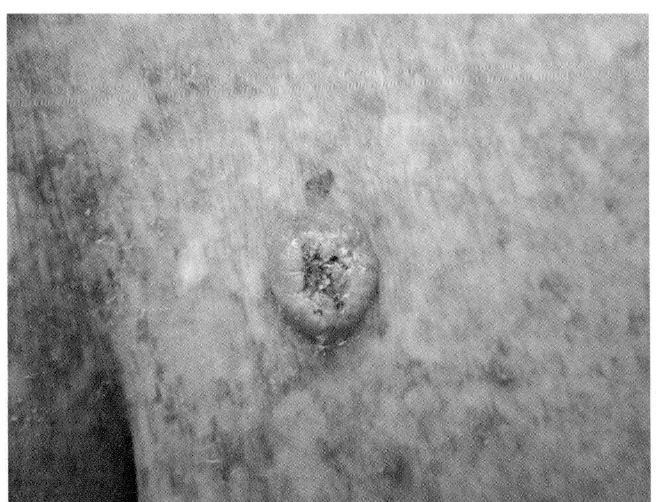

Figure 35.3 Keratoacanthoma: a volcano-like pink nodule with central keratotic plug. Note the background of sun-damaged skin.

The *giant* type of KAC, also known as keratoacanthoma centrifugum marginatum, is a rare condition in which large KACs can occur. Typically, lesions can grow up to 30 cm in diameter, with central ulceration and crusting. Unlike solitary KACs, the lesions do not spontaneously regress. Although keratoacanthoma centrifugum marginatum can appear on any site, the dorsal hands and pretibial regions are most commonly involved.

Differential Diagnosis

The differential diagnosis for KACs includes SCC, cutaneous horn, hypertrophic actinic keratosis, verruca vulgaris, and verrucous carcinoma. These lesions can be differentiated based on clinical history and histopathology review. KACs have a rapid onset within weeks to months, and may spontaneously involute.

Diagnosis

The gold standard for diagnosing these lesions remains skin biopsy.

Pathology

On histologic examination, KACs have a volcano-like architecture with central invagination. Keratinocytes are well differentiated with glassy cytoplasm. Eosinophils and lymphocytes can both be found at the periphery of the volcano-like structure. Cytologic atypia, such as mitosis or hyperchromatic nuclei, is rare, and the presence of numerous cells with atypia should warrant consideration of SCC. On molecular analysis, increased epidermal growth factor receptors and MYC genomic mutations can be detected [46].

Treatment

Currently, KACs are thought to represent low-grade SCCs. Therefore, they are typically treated with surgical excision or Mohs surgery. For conditions with multiple KACs, such as the Ferguson Smith type, Grzybowski variant, and keratoacanthoma centrifugum marginatum, oral retinoids, oral methotrexate, and oral cyclophosphamide may prove beneficial in preventing the onset of new lesions.

Merkel Cell Carcinoma (MCC)

Merkel cell carcinoma, also known as primary cutaneous neuroendocrine carcinoma, was first described in the 1970s, and was recently recognized to be caused by polyomavirus [47]. The viral DNA integrates within the tumor genome clonally, with expansion of these cells leading to development of MCC. This tumor is aggressively metastatic, with high rates of recurrence and associated risk of mortality.

Incidence and Mortality

Although the incidence rate is only 0.44/100,000, this tumor's age-adjusted incidence increased annually by 8% from 1986 to 2001 [48]. The increase was thought to be related to improved diagnosis over this time period and other factors. The age-adjusted mortality rate is estimated to be 0.031/100,000, but it is increasing annually [49, 50].

Etiology and Risk Factors

In 2010, the cause of MCC was linked to the polyomavirus and its exact role in immune dysfunction is currently being investigated [51]. Infection with the polyomavirus appears widespread, with lymphoid tissue acting as the reservoir. The virus is more commonly found in immunosuppressed individuals, providing a possible explanation for the increased frequency of MCC in these individuals. The majority of patients affected are men, with tumors located on the head and neck areas. Immunosuppression is a poor prognostic indicator, with a 3-year survival rate of 43% compared to 68% in immunocompetent patients [52, 53]. Tumors located on the scalp are at greatest risk of presenting with distant metastasis, while tumors of the lip had the highest rate of invasion into underlying muscle or bone [54]. The most common site of metastasis is the draining lymph node basin, followed by skin, lung, central nervous system, bone, and liver [48]. There are no known genetic syndromes associated with MCC.

Clinical Features

Clinically, MCC presents as a rapidly growing, well-defined, red to pink nodule or cystic papule. Overlying telangiectasias are frequently present. Although it starts out small, it can rapidly increase in size over weeks to months. Despite its aggressive nature, most lesions are asymptomatic. Ulcerations can occur with advanced tumors. At initial presentation up to 27% of patients have lymph node involvement and 7% have distant metastatic disease [55].

Due to MCC's aggressive nature and nonspecific appearance, the acronym AEIOU has been suggested for diagnosis: *A*symptomatic/lack of tenderness, *E*xpanding rapidly, *I*mmunosuppression, *O*lder than 50 years, *UV*-exposed location [56].

Differential Diagnosis

Due to the nondescript clinical features of MCC, the differential diagnosis is broad and includes BCC, SCC, amelanotic melanoma, metastatic small cell carcinoma, leukemia cutis, lymphoma cutis, melanoma, pyogenic granuloma, cysts, and clear cell acanthomas.

Diagnosis

The gold standard for diagnosis of MCC is skin biopsy. Immunohistochemistry is routinely performed to differentiate MCC from other small blue tumors of the skin. A sentinel lymph node biopsy (SLNB) may help predict survival; even small MCCs can have regional lymph node involvement. Therefore, SLNB is commonly recommended for patients diagnosed with MCC [57, 58]. In sentinel lymph node negative patients, there is the potential for a false-negative SLNB. Hence, patients warrant careful follow-up.

In cases where distant metastasis is suspected, fluorodeoxyglucose-positron emission tomography (FDG-PET) imaging is the radiographic modality of choice. When used in conjunction with computed tomographic (CT) scan, it can provide a whole-body survey for possible distant metastasis. CT scan alone has poor sensitivity for detecting nodal disease and is not recommended for use as a single modality for staging of disease [48]. Staging requires knowing the size of the tumor, presence or absence of nodal metastasis (either on histopathologic or clinical examination), and presence or absence of distant metastasis (Table 35.2).

Investigation for viral markers may also be warranted. Recent studies have shown that mutated forms of polyomavirus found in peripheral blood mononuclear cells are indications of tumor dissemination and associated with a worse prognosis [59].

Pathology

The histology of MCC demonstrates small, round, blue cells and may also be confused with extraosseous Ewing sarcoma. Ewing sarcoma is generally CK20−, CD99+, vimentin+, and NSE+. Melanoma can be distinguished from MCC, as melanoma will be S100+, HMB45+, melan-A+, tyrosinase+, and MITF+.

Immunohistochemistry is necessary for differentiating this tumor from metastatic small cell lung cancer, which can look clinically and histologically similar. MCC displays positive CK20 perinuclear dot staining, although this marker can be positive in 7% of small cell lung cancers. TTF-1 is a more useful marker for distinguishing the two tumors, as small cell lung cancer is positive for this marker whereas MCC is not. Small cell lung cancer is also positive for CD56, and chromogranin and synaptophysin in two-thirds of cases [48].

Treatment

Proper staging can help guide treatment for MCC (Table 35.2). The staging table divides tumor staging by absence (stage I–II) or presence (stage III) of regional lymph node metastasis and by presence of distant metastasis (stage IV).

Surgical resection with SLNB is the first-line choice for treatment and diagnosis. However, local recurrence after surgical excision can be as high as 75%. Regional lymph node involvement is found in 30–80%, and distant metastasis (stage IV disease) is found in 20–75%. Mortality can be as high as 20–55% [48, 56]. Survival rates are poor for MCC, especially for patients with regional or distant metastasis. The 5-year survival is 75%, 59%, and 25% for stage I/II, stage III, and stage IV disease, respectively. Recurrences are common within the first 3 years after diagnosis [48, 60].

Aside from surgical resection with SLNB, there is no standard protocol for treatment of MCC. Even with surgical resection, there is poor evidence for understanding the appropriate surgical margins. Historically, wide local margins of at least 3 cm have been recommended, although there are few clinical trials to prove the efficacy of these margins. Mohs micrographic surgery performed by dermatologic surgeons is an intriguing option given the ability for tissue conservation and the identification of tumors that may require extremely wide margins of excision [61]. However, the need for concurrent sentinel node mapping (and/or neck dissection) suggests that surgical excision of the primary tumor in the same setting may be a better choice in certain circumstances.

Table 35.2 Merkel cell carcinoma staging, from the American Joint Committee on Cancer (AJCC) and the Union for International Cancer Control (UICC).

Definitions of AJCC TNM	
Definition of primary tumor (T)	
T category	**T criteria**
TX	Primary tumor cannot be assessed (e.g., curetted)
T0	No evidence of primary tumor
Tis	*In situ* primary tumor
T1	Maximum clinical tumor diameter ≤2 cm
T2	Maximum clinical tumor diameter >2 but ≤5 cm
T3	Maximum clinical tumor diameter >5 cm
T4	Primary tumor invades fascia, muscle, cartilage, or bone
Definition of regional lymph node (N)	
Clinical (N)	
N category	**N criteria**
NX	Regional lymph nodes cannot be clinically assessed (e.g., previously removed for another reason, or because of body habitus)
N0	No regional lymph node metastasis detected on clinical and/or radiologic examination
N1	Metastasis in regional lymph node(s)
N2	In-transit metastasis (discontinuous from primary tumor; located between primary tumor and draining regional nodal basin, or distal to the primary tumor) *without* lymph node metastasis
N3	In-transit metastasis (discontinuous from primary tumor; located between primary tumor and draining regional nodal basin, or distal to the primary tumor) *with* lymph node metastasis
Pathological (pN)	
pN category	**pN criteria**
pNX	Regional lymph nodes cannot be assessed (e.g., previously removed for another reason or *not* removed for pathological evaluation)
pN0	No regional lymph node metastasis detected on pathological evaluation
pN1	Metastasis in regional lymph node(s)
pN1a(sn)	Clinically occult regional lymph node metastasis identified only by sentinel lymph node biopsy
pN1a	Clinically occult regional lymph node metastasis following lymph node dissection
pN1b	Clinically and/or radiologically detected regional lymph node metastasis
pN2	In-transit metastasis (discontinuous from primary tumor; located between primary tumor and draining regional nodal basin, or distal to the primary tumor) *without* lymph node metastasis
pN3	In-transit metastasis (discontinuous from primary tumor; located between primary tumor and draining regional nodal basin, or distal to the primary tumor) *with* lymph node metastasis
Definition of distant metastasis (M)	
Clinical (M)	
M category	**M criteria**
M0	No distant metastasis detected on clinical and/or radiologic examination
M1	Distant metastasis detected on clinical and/or radiologic examination
M1a	Metastasis to distant skin, distant subcutaneous tissue, or distant lymph node(s)
M1b	Metastasis to lung
M1c	Metastasis to all other visceral sites

(Continued)

Table 35.2 (Continued)

Pathological (M)			
M category	**M criteria**		
M0	No distant metastasis detected on clinical and/or radiologic examination		
pM1	Distant metastasis microscopically confirmed		
pM1a	Metastasis to distant skin, distant subcutaneous tissue, or distant lymph node(s), microscopically confirmed		
pM1b	Metastasis to lung, microscopically confirmed		
pM1c	Metastasis to all other distant sites, microscopically confirmed		
AJCC prognostic stage groups			
Clinical stage group (cTNM)			
When T is...	**And N is...**	**And M is...**	**Then the stage group is...**
Tis	N0	M0	0
T1	N0	M0	I
T2–3	N0	M0	IIA
T4	N0	M0	IIB
T0–4	N1–3	M0	III
T0–4	Any N	M1	IV
Pathological stage group (pTNM)			
When T is...	**And N is...**	**And M is...**	**Then the stage group is...**
Tis	N0	M0	0
T1	N0	M0	I
T2–3	N0	M0	IIA
T4	N0	M0	IIB
T1–4	N1a(sn) or N1a	M0	IIIA
T0	N1b	M0	IIIA
T1–4	N1b–3	M0	IIIB
T0–4	Any N	M1	IV

Source: Amin MB *et al.*, eds [23]. Used with permission of the American College of Surgeons, Chicago, Illinois. The original source for this information is the AJCC Cancer Staging Manual, Eighth Edition (2016), which is published by Springer Science + Business Media.

Treatment regimens are typically based on stage of disease. Several guidelines published on treatment of MCC by the German and American groups disagreed on several points, and a set of guidelines was developed by the French Society of Dermatology to reconcile these discrepancies [62]. These guidelines clearly illustrate the need for MCC to be managed in a multidisciplinary fashion.

For localized disease (stage I/II), several studies have suggested that adjuvant radiotherapy may not be necessary for lesions <2 cm in diameter [63–66]. For tumors ≥2 cm in diameter, or in cases where clear surgical margins are difficult to obtain due to the location of the tumor, adjuvant radiotherapy to the site of the tumor should strongly be considered [66].

Regional lymph node involvement is the most consistent predictor of survival, and those with absence of lymph node disease do better than those with presence of lymph node disease. For tumors with regional lymph node metastasis (stage III) on SLNB, a complete lymph node dissection (CLND) is recommended based on limited data and multidisciplinary consensus. In one study, patients had a recurrence rate of 0% after undergoing CLND. Other studies have supported these results, demonstrating high recurrence rates after a positive SLNB without CLND [65, 67]. For those with extensive lymph node disease seen on SLNB or CLND, adjuvant radiotherapy should be considered, based on survival studies. Adjuvant radiotherapy to the lymph node basin, combined with surgery, provides the best disease-free survival [68–70]. The role of chemotherapy for tumors with local metastasis is still being investigated, as use of carboplatin and etoposide has failed to demonstrate survival benefit in patients with MCC [71].

For patients with distant metastasis, chemotherapy may be effective. There is currently no standard therapeutic regimen for distant metastasis, although typical regimens are based on those designed for small cell carcinoma. Agents such as anthracyclines, antimetabolites, bleomycin, cyclophosphamide, etoposide, and platinums have been used alone or in combination for treatment of stage IV MCC [48, 60].

Due to the high rates of local recurrence and regional or distant metastasis, close clinical follow-up is recommended at

6-week intervals during the first year of diagnosis. Pembrolizumab, a monoclonal antibody against the programmed death 1 (PD-1) receptor, has recently demonstrated efficacy in patients with advanced MCC [72].

Dermatofibrosarcoma Protuberans (DFSP)

Dermatofibrosarcoma protuberans is a rare sarcoma that is locally aggressive.

Incidence and Mortality

The incidence rate of DFSP is estimated to be 0.42 per 100,000 in the general population. By race, Whites had an incidence rate of 0.39 per 100,000 while Blacks had an incidence rate of 0.65 per 100,000. Between 1973 and 2002, overall incidence increased by 43%, with women demonstrating slightly higher incidence rates than men. The 5-year survival for this period was 99.2% [73].

Etiology and Risk Factors

DFSP typically appears on young to middle-aged individuals. However, DFSP in children has also been reported [74]. Lesions favor the trunk in 50–60% of cases, although the proximal extremities (20–30%) and head and neck (10–15%) areas can also be affected. On truncal areas, DFSP typically presents on the shoulder or pelvic region. The tumor is slowly progressive but becomes painful and more prominent as it grows in size. The etiology of this tumor is unclear, as are risk factors for developing DFSP. There are no known genetic syndromes associated with development of DFSP.

Clinical Features

Clinically, lesions present as skin-colored to pink indurated plaques. These plaques may grow into asymmetric violaceous to red-brown nodules with tenderness to palpation. The tumor appears attached to the underlying subcutaneous tissue.

In contrast, childhood-onset DFSP typically has an atrophic appearance with a blue-red color. Lesions may also appear hypopigmented in some cases.

Differential Diagnosis

During the early stages, DFSP can resemble a keloid or dermatofibroma. For childhood-onset DFSP, the blue-red color may be mistaken for a hemangioma or other vascular malformation.

Diagnosis

A skin biopsy is recommended for diagnosis of this tumor. A punch or deep shave biopsy is recommended.

Pathology

Skin biopsy shows a deep tumor with uniform, storiform arrangement of spindle cells. There is minimal nuclear atypia with mitotic figures. Adnexal structures and adipose tissue are infiltrated with spindle cells or can appear completely obliterated. Immunohistochemical staining is usually CD34+ and factor XIIIa−. Cytogenetic studies may reveal a t(17;22)(22;q13) fusion of the collagen 1A1 promoter (*COL1A1*) on chromosome 17 and the platelet-derived growth factor β-chain (*PDGFB*) gene on chromosome 22.

Treatment

Complete surgical excision is recommended, and Mohs micrographic surgery is typically used due to the benefit of margin control. For those undergoing excision, wide margins are required (2.8–4 cm) [75, 76]. Due to the difficulty in obtaining clear surgical margins, Mohs surgery should be considered and can lead to significantly lower recurrence rates [77, 78].

Conservative surgery plus adjuvant radiotherapy is another option for treatment of DFSP. In a study of 53 patients with a median tumor size of 4 cm, radiotherapy was used either pre- or post-operatively to shrink the size of the tumor or to treat positive margins, respectively. Overall survival for both pre- and post-operative radiotherapy patients was 98% at 5 and 10 years. One patient was found to have a recurrence 10 years after initial treatment, demonstrating the importance of long-term surveillance after tumor removal [79]. Other studies have also found similar overall survival rates at 5 years [80].

Additionally, due to the t(17;22) reciprocal translocation, imatinib mesylate, which targets the PDGF receptor, is approved by the FDA for unresectable, recurrent, and/or metastatic DFSP [81].

Atypical Fibroxanthoma (AFX)

This rare tumor represents a low-grade malignancy and is often thought of as a superficial variant of malignant fibrous histiocytoma.

Incidence and Mortality

Due to the rarity of AFX, there are no clear estimates of its true incidence and mortality rates. A New Zealand study examining 50,411 cases of NMSC surgically excised over a 10-year period found that only 101 of these tumors were AFX, representing much less than 1% of all NMSC treated [82]. Similarly, in a study of 42,279 NMSC treated with Mohs, less than 1% were AFX [83].

Etiology and Risk Factors

This low- to intermediate-grade malignancy is considered a sarcoma, and commonly occurs on sun-damaged skin of elderly patients. The head and neck area is most commonly affected. Although the pathogenesis and risk factors for AFX are unclear, UVR exposure seems to play a significant role in the development of this lesion. *TP53* mutations are also thought to have a role in the pathogenesis of this tumor [84, 85]. Additionally, studies have described the occurrence of AFX on sites treated with radiotherapy, as well as in immunosuppressed individuals [86–88].

Clinical Features

This indolent tumor starts as a pink to skin-colored papule which rapidly enlarges to form a dome-shaped and well-circumscribed nodule. Ulceration and serosanguineous crusting may also be present. Bleeding on minor trauma is a common finding [89].

Differential Diagnosis

The differential diagnosis for AFX includes BCC, SCC, MCC, cutaneous tumor metastasis, undifferentiated pleomorphic sarcoma, malignant fibrous histiocytoma, and amelanotic melanoma.

Diagnosis

Skin biopsy of the lesion is diagnostic. A punch biopsy or deep shave is recommended.

Pathology

Histopathologic examination shows a thin epidermis with a dome-shaped nodule high in the dermis. The nodule is composed of atypical spindle cells, as well as pale-staining vacuolated cytoplasm. Mitoses are frequently present. The tumor is vimentin+, muscle-specific actin+, CD68+, and CD10+.

Treatment

Treatment of this superficial sarcoma consists of surgical excision. Mohs micrographic surgery can be considered, as it offers complete margin clearance.

Kaposi Sarcoma (KS)

Kaposi sarcoma has been definitively associated with human herpes virus 8 (HHV-8). Initially described in the Mediterranean population, KS experienced a surge in incidence due to its epidemic appearance among those with human immunodeficiency virus (HIV). However, with the advent of antiretroviral therapy (ART), HIV-related KS has markedly diminished in developed countries.

Incidence and Mortality

Between 1980 and 2005, the incidence of AIDS-related KS was approximately 1.9 per 100,000, compared to classic KS with an incidence of 1.4 per 100,000. Since the early 1990s the incidence of AIDS-related KS has steadily declined, from 4.6 per 100,000 in the early 1990s to 0.3 per 100,000 in the late 1990s. In contrast, the incidence for classic Mediterranean KS has been steady over this period of time (1.7 per 100,000) [90].

The 5-year survival rate for AIDS-related KS also improved over the past decades, from 12.1% between 1980 and 1995, to 54% between 1996 and 2005. The 5-year survival rate for classic Mediterranean KS patients has been stable, with a range of 76–89% since the 1980s [90].

Etiology and Risk Factors

Clinically there are four major types of KS: classic Mediterranean type, African endemic, immunosuppressed, and AIDS-related [91, 92].

Patients with the classic Mediterranean type are most often of Ashkenazi Jewish or Mediterranean descent. There is a slight male predominance, and most patients present after 50 years of age.

For the African endemic type, there is a clear male predominance, although a lymphadenopathic variant can have an equal gender ratio in children. This variant rapidly disseminates in children and causes high mortality.

For the immunosuppression type, not to be confused with the HIV-associated type, individuals are typically immunosuppressed secondary to systemic therapies. Those on cyclosporine typically have a higher incidence of disease. In addition to cyclosporine, KS has also been reported after initiation of systemic prednisone, cytotoxic chemotherapeutics, and calcineurin inhibitors for solid-organ transplants.

For the AIDS-related type, KS is considered an AIDS-defining illness.

HHV-8 was first identified within KS lesions of AIDS patients and has now been shown to be present in the majority of KS lesions. HHV-8 is thought to play a key role in stimulating proliferation, inducing the inflammatory response, and promoting angiogenesis [92–94]. The host immune response to HHV-8 viral particles may also contribute to the development of KS, as pre-existing KS plaques can worsen with treatment of AIDS and initiation of the immune reconstitution inflammatory syndrome.

Clinical Features

The *classic* type presents as slowly growing violaceous macules and papules on the distal lower extremities of elderly men of Ashkenazi Jewish or Mediterranean descent. Without treatment, these papules can coalesce or enlarge to form large nodules and plaques. Some lesions may regress, leading to the presence of multiple lesions at various stages.

The *African endemic* type can range in clinical presentation. Some lesions present as classic KS, with violaceous papules on the lower extremities. These tumors act similarly to classic KS. In contrast, the lymphadenopathic type of African endemic KS typically affects children, with rapid involvement of lymph nodes and a high fatality rate.

The *immunosuppression* type is frequently associated with systemic medications used for solid-organ transplants. Clinically, lesions resemble classic KS, with violaceous nodules and plaques. These lesions typically resolve without therapy upon cessation of the immunosuppressive systemic mediation. Those on prolonged immunosuppression are at increased risk of aggressive spread of KS to internal organs.

The *AIDS-related* type affects HIV-infected patients with CD4 T-cell counts ≤500 cells/mm^3. Clinically, lesions can look like those of classic KS, although they can have a more aggressive course with wide dissemination over the body. The trunk and face are commonly involved, and lesions can lead to significant cosmetic disfigurement. Lesions can also range in appearance from pink macules to purple-black tumors. In the oral cavity and other mucosal membrane sites, violaceous papules may also be appreciated. Systemic involvement of the lymph nodes, gastrointestinal tract, and lungs has also been reported. Although any systemic involvement of internal organs is considered a poor prognostic indicator, metastasis involving the lungs portends a worse prognosis than involvement of other organs.

Diagnosis

A punch biopsy of the skin is recommended for diagnosis of cutaneous KS. Individuals with risk factors for HIV should also be consented and tested for this virus. Patients suspected of having pulmonary or gastrointestinal involvement may need a bronchoscopy for visualization, as well as an esophagogastroduodenoscopy or colonoscopy.

There are no staging guidelines for KS, although the AIDS Clinical Trial Group has proposed a staging system for AIDS-related KS. This staging system has not been prospectively evaluated for prognostic significance.

Pathology

Despite the four different clinical variants of KS, lesions appear similar on histopathologic examination. Skin biopsies of KS can vary significantly based on the stage of the lesions. Three distinct histological types are recognized: patch, plaque, and nodular.

In the *patch* stage, superficial dermal proliferations of small vessels can be seen between collagen bundles. A sparse lymphoplasmacytic infiltrate may also be present. In the *plaque* stage, the vascular proliferation of the upper dermis expands into the deep dermis and may even invade the subcutis. There is a greater prominence of spindle-shaped endothelial cells around the vessels. In the *nodular* phase, dermal collagen is replaced by proliferations of spindled endothelial cells. These spindle cells can create intersecting slit-like spaces with erythrocytes, often creating a sieve-like pattern. Hemosiderin deposits, lymphocytes, and plasma cells can be present. Mitotic figures and pleomorphism are rare. In the late phase, increased mitotic activity may be present. HHV-8 immunostaining is positive during all stages of the disease.

Differential Diagnosis

The differential diagnosis for KS includes angiosarcoma, cutaneous metastasis, and polyarteritis nodosa. Given the violaceous appearance, vascular malformations such as hobnail hemangiomas may also be considered. These lesions can be differentiated based on histologic differences.

Treatment

Currently, there is no standard of care or national guideline recommendations for treatment of KS [53]. Treatment ranges from surgical excision of small lesions to treatment with various chemotherapeutics. Surgical resection of solitary lesions can preserve cosmesis while also providing tumor clearance. For multicentric lesions, adjuvant chemotherapy and/or radiation may be appropriate [95]. Rapidly progressive KS tumors or symptomatic visceral involvement are indications for initiation of systemic chemotherapy.

In contrast to the other types of KS, removing the patient from the offending immunosuppressive medication for the immunosuppressed type of KS can often bring about an improvement. For the AIDS-related type, improvement in CD4 count may at first worsen the burden of disease as part of the immune reconstitution syndrome. However, lesions will eventually resolve with increased CD4 counts.

Conclusion

Non-melanoma skin cancers (NMSC) affect all populations, from children to adults, and vary in their degree of morbidity and mortality. The incidence of the most common NMSCs continues to rise, and subsequently these neoplasms represent a significant burden on patient well-being and healthcare expenditures. The clinician should be aware of the clinical characteristics of each tumor type, particularly keratinocyte carcinomas, and the associated risk factors that place patients at greatest risk for their development.

References

1 Roewert-Huber J, Lange-Asschenfeldt B, Stockfleth E, Kerl H. Epidemiology and aetiology of basal cell carcinoma. *Br J Dermatol* 2007;157 Suppl 2:47–51.

2 Berlin JM, Warner MR, Bailin PL. Metastatic basal cell carcinoma presenting as unilateral axillary lymphadenopathy: report of a case and review of the literature. *Dermatol Surg* 2002;28:1082–4.

3 Gropper AB, Girouard SD, Hojman LP, *et al.* Metastatic basal cell carcinoma of the posterior neck: case report and review of the literature. *J Cutan Pathol* 2012;39:526–34.

4 Lo JS, Snow SN, Reizner GT, *et al.* Metastatic basal cell carcinoma: report of twelve cases with a review of the literature. *J Am Acad Dermatol* 1991;24:715–9.

5 Ting PT, Kasper R, Arlette JP. Metastatic basal cell carcinoma: report of two cases and literature review. *J Cutan Med Surg* 2005;9:10–5.

6 Scrivener Y, Grosshans E, Cribier B. Variations of basal cell carcinomas according to gender, age, location and histopathological subtype. *Br J Dermatol* 2002;147:41–7.

7 Dessinioti C, Tzannis K, Sypsa V, *et al.* Epidemiologic risk factors of basal cell carcinoma development and age at onset in a Southern European population from Greece. *Exp Dermatol* 2011;20:622–6.

8 Marcil I, Stern RS. Risk of developing a subsequent nonmelanoma skin cancer in patients with a history of nonmelanoma skin cancer: a critical review of the literature and meta-analysis. *Arch Dermatol* 2000;136:1524–30.

9 Graells J. The risk and risk factors of a second non-melanoma skin cancer: a study in a Mediterranean population. *J Eur Acad Dermatol Venereol* 2004;18:142–7.

10 Tessari G, Girolomoni G. Nonmelanoma skin cancer in solid organ transplant recipients: update on epidemiology, risk factors, and management. *Dermatol Surg* 2012;38:1622–30.

11 Gorlin RJ, Goltz RW. Multiple nevoid basal-cell epithelioma, jaw cysts and bifid rib. *A syndrome. N Engl J Med* 1960;262:908–12.

12 Love WE, Bernhard JD, Bordeaux JS. Topical imiquimod or fluorouracil therapy for basal and squamous cell carcinoma: a systematic review. *Arch Dermatol* 2009;145:1431–8.
13 Connolly SM, Baker DR, Coldiron BM, *et al.* AAD/ACMS/ASDSA/ASMS 2012 appropriate use criteria for Mohs micrographic surgery: a report of the American Academy of Dermatology, American College of Mohs Surgery, American Society for Dermatologic Surgery Association, and the American Society for Mohs Surgery. *J Am Acad Dermatol* 2012;67:531–50.
14 Sekulic A, Migden MR, Lewis K, *et al.* Pivotal ERIVANCE basal cell carcinoma (BCC) study: 12-month update of efficacy and safety of vismodegib in advanced BCC. *J Am Acad Dermatol* 2015;72(6):1021–6.
15 Danial C, Sarin KY, Oro AE, Chang AL. An investigator-initiated open-label trial of sonidegib in advanced basal cell carcinoma patients resistant to vismodegib. *Clin Cancer Res* 2016;22(6):1325–9.
16 Brantsch KD, Meisner C, Schonfisch B, *et al.* Analysis of risk factors determining prognosis of cutaneous squamous-cell carcinoma: a prospective study. *Lancet Oncol* 2008;9:713–20.
17 Lomas A, Leonardi-Bee J, Bath-Hextall F. A systematic review of worldwide incidence of nonmelanoma skin cancer. *Br J Dermatol* 2012;166:1069–80.
18 Aldabagh B, Angeles JG, Cardones AR, Arron ST. Cutaneous squamous cell carcinoma and human papillomavirus: is there an association? *Dermatol Surg* 2013;39:1–23.
19 Zwald FO, Brown M. Skin cancer in solid organ transplant recipients: advances in therapy and management: part I. Epidemiology of skin cancer in solid organ transplant recipients. *J Am Acad Dermatol* 2011;65:253–61; quiz 62.
20 Mattei PL, Alora-Palli MB, Kraft S, *et al.* Cutaneous effects of BRAF inhibitor therapy: a case series. *Ann Oncol* 2013;24:530–7.
21 Chu EY, Wanat KA, Miller CJ, *et al.* Diverse cutaneous side effects associated with BRAF inhibitor therapy: a clinicopathologic study. *J Am Acad Dermatol* 2012;67:1265–72.
22 Huang V, Hepper D, Anadkat M, Cornelius L. Cutaneous toxic effects associated with vemurafenib and inhibition of the BRAF pathway. *Arch Dermatol* 2012;148:628–33.
23 Amin MB, Edge SB, Greene FL, *et al.* (eds). *AJCC Cancer Staging Manual*, 8th edn. New York: Springer, 2017.
24 Jambusaria-Pahlajani A, Hess SD, Katz KA, Berg D, Schmults CD. Uncertainty in the perioperative management of high-risk cutaneous squamous cell carcinoma among Mohs surgeons. *Arch Dermatol* 2010;146:1225–31.
25 Veness MJ. Defining patients with high-risk cutaneous squamous cell carcinoma. *Australas J Dermatol* 2006;47:28–33.
26 Veness MJ. Treatment recommendations in patients diagnosed with high-risk cutaneous squamous cell carcinoma. *Australas Radiol* 2005;49:365–76.
27 Veness MJ, Palme CE, Smith M, *et al.* Cutaneous head and neck squamous cell carcinoma metastatic to cervical lymph nodes (nonparotid): a better outcome with surgery and adjuvant radiotherapy. *Laryngoscope* 2003;113:1827–33.
28 Brash DE, Rudolph JA, Simon JA, *et al.* A role for sunlight in skin cancer: UV-induced p53 mutations in squamous cell carcinoma. *Proc Natl Acad Sci U S A* 1991;88:10124–8.
29 Pierceall WE, Mukhopadhyay T, Goldberg LH, Ananthaswamy HN. Mutations in the p53 tumor suppressor gene in human cutaneous squamous cell carcinomas. *Mol Carcinog* 1991;4:445–9.
30 van der Schroeff JG, Evers LM, Boot AJ, Bos JL. Ras oncogene mutations in basal cell carcinomas and squamous cell carcinomas of human skin. *J Invest Dermatol* 1990;94:423–5.
31 Shimizu I, Cruz A, Chang KH, Dufresne RG. Treatment of squamous cell carcinoma in situ: a review. *Dermatol Surg* 2011;37:1394–411.
32 Lovett RD, Perez CA, Shapiro SJ, Garcia DM. External irradiation of epithelial skin cancer. *Int J Radiat Oncol Biol Phys* 1990;19:235–42.
33 Yin VT, Pfeiffer ML, Esmaeli B. Targeted therapy for orbital and periocular basal cell carcinoma and squamous cell carcinoma. *Ophthal Plast Reconstr Surg* 2013;29:87–92.
34 Benasso M, Merlano M, Sanguineti G, *et al.* Gemcitabine, cisplatin, and radiation in advanced, unresectable squamous cell carcinoma of the head and neck: a feasibility study. *Am J Clin Oncol* 2001;24:618–22.
35 Brizel DM, Albers ME, Fisher SR, *et al.* Hyperfractionated irradiation with or without concurrent chemotherapy for locally advanced head and neck cancer. *N Engl J Med* 1998;338:1798–804.
36 Wendt TG, Grabenbauer GG, Rodel CM, *et al.* Simultaneous radiochemotherapy versus radiotherapy alone in advanced head and neck cancer: a randomized multicenter study. *J Clin Oncol* 1998;16:1318–24.
37 Forastiere AA. Head and neck cancer: overview of recent developments and future directions. *Semin Oncol* 2000;27:1–4.
38 Jacobs C, Makuch R. Efficacy of adjuvant chemotherapy for patients with resectable head and neck cancer: a subset analysis of the Head and Neck Contracts Program. *J Clin Oncol* 1990;8:838–47.
39 de Braud F, Heilbrun LK, Ahmed K, *et al.* Metastatic squamous cell carcinoma of an unknown primary localized to the neck. Advantages of an aggressive treatment. *Cancer* 1989;64:510–5.
40 Cranmer LD1, Engelhardt C, Morgan SS. Treatment of unresectable and metastatic cutaneous squamous cell carcinoma. *Oncologist* 2010;15(12):1320–8.
41 Paccagnella A, Orlando A, Marchiori C, *et al.* Phase III trial of initial chemotherapy in stage III or IV head and neck cancers: a study by the Gruppo di Studio sui Tumori della Testa e del Collo. *J Natl Cancer Inst* 1994;86:265–72.
42 Curry JL, Torres-Cabala CA, Kim KB, *et al.* Dermatologic toxicities to targeted cancer therapy: shared clinical and histologic adverse skin reactions. *Int J Dermatol* 2014;53(3):376–84.
43 Kim S, Eleff M, Nicolaou N. Cetuximab as primary treatment for cutaneous squamous cell carcinoma to the neck. *Head Neck* 2011;33(2):286–8.
44 Schwartz RA. Keratoacanthoma: a clinico-pathologic enigma. *Dermatol Surg* 2004;30:326–33; discussion 33.
45 Sullivan JJ. Keratoacanthoma: the Australian experience. *Australas J Dermatol* 1997;38 Suppl 1:S36–9.
46 Jacobs MS, Persons DL, Fraga GR. EGFR and MYC gene copy number aberrations are more common in squamous cell carcinoma than keratoacanthoma: a FISH study. *J Cutan Pathol* 2013;40:447–54.

47 Feng H, Shuda M, Chang Y, Moore PS. Clonal integration of a polyomavirus in human Merkel cell carcinoma. *Science* 2008;319:1096–100.

48 Prieto Munoz I, Pardo Masferrer J, Olivera Vegas J, *et al.* Merkel cell carcinoma from 2008 to 2012: Reaching a new level of understanding. *Cancer Treat Rev* 2013;39(5):421–9.

49 Ascoli V, Minelli G, Kanieff M, Frova L, Conti S. Merkel cell carcinoma: a population-based study on mortality and the association with other cancers. *Cancer Causes Control* 2011;22:1521–7.

50 Becker JC. Merkel cell carcinoma. *Ann Oncol* 2010;21 Suppl 7:vii81–5.

51 Amber K, McLeod MP, Nouri K. The Merkel cell polyomavirus and its involvement in Merkel cell carcinoma. *Dermatol Surg* 2013;39:232–8.

52 Smith VA, Camp ER, Lentsch EJ. Merkel cell carcinoma: identification of prognostic factors unique to tumors located in the head and neck based on analysis of SEER data. *Laryngoscope* 2012;122:1283–90.

53 Tarantola TI, Vallow LA, Halyard MY, *et al.* Prognostic factors in Merkel cell carcinoma: analysis of 240 cases. *J Am Acad Dermatol* 2013;68:425–32.

54 Smith VA, MaDan OP, Lentsch EJ. Tumor location is an independent prognostic factor in head and neck Merkel cell carcinoma. *Otolaryngology* 2012;146:403–8.

55 Lemos BD, Storer BE, Iyer JG, *et al.* Pathologic nodal evaluation improves prognostic accuracy in Merkel cell carcinoma: analysis of 5823 cases as the basis of the first consensus staging system. *J Am Acad Dermatol* 2010;63:751–61.

56 Heath M, Jaimes N, Lemos B, *et al.* Clinical characteristics of Merkel cell carcinoma at diagnosis in 195 patients: the AEIOU features. *J Am Acad Dermatol* 2008;58:375–81.

57 Kouzmina M, Leikola J, Bohling T, Koljonen V. Positive sentinel lymph node biopsy predicts local metastases during the course of disease in Merkel cell carcinoma. *J Plast Surg Hand Surg* 2013;47:139–43.

58 Santamaria-Barria JA, Boland GM, Yeap BY, *et al.* Merkel cell carcinoma: 30-year experience from a single institution. *Ann Surg Oncol* 2013;20:1365–73.

59 Laude HC, Jonchere B, Maubec E, *et al.* Distinct merkel cell polyomavirus molecular features in tumour and non tumour specimens from patients with merkel cell carcinoma. *PLoS Pathog* 2010;6(8):e1001076.

60 Bichakjian CK, Lowe L, Lao CD, *et al.* Merkel cell carcinoma: critical review with guidelines for multidisciplinary management. *Cancer* 2007;110:1–12.

61 O'Connor WJ, Roenigk RK, Brodland DG. Merkel cell carcinoma. Comparison of Mohs micrographic surgery and wide excision in eighty-six patients. *Dermatol Surg* 1997;23:929–33.

62 Boccara O, Girard C, Mortier L, *et al.* Guidelines for the diagnosis and treatment of Merkel cell carcinoma – Cutaneous Oncology Group of the French Society of Dermatology. *Eur J Dermatol* 2012;22:375–9.

63 Allen PJ, Bowne WB, Jaques DP, *et al.* Merkel cell carcinoma: prognosis and treatment of patients from a single institution. *J Clin Oncol* 2005;23:2300–9.

64 Medina-Franco H, Urist MM, Fiveash J, *et al.* Multimodality treatment of Merkel cell carcinoma: case series and literature review of 1024 cases. *Ann Surg Oncol* 2001;8:204–8.

65 Senchenkov A, Barnes SA, Moran SL. Predictors of survival and recurrence in the surgical treatment of merkel cell carcinoma of the extremities. *J Surg Oncol* 2007;95:229–34.

66 Veness MJ, Perera L, McCourt J, *et al.* Merkel cell carcinoma: improved outcome with adjuvant radiotherapy. *ANZ J Surg* 2005;75:275–81.

67 Mehrany K, Otley CC, Weenig RH, *et al.* A meta-analysis of the prognostic significance of sentinel lymph node status in Merkel cell carcinoma. *Dermatol Surg* 2002;28:113–7; discussion 7.

68 Clark JR, Veness MJ, Gilbert R, O'Brien CJ, Gullane PJ. Merkel cell carcinoma of the head and neck: is adjuvant radiotherapy necessary? *Head Neck* 2007;29:249–57.

69 Lawenda BD, Arnold MG, Tokarz VA, *et al.* Analysis of radiation therapy for the control of Merkel cell carcinoma of the head and neck based on 36 cases and a literature review. *Ear Nose Throat J* 2008;87:634–43.

70 Poulsen M. Merkel-cell carcinoma of the skin. *Lancet Oncol* 2004;5:593–9.

71 Poulsen MG, Rischin D, Porter I, *et al.* Does chemotherapy improve survival in high-risk stage I and II Merkel cell carcinoma of the skin? *Int J Radiat Oncol Biol Phys* 2006;64:114–9.

72 Nghiem PT, Bhatia S, Lipson EJ, *et al.* PD-1 Blockade with pembrolizumab in advanced Merkel-cell carcinoma. *N Engl J Med* 2016;374:2542–52.

73 Criscione VD, Weinstock MA. Descriptive epidemiology of dermatofibrosarcoma protuberans in the United States, 1973 to 2002. *J Am Acad Dermatol* 2007;56:968–73.

74 Manganoni AM, Pavoni L, Gualdi G, *et al.* Dermatofibrosarcoma protuberans in an adolescent: a case report and review of the literature. *J Pediatr Hematol Oncol* 2013;35(5):383–7.

75 Akram J, Wooler G, Lock-Andersen J. Dermatofibrosarcoma protuberans: Clinical series, national Danish incidence data and suggested guidelines. *J Plast Surg Hand Surg* 2014;48(1):67–73.

76 Goldberg C, Hoang D, McRae M, *et al.* A strategy for the successful management of dermatofibrosarcoma protuberans. *Ann Plast Surg* 2015;74(1):80–4.

77 Snow SN, Gordon EM, Larson PO, *et al.* Dermatofibrosarcoma protuberans: a report on 29 patients treated by Mohs micrographic surgery with long-term follow-up and review of the literature. *Cancer* 2004;101:28–38.

78 Paradisi A, Abeni D, Rusciani A, *et al.* Dermatofibrosarcoma protuberans: wide local excision vs. Mohs micrographic surgery. *Cancer Treat Rev* 2008;34:728–36.

79 Castle KO, Guadagnolo BA, Tsai CJ, Feig BW, Zagars GK. Dermatofibrosarcoma protuberans: long-term outcomes of 53 patients treated with conservative surgery and radiation therapy. *Int J Radiat Oncol Biol Phys* 2013;86:585–90.

80 Uysal B, Sager O, Gamsiz H, *et al.* Evaluation of the role of radiotherapy in the management of dermatofibrosarcoma protuberans. *J BUON* 2013;18:268–73.

81 Rutkowski P, Van Glabbeke M, Rankin CJ, *et al.* Imatinib mesylate in advanced dermatofibrosarcoma protuberans:

pooled analysis of two phase II clinical trials. *J Clin Oncol* 2010;28:1772–9.

82 Withers AH, Brougham ND, Barber RM, Tan ST. Atypical fibroxanthoma and malignant fibrous histiocytoma. *J Plast Reconstr Aesthet Surg* 2011;64:e273–8.

83 Anderson HL, Joseph AK. A pilot feasibility study of a rare skin tumor database. *Dermatol Surg* 2007;33:693–6.

84 Lee CS, Chou ST. p53 protein immunoreactivity in fibrohistiocytic tumors of the skin. *Pathology* 1998;30:272–5.

85 Westermann FN, Langlois NE, Simpson JG. Apoptosis in atypical fibroxanthoma and pleomorphic malignant fibrous histiocytoma. *Am J Dermatopathol* 1997;19:228–31.

86 Ang GC, Roenigk RK, Otley CC, Kim Phillips P, Weaver AL. More than 2 decades of treating atypical fibroxanthoma at mayo clinic: what have we learned from 91 patients? *Dermatol Surg* 2009;35:765–72.

87 Fretzin DF, Helwig EB. Atypical fibroxanthoma of the skin. A clinicopathologic study of 140 cases. *Cancer* 1973;31:1541–52.

88 Hudson AW, Winkelmann RK. Atypical fibroxanthoma of the skin: a reappraisal of 19 cases in which the original diagnosis was spindle-cell squamous carcinoma. *Cancer* 1972;29:413–22.

89 Iorizzo LJ, 3rd, Brown MD. Atypical fibroxanthoma: a review of the literature. *Dermatol Surg* 2011;37:146–57.

90 Armstrong AW, Lam KH, Chase EP. Epidemiology of classic and AIDS-related Kaposi's sarcoma in the USA: incidence, survival, and geographical distribution from 1975 to 2005. *Epidemiol Infect* 2013;141(1):200–6.

91 Akasbi Y, Awada A, Arifi S, Mellas N, El Mesbahi O. Non-HIV Kaposi's sarcoma: a review and therapeutic perspectives. *Bull Cancer* 2012;99:92–9.

92 Martin JN. Kaposi sarcoma-associated herpesvirus/human herpesvirus 8 and Kaposi sarcoma. *Adv Dental Res* 2011;23:76–8.

93 Moore PS, Chang Y. Kaposi's sarcoma-associated herpesvirus-encoded oncogenes and oncogenesis. *J Natl Cancer Inst* Monographs 1998:65–71.

94 Muralidhar S, Veytsmann G, Chandran B, *et al.* Characterization of the human herpesvirus 8 (Kaposi's sarcoma-associated herpesvirus) oncogene, kaposin (ORF K12). *J Clin Virol* 2000;16:203–13.

95 Regnier-Rosencher E, Guillot B, Dupin N. Treatments for classic Kaposi sarcoma: a systematic review of the literature. *J Am Acad Dermatol* 2013;68:313–31.

Section 10

Endocrine Cancers

36

Thyroid Cancer

Maria E. Cabanillas[1], Steven P. Weitzman[1], Ramona Dadu[1], Ted Gansler[2], and Mark Zafereo[1]

[1] The University of Texas MD Anderson Cancer Center, Houston, Texas, USA
[2] American Cancer Society, Atlanta, Georgia, USA

Introduction

Thyroid cancer is quite common, especially among women in developed countries such as the United States (US), and has been increasing substantially during recent decades. Benign thyroid disorders are much more common, and must be distinguished from cancer. Although most cases of thyroid cancer are papillary and follicular carcinomas with a favorable prognosis, management of medullary and anaplastic carcinomas is more challenging. Several hereditary predisposition syndromes, particularly for medullary thyroid cancer (MTC), have been described and their molecular bases elucidated; this information has been applied to genetic testing that permits prevention of MTC through prophylactic surgery. Progress in understanding the molecular pathology of thyroid cancer has led to a number of targeted therapies with greater efficacy than older cytotoxic regimens.

Incidence, Mortality, and Survival

Approximately 56,870 new cancers of the thyroid are diagnosed annually (3.4% of cancer diagnoses) and approximately 2,010 deaths from thyroid cancers occur each year (0.3% of cancer deaths) in the US [1]. The incidence rate of thyroid cancer in the US has increased more rapidly than that of any other malignancy [2]. Thyroid cancer is the most common endocrine malignancy among men and women and is the fifth most common malignancy among females in the US, accounting for 5% of estimated cancer diagnoses in females in 2016 [1].

The incidence rate of thyroid cancers in the US, based on cases diagnosed in 2009–2013, was approximately 13.9 per 100,000 men and women per year. During the same time period, the age-adjusted death rate was 0.5 per 100,000 individuals per year. The lifetime risk of developing thyroid cancer (considering data for men and women together) is approximately 1.2% [3].

The incidence rate of thyroid cancer increased by an average of 6.6% annually from 1998 to 2009. This increase has been attributed largely, but not entirely, to the more frequent incidental detection of thyroid cancer by increased use of diagnostic imaging tests [4,5]. The rate of increase has since slowed to an average increase of 2.1% from 2009 to 2013, after changes in clinical practice such as more conservative indications for biopsy were instituted [4,5].

Fortunately, thyroid cancer is generally an indolent malignancy, and many patients with thyroid cancer live unknowingly with disease for many years. The prognosis for most patients with thyroid cancer is very favorable, with 98.1% surviving at least 5 years after diagnosis [3]. However, survival varies substantially by histological type. Death from thyroid cancer occurs most commonly in patients with aggressive histopathology, high tumor burden, and/or distant metastases. The 5-year survival rates for individuals with papillary or follicular carcinoma are in the range of 91.5–96.2% and 88.4–90.5%. Corresponding ranges for patients with MTC or anaplastic thyroid carcinoma (ATC) are 73.5–88.7% and 5.6–11.4%, respectively [6].

Types of Thyroid Cancer

The classification of thyroid cancer includes three major types – differentiated thyroid cancer (DTC), MTC, and ATC – with several subtypes thereof, and a few extremely rare types. DTC is, by far, the most common type of thyroid cancer. The cells of DTC retain many morphological and metabolic characteristics of normal follicular epithelium including, in many cases, the ability to concentrate iodine. The most common subtypes of DTC are papillary thyroid carcinoma (PTC), follicular carcinoma (FTC), and Hurthle cell (oxyphilic) carcinoma, comprising 89.1%, 4.8%, and 2.1% of all thyroid cancers, respectively [4]. In addition, there are variants of subtypes, most of which are beyond the scope of this chapter.

The American Cancer Society's Oncology in Practice: Clinical Management, First Edition. Edited by The American Cancer Society.

However, some variants have profound diagnostic and therapeutic implications. In the follicular variant of PTC, cells have nuclear morphology typical of PTC but are arranged in follicles (similar to those of follicular carcinoma) rather than fibrovascular papillary structures. Their behavior is similar to that of classic PTC but there is a subgroup of encapsulated, noninvasive lesions which were previously considered PTC that have recently been reclassified as "noninvasive follicular thyroid neoplasm with papillary-like nuclear features" or "NIFTP" based upon recognition of their indolent behavior and the importance of avoiding overtreatment [7]. The morphology and prognosis of poorly differentiated thyroid carcinoma (PDTC; including lesions previously classified as insular thyroid cancer) are intermediate between those of DTC and ATC, and this tumor is thought to represent a stage in the evolution from DTC to ATC [8]. Approximately 1.7% of thyroid cancers are classified as MTC [4]. These cancers produce and secrete calcitonin, as do the parafollicular C cells from which they arise. ATC is uncommon, accounting for only 0.8% of thyroid cancers [4]. This disease may evolve by de-differentiation of pre-existing DTC or may be diagnosed in individuals as the initial presentation of their thyroid cancer.

Etiology and Risk Factors

Demographic Factors

The vast majority of thyroid cancers are not associated with any known risk factor, such as ionizing radiation exposure or heritable condition. The median age at diagnosis is 51 years, and 63.5% of patients are aged between 35 and 64 years at the time of their diagnosis. Thyroid cancer is also highly represented among cancers in adolescents, making up 11% of overall US cancer diagnoses among persons aged 14–19 years [1]. Incidence rates among women and men are 20.6 and 6.9 per 100,000 individuals per year. This prominent female predisposition appears limited to nonfatal cases, with mortality rates for both sexes being the same – 0.5 deaths per 100,000 individuals per year. Similarly, incidence rates are much lower among African Americans (9.09) relative to Caucasians (16.52) in the US, but differences in mortality rates are much smaller (0.52 and 0.51, respectively) [3,4]. It is important to keep in mind that these statistics reflect data for all types of thyroid cancer combined. Since DTC is by far the most common type (>95% of all thyroid cancer), these numbers largely reflect patients with DTC and not those with less common types [4]. For example, the striking female predominance described for DTC has not been observed with MTC or ATC [9].

Heritable Genetic Conditions

Medullary Carcinoma

About 25% of MTC diagnoses occur in individuals with multiple endocrine neoplasia (MEN) type 2a, MEN type 2b, or familial medullary thyroid cancer (FMTC, now considered a subtype of MEN2a). MEN2a accounts for approximately 95% of MEN2 cases (of which 10–20% are FMTC), and MEN2b accounts for 5% [10]. These conditions are the result of germline mutations in various positions on the *RET* proto-oncogene. Although these germline mutations are heritable in an autosomal dominant fashion, approximately 5–9% of MEN2a cases and 75% of MEN2b cases are due to *de novo* mutations [11]. Thus, all patients diagnosed with MTC should be tested for germline *RET* mutations. *RET* mutations also occur in most sporadic MTCs, but these are somatic (involving only the tumor) rather than germline mutations and are therefore not heritable. The main clinical components of MEN2a are MTC (70–95% penetrance), pheochromocytoma (4–50% penetrance), and hyperparathyroidism (2–30% penetrance). The penetrance is variable in MEN2a, and depends on the specific *RET* mutation [11].

In MEN2b, MTC penetrance is virtually 100% but pheochromocytoma penetrance is approximately 50%. Those with MEN2b tend to develop MTC at a younger age and it follows a more aggressive course than is seen in MEN2a. Additional components of MEN2b include mucosal neuromas, diffuse ganglioneuromatosis of the gastrointestinal tract (40% penetrance), and physical characteristics similar to Marfan syndrome (75% penetrance). FMTC is a variant of MEN2a with a very low penetrance of pheochromocytoma and MTC being the only neoplastic manifestation.

Management of individuals who have inherited a *RET* allele but do not have clinically apparent MTC includes early screening for MTC with serum calcitonin levels and eventual prophylactic thyroidectomy. The timing of prophylactic thyroidectomy is based on the American Thyroid Association risk category (which is based on the type of *RET* mutation) [11,12] and is beyond the scope of this chapter. Screening for and management of other associated neoplasms and non-neoplastic disorders is essential [13,14].

Non-Medullary carcinoma

The hereditary conditions associated with FTC and PTC are quite diverse. They include non-syndromic familial non-medullary thyroid cancer (FNMTC) as well as several syndromes in which thyroid cancer is a component, albeit not the most prominent manifestation.

FNMTC is defined by the presence of two or more first-degree relatives with DTC in the absence of a strong non-genetic risk factor such as radiation exposure. Associations of several known genes (*SRGAP1*, *TITF-1/NKX2.1*, *FOXE1*, and *HABP2*) with FNMTC have been proposed, as have associations with yet-unknown genes at several other loci. Penetrance is variable, suggesting interaction with other genes and with non-genetic exposures. Approximately 3.2–6.2% of thyroid cancer cases are thought to be due to FNMTC [14]. Unfortunately, genetic testing for non-syndromic FNMTC is currently not available. Screening by ultrasonography is therefore recommended for members of affected families. Genetic syndromes with increased risk of non-medullary thyroid cancer include Cowden syndrome (associated with FTC and benign nodular thyroid disease), familial adenomatous polyposis (2–12% papillary thyroid cancer penetrance), Carney complex type 1 (15% penetrance of non-medullary thyroid cancer), and Werner syndrome (increased risk for FTC, PTC, and ATC) [14].

Ionizing Radiation

Exposure to ionizing radiation from external beam head and neck radiotherapy or radiation released from nuclear weapons has been shown to increase the incidence of DTC. Iodine radioisotopes released by other means, such as a result of nuclear power plant accidents, and from medical use, are also a cause of DTC. These sources of radiation exposure have a greater effect on children and adolescents compared to adults [15,16].

Iodine Deficiency

FTC is more common in areas of the world where diets are low in iodine. In most high-resource nations, individuals consume sufficient dietary iodine following the supplementation of table salt with iodine [17].

Diagnosis

The prevalence of thyroid nodules increases with age and is higher in females. In the general population, the prevalence of thyroid nodules is 2–6% based on palpation, and 19–35% using ultrasound [18]. In contrast, the lifetime risk of being diagnosed with thyroid cancer is 1.2% [3], so the prevalence of thyroid cancer that is both undiagnosed and clinically diagnosable is undoubtedly much lower. These numbers illustrate the challenge in distinguishing thyroid cancers (which are relatively rare, comprising approximately 5% of thyroid nodules) from non-neoplastic lesions and benign neoplasms (which are very common), while limiting patient morbidity during the diagnostic process. The algorithms for the evaluation of thyroid nodules are continually evolving. They currently involve a combination of sonographic appearance, determination of serum thyroid stimulating hormone (TSH) levels, radioiodine imaging, and fine-needle aspiration (FNA) [19].

Symptoms and Presentation

The most common presentations of thyroid cancer are as an asymptomatic thyroid mass identified by the patient or by a clinician in the course of physical examination or incidentally through diagnostic imaging for evaluation of an unrelated health condition. Occasionally, palpable involvement of regional lymph nodes can be the first sign of thyroid cancer. Head and neck pain, dyspnea, dysphagia, and voice changes are uncommon presentations of DTC but often result from compression and/or invasion of adjacent organs and tissues by more aggressive forms of the disease (i.e., PDTC and ATC). Patients with MTC may also present with diarrhea and flushing due to secretion of substances such as calcitonin, prostaglandins, and vasoactive intestinal peptide (VIP), among others. Those who are germline carriers of a *RET* mutation (MEN2) are often diagnosed during screening or prophylactic thyroidectomy.

FNA or No FNA?

The initial question in evaluating a thyroid nodule is whether FNA should be performed. The answer is based on the TSH level and ultrasound findings (which include evaluation of the thyroid, central neck, and lateral neck). A low TSH level may be seen as a result of suppression by thyroid hormone released from an autonomously functioning thyroid nodule ("hot nodule"). Thus, patients with low TSH in the setting of a thyroid nodule should undergo radionuclide scan instead of proceeding to FNA. These patients' hyperthyroidism should first be managed medically, or surgically in some cases. These hyperfunctioning nodules are rarely malignant. If the TSH level is normal or increased, FNA is recommended when ultrasound finding are worrisome. In general, larger size (>1 cm, as measured on ultrasound), microcalcifications, irregular contour, hypoechogenicity, shape taller than wide, and suspicious cervical lymph nodes support a decision to perform FNA [20]. Additional criteria have been described for selecting which of several nodules to sample by FNA. Non-worrisome nodules should be followed serially to monitor for growth, which may indicate the need for FNA. Further details are beyond the scope of this chapter and decisions should be guided by the recommendations of contemporary guidelines [19–21].

FNA Results

Cytologic interpretations of thyroid FNA samples are reported according to the Bethesda System for Reporting Thyroid Cytopathology (BSRTC). The BSRTC results can be used together with the ultrasound findings to guide management of thyroid nodules. The six categories in BSRTC are (I) non-diagnostic/unsatisfactory, (II) benign, (III) atypical cells of undetermined significance/follicular lesion of undetermined significance, (IV) follicular neoplasm/suspicious for follicular neoplasm, (V) suspicious for malignancy, and (VI) malignant [22,23]. Cytologically "indeterminate" categories refer specifically to categories III, IV, and V because the pathologic features encountered cannot reliably differentiate between benign and malignant. For example, Bethesda categories III, IV, and V carry a risk of malignancy of 14%, 25%, and 70%, respectively. Conversely, categories II and VI cytopathology can reliably distinguish between benign and malignant, as these carry a 2.5% and 99% risk of malignancy, respectively [22,23]. However, FTC cannot be diagnosed by cytopathology because capsular penetration, the histological feature which distinguishes follicular adenomas from FTC, cannot be evaluated in cytologic specimens. Thus, FTC cannot be definitively diagnosed without surgical excision of these tumors. Table 36.1 shows the follow-up and surgical management recommended by BSRTC category.

It is important to identify the specific type of thyroid cancer by FNA (when possible) and subsequently confirm a final diagnosis based upon the histopathology of the surgical specimen. In general, classification is based on tumor architecture, features of individual cells, and histochemical or immunohistochemical identification of differentiation/lineage-specific substances. Examples of architectural features include the fibrovascular cores covered by neoplastic epithelial cells in papillary carcinoma and the colloid-containing/epithelial-lined spaces of follicular carcinoma. The nuclear inclusions and grooves/folds of papillary carcinoma and the granular mitochondria-rich cytoplasm of Hurthle cell carcinoma are examples of cellular features. Identification of amyloid, calcitonin, carcinoembryonic antigen, chromogranin-A, etc., can be extremely valuable in distinguishing MTC from other thyroid cancers [24,25]. A detailed discussion of specific morphologic criteria is beyond the scope of this chapter.

Progress in understanding the molecular pathology of thyroid neoplasia has led to the development of several molecular diagnostic tests. These tests may assess for gene mutations/fusions,

Table 36.1 Evaluation of thyroid nodules. The cytopathologic diagnosis of thyroid nodules is based on the Bethesda System for Reporting Thyroid Cytopathology (BSRTC). Categories III, IV, and V are considered "indeterminate" cytopathology, as distinguishing benign from malignant nodules is unreliable. The risk of malignancy in these categories is 14%, 25%, and 70%, respectively, whereas in categories II and V, the risk of malignancy is 2.5% and 99%, respectively [22,23]. Management of thyroid nodules relies heavily on BSRTC in addition to other clinical factors (such as size of the nodule, multifocality, lymph node involvement, and invasiveness on imaging). Thus, all patients being evaluated for thyroid nodules should undergo comprehensive neck ultrasound (including lateral neck), and for those with invasive and/or extensive disease, cross-sectional imaging with contrast. "Thyroid surgery" refers to lobectomy or total thyroidectomy, where lobectomy is reserved for patients with well-differentiated tumors who are suspected to have low risk of disease recurrence. Molecular diagnostic tests may aid in management of Bethesda category III–V "indeterminate" thyroid nodules; however, some would argue that category V carries a high enough risk of malignancy that molecular testing is not warranted.

BSRTC category	Management recommendations
I. Non-diagnostic or unsatisfactory	Repeat FNA under ultrasound guidance
II. Benign	Serial ultrasound follow-up may be indicated
III. Atypical cells of undetermined significance/follicular lesion of undetermined significance	Repeat FNA and/or serial ultrasound follow-up
IV. Suspicious for follicular neoplasm	Surgical (diagnostic) lobectomy
V. Suspicious for malignancy	Thyroid surgery
VI. Malignant	Thyroid surgery

FNA, fine-needle aspiration.

mRNA gene expression, and miRNA gene expression. They are meant to help guide the management of cytologically indeterminate thyroid nodules using a variety of approaches. Some attempt to "rule out" malignancy and thereby avoid unnecessary diagnostic surgery. When positive, these tests do not indicate the presence of cancer because they lack sufficient positive predictive value. Other tests look to "rule in" cancer thereby supporting the decision to perform diagnostic surgery and, in some cases, may even guide the extent of surgery. However, these tests may lack the negative predictive value to avoid surgery in those with no abnormality detected. Finally, some have developed tests which attempt to achieve the ideal of accurately identifying those nodules which are cancerous as well as those which are benign [26]. As this technology is rapidly evolving, ensure that you are familiar with the positive and negative predictive value of any molecular test considered for indeterminate nodules, especially as they apply to a specific patient.

Molecular Pathology

In addition to the germline mutations noted in the previous discussion of heritable genetic conditions, several somatic (non-heritable) mutations are commonly present in thyroid cancer. Mutations along the mitogen-activated protein kinase pathway are common in thyroid cancer [27]. The most common mutation in PTC, occurring in 50–70% of tumors, is *BRAF*V600E [28,29]. This mutation also occurs in approximately 25% of ATC tumors. *BRAF* mutations have been associated with a reduced ability to concentrate radioactive iodine, and the occurrence of *BRAF*, particularly with coexisting *TERT* mutations, leads to more aggressive tumor behavior [30,31]. Genetic rearrangements, most commonly *RET/PTC*, also occur in PTC. Of all thyroid cancers, ATC tumors have the highest mutation burden and often harbor *TP53* mutations. *RAS* mutations occur in FTC, ATC and, rarely, MTC. Somatic *RET* mutations are frequent in MTC [29].

Staging

Thyroid cancer is staged according to the American Joint Committee on Cancer (AJCC)/Union for International Cancer Control (UICC) system. The Eighth Edition of this system for staging PTC, FTC, PDTC, Hurthle cell, and ATC (Table 36.2) and MTC (Table 36.3), has been published and can be used by clinicians to support patient care decisions starting in January 2017. However, until 1 January 2018, documentation of stage information in medical records should be based on the Seventh Edition [32,33].

One notable change in thyroid cancer staging is the change in the age cut-off from 45 to 55 years old for up-staging DTC patients. DTC patients younger than age 55 years with distant metastatic disease are never staged higher than stage II because their risk of dying from thyroid cancer is relatively low. However, DTC patients aged 55 or older with metastatic disease are classified as stage IV. Furthermore, patients with ATC are always classified as stage IV, regardless of T, N, and M categories. However, TNM information determines whether the prognostic stage group is IVA, IVB, or IVC.

Treatment and Follow-Up of Differentiated Thyroid Cancer

Surgery

The usual surgical treatment of known DTC is thyroid surgery, either thyroid lobectomy or total thyroidectomy depending upon the clinical factors. As already noted, cytomorphology of FNA samples cannot reliably distinguish cells of follicular adenomas from those of follicular carcinomas. For this reason, the initial surgery for indeterminate nodules may consist of diagnostic lobectomy. If histopathology demonstrates malignancy with greater than minimal invasion, then a completion thyroidectomy may be considered, depending upon several patient and prognostic factors. Total thyroidectomy may be chosen up front in those with Bethesda III or IV cytopathology based on patient preference for avoiding two procedures, or molecular testing indicating a high likelihood of thyroid cancer.

Lobectomy may be considered as definitive surgery for selected patients with small PTCs, if physical examination and imaging indicate no evidence of spread beyond the thyroid (locally, to regional lymph nodes, or to distant sites) or with only microscopic lymph node metastases [19].

Table 36.2 AJCC staging of papillary, follicular, poorly differentiated, Hurthle cell, and anaplastic thyroid carcinoma. Used with permission of the American College of Surgeons, Chicago, Illinois. The original source for this information is the AJCC Cancer Staging Manual, Eighth Edition (2016), which is published by Springer Science + Business Media.

Definition of primary tumor (T)

T Category	T Criteria
TX	Primary tumor cannot be assessed
T0	No evidence of primary tumor
T1	Tumor ≤2 cm in greatest dimension limited to the thyroid
T1a	Tumor ≤1 cm in greatest dimension limited to the thyroid
T1b	Tumor >1 cm but ≤2 cm in greatest dimension limited to the thyroid
T2	Tumor >2 cm but ≤4 cm in greatest dimension limited to the thyroid
T3	Tumor >4 cm limited to the thyroid, or gross extrathyroidal extension invading only strap muscles
T3a	Tumor >4 cm limited to the thyroid
T3b	Gross extrathyroidal extension invading only strap muscles (sternohyoid, sternothyroid, thyrohyoid, or omohyoid muscles) from a tumor of any size
T4	Includes gross extrathyroidal extension
T4a	Gross extrathyroidal extension invading subcutaneous soft tissues, larynx, trachea, esophagus, or recurrent laryngeal nerve from a tumor of any size
T4b	Gross extrathyroidal extension invading prevertebral fascia or encasing the carotid artery or mediastinal vessels from a tumor of any size

Note: All categories may be subdivided: (s) solitary tumor and (m) multifocal tumor (the largest tumor determines the classification).

Definition of regional lymph node (N)

N Category	N Criteria
NX	Regional lymph nodes cannot be assessed
N0	No evidence of locoregional lymph node metastasis
N0a	One or more cytologically or histologically confirmed benign lymph nodes
N0b	No radiologic or clinical evidence of locoregional lymph node metastasis
N1	Metastasis to regional nodes
N1a	Metastasis to level VI or VII (pretracheal, paratracheal, or prelaryngeal/Delphian, or upper mediastinal) lymph nodes. This can be unilateral or bilateral disease
N1b	Metastasis to unilateral, bilateral, or contralateral lateral neck lymph nodes (levels I, II, III, IV, or V) or retropharyngeal lymph nodes

Definition of distant metastasis (M)

M Category	M Criteria
M0	No distant metastasis
M1	Distant metastasis

(Continued)

Table 36.2 (Continued)

AJCC prognostic stage groups				
Differentiated				
When age at diagnosis is…	**And T is…**	**And N is…**	**And M is…**	**Then the stage group is…**
<55 years	Any T	Any N	M0	I
<55 years	Any T	Any N	M1	II
≥55 years	T1	N0/NX	M0	I
≥55 years	T1	N1	M0	II
≥55 years	T2	N0/NX	M0	I
≥55 years	T2	N1	M0	II
≥55 years	T3a/T3b	Any N	M0	II
≥55 years	T4a	Any N	M0	III
≥55 years	T4b	Any N	M0	IVA
≥55 years	Any T	Any N	M1	IVB

Anaplastic			
When T is…	**And N is…**	**And M is…**	**Then the stage group is…**
T1–T3a	N0/NX	M0	IVA
T1–T3a	N1	M0	IVB
T3b	Any N	M0	IVB
T4	Any N	M0	IVB
Any T	Any N	M1	IVC

Table 36.3 AJCC staging of medullary thyroid carcinoma. Used with permission of the American College of Surgeons, Chicago, Illinois. The original source for this information is the AJCC Cancer Staging Manual, Eighth Edition (2016), which is published by Springer Science + Business Media.

Definition of primary tumor (T)	
T Category	**T Criteria**
TX	Primary tumor cannot be assessed
T0	No evidence of primary tumor
T1	Tumor ≤2 cm in greatest dimension limited to the thyroid
T1a	Tumor ≤1 cm in greatest dimension limited to the thyroid
T1b	Tumor >1 cm but ≤2 cm in greatest dimension limited to the thyroid
T2	Tumor >2 cm but <4 cm in greatest dimension limited to the thyroid
T3	Tumor ≥4 cm or with extrathyroidal extension
T3a	Tumor ≥4 cm in greatest dimension limited to the thyroid
T3b	Tumor of any size with gross extrathyroidal extension invading only strap muscles (sternohyoid, sternothyroid, thyrohyoid, or omohyoid muscles)
T4	Advanced disease
T4a	Moderately advanced disease; tumor of any size with gross extrathyroidal extension into the nearby tissues of the neck, including subcutaneous soft tissue, larynx, trachea, esophagus, or recurrent laryngeal nerve
T4b	Very advanced disease; tumor of any size with extension toward the spine or into nearby large blood vessels, invading the prevertebral fascia, or encasing the carotid artery or mediastinal vessels

Table 36.3 (Continued)

Definition of regional lymph node (N)

N Category	N Criteria
NX	Regional lymph nodes cannot be assessed
N0	No evidence of locoregional lymph node metastasis
N0a	One or more cytologically or histologically confirmed benign lymph nodes
N0b	No radiologic or clinical evidence of locoregional lymph node metastasis
N1	Metastasis to regional nodes
N1a	Metastasis to level VI or VII (pretracheal, paratracheal, or prelaryngeal/Delphian, or upper mediastinal) lymph nodes. This can be unilateral or bilateral disease
N1b	Metastasis to unilateral, bilateral, or contralateral lateral neck lymph nodes (levels I, II, III, IV, or V) or retropharyngeal lymph nodes

Definition of distant metastasis (M)

M Category	M Criteria
M0	No distant metastasis
M1	Distant metastasis

AJCC prognostic stage groups

When T is...	And N is...	And M is...	Then the stage group is...
T1	N0	M0	I
T2	N0	M0	II
T3	N0	M0	II
T1–3	N1a	M0	III
T4a	Any N	M0	IVA
T1–3	N1b	M0	IVA
T4b	Any N	M0	IVB
Any T	Any N	M1	IVC

Lymph node dissection is usually recommended for compartments with clinical or imaging findings suggestive of involvement or if there is documented involvement based on FNA. This occurs considerably more often with PTC compared to FTC, because the prevalence of nodal involvement is much higher for the former. Depending upon the prognostic features of individual cases, prophylactic central compartment dissection can be considered for some patients with PTC [19].

Radioactive Iodine Ablation for DTC

Radioactive iodine (RAI) ablation takes advantage of the fact that only thyroid follicular epithelium, both normal and malignant, concentrates iodine. Orally administered iodine-131 (^{131}I; a radioisotope of iodine) is taken up by any residual thyroid tissue remaining following total thyroidectomy and by DTC cells, which are subsequently destroyed by the emitted radiation. This serves a dual purpose. The most obvious is destroying residual DTC cells in local, regional, or distant locations. In addition, destroying residual normal thyroid tissue eliminates the production of thyroglobulin, so that it can be used as a serum marker of persistent or recurrent DTC. RAI ablation is feasible only for patients who have undergone total thyroidectomy and have small amounts of normal and neoplastic thyroid tissue. If ^{131}I is administered to patients following lobectomy alone, it will be taken up by the remaining lobe but the dose will be inadequate to destroy DTC cells.

Because uptake of iodine (including stable and radioactive isotopes) is regulated by thyroid stimulating hormone/thyrotropin (TSH), two strategies may be used to increase TSH levels prior to RAI ablation. Withholding thyroid hormone replacement for several weeks will induce pituitary TSH production. Alternatively, recombinant TSH can be administered by injection 2 days prior to RAI ablation [19]. The advantage of the latter approach is that patients can avoid the symptoms of hypothyroidism. A low-iodine diet is also recommended prior to RAI ablation to maximize uptake of ^{131}I.

A diagnostic RAI scan with a tracer dose of ^{123}I is also recommended to determine the optimal treatment dose of ^{131}I.

Current thyroid cancer guidelines recommend a risk-adapted approach to the selection of patients for postoperative RAI treatment [20]. Patients with DTC are classified as at low, intermediate, or high risk of recurrence based on their clinicopathological characteristics. ^{131}I treatment will likely decrease recurrence and disease-specific mortality, and may facilitate initial staging/follow-up for patients with high-risk DTC. Low-risk patients are unlikely to obtain additional benefit from ^{131}I treatment and could be monitored with serial images and thyroglobulin panel [20,34,35].

TSH Suppression

Oral thyroxine replacement is necessary after total thyroidectomy to maintain a euthyroid state.

TSH is a growth factor produced by the pituitary which increases proliferation of normal and neoplastic follicular epithelium. Thyroxine replacement can therefore be used to inhibit pituitary TSH production, thereby reducing DTC cell proliferation. The degree of TSH suppression is determined by the risk of disease recurrence and the patient's comorbidities. TSH suppression is not recommended for patients with MTC or ATC as they are not responsive to TSH.

A more dynamic rather than a static staging system is now used for the management of patients with DTC. Following initial treatment with surgery ± ^{131}I and thyroid hormone suppression, patients' disease status is classified as excellent response to therapy, structural incomplete response, biochemical incomplete response, and intermediate response to therapy. Additional treatment and the follow-up are decided based on this evaluation, usually performed 6 months after initial therapy [20,29].

Treatment of RAI-Refractory Disease

RAI-refractory DTC is defined as a patient with metastatic lesions that have no RAI uptake, one or more lesions that do not have any RAI uptake, or progression of lesions despite RAI uptake [29]. Depending on the location of lesions, recurrences are preferably approached surgically (particularly those in the neck). Unresectable disease is addressed either with localized therapies (such as laser or thermal ablation techniques, embolization, and a variety of external radiotherapy techniques) or with pharmacotherapy. Bone metastases can be treated with a bisphosphonate or a receptor activator of nuclear factor kappa-B ligand (RANKL) inhibitor. These agents may reduce the incidence of skeletal events such as pathological fracture and spinal cord compression. Sorafenib and lenvatinib are both tyrosine kinase inhibitors (TKIs) that are FDA approved for RAI-refractory DTC [24,36]. Other targeted agents have been studied in RAI-refractory DTC, particularly the selective BRAF inhibitors in patients with *BRAF*V600E mutated PTC [37]. Vandetanib and cabozantinib are approved for treatment of progressive MTC but have also been studied in RAI-refractory DTC [24,38,39,40].

Follow-Up and Survivorship

Depending on initial treatments, routine follow-up after curative-intent treatment should include blood tests for thyroglobulin levels, anti-thyroglobulin antibodies levels (these antibodies interfere with the thyroglobulin assay), and TSH. Neck ultrasound is also necessary to detect local recurrence or new primary tumors in a residual lobe. RAI imaging should be mostly limited to detecting metastases in the face of unexplained (normal ultrasound) and rising thyroglobulin [19]. Care of DTC survivors should also include surveillance and management of long-term and late effects of treatment. Surgery may cause hypoparathyroidism and voice problems. RAI ablation can damage the salivary and lacrimal glands leading to xerostomia, sialoadenitis, and keratoconjunctivitis sicca [41].

Treatment and Follow-Up of Medullary Thyroid Cancer

Genetic Testing

Genetic testing for MEN2 syndromes occurs in two contexts. As noted earlier, at-risk relatives of known cases should receive genetic counseling and testing. This allows for appropriate screening and eventual prophylactic thyroidectomy in addition to management of the other neoplastic and non-neoplastic components of the syndrome. The second context is all patients with newly diagnosed MTC. They should be tested for a germline *RET* mutation since germline mutations can occur *de novo*.

Surgery

If genetic testing detects a MEN2 mutation, the patient should be evaluated for pheochromocytoma and primary hyperparathyroidism. Because the former can complicate anesthetic management, this tumor should be resected before addressing the MTC. If a parathyroid adenoma is present, parathyroidectomy should be performed at the time of thyroidectomy [24].

Treatment of the primary tumor is total thyroidectomy. Baseline calcitonin and carcinoembryonic antigen (CEA), the tumor markers for MTC, should be obtained preoperatively. Central neck dissection should be performed regardless of imaging results because most patients have involvement of the central compartment at diagnosis. Lateral neck lymph node compartment dissections are performed if metastatic lymph nodes are demonstrated (by FNA) or suspected by clinical examination or imaging, although some surgeons recommend prophylactic ipsilateral or bilateral lateral neck dissections for patients with high serum calcitonin [19].

Lymph node dissection is not recommended for individuals with MEN2a undergoing prophylactic thyroidectomy. There is some controversy as to whether central lymph node dissection should accompany prophylactic total thyroidectomy for young children with MEN2b, however the American Thyroid Association recommends central neck dissection if the surgeon is able to identify and preserve the parathyroid glands. Older children and adults should undergo central neck dissection, since the risk of nodal metastasis is high [11].

Treatment of Persistent and Recurrent MTC

Most cases of metastatic MTC have an indolent course with slow disease progression over many years. Initially a "watch and wait" approach is appropriate in most cases. As described for DTC, locally persistent or recurrent MTC is preferably treated with surgery. Unresectable, distant metastatic disease may be treated with localized therapies such as laser or thermal ablation techniques, embolization, and a variety of external radiotherapy techniques [29]. Bone is a fairly common site of metastasis in MTC patients; bone metastases can be treated with a bisphosphonate or a receptor activator of nuclear factor kappa-B ligand (RANKL) inhibitor [42]. Vandetanib and cabozantinib are TKIs approved for treatment of progressive MTC. Determining which drug to treat patients with first is beyond the scope of this chapter but has been well described previously [43].

Follow-Up and Survivorship

Follow-up after treatment of MTC consists of neck ultrasonography and testing for serum levels of calcitonin and CEA. If calcitonin levels are high, cross-sectional imaging can be helpful in identifying metastatic disease [24]. Follow-up also depends upon whether genetic evaluation indicates risk for other components of MEN2 syndromes. As in DTC, care of MTC survivors should also include surveillance and management of long-term and late effects of surgery, such as hypoparathyroidism and voice problems.

Treatment and Follow-Up of Anaplastic Thyroid Cancer

Surgery

The clinical approach to treating ATC is first based on resectability. Patients with potentially resectable disease at presentation (or after neoadjuvant radiotherapy or chemoradiotherapy) are considered as candidates for curative-intent treatment, whereas the goals for patients with unresectable disease are palliation of symptoms and in some cases, life-extending cancer-directed therapy [44,45]. Thus, total thyroidectomy with therapeutic lymph node dissection is recommended for patients with primary tumors that are potentially resectable. Unfortunately, due to the rapid growth and high propensity for invasion of ATC, patients often present with surgically unresectable disease. Locally unresectable disease is best treated with external beam radiation therapy in order to relieve symptoms and to prevent or treat life-threatening airway obstruction or compression. Tracheostomy is sometimes necessary but diminishes quality of life and therefore a frank discussion of the pros and cons of tracheostomy is recommended. However, patients who present with distant metastatic disease may be best served by systemic therapies (see section "Systemic Therapies").

Radiation Therapy

External radiation therapy (external beam radiotherapy or intensity modulated radiotherapy) with radiosensitizing chemoradiotherapy is recommended after complete or incomplete resection [46,47]. Radiation therapy is also used in palliation of local disease or symptomatic metastases (e.g., to bones or the brain).

Systemic Therapies

Adjuvant cytotoxic chemotherapy can be used with the intent of improving prognosis. More often, cytotoxic chemotherapy is administered with palliative intent. Common agents include taxanes, carboplatin, and doxorubicin [45]. Several targeted therapies have been studied in ATC with mixed results [44,46]. However, lenvatinib appears to be the most promising agent thus far and is approved in Japan for this indication [47]. Other promising targeted therapies include the selective BRAF inhibitors (vemurafenib and dabrafenib [46,48,49]) alone or in combination with MEK inhibitors [46]. Clinical trials of investigational targeted therapies are ongoing and relatively healthy patients should be referred for consideration of participation. Referral to a tertiary center with expertise in this rare cancer is recommended.

Palliative Care

Early referral to palliative care programs is recommended for pain management and discussion of advanced directives given the aggressive nature of ATC.

References

1 Siegel RL, Miller KD, Jemal A. Cancer statistics, 2017. *CA Cancer J Clin* 2017;67(1):7–30.

2 Simard EP, Ward EM, Siegel R, Jemal A. Cancers with increasing incidence trends in the United States: 1999 through 2008. *CA Cancer J Clin* 2012;62(2):118–28.

3 SEER Cancer Statistics Factsheets: Thyroid Cancer. National Cancer Institute Bethesda, MD. Available from: http://seer.cancer.gov/statfacts/html/thyro.html (accessed 5 October 2017).

4 Howlader N, Noone AM, Krapcho M, *et al.* SEER Cancer Statistics Review, 1975-2013, National Cancer Institute. Bethesda, MD (updated April 2016). Available from: http://seer.cancer.gov/csr/1975_2013/, based on November 2015 SEER data submission, posted to the SEER web site.

5 Morris LG, Tuttle RM, Davies L. Changing trends in the incidence of thyroid cancer in the United States. *JAMA Otolaryngol Head Neck Surg* 2016;142(7): 709–11.

6 Yu GP, Li JC, Branovan D, McCormick S, Schantz SP. Thyroid cancer incidence and survival in the national cancer institute surveillance, epidemiology, and end results race/ethnicity groups. *Thyroid* 2010;20(5):465–73.

7 Nikiforov YE, Seethala RR, Tallini G, *et al.* Nomenclature revision for encapsulated follicular variant of papillary thyroid carcinoma: a paradigm shift to reduce overtreatment of indolent tumors. *JAMA Oncol* 2016;2(8):1023–9.

8 Volante M, Collini P, Nikiforov YE, *et al.* Poorly differentiated thyroid carcinoma: the Turin proposal for the use of uniform diagnostic criteria and an algorithmic diagnostic approach. *Am J Surg Pathol* 2007;31(8):1256–64.

9 Aschebrook-Kilfoy B, Ward MH, Sabra MM, Devesa SS. Thyroid cancer incidence patterns in the United States by histologic type, 1992-2006. *Thyroid* 2011;21(2):125–34.

10 Marquard J, Eng C. Multiple Endocrine Neoplasia Type 2: University of Washington Seattle; 2015 (updated 25 June 2015). Available from: https://www.ncbi.nlm.nih.gov/books/NBK1257/ (accessed 5 October 2017).

11 Wells SA, Jr, Asa SL, Dralle H, *et al.* Revised American Thyroid Association guidelines for the management of medullary thyroid carcinoma. *Thyroid* 2015;25(6):567–610.

12 Waguespack SG, Rich TA, Perrier ND, Jimenez C, Cote GJ. Management of medullary thyroid carcinoma and MEN2 syndromes in childhood. *Nat Rev Endocrinol* 2011;7(10):596–607.

13 Moline J, Eng C. Multiple endocrine neoplasia type 2: an overview. *Genet Med* 2011;13(9):755–64.

14 Rowland KJ, Moley JF. Hereditary thyroid cancer syndromes and genetic testing. *J Surg Oncol* 2015;111(1):51–60.

15 Takamura N, Orita M, Saenko V, *et al.* Radiation and risk of thyroid cancer: Fukushima and Chernobyl. *Lancet Diabetes Endocrinol* 2016;4(8):647.

16 Furukawa K, Preston D, Funamoto S, *et al.* Long-term trend of thyroid cancer risk among Japanese atomic-bomb survivors: 60 years after exposure. *Int J Cancer* 2013;132(5):1222–6.

17 Zimmermann MB, Galetti V. Iodine intake as a risk factor for thyroid cancer: a comprehensive review of animal and human studies. *Thyroid Res* 2015;8:8.

18 Dean DS, Gharib H. Epidemiology of thyroid nodules. *Best Pract Res Clin Endocrinol Metab* 2008;22(6):901–11.

19 Haddad R. Thyroid Carcinoma Version 1.2016: National Comprehensive Cancer Network; 2016 (cited 1 November 2016). Available from: nccn.org.

20 Haugen BR, Alexander EK, Bible KC, *et al.* 2015 American Thyroid Association Management Guidelines for Adult Patients with Thyroid Nodules and Differentiated Thyroid Cancer: The American Thyroid Association Guidelines Task Force on Thyroid Nodules and Differentiated Thyroid Cancer. *Thyroid* 2016;26(1):1–133.

21 Gharib H, Papini E, Garber JR, *et al.* American Association of Clinical Endocrinologists, American College of Endocrinology, and Associazione Medici Endocrinologi Medical guidelines for clinical practice for the diagnosis and management of thyroid nodules – 2016 update. *Endocr Pract* 2016;22(5):622–39.

22 Ali SZ, Cibas ES. *The Bethesda system for reporting thyroid cytopathology : definitions, criteria, and explanatory notes.* New York: Springer, 2010: xiv, 171 pp.

23 Bongiovanni M, Spitale A, Faquin WC, Mazzucchelli L, Baloch ZW. The Bethesda System for Reporting Thyroid Cytopathology: a meta-analysis. *Acta Cytol* 2012;56(4):333–9.

24 Cabanillas ME, Dadu R, Hu MI, *et al.* Thyroid gland malignancies. *Hematol Oncol Clin North Am* 2015;29(6):1123–43.

25 DeLellis R, Lloyd R, Heitz P, Eng C. *Pathology and Genetics of Tumours of Endocrine Organs.* Lyon: IARC Press, 2004.

26 Ferris RL, Baloch Z, Bernet V, *et al.* American Thyroid Association Statement on Surgical Application of Molecular Profiling for Thyroid Nodules: Current Impact on Perioperative Decision Making. *Thyroid* 2015;25(7):760–8.

27 Nikiforov YE, Nikiforova MN. Molecular genetics and diagnosis of thyroid cancer. *Nat Rev Endocrinol* 2011;7(10):569–80.

28 Cancer Genome Atlas Research Network. Integrated genomic characterization of papillary thyroid carcinoma. *Cell* 2014;159(3):676–90.

29 Cabanillas ME, McFadden DG, Durante C. Thyroid cancer. *Lancet* 2016;388(10061):2783–95.

30 Landa I, Ganly I, Chan TA, *et al.* Frequent somatic TERT promoter mutations in thyroid cancer: higher prevalence in advanced forms of the disease. *J Clin Endocrinol Metab* 2013;98(9):E1562–6.

31 Melo M, da Rocha AG, Vinagre J, Sobrinho-Simoes M, Soares P. Coexistence of TERT promoter and BRAF mutations in papillary thyroid carcinoma: added value in patient prognosis? *J Clin Oncol* 2015;33(6):667–8.

32 Edge S, Byrd D, Compton C, *et al. AJCC Cancer Staging Manual 7th Edition.* American Joint Committee on Cancer (ed.). New York: Springer, 2010.

33 Amin M, Edge S, Greene R, Byrd D, Brookland R. *Cancer Staging Manual 8th Edition.* American Joint Committee on Cancer (ed.). New York: Springer, 2017.

34 Ruel E, Thomas S, Dinan M, *et al.* Adjuvant radioactive iodine therapy is associated with improved survival for patients with intermediate-risk papillary thyroid cancer. *J Clin Endocrinol Metab* 2015;100(4):1529–36.

35 Jonklaas J, Cooper DS, Ain KB, *et al.* Radioiodine therapy in patients with stage I differentiated thyroid cancer. *Thyroid* 2010;20(12):1423–4.

36 Sacks W, Braunstein GD. Evolving approaches in managing radioactive iodine-refractory differentiated thyroid cancer. *Endocr Pract* 2014;20(3):263–75.

37 Brose MS, Cabanillas ME, Cohen EE, *et al.* Vemurafenib in patients with BRAF(V600E)-positive metastatic or unresectable papillary thyroid cancer refractory to radioactive iodine: a non-randomised, multicentre, open-label, phase 2 trial. *Lancet Oncol* 2016;17(9):1272–82.

38 Leboulleux S, Bastholt L, Krause T, *et al.* Vandetanib in locally advanced or metastatic differentiated thyroid cancer: a randomised, double-blind, phase 2 trial. *Lancet Oncol* 2012;13(9):897–905.

39 Cabanillas ME, Brose MS, Holland J, Ferguson KC, Sherman SI. A phase I study of cabozantinib (XL184) in patients with differentiated thyroid cancer. *Thyroid* 2014;24(10):1508–14.

40 Cabanillas ME, de Souza JA, Geyer S, *et al.* Cabozantinib As Salvage Therapy for Patients With Tyrosine Kinase Inhibitor-Refractory Differentiated Thyroid Cancer: Results of a Multicenter Phase II International Thyroid Oncology Group Trial. *J Clin Oncol* 2017;35(29):3315–3321.

41 Flores S, Habra M. Thyroid cancer survivorship management. In: *Advances in Cancer Survivorship Management.* New York: Springer, 2015:241–53.

42 Xu JY, Murphy WA, Jr, Milton DR, *et al.* Bone metastases and skeletal-related events in medullary thyroid carcinoma. *J Clin Endocrinol Metab* 2016;101(12):4871–77

43 Cabanillas ME, Hu MI, Jimenez C. Medullary thyroid cancer in the era of tyrosine kinase inhibitors: to treat or not to treat – and with which drug – those are the questions. *J Clin Endocrinol Metab* 2014:99(12):4390–6.

44 Cabanillas ME, Zafereo M, Gunn GB, Ferrarotto R. Anaplastic thyroid carcinoma: treatment in the age of molecular targeted therapy. *J Oncol Pract* 2016;12(6):511–8.

45 Smallridge RC, Ain KB, Asa SL, *et al.* American Thyroid Association guidelines for management of patients with anaplastic thyroid cancer. *Thyroid* 2012;22(11):1104–39.

46 Cabanillas ME, Busaidy N, Khan SA, *et al.* Molecular diagnostics and anaplastic thyroid carcinoma: the time has come to harvest the high hanging fruit. *Int J Endocr Oncol* 2016;3(3):221–33.

47 Takahashi S, Kiyota N, Yamazaki T, *et al.* Phase II study of lenvatinib in patients with differentiated, medullary, and anaplastic thyroid cancer: Final analysis results. *J Clin Oncol* 2016;34(suppl):abstr 6088.

48 Hyman DM, Puzanov I, Subbiah V, *et al.* Vemurafenib in multiple nonmelanoma cancers with BRAF V600 mutations. *N Engl J Med* 2015;373(8):726–36.

49 Subbiah V, Kreitman RJ, Wainberg ZA, *et al.* Dabrafenib and Trametinib Treatment in Patients With Locally Advanced or Metastatic BRAF V600-Mutant Anaplastic Thyroid Cancer. *J Clin Oncol* doi: 10.1200/JCO.2017.73.6785. [Epub ahead of print].

37

Adrenal Cortical Carcinoma and Pheochromocytoma

Robert Dreicer[1], Moshe C. Ornstein[2], Kriti Mittal[3], Jordan Reynolds[4], Joseph Klink[5], Christopher Przybycin[4], and Jorge A. Garcia[6]

[1] University of Virginia School of Medicine, Charlottesville, Virginia, USA
[2] Taussig Cancer Institute, Cleveland, Ohio, USA
[3] University of Massachusetts Medical School, Worcester, Massachusetts, USA
[4] Robert J Tomsich Pathology and Laboratory Medicine Institute, Cleveland, Ohio, USA
[5] Deaconess Clinic Gateway Health Center, Newburgh, Indiana, USA
[6] Cleveland Clinic Lerner College of Medicine, Cleveland, Ohio, USA

Incidence and Mortality

Adrenal Cancer

Primary tumors of the adrenal gland can arise from the cortex (such as adrenal adenoma and adrenal cortical carcinoma) or from the medulla (including pheochromocytoma and neuroblastoma). Adrenal cortical carcinoma (ACC) is a rare endocrine malignancy with an estimated age-adjusted incidence rate of 0.72 per million in the United States (US) [1]. With approximately 300 new cases annually in the US, it is a prototypical orphan malignancy. The age distribution of ACC is bimodal, with one peak in childhood and the other in the fourth and fifth decades of life, with an average age at diagnosis of 55 years [2]. The female to male ratio is 4:3. Left-sided tumors appear to be more frequent than right-sided ones, and bilateral ACCs have been reported [2]. Hormone-secreting ACCs occur more commonly than nonfunctional ACCs, with approximately 60% of patients demonstrating hypersecretion of adrenal cortical hormones, commonly cortisol, aldosterone, and other early androgens [3]. Nonfunctional tumors occur at a greater frequency in patients older than 30 years and are often discovered by imaging [4]. This highly aggressive malignancy accounts for 0.2% of cancer deaths in the US and 5-year survival rates reported in case series vary from 16 to 60% [5,6].

Pheochromocytoma

The vast majority of pheochromocytomas arise from chromaffin cells in the adrenal medulla. Paraganglioma refers to the same neoplasm arising in extra-adrenal sites. Pheochromocytomas are extremely rare with an incidence of 2–8 per 1,000,000 adults. These tumors secrete a variety of neurotransmitters, especially catecholamines. Patients with malignant pheochromocytoma have 5-year survival rates that range from 20 to 70% [7].

Risk Factors

Adrenal Cancer

In case control studies, smoking has been identified as a potential risk factor for ACC, as has the use of oral contraceptives, especially if used prior to the age of 25 years [8].

Genetic alterations identified in familial syndromes such as Li–Fraumeni and Beckwith–Weidemann syndromes, multiple endocrine neoplasia (MEN)-1, and Carney syndrome have also been associated with a predisposition to develop ACC [9]. Germline mutations in the *TP53* gene (as in Li–Fraumeni syndrome) have been identified in a majority of sporadic childhood ACC cases in southern Brazil, which may explain the disproportionately higher incidence of ACC seen in this region [10].

Pheochromocytoma

Ten percent of pheochromocytomas are associated with MEN syndromes 2A or 2B, neurofibromatosis type I, or von Hippel–Lindau disease. While the majority of hereditary cases are benign, approximately 10% are malignant. Approximately 50% of patients with malignant pheochromocytomas carry hereditary germline mutations in the succinate dehydrogenase subunit B gene (*SDHB*) [11].

Pathology

Adrenal Cancer

The most common strategy employed in making a diagnosis of ACC is the Weiss system [12]. The system uses nine histologic features which were found to be associated with adverse

The American Cancer Society's Oncology in Practice: Clinical Management, First Edition. Edited by The American Cancer Society.

behavior (recurrence and/or metastasis): nuclear grade 3 or 4, greater than 5 mitotic figures per 50 high-power fields, atypical mitoses, clear cells comprising less than 25% of the tumor, diffuse tumor cell architecture involving at least one-third of the tumor, necrosis, venous invasion, sinusoidal vessel invasion, and invasion of the tumor capsule. These features are weighted equally, each receiving 1 point if present. The sum is the Weiss score, ranging from 0 to 9. In the original study, scores greater than 4 were associated with recurrence and/or metastasis [12]. Subsequent validations of the Weiss system [13,14] showed that a score of 3 or higher predicts malignant behavior; therefore, a score of 3 is the threshold currently used.

Other systems have been proposed, often with comparable predictive capacity, but have not achieved the widespread use of the Weiss system [15–17]. A modification of the Weiss system proposed in 2002 [13] simplified the analysis by incorporating only five of the original histologic parameters, those considered to be the easiest and most reproducibly interpreted: mitotic rate greater than 5 per 50 high-power fields, clear cells comprising less than 25% of the tumor, abnormal mitoses, necrosis, and capsular invasion [13,16]. The conventional Weiss system is less useful for certain histologic variants of adrenocortical neoplasms, such as those with extensive myxoid change [18].

A specific model for use with adrenocortical tumors in children has been proposed [19] because clinically benign behavior has been observed frequently in tumors containing histologically worrisome features according to Weiss criteria (e.g., necrosis, nuclear atypia, vascular invasion, etc.) [20].

Immunohistochemistry staining can be helpful in distinguishing ACC from other entities. The closest morphologic mimic and most difficult differential diagnosis is metastases from clear cell renal cell carcinoma. Calretinin, D2-40, inhibin, melanA, and S-100 positivity is seen in ACC. ACC are typically negative for low and high molecular weight keratins, and epithelial membrane antigen. They can rarely be positive for chromogranin and synaptophysin [21]. To date, immunohistochemistry stain usage yields mixed results because adrenal-derived neoplasms may exhibit variable immunostaining patterns. A promising immunohistochemistry stain for steroidogenic factor 1 (SF1) is a recent marker found to be very helpful in differentiating ACC from metastatic renal cell carcinoma and germ cell tumors [22].

Comparative genomic hybridization (CGH) demonstrates widespread chromosomal changes in carcinomas and fewer in adenomas. The most common gains are chromosome 5, 12, and 19 while loss of heterozygosity (LOH) at 2p16 is found in 92% of tumors as well as 11q13 (90%) and 17p13 (85%) [23]. Despite frequent LOH of 17p13 (including the *TP53* locus), somatic *TP53* mutations are only found in 25% of sporadic adult carcinomas [24] while LOH of the *TP53* locus is found in 50% of cases [25].

Expression profiling studies show up-regulation of proliferation genes such as *TOP2A* and *Ki-67* in ACC [26]. Adenomas and ACC showed up-regulation of ubiquitin-related genes and insulin-like growth factor-related (IGF) genes, but a cytokine gene (*CXCL10*) and cadherin 2 gene (*CDH2*) were down-regulated in carcinomas compared with adenomas [27]. Microarray analysis of gene expression in ACC demonstrated up-regulation of *IGF2* in 10% of adrenal adenomas and 90% of ACCs [26]. *IGF2* is located at 11p15, and is the same gene altered in Beckwith–Wiedemann syndrome [28] and in patients with sporadic ACC.

The Wnt/β-catenin pathway is involved in the spectrum of adrenal disease from adrenal hyperplasia to adenoma to carcinoma. Accumulation of β-catenin leads to expression of proliferation factors. Wnt/β-catenin alterations are present in 50% of ACCs [29].

MicroRNA (miRNA) studies reveal that up- or down-regulation of 17 miRNAs is associated with benign adrenocortical tumors. Mir483-5p has been the miRNA most commonly associated with malignancy [30]. In addition, MiR-483 is expressed from intron 2 of the *IGF2* gene, further highlighting the diagnostic and therapeutic potential for *IGF2*.

Pheochromocytoma

Pheochromocytoma is a neoplasm of the neural crest-derived chromaffin cells of the adrenal medulla; in current usage the term is restricted to paragangliomas arising within the adrenal medulla. Prediction of the clinical outcome of pheochromocytomas by pathologic criteria is inherently problematic; indeed, the presence of metastasis is the only definitive feature of malignancy. Attempts have been made, however, to identify tumor characteristics that could provide at least some estimate of the likelihood of an aggressive course, and initial findings suggest that molecular profiling may contribute meaningful prognostic information.

The most comprehensive pathologic scoring system for pheochromocytomas is the Pheochromocytoma of Adrenal gland Scaled Score (PASS), proposed by Thompson [31]. PASS has two chief limitations. The first is the significant overlap of scores between clinically benign and clinically malignant tumors and the significant interobserver and intraobserver variability in assignment of PASS to individual cases, even among experienced endocrine pathologists.

Immunohistochemistry for proliferation/cell cycle markers has not been shown to discriminate reliably between benign and malignant pheochromocytomas. While increased expression of the proliferation marker Ki-67 has been found more frequently in malignant tumors, relatively few malignant pheochromocytomas have this characteristic [32]. Other cell cycle/apoptosis markers have been studied (e.g., p53, Bcl-2, mdm-2, cyclin D1, p21, p27) but reproducible significant differences in expression between benign and malignant pheochromocytomas have not been found [31,32].

Immunohistochemistry may play a role, however, in identifying those patients whose tumors are associated with the familial pheochromocytoma/paraganglioma syndromes, caused by germline mutations in the genes encoding the succinate dehydrogenase complex (*SDHD, SDHAF2, SDHC,* and *SDHB*). Identifying these patients is important, not only because of the implications for family members but also because tumors associated with *SDHB* mutations often show aggressive behavior [33].

Prognostic and Predictive Factors

Adrenal Cancer

Older age, American Joint Committee on Cancer (AJCC) stage III or IV disease, cortisol hypersecretion, high mitotic counts, and Ki-67 index, as well as lack of surgical resectability, are adverse prognostic factors in ACC [34]. In patients with ACC undergoing surgical resection, age ≥55 years, positive resection margins, lymph node involvement, poorly differentiated tumors, and distant metastases portend a worse prognosis [2].

Diagnosis

While 60% of ACCs are hypersecreting tumors, clinical and biochemical evidence of increased steroid secretion aid in localizing tumor origin to the adrenal cortex. Cushing syndrome as well as aldosterone- and, less commonly, androgen-excess states have been described in patients with benign adenomas. In the setting of an incidentally diagnosed adrenal mass, the likelihood of the lesion being ACC increases with tumor size. ACC accounts for 2% of lesions ≤4 cm, 6% of tumors measuring 4.1–6 cm, and 25% of tumors over 6 cm [35]. Thus, establishing a diagnosis of ACC requires a combination of clinical, laboratory, and radiographic features. The differential diagnosis of an adrenal mass is listed in Table 37.1.

Malignancy should be suspected in patients with adrenal tumors who develop rapid progression of hormonal secretion and those who demonstrate co-secretion of multiple adrenal hormones. In a series of 105 ACC patients, the mean duration of symptoms prior to diagnosis was reported to be 8.7 months [36]. A series of 205 ACC cases revealed that amongst the patients with secreting tumors, the percentage with overproduction of both cortisol and androgens or cortisol alone was 47% and 27%, respectively [37]. Clinical features of cortisol excess include central obesity, buffalo hump, dermal striae with thinning of skin, osteoporosis, hypertension, myopathy, glucose intolerance, and gonadal dysfunction. While females with excess secretion of androgens can develop hirsutism, virilization, deepening of voice, male pattern baldness, and menstrual disturbances, males can present with gynecomastia and testicular atrophy. Systemic symptoms may also include fever and, less commonly, weight loss [38].

Functional ACCs may autonomously elaborate hormones associated with the hypothalamus–pituitary–adrenal (HPA) axis (cortisol, androgens) or the renin–angiotensin–aldosterone (RAA) axis. Besides basal levels of cortisol, dynamic assessment of the HPA axis through the dexamethasone or adrenocorticotropic hormone (ACTH) test should be performed. In addition to terminal steroid hormones, steroid precursors such as 11-hydroxyprogesterone should be measured during the initial hormonal evaluation. Blood pressure and serum potassium levels are assessed to indicate the potential for excessive aldosterone production. Additionally, urinary or plasma catecholamine levels should be measured to rule out underlying pheochromocytoma. Table 37.2 outlines the initial hormonal workup for evaluation of adrenal tumors.

Adrenal biopsies are not always helpful in distinguishing between adrenal adenomas and carcinomas, with the likelihood of identifying a primary adrenal malignancy being about 30% [39]. Adrenal biopsies also incur the theoretical risk of needle-track metastasis and rarely, hemorrhage, pain, and tumor spillage [3]. Furthermore, adrenal biopsies are contraindicated in patients with suspected pheochromocytoma due to the risk of precipitation of hypertensive crisis. In most patients with limited-stage disease, completion of biochemical evaluation is followed by diagnostic adrenalectomy for histopathologic assessment.

Pheochromocytoma

Hypertension is the most common feature of pheochromocytoma, with cardiovascular complications, hypertensive crisis, heart failure, and cerebrovascular accidents representing the most frequent causes of mortality. Increased plasma or urinary levels of catecholamines and their metabolites are perhaps the defining presentation of pheochromocytoma, as greater than 90% of patients will have elevated 24-hour urine levels of catecholamines, vanillylmandelic acid (VMA), and metanephrines [11]. Malignancy is defined by the presence of metastases, given

Table 37.1 Differential diagnosis of an adrenal incidentaloma.

Neoplastic etiologies		Non-neoplastic etiologies
Adrenal cortical neoplasms	• Adenoma • Nodular hyperplasia • Adrenal cortical carcinoma	Cysts Pseudocysts Hemorrhage
Adrenal medullary neoplasms	• Pheochromocytoma • Neuroblastoma • Ganglioneuroma • Ganglioneuroblastoma	Hemangioma Lipoma Angiomyolipoma Fibroma
Secondary metastatic deposits	• Renal cell carcinoma • Breast carcinoma • Lung carcinoma • Ovarian carcinoma • Melanoma • Others	Neurofibroma Teratoma Granulomatosis Infections Others
Other neoplasms	Lymphoma • Leiomyosarcoma • Angiosarcoma • Others	

Table 37.2 Hormonal workup for adrenal neoplasms.

Adrenal cortical hormones		Medullary catecholamines
Glucocorticoids	• Basal serum cortisol, plasma ACTH • Dexamethasone suppression test • 24-hour urinary free cortisol	• Plasma norepinephrine • Plasma metanephrine • 24-hour urinary fractionated metanephrine
Mineralocorticoids	• Serum potassium • Aldosterone/renin ratio	
Androgens	• DHEA-S • 17-OH-progesterone • Testosterone • 17-beta-estradiol • 24-hour urine steroid metabolites	

ACTH, adrenocorticotropic hormone; DHEA-S, dehydroepiandrosterone sulfate.

the inability to make this distinction pathologically, however there are several relatively well-described predictors of metastasis including tumors greater than 5 cm and germline mutations of the *SDHB* gene [40].

Adrenal Cancer

Imaging

Incidental adrenal lesions (incidentalomas) may be identified in 5% of the population by routine computed tomography (CT) scan [41]. Given the high lipid content of most adenomas, they usually have attenuation values of less than 10 Hounsfield units (HU) on unenhanced CT, or less than 30 HU on enhanced CT [42]. Lesions that demonstrate washout of less than 50% with a delayed attenuation of greater than 35 HU on enhanced CT are more likely to be malignant. Classic magnetic resonance imaging (MRI) features of ACC include heterogeneous signal intensity, peripheral nodular enhancement, and central hypoperfusion. Given absence of evidence favoring one technique, either CT or MRI can be used for diagnostic purposes because both approach a sensitivity and specificity of 90% [6]. Size is another characteristic that may be helpful; most lesions less than 4 cm are likely to be benign, whereas most ACCs are greater than 5 cm, with a reported median tumor size of 11–13 cm [2]. The utility of PET-CT was assessed prospectively in a multicenter study of 77 patients, wherein an adrenal to liver maximum standardized uptake value (SUV) ratio less than 1.45 was highly predictive of a benign lesion [43]. A large meta-analysis estimated the sensitivity and specificity of ^{18}F-fluorodeoxyglucose–positron emission tomography (FDG-PET) in distinguishing benign from malignant adrenal lesions at 97% and 91%, respectively [44]. Besides the higher cost, other limitations of this modality include mild FDG uptake reported in benign, lipid-poor adenomas as well as decreased uptake by subcentimeter adrenal lesions [44]. Nevertheless, in patients without a known malignancy, FDG-negativity is highly predictive of a benign adrenal lesion, and combining attenuation values with SUV measurements can improve the specificity [44,45].

Pheochromocytoma

Localization and characterization of pheochromocytoma relies upon conventional imaging modalities such as CT and MRI. Metaiodobenzylguanidine (MIBG) shares structural features with norepinephrine and ^{131}I/^{123}I and has high overall sensitivity for imaging pheochromocytoma. Newer PET agents such as ^{18}F-fluorodopamine may provide even better imaging characteristics than MIBG [45].

Staging

Adrenal Cancer

In the AJCC Eighth Edition staging system [46], localized tumors confined to the adrenal gland measuring ≤5 cm are classified as stage I and those measuring >5 cm as stage II. Tumors that infiltrate surrounding adipose tissue (T3), invade adjacent organs/vessels (liver, spleen, kidney, diaphragm, pancreas, renal vein, or vena cava) (T4), or involve at least one lymph node (N1) qualify as stage III. Tumors of any size, invasion, or lymph node involvement that have distant metastases (M1) are categorized as stage IV. These definitions are similar to the UICC Seventh Edition staging for adrenal cancer [47]. The European Network for the Study of Adrenal Tumors (ENSAT) proposed a modification to this system that has also been subsequently validated [48].

Approximately 40.6% of patients initially present with localized tumors, while 21.6% of patients present with distant metastatic disease [2,34]. Liver (10.9%) and lungs (9%) are the most common sites of metastases, followed by bones and lymph nodes [2]. The 5-year disease-specific survival rates of 416 patients from the German registry range from 82% for TNM stage I to 18% for patients presenting with stage IV disease [48].

For completion of staging, CT of the chest is recommended in addition to abdominopelvic imaging in newly diagnosed patients. Bone imaging may be performed when skeletal metastases are clinically suspected. The role of FDG-PET in distinguishing benign from malignant adrenal lesions is well established, both in patients with known extra-adrenal malignancy or isolated adrenal lesions without known malignancy.

Pheochromocytoma

Prior to the publication of the Eighth Edition of the *AJCC Cancer Staging Manual*, there was no standard staging system for pheochromocytoma and patients were generally divided according to whether they had localized, regional, or metastatic disease. Some advocated the use of adrenal cancer staging criteria for pheochromocytoma as well. With the eighth AJCC staging manual, traditional TNM staging has been applied to pheochromocytoma [46]. Of note, in this staging system, primary tumors are staged from T1 to T3. Tumors that are <5 cm in greatest dimension (T1) are categorized as stage I, while those ≥5 cm (T2) are classified as stage II. Stage III tumors are those that invade into surrounding tissue (T3) or involve at least one regional lymph node (N1). Tumors of any size, local invasion, or nodal status that have distant metastases are classified as M1 and stage IV. They are further subclassified based on bone involvement only (M1a), distant metastases limited to distant lymph node, liver, or lung (M1b), and distant metastases to bone and multiple other sites (M1c) [46].

Surgical Management

Adrenal Cancer

The variable presentation of ACC leads to unique challenges in surgical planning. Issues include the inability to use imaging to definitively rule out malignancy, for while the presence of an adrenal tumor greater than 4 cm in diameter on cross-sectional imaging raises the suspicion for ACC, occasionally adrenal tumors as small as 2 cm will harbor ACC [49]. Additional concerns include special presentations such as tumor thrombus that can extend as high as the right atrium and the potential for ACC to invade local structures making complete resection impossible [50]. Some ACCs are functioning, producing a variety of adrenal hormones. As much information as possible should be obtained about each of these possibilities before taking a patient with ACC to the operating room in order to avoid complications from intraoperative manifestations of hormonal excess.

Either an adrenal protocol CT or an adrenal protocol MRI is acceptable. If the mass is highly suspicious for ACC and anatomic details are clearly visible on CT, there appears to be no additional information to be gleaned from a dedicated adrenal MRI. The factors that must be elucidated on preoperative imaging include the size of the mass, potential invasion into surrounding structures, including the great vessels, the presence of a tumor thrombus, and the presence of intra-abdominal metastasis; attention should be also directed to the presence of a normal, uninvolved contralateral adrenal gland, as bilateral adrenalectomy has significant implications for postoperative management.

The surgical approach is dictated by the tumor's size and location as well as surgeon experience. Complete tumor resection with negative surgical margins is critical to long-term survival [51]. While laparoscopic adrenalectomy is associated with less pain, less perioperative morbidity, and shorter hospitalization, questions have been raised about the oncologic efficacy of this approach, especially for tumors greater than 10 cm in diameter [49,52]. The inferior oncologic outcomes of laparoscopic versus open adrenalectomy for ACC may be due in part to a higher rate of positive surgical margins in the laparoscopic group. Nonetheless, laparoscopic adrenalectomy may be considered for ACCs less than 10 cm in diameter that are amenable to complete laparoscopic resection with negative surgical margins, when the surgeon has technical expertise in this procedure.

While both sides can be approached either transperitoneally or retroperitoneally, transperitoneal laparoscopy is usually used for left adrenalectomy and retroperitoneal laparoscopy typically employed for right adrenalectomy. The robotic adrenalectomy is similar to the laparoscopic approach. The magnification, three-dimensional vision, and precise motion of the robot can be beneficial for adrenalectomy. An experienced laparoscopist may choose to perform routine adrenalectomies using a pure laparoscopic (nonrobotic) technique and reserve the robotic technique for more complex cases and partial adrenalectomies.

Larger and more complex adrenal tumors may require open adrenalectomy. The exact approach will be dictated by tumor location, size, complexity, patient anatomy, and surgeon preference.

Postoperatively, the adrenalectomy patient is managed in most aspects like a patient having major intra-abdominal surgery. A concern unique to the postoperative adrenalectomy patient is adrenal insufficiency. In the first few hours to days after adrenalectomy, the patient must be monitored closely for signs of adrenal insufficiency, including hypotension, vomiting, diarrhea, confusion, or electrolyte disturbances. Stress dose steroids may be required, and in some cases fludrocortisone may be necessary.

Pheochromocytoma

Additional surgical considerations for management of pheochromocytomas include the absolute requirement for a metabolic evaluation to rule out a hormonally active tumor. A long list of serum and urine tests are available to test for excess adrenal hormone production, however the following simplified scheme can save time and expense, avoiding the requirement for a 24-hour urine sample while covering all surgically significant hormonal abnormalities: electrolytes, fractionated plasma metanephrines, serum testosterone, serum aldosterone, serum cortisol, and a low-dose dexamethasone suppression test. Failure to identify and properly compensate for epinephrine or norepinephrine overproduction by the tumor may lead to severe intraoperative hyper- and hypotension. The patient should begin phenoxybenzamine 2 weeks before scheduled surgery and increase the dose gradually as tolerated. A beta blocker may be added a couple of days before surgery, but only after complete alpha blockade has been achieved. The anesthesia team must be alerted before starting the adrenalectomy if pheochromocytoma is suspected. Before inducing anesthesia, they will often prepare a set of antihypertensive infusions for the first part of the surgical procedure and vasopressors to begin when the tumor is out. With proper preparation, the blood pressure can be maintained in an acceptable range throughout the operation and adverse sequelae may be avoided.

Surgical Management of Metastatic Disease

The variable natural history of some patients with metastatic ACC and the absence of effective systemic therapy have led to an experience with the selected use of metastasectomy. Investigators recently reported their experience with surgical resection of either recurrent or metastatic disease [53]. Sites of resection were primarily for liver, lung, and other abdominal disease including local recurrences. Median and 5-year survivals from time of first metastasectomy were 2.5 years and 41%, respectively. Nearly 80% of patients were rendered disease free by their initial surgical intervention and the disease-free interval ranged from 2.8 months to more than 12 years. Although this and other published experiences demonstrate the plausibility of this approach, it is important to consider that many patients for whom surgical resection of recurrent or metastatic disease is felt a reasonable option are likely to have more favorable disease biology, thus careful selection of patients at centers with reasonable experience with this approach seems most appropriate.

Systemic Therapy

Adrenal Cancer

Mitotane

Although its precise mechanism of antitumor activity remains undefined, mitotane is believed to require metabolic transformation within the tumor by an unidentified cytochrome P450 enzyme(s), with the resultant acyl chloride derivative causing cytotoxicity through covalent binding to adrenocortical macromolecules [54].

Mitotane is poorly absorbed and highly lipophilic. Following oral administration, 60% is excreted in stool with 40% concentrating in liver, brain, adipose, and adrenal tissues thus prolonging achievement of therapeutic serum levels and clearance after drug discontinuation [54,55]. Gastrointestinal side effects include nausea, vomiting, anorexia, and diarrhea, however in most cases dose-limiting side effects include fatigue, somnolence, ataxia, and confusion [56]. Most patients are safely managed by initiating therapy at 1–2 g/day, increasing the total daily dose by 1 g every 1–2 weeks to the maximum tolerated dose, typically in the 4–6 g/day range [54,57]. At doses over 2 g/day, corticosteroid replacement is typically necessary, as a result of both the inhibition of adrenocortical steroidogenesis and increased metabolic clearance of corticosteroids secondary to the induction of hepatic cytochrome P450 enzymes [54,58]. Despite limited data demonstrating improvement in outcomes, some clinicians routinely obtain mitotane levels and attempt to maintain blood levels between 10 and 14 mg/L [54,57].

In an early study of 138 patients with metastatic ACC treated with maximal doses of 8–10 g/day, 34% of the 59 patients with evaluable disease had objective tumor regression with a median duration of about 7 months. A greater than 50% reduction in urinary hormone excretion was observed in 69% of patients with frequent improvement in endocrine-related symptoms; clinical benefit lasted an average of 4.8 months [59].

The role of mitotane in the adjuvant setting has been a focus of a number of groups [60]. Taking advantage of diverse practice patterns within European centers, with some routinely using adjuvant mitotane and others observing patients following adrenalectomy, investigators retrospectively compared outcomes of 47 patients, whose treatment at four Italian centers included adjuvant mitotane, with those of two independent control groups of patients who did not receive adjuvant mitotane. The first control group was comprised of 55 patients from four other Italian centers. The second control group, with 75 patients, was recruited from 47 German centers. Although baseline features of the two groups of patients from Italy were similar, the patients from the German control group tended to be older with earlier-stage disease. Recurrence-free survival was significantly prolonged in the mitotane group, as compared with the two control groups (median recurrence-free survival, 42 months, as compared with 10 months in control group 1 and 25 months in control group 2) [61].

The ongoing Efficacy of Adjuvant Mitotane Treatment (ADIUVO) study (NLM Identifier: NCT00777244) plans to randomize 200 patients to observation versus mitotane (administered until progression or unacceptable toxicity for a minimum of 2 years) with doses adjusted by blood concentration and tolerability; the primary endpoint is disease-free survival.

Chemotherapy

Adrenal Cancer

Cytotoxic agents, both as single agents and in combination, have been utilized in the management of advanced ACC, albeit with very limited prospective evidence published in the literature [62].

Cisplatin is the most widely utilized systemic chemotherapy agent in advanced ACC, with both objective and clinical responses reported with its use as a single agent [63]. In a Southwest Oncology Group study of patients with advanced mitotane-naïve ACC treated with cisplatin 75–100 mg/m^2 administered every 21 days and mitotane up to 4 g/day, objective responses were reported in 11 of 37 eligible patients (one complete response (CR), 10 partial response (PR)) for an overall response rate of 30%. The median response duration was 7.9 months [64].

One of the largest prospective trials conducted in advanced ACC enrolled 72 patients with metastatic ACC [65]. Patients received etoposide (100 mg/m^2 on days 5–7), doxorubicin (20 mg/m^2 on days 1 and 8), and cisplatin (40 mg/m^2 on days 2 and 9), repeated every 4 weeks. Mitotane was administered daily at the maximum tolerated dose. An objective response was observed in 15 patients (5 CR, 10 PR). The median time to disease progression and overall survival were 9.1 and 28.5 months, respectively. Therapy-related toxicity was primarily hematologic and gastrointestinal, with one treatment-related septic death.

The efficacy of streptozocin (1 g/day for 5 days as a loading dose followed by 2 g every 3 weeks) with mitotane (1–4 g/day) was studied as adjuvant therapy for patients with stage I and II disease, and as treatment for patients with overt metastatic disease. The investigators reported an overall response rate of 36.4% in patients with measurable metastatic disease, with the majority of patients having a partial response [66].

A phase 2 trial of patients with advanced ACC studied a regimen of mitotane, doxorubicin10 mg/m^2/day, vincristine 0.4 mg/m^2/day, and etoposide 75 mg/m^2 administered as a continuous intravenous infusion over 96 hours with treatment repeated every 3 weeks. Five of 36 patients achieved an objective response (1 CR, 4 PR). The mean duration of response was 12.4months and the median survival for the group as a whole was 13.5 months [67].

More recently an international consortium group of investigators initiated the "First International Randomized trial in locally advanced and Metastatic Adrenocortical Carcinoma Treatment" (FIRM-ACT) which randomized patients to receive either the etoposide, doxorubicin, and cisplatin plus mitotane (EDP-M) regimen or the streptozocin plus mitotane (S-M) regimen as first-line treatment for patients with unresectable or metastatic ACC [65–67]. The primary endpoint was overall survival; secondary endpoints included progression-free survival (PFS), objective response, quality of life, and the effect of a blood mitotane level of 14–20 mg/L on clinical outcome. Patients randomized to EDP-M had a higher objective response rate than those treated with S-M (23.2% vs 9.2%, P <0.001) and a longer median PFS (5.0 months vs 2.1 months), however there was no significant between-group difference in overall survival (14.8 months and 12.0 months), respectively (P = 0.07). There was a nonsignificant (P = 0.13) trend towards longer survival in those patients with mitotane levels of 14 mg/L or higher. Quality of life measures and serious adverse events were similar between the two treatment arms [68].

Pheochromocytoma

Systemic chemotherapy has been utilized for several decades, with some antitumor activity reported. The most commonly used agents are cyclophosphamide, doxorubicin, vincristine, and dacarbazine. The rarity of this entity has precluded prospective assessment of the role of chemotherapy [40].

Targeted Therapies and Immunotherapy

Adrenal Cancer

Potentially targetable molecular pathways that may play a role in ACC tumorigenesis include, but are not limited, to vascular endothelial growth factor (VEGF), insulin-like growth 1 factor receptor (IGF-1R), and epidermal growth factor receptor (EGFR) receptor signaling [69].

A recent multicenter phase 2 trial tested the role of sunitinib, a multitargeted tyrosine kinase inhibitor with activity against VEGFR1 and VEGFR2 among others [70]. All patients had been heavily pretreated with both mitotane and chemotherapy. Sunitinib was administered in a schedule of 50 mg/day for 4 weeks on and 2 weeks off. None of the 35 evaluable patients demonstrated an objective response; only 5 patients had stable disease at 12 weeks and the median PFS was 2.8 months. Toxicity was typical of that anticipated with sunitinib.

Dovitinib is a fibroblast growth factor receptor (FGFR) tyrosine kinase inhibitor (TKI) investigated in ACC based on preclinical data implicating FGFR in ACC pathogenesis. In a phase 2 trial of ACC patients with no prior therapy other than mitotane, 17 patients were treated with dovitinib. With a median follow-up of 5.2 months, only one partial response was noted although 23% demonstrated stable disease for more than 6 months while on therapy, suggesting a possible role for FGFR inhibition in the management of ACC [71].

Ten heavily pretreated patients with ACC received bevacizumab (5 mg/kg every 21 days) plus capecitabine (950 mg/m^2) twice daily for 14 days of a 21-day schedule. No clinical activity was observed [72].

Insulin-like growth factor 2 (IGF-2) is up-regulated in as many as 80–90% of ACCs and is known to activate the IGF-1 receptor (IGF-1R). A recent study of 26 pretreated ACC patients evaluated the combination of cixutumumab, a monoclonal antibody directed against the IGF-1R, dosed at 3–6 mg/kg intravenously (IV) weekly, and temsirolimus, 25–37.5 mg IV weekly. Toxicities including thrombocytopenia, mucositis, hypercholesterolemia, hypertriglyceridemia, and hyperglycemia were common. Eleven of 26 patients (42%) achieved stable disease persisting for ≥6 months [73].

The EGFR is expressed in 76% of ACCs, and remains an intriguing target, although in the largest experience reported to date there is no evidence of mutations in the EGFR gene [22]. The oral EGFR inhibitor gefitinib, 250 mg daily, was evaluated in a phase 2 trial of 19 patients with advanced ACC and disease progression following either mitotane or chemotherapy. No patient had an objective response or stable disease [74].

The immune checkpoint inhibitors are being investigated for the treatment of ACC. A phase 2 trial of nivolumab, an anti-programmed death-1 (PD-1) monoclonal antibody, is currently enrolling patients with ACC to investigate efficacy in this setting (NLM identifier: NCT02720484). Similarly, the safety of avelumab, a fully human anti-programmed death ligand-1 (PD-L1) antibody, is currently under study in an expanded phase 1 trial with a goal accrual of 50 patients with ACC [75].

Pheochromocytoma

Limited reports in the literature demonstrate some antitumor activity with sunitinib used in the conventional dose and schedule of this agent. The mechanistic target of rapamycin (mTOR) inhibitor everolimus has also been reported to have disease-stabilizing activity. Two prospective phase 2 trials have been launched in North America testing the activity of sunitinib and pazopanib respectively. A larger randomized double-blind phase 2 trial of sunitinib has been activated in Europe [40].

Axitinib, a VEGFR TKI, has recently been studied in 9 patients with malignant pheochromocytoma and paraganglioma. Only one patient had had response evaluation criteria in solid tumors (RECIST) progressive disease, with 3 patients demonstrating a partial response (PR) and 5 having a reduction in tumor burden that did not achieve a PR. Toxicities were typical of axitinib [76]. These data suggest a potential role for axitinib in this setting [76].

Conclusions

Despite the challenges presented by its rarity and biological aggressiveness, the rapid introduction of next-generation sequencing and the potential to identify targetable mutations with novel agents sets the stage for a different approach to the management of advanced ACC. A paradigm to conduct novel agent trials that focus on the target, not the underlying histology, is in the early stages. This approach, along with improvement in the understanding of ACC biology, may lead to improvements in therapeutic options for patients.

References

1 Golden S, Robinson K, Saldanha I, *et al.* Prevalence and incidence of endocrine and metabolic disorders in the United States: a comprehensive review. *J Clin Endocrinol Metab* 2009;94:1853–78.

2 Bilimoria K, Shen W, Elaraj D, *et al.* Adrenocortical carcinoma in the United States.Treatment utilization and prognostic factors. *Cancer* 2008;113:2130–6.

3 Phan A. Adrenal cortical carcinoma – review of current knowledge and treatment practices. *Hematol Oncol Clin N Am* 2007;21:489–507.

4 Wooten M, King D. Adrenal cortical carcinoma. Epidemiology and treatment with mitotane and a review of the literature. *Cancer* 1993;72:3145–55.

5 Lafemina J, Brennan M. Adrenocortical carcinoma: past, present, and future. *J Surg Oncol* 2012;106:586–94.

6 Schteingart D, Doherty G, Gauger P, *et al.* Management of patients with adrenal cancer: recommendations of an international consensus conference. *Endocrine-Related Cancer* 2005;12:667–80.

7 Goffredo P, Sosa JA, Roman SA. Malignant pheochromocytoma and paraganglioma: A population level

analysis of long-term survival over two decades. *J Surg Oncol* 2013;107:659–64.

8 Hsing A, Nam J, Co Chien H, McLaughlin J, Fraumeni J. Risk factors for adrenal cancer: an exploratory study. *Int J Cancer* 1996;65:432–6.

9 Ganeshan D, Bhosale P, Kundra V. Current update on cytogenetics, taxonomy,diagnosis, and management of adrenocortical carcinoma: what radiologists should know. *Am J Radiol* 2012;199:1283–93.

10 Latronico A, Pinto E, Domenice S, *et al.* An inherited mutation outside the highly conserved DNA-binding domain of the p53 tumor suppressor protein in children and adults with sporadic adrenocortical tumors. *J Clin Endocrinol Metab* 2001;86:4970–3.

11 Harari A, Inabnet WB. Malignant pheochromocytoma: a review. *Am J Surg* 2011;201:700–8.

12 Weiss LM. Comparative histologic study of 43 metastasizing and nonmetastasizing adrenocortical tumors. *Am J Surg Pathol* 1984;8:163–9.

13 Aubert S, Wacrenier A, Leroy X, *et al.* Weiss system revisited: a clinicopathologic and immunohistochemical study of 49 adrenocortical tumors. *Am J Surg Pathol* 2002;26:1612–9.

14 Saez R, Craig J, Kuhn J, *et al.* Phase I clinical investigation of amonafide. *J Clin Oncol* 1989;7:1351–8.

15 van Slooten H, Schaberg A, Smeenk D, Moolenaar AJ. Morphologic characteristics of benign and malignant adrenocortical tumors. *Cancer* 1985;55:766–73.

16 van't Sant HP, Bouvy ND, Kazemier G, *et al.* The prognostic value of two different histopathological scoring systems for adrenocortical carcinomas. *Histopathology* 2007;51:239–45.

17 Hough AJ, Hollifield JW, Page DL, Hartmann WH. Prognostic factors in adrenal cortical tumors. A mathematical analysis of clinical and morphologic data. *Am J Clin Pathol* 1979;72:390–9.

18 Papotti M, Volante M, Duregon E, *et al.* Adrenocortical tumors with myxoid features: a distinct morphologic and phenotypical variant exhibiting malignant behavior. *Am J Surg Pathol* 2010;34:973–83.

19 Wieneke JA, Thompson LD, Heffess CS. Adrenal cortical neoplasms in the pediatric population: a clinicopathologic and immunophenotypic analysis of 83 patients. *Am J Surg Pathol* 2003;27:867–81.

20 Dehner LP, Hill DA. Adrenal cortical neoplasms in children: why so many carcinomas and yet so many survivors? *Pediatr Dev Pathol* 2009;12:284–91.

21 Sangoi AR, Fujiwara M, West RB, *et al.* Immunohistochemical distinction of primary adrenal cortical lesions from metastatic clear cell renal cell carcinoma: a study of 248 cases. *Am J Surg Pathol* 2011;35:678–86.

22 Adam P, Hahner S, Hartmann M, *et al.* Epidermal growth factor receptor in adrenocortical tumors: analysis of gene sequence, protein expression and correlation with clinical outcome. *Mod Pathol* 2010;23:1596–604.

23 Sidhu S, Marsh DJ, Theodosopoulos G, *et al.* Comparative genomic hybridization analysis of adrenocortical tumors. *J Clin Endocrinol Metab* 2002;87:3467–74.

24 Libe R, Groussin L, Tissier F, *et al.* Somatic TP53 mutations are relatively rare among adrenocortical cancers with the frequent 17p13 loss of heterozygosity. *Clin Cancer Res* 2007;13:844–50.

25 Soon PSH, Libe R, Benn DE, *et al.* Loss of heterozygosity of 17p13, with possible involvement of ACADVL and ALOX15B, in the pathogenesis of adrenocortical tumors. *Ann Surg* 2008;247:157–64.

26 Giordano TJ, Thomas DG, Kuick R, *et al.* Distinct transcriptional profiles of adrenocortical tumors uncovered by DNA microarray analysis. *Am J Pathol* 2003;162:521–31.

27 Velazquez-Fernandez D, Laurell C, Geli J, *et al.* Expression profiling of adrenocortical neoplasms suggests a molecular signature of malignancy. *Surgery* 2005;138:1087–94.

28 Weksberg R, Smith AC, Squire J, Sadowski P. Beckwith-Wiedemann syndrome demonstrates a role for epigenetic control of normal development. *Hum Mol Genet* 2003;12:R61–8.

29 Bonnet S, Gaujoux S, Launay P, *et al.* Wnt/β-catenin pathway activation in adrenocortical adenomas is frequently due to somatic CTNNB1-activating mutations, which are associated with larger and nonsecreting tumors: a study in cortisol-secreting and -nonsecreting tumors. *J Clin Endocrinol Metab* 2011;96:E419–26.

30 Patterson EE, Holloway AK, Weng J, Fojo T, Kebebew E. MicroRNA profiling of adrenocortical tumors reveals miR-483 as a marker of malignancy. *Cancer* 2011;117:1630–9.

31 Thompson L. Pheochromocytoma of the Adrenal gland Scaled Score (PASS) to separate benign from malignant neoplasms: a clinicopathologic and immunophenotypic study of 100 cases. *Am J Surg Pathol* 2002;26:551–66.

32 Strong V, Kennedy T, Al-Ahmadie H, *et al.* Prognostic indicators of malignancy in adrenal pheochromocytomas: clinical, histopathologic, and cell cycle/apoptosis gene expression analysis. *Surgery* 2008;143:759–68.

33 Amar L, Baudin E, Burnichon N, *et al.* Succinate dehydrogenase B gene mutations predict survival in patients with malignant pheochromocytomas or paragangliomas. *J Clin Endocrinol Metab* 2007;92:3822–8.

34 Kebebew E, Reiff E, Duh Q, Clark O, McMillan A. Extent of disease at presentation and outcome for adrenocortical carcinoma: have we made progress? *World J Surg* 2006;30:872–8.

35 NIH state-of-the-science statement on management of the clinically inapparent adrenal mass ("incidentaloma"). *NIH Consens State Sci Statements* 2002;19:1–25.

36 Luton J, Cerdas S, Billaud L, *et al.* Clinical features of adrenocortical carcinoma, prognostic factors, and the effect of mitotane therapy. *N Engl J Med* 1990;322:1195–201.

37 Abiven G, Coste J, Groussin L, *et al.* Clinical and biological features in the prognosis of adrenocortical cancer: poor outcome of cortisol-secreting tumors in a series of 202 consecutive patients. *J Clin Endocrinol Metab* 2006;91:2650–5.

38 Fassnacht M, Libé R, Kroiss M, Allolio B. Adrenocortical carcinoma: a clinician's update. *Nat Rev Endocrinol* 2011;7:323–35.

39 Mazzaglia P, Monchik J. Limited value of adrenal biopsy in the evaluation of adrenal neoplasm. *Arch Surg* 2009;144:465–70.

40 Jimenez C, Rohren E, Habra M, *et al.* Current and future treatments for malignant pheochromocytoma and sympathetic paraganglioma. *Curr Oncol Rep* 2013;15:356–71.
41 Song J, Chaudhry F, Mayo-Smith W. The incidental adrenal mass on CT: prevalence of adrenal disease in 1,049 consecutive adrenal masses in patients with no known malignancy. *Am J Roentgenol* 2008;190:1163–8.
42 Caoili E, Korobkin M, Francis I, *et al.* Adrenal masses: characterization with combined unenhanced and delayed enhanced CT. *Radiology* 2002;222:629–33.
43 Groussin L, Bonardel G, Silvéra S, *et al.* 18 F-Fluorodeoxyglucose positron emission tomography for the diagnosis of adrenocortical tumors: a prospective study in 77 operated patients. *J Clin Endocrinol Metab* 2009;94:1713–22.
44 Boland G, Dwamena B, Jagtiani S, *et al.* Characterization of adrenal masses by using FDG PET: a systematic review and meta-analysis of diagnostic test performance. *Radiology* 2011;259:117–26.
45 Chen C, Carrasquillo J. Molecular imaging of adrenal neoplasms. *J Surg Oncol* 2012;106:532–42.
46 Jimenez C, Libutti SK, Landry CS, *et al.* Adrenal – neuroendocrine tumors. In: MB Amin, SB Edge, FL Greene, *et al.* (eds) *AJCC Cancer Staging Manual*, 8th edn. New York: Springer Nature, 2017.
47 Sobin LH, Gospodarowicz MK, Wittekind Ch (eds) *TNM Classification of Malignant Tumours*, 7th edn. New York: Wiley, 2009.
48 Fassnacht M, Johanssen S, Quinkler M, *et al.* Limited prognostic value of the 2004 International Union Against Cancer staging classification for adrenocortical carcinoma: proposal for a Revised TNM Classification. *Cancer* 2009;115:243–50.
49 Mir M, Klink J, Guillotreau J, *et al.* Comparative outcomes of laparoscopic and open adrenalectomy for adrenocortical carcinoma: single, high-volume center experience. *Ann Surg Oncol* 2013;20:1456–61.
50 Gaujoux S, Brennan M. Recommendation for standardized surgical management of primary adrenocortical carcinoma. *Surgery* 2012;152:123–32.
51 Schulick R, Brennan M. Long-term survival after complete resection and repeat resection in patients with adrenocortical carcinoma. *Ann Surg Oncol* 1999;6:719–26.
52 Lee J, El-Tamer M, Schifftner T, *et al.* Open and laparoscopic adrenalectomy: analysis of the National Surgical Quality Improvement Program. *J Am Coll Surg* 2008;206:953–9.
53 Dartrice N, Langan R, Ripley R, *et al.* Operative management for recurrent and metastatic adrenocortical carcinoma. *J Surg Oncol* 2012;105:709–13.
54 Veytsman I, Nieman L, Fojo T. Management of endocrine manifestations and the use of mitotane as a chemotherapeutic agent for adrenocortical carcinoma. *J Clin Oncol* 2009;27:4619–29.
55 Maluf D, de Oliveira B, Lalli E. Therapy of adrenocortical cancer: present and future. *Am J Cancer Res* 2011;1:222–23.
56 Tacon L, Prichard R, Soon P, *et al.* Current and emerging therapies for advanced adrenocortical carcinoma. *Oncologist* 2011;16:36–48.
57 Terzolo M, Pia A, Berruti A, *et al.* Low-dose monitored mitotane treatment achieves the therapeutic range with manageable side effects in patients with adrenocortical cancer. *J Clin Endocrinol Metab* 2000;85:2234–8.
58 Robinson B, Hales I, Henniker A, *et al.* The effect of o,p'-DDD on adrenal steroid replacement therapy requirements. *Clin Endocrinol* 1987;27:437–44.
59 Hutter A, Kayhoe D. Adrenal cortical carcinoma. Results of treatment with o,p ′ DDD in 138 patients. *American J Med* 1966;41:581–92.
60 Terzolo M, Fassnacht M, Ciccone G, Allolio B, Berruti A. Adjuvant mitotane for adrenocortical cancer – working through uncertainty. *J Clin Endocrinol Metab* 2009;94:1879–80.
61 Terzolo M, Angeli A, Fassnacht M, *et al.* Adjuvant mitotane treatment for adrenocortical carcinoma. *N Engl J Med* 2007;356:2372–80.
62 Ahlman H, Khorram-Manesh A, Jansson S, *et al.* Cytotoxic treatment of adrenocortical carcinoma. *World J Surg* 2001;25:927–33.
63 Tattersall M, Lander H, Bain B, *et al.* Cis-platinum treatment of metastatic adrenal carcinoma. *Med J Aust* 1980;1:419–21.
64 Bukowski R, Wolfe M, Levine H, *et al.* Phase II trial of mitotane and cisplatin in patients with adrenal carcinoma: a Southwest Oncology Group study. *J Clin Oncol* 1993;11:161–5.
65 Berruti A, Terzolo M, Sperone P, *et al.* Etoposide, doxorubicin and cisplatin plus mitotane in the treatment of advanced adrenocortical carcinoma: a large prospective phase II trial. *Endocr Relat Cancer* 2005;12:657–66.
66 Khan T, Imam H, Juhlin C, *et al.* Streptozocin and o,p′DDD in the treatment of adrenocortical cancer patients: Long-term survival in its adjuvant use. *Ann Oncol* 2000;11:1281–7.
67 Abraham J, Bakke S, Rutt A, *et al.* A phase II trial of combination chemotherapy and surgical resection for the treatment of metastatic adrenocortical carcinoma: Continuous infusion doxorubicin, vincristine, and etoposide with daily mitotane as a P-glycoprotein antagonist. *Cancer* 2002;94:2333–43.
68 Fassnacht M, Terzolo M, Allolio B, *et al.* Combination chemotherapy in advanced adrenocortical carcinoma. *N Engl J Med* 2012;366:2189–97.
69 Hubalewska-Dydejczyk A, Jabrocka-Hybel A, Pach D, Gilis-Januszewska A, Sokołowski G. Current and future medical therapy, and the molecular features of adrenocortical cancer. *Recent Pat Anticancer Drug Discov* 2012;7:132–45.
70 Kroiss M, Quinkler M, Johanssen S, *et al.* Sunitinib in refractory adrenocortical carcinoma: a phase II, single-arm, open-label trial. *J Clin Endocrinol Metab* 2012;97:3495–503.
71 García-Donas J, Hernando Polo S, Guix M, *et al.* Phase II study of dovitinib in first line metastatic or (non resectable primary) adrenocortical carcinoma (ACC): SOGUG study 2011-03. *J Clin Oncol* 2013;31(15 suppl):4587.
72 Wortmann S, Quinkler M, Ritter C, *et al.* Bevacizumab plus capecitabine as a salvage therapy in advanced adrenocortical carcinoma. *Eur J Endocrinol* 2010;162:349–56.
73 Naing A, Lorusso P, Fu S, *et al.* Insulin growth factor receptor (IGF-1R) antibody cixutumumab combined with the mTOR

inhibitor temsirolimus in patients with metastatic adrenocortical carcinoma. *Br J Cancer* 2013;108:826–30.
74 Samnotra V, Vassilopoulou-Sellin R, Fojo A, *et al.* A phase II trial of gefitinib monotherapy in patients with unresectable adrenocortical carcinoma. *J Clin Oncol* 2007;25:15527 (abstr).
75 Heery CR, Infante JR, Iannotti N, *et al.* Phase I expansion cohort trial to investigate the safety and clinical activity of avelumab (MSB0010718C) in patients with metastatic or locally advanced solid tumors. *J Clin Oncol* 2015;33(15 suppl):abstr TPS3101.
76 Burotto Pichun ME, Edgerly M, Velarde M, *et al.* Phase II clinical trial of axitinib in metastatic pheochromocytomas and paraganlgiomas (P/PG): Preliminary results. *J Clin Oncol* 2015;33(7) suppl:457.

38

Pituitary Tumors

Adriana G. Ioachimescu and Nelson M. Oyesiku

Emory Pituitary Center, Emory University School of Medicine, Atlanta, Georgia, USA

Incidence and Mortality

Tumors arising from the pituitary gland account for approximately 15% of intracranial tumors and are almost always benign adenomas. Pituitary adenomas are identified in 20% of the general population at autopsy and 10–20% incidentally by brain imaging [1]. The actual incidence, including undiagnosed and subclinical cases, is therefore likely to be substantially higher than the reported incidence rate in the Central Brain Tumor Registry of the United States (CBTRUS) from 2004 to 2009 of approximately 3.13 [2]. They are classified into nonfunctioning and functioning pituitary adenomas based on hormonal activity. The following types of functioning pituitary adenomas are recognized based on clinical presentation and biochemical activity: prolactinomas (lactotroph tumors), growth hormone (GH)-secreting tumors (somatotropinomas), adrenocorticotrophic hormone (ACTH)-secreting tumors (corticotropinomas), thyroid stimulating hormone (TSH)-secreting tumors (TSHomas), and gonadotroph-secreting tumors (functioning gonadotropinomas).

The incidence of pituitary adenomas increases with age with the exception of prolactin- and ACTH-secreting adenomas which peak in the third to fifth life decades. Also, prolactin- and ACTH-secreting adenomas affect women more frequently than men, with a male to female incidence rate ratio of 0.89. In contrast to most other intracranial neoplasms, the White to Black incidence rate ratio for pituitary tumors is 0.55. The nonfunctioning pituitary adenomas (NFPA) represent 35% of pituitary tumors. The most frequent functioning types of pituitary tumors are prolactinomas, which represent 35% of all pituitary tumors. GH-secreting adenomas represent 15% of pituitary adenomas, have an annual incidence of 3–4/million, and cause acromegaly. Mixed somatolactotroph tumors represent 5% of pituitary tumors. ACTH-secreting tumors represent 10% of pituitary adenomas, have an annual incidence of 2–3/million/year, and cause Cushing disease. TSHomas and hormonally-efficient gonadotropinomas are rare, encompassing less than 2% of pituitary tumors. Primary pituitary carcinomas are extraordinarily rare, with an incidence rate of 0.01 per 100,000 person-years, representing 0.1% of all pituitary tumors [3]. Craniopharyngioma is a common sellar/suprasellar tumor with incidence of 0.18/100,000 person-years, representing 5–15% of intracranial tumors in children and 2–5% in adults. Metastatic lesions of breast and lung cancers in the sellar region are rare, representing only 1.8% of all metastases and 1% of pituitary masses. Table 38.1 shows other possible causes of masses in the pituitary region as indicated by pathology after their surgical removal.

All-cause mortality is increased in patients with pituitary adenomas, especially from vascular diseases. Patients with acromegaly have mortality 2–3 times above the general population from cardiovascular and respiratory causes and possibly malignant diseases. Mortality has improved with modern treatment that achieves biochemical control (GH levels lower than 1 ng/mL and normal IGF-1), but remains higher than for the general population. Confounding factors include hypopituitarism associated with large adenomas, surgery, and radiation therapy [4]. Cushing disease leads to more than double mortality risk from macrovascular diseases, uncontrolled diabetes mellitus, and infections [5]. Biochemical control improves survival, which becomes similar to the general population. Patients with craniopharyngiomas have mortality 3–5 times above the general population. Some studies suggest that patients with NFPA and incomplete resection or those who receive radiation have increased mortality compared with those with gross–total resection [6]. In pituitary carcinomas prognosis is poor with survival of only a few months or 1–2 years despite surgery, radiation, and chemotherapy [7]. Conventional high-dose external-beam radiation administered for pituitary tumors has been associated with increased cerebrovascular events, but is no longer recommended today. Even with lower-dose conformal radiation, some degree of hypopituitarism may occur in up to 50% patients. The risk of secondary malignancies (glioma, meningioma) is very small.

The American Cancer Society's Oncology in Practice: Clinical Management, First Edition. Edited by The American Cancer Society.

Table 38.1 Classification of pituitary pathology[1].

Neoplastic
Benign[2]
Pituitary adenoma
Craniopharyngioma
Gangliocytoma/ganglioglioma
Granular cell tumor
Meningioma
Schwannoma
Chordoma
Vascular and mesenchymal tumors
Malignant
Pituitary carcinoma
Gliomas
Germ cell tumor
Lymphoma/leukemia/Langerhans cell histiocytosis
Vascular and mesenchymal tumors
Metastases
Miscellaneous (salivary gland lesions, melanoma, etc.)
Non-neoplastic
Hyperplasia
Inflammatory lesions
Infectious
Immune
Cysts
Rathke cleft cysts
Arachnoid
Dermoid/epidermoid
Aneurysms
Meningoencephalocele
Hamartoma
Brown tumor of bone

Source: Asa S. Practical Pituitary Pathology. What does the pathologist need to know? Arch Pathol Med, vol 132, Aug 2008. Reproduced with permission of College of American Pathologists.

[1] Surgical pathology only, not including developmental and metabolic lesions that are not biopsied.

[2] Although classified as benign, many of these lesions are locally invasive and cause significant morbidity and mortality.

Etiology and Risk Factors

Pathogenesis involves a combination of genetic events, epigenetic silencing of tumor suppressors, oncogenic factors, hormone stimulation, and growth factors. Pituitary adenomas are monoclonal neoplasms. However, the extraordinary cases of pituitary adenoma progression into malignancy may involve a different clone profile in the metastasis and primary tumor [8]. Some microRNAs have been found to be down-regulated compared with the normal pituitary gland and may play a role in tumorigenesis [9].

Gene expression studies have identified unique and specific molecular markers for different types of pituitary adenomas. The folate receptor (gp38), a glycosyl-phosphatidylinositol linked membrane protein that initiates cellular accumulation of 5-methyltetrahydrofolic acid in epithelial cells, is preferentially expressed in nonfunctioning adenomas. Folic acid is an essential vitamin and a precursor for cofactors that regulate metabolism and it plays an integral role in cellular growth and development. Overexpression of the folate receptor is thought to confer a growth advantage to cells exposed to a limited concentration of 5-methyltetrahydrofolic acid by providing a means for enhanced uptake of this vital metabolite [10,11].

Ornithine decarboxylase (ODC) is preferentially expressed in GH adenomas. ODC is the first and a key (rate-limiting) enzyme in the biosynthesis of polyamines that are essential for cell proliferation, differentiation, and transformation. Overexpression of ODC is characteristic of neoplastic development and progression and ODC activity correlates with aggressiveness of several types of neoplasms, including pituitary adenomas [11].

C-mer proto-oncogene expression is preferentially expressed in ACTH adenomas. The CMP-tk is a transmembrane receptor containing intrinsic tyrosine kinase activity and is a member of the Axl subfamily of receptor tyrosine kinases (RTK). These RTKs are involved in control of cellular growth and differentiation, and when aberrantly expressed can result in neoplasia. The overexpression of CMP-tk in ACTH adenomas suggests that it may serve an important functional role in tumor initiation or progression [11].

Familial Pituitary Adenomas

Most pituitary adenomas are sporadic, although familial predisposition is rarely encountered. Some patients have autosomal-dominant syndromic conditions like multiple endocrine neoplasia type 1 (MEN-1) and Carney complex. MEN-1 is caused by a germline mutation of the tumor suppressor *MEN1* gene (encoding menin) on chromosome 11q13 and is associated with parathyroid hyperplasia, pituitary adenomas (most frequently prolactinomas), and pancreatic neuroendocrine tumors. Carney complex is caused by a protein kinase A-regulatory subunit 1 (*PRKAR1*) mutation and is associated with atrial myxomas, pigmented nodular adrenal hyperplasia, pituitary adenomas, and cutaneous lesions. Other patients have familial isolated pituitary adenomas (FIPA) that occur in two or more members of the same family outside of the setting of syndromic conditions. FIPA comprises approximately 2% of pituitary adenomas and 20% of these families have germline aryl hydrocarbon receptor interacting protein (*AIP*) gene mutations or deletions. In patients younger than 30 years with sporadic pituitary adenomas, *AIP* mutations were detected in 8.6% cases and MEN1 mutation in 3.4% [12]. Most tumors due to *AIP* mutations are large somatotropinomas that lead to gigantism and are often relatively resistant to somatostatin analog treatment; however prolactinomas, NFPA, and ACTH-secreting tumors have been described [13]. Currently, there are no known measures to prevent the development of pituitary adenomas.

Pathology

Immunohistochemical Classification

The anterior pituitary secretes prolactin, ACTH, GH, TSH, FSH, and LH, and the posterior pituitary stores contain vasopressin and oxytocin secreted in the supraoptic and paraventricular hypothalamic nuclei. Pituitary adenomas arise from cells of the anterior pituitary gland and are characterized by immunohistochemistry based on hormone content as somatotroph, lactotroph, thyrotroph, gonadotroph, or null-cell. Clinical–pathological classification takes into account both pathology and endocrine phenotype. NFPA are either null-cell adenomas or "hormonally-inefficient" gonadotropinomas that stain for alpha subunit, LH, or FSH. On the other hand, functioning gonadotropinomas that cause elevated plasma levels of gonadotrophs and gonadal hormones are extremely rare.

Atypical Pituitary Adenomas

The 2004 World Health Organization (WHO) classification of pituitary adenomas introduced the "atypical" variant, defined by three characteristics: Ki-67 labeling index (a measure of proliferation rate) greater than 3%, diffuse p53 immunoreactivity, and increased mitotic activity. Atypical pituitary adenomas are usually macroadenomas invasive at the time of diagnosis, but long-term studies are needed to clarify whether they have a worse prognosis than the remainder of the adenomas [14,15]. Pituitary carcinomas are diagnosed based on subarachnoid, brain, or systemic spread, usually to the liver or bone [3].

Diagnosis

General Considerations on Diagnosis of Pituitary Masses

Pituitary adenomas are classified into macro- and microadenomas based on a threshold diameter of 1 cm. Presence of a pituitary mass is suspected based on mass effect symptoms or endocrine abnormalities.

Knowledge of the anatomy of the region is important to understanding the mass effect symptoms caused by pituitary tumors. The pituitary gland is located in the sella turcica, immediately superior to the sphenoid sinus, and is connected to the hypothalamus by the infundibulum or stalk. Cavernous sinuses that include the internal carotid artery and cranial nerves III, IV, V1, V2, and VI are located laterally to the pituitary gland on each side and the optic chiasm is located above the pituitary gland. Thus, symptoms of mass effect from direct compression of these structures include headache, vision loss (bitemporal hemianopia or supero-temporal quadrantopia) from optic chiasm compression, ophthalmoparesis (diplopia and ptosis) from compression of the cavernous sinus, cerebrospinal fluid (CSF) rhinorrhea, and rarely hydrocephalus from giant tumors. Visual field testing is indicated in patients with macroadenomas.

Endocrine abnormalities may be hypersecretion functioning pituitary adenomas or various degrees of anterior pituitary hormone deficits with pituitary macroadenomas. Posterior pituitary gland deficits like diabetes insipidus are not typical clinical manifestations of pituitary adenomas. Diabetes insipidus may occur with craniopharyngiomas or tumors that infiltrate the infundibulum (e.g., metastases) or as a postoperative complication of stalk injury. Rarely, pituitary adenomas present with apoplexy (i.e., an ischemic event or hemorrhage that leads to sudden increase in tumor size accompanied by severe headaches, vision loss, nausea, vomiting, and pituitary hormone deficiencies). Clinical suspicion of pituitary apoplexy requires urgent confirmation by computed tomography (CT) or magnetic resonance imaging (MRI), clinical and hormonal evaluation, and management, including correction of potentially life-threatening ACTH deficiency [16,17]. Evaluation by an endocrinologist is essential in patients diagnosed with pituitary masses in order to determine the tumor type and to guide further treatment, as well as to optimize hormonal status preoperatively.

Diagnosis of Nonfunctioning Pituitary Adenomas (NFPA)

Patients with nonfunctioning macroadenomas usually present with mass effect and pituitary hormone deficiencies. The only pituitary hormone potentially mildly elevated is prolactin, due to pituitary stalk compression and diminished inhibitory dopaminergic tone. NFPA can also present as an incidentaloma during imaging for an unrelated reason (most frequently headaches, trauma, or suspicion of cerebrovascular ischemic event). If the diagnosis of incidentaloma is made by CT scan, evaluation by contrast-enhanced MRI is recommended to further delineate the tumor and related anatomy. Immunohistochemical analysis of incidentalomas shows that the majority are nonfunctioning gonadotroph adenomas. Pituitary incidentaloma patients should undergo evaluation for hormone excess (insulin-like growth factor 1 and prolactin level) and hormone deficiencies. Patients with macroincidentalomas should have MRI scan and hormonal evaluation repeated after 6 months and subsequently annually, and also visual field testing if the tumor is close to the optic chiasm. Patients with microincidentalomas should have MRI scan repeated after 1 year and subsequently every 1–2 years, while biochemical evaluation should be repeated only in suggestive clinical situations [1].

Diagnosis of Prolactinomas

Patients with prolactinomas present with clinical manifestations related to hormone excess with or without mass effect symptoms. Hyperprolactinemia leads to gonadal inhibition (hypogonadism) and sometimes galactorrhea. Premenopausal women usually present with irregular periods, amenorrhea, infertility, and galactorrhea and harbor microadenomas. Men tend to present late with mass effect symptoms, although symptoms of hypogonadism (decreased libido, impotence, infertility, hot flashes, decreased muscle strength, and gynecomastia) may have been present for many years. Diagnostic tests show significantly elevated prolactin levels at least five times above normal which usually parallel the size of the tumor [18]. If a large pituitary tumor is associated with a mild degree of hyperprolactinemia, prolactin measurement after serial dilution is indicated to exclude the hook effect, in which very high prolactin levels saturate the assay's reagent antibodies and cause a falsely low result [19].

Central hypogonadism is a consequence of significant hyperprolactinemia. In men, it is characterized by low testosterone along with low levels of gonadotroph hormones (LH and FSH). In women, low estradiol and low LH and FSH are characteristics, even in postmenopausal women. Decreased bone strength and increased risk for fracture is a long-term complication of untreated hypogonadism in both genders.

Diagnosis of Acromegaly

Patients with acromegaly exhibit consequences of GH excess as well as mass effect symptoms, since the tumor is a macroadenoma in 65% of cases. Oversecretion of GH leads to phenotypical changes (acral enlargement, facial and teeth changes), increased sweating, arthralgias, headaches, hypertension, glucose intolerance, carpal tunnel syndrome, hypogonadism, and sleep apnea. Although phenotypical changes can be pronounced, acromegaly has a slow progressive course and diagnosis is usually made almost 10 years after onset of manifestations. Therefore, cardiovascular, respiratory, metabolic, and musculoskeletal complications ensue, which decrease patients' survival and quality of life. The screening test for acromegaly is measurement of serum insulin-like growth factor 1 (IGF 1, also known as somatomedin-C) level. If age- and gender-adjusted IGF-1 is elevated, the 2-hour GH suppression after an oral glucose load is indicated to confirm the diagnosis. A GH threshold of 0.4 or 1 ng/mL should be used depending on sensitivity of the GH assay [20]. Other biochemical abnormalities in patients with acromegaly may include hyperprolactinemia (as a result of a co-secreting tumor that secretes prolactin or due to stalk effect) and central hypogonadism.

Diagnosis of Cushing Disease

Cushing disease is part of a heterogeneous group of conditions called Cushing syndrome that includes pituitary and "ectopic" ACTH-secreting tumors as well as corticosteroid-secreting adrenal tumors. Cushing disease is defined as Cushing syndrome caused by an ACTH-secreting (corticotroph) pituitary adenoma.

Patients with Cushing syndrome present with centripetal weight gain (abdominal, supraclavicular and dorso-cervical fat accumulation), skin changes (dark striae, easy bruising, hirsutism), proximal muscle weakness, hypertension, hypogonadism, and impaired glucose tolerance. The long-term consequences of untreated hypercortisolemia (accelerated atherosclerosis, opportunistic infections, deep vein thromboses, and bone fractures) are devastating and lead to increased mortality. Differential diagnosis includes reactive hypercortisolemia (or pseudoCushing) that occurs in patients with psychiatric conditions (depression, anxiety, anorexia nervosa, and obsessive compulsive disorder), uncontrolled diabetes mellitus, chronic alcoholism, and morbid obesity.

The biochemical diagnosis of Cushing syndrome includes a combination of screening tests: bedtime salivary cortisol measurements, 24-hour urinary cortisol levels, and low-dose dexamethasone suppression tests [21,22]. Once the diagnosis of hypercortisolemia is firmly established by a combination of abnormal screening tests, ACTH levels should be measured. ACTH is normal or high in patients with Cushing disease and low in patients with adrenal tumors [21]. If ACTH levels are normal or elevated, a high-dose dexamethasone suppression test is usually helpful. As functioning corticotropinomas are usually small and sometimes not even visible on the MRI scan, many patients also require inferior petrosal sinus sampling to differentiate between pituitary and ectopic Cushing syndrome [23]. Ectopic Cushing syndrome occurs in rare cases of paraneoplastic ACTH secretion from neuroendocrine tumors located in the lung, thymus, or gastrointestinal tract.

Diagnosis of Rare Functioning Tumors

Patients with TSHomas present with manifestations of hyperthyroidism (palpitations, tremor, insomnia, tachycardia, and loose bowel movements), increased thyroid size (goiter) and mass effect symptoms characteristic of a pituitary macroadenoma [24]. Biochemical evaluation shows normal or mildly elevated TSH levels along with elevated thyroid hormone levels. The main differential diagnosis is the syndrome of resistance to thyroid hormone, which is usually associated with a family history of thyroid disease. Measurement of alpha subunit is helpful in making the diagnosis, as are dynamic endocrine and genetic testing [25].

Functioning gonadotropinomas are rare, as the FSH and LH secretion is usually not sufficient to result in gonadal hormone hypersecretion. The diagnosis of functioning gonadotropinoma in men is suggested by elevated gonadotroph level, alpha subunit, and testosterone. In premenopausal women, the diagnosis is suggested by a markedly elevated FSH, alpha subunit, and estradiol with lower than normal LH along with endometrial hyperplasia and polycystic ovaries on ultrasound.

Craniopharyngiomas present with mass effect symptoms, diabetes insipidus, and multiple anterior pituitary hormone deficiencies. Due to their suprasellar location, they may cause hypothalamic syndrome with increased appetite, morbid obesity, and sleep dysregulation. As many craniopharyngiomas present in childhood, linear growth and sexual development are often affected.

Treatment

General Considerations

Pituitary tumors are best treated in tertiary referral centers by multidisciplinary collaboration between experienced neurosurgeons, endocrinologists, and radiation oncologists.

Surgical resection of pituitary adenomas is almost exclusively done by the transsphenoidal approach, while staged or combined transsphenoidal–transcranial approaches are used for giant tumors with large temporal suprasellar components, especially dumbbell configuration. Transsphenoidal surgery (TSS) is done with endoscopic or microscopic techniques [21]. Most recently, three-dimensional endoscopic pituitary surgery is being used in some centers as it provides improved depth perception [26].

The floor of the sella is often thinned considerably by the tumor within the sella. Once an opening has been made, the round blade can be used to develop the plane between the sellar dura and the bony floor, and the foot plate of the Kerrison can then be used to further remove the bone. For conchal-type sphenoid sinuses, more bony removal with a drill or ultrasonic bone tip may be required to remove enough bone to view the sella. Great care is taken at the "10 o'clock" and "2 o'clock" positions in the sella to avoid injury to the carotid arteries as they swing medially and anteriorly at the top of the sella. If an extended transsphenoidal approach to suprasellar pathology is indicated, the opening can be extended superiorly and anteriorly into the planum sphenoidale, exposing the dura of the anterior cranial fossa.

Sellar reconstruction may involve harvesting a small piece of fat from the abdomen which is placed in the sphenoid sinus and sella. If there is a sign of a CSF leak, a small piece of fat is placed into the defect for repair and sealed with Tisseel™ tissue sealant or a nasoseptal flap. In cases without a CSF leak, sellar reconstruction may simply consist of placing Durafoam® dural graft over the opening of the sella. Dry gelfoam is then used to pack the sphenoid sinus, supporting this dural graft. Although some rhinologists prefer to place packing within the nasal cavity, we have found no increase in scarring with no packing at all, and this is much appreciated by the patient.

Main postoperative complications of TSS consist of transient diabetes insipidus (up to 20% of cases), while CSF leak and meningitis are exceptional. Permanent postoperative diabetes insipidus is rare in case of pituitary adenomas (1% at one year) but frequent after surgery for craniopharyngiomas. Perioperative TSS mortality is less than 1% in experienced centers.

Radiation Therapy

Radiation therapy is indicated as adjuvant therapy for control of the postoperative tumor residual and achievement or improvement of biochemical control, the latter in patients with functioning tumors. Pituitary radiation can be delivered in two main modalities. Stereotactic radiosurgery (Gamma Knife®, linear accelerator, CyberKnife, or proton beam) consists of high-dose radiation delivered in a single treatment. When normal tissue cannot be safely separated from the tumor, fractionated radiation is used and involves delivery of small doses of radiation daily, over the course of a few weeks. For pituitary tumors, the decisive factor is proximity to the optic nerve in order to reduce the risk of optic neuropathy. Results of radiation treatment vary across published series to continuous technological advances, different radiation doses, as well as different definitions of biochemical cure in different studies. In general, patients with smaller tumors respond better to radiation and have lower risks of complications, which supports the role of debulking surgery before radiation [27]. The main complication of radiotherapy consists of long-term isolated or multiple anterior pituitary hormone deficiencies in 30–50% of patients [28]. Hypopituitarism has been associated with increased cardiovascular and cerebrovascular mortality [29]. This issue has to be revisited in future prospective studies, as glucocorticoid doses used currently are smaller and closer to physiologic production. Also, progress has been made in treatment of hypogonadism and GH deficiency. Secondary tumor formation after pituitary radiation (meningiomas, gliomas) is low (<2%), but higher than in the general population, although there is a bias related to frequent imaging of pituitary tumor patients and there is a lack of proper comparative epidemiological studies [28].

Treatment of NFPA is aimed at controlling tumor growth and decreasing mass effect. TSS is first-line therapy for NFPA and leads to improvement of visual field deficits in 85% of patients. Pituitary microadenomas discovered incidentally can be followed conservatively as their risk of growth is lower than 10% at 10 years. Nonfunctioning macroadenomas that do not cause mass effect symptoms can also be followed with serial MRI scans, but the tumor growth risk is 50% at 5 years [30]. Pituitary incidentalomas that cause significant hormonal abnormalities or vision loss should be treated. Also, surgery should be considered if subsequent evaluation during follow-up indicates tumor enlargement or hormone deficits. TSS improves mass effect symptoms and hormone deficiencies. The main prognostic factor for gross-total tumor resection is lack of invasion of cavernous sinuses preoperatively [6]. Postoperatively, MRI surveillance is recommended at 3 months (Figure 38.1) and periodically thereafter in order to detect possible recurrences.

The recurrence rate after gross-total tumor resection of NFPA is lower than 10% [31]. However, when both progression of postoperative tumor residual and recurrence are considered, the postoperative re-growth rate ranges between 6 and 46% in different studies [30]. Adjuvant radiation is employed in the following situations: significant amount of tumor residual that cannot be safely removed by a reoperation, and aggressive tumors with previous recurrence or histological features of atypia. Both stereotactic radiation in doses of 14–18 Gy and fractionated stereotactic radiation (45–54 Gy) have been successfully used to control the postoperative tumor residual. Studies show that radiation decreases tumor growth to less than 10% [27]. No medical treatment is approved for patients with NFPA although the dopamine agonist cabergoline has been used in small studies with variable results [32].

Treatment of prolactinomas is aimed at normalization of hyperprolactinemia and its consequences, as well as tumor control for macroadenomas. First-line treatment is usually medical with oral dopamine agonists, while surgery is reserved for apoplexy with vision loss, intolerance or resistance to dopamine agonists, women with macroadenomas who wish to pursue pregnancy, or patients who choose to have surgery [18]. Radiation is reserved for rare cases of tumor progression despite treatment with dopamine agonists and surgery. Prolactinomas are the least radiosensitive pituitary adenomas. Currently, in the US, two dopamine agonists are approved, bromocriptine and cabergoline. Cabergoline may result in biochemical control in some tumors resistant to bromocriptine [33] and has a better side effect profile. Although high-dose cabergoline treatment is associated with valvular heart abnormalities in patients with Parkinson disease, studies done in patients with prolactinomas have not raised significant concerns [34]. Further long-term follow-up studies are needed. Echocardiogram should be considered in patients treated for many years with high-dose cabergoline. Recurrence of hyperprolactinemia after stopping the dopamine agonist treatment is a risk; use of cabergoline for more than 2 years and normal MRI scan at the time of discontinuation are potential predictors of normoprolactinemia [35], but should be interpreted with caution. Women successfully treated with dopamine agonists are usually able to achieve pregnancy, which poses a risk for tumor growth due to elevated estrogen levels. With microprolactinoma, the risk of clinical consequences from tumor enlargement is very small (less than 5%), but macroprolactinomas may cause mass effect symptoms in 25–30% of cases. Current recommendations are to stop the dopamine agonist after pregnancy is confirmed and follow the patient clinically and with serial visual fields. If mass effect symptoms occur, MRI should be performed and a decision regarding restarting the dopamine agonist should be taken depending on findings. TSS can also be performed in the second trimester of pregnancy in case of lack of response or intolerance to dopamine agonists [36]. Bromocriptine and cabergoline have not been associated with significant risks to the mother and fetus, but experience with cabergoline is limited [37]. Breastfeeding has not been shown to increase the risk of tumor growth and can be safely pursued in women who do not need dopamine agonists.

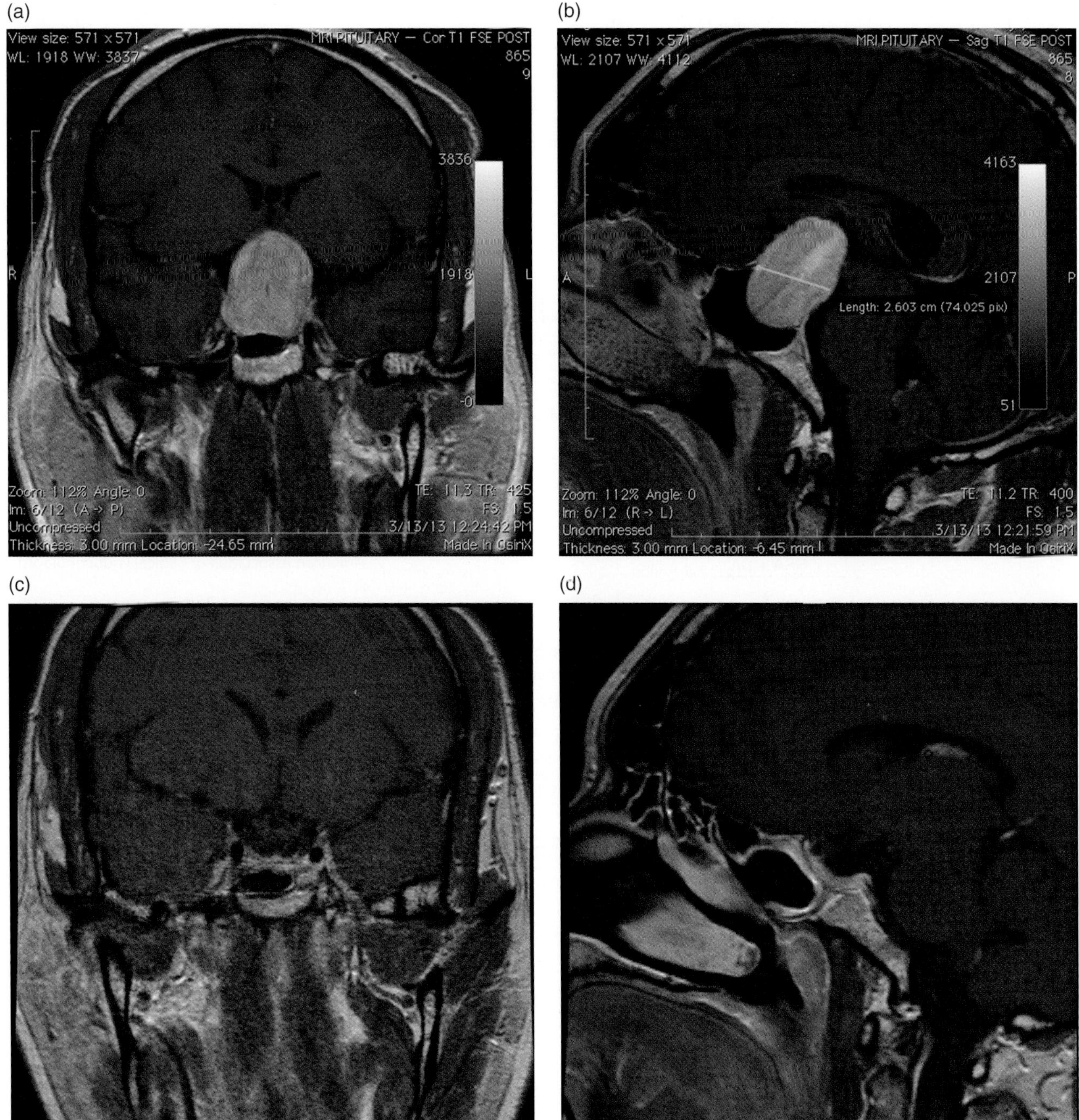

Figure 38.1 MRI scan preoperatively (a, b) and postoperatively (c, d) in a patient with NFPA.

Treatment for acromegaly aims for normalization of biochemical parameters and control/reduction of tumor burden [38]. Biochemical control is associated with improvement of cardiac function, glucose metabolism, sweating, joint pain, and sleep apnea. TSS is the first line of treatment and results in biochemical control in 75–95% of intrasellar adenomas and less than 50% of large and invasive tumors [39–42]. Biochemical recurrence defined by elevated IGF-1 levels occurs in less than 12% of cases after postoperative remission. In patients without postoperative biochemical remission or poor surgical candidates, treatment involves medical treatment with somatostatin analogs, GH-receptor antagonist, and dopamine agonists (Figures 38.2 and 38.3) [20]. As many patients with acromegaly are diagnosed late, they harbor invasive macroadenomas and require multimodality treatment (Figure 38.3).

Medical treatment with long-acting somatostatin analogs (octreotide LAR and lanreotide depot) leads to biochemical normalization in approximately 30% of patients, and tumor reduction by more than 20% in up to 30% of patients [38,43]. These medications are administered monthly as an injection and are usually well tolerated. Main side effects are gastrointestinal in the first few days of treatment, with other side effects including gallstones or biliary sludge formation, glucose metabolism perturbations (hypo- and hyperglycemia), bradycardia,

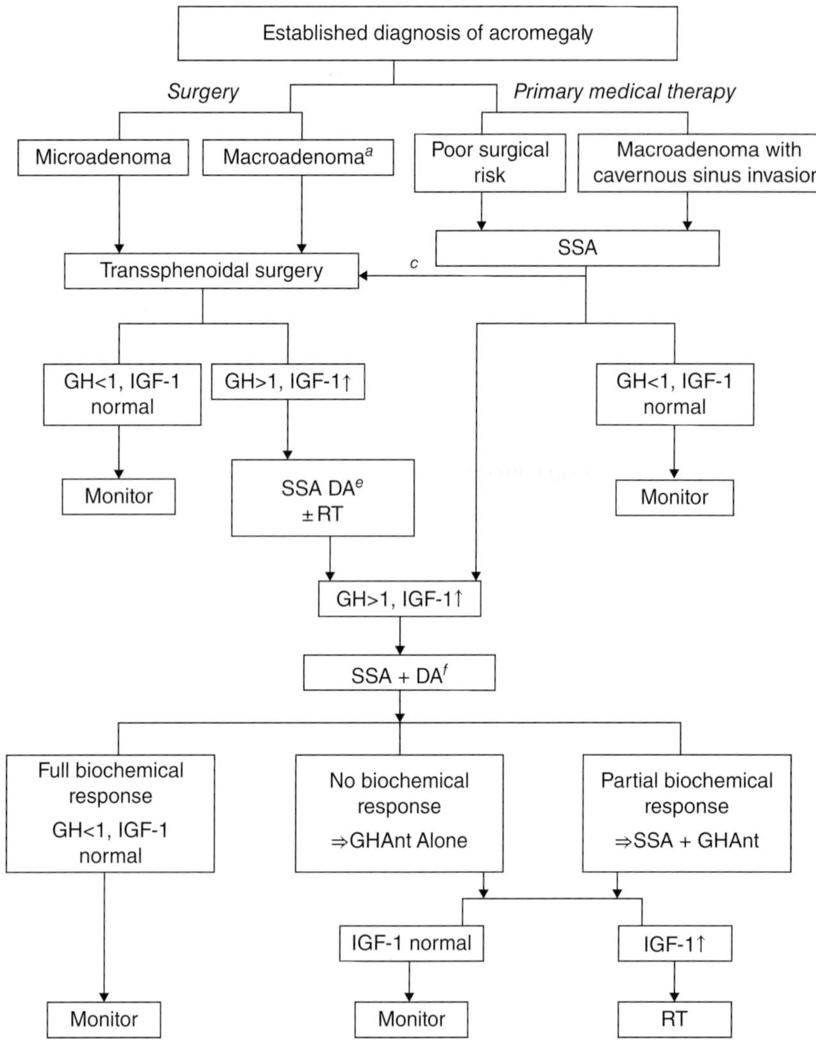

Figure 38.2 American Association of Clinical Endocrinologists guidelines for treatment of acromegaly. *a*, Visual field compromise is absolute indication for surgery. *b*, Primary medical therapy can be considered if there is no visual field deficit and there is no possibility of surgical cure because of cavernous sinus involvement. *c*, Reconsider surgery to debulk tumor to improve response to medical therapy, to reduce medical comorbidities, or to comply with patient preference. *d*, Consider a dopamine agonist (DA) in the setting of modest disease. *e*, Consider radiotherapy (RT) in patients with residual tumor after surgery. This decision is based on several factors, including age, reproductive status, pituitary function, insurance coverage, and patient preference regarding long-term medical therapy. *f*, Addition of a DA in the setting of modest disease. GH, growth hormone; GHant, growth hormone antagonist; IGF-1, insulin-like growth factor; SSA, somatostatin analog. *Source:* Katznelson L, Atkinson JL, Cook DM, Ezzat SZ, Hamrahian AH, Miller KK. American Association of Clinical Endocrinologists medical guidelines for clinical practice for the diagnosis and treatment of acromegaly – 2011 update. *Endocr Pract* 2011;17 Suppl 4:1–44. Reproduced with permission of American Association of Clinical Endocrinologists.

hypothyroidism, and pain at the injection site. Daily subcutaneous injections of the GH-receptor antagonist pegvisomant normalize IGF-1 levels in 63% of patients [44]. GH levels should not be followed during treatment with pegvisomant. The tumor may increase in size while on pegvisomant alone in less than 7% of cases, especially if previous treatment with somatostatin analogs was stopped [45]. Even though combination treatment of somatostatin analogs and pegvisomant is not currently approved by the US Food and Drug Administration (FDA) for treatment of acromegaly, this combination is frequently used in clinical practice with good biochemical results and allows a lower dose of each medication to be used [46]. Side effects from pegvisomant include abnormal liver tests, which should be followed closely in the first few months of therapy, and lipoatrophy at injection sites. Dopamine agonists have not been approved by the FDA for treatment of acromegaly. However, they have been used for many years with varying results. Hyperprolactinemia or prolactin immunostaining are not important in predicting the response. Cabergoline is effective in 33% of patients with acromegaly; mild elevation of IGF-1 level (1–1.5 times above the normal limit) seems to be the most important predictor of success [47]. The combination of cabergoline with somatostatin analogs increases the response rate to 50%. One caveat of cabergoline treatment in acromegaly is that higher doses are necessary compared with prolactinomas, which leads to the need for echocardiographic monitoring. Radiotherapy offers patients with acromegaly the potential for cure or at least reduction of the doses used for medical treatment. Stereotactic radiosurgery in doses of 10–35 Gy has been associated with 48–53% normalization of IGF-1 at 3–10 years [27]. Radiosurgery seems to be more effective with effect occurring earlier than with fractionated radiation. This underlines the role of surgical debulking and tumor shrinkage with somatostatin analogs prior to radiation. Somatostatin analogs should be stopped for 1 month prior to and during radiation treatment to allow maximal uptake of radiation into the tumor.

Treatment for Cushing disease aims for definitive normalization of cortisol levels and tumor growth control. TSS in the hands of an expert neurosurgeon is the first-line therapy and achieves biochemical control in 70–90% cases. Remission rates are excellent for microadenomas (85–90%) and 50–65% for macroadenomas [48]. Postoperative recurrence occurs however in 20–30% of patients, so reoperation or adjuvant treatment with medications or radiation may be necessary. Stereotactic radiosurgery (20–25 Gy) has been associated with 35–80% biochemical remission at 7.5–33 months in different studies. The effect seems to occur

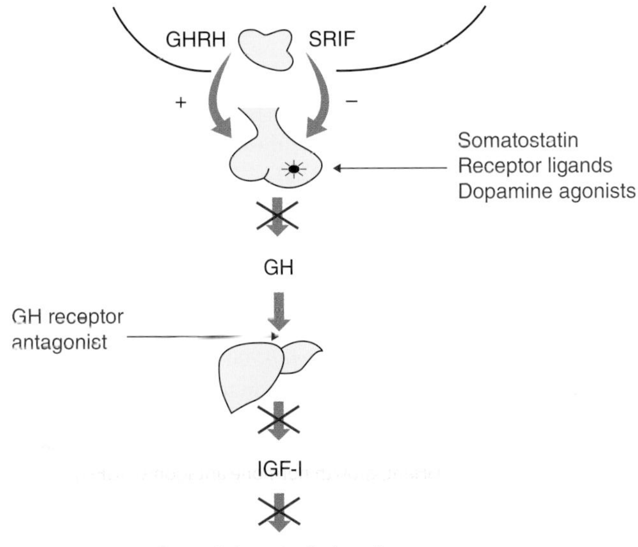

Figure 38.3 Mechanism of action for drugs used to treat acromegaly. Somatostatin receptor ligands and dopamine agonist medications target GH secretion from the pituitary. GH receptor antagonists block GH action at the hepatic receptor. Both therapies act to decrease serum IGF-1 levels. GH, growth hormone; GHRH, growth hormone releasing hormone; IGF-1, insulin-like growth factor; SRIF, somatostatin. *Source:* Carmichael JD, Bonert VS. Medical therapy: options and uses. *Rev Endocr Metab Disord* 2008;9(1):71–81. Reproduced with permission of Springer.

earlier compared to fractionated stereotactic radiation (50–80% at 18–42 months). Local control of tumor growth is excellent for both techniques (less than 10% tumor regrowth) [27]. Although not approved by the FDA for this indication, inhibitors of steroidogenesis have been used for a long time in treatment of Cushing disease while waiting for the effect of radiation. Problems with these medications include potential adrenal insufficiency, adverse effects, and potential for escape and recurrence of hypercortisolemia [49]. Ketoconazole, an imidazole antifungal compound that inhibits several steps of adrenal steroidogenesis, has been used most frequently in patients with Cushing disease and normalizes cortisol in 70% of cases [50]. It may also have a possible direct effect of ACTH inhibition. Side effects include hepatotoxicity, nausea, headaches, and hypogonadism. Metyrapone is not readily available in the US but can be obtained from the manufacturer. It reduces cortisol levels in 75% of patients with Cushing disease. Adverse effects include hypertension, edema, hirsutism, nausea, and dizziness. Mitotane is rarely used for patients with Cushing disease due to gastrointestinal and neurological dose-dependent adverse effects. Etomidate is an intravenous anesthetic agent that rapidly blocks adrenal steroidogenesis and is used in acutely ill hospitalized Cushing patients. Bilateral adrenalectomy has been the last resource for patients with Cushing disease who are not in remission after surgery and radiation. It carries a risk of Nelson syndrome (pituitary tumor growth with mass effect symptoms and skin hyperpigmentation), especially for postoperative tumor residual not treated with radiation. Rising ACTH levels in the first few months after adrenalectomy predict the risk of Nelson syndrome [51]. Recent pharmacological advances have changed the therapeutic paradigm in Cushing disease. Two medications were approved in 2012 for treatment of Cushing disease, including a somatostatin analog with affinity for somatostatin receptor 5 expressed in corticotroph tumors (pasireotide) and a glucocorticoid-receptor blocker (mifepristone). Their place in the Cushing disease treatment algorithm is still to be clarified. Pasireotide administered as twice-a-day subcutaneous injection has been approved after a study of 162 adults with Cushing disease showed significant decrease in urine free cortisol levels and improvement in symptoms [52]. The main side effect of pasireotide is new-onset or worsening hyperglycemia in 70% of patients. Other side effects are similar to the other somatostatin analogs, octreotide and lanreotide. Mifepristone was approved after a 24-week trial of 50 patients with Cushing syndrome, of whom 43 had Cushing disease. Mifepristone significantly improved glucose levels in 60% of patients, as well as diastolic blood pressure, weight, waist circumference, moods, cognition, and quality of life [53]. Although almost 90% of patients experienced side effects (nausea, fatigue, headache, hypokalemia, and endometrial thickening in women), these were mild or moderate and did not lead to discontinuation of the drug in most cases. Important to note, cortisol levels increase significantly during treatment with mifepristone and have no role in dosage adjustments.

Treatment of Aggressive Pituitary Adenomas

Although rare, locally aggressive pituitary adenomas and pituitary carcinomas are challenging to treat and carry a poor prognosis. They are characterized by an increased cell proliferation rate and regrowth despite multimodality treatment. Surgery is the mainstay for management, although repeated attempts at debulking are usually necessary as tumor regrowth and cavernous tumor invasion are usually present [54]. Radiotherapy is often used but with less success to prevent tumor regrowth in these patients compared to the non-aggressive adenomas. Dopamine agonists have been tried and some case reports suggest tumor arrest or shrinkage with high-dose cabergoline, but others showed no response. Temozolomide is a second-generation oral alkylating agent that impairs DNA replication and induces apoptosis by methylating DNA. Although only approved for treatment of glioblastoma, temozolomide has been used anecdotally in pituitary tumors resistant to multimodality therapy [55]. In general, tumors with high levels of O^6-methylguanine-DNA methyltransferase (*MGMT*) expression seem to be less responsive to temozolomide, although recent studies in patients with pituitary tumors seem to show a predictive value of only 53% [55]. Craniopharyngiomas can be locally aggressive with potential for regrowth and may require multiple surgeries and radiation. The hormonal deficiencies present preoperatively usually do not resolve as a result of surgery, and postoperative recurrences decrease the patient's survival [56].

Regardless of pituitary tumor type, isolated or multiple pituitary hormone deficiencies may occur in up to 50% of patients 5–10 years after pituitary radiation.

Conclusion

In summary, pituitary tumors require a multidisciplinary approach to achieve hormonal and tumor control and to detect recurrences in a timely fashion.

References

1 Freda PU, Beckers AM, Katznelson L, *et al.* Pituitary incidentaloma: an endocrine society clinical practice guideline. *J Clin Endocrinol Metab* 2011;96(4):894–904.

2 Gittleman H, Ostrom QT, Farah PD, *et al.* Descriptive epidemiology of pituitary tumors in the United States, 2004-2009. *J Neurosurg* 2014;121(3):527–35.

3 Heaney AP. Clinical review: Pituitary carcinoma: difficult diagnosis and treatment. *J Clin Endocrinol Metab* 2011;96(12):3649–60.

4 Sherlock M, Ayuk J, Tomlinson JW, *et al.* Mortality in patients with pituitary disease. *Endocr Rev* 2010;31(3):301–42.

5 Clayton RN, Raskauskiene D, Reulen RC, Jones PW. Mortality and morbidity in Cushing's disease over 50 years in Stoke-on-Trent, UK: audit and meta-analysis of literature. *J Clin Endocrinol Metab* 2011;96(3):632–42.

6 Chang EF, Zada G, Kim S, Lamborn KR, *et al.* Long-term recurrence and mortality after surgery and adjuvant radiotherapy for nonfunctional pituitary adenomas. *J Neurosurg* 2008;108(4):736–45.

7 Pasquel FJ, Vincentelli C, Brat DJ, Oyesiku NM, Ioachimescu AG. Pituitary carcinoma in situ. Endocr Pract 2013:1–15.

8 Asa SL, Ezzat S. The pathogenesis of pituitary tumors. *Annu Rev Pathol* 2009;4:97–126.

9 D'Angelo D, Palmieri D, Mussnich P, *et al.* Altered microRNA expression profile in human pituitary GH adenomas: down-regulation of miRNA targeting HMGA1, HMGA2, and E2F1. *J Clin Endocrinol Metab* 2012;97(7):E1128–38.

10 Evans CO, Reddy P, Brat DJ, *et al.* Differential expression of folate receptor in pituitary adenomas. *Cancer Res* 2003;63(14):4218–24.

11 Evans CO, Young AN, Brown MR, *et al.* Novel patterns of gene expression in pituitary adenomas identified by complementary deoxyribonucleic acid microarrays and quantitative reverse transcription-polymerase chain reaction. *J Clin Endocrinol Metab* 2001;86(7):3097–107.

12 Cuny T, Pertuit M, Sahnoun-Fathallah M, *et al.* Genetic analysis in young patients with sporadic pituitary macroadenomas: besides AIP don't forget MEN1 genetic analysis. *Eur J Endocrinol* 2013;168(4):533–41.

13 Daly AF, Beckers A. Familial isolated pituitary adenomas (FIPA) and mutations in the aryl hydrocarbon receptor interacting protein (AIP) gene. *Endocrinol Metab Clin North Am* 2015;44(1):19–25.

14 Zada G, Woodmansee WW, Ramkissoon S, *et al.* Atypical pituitary adenomas: incidence, clinical characteristics, and implications. *J Neurosurg* 2011;114(2):336–44.

15 Sav A, Rotondo F, Syro LV, *et al.* Invasive, atypical and aggressive pituitary adenomas and carcinomas. *Endocrinol Metab Clin North Am* 2015;44(1):99–104.

16 Briet C, Salenave S, Chanson P. Pituitary apoplexy. *Endocrinol Metab Clin North Am* 2015;44(1):199–209.

17 Randeva HS, Schoebel J, Byrne J, *et al.* Classical pituitary apoplexy: clinical features, management and outcome. *Clin Endocrinol (Oxf)* 1999;51(2):181–8.

18 Melmed S, Casanueva FF, Hoffman AR, *et al.*Diagnosis and treatment of hyperprolactinemia: an Endocrine Society clinical practice guideline. *J Clin Endocrinol Metab* 2011;96(2):273–88.

19 Fleseriu M, Lee M, Pineyro MM, Skugor M, Reddy SK, Siraj ES, Hamrahian AH: Giant invasive pituitary prolactinoma with falsely low serum prolactin: the significance of 'hook effect'. *J Neurooncol* 2006, 79(1):41–43.

20 Katznelson L, Laws ER, Jr, Melmed S, *et al.* Acromegaly: an Endocrine Society clinical practice guideline. *J Clin Endocrinol Metab* 2014;99(11):3933–51.

21 Nieman LK, Biller BM, Findling JW, *et al.* The diagnosis of Cushing's syndrome: an Endocrine Society Clinical Practice Guideline. *J Clin Endocrinol Metab* 2008;93(5):1526–40.

22 Raff H. Cushing syndrome: update on testing. *Endocrinol Metab Clin North Am* 2015;44(1):43–50.

23 Utz A, Biller BM. The role of bilateral inferior petrosal sinus sampling in the diagnosis of Cushing's syndrome. *Arq Bras Endocrinol Metabol* 2007;51(8):1329–38.

24 Azzalin A, Appin CL, Schniederjan MJ, *et al.* Comprehensive evaluation of thyrotropinomas: single-center 20-year experience. *Pituitary* 2016;19(2):183–93.

25 Beck-Peccoz P, Persani L, Mannavola D, Campi I. Pituitary tumours: TSH-secreting adenomas. *Best Pract Res Clin Endocrinol Metab* 2009;23(5):597–606.

26 Kari E, Oyesiku NM, Dadashev V, Wise SK. Comparison of traditional 2-dimensional endoscopic pituitary surgery with new 3-dimensional endoscopic technology: intraoperative and early postoperative factors. *Int Forum Allergy Rhinol* 2012;2(1):2–8.

27 Loeffler JS, Shih HA. Radiation therapy in the management of pituitary adenomas. *J Clin Endocrinol Metab* 2011;96(7):1992–2003.

28 Gittoes NJ. Pituitary radiotherapy: current controversies. *Trends Endocrinol Metab* 2005;16(9):407–13.

29 Tomlinson JW, Holden N, Hills RK, *et al.* Association between premature mortality and hypopituitarism. West Midlands Prospective Hypopituitary Study Group. *Lancet* 2001;357(9254):425–31.

30 Dekkers OM, Pereira AM, Romijn JA. Treatment and follow-up of clinically nonfunctioning pituitary macroadenomas. *J Clin Endocrinol Metab* 2008;93(10):3717–26.

31 Ioachimescu AG, Eiland L, Chhabra VS, *et al.* Silent corticotroph adenomas: Emory University cohort and comparison with ACTH-negative nonfunctioning pituitary adenomas. *Neurosurgery* 2012;71(2):296–303; discussion 304.

32 Garcia EC, Naves LA, Silva AO, *et al.* Short-term treatment with cabergoline can lead to tumor shrinkage in patients with nonfunctioning pituitary adenomas. *Pituitary* 2013;16(2):189–94.

33 Colao A, Di Sarno A, Sarnacchiaro F, *et al.* Prolactinomas resistant to standard dopamine agonists respond to chronic cabergoline treatment. *J Clin Endocrinol Metab* 1997;82(3):876–83.

34 Kars M, Pereira AM, Bax JJ, Romijn JA. Cabergoline and cardiac valve disease in prolactinoma patients: additional studies during long-term treatment are required. *Eur J Endocrinol* 2008;159(4):363–7.

35 Dekkers OM, Lagro J, Burman P, *et al.* Recurrence of hyperprolactinemia after withdrawal of dopamine agonists:

systematic review and meta-analysis. *J Clin Endocrinol Metab* 2010;95(1):43–51.

36 Molitch ME. Pituitary disorders during pregnancy. *Endocrinol Metab Clin North Am* 2006;35(1):99–116, vi.

37 Colao A, Abs R, Barcena DG, *et al.* Pregnancy outcomes following cabergoline treatment: extended results from a 12-year observational study. *Clin Endocrinol (Oxf)* 2008;68(1):66–71.

38 Plockinger U. Medical therapy of acromegaly. *Int J Endocrinol* 2012;2012:268957.

39 Anthony JR, Ioachimescu AG. Acromegaly and bone disease. *Curr Opin Endocrinol Diabetes Obes* 2014;21(6):476–82.

40 Biermasz NR, van Dulken H, Roelfsema F. Ten-year follow-up results of transsphenoidal microsurgery in acromegaly. *J Clin Endocrinol Metab* 2000;85(12):4596–602.

41 Kreutzer J, Vance ML, Lopes MB, Laws ER, Jr. Surgical management of GH-secreting pituitary adenomas: an outcome study using modern remission criteria. *J Clin Endocrinol Metab* 2001;86(9):4072–7.

42 Marquez Y, Tuchman A, Zada G. Surgery and radiosurgery for acromegaly: a review of indications, operative techniques, outcomes, and complications. *Int J Endocrinol* 2012;2012:386401.

43 Colao A, Bronstein MD, Freda P, *et al.* Pasireotide versus octreotide in acromegaly: a head-to-head superiority study. *J Clin Endocrinol Metab* 2014;99(3):791–9.

44 van der Lely AJ, Biller BM, Brue T, *et al.* Long-term safety of pegvisomant in patients with acromegaly: comprehensive review of 1288 subjects in ACROSTUDY. *J Clin Endocrinol Metab* 2012;97(5):1589–97.

45 Marazuela M, Paniagua AE, Gahete MD, *et al.* Somatotroph tumor progression during pegvisomant therapy: a clinical and molecular study. *J Clin Endocrinol Metab* 2011;96(2):E251–9.

46 Neggers SJ, de Herder WW, Janssen JA, Feelders RA, van der Lely AJ. Combined treatment for acromegaly with long-acting somatostatin analogs and pegvisomant: long-term safety for up to 4.5 years (median 2.2 years) of follow-up in 86 patients. *Eur J Endocrinol* 2009;160(4):529–33.

47 Sandret L, Maison P, Chanson P. Place of cabergoline in acromegaly: a meta-analysis. *J Clin Endocrinol Metab* 2011;96(5):1327–35.

48 Buchfelder M, Schlaffer S. Pituitary surgery for Cushing's disease. *Neuroendocrinology* 2010;92 Suppl 1:102–6.

49 Tritos NA, Biller BM. Advances in medical therapies for Cushing's syndrome. *Discov Med* 2012;13(69):171–9.

50 Feelders RA, Hofland LJ, de Herder WW. Medical treatment of Cushing's syndrome: adrenal-blocking drugs and ketaconazole. *Neuroendocrinology* 2010;92 Suppl 1:111–5.

51 Assie G, Bahurel H, Coste J, *et al.* Corticotroph tumor progression after adrenalectomy in Cushing's Disease: A reappraisal of Nelson's Syndrome. *J Clin Endocrinol Metab* 2007;92(1):172–9.

52 Colao A, Petersenn S, Newell-Price J, *et al.* A 12-month phase 3 study of pasireotide in Cushing's disease. *N Engl J Med* 2012;366(10):914–24.

53 Fleseriu M, Biller BM, Findling JW, *et al.* Mifepristone, a glucocorticoid receptor antagonist, produces clinical and metabolic benefits in patients with Cushing's syndrome. *J Clin Endocrinol Metab* 2012;97(6):2039–49.

54 Miller BA, Rutledge WC, Ioachimescu AG, Oyesiku NM. Management of large aggressive nonfunctional pituitary tumors: experimental medical options when surgery and radiation fail. *Neurosurg Clin N Am* 2012;23(4):587–94.

55 Syro LV, Ortiz LD, Scheithauer BW, *et al.* Treatment of pituitary neoplasms with temozolomide: a review. *Cancer* 2011;117(3):454–62.

56 Karavitaki N, Brufani C, Warner JT, *et al.* Craniopharyngiomas in children and adults: systematic analysis of 121 cases with long-term follow-up. *Clin Endocrinol (Oxf)* 2005;62(4):397–409.

39

Gastroenteropancreatic Neuroendocrine Tumors

Jonathan Strosberg

H. Lee Moffitt Cancer Center and Research Institute, Tampa, Florida, USA

Introduction

Neuroendocrine tumors (NETs) arise in the diffuse neuroendocrine system and are characterized by the ability to synthesize, store, and secrete a variety of neuroamines and peptides. Gastroenteropancreatic neuroendocrine tumors (GEP-NETs) include carcinoid tumors of the luminal gastrointestinal tract and pancreatic neuroendocrine tumors. Carcinoid tumors originate from endocrine (enterochromaffin) cells of the gut. The name "carcinoid" means "cancer-like," although it is now clear that "carcinoid" is a misnomer given the malignant potential of most small bowel NETs. Pancreatic neuroendocrine tumors are thought to arise in the islets of Langerhans, although recent evidence suggests that some originate in ductal cells and acquire neuroendocrine differentiation [1].

Efforts to replace the term "carcinoid tumor" with "neuroendocrine tumor" have been somewhat unsuccessful: the term "carcinoid" continues to be used to describe NETs originating in the gastrointestinal tract. However, the terms "pancreatic carcinoid" and "islet cell tumor' have largely disappeared from the literature, and have been replaced by the term "pancreatic neuroendocrine tumor," or pNET [2].

There has also been much debate over use of the term "tumor" versus "carcinoma." This controversy arises from the fact that there are no reliable pathologic criteria to distinguish benign from malignant low-grade NETs. A concern is that "carcinoma" may be an inappropriate description for localized tumors of low malignant potential, whereas "tumor" or "neoplasm" may be an inadequate term to describe malignant tumors that have metastasized. The current World Health Organization (WHO) guidelines recommend use of the term "neuroendocrine tumor" for patients with well-differentiated tumors regardless of stage, and "neuroendocrine carcinoma" for patients with poorly differentiated or high-grade cancers [3].

Multiple classifications have been developed for GEP-NETs. In 1963, Williams and Sandler categorized carcinoid tumors based on embryonic derivation, distinguishing between foregut (gastroduodenal), midgut (jejunal, ileal, cecal), and hindgut (distal colic and rectal) tumors [4]. As a rule of thumb, midgut carcinoid tumors are associated with the classical carcinoid syndrome whereas hindgut tumors are hormonally silent. Foregut tumors may be associated with atypical hormonal syndromes. While this embryological classification has some utility, it is somewhat oversimplified. For example, carcinoid tumors of the ileocecum have a substantially higher metastatic potential than carcinoid tumors of the appendix despite sharing a midgut origin. Likewise, colonic neuroendocrine tumors are, on average, more aggressive than rectal NETs which tend to be small and superficial.

Another classification scheme is based on hormonal output. Functional tumors are defined by the presence of a clinical syndrome caused by excess hormone secretion, whereas nonfunctional tumors are nonsecretory. For example, a pancreatic NET that produces insulin resulting in hypoglycemia is called an "insulinoma." It is important to note that tumors should only be described as functional if they produce signs and symptoms consistent with hormonal secretion. It is a common error of terminology to define a tumor as functional (e.g., "insulinoma" or "gastrinoma") simply because insulin or gastrin is detected by immunohistochemical (IHC) staining [5].

Tumor differentiation and grade are important prognostic and predictive factors. While used interchangeably in characterizing many other neoplasms, differentiation and grade have different meanings in the context of NETs: differentiation refers to the resemblance between the morphology of the tumor and tissue of origin, whereas tumor grade of a NET is measured through markers of cell proliferation such as mitotic rate and Ki-67 index. Well-differentiated NETs consist of small monomorphic cells arranged in islets or trabeculae with a "salt and pepper" chromatin pattern. In contrast, poorly differentiated NETs are often characterized as sheets of pleomorphic cells with extensive necrosis. Tumor grades are defined numerically with low-grade tumors having a mitotic rate of 0–1 per 10 high powered fields (HPF) or Ki-67 index of 0–2%, intermediate-grade tumors having a mitotic rate of 2–20 or Ki-67 index of 3–20%, and high-grade tumors having a mitotic rate or Ki-67 index >20 [2]. In the 2010 WHO classification, well-differentiated tumors are subdivided as either low- or intermediate-grade

The American Cancer Society's Oncology in Practice: Clinical Management, First Edition. Edited by The American Cancer Society.

whereas poorly differentiated tumors are considered equivalent to high-grade. There are several pitfalls in this classification. One is that it negates the possibility of a well-differentiated high-grade tumor, an entity which clearly exists (poorly differentiated low-grade tumors are less common) [6]. Another flaw of a numerical grading classification is that there can be significant heterogeneity in mitotic activity between different tumors within the same patient and even within a particular tumor [7]. Despite these concerns, current grading systems have proven to be prognostic in multiple studies.

Formal TNM staging classifications have recently been introduced for GEP-NETs [8–10]. The European Neuroendocrine Tumor Society (ENETS) and the American Joint Committee on Cancer (AJCC) have designed staging systems that are similar but not identical. Validations of both staging systems have been performed on population and institutional databases with some evidence suggesting that the ENETS classification may have a slightly higher prognostic relevance [11]. As a general rule, early-stage tumors of all primary sites are associated with a very favorable long-term prognosis whereas the prognosis of patients with distant metastases (stage IV) depends both on tumor grade and primary site. Stage IV NETs originating in the midgut (ileocecum) tend to have significantly higher 5- and 10-year survival rates compared to stage IV colorectal or pancreatic NETs.

Clinical Features of GEP-NETs

GEP-NETs are heterogeneous neoplasms. Rates and locations of metastatic spread, patterns of hormonal secretion, and survival outcomes vary significantly between tumors of different primary sites. It is increasingly apparent that underlying differences in tumor biology explain this variability.

Midgut Neuroendocrine (Carcinoid) Tumors

Jejunal and ileocecal NETs arise from epithelial enterochromaffin cells. Most small intestinal NETs originate within 60 cm of the ileocecal valve where the concentration of enterochromaffin cells is highest [12]. Approximately 25% of patients have multifocal tumors at time of diagnosis, often clustered in close proximity to each other [13]. Malignant potential correlates strongly with tumor size, however even tumors smaller than 1 cm can metastasize [14]. The most frequent sites of distant spread are the liver, mesentery, bone, and peritoneum [15]. Lymph node metastases at the root of the mesentery are common, and may be associated with dense desmoplastic fibrosis, causing tethering of the bowel and mesenteric ischemia [16].

Most midgut NETs produce serotonin and other vasoactive substances which can result in the typical carcinoid syndrome [17]. Serotonin is derived from the amino acid tryptophan, and is enzymatically inactivated in the liver into 5-hydroxyindoleacetic acid (5-HIAA), a urinary metabolite [18,19]. Consequently, the carcinoid syndrome occurs in patients with metastatic tumors that secrete serotonin directly into the systemic (rather than portal) circulation. Other vasoactive substances elaborated by carcinoid tumors include biogenic amines (e.g., dopamine, histamine, and hydroxytryptophan), tachykinins (substance P, kallikrein), and prostaglandins [20].

In an analysis of 91 patients with the carcinoid syndrome, diarrhea, flushing, and bronchospasm occurred in 73%, 65%, and 8% of patients, respectively [21]. Diarrhea is thought to be a direct effect of serotonin which stimulates peristalsis and affects electrolyte and fluid secretion via 5-HT2A receptors [22]. The flushing phenomenon is attributable to multiple vasoactive substances including prostaglandins and tachykinins [23–25]. Flushing typically involves the face, neck, and upper torso, and may be precipitated by stress, alcohol, and tyramine-containing foods or spices. Patients with chronic flushing may develop facial telangiectasias resembling rosacea.

Carcinoid heart disease (CHD) typically occurs in patients with high levels of circulating serotonin. Fibrosis and thickening of right-sided cardiac valves results in tricuspid regurgitation and pulmonary valve stenosis [26]. The right heart is usually affected due to its direct exposure to serotonin secreted by liver metastases, whereas left heart valves are clinically involved in fewer than 10% of CHD cases [27]. The incidence of CHD appears to be diminishing, possibly due to use of serotonin-inhibiting therapies [15,28].

Common symptoms related to primary intestinal tumors include abdominal pain, which can be crampy and intermittent, or bowel obstruction [29]. Patients with liver metastases can present with hormonal symptoms such as flushing and diarrhea, or tumor-burden related symptoms such as abdominal pain, weight loss, fatigue, and early satiety. Increasing numbers of patients are diagnosed incidentally after undergoing radiographic or endoscopic procedures for other indications [13]. The slowly progressive nature of midgut NETs can result in delayed diagnoses occurring years after onset of symptoms; however some sources document a median time to diagnosis of less than 6 months [30].

The large majority of midgut NETs are well-differentiated with low mitotic activity. Despite their high propensity to metastasize, ileocecal NETs are associated with a relatively favorable long-term prognosis, even among patients with stage IV disease. Early-stage tumors have 5-year survival rates approaching 100% after potentially curative resection [13,31–34]. Patients with metastatic tumors have 5-year survival rates ranging from 50% in national databases such as Surveillance, Epidemiology and End Results (SEER) registry to roughly 75% in large institutional databases [13,32,33].

Gastroduodenal Carcinoid Tumors

Gastric carcinoid tumors arise from subepithelial histamine-secreting endocrine cells termed "enterochromaffin-like" (ECL) cells [35]. Gastric carcinoid tumors can develop sporadically, but more commonly develop due to the trophic effects of elevated serum gastrin. Three distinct types have been identified.

Type I tumors occur in patients with chronic atrophic gastritis and account for about 80% of gastric carcinoids [36–38]. In this condition, chronic gastric achlorhydria stimulates G cells of the antrum to produce excess serum gastrin. Gastrin, in turn, simulates ECL hyperplasia and development of multifocal, polypoid carcinoid tumors. These tumors generally behave in a benign fashion; however metastases have been reported to occur in approximately 5% of patients [39]. The diagnosed incidence of type I gastric carcinoid tumors has been rising as rates of upper endoscopy in the general population increase [36]. Most guidelines recommend a conservative approach to type I gastric carcinoid tumors and favor endoscopic surveillance every 6–12 months with snare polypectomy of tumors [40–42]. Rarely, antrectomy is recommended to eliminate the underlying gastrin stimulus in patients with widespread progressive tumors [43]. Given the indolent natural history of type I gastric carcinoid tumors, it is unclear whether any surveillance or intervention truly improves outcomes.

Type II gastric carcinoid tumors also arise in the setting of elevated serum gastrin. In these rare tumors, elevated gastrin is produced by pancreatic or duodenal gastrinomas, typically in the setting of multiple endocrine neoplasia type 1 (MEN1) [44]. As is the case with type I disease, tumors tend to be small, multifocal, and clinically indolent. Patients with type II gastric NETs will usually have underlying symptoms of Zollinger–Ellison syndrome such as diarrhea, heartburn, and peptic ulceration as well as radiographic evidence of an underlying gastrinoma. However, it is occasionally difficult to distinguish type I from type II tumors since both are associated with elevated serum gastrin. Biopsy of non-neoplastic mucosa to document presence or absence of atrophic gastritis, and measurement of gastric pH (high in type I, low in type II) can be useful [45]. Management of type II gastric carcinoid tumors is also conservative. Tumors often regress with successful treatment of the underlying gastrinoma.

Sporadic gastric carcinoid tumors (type III) occur in fewer than 15% of cases and are not associated with elevated gastrin levels. These tumors have a much higher malignant potential than type I or type II tumors. Locally advanced cases are usually managed with radical gastrectomy. Recent data suggest that small, superficial type III tumors can be managed with endoscopic resections and careful surveillance [46].

There are relatively few data describing duodenal carcinoid tumors. They are often detected incidentally and are usually located in the duodenal bulb [47,48]. Hormonally functioning duodenal carcinoid tumors are uncommon.

Appendiceal Carcinoid Tumors

Carcinoid tumors of the appendix are found in approximately 1 in 300 appendectomy specimens, nearly always incidentally during surgery for appendicitis [49,50]. They typically arise from submucosal endocrine cells at the tip of the appendix. Median age at presentation is approximately 40 with a female predominance. Tumor size is the most important prognostic factor for development of metastases. In one large series of patients, no metastases were observed in 127 patients whose tumors were smaller than 2 cm in diameter [49]. Consequently, simple appendectomy was considered sufficient treatment for patients with tumors <2 cm in size, whereas completion right hemicolectomy was recommended for larger tumors. In recent years, there have been reports of patients with tumors 1–2 cm in diameter who developed locoregional or distant metastases [51]. The risk of malignant spread appears to correlate with invasion into the mesoappendix. Consequently, hemicolectomy can be considered for select patients with tumors of intermediate size (1–2 cm) based on depth of invasion [52].

Colorectal Carcinoid Tumors

More than half of rectal carcinoid tumors are detected incidentally during lower endoscopy [53]. The remainder present with rectal bleeding, pain, or change in bowel habits. Rectal carcinoid tumors are hormonally inactive and almost never produce the carcinoid syndrome. Most arise in the mid-rectum approximately 5–10 cm from the anal verge and are submucosal in location. Malignant potential closely correlates with size; tumors under 1 cm in diameter rarely metastasize and can usually be resected endoscopically or transanally, whereas tumors larger than 2 cm metastasize in over 50% of cases [54,55]. The metastatic potential of intermediate size tumors appears to correlate with invasion of the muscularis propria.

Colonic NETs distal to the cecum tend to be more aggressive than rectal tumors and are often poorly differentiated [56]. Unlike rectal carcinoid tumors which are usually localized, colonic NETs are distributed in roughly equal numbers between local, regional, and metastatic stage. Once they have metastasized, NETs of the colon and rectum tend to behave more aggressively than midgut NETs [57].

Pancreatic Neuroendocrine Tumors

Pancreatic NETs are heterogeneous neoplasms that can secrete a variety of peptide hormones and biogenic amines including insulin, gastrin, glucagon, vasoactive intestinal peptide (VIP), serotonin, somatostatin, and parathyroid hormone. In contemporary clinical series, fewer than 25% of tumors are hormonally functional [58,59]. Insulinomas and gastrinomas are the most common functional subtypes with an annual incidence of 1–4 cases per million. The incidence of rarer subtypes such as VIPomas and glucagonomas is estimated to be less than one per 10 million [60].

Insulinomas

About 90% of insulinomas are smaller than 2 cm and fewer than 10% are considered malignant, although it is unclear whether the remainder are truly benign, or of very low malignant potential [61]. Patients typically present with neuroglycopenic symptoms such as lethargy, confusion, dizziness, diplopia, palpitations, and diaphoresis. The classical diagnostic "Whipple triad" consists of symptomatic hypoglycemia, low blood glucose levels, and relief of symptoms with glucose administration [62]. Diagnosis often requires a monitored fast where serum glucose is measured along with insulin, proinsulin, and C-peptide in order to demonstrate hypoglycemia (glucose <45 mg/dL) associated with inappropriate levels of insulin or proinsulin and C-peptide [61].

Gastrinomas

Gastrinomas originate in the duodenum and the pancreas, typically within the "gastrinoma triangle" bounded by the porta hepatis, the border of the second and third parts of the duodenum, and pancreatic head and neck. Tumors of pancreatic origin are more likely to metastasize than duodenal ones [63–65]. The MEN1 syndrome is implicated in about 20% of cases and is associated with tumor multifocality. The gastrinoma syndrome, characterized by peptic ulceration, heartburn, and diarrhea, was first described in 1955 by Zollinger and Ellison [66]. The syndrome is caused by secretion of gastrin, which stimulates the parietal cells of the stomach to produce excess gastric acid. Peptic ulcerations primarily impact the first part of the duodenum, but can also affect atypical locations such as the distal duodenum and upper jejunum. Severe and persistent diarrhea may occur due to the passage of excess gastric acid into the small intestine, neutralizing pancreatic bicarbonate secretion and causing malabsorption [67].

The diagnosis of gastrinoma can be established with measurement of fasting serum gastrin exceeding ten times the upper limit of normal (i.e., >1,000 pg/mL). It is important to note that proton pump inhibitors elevate serum gastrin levels leading to false positive diagnoses. In cases where the diagnosis is equivocal, a secretin stimulation test can help identify gastrinomas: a serum gastrin rise of >200 pg/mL is considered diagnostic [68]. Prior to the advent of acid-blocking medications, the Zollinger–Ellison syndrome was a highly morbid condition necessitating palliative gastrectomy or vagotomy. Today, high-dose proton pump inhibitors effectively control symptoms in the majority of cases [69].

VIPomas

VIPomas typically originate in the tail of the pancreas and secrete vasoactive intestinal peptide (VIP). VIP stimulates intestinal secretion and inhibits electrolyte and water absorption. The resulting syndrome (also known as the Verner–Morrison syndrome) is characterized by profuse watery diarrhea, often exceeding 3 L/day [70]. Other complications include hypochlorhydria, hypokalemia, and dehydration [71,72].

Glucagonomas

Glucagonomas originate in the alpha cells of the pancreas. Clinical manifestations include hyperglycemia, weight loss, venous thromboses, cheilitis, glossitis, and an unusual rash called necrolytic migratory erythema (NME) [73,74]. NME characteristically manifests as erythematous papules or plaques involving the face, lower extremities, perineum, and flexural regions [75]. The underlying cause of NME is uncertain, but may be related to amino-acid or zinc deficiency [76,77]. Cachexia and hyperglycemia are attributable to the catabolic effects of glucagon.

Nonfunctioning Pancreatic NETs

In modern clinical series, the majority of pancreatic NETs are not associated with a hormonal syndrome. Primary tumors may be detected as a result of tumor growth causing impingement of adjacent structures and leading to symptoms such as weight loss, abdominal pain, and jaundice [60]. Most patients are diagnosed in the metastatic setting with the liver being the most common site of distant spread, followed by retroperitoneum and bone [78]. Increasingly, nonfunctioning tumors are discovered incidentally in patients who undergo radiographic or endoscopic evaluations for unrelated conditions [79]. Incidentally detected tumors are often small, localized, and of uncertain clinical significance.

Incidence

In a series of 35,618 carcinoid tumors reported to the United States National Cancer Institute's SEER registry, the reported annual age-adjusted incidence rate grew from 1.1/100,000 in 1973 to 5.25/100,000 in 2004 [33]. The expansion in diagnoses is likely related to an increase in imaging and endoscopic procedures as well as improved recognition of neuroendocrine histology. Similar increases in incidence rates were found in a Swedish national database [80].

In the SEER database, carcinoid tumors of the midgut and rectum were the most common primary site within the gastrointestinal tract with an annual incidence rate of nearly 1/100,000 [33]. Midgut carcinoid tumors occurred most commonly in Caucasian patients whereas rectal tumors developed predominantly in African American, Asian, and Native American patients. Female patients were more likely to develop carcinoid tumors in the stomach, appendix, or cecum, whereas male patients were more likely to develop tumors in the jejunum-ileum, thymus, duodenum, and rectum. The median age at diagnosis was 66 for midgut NETs, 56 for rectal NETs, and 47 for appendiceal NETs.

In the SEER database, 29% of patients with jejunal/ileal tumors had localized disease, 41% had locoregional disease, and 30% had distant metastases at time of diagnosis. In sharp contrast, 92% of rectal tumors, 76% of gastric tumors, and 60% of appendiceal tumors were localized at diagnosis. The frequency of local tumors in locations such as the appendix may have been underestimated in the SEER registry given the fact that many tumors were considered benign and therefore not reported.

The incidence of pancreatic NETs reported to the SEER registry also increased between 1973 and 2000 [59]. The crude annual incidence rate per 1,000,000 was 1.8 in females and 2.6 in males. At diagnosis 11% of tumors were localized, 21% were locally advanced, and 60% were metastatic. However, it is important to note that small localized tumors may have been considered benign and were therefore underreported. The majority of tumors (90%) were considered hormonally nonfunctional.

Tumor Biology and Genetic Syndromes

Although the large majority of GEP-NETs are sporadic, several hereditary syndromes have been identified which illuminate underlying oncogenic pathways associated with both familial and sporadic tumors. Multiple endocrine neoplasia type 1 (MEN1) is an autosomal dominant syndrome characterized by a predisposition to tumors of the anterior pituitary, parathyroid glands, and pancreaticoduodenal neuroendocrine cells [81]. The underlying tumor suppressor gene mutation has been identified in the long arm of chromosome 11 (11q13) [82,83]. *MEN1* encodes for menin, a nuclear protein that is a component of the histone methyltransferase (HMT) complex and regulates gene transcription through chromatin remodeling [84].

The most common manifestation of MEN1 is parathyroid hyperplasia, which typically develops around the third decade. Pituitary adenomas are observed in roughly 20% of patients. Pancreatic NETs, most commonly gastrinomas and nonfunctioning tumors, become clinically apparent in about one-third of patients, with a higher rate of subclinical disease. Tumors are almost invariably multifocal; consequently, the role of curative surgical therapy is controversial [85,86]. Most pancreatic tumors associated with MEN1 are exceptionally slow-growing and life expectancy appears to be only modestly diminished by this syndrome [87,88].

Von Hippel–Lindau syndrome (VHL) is an autosomal dominant syndrome caused by mutations in the *VHL* gene located on chromosome 3p25 [89]. This gene regulates hypoxia-inducible gene (HIF-1α) expression which stimulates hypoxia-associated cytokines, including erythropoietin, vascular endothelial growth factor (VEGF), and platelet-derived growth factor (PDGF). VHL syndrome is linked to several different benign and malignant tumors including renal cell carcinomas, hemangioblastomas, pheochromocytomas, and pancreatic NETs, the last developing in only 10% of cases [90].

Tuberous sclerosis is an autosomal dominant syndrome caused by mutations in either of two tumor suppressor genes: *TSC1* on chromosome 9q34 which encodes the protein hamartin or *TSC2* on chromosome 16p13 which encodes tuberin [91]. Hamartin and tuberin function as a complex which inhibits mechanistic target of rapamycin (mTOR) pathway signaling. Tuberous sclerosis is characterized by low-grade neoplasms and hamartomas in multiple organs including skin, brain, and kidney. Pancreatic NETs occur in only 1–5% of cases [92].

Genetic syndromes provide insight into oncogene pathway aberrations in sporadic tumors. Somatic mutations of the *MEN1* gene occur in roughly 30–45% of sporadic pancreatic NETs, likely causing epigenetic changes associated with chromatin remodeling [93,94]. The association between VHL and pancreatic NETs highlights the importance of angiogenesis in progression of NETs. The link between tuberous sclerosis and pancreatic NETs illustrates the critical role played by the mTOR pathway in NET development.

In recent years, whole exome sequencing has provided a more detailed picture of the genetic basis of pancreatic NETs. In one analysis of 68 sporadic pancreatic NET specimens, 44% of tumors had somatic inactivating mutations in *MEN1*, 43% had mutations in either *DAXX* or *ATRX* (genes encoding subunits of a chromatin remodeling complex), and 14% had mutations in genes associated with the mTOR pathway including *TSC2*, *PTEN*, and *PIK3CA* [94]. Common tumor suppressor and oncogenes such as *TP53*, or *KRAS* were not mutated.

New research sheds some light on the functions of *DAXX*/*ATRX*. Both gene products act together in a chromatin assembly pathway that deposits the histone variant H3.3 in telomeres [95]. Mutations in either gene are strongly associated with development of a telomere maintenance pathway known as alternative lengthening of telomeres (ALT). ALT can be identified on fluorescent *in situ* hybridization (FISH), and is associated with marked genomic instability, defects in the G2/M checkpoint, and altered double-strand break (DSB) repair.

The genetic underpinnings of small bowel carcinoid tumors are poorly understood. Chromosome 18 deletions are frequently observed on comparative genomic hybridization but are of uncertain significance [96]. Massively parallel DNA sequencing of 48 small bowel carcinoid specimens has confirmed a low mutational rate of 0.1 somatic single nucleotide variants (SNVs) per 10^6 nucleotides [97]. Somatic gene copy number alterations (SCNAs) were more common, with an average of 12.6 amplifications and 8.7 deletions per tumor. Genes affected by deletions and amplifications included *AKT*, *SMAD4*, *AURKA*, *MAP2K*, *PDGFR*, and *SRC*.

Diagnostic Procedures

Diagnostic evaluations of GEP-NETs are aided by specific serum markers and imaging modalities. For patients who present with a hormonal syndrome, identification and measurement of the specific hormone associated with the syndrome is recommended. In patients with nonfunctional tumors, nonhormonal tumor marker(s) such as chromogranin A (CgA) can occasionally be useful. Due to their lack of specificity, tumor markers should only be obtained after pathologic diagnosis and not as part of an initial evaluation.

Immunohistochemical (IHC) Markers

Markers of neuroendocrine differentiation include chromogranin, synaptophysin, neuron-specific enolase (NSE), and CD56. CgA is a glycoprotein which is associated with dense-core secretory vesicles within endocrine and neuronal tissues [98]. Synaptophysin is a synaptic vesicle membrane protein also found in nervous and endocrine organs. Well-differentiated GEP-NETs tend to stain strongly and diffusely for both CgA and synaptophysin on IHC whereas poorly differentiated tumors often maintain synaptophysin expression while staining weakly for CgA. While some guidelines recommend testing with CgA and synaptophysin for diagnosis of GEP-NET, it is not clear that immunolabeling is necessary in histologically typical cases [2]. For NETs of unknown origin, certain IHC markers can aid in identification of primary site. These include CDX2 for primary intestinal tumors, and PDS1 or Isl1 for pancreatic NETs.

Tumor grade is an essential component of a pathological report, providing important prognostic information. Guidelines suggest that the mitotic rate and Ki-67 index be measured in the most mitotically active areas of the tumor. There is some controversy as to whether both mitotic rate and Ki-67 need to be reported, since evidence suggests that they correlate closely with each other [99]. Ki-67 index is probably most useful in cases where the amount of tumor tissue is limited and an accurate mitotic count cannot be ascertained.

Serum and Urine Markers

Patients who present with chronic diarrhea and/or flushing should undergo measurement of 24-hour urinary excretion of 5-HIAA [100]. 5-HIAA is an end product of serotonin metabolism and has a fairly high specificity when patients are instructed to avoid tryptophan- and serotonin-rich foods [101–103]. Normal ranges vary by assay but are typically under 15 mg/day. False positive values may be seen in patients with malabsorptive syndromes such as celiac sprue. Although there is often no clear correlation between 5-HIAA results and severity of carcinoid syndrome, patients with very high levels (>100 mg/day) are especially prone to develop significant flushing and/or diarrhea and carcinoid heart disease. Measurement of urinary 5-HIAA excretion is generally not useful in gastroduodenal carcinoid tumors which lack aromatic amino acid decarboxylase needed to convert 5-hydroxytryptophan to serotonin [104]. Distal colon and rectal NETs rarely produce serotonin; therefore, 5-HIAA measurement is rarely of benefit [57].

Assays have been developed for serotonin levels of whole blood, platelet-poor plasma, and platelet-rich plasma [105,106]. However, the sensitivities and specificities of these tests are not well established and levels can be affected by platelet serotonin release. In recent years, a plasma 5-HIAA assay has been described which appears to be equivalent in accuracy to 24-hour urine 5-HIAA measurement and superior to blood serotonin [105].

Chromogranin A (CgA)

Chromogranin A is a protein that is stored and released with peptides and amines in a variety of neuroendocrine tissues [106]. False positive elevations of CgA are invariably observed in patients with chronic atrophic gastritis and with use of proton pump inhibitors (PPIs) [107]. The sensitivity and specificity of CgA depend on the cut-off value: in one series of patients, the optimal cut-off was 32 U/L, with a sensitivity and specificity of 75% and 84%, respectively. When specificity was set at 95%, the cut-off range was 84–87 U/L, and sensitivity was only 55% [108]. In the US, multiple different CgA assays limit reproducibility across treatment centers. Due to its relatively low positive predictive value, CgA should not be used as a screening test for diagnosis of GEP-NET. It is more appropriately used as a tumor marker in patients with an established diagnosis in order to assess response to therapy or recurrence after surgical resection.

Other Tumor Markers

Other circulating proteins that can be elaborated by NETs and can therefore serve as potential tumor markers include pancreatic polypeptide (PP), pancreastatin, β-hCG, substance P, and NSE [101]. In a phase 3 study, elevations in both CgA and NSE were prognostic for progression-free and overall survival, and reductions in both serum biomarkers were predictive for radiographic response [109]. Pancreastatin is a breakdown fragment of CgA [110]. In several studies, pancreastatin was more specific and sensitive than its parent molecule and was not falsely elevated by PPI use [111]. At this time, there are insufficient data from large studies to select one particular tumor marker as a gold standard. CgA remains widely used for historical reasons. In general, selection of a particular biomarker, rather than a panel of markers, is advisable for monitoring of patients over time.

Diagnostic Imaging

GEP-NETs develop and tend to metastasize within the abdominal cavity. Cross-sectional imaging studies should therefore focus on the abdomen for patients with pancreatic NETs, and abdomen/pelvis for small bowel NETs. Somatostatin-receptor scintigraphy (SRS; OctreoScan®) is a nuclear medicine scan that localizes somatostatin-receptor expressing tumors and is therefore useful for evaluating GEP-NETs. Novel positron emission tomography (PET) scans, including the recently approved gallium-68-DOTATATE PET, can also image somatostatin-receptor expressing tumors.

Computed Tomography (CT)

Metastatic GEP-NETs to the liver are often vascular and tend to enhance during early arterial phases of imaging, with washout during the portal venous imaging phase. Therefore, three-phase CT scans are recommended which include noncontrast images, arterial phase sequences (approximately 20 seconds after contrast injection), and portal venous phase sequences (approximately 70 seconds after contrast injection) [112]. The use of multiple phases maximizes the conspicuity of liver metastases and improves the sensitivity of CT scanning.

CT scans are useful for localizing primary small intestinal carcinoid tumors. These tumors often involve the adjacent mesentery, producing desmoplastic fibrosis. They often appear as infiltrative masses with a circumferential pattern of soft-tissue strands which tether surrounding bowel. Small carcinoid tumors of the intestine can be difficult to visualize with standard barium contrast. Visualization of small lesions can be aided by use of a negative intraluminal gastrointestinal contrast agent following a rapid bolus of intravenous contrast and multiplanar reconstruction [113].

Pancreatic NETs are often detected on multiphasic CT scans and appear as homogeneous enhancing masses during arterial and pancreatic or portal venous phases of imaging [114]. Pancreatic NETs can occasionally be cystic.

Magnetic Resonance Imaging (MRI)

MRI scans are an alternative to CT scans and may represent a more sensitive technique for detection of liver metastases. In one study of 64 patients with metastatic GEP-NETs, the number of detected metastases was higher with MRI than with CT scan ($P = 0.02$) or with SRS ($P < 0.0001$) [115]. In this series, MRI detected 190 metastases missed by SRS and 69 missed by CT. The optimal MRI sequences were T2-weighted images and arterial phase enhanced T1-weighted images. In another study of 37 patients with liver metastases, the most sensitive sequences were hepatic arterial phase and fast spin-echo T2-weighted images [116]. Gadoxetic acid is a relatively new gadolinium-based MRI contrast enhancing agent which is taken up by hepatocytes and is particularly sensitive for detection of small liver metastases.

Somatostatin-Receptor Scintigraphy (OctreoScan®)

Well-differentiated GEP-NETs express high levels of somatostatin receptors and therefore can be imaged with radiolabeled somatostatin analogs. Indium-111 labeled octreotide (^{111}In pentetreotide; OctreoScan®) is widely used for staging of GEP-NETs. This whole-body scanning technique enables detection of metastases outside the abdominal region. It also provides *in vivo* information on levels of tumoral somatostatin-receptor expression. Images are generally performed 4 hours and 24 hours after contrast administration [117,118]. Tumor uptake is often graded on the 4-point Krenning scale: grade 1, lower uptake than normal liver; grade 2, uptake equal to liver; grade 3, uptake greater than liver tissue; grade 4 higher than splenic/renal uptake. This information is both prognostic (aggressive tumors are often somatostatin-receptor negative) and predictive for response to somatostatin-receptor targeting therapies (see "Systemic Therapy").

The accuracy of SRS has increased with the addition of single photon emission computed tomography (SPECT) to planar imaging, since SPECT permits more accurate differentiation between areas of pathologic and physiologic uptake [119]. In one report describing 72 patients with neuroendocrine tumors who were examined with SPECT-CT hybrid imaging, the combination improved localization in 23 of 44 SRS positive studies and affected clinical management in 10 patients [120].

Advancements in CT and MRI technology over the past several decades have generated doubts as to whether SRS remains a necessary component of the staging workup for GEP-NETs. In one series of 121 NET patients, multiphase CT and MRI scans detected more tumors than SPECT-OctreoScan® [121]. None of the patients had soft-tissue metastases or primary tumors identified on SRS that were not seen on CT or MRI scans. However, SRS did identify skeletal metastases that were not observed on cross-sectional imaging. The authors concluded that routine use of SRS was not recommended for GEP-NET staging. In another study, CT and MRI were more sensitive than SRS for detection of liver metastases [115]. SRS was found to be particularly insensitive (<35%) for detection of lesions smaller than 1.5 cm in diameter.

Functional Positron Emission Tomography (PET) Scans

Conventional fluorodeoxyglucose (FDG) PET scans are not useful for imaging patients with low-grade GEP-NETs, which are relatively slow-growing and metabolically inactive. Tumors with higher proliferative activity, however, take up high levels of glucose; consequently FDG-PET scans are considered standard for imaging high-grade or poorly differentiated tumors.

Several novel PET radiotracers that are available at specialized centers exploit NET expression of somatostatin receptors and uptake of biogenic amines. These tracers include ^{18}F-dihydroxyphenylalanine (^{18}F-DOPA), ^{11}C-5-hydroxytryptophan (^{11}C-5-HTP), ^{68}Ga DOTA- D-Phe^{1}-Tyr^{3}-octreotide (68-Ga-DOTATOC), and ^{68}Ga DOTA-D-Phe^{1}-Tyr^{3}-Thr^{8}-octreotate (^{68}Ga-DOTATATE) [122–125]. These PET modalities offer higher spatial resolution than conventional SRS and improved sensitivity for detection of small lesions. In a study of 47 patients with GEP-NETs who had at least one lesion on conventional imaging, ^{11}C-5-HTP PET had a sensitivity of 96%, compared to 46%, 77%, and 68% for SRS, SRS-CT, and CT alone [122]. In another study of 27 patients comparing ^{68}Ga-DOTATOC PET to conventional SRS, PET imaging was superior for detection of pulmonary and skeletal metastases [123]. Perhaps the most rigorously studied novel imaging modality is the ^{68}Ga-DOTATATE PET scan which was recently approved by the US Food and Drug Administration (FDA) for evaluation of somatostatin-receptor positive NETs. In one study of 131 patients with known or suspected NET, a ^{68}Ga-DOTATATE PET-CT detected 95% of lesions, compared to 45% with cross-sectional imaging and 31% with SRS. More importantly, 33% of patients had a change in management as a result of the scan [125].

Endoscopic Ultrasonography (EUS)

EUS is a highly sensitive imaging modality for pancreatic tumors, detecting lesions as small as 3 mm in diameter [126,127]. It also enables diagnostic needle aspiration during a single procedure. In one study of 37 patients who had negative CT scans and transabdominal ultrasounds but were eventually diagnosed with pancreatic NET, EUS detected the tumors with a high degree of sensitivity and specificity (82% and 95%, respectively) [127]. In another study of 56 patients, EUS had a higher sensitivity for detection of pancreatic NETs than CT scan (92% vs. 63%) [126]. The main role of EUS is for preoperative diagnosis of localized pancreatic NETs. EUS should also be considered in cases of metastatic NET of unknown primary where identification of a primary tumor in the pancreas might impact choice of systemic therapy.

Arterial Stimulation with Venous Sampling (ASVS)

This complex and invasive procedure is occasionally performed in patients with hormonal symptoms which are thought to originate in an occult pancreatic NET. ASVS involves selective intra-arterial administration of a secretagogue (such as calcium for insulinomas or secretin for gastrinomas) [128,129] into pancreatic arteries with subsequent sampling of the hepatic veins. It thus enables localization of a tumor to a particular region of the pancreas (i.e., head/neck vs. body/tail). Due to improvements in noninvasive localization techniques such as multiphase CT scan and EUS, ASVS is seldom performed.

Treatment of Localized Tumors

Patients who are diagnosed with localized tumors are usually treated surgically. The approach to surgery depends largely on the primary tumor site. There is increasing awareness that surveillance, or "watchful waiting," may be appropriate for select patients with incidentally detected tumors [130].

Pancreatic Neuroendocrine Tumors

Patients with pNETs that are symptomatic, mitotically active, or larger than 2 cm in diameter should generally undergo formal oncologic surgery (i.e., pancreaticoduodenectomy or distal pancreatectomy for neoplasms involving the head or body/tail of the pancreas, respectively). There is some controversy regarding the approach to incidentally detected pNETs <2 cm. In fact, recent evidence has demonstrated a 5-year overall survival (OS) of 100% [131], leading several guidelines to endorse a "wait and see" policy in select patients. However, this approach should be considered only for patients with low-grade tumors, thus rendering mandatory fine-needle aspiration or biopsy. Enucleation is another option for patients with small, low-risk tumors which do not involve the pancreatic duct.

Midgut Carcinoid Tumors

Most carcinoid tumors of the jejunum and ileocecum exhibit malignant behavior despite their slow rate of growth and should therefore be resected with appropriate oncologic resection of the involved segment and small bowel mesentery [41,52]. Due to the high frequency of multifocal tumors (approximately 25% of cases), the entire bowel should be palpated to rule out additional primary tumors.

Recommendations on surveillance after surgery are not based on evidence and can therefore vary significantly [41,131]. As a general principle, a long duration of surveillance (e.g., up to

5–10 years) is more important than frequent surveillance in these indolent tumors. Many patients can be seen and scanned as infrequently as once yearly. There is some disagreement on specific imaging modalities. The National Comprehensive Cancer Network (NCCN) recommends standard cross-sectional imaging studies such as multiphasic CT or MRI of the abdomen/pelvis rather than SRS for postoperative surveillance [41].

Appendiceal Carcinoid Tumors

Carcinoid tumors of the appendix are nearly always detected incidentally during appendectomies for acute appendicitis or during intra-abdominal surgery for other indications. After the initial appendectomy, most guidelines suggest that a completion formal right hemicolectomy be performed for tumors larger than 2 cm [41,131]. There is some controversy over the role of completion right hemicolectomy for tumors between 1 and 2 cm [51]. Other factors such as mesoappendiceal invasion and location in the base of the appendix as well as patient age and comorbidities should be considered prior to recommending further surgery. Patients with tumors smaller than 1 cm do not generally require any further surgery or surveillance after appendectomy.

Colorectal Carcinoid Tumors

Most rectal carcinoid tumors are small and submucosal in location. Tumors that are smaller than 1 cm and confined to the mucosa or submucosa (T1) can often be managed with endoscopic resection [57]. In one study, no recurrences were detected after endoscopic or transanal resection of T1 tumors [132,133]. Another study reported a positive resection margin in 17% of patients undergoing endoscopic polypectomy, however the clinical significance was unclear since only one patient with a positive margin had a local recurrence which occurred 16 years later [134]. Numerous endoscopic resection techniques have been described including band snares [135], band ligation [136], and aspiration lumpectomy [137].

Tumors between 1 and 2 cm in size can often be treated with transanal surgical resection or transanal endoscopic microsurgery (TEM) [138]. Patients with tumors that are larger than 2 cm, invasive beyond the muscularis propria (i.e., T3 or T4), or involving regional lymph nodes should generally undergo a formal oncologic resection with lymph node sampling [57,139,140].

Carcinoid tumors of the colon tend to be relatively aggressive compared to rectal carcinoid tumors. Most are relatively large and invasive; consequently a formal partial colectomy is performed in most cases.

Gastric Carcinoid Tumors

Type I and II gastric carcinoid tumors are of very low malignant potential and are usually managed conservatively. For type I tumors, endoscopic surveillance with endoscopic resection is generally recommended roughly every 6–12 months, although lower frequency of surveillance may be appropriate in some cases [41,141,142]. Antrectomy to remove the gastrin stimulus is occasionally performed for patients with multifocal tumors that are enlarging or proliferating relatively rapidly. Sporadic tumors (type III) are often treated with partial gastrectomy and regional lymphadenectomy. Recent data suggest that endoscopic resection may be sufficient for select patients with small tumors invading the submucosa (T1) [46].

Systemic Therapy

Somatostatin Analogs

The human hormone somatostatin has two bioactive forms consisting of 14 and 28 amino acids [143]. It interacts with somatostatin receptors which belong to a family of G-protein coupled receptors with seven transmembrane domains [144]. Somatostatin was initially identified as an inhibitor of growth hormone, and was subsequently found to perform numerous other inhibitory functions within the diffuse endocrine system. Somatostatin's actions in the digestive tract include inhibition of bowel motility, reduction of mesenteric blood flow, and suppression of other hormones such as gastrin, cholecystokinin, and serotonin. In the 1970s, case reports documented successful use of somatostatin-14 for palliation of the carcinoid syndrome. Unfortunately, native human somatostatin could only be administered as a continuous infusion due to its half-life of 2 minutes. In order to improve the pharmacokinetics of somatostatin, synthetic somatostatin analogs (SSAs) were developed in the 1980s by elimination of enzymatic cleavage sites within the polypeptide chain.

Octreotide and lanreotide are both synthetic octapeptides which share similar somatostatin receptor affinities, binding avidly to sst_2 and moderately to sst_5 [145]. The first clinical trial of octreotide evaluated the drug in 25 patients with malignant carcinoid syndrome [146]. Rapid improvements in flushing and diarrhea were observed in 22 patients (88%) and major reductions in urine 5-HIAA were reported in 18 cases (72%), leading to the approval of octreotide by the FDA for management of the carcinoid syndrome. A subsequent crossover trial comparing octreotide versus lanreotide in 33 patients with carcinoid syndrome demonstrated no significant differences between the two analogs in terms of symptom control or biochemical responses [147]. Other small trials and clinical series have demonstrated that both octreotide and lanreotide can palliate hormonal syndromes associated with functioning pancreatic NETs, particularly VIPomas and glucagonomas [148]. The insulinoma syndrome is somewhat refractory to octreotide and lanreotide, likely due to the fact that most insulinomas express relatively low levels of the sst_2 receptor. The gastrinoma syndrome can also be palliated with SSAs, however high-dose proton pump inhibitors (PPIs) are even more essential for control of gastric acid secretion [63].

Octreotide was originally developed as an immediate-release subcutaneous (SC) formulation and studied at doses of 100 mcg to 500 mcg administered 3 times daily. In the 1990s, long-acting depot formulations of both octreotide and lanreotide were developed, enabling monthly dosing. The registration trial of octreotide long-acting repeatable (LAR) for treatment of the carcinoid syndrome compared intramuscular (IM) doses of 10 mg, 20 mg, and 30 mg every 4 weeks with open-label SC octreotide administered every 8 hours [149]. Octreotide LAR was found to be at least as effective as SC octreotide. Control of diarrhea was equivalent for all doses of octreotide LAR, but control of flushing and suppression of urine 5-HIAA was mildly inferior in the 10 mg cohort. As a result, a 20 mg starting dose of octreotide LAR was recommended for treatment of the carcinoid syndrome with titration to 30 mg in patients with suboptimal symptom control. Depot lanreotide is administered as a deep SC injection at doses ranging from 60 mg to 120 mg every 4 weeks [150]. The formulation is available as a prefilled syringe and yields therapeutic plasma levels within 24 hours.

Both octreotide and lanreotide are exceptionally well tolerated. Side effects include steatorrhea and bloating which are caused by suppression of pancreatic exocrine activity. Supplemental use of digestive enzymes can occasionally alleviate these side effects. Long-term use of SSAs can cause cholelithiasis due to inhibition of physiologic gallbladder contractions. Above-label doses and frequencies of SSAs are often prescribed for patients who experience suboptimal control of their hormonal syndromes [151]. In some cases, supplemental dosing of SC octreotide may alleviate breakthrough symptoms such as flushing or diarrhea. Evidence suggests that somatostatin receptors may be saturated at octreotide LAR doses above 60 mg; thus higher doses may be of minimal marginal benefit [152].

Treatment and Prophylaxis of the Carcinoid Crisis

Carcinoid crisis is a term that refers to acute flushing and hypotension caused by massive release of serotonin and other vasoactive substances into the circulation [153]. Common triggers of carcinoid crisis include general anesthesia, epinephrine, and physical manipulation of tumors; therefore carcinoid crisis is typically an intraoperative emergency. Patients with pre-existing carcinoid syndrome are most prone to develop carcinoid crisis, however there have been reports of intraoperative hypotension occurring in patients without prior evidence of serotonin secretion. Most guidelines call for bolus intravenous administrations of octreotide, typically at doses of 500 mcg, for patients who develop carcinoid crisis [131]. Continuous intravenous infusion of octreotide can also be initiated after a bolus dose. Prophylactic doses of IV or SC octreotide are typically administered prior to surgery for at-risk patients, however one study has questioned the efficacy of prophylaxis [154].

The Antiproliferative Effect of Somatostatin Analogs

In recent years, high-level evidence has emerged that SSAs can significantly inhibit growth of well-differentiated GEP-NETs, via both direct and indirect mechanisms [155]. The direct effect involves interaction between SSAs and somatostatin receptors on tumor cells, although the precise signaling transduction pathways are not fully understood [156]. The indirect antiproliferative effect is mediated through suppression of circulating growth factors [157].

Until recently, evidence of the antiproliferative effects of SSAs derived from single-arm phase 2 trials documenting disease stabilization in roughly 50% of patients treated with either octreotide or lanreotide. Proof of the antiproliferative effect of SSAs emerged with publication of the PROMID trial [158]. This randomized phase 3 study compared octreotide LAR 30 mg versus placebo in 85 patients with advanced carcinoid tumors originating in the midgut. Time to tumor progression (TTP) increased from 6 months in the placebo arm to 14.3 months in the octreotide LAR arm ($P = 0.000072$). Serious adverse events were evenly balanced. On subset analysis, patients with low tumor burden (<10% hepatic involvement) and resected primary tumors benefitted most significantly from treatment with octreotide LAR versus placebo. More recently, results of the CLARINET trial were reported [159]. This randomized phase 3 study compared depot lanreotide 120 mg to placebo in 204 patients with hormonally nonfunctioning GEP-NETs. The study met its primary endpoint with a 53% improvement in progression-free survival (PFS; $P = 0.0002$). The most common adverse effects associated with lanreotide were diarrhea, abdominal pain, and cholelithiasis. These studies demonstrate that SSAs can significantly inhibit tumor growth in patients with advanced GEP-NETs. Objective response rates, however, are quite rare. Tumors with low proliferative activity, slow progression, and high expression of somatostatin receptors are most likely to be controlled with SSAs.

Interferon-α

Interferons (IFNs) are a complex array of cytokines with antiviral and antitumor properties.

Interferon-α (IFN-α) was first introduced to treatment of midgut NETs in the early 1980s when symptomatic responses were reported in a small series of patients with malignant carcinoid syndrome. A larger study of IFN-α 3–6 million units/day reported objective tumor responses in 4 of 36 patients (11%) with advanced carcinoid tumors and major reductions in urine 5-HIAA in 16 patients (53%) [160]. A subsequent phase 2 study of 49 patients with advanced NETs evaluated IFNα-2a at a daily dose of 6 million units daily for 8 weeks followed by the same dose 3 times a week thereafter. Among 34 patients with carcinoid tumors, partial radiographic responses were observed in 4 patients (12%) and major improvements in carcinoid syndrome were reported in 64% of cases [161]. Higher doses of IFN-α proved to be much less tolerable. A study evaluating a dose of 24 million units/m^2 3 times a week reported high rates of fevers/chills, anorexia, weight loss, leukopenia, and liver function abnormalities [162].

Studies of IFN-α Combined with SSAs

In vitro data demonstrating that IFN-α potentiates expression of somatostatin receptors in NET cells have led to several clinical studies evaluating the combination of IFN with SSAs. In one clinical study, addition of IFN-α to octreotide resulted in symptomatic improvement in 49% of patients with carcinoid syndrome whose symptoms were not controlled with octreotide monotherapy [163]. A more recent trial investigated pegylated IFN, a long-acting formulation which enables weekly dosing. Of 17 patients who progressed on SSA therapy, inhibition of tumor growth was observed in 13 [164].

Several randomized clinical trials have investigated SSAs alone versus in combination with IFN-α. One study of 68 patients with metastatic midgut carcinoid tumors compared octreotide alone versus combination with IFN-α 3 million units administered 5 times per week. The 5-year survival rate in the combination arm was 57% versus 37% in the octreotide monotherapy arm ($P = 0.13$) [165]. Time to tumor progression was significantly improved with a hazard ratio of 0.28 ($P = 0.008$). Another randomized study of 109 GEP-NET patients compared octreotide alone versus octreotide combined with IFN-α 4.5 million units administered 3 times per week [166]. The median survival was prolonged in the combination arm (51 vs. 35 months) but results did not achieve statistical significance ($P = 0.38$). A three-arm trial of 80 therapy-naïve patients with advanced GEP-NETs evaluated SC lanreotide alone versus IFN-α 5 million units 3 times weekly, or the combination of the two drugs. In this trial, time to tumor progression was similar in all three arms [167].

Given the underpowered nature of these randomized trials, it is difficult to draw definitive conclusions regarding the benefits of IFN-α. The most compelling data are in midgut NETs where combination therapy with SSAs appears to palliate symptoms and control tumor growth.

Everolimus

The mTOR enzyme regulates cell proliferation and metabolism in response to environmental stimuli. Germline mutations of *TSC2*, an endogenous inhibitor of mTOR, are a risk factor for development of pancreatic NETs. Somatic mutations in mTOR pathway genes, including *PTEN* and *PIK3CA*, and *TSC2* occur in roughly 15% of pancreatic NETs [94]. Other alterations in mTOR pathway genes, including amplifications of *AKT1/2*, are observed in nearly one-third of small bowel carcinoid tumors [97].

The oral mTOR inhibitor everolimus has been studied extensively in GEP-NETs. A phase 2 study of 160 patients with pancreatic NETs evaluated patients in two strata: everolimus monotherapy ($n = 115$) or everolimus plus octreotide ($n = 45$) [168]. Response rates and median PFS were 9% and 9.7 months in the monotherapy arm versus 4% and 16.7 months in the combined therapy arm respectively. A subsequent phase 3 trial (RADIANT 3) randomly assigned 410 patients with low- and intermediate-grade pancreatic NETs to treatment with everolimus 10 mg versus placebo [169]. Concurrent SSA therapy was allowed. Despite an objective response rate of only 5% in the everolimus arm, the study demonstrated a clinically and statistically significant improvement in PFS. Median PFS increased from 4.6 months on the placebo arm to 11 months on the everolimus arm (hazard ratio (HR) 0.35, $P < 0.001$). Overall survival differences were not observed, possibly due to the crossover design. Everolimus has since been approved by the FDA for treatment of patients with advanced pancreatic NETs.

Another phase 3 study (RADIANT 2) randomly assigned 429 patients with hormonally functional (predominantly midgut) carcinoid tumors to treatment with everolimus 10 mg plus octreotide versus placebo plus octreotide. Median PFS increased from 11.3 months on the placebo arm to 16.4 months on the everolimus arm (HR 0.77, $P = 0.026$) [170]. While clinically significant, the primary endpoint fell short of its prespecified statistical significance threshold of $P < 0.0246$. There was no trend towards improvement in overall survival in the everolimus arm, possibly due to the high rate of crossover to everolimus in the placebo arm.

The third phase 3 study of everolimus in NET (RADIANT 4) compared everolimus versus placebo in 302 nonfunctioning NETs of the gastrointestinal tract and lungs [171]. In this study, concurrent octreotide was prohibited, and crossover from placebo did not occur at time of progression. Median PFS improved from 3.9 on the placebo arm to 11.0 months on the everolimus arm (HR 0.48, $P < 0.000001$). As a result of this study, everolimus was approved for treatment of nonfunctioning gastrointestinal and lung NETs (in addition to its prior indication for pancreatic NET).

Although the RADIANT 2 study was technically negative whereas the RADIANT 4 study in nonfunctioning NETs was positive, it is unlikely that tumor functionality (i.e., history of carcinoid syndrome) influences response to everolimus. It is more likely that the benefits of everolimus were more difficult to demonstrate in a study evaluating patients with slow-growing midgut NETs (the RADIANT 2 population) compared to more aggressive NETs evaluated in the RADIANT 4 study. In general, everolimus should be considered in patients with clinically significant disease progression, regardless of hormonal output.

Side effects of everolimus include aphthous oral ulcers, rash, diarrhea, hyperglycemia, and cytopenias. Pneumonitis is relatively rare but potentially serious. Everolimus is an immunosuppressive drug and atypical infections such as tuberculosis or aspergillosis are occasionally observed. While most toxicities are mild, chronic side effects may adversely impact patient quality of life.

Angiogenesis Inhibitors

Neuroendocrine tumors are highly vascular and frequently express the vascular endothelial growth factor (VEGF) ligand and receptor (VEGFR). Increased levels of circulating VEGF have been associated with tumor progression. Consequently, inhibition of the VEGF pathway has been identified as a therapeutic strategy.

The tyrosine kinase inhibitor (TKI) sunitinib targets VEGFRs 1, 2, and 3, as well as platelet-derived growth factor receptor (PDGFR). In a phase 2 trial, treatment with sunitinib yielded objective response rates of 2.4% and 16.7% in patients with advanced carcinoid tumors and pancreatic NETs, respectively [172]. Based on the relatively high response rates in the latter cohort, a multinational phase 3 trial randomly assigned patients with low- and intermediate-grade pancreatic NETs to sunitinib 37.5 mg daily versus placebo. The study enrolled 171 patients, and demonstrated a statistically significant improvement in median PFS from 5.5 months on the placebo arm to 11.1 months on the sunitinib arm [173]. The hazard ratio of 0.42 was highly significant ($P < 0.001$). There was a nonsignificant trend towards improvement in overall survival. The objective response rate associated with sunitinib was 9.3%. Side effects of sunitinib included nausea, diarrhea, fatigue, cytopenias, palmar-plantar erythrodysesthesia, and hypertension. Based on results of this study, sunitinib is FDA approved for treatment of pancreatic NETs. Other VEGFR-targeting TKIs, including pazopanib and axitinib, are being investigated in clinical trials of GEP-NET patients.

Bevacizumab is a humanized monoclonal antibody to circulating VEGF-A. In a randomized phase 2 trial, 44 patients with metastatic carcinoid tumors were randomly assigned to treatment with bevacizumab or PEG-IFN for 18 weeks, followed by both agents in combination [174]. At the week 18 time point, the rate of PFS was 95% on the bevacizumab arm versus 68% on the PEG-IFN arm. However these promising results were not confirmed in a subsequent phase 3 study comparing bevacizumab to IFN-α in patients with high-risk carcinoid tumors. In this trial, which was sponsored by the Southwest Oncology Group (SWOG), no improvement in PFS was observed with bevacizumab [175].

Cytotoxic Chemotherapy

Cytotoxic agents are particularly active in poorly-differentiated or high-grade neuroendocrine cancers as well as in pancreatic NETs. Poorly-differentiated neuroendocrine cancers are aggressive malignancies which are treated similarly to small cell lung cancer. In a study evaluating cisplatin and etoposide in GEP-NETs, a response rate of 67% was observed in poorly-differentiated cancers versus 7% in well-differentiated tumors [176]. Another study of cisplatin and etoposide in poorly-differentiated GEP-NETs demonstrated a response rate of 42% [177]. The durations of response in both studies were short (8–9 months) with median overall survivals of roughly 1.5 years. A recent retrospective analysis of patients with high-grade carcinomas demonstrated that carboplatin was interchangeable with cisplatin. Moreover, tumors with very high Ki-67 proliferation rates (>55%) appeared to be more sensitive to platinum-based combinations than tumors with lower Ki-67 rates (20–55%) [178].

Pancreatic NETs are often treated with alkylating agents as well as with fluoropyrimidines such as 5-fluorouracil (5-FU) or capecitabine. One of the first cytotoxic drugs tested in pancreatic NETs was the nitrosourea streptozocin, an agent that is specifically toxic to pancreatic beta cells. Based on encouraging phase 2 data, two randomized trials were conducted in the 1970s and 1980s. One reported response rates of 63% with streptozocin plus 5-FU versus 36% with streptozocin monotherapy [179]. The second trial evaluated streptozocin plus doxorubicin versus streptozocin plus 5-FU and reported response rates and time to tumor progression of 69% and 20 months versus 45% and 6.9 months, respectively [180]. It is important to note that these trials did not employ strict radiographic criteria for measurement of response rates. A more recent retrospective study investigating the combination of streptozocin, 5-FU, and doxorubicin in 84 pancreatic NETs reported a response rate of 39% using objective radiographic parameters [181].

In recent years, the oral alkylating agent temozolomide has been studied in pancreatic NETs. A phase 2 study evaluating the combination of temozolomide and thalidomide reported an objective response rate of 45% in the pancreatic NET subset which consisted of 11 patients [182]. A phase 2 trial of temozolomide combined with bevacizumab reported a response rate of 33% and median PFS of 14.3 months in the pancreatic NET cohort of 15 patients [183]. The combination of capecitabine with temozolomide has been investigated in several retrospective studies. In one institutional series of 30 chemotherapy-naïve patients with pancreatic NETs, a radiographic response rate of 70% was observed with a median PFS of 18 months [184]. Another institutional series consisting primarily of pancreatic NETs reported a response rate of 61% with capecitabine and temozolomide [185]. An ongoing clinical trial sponsored by the Eastern Cooperative Oncology Group (ECOG) is designed to compare capecitabine plus temozolomide to temozolomide monotherapy.

Well-differentiated carcinoid tumors are substantially more resistant to chemotherapy than pancreatic NETs. A randomized clinical trial of streptozocin plus fluorouracil compared to doxorubicin plus fluorouracil in patients with advanced carcinoid tumors demonstrated response rates of 16% and a disappointing median PFS of 5 months in both arms of the study [186]. In the phase 2 study of temozolomide plus thalidomide, the response rate in the carcinoid tumor cohort was only 7% (compared to 45% in the pancreatic NET cohort) [182]. In the phase 2 study of temozolomide plus bevacizumab, the response rate in the carcinoid tumor cohort was 0% (compared to 33% in the pancreatic NET cohort) [183].

Radiolabeled Somatostatin Analogs

An emerging form of therapy known as peptide receptor radiotherapy (PRRT) enables delivery of radioactive isotopes to somatostatin-receptor expressing tumors. Radiolabeled SSAs consist of a radionuclide isotope, a somatostatin analog (peptide), and a chelator which binds them. SSAs include octreotide as well as octreotate, an analog with enhanced binding to sst_2. The activity of PRRT correlates with levels of somatostatin receptor uptake on somatostatin-receptor scintigraphy. Consequently, the main selection criterion for PRRT is evidence of high radiotracer expression on OctreoScan®.

Early clinical trials of PRRT used octreotide radiolabeled with high doses of indium-111 [187]. Although ^{111}In-octreotide palliated symptoms in many cases, objective radiographic responses were rare. The next generation of radiolabeled SSAs used yttrium (^{90}Y), a high-energy β-emitting isotope with greater tissue penetration. In one study, objective responses associated with ^{90}Y-DOTA-Tyr^3-octreotide (^{90}Y-DOTATOC) were observed in 28% of 87 patients [188]. More recently, a multicenter phase 2 trial of 90 patients with metastatic carcinoid tumors reported a high stable disease rate of 70%, but an objective response rate of only 4%, possibly due to the preponderance of heavily pretreated midgut carcinoid tumors [189]. Toxicities associated with ^{90}Y-DOTATOC include renal insufficiency, which is partially ameliorated by concurrent amino acid infusions. In one large institutional series of 1,109 patients, 102 patients (9%) had severe permanent renal toxicity [190]. Acute gastrointestinal toxicities, including nausea and vomiting, are primarily attributable to the amino acid infusions. Myelosuppression is another side effect of PRRT, with grade 3 and 4 hematological toxicities occurring in approximately 13% of cases. Rare cases of leukemia and myelodysplastic syndrome have been reported.

The latest generation of radiolabeled SSAs utilizes ^{177}lutetium-DOTATATE (^{177}Lu-DOTA-Tyr^3-octreotate), a β and γ particle emitter with high affinity for sst_2. In one series of 310 patients with GEP-NETs, an objective response rate of 30% was reported. Predictive factors for response included high radiotracer uptake on SRS and pancreatic primary site. Median OS was 46 months [191]. Adverse events associated with ^{177}Lu-DOTATATE, including nephrotoxicity, appear to be mild compared to ^{90}Y-DOTATOC.

The efficacy of PRRT was recently confirmed in the international phase 3 NETTER-1 study which compared ^{177}Lu-DOTATATE to high-dose octreotide LAR (60 mg) in patients with midgut NETs progressing radiographically on standard dose octreotide LAR [192]. The study demonstrated a marked 79% improvement in PFS associated with ^{177}Lu-DOTATATE (*P* <0.00001). Median PFS was 8 months on the control arm of the study and not reached with ^{177}Lu-DOTATATE at the time of primary analysis. Objective response was 18% on the investigational arm of the study versus 3% on the control arm. Treatment was well tolerated, with the most common side effects being grade 1–2 nausea and vomiting associated with amino acid infusion concurrent with the ^{177}Lu-DOTATATE administration. Grade 3 or 4 neutropenia and thrombocytopenia occurred in only 1% and 2% of patients treated with ^{177}Lu-DOTATATE respectively.

Liver-Targeted Therapies

The liver is the predominant site of metastases in patients with GEP-NETs. Liver-directed therapies are designed to palliate or prevent symptoms related to tumor growth and hormonal secretion. Treatment options include resection or ablation, hepatic arterial embolization, and transplantation. Data supporting liver-directed therapy derive primarily from retrospective studies. In the absence of randomized data, the effects of liver-directed therapy on survival remain unproven.

Hepatic cytoreductive surgery is generally recommended if at least 90% of disease can be resected [193,194]. This is contrary to the paradigm in many cancers where metastasectomy is only performed with curative intent. Various ablative techniques have also been described, including alcohol ablation, cryoablation, and radiofrequency ablation (RFA) [194–196]. Percutaneous or operative ablation methods are appropriate for tumors smaller than 5–7 cm in diameter. Data supporting a cytoreductive surgical approach derive from institutional series which document relatively long survival durations among patients undergoing operative treatment. However, there are no randomized studies comparing surgical to nonsurgical approaches, and it is possible that encouraging outcomes are more strongly related to favorable baseline factors than to aggressive surgical treatment.

Hepatic transarterial embolization (TAE) is typically performed in patients with progressive unresectable liver metastases. The rationale for embolization is that liver metastases are primarily vascularized from the hepatic arterial circulation, whereas normal liver parenchyma is supplied primarily from the portal vein. The intense vascularity of GEP-NETs renders them particularly sensitive to embolic therapies. Various particulate and occlusive materials have been used including polyvinyl alcohol (PVA), Gelfoam® (Pharmacia and Upjohn Co, Kalamazoo, MI), and trisacryl gelatin microspheres (Embosphere®; BioSphere Medical Inc. Rockland, MA) [197–199]. Transarterial chemoembolization (TACE) can also be performed by infusing an emulsion of cytotoxic drugs, such as doxorubicin or cisplatin, with lipiodol until complete or near-complete stasis of flow is achieved [200,201]. Among patients with disseminated metastases, a series of two or three staged lobar embolizations is usually needed to treat the entire liver. Short-term toxicities caused by transient liver ischemia include nausea, abdominal pain, and fevers. Serum transaminases typically increase significantly, peaking 2–3 days after each embolization. Severe complications are quite rare; however patients who have undergone prior Whipple resection are particularly prone to develop liver abscesses after embolization. Contraindications to transarterial embolization include significant underlying liver dysfunction, portal venous thrombosis, and moderate to severe ascites.

Nearly all published data on transarterial embolization have been drawn from retrospective institutional series. The majority of institutions report partial radiographic response rates of approximately 50% and symptomatic responses in the majority of cases. In one prospective phase 2 trial of transarterial embolization followed by sunitinib, a response rate of 72% with a median PFS of 15.2 months was observed [202]. Randomized trials comparing "bland" embolization to chemoembolization have not been completed. A randomized trial that was halted early due to poor accrual did not demonstrate a significant difference in outcomes; however toxicities were slightly higher in the chemoembolization arm [203].

A novel liver-directed therapy consists of arterial infusion of ^{90}Y embedded either in a resin microsphere (Sir-Spheres®, Sirtex Medical Limited, Lane Cove, Australia) or a glass microsphere (TheraSphere®, MDS-Nordion Inc., Ontario, Canada). This procedure, also known as selective internal radiotherapy (SIRT), enables direct delivery of radionuclides to hepatic metastases. Unlike other embolotherapies, the ^{90}Y microspheres are not infused until stasis of blood flow due to the fact that radiotherapy requires normal oxygen tension. Consequently, patients with mild to moderate liver dysfunction or portal vein thrombosis who are ineligible for bland embolization or chemoembolization may be able to tolerate radioembolization.

Response rates associated with SIRT have been somewhat encouraging. In one retrospective study of 148 patients treated with Sir-Spheres®, the objective radiographic response rate was 63% with a median survival of 70 months [204]. Another study of 42 patients treated with either TheraSphere® or Sir-Spheres® reported a response rate of 51%; however only 29 of the 42 enrolled patients were evaluable for response [205]. Short-term toxicities associated with SIRT are relatively mild due to the fact that the procedure does not induce ischemic hepatitis. Consequently, SIRT can be performed on an outpatient basis. However, there are reasons to be cautious about routine use of SIRT in the absence of data from prospective trials with long-term follow-up. For example, radiation-associated changes in liver function can emerge long after SIRT treatment. Other concerns include the risk of radiation enteritis, which can occur if particles are accidentally infused into arteries supplying the digestive tract. Moreover, the cost differential between SIRT and more traditional embolization techniques is considerable.

Liver transplantation has been described in metastatic NET patients; however it is performed uncommonly. Most transplantation centers report a high postoperative mortality rate of 10–20%. In the largest meta-analysis of 103 patients, the 5-year survival rate was 47% with only 24% of patients free of recurrence [206]. Another multicenter analysis of 85 cases reported a 5-year survival of 47% and recurrence-free survival of 20% [207]. Since recurrence-free survival curves have not reached a plateau, it appears that transplantation can be considered potentially curative only in very select patients. Adverse prognostic factors for early recurrence have included high tumor burden, pancreatic primary site, and elevated Ki-67 index.

Prognosis of Patients with GEP-NETs

Many factors impact the prognosis of patients with GEP-NETs including tumor stage, differentiation, histological grade, and primary site. Patient-specific factors such as age and comorbidities are also important prognostic factors given the relatively favorable natural history of most GEP-NETs.

There is agreement across studies that patients with well-differentiated localized tumors have disease-specific survival rates approaching 100%. Patients with distant metastases have substantially lower survival rates which vary significantly based on primary tumor site. In an analysis of the SEER registry, 5-year survival rates were significantly higher for patients with metastatic small bowel tumors (51%) versus gastric (18%), appendiceal (27%), or rectal tumors (13%) [31]. Tumor differentiation is an even more important prognostic factor than stage. In the SEER database, patients with poorly-differentiated tumors had 5-year survival rates of only 38%, 21%, and 4% in the local, locoregional, and metastatic stages [33].

Interestingly, there are large discrepancies in prognosis between institutional databases and national registries such as SEER. It is unclear whether these variances are related to differences in reporting, selection biases, or differences in treatments offered in community hospitals versus centers of expertise.

Conclusions

The study of NETs, once an esoteric branch of oncology, has advanced substantially in recent years. New grading and staging classifications have been standardized over the past decade enabling stratification of patients into well-defined prognostic groups. Large randomized clinical trials have led to approval of drugs based on high-level evidence of efficacy, and recent advances in genetic sequencing shed light on new potential targets for therapy. In this era of expanding treatment options, it is essential that future studies identify prognostic and predictive biomarkers which will enable a more rational and personalized approach to patient care.

References

1 Vortmeyer AO, Huang S, Lubensky I, Zhuang Z. Non-islet origin of pancreatic islet cell tumors. *J Clin Endocrinol Metab* 2004;89:1934–38.

2 Klimstra DS, Modlin IR, Coppola D, *et al.* The pathologic classification of neuroendocrine tumors: a review of nomenclature, grading, and staging systems. *Pancreas* 2010;39:707–12.

3 Bosman F, Carneiro F, Hruban R, Theise N. *WHO Classification of Tumours of the Digestive System.* Lyon: IARC Press, 2010.

4 Williams ED, Sandler M. The classification of carcinoid tum ours. *Lancet* 1963;1:238–9.

5 Kloppel G, Heitz PU, Capella C, Solcia E. Pathology and nomenclature of human gastrointestinal neuroendocrine (carcinoid) tumors and related lesions. *World J Surg* 1996;20:132–41.

6 Velayoudom-Cephise FL, Duvillard P, Foucan L, *et al.* Are G3 ENETS neuroendocrine neoplasms heterogeneous? *Endocr Relat Cancer* 2013;20:649–57.

7 Yang Z, Tang LH, Klimstra DS. Effect of tumor heterogeneity on the assessment of Ki67 labeling index in well-differentiated neuroendocrine tumors metastatic to the liver: implications for prognostic stratification. *Am J Surg Pathol* 2011;35:853–60.

8 Bergsland EK, Woltering EA, Rindi G, *et al.* Neuroendocrine tumors of the pancreas. In: MB Amin (ed.) *AJCC Cancer Staging Manual*, 8th edn. New York: Springer, 2017.

9 Rindi G, Kloppel G, Alhman H, *et al.* TNM staging of foregut (neuro)endocrine tumors: a consensus proposal including a grading system. *Virchows Arch* 2006;449:395–401.

10 Rindi G, Kloppel G, Couvelard A, *et al.* TNM staging of midgut and hindgut (neuro) endocrine tumors: a consensus proposal including a grading system. *Virchows Arch* 2007;451:757–62.

11 Rindi G, Falconi M, Klersy C, *et al.* TNM staging of neoplasms of the endocrine pancreas: results from a large international cohort study. *J Natl Cancer Inst* 2012;104:764–77.

12 Moertel CG. Karnofsky memorial lecture. An odyssey in the land of small tumors. *J Clin Oncol* 1987;5:1502–22.

13 Strosberg JR, Weber JM, Feldman M, *et al.* Prognostic validity of the American Joint Committee on Cancer staging classification for midgut neuroendocrine tumors. *J Clin Oncol* 2013;31:420–5.

14 Makridis C, Oberg K, Juhlin C, *et al.* Surgical treatment of mid-gut carcinoid tumors. *World J Surg* 1990;14:377–83; discussion 384–5.

15 Strosberg J, Gardner N, Kvols L. Survival and prognostic factor analysis of 146 metastatic neuroendocrine tumors of the mid-gut. *Neuroendocrinology* 2009;89:471–6.

16 Eckhauser FE, Argenta LC, Strodel WE, *et al.* Mesenteric angiopathy, intestinal gangrene, and midgut carcinoids. *Surgery* 1981;90:720–8.

17 Thorson A, Biorck G, Bjorkman G, Waldenstrom J. Malignant carcinoid of the small intestine with metastases to the liver, valvular disease of the right side of the heart (pulmonary stenosis and tricuspid regurgitation without septal defects), peripheral vasomotor symptoms, bronchoconstriction, and an unusual type of cyanosis; a clinical and pathologic syndrome. *Am Heart J* 1954;47:795–817.

18 Lembeck F. [Detection of 5-hydroxytryptamine in carcinoid metastases.]. *Naunyn Schmiedebergs Arch Exp Pathol Pharmakol* 1954;221:50–66.

19 Erspamer V, Asero B. Identification of enteramine, the specific hormone of the enterochromaffin cell system, as 5-hydroxytryptamine. *Nature* 1952;169:800–1.

20 Vinik AI, Silva MP, Woltering EA, *et al.* Biochemical testing for neuroendocrine tumors. *Pancreas* 2009;38:876–89.

21 Davis Z, Moertel CG, McIlrath DC. The malignant carcinoid syndrome. *Surg Gynecol Obstet* 1973;137:637–44.

22 von der Ohe MR, Camilleri M, Kvols LK, Thomforde GM. Motor dysfunction of the small bowel and colon in patients with the carcinoid syndrome and diarrhea. *N Engl J Med* 1993;329:1073–8.

23 Cunningham JL, Janson ET, Agarwal S, *et al.* Tachykinins in endocrine tumors and the carcinoid syndrome. *Eur J Endocrinol* 2008;159:275–82.

24 Smith AG, Greaves MW. Blood prostaglandin activity associated with noradrenaline-provoked flush in the carcinoid syndrome. *Br J Dermatol* 1974;90:547–51.

25 Matuchansky C, Launay JM. Serotonin, catecholamines, and spontaneous midgut carcinoid flush: plasma studies from flushing and nonflushing sites. *Gastroenterology* 1995;108:743–51.

26 Pellikka PA, Tajik AJ, Khandheria BK, *et al.* Carcinoid heart disease. Clinical and echocardiographic spectrum in 74 patients. *Circulation* 1993;87:1188–96.

27 Connolly HM, Schaff HV, Mullany CJ, *et al.* Surgical management of left-sided carcinoid heart disease. *Circulation* 2001;104:I36–40.

28 Zuetenhorst JM, Taal BG. Carcinoid heart disease. *N Engl J Med* 2003;348:2359–61; author reply 2359–61.

29 Moertel CG, Sauer WG, Dockerty MB, Baggenstoss AH. Life history of the carcinoid tumor of the small intestine. *Cancer* 1961;14:901–12.

30 Ter-Minassian M, Chan JA, Hooshmand SM, *et al.* Clinical presentation, recurrence, and survival in patients with neuroendocrine tumors: results from a prospective institutional database. *Endocr Relat Cancer* 2013;20:187–96.

31 Maggard MA, O'Connell JB, Ko CY. Updated population-based review of carcinoid tumors. *Ann Surg* 2004;240:117–22.

32 Jann H, Roll S, Couvelard A, *et al.* Neuroendocrine tumors of midgut and hindgut origin: Tumor-node-metastasis classification determines clinical outcome. *Cancer* 2011;117:3332–41.

33 Yao JC, Hassan M, Phan A, *et al.* One hundred years after "carcinoid": epidemiology of and prognostic factors for neuroendocrine tumors in 35,825 cases in the United States. *J Clin Oncol* 2008;26:3063–72.

34 Modlin IM, Sandor A. An analysis of 8305 cases of carcinoid tumors. *Cancer* 1997;79:813–29.

35 Rindi G, Bordi C, Rappel S, *et al.* Gastric carcinoids and neuroendocrine carcinomas: pathogenesis, pathology, and behavior. *World J Surg* 1996;20:168–72.

36 Modlin IM, Gilligan CJ, Lawton GP, *et al.* Gastric carcinoids. *The Yale Experience. Arch Surg* 1995;130:250–5; discussion 255–6.

37 Thomas RM, Baybick JH, Elsayed AM, Sobin LH. Gastric carcinoids. An immunohistochemical and clinicopathologic study of 104 patients. *Cancer* 1994;73:2053–8.

38 Moses RE, Frank BB, Leavitt M, Miller R. The syndrome of type A chronic atrophic gastritis, pernicious anemia, and multiple gastric carcinoids. *J Clin Gastroenterol* 1986;8:61–5.

39 Spampatti MP, Massironi S, Rossi RE, *et al.* Unusually aggressive type 1 gastric carcinoid: a case report with a review of the literature. *Eur J Gastroenterol Hepatol* 2012;24:589–93.

40 Ahlman H, Kolby L, Lundell L, *et al.* Clinical management of gastric carcinoid tumors. *Digestion* 1994;55 Suppl 3:77–85.

41 Kulke MH, Benson AB, 3rd, Bergsland E, *et al.* Neuroendocrine tumors. *J Natl Compr Canc Netw* 2012;10:724–64.

42 Kulke MH, Anthony LB, Bushnell DL, *et al.* NANETS treatment guidelines: well-differentiated neuroendocrine tumors of the stomach and pancreas. *Pancreas* 2010;39:735–52.

43 Hirschowitz BI, Griffith J, Pellegrin D, Cummings OW. Rapid regression of enterochromaffinlike cell gastric carcinoids in pernicious anemia after antrectomy. *Gastroenterology* 1992;102:1409–18.

44 Delle Fave G, Capurso G, Milione M, Panzuto F. Endocrine tumours of the stomach. *Best Pract Res Clin Gastroenterol* 2005;19:659–73.

45 Shah P, Singh MH, Yang YX, Metz DC. Hypochlorhydria and achlorhydria are associated with false-positive secretin stimulation testing for Zollinger-Ellison syndrome. *Pancreas* 2013;42:932–6.

46 Saund MS, Al Natour RH, Sharma AM, *et al.* Tumor size and depth predict rate of lymph node metastasis and utilization of lymph node sampling in surgically managed gastric carcinoids. *Ann Surg Oncol* 2011;18:2826–32.

47 Waisberg J, Joppert-Netto G, Vasconcellos C, *et al.* Carcinoid tumor of the duodenum: a rare tumor at an unusual site. Case series from a single institution. *Arq Gastroenterol* 2013;50:3–9.

48 Kim GH, Kim JI, Jeon SW, *et al.* Endoscopic resection for duodenal carcinoid tumors: A multicenter, retrospective study. *J Gastroenterol Hepatol* 2014;29:318–24.

49 Moertel CG, Weiland LH, Nagorney DM, Dockerty MB. Carcinoid tumor of the appendix: treatment and prognosis. *N Engl J Med* 1987;317:1699–701.

50 Shaw PA. Carcinoid tumours of the appendix are different. *J Pathol* 1990;162:189–90.

51 Grozinsky-Glasberg S, Alexandraki KI, Barak D, *et al.* Current size criteria for the management of neuroendocrine tumors of the appendix: are they valid? Clinical experience and review of the literature. *Neuroendocrinology* 2013;98:31–7.

52 Pape UF, Perren A, Niederle B, *et al.* ENETS Consensus Guidelines for the management of patients with neuroendocrine neoplasms from the jejuno-ileum and the appendix including goblet cell carcinomas. *Neuroendocrinology* 2012;95:135–56.

53 Jetmore AB, Ray JE, Gathright JB, Jr., *et al.* Rectal carcinoids: the most frequent carcinoid tumor. *Dis Colon Rectum* 1992;35:717–25.

54 Naunheim KS, Zeitels J, Kaplan EL, *et al.* Rectal carcinoid tumors – treatment and prognosis. *Surgery* 1983;94:670–6.

55 Fahy BN, Tang LH, Klimstra D, *et al.* Carcinoid of the rectum risk stratification (CaRRs): A strategy for preoperative outcome assessment. *Ann Surg Oncol* 2007;14:1735–43.

56 Federspiel BH, Burke AP, Sobin LH, Shekitka KM. Rectal and colonic carcinoids. A clinicopathologic study of 84 cases. *Cancer* 1990;65:135–40.

57 Anthony LB, Strosberg JR, Klimstra DS, *et al.* The NANETS consensus guidelines for the diagnosis and management of gastrointestinal neuroendocrine tumors (nets): well-differentiated nets of the distal colon and rectum. *Pancreas* 2010;39:767–74.

58 Strosberg JR, Cheema A, Weber J, *et al.* Prognostic validity of a novel American Joint Committee on Cancer Staging Classification for pancreatic neuroendocrine tumors. *J Clin Oncol* 2011;29:3044–9.

59 Halfdanarson TR, Rubin J, Farnell MB, *et al.* Pancreatic endocrine neoplasms: epidemiology and prognosis of pancreatic endocrine tumors. *Endocr Relat Cancer* 2008;15:409–27.

60 Oberg K, Eriksson B. Endocrine tumours of the pancreas. *Best Pract Res Clin Gastroenterol* 2005;19:753–81.
61 Service FJ, McMahon MM, O'Brien PC, Ballard DJ. Functioning insulinoma – incidence, recurrence, and long-term survival of patients: a 60-year study. *Mayo Clin Proc* 1991;66:711–9.
62 Whipple AO. Islet cell tumors of the pancreas. *Can Med Assoc J* 1952;66:334–42.
63 Jensen RT. Gastrinomas: advances in diagnosis and management. *Neuroendocrinology* 2004;80 Suppl 1:23–7.
64 Gibril F, Jensen RT. Advances in evaluation and management of gastrinoma in patients with Zollinger-Ellison syndrome. *Curr Gastroenterol Rep* 2005;7:114–21.
65 Wolfe MM, Jensen RT. Zollinger-Ellison syndrome. Current concepts in diagnosis and management. *N Engl J Med* 1987;317:1200–9.
66 Zollinger RM, Ellison EH. Primary peptic ulcerations of the jejunum associated with islet cell tumors of the pancreas. *Ann Surg* 1955;142:709–23; discussion, 724–8.
67 Zollinger RM, Ellison EC, Fabri PJ, *et al.* Primary peptic ulcerations of the jejunum associated with islet cell tumors. *Twenty-five-year appraisal. Ann Surg* 1980;192:422–30.
68 Berna MJ, Hoffmann KM, Long SH, *et al.* Serum gastrin in Zollinger-Ellison syndrome: II. Prospective study of gastrin provocative testing in 293 patients from the National Institutes of Health and comparison with 537 cases from the literature. evaluation of diagnostic criteria, proposal of new criteria, and correlations with clinical and tumoral features. *Medicine (Baltimore)* 2006;85:331–64.
69 Metz DC, Strader DB, Orbuch M, *et al.* Use of omeprazole in Zollinger-Ellison syndrome: a prospective nine-year study of efficacy and safety. *Aliment Pharmacol Ther* 1993;7:597–610.
70 Verner JV, Morrison AB. Islet cell tumor and a syndrome of refractory watery diarrhea and hypokalemia. *Am J Med* 1958;25:374–80.
71 Bloom SR, Polak JM, Pearse AG. Vasoactive intestinal peptide and watery-diarrhoea syndrome. *Lancet* 1973;2:14–16.
72 Grier JF. WDHA (watery diarrhea, hypokalemia, achlorhydria) syndrome: clinical features, diagnosis, and treatment. *South Med J* 1995;88:22–4.
73 McGavran MH, Unger RH, Recant L, *et al.* A glucagon-secreting alpha-cell carcinoma of the pancreas. *N Engl J Med* 1966;274:1408–13.
74 Wermers RA, Fatourechi V, Wynne AG, *et al.* The glucagonoma syndrome. Clinical and pathologic features in 21 patients. *Medicine (Baltimore)* 1996;75:53–63.
75 Wilkinson DS. Necrolytic migratory erythema with carcinoma of the pancreas. *Trans St Johns Hosp Dermatol Soc* 1973;59:244–50.
76 Sinclair SA, Reynolds NJ. Necrolytic migratory erythema and zinc deficiency. *Br J Dermatol* 1997;136:783–5.
77 Alexander EK, Robinson M, Staniec M, Dluhy RG. Peripheral amino acid and fatty acid infusion for the treatment of necrolytic migratory erythema in the glucagonoma syndrome. *Clin Endocrinol (Oxf)* 2002;57:827–31.
78 Strosberg J, Gardner N, Kvols L. Survival and prognostic factor analysis in patients with metastatic pancreatic endocrine carcinomas. *Pancreas* 2009;38:255–8.
79 Cheema A, Weber J, Strosberg JR. Incidental detection of pancreatic neuroendocrine tumors: an analysis of incidence and outcomes. *Ann Surg Oncol* 2012;19:2932–6.
80 Hemminki K, Li X. Incidence trends and risk factors of carcinoid tumors: a nationwide epidemiologic study from Sweden. *Cancer* 2001;92:2204–10.
81 Wermer P. Genetic aspects of adenomatosis of endocrine glands. *Am J Med* 1954;16:363–71.
82 Scacheri PC, Davis S, Odom DT, *et al.* Genome-wide analysis of menin binding provides insights into MEN1 tumorigenesis. *PLoS Genet* 2006;2:e51.
83 Larsson C, Skogseid B, Oberg K, *et al.* Multiple endocrine neoplasia type 1 gene maps to chromosome 11 and is lost in insulinoma. *Nature* 1988;332:85–7.
84 Agarwal SK, Lee Burns A, Sukhodolets KE, *et al.* Molecular pathology of the MEN1 gene. *Ann N Y Acad Sci* 2004;1014:189–98.
85 Thompson NW. Current concepts in the surgical management of multiple endocrine neoplasia type 1 pancreatic-duodenal disease. Results in the treatment of 40 patients with Zollinger-Ellison syndrome, hypoglycaemia or both. *J Intern Med* 1998;243:495–500.
86 Norton JA, Fraker DL, Alexander HR, *et al.* Surgery to cure the Zollinger-Ellison syndrome. *N Engl J Med* 1999;341:635–44.
87 Ebeling T, Vierimaa O, Kytola S, *et al.* Effect of multiple endocrine neoplasia type 1 (MEN1) gene mutations on premature mortality in familial MEN1 syndrome with founder mutations. *J Clin Endocrinol Metab* 2004; 89:3392–6.
88 Dean PG, van Heerden JA, Farley DR, *et al.* Are patients with multiple endocrine neoplasia type I prone to premature death? *World J Surg* 2000;24:1437–41.
89 Richards FM, Maher ER, Latif F, *et al.* Detailed genetic mapping of the von Hippel-Lindau disease tumour suppressor gene. *J Med Genet* 1993;30:104–7.
90 Hammel PR, Vilgrain V, Terris B, *et al.* Pancreatic involvement in von Hippel-Lindau disease. The Groupe Francophone d'Etude de la Maladie de von Hippel-Lindau. *Gastroenterology* 2000;119:1087–95.
91 van Slegtenhorst M, de Hoogt R, Hermans C, *et al.* Identification of the tuberous sclerosis gene TSC1 on chromosome 9q34. *Science* 1997;277:805–8.
92 Verhoef S, van Diemen-Steenvoorde R, Akkersdijk WL, *et al.* Malignant pancreatic tumour within the spectrum of tuberous sclerosis complex in childhood. *Eur J Pediatr* 1999;158:284–7.
93 Gortz B, Roth J, Krahenmann A, *et al.* Mutations and allelic deletions of the MEN1 gene are associated with a subset of sporadic endocrine pancreatic and neuroendocrine tumors and not restricted to foregut neoplasms. *Am J Pathol* 1999;154:429–36.
94 Jiao Y, Shi C, Edil BH, *et al.* DAXX/ATRX, MEN1, and mTOR pathway genes are frequently altered in pancreatic neuroendocrine tumors. *Science* 2011;331:1199–203.
95 Lovejoy CA, Li W, Reisenweber S, *et al.* Loss of ATRX, genome instability, and an altered DNA damage response are hallmarks of the alternative lengthening of telomeres pathway. *PLoS Genet* 2012;8:e1002772.

96 Cunningham JL, Diaz de Stahl T, Sjoblom T, *et al.* Common pathogenetic mechanism involving human chromosome 18 in familial and sporadic ileal carcinoid tumors. *Genes Chromosomes Cancer* 2011;50:82–94.

97 Banck MS, Kanwar R, Kulkarni AA, *et al.* The genomic landscape of small intestine neuroendocrine tumors. *J Clin Invest* 2013;123:2502–8.

98 Taupenot L, Harper KL, O'Connor DT. The chromogranin-secretogranin family. *N Engl J Med* 2003;348:1134–49.

99 Strosberg J, Nasir A, Coppola D, *et al.* Correlation between grade and prognosis in metastatic gastroenteropancreatic neuroendocrine tumors. *Hum Pathol* 2009;40:1262–8.

100 O'Toole D, Grossman A, Gross D, *et al.* ENETS Consensus Guidelines for the Standards of Care in Neuroendocrine Tumors: biochemical markers. *Neuroendocrinology* 2009;90:194–202.

101 Bajetta E, Ferrari L, Martinetti A, *et al.* Chromogranin A, neuron specific enolase, carcinoembryonic antigen, and hydroxyindole acetic acid evaluation in patients with neuroendocrine tumors. *Cancer* 1999;86:858–65.

102 Haverback BJ, Sjoerdsma A, Terry LL. Urinary excretion of the serotonin metabolite, 5-hydroxyindoleacetic acid, in various clinical conditions. *N Engl J Med* 1956;255:270–2.

103 Kema IP, Schellings AM, Meiborg G, *et al.* Influence of a serotonin- and dopamine-rich diet on platelet serotonin content and urinary excretion of biogenic amines and their metabolites. *Clin Chem* 1992;38:1730–6.

104 Feldman JM, O'Dorisio TM. Role of neuropeptides and serotonin in the diagnosis of carcinoid tumors. *Am J Med* 1986;81:41–8.

105 Degg TJ, Allen KR, Barth JH. Measurement of plasma 5-hydroxyindoleacetic acid in carcinoid disease: an alternative to 24-h urine collections? *Ann Clin Biochem* 2000;37 (Pt 5):724–6.

106 O'Connor DT, Deftos LJ. Secretion of chromogranin A by peptide-producing endocrine neoplasms. *N Engl J Med* 1986;314:1145–51.

107 Pregun I, Herszenyi L, Juhasz M, *et al.* Effect of proton-pump inhibitor therapy on serum chromogranin a level. *Digestion* 2011;84:22–8.

108 Campana D, Nori F, Piscitelli L, *et al.* Chromogranin A: is it a useful marker of neuroendocrine tumors? *J Clin Oncol* 2007;25:1967–73.

109 Yao JC, Pavel M, Phan AT, *et al.* Chromogranin A and neuron-specific enolase as prognostic markers in patients with advanced pNET treated with everolimus. *J Clin Endocrinol Metab* 2011;96:3741–9.

110 Desai DC, O'Dorisio TM, Schirmer WJ, *et al.* Serum pancreastatin levels predict response to hepatic artery chemoembolization and somatostatin analogue therapy in metastatic neuroendocrine tumors. *Regul Pept* 2001;96:113–7.

111 Raines D, Chester M, Diebold AE, *et al.* A prospective evaluation of the effect of chronic proton pump inhibitor use on plasma biomarker levels in humans. *Pancreas* 2012;41:508–11.

112 Paulson EK, McDermott VG, Keogan MT, *et al.* Carcinoid metastases to the liver: role of triple-phase helical CT. *Radiology* 1998;206:143–50.

113 Paulsen SR, Huprich JE, Fletcher JG, *et al.* CT enterography as a diagnostic tool in evaluating small bowel disorders: review of clinical experience with over 700 cases. *Radiographics* 2006;26:641–57; discussion 657–62.

114 Legmann P, Vignaux O, Dousset B, *et al.* Pancreatic tumors: comparison of dual-phase helical CT and endoscopic sonography. *AJR Am J Roentgenol* 1998;170:1315–22.

115 Dromain C, de Baere T, Lumbroso J, *et al.* Detection of liver metastases from endocrine tumors: a prospective comparison of somatostatin receptor scintigraphy, computed tomography, and magnetic resonance imaging. *J Clin Oncol* 2005;23:70–8.

116 Dromain C, de Baere T, Baudin E, *et al.* MR imaging of hepatic metastases caused by neuroendocrine tumors: comparing four techniques. *AJR Am J Roentgenol* 2003;180:121–8.

117 Krenning EP, Bakker WH, Kooij PP, *et al.* Somatostatin receptor scintigraphy with indium-111-DTPA-D-Phe-1-octreotide in man: metabolism, dosimetry and comparison with iodine-123-Tyr-3-octreotide. *J Nucl Med* 1992;33:652–8.

118 Krenning EP, Kwekkeboom DJ, Bakker WH, *et al.* Somatostatin receptor scintigraphy with [111In-DTPA-D-Phe1]- and [123I-Tyr3]-octreotide: the Rotterdam experience with more than 1000 patients. *Eur J Nucl Med* 1993;20:716–31.

119 Schillaci O, Corleto VD, Annibale B, *et al.* Single photon emission computed tomography procedure improves accuracy of somatostatin receptor scintigraphy in gastro-entero pancreatic tumours. *Ital J Gastroenterol Hepatol* 1999;31 Suppl 2:S186–9.

120 Krausz Y, Keidar Z, Kogan I, *et al.* SPECT/CT hybrid imaging with 111In-pentetreotide in assessment of neuroendocrine tumours. *Clin Endocrinol (Oxf)* 2003;59:565–73.

121 Reidy-Lagunes DL, Gollub MJ, Saltz LB. Addition of octreotide functional imaging to cross-sectional computed tomography or magnetic resonance imaging for the detection of neuroendocrine tumors: added value or an anachronism? *J Clin Oncol* 2011;29:e74–5.

122 Koopmans KP, Neels OC, Kema IP, *et al.* Improved staging of patients with carcinoid and islet cell tumors with 18F-dihydroxy-phenyl-alanine and 11C-5-hydroxy-tryptophan positron emission tomography. *J Clin Oncol* 2008;26:1489–95.

123 Buchmann I, Henze M, Engelbrecht S, *et al.* Comparison of 68Ga-DOTATOC PET and 111In-DTPAOC (Octreoscan) SPECT in patients with neuroendocrine tumours. *Eur J Nucl Med Mol Imaging* 2007;34:1617–26.

124 Nanni C, Rubello D, Fanti S. 18F-DOPA PET/CT and neuroendocrine tumours. *Eur J Nucl Med Mol Imaging* 2006;33:509–13.

125 Sadowski SM, Neychev V, Millo C, *et al.* Prospective study of 68Ga-DOTATATE Positron emission tomography/computed tomography for detecting gastro-entero-pancreatic neuroendocrine tumors and unknown primary sites. *J Clin Oncol* 2016;34:588–96.

126 Khashab MA, Yong E, Lennon AM, *et al.* EUS is still superior to multidetector computerized tomography for detection of pancreatic neuroendocrine tumors. *Gastrointest Endosc* 2011;73:691–6.

127 Rosch T, Lightdale CJ, Botet JF, *et al.* Localization of pancreatic endocrine tumors by endoscopic ultrasonography. *N Engl J Med* 1992;326:1721–6.

128 Doppman JL, Miller DL, Chang R, *et al.* Intraarterial calcium stimulation test for detection of insulinomas. *World J Surg* 1993;17:439–43.

129 Thom AK, Norton JA, Doppman JL, *et al.* Prospective study of the use of intraarterial secretin injection and portal venous sampling to localize duodenal gastrinomas. *Surgery* 1992;112:1002–8; discussion 1008–9.

130 Lee LC, Grant CS, Salomao DR, *et al.* Small, nonfunctioning, asymptomatic pancreatic neuroendocrine tumors (PNETs): role for nonoperative management. *Surgery* 2012;152:965–74.

131 Boudreaux JP, Klimstra DS, Hassan MM, *et al.* The NANETS consensus guideline for the diagnosis and management of neuroendocrine tumors: well-differentiated neuroendocrine tumors of the jejunum, ileum, appendix, and cecum. *Pancreas* 2010;39:753–66.

132 Onozato Y, Kakizaki S, Iizuka H, *et al.* Endoscopic treatment of rectal carcinoid tumors. *Dis Colon Rectum* 2010;53:169–76.

133 Murray SE, Sippel RS, Lloyd R, Chen H. Surveillance of small rectal carcinoid tumors in the absence of metastatic disease. *Ann Surg Oncol* 2012;19:3486–90.

134 Kobayashi K, Katsumata T, Yoshizawa S, *et al.* Indications of endoscopic polypectomy for rectal carcinoid tumors and clinical usefulness of endoscopic ultrasonography. *Dis Colon Rectum* 2005;48:285–91.

135 Berkelhammer C, Jasper I, Kirvaitis E, *et al.* "Band-snare" resection of small rectal carcinoid tumors. *Gastrointest Endosc* 1999;50:582–5.

136 Okamoto Y, Fujii M, Tateiwa S, *et al.* Treatment of multiple rectal carcinoids by endoscopic mucosal resection using a device for esophageal variceal ligation. *Endoscopy* 2004;36:469–70.

137 Imada-Shirakata Y, Sakai M, Kajiyama T, *et al.* Endoscopic resection of rectal carcinoid tumors using aspiration lumpectomy. *Endoscopy* 1997;29:34–8.

138 Kinoshita T, Kanehira E, Omura K, *et al.* Transanal endoscopic microsurgery in the treatment of rectal carcinoid tumor. *Surg Endosc* 2007;21:970–4.

139 Schindl M, Niederle B, Hafner M, *et al.* Stage-dependent therapy of rectal carcinoid tumors. *World J Surg* 1998;22:628–33; discussion 634.

140 Caplin M, Sundin A, Nillson O, *et al.* ENETS Consensus Guidelines for the management of patients with digestive neuroendocrine neoplasms: colorectal neuroendocrine neoplasms. *Neuroendocrinology* 2012;95:88–97.

141 Kulke MH, Anthony LB, Bushnell DL, *et al.* NANETS treatment guidelines: well-differentiated neuroendocrine tumors of the stomach and pancreas. *Pancreas* 2010;39:735–52.

142 Schindl M, Kaserer K, Niederle B. Treatment of gastric neuroendocrine tumors: the necessity of a type-adapted treatment. *Arch Surg* 2001;136:49–54.

143 Reichlin S. Somatostatin. *N Engl J Med* 1983;309:1495–501.

144 Lamberts SW, van der Lely AJ, de Herder WW, Hofland LJ. Octreotide. *N Engl J Med* 1996;334:246–54.

145 Maurer R, Reubi JC. Somatostatin receptors. *Jama* 1985;253:2741.

146 Kvols LK, Moertel CG, O'Connell MJ, *et al.* Treatment of the malignant carcinoid syndrome. Evaluation of a long-acting somatostatin analogue. *N Engl J Med* 1986;315:663–6.

147 O'Toole D, Ducreux M, Bommelaer G, *et al.* Treatment of carcinoid syndrome: a prospective crossover evaluation of lanreotide versus octreotide in terms of efficacy, patient acceptability, and tolerance. *Cancer* 2000;88:770–6.

148 Maton PN. Use of octreotide acetate for control of symptoms in patients with islet cell tumors. *World J Surg* 1993;17:504–10.

149 Rubin J, Ajani J, Schirmer W, *et al.* Octreotide acetate long-acting formulation versus open-label subcutaneous octreotide acetate in malignant carcinoid syndrome. *J Clin Oncol* 1999;17:600–6.

150 Ruszniewski P, Ducreux M, Chayvialle JA, *et al.* Treatment of the carcinoid syndrome with the longacting somatostatin analogue lanreotide: a prospective study in 39 patients. *Gut* 1996;39:279–83.

151 Strosberg J, Weber J, Feldman M, *et al.* Above-label doses of octreotide-LAR in patients with metastatic small intestinal carcinoid tumors. *Gastrointest Cancer Res* 2013;6:81–5.

152 Woltering EA, Mamikunian PM, Zietz S, *et al.* Effect of octreotide LAR dose and weight on octreotide blood levels in patients with neuroendocrine tumors. *Pancreas* 2005;31:392–400.

153 Kahil ME, Brown H, Fred HL. The carcinoid crisis. *Arch Intern Med* 1964;114:26–8.

154 Massimino K, Harrskog O, Pommier S, Pommier R. Octreotide LAR and bolus octreotide are insufficient for preventing intraoperative complications in carcinoid patients. *J Surg Oncol* 2013;107:842–6.

155 Strosberg J, Kvols L. Antiproliferative effect of somatostatin analogs in gastroenteropancreatic neuroendocrine tumors. *World J Gastroenterol* 2010;16:2963–70.

156 Reardon DB, Dent P, Wood SL, *et al.* Activation in vitro of somatostatin receptor subtypes 2, 3, or 4 stimulates protein tyrosine phosphatase activity in membranes from transfected Ras-transformed NIH 3T3 cells: coexpression with catalytically inactive SHP-2 blocks responsiveness. *Mol Endocrinol* 1997;11:1062–9.

157 Weckbecker G, Lewis I, Albert R, *et al.* Opportunities in somatostatin research: biological, chemical and therapeutic aspects. *Nat Rev Drug Discov* 2003;2:999–1017.

158 Rinke A, Muller HH, Schade-Brittinger C, *et al.* Placebo-controlled, double-blind, prospective, randomized study on the effect of octreotide LAR in the control of tumor growth in patients with metastatic neuroendocrine midgut tumors: a report from the PROMID Study Group. *J Clin Oncol* 2009;27:4656–63.

159 Caplin M, Pavel M, Ćwikła JB, *et al.* Lanreotide in metastatic enteropancreatic neuroendocrine tumors. *N Engl J Med* 2014;371(3):224–33. Available at: https://www.ncbi.nlm.nih.gov/pubmed/25014687 [accessed 18 December 2017].

160 Oberg K, Norheim I, Lind E, *et al.* Treatment of malignant carcinoid tumors with human leukocyte interferon: long-term results. *Cancer Treat Rep* 1986;70:1297–304.

161 Bajetta E, Zilembo N, Di Bartolomeo M, *et al.* Treatment of metastatic carcinoids and other neuroendocrine tumors with recombinant interferon-alpha-2a. A study by the Italian

Trials in Medical Oncology Group. *Cancer* 1993;72:3099–105.
162 Moertel CG, Rubin J, Kvols LK. Therapy of metastatic carcinoid tumor and the malignant carcinoid syndrome with recombinant leukocyte A interferon. *J Clin Oncol* 1989;7:865–8.
163 Janson ET, Oberg K. Long-term management of the carcinoid syndrome. Treatment with octreotide alone and in combination with alpha-interferon. *Acta Oncol* 1993;32:225–9.
164 Pavel ME, Baum U, Hahn EG, *et al.* Efficacy and tolerability of pegylated IFN-alpha in patients with neuroendocrine gastroenteropancreatic carcinomas. *J Interferon Cytokine Res* 2006;26:8–13.
165 Kolby L, Persson G, Franzen S, Ahren B. Randomized clinical trial of the effect of interferon alpha on survival in patients with disseminated midgut carcinoid tumours. *Br J Surg* 2003;90:687–93.
166 Arnold R, Rinke A, Klose KJ, *et al* l. Octreotide versus octreotide plus interferon-alpha in endocrine gastroenteropancreatic tumors: a randomized trial. *Clin Gastroenterol Hepatol* 2005;3:761–71.
167 Faiss S, Pape UF, Bohmig M, *et al.* Prospective, randomized, multicenter trial on the antiproliferative effect of lanreotide, interferon alfa, and their combination for therapy of metastatic neuroendocrine gastroenteropancreatic tumors – the International Lanreotide and Interferon Alfa Study Group. *J Clin Oncol* 2003;21:2689–96.
168 Yao JC, Lombard-Bohas C, Baudin E, *et al.* Daily oral everolimus activity in patients with metastatic pancreatic neuroendocrine tumors after failure of cytotoxic chemotherapy: a phase II trial. *J Clin Oncol* 2010;28:69–76.
169 Yao JC, Shah MH, Ito T, *et al.* Everolimus for advanced pancreatic neuroendocrine tumors. *N Engl J Med* 2011;364:514–23.
170 Pavel ME, Hainsworth JD, Baudin E, *et al.* Everolimus plus octreotide long-acting repeatable for the treatment of advanced neuroendocrine tumours associated with carcinoid syndrome (RADIANT-2): a randomised, placebo-controlled, phase 3 study. *Lancet* 2011;378:2005–12.
171 Yao JC, Fazio N, Singh S, *et al.* Everolimus for the treatment of advanced, non-functional neuroendocrine tumours of the lung or gastrointestinal tract (RADIANT-4): a randomised, placebo-controlled, phase 3 study. *Lancet* 2016;387:968–77.
172 Kulke MH, Lenz HJ, Meropol NJ, *et al.* Activity of sunitinib in patients with advanced neuroendocrine tumors. *J Clin Oncol* 2008;26:3403–10.
173 Raymond E, Dahan L, Raoul JL, *et al.* Sunitinib malate for the treatment of pancreatic neuroendocrine tumors. *N Engl J Med* 2011;364:501–13.
174 Yao JC, Phan A, Hoff PM, *et al.* Targeting vascular endothelial growth factor in advanced carcinoid tumor: a random assignment phase II study of depot octreotide with bevacizumab and pegylated interferon alpha-2b. *J Clin Oncol* 2008;26:1316–23.
175 Yao JC, Guthrie KA, Moran C, *et al.* Phase III prospective randomized comparison trial of depot octreotide plus interferon alfa-2b versus depot octreotide plus bevacizumab in patients with advanced carcinoid tumors: SWOG S0518. *J Clin Oncol* 2017;35(15):1695–703.
176 Moertel CG, Kvols LK, O'Connell MJ, Rubin J. Treatment of neuroendocrine carcinomas with combined etoposide and cisplatin. Evidence of major therapeutic activity in the anaplastic variants of these neoplasms. *Cancer* 1991;68:227–32.
177 Mitry E, Baudin E, Ducreux M, *et al.* Treatment of poorly differentiated neuroendocrine tumours with etoposide and cisplatin. *Br J Cancer* 1999;81:1351–5.
178 Sorbye H, Welin S, Langer SW, *et al.* Predictive and prognostic factors for treatment and survival in 305 patients with advanced gastrointestinal neuroendocrine carcinoma (WHO G3): the NORDIC NEC study. *Ann Oncol* 2013;24:152–60.
179 Moertel CG, Hanley JA, Johnson LA. Streptozocin alone compared with streptozocin plus fluorouracil in the treatment of advanced islet-cell carcinoma. *N Engl J Med* 1980;303:1189–94.
180 Moertel CG, Lefkopoulo M, Lipsitz S, *et al.* Streptozocin-doxorubicin, streptozocin-fluorouracil or chlorozotocin in the treatment of advanced islet-cell carcinoma. *N Engl J Med* 1992;326:519–23.
181 Kouvaraki MA, Ajani JA, Hoff P, *et al.* Fluorouracil, doxorubicin, and streptozocin in the treatment of patients with locally advanced and metastatic pancreatic endocrine carcinomas. *J Clin Oncol* 2004;22:4762–71.
182 Kulke MH, Stuart K, Enzinger PC, *et al.* Phase II study of temozolomide and thalidomide in patients with metastatic neuroendocrine tumors. *J Clin Oncol* 2006;24:401–6.
183 Chan JA, Stuart K, Earle CC, *et al.* Prospective study of bevacizumab plus temozolomide in patients with advanced neuroendocrine tumors. *J Clin Oncol* 2012;30:2963–8.
184 Strosberg JR, Fine RL, Choi J, *et al.* First-line chemotherapy with capecitabine and temozolomide in patients with metastatic pancreatic endocrine carcinomas. *Cancer* 2011;117:268–75.
185 Fine RL, Gulati AP, Krantz BA, *et al.* Capecitabine and temozolomide (CAPTEM) for metastatic, well-differentiated neuroendocrine cancers: The Pancreas Center at Columbia University experience. *Cancer Chemother Pharmacol* 2013;71:663–70.
186 Sun W, Lipsitz S, Catalano P, *et al.* Phase II/III study of doxorubicin with fluorouracil compared with streptozocin with fluorouracil or dacarbazine in the treatment of advanced carcinoid tumors: Eastern Cooperative Oncology Group Study E1281. *J Clin Oncol* 2005;23:4897–904.
187 Valkema R, De Jong M, Bakker WH, *et al.* Phase I study of peptide receptor radionuclide therapy with [In-DTPA] octreotide: the Rotterdam experience. *Semin Nucl Med* 2002;32:110–22.
188 Paganelli G, Bodei L, Handkiewicz Junak D, *et al.* 90Y-DOTA-D-Phe1-Try3-octreotide in therapy of neuroendocrine malignancies. *Biopolymers* 2002;66:393–8.
189 Bushnell DL, Jr., O'Dorisio TM, O'Dorisio MS, *et al.* 90Y-edotreotide for metastatic carcinoid refractory to octreotide. *J Clin Oncol* 2010;28:1652–9.
190 Imhof A, Brunner P, Marincek N, *et al.* Response, survival, and long-term toxicity after therapy with the radiolabeled somatostatin analogue [90Y-DOTA]-TOC in metastasized neuroendocrine cancers. *J Clin Oncol* 2011;29:2416–23.

191 Kwekkeboom DJ, de Herder WW, Kam BL, *et al.* Treatment with the radiolabeled somatostatin analog [177 Lu-DOTA 0,Tyr3]octreotate: toxicity, efficacy, and survival. *J Clin Oncol* 2008;26:2124–30.

192 Strosberg J, El-Haddad G, Wolin E, *et al.* Phase 3 Trial of 177Lu-Dotatate for Midgut Neuroendocrine Tumors. *N Engl J Med* 2017;376(2):125–135. Available at: https://www.ncbi.nlm.nih.gov/pubmed/28076709 [accessed 18 December 2017].

193 Que FG, Nagorney DM, Batts KP, *et al.* Hepatic resection for metastatic neuroendocrine carcinomas. *Am J Surg* 1995;169:36–42; discussion 42–3.

194 Sarmiento JM, Heywood G, Rubin J, *et al.* Surgical treatment of neuroendocrine metastases to the liver: a plea for resection to increase survival. *J Am Coll Surg* 2003;197:29–37.

195 Hellman P, Ladjevardi S, Skogseid B, *et al.* Radiofrequency tissue ablation using cooled tip for liver metastases of endocrine tumors. *World J Surg* 2002;26:1052–6.

196 Kvols LK, Turaga KK, Strosberg J, Choi J. Role of interventional radiology in the treatment of patients with neuroendocrine metastases in the liver. *J Natl Compr Canc Netw* 2009;7:765–72.

197 Strosberg JR, Choi J, Cantor AB, Kvols LK. Selective hepatic artery embolization for treatment of patients with metastatic carcinoid and pancreatic endocrine tumors. *Cancer Control* 2006;13:72–8.

198 Gupta S, Yao JC, Ahrar K, *et al.* Hepatic artery embolization and chemoembolization for treatment of patients with metastatic carcinoid tumors: the M.D. Anderson experience. *Cancer J* 2003;9:261–7.

199 Eriksson BK, Larsson EG, Skogseid BM, *et al.* Liver embolizations of patients with malignant neuroendocrine gastrointestinal tumors. *Cancer* 1998;83:2293–301.

200 Therasse E, Breittmayer F, Roche A, *et al.* Transcatheter chemoembolization of progressive carcinoid liver metastasis. *Radiology* 1993;189:541–7.

201 Ruszniewski P, Rougier P, Roche A, *et al.* Hepatic arterial chemoembolization in patients with liver metastases of endocrine tumors. A prospective phase II study in 24 patients. *Cancer* 1993;71:2624–30.

202 Strosberg JR, Weber JM, Choi J, *et al.* A phase II clinical trial of sunitinib following hepatic transarterial embolization for metastatic neuroendocrine tumors. *Ann Oncol* 2012;23:2335–41.

203 Maire F, Lombard-Bohas C, O'Toole D, *et al.* Hepatic arterial embolization versus chemoembolization in the treatment of liver metastases from well-differentiated midgut endocrine tumors: a prospective randomized study. *Neuroendocrinology* 2012;96:294–300.

204 Kennedy AS, Dezarn WA, McNeillie P, *et al.* Radioembolization for unresectable neuroendocrine hepatic metastases using resin 90Y-microspheres: early results in 148 patients. *Am J Clin Oncol* 2008;31:271–9.

205 Rhee TK, Lewandowski RJ, Liu DM, *et al.* 90Y Radioembolization for metastatic neuroendocrine liver tumors: preliminary results from a multi-institutional experience. *Ann Surg* 2008;247:1029–35.

206 Lehnert T. Liver transplantation for metastatic neuroendocrine carcinoma: an analysis of 103 patients. *Transplantation* 1998;66:1307–12.

207 Le Treut YP, Gregoire E, Belghiti J, *et al.* Predictors of long-term survival after liver transplantation for metastatic endocrine tumors: an 85-case French multicentric report. *Am J Transplant* 2008;8:1205–13.

Section 11

Cancer of the Nervous System and Eye

40

Central Nervous System and Peripheral Nerves

D. Ryan Ormond[1], Alexandros Bouras[2], Michael Moore[3], Matthew Gary[4], Paula Province Warren[5], Roshan Prabhu[6], Kathleen M. Egan[7], Srikant Rangaraju[4], Christina Appin[8], Constantinos Hadjipanayis[2], Burt Nabors[5], Alfredo Voloschin[9], and Jeffrey J. Olson[3]

[1] University of Colorado School of Medicine, Aurora, Colorado, USA
[2] Icahn School of Medicine at Mount Sinai, New York, New York, USA
[3] Emory University School of Medicine, Atlanta, Georgia, USA
[4] Emory Clinic, Atlanta, Georgia, USA
[5] University of Alabama at Birmingham, Birmingham, Alabama, USA
[6] Southeast Radiation Oncology Group, Charlotte, North Carolina, USA
[7] H. Lee Moffitt Cancer Center, Tampa, Florida, USA
[8] Northwestern University, Feinberg School of Medicine, Chicago, Illinois, USA
[9] Winship Cancer Institute, Emory University School of Medicine, Atlanta, Georgia, USA

Introduction

Involvement of the nervous system by tumors originating within or adjacent to it is not common in the overall landscape of human cancers. Though these tumors are uncommon, the therapy of the different lesions differs considerably and the treating physician cannot assume that applicability of a given regimen or modality can be generalized across tumor types. One can compartmentalize thought regarding the therapy of this set of tumors in terms of surgery, chemotherapy, targeted therapy, and radiation therapy.

Surgery is still necessary for definitive diagnosis in most tumors involving the nervous system. In some cases, surgery by itself is curative. To improve preservation of normal structures and maximize postoperative quality of life, efforts have been made to simplify and standardize intraoperative electrophysiological monitoring and enhance intraoperative tumor visualization [1–3]. Advances in imaging such as magnetic resonance spectroscopy and laboratory techniques such as quantification and characterization of circulating tumor-related DNA may ultimately provide alternatives to surgically obtained tissue for diagnostic purposes [4–6].

Systemic chemotherapy, an important therapeutic component for many cancers, has a substantial role in primary central nervous system lymphomas and a more limited but positive role in primary malignant tumors of the brain with agents such as temozolomide that cross the blood–brain barrier [7, 8]. However, it is less effective in the common circumstance of metastatic disease involving the central nervous system and in most of the rarer histologic subtypes of brain tumors [9].

Rapid advances in uncovering the biological mechanisms behind nervous system tumors may make targeted agents a promising treatment in the future. To date, only a few targeted agents have significant clinical data for treatment of CNS malignancies [10–16].

After surgical diagnosis the cornerstone of brain tumor therapy continues to be radiation therapy. The physics of the X-ray itself has not changed since its discovery but ability to tailor the dose to the conformation of the pathologic tissue is clearly advancing and becoming broadly available. Techniques such as intensity-modulated and image-guided planning are becoming more automated, which facilitates dissemination beyond specialized centers, in turn maximizing safety for all individuals with tumors of the nervous system [17, 18].

The presentation in this chapter is primarily aimed at the management of adult brain tumors. First, it provides brief general background comments. Then it discusses the use of the primary treatment modalities in general and finally their more specific application by tumor type.

Incidence and Mortality

CNS tumors are the fourteenth most common cancer diagnosis in US men and fifteenth most common cancer diagnosis in US women [19]. CNS cancers will kill nearly 17,000 persons in 2017 and are the leading cause of cancer death in men aged 20–39 and the fifth in women of that age [20].

During 2004–2007, more than 213,500 CNS tumors were diagnosed in the US, of which approximately one-third were

The American Cancer Society's Oncology in Practice: Clinical Management, First Edition. Edited by The American Cancer Society.

malignant. Neuroepithelial tumors (primarily gliomas) are the most common histological group of malignant brain tumor, occurring more frequently in men than women. Meningiomas comprise the most common nonmalignant adult brain tumor, occurring twice as often in women than in men. CNS tumors can occur at any age. Overall, primary brain tumors have a bimodal incidence, with a small peak in infancy and childhood and then a consistent rise with age. Some tumors, such as medulloblastoma and brainstem glioma, are more common in children than in adults, whereas others, such as glioblastoma multiforme and meningioma, are more common in adults. Tumors of the CNS represent the second most common cancer type in children aged 0–14 (behind only leukemias), comprising 25% of all cancers in children. Overall incidence rates are lower in children than in adults but tumors in children are more likely to be malignant [19].

As a cause of disability and death, metastases to the CNS are far more common than are primary CNS tumors [21]. Although exact data are not available, one estimate suggests that in excess of 100,000 individuals a year will die having suffered from symptomatic intracranial metastases and that as many as 80,000 patients a year will suffer spinal cord compression as a result of metastatic tumor [4, 22]. Survival rates in CNS tumors are strongly related to age at diagnosis as well as histological type and era of diagnosis. Overall survival has improved over the last 30 years of available data, from 22% during 1975–1977 to 35% during 2005–2011 [20].

Etiologic Factors

Environmental Risk Factors

Although a relatively large number of studies have examined the relationship between the environment and occurrence of brain tumors, environmental risk factors remain poorly understood. Only two unequivocal risk factors have been identified: ionizing radiation [23] and immunosuppression [24].

Genetic Risk

A few inherited diseases predispose to the development of primary CNS tumors (Table 40.1) [25–28], the majority with an autosomal dominant mode of inheritance. Familial occurrence of glioma in one or more blood relatives is associated with approximately a doubling of risk in the individual [29]. Hereditary diseases are extremely rare and much of the excess familial risk is now thought to be a consequence of multiple low-risk genetic polymorphisms.

Classification of Tumors

The cells of the CNS include neurons and glia, as well as several other neuroepithelial and non-neuroepithelial cell types. Glia account for approximately 90% of the cells in the CNS and include astrocytes, oligodendrocytes, ependymal cells, and

Table 40.1 Hereditary syndromes associated with brain tumors.

Syndrome	Tumor type	Involved chromosomes	Gene	Reference [#]
Li–Fraumeni syndrome	Glioma, medulloblastoma	17p13	*TP53*	[315]
Tuberous sclerosis	Subependymal giant-cell astrocytoma, cortical tubers, glioma	9q34, 16p13	*TSC1, TSC2*	[316]
Neurofibromatosis type 1 (von Recklinghausen disease; NF1)	Glioma (optic nerve) astrocytoma, glioblastoma	17q11	*NF1*	[317], [318]
Neurofibromatosis type 2 (NF2)	Meningioma, schwannoma (bilateral acoustic neuroma), ependymomas	22q12	*NF2*	[319]
Multiple endocrine neoplasia type 1 (MEN1)	Pituitary	11q13	*MEN1*	[26]
Retinoblastoma	Retinoblastoma	13q14	*RB1*	[27]
Basal cell nevus syndrome (Gorlin syndrome)	Medulloblastoma	9q22	*PTCH*	[320]
Turcot syndrome (hereditary nonpolyposis colorectal cancer syndrome (HNPCC))	Brain tumors of diverse histology, including glioblastoma and medulloblastoma	5q21	*APC*	[321]
		2p16	*hMLH2*	
		3p21	*hMLH1*	
		7p22	*hPMS2*	
von Hippel–Lindau disease	Hemangioblastoma	3p25-20	*VHL*	[322]
Cowden syndrome	Dysplastic cerebellar gangliocytoma, meningioma, astrocytoma	10p23	*PTEN (MMACI)*	[323]
Rhabdoid predisposition syndrome	Choroid plexus carcinoma, medulloblastoma, primitive neuroectodermal tumors	22q11	*hSNFS/INI1*	[28]

microglia [30]. Tumors can originate from any of these cells, with the exception of microglia, and are called gliomas. Astrocytomas can be either diffusely infiltrative or solid and well-circumscribed, whereas oligodendrogliomas are purely infiltrative and ependymomas are noninfiltrative. The diffuse gliomas are the most common primary brain neoplasms, with diffuse astrocytomas constituting 60% of such tumors [30]. Unlike diffuse gliomas, neuronal and glioneuronal tumors, as a group, tend to be well-circumscribed and poorly or non-infiltrative. The choroid plexus and pineal gland also produce neuroepithelial tumors. In addition to neuroepithelial tissues, CNS tumors may also arise from other tissues, such as adenohypophysis, meningothelia, and peripheral nerve sheath, among many others.

CNS tumors have, until recently, been classified primarily based on the cell of origin and pattern of differentiation, with the World Health Organization (WHO) system of classification being the most widely used [31]. In recent years, however, numerous studies have shown that molecular alterations can have a significant impact on prognosis and perhaps response to treatment. One of the most important examples of this in CNS tumors is the *IDH* mutation in infiltrating gliomas. A number of studies have shown the positive prognostic significance of an *IDH* mutation in an infiltrating glioma [32–34] and a study published in 2015 in the *New England Journal of Medicine* (NEJM) has shown that infiltrating gliomas can be classified based on their *IDH* mutation status and whether or not the tumor is 1p/19q co-deleted [35]. Stratification by these molecular alterations was shown to more accurately reflect the biological behavior of these tumors than stratification by histology [35]. A new WHO edition, published in 2016, incorporates the results of molecular studies into the diagnosis of these tumors, along with the histologic appearance and grade [36].

There are other factors to consider when classifying CNS tumors. Tumors located in the sellar region, pineal region, cerebellopontine angle, and meninges each have unique differential diagnoses. Tumors from these locations can arise from a more than one cell type, contributing to the challenge in making a diagnosis. Some primary CNS tumors, such as germ cell tumors and hematolymphoid neoplasms, have systemic homologous counterparts. Other groups of tumors exhibit similar appearance and behavior, such as embryonal tumors which are all poorly differentiated, primitive appearing, and demonstrate malignant behavior. And finally, there are metastatic tumors from other sites in the body (the most frequent being lung), which are the most common CNS tumors overall.

Table 40.2 lists tumors of neuroepithelial origin with corresponding WHO grades, while Table 40.3 lists tumors of non-neuroepithelial origin also with WHO grades (where applicable) [36].

Central Nervous System Tumor Signs and Symptoms

Neurologic symptoms are primarily related to two key factors: the size of the tumor and the location of the tumor. Interestingly, increased tumor size does not always correlate with symptom severity, as this is relative to the region affected, particularly in the

Table 40.2 Tumors of neuroepithelial origin and their WHO grade [36].

Gliomas
Infiltrative
Astrocytomas
Diffuse astrocytoma II
Anaplastic astrocytoma III
Glioblastoma IV
Diffuse midline glioma, *H3K27M*-mutant IV
Oligodendrogliomas
Oligodendroglioma II
Anaplastic oligodendroglioma III
Note: Diffuse astrocytomas, anaplastic astrocytomas and glioblastomas can be further classified as *IDH*-mutant, *IDH*-wildtype or NOS. Oligodendrogliomas (grade II and III) can be further classified as *IDH*-mutant and 1p/19q-codeleted, or NOS.
Noninfiltrative/poorly infiltrative (circumscribed)
Astrocytomas
Pilocytic astrocytoma I
Subependymal giant cell astrocytoma I
Pilomyxoid astrocytoma II
Pleomorphic xanthoastrocytoma II
Ependymal tumors
Subependymoma I
Myxopapillary ependymoma I
Ependymoma II
Anaplastic ependymoma III
Ependymoma, RELA-fusion positive II-III
Neuronal and glioneuronal tumors
Neuronal
Gangliocytoma I
Dysplastic gangliocytoma of cerebellum (Lhermitte–Duclos) I
Central neurocytoma II
Extraventricular neurocytoma II
Cerebellar liponeurocytoma II
Mixed glioneuronal
Ganglioglioma I
Anaplastic ganglioglioma III
Desmoplastic infantile astrocytoma/ganglioglioma I
Dysembryoplastic neuroepithelial tumor I
Papillary glioneuronal tumor I
Rosette-forming glioneuronal tumor of the fourth ventricle I
Choroid plexus tumors
Choroid plexus papilloma I
Atypical choroid plexus papilloma II
Choroid plexus carcinoma III

(*Continued*)

Table 40.2 (Continued)

Pineal region tumors
Pineocytoma I
Pineal parenchymal tumor of intermediate differentiation II or III
Pineoblastoma IV
Papillary tumor of the pineal region II-III
Embryonal tumors
Medulloblastoma IV
CNS primitive neuroectodermal tumor (PNET) IV
Atypical teratoid/rhabdoid tumor (AT/RT) IV

brain. For example, a neoplasm in the frontal lobe may remain somewhat clinically silent for a relatively long time period, whereas a neoplasm in the primary motor cortex or brainstem may present with acute neurologic dysfunction much sooner.

There are several mechanisms by which CNS tumors cause neurologic symptoms. Invasion is a mechanism by which tumors can infiltrate and replace normal tissue. Tumors can also cause neurologic symptoms by compression and dislocation of normal tissue. This can happen by way of tumor-associated edema or by obstruction of normal cerebrospinal fluid (CSF) pathways by the tumor itself, resulting in hydrocephalus. Additionally, as a result of the combination of edema, compression, and hydrocephalus, large brain tumors can sometimes result in herniation of normal cerebral structures and therefore cause acute neurologic deterioration or death.

Generalized Symptoms and Signs

Generalized symptoms and signs of brain tumors are numerous and most often reflect an increase in intracerebral pressure (ICP). Headache is the most common symptom associated with elevated ICP and can occur as one of the first symptoms in patients with brain tumors. The location of the tumor is predictive on the presence of headache, with approximately 3% of patients with supratentorial tumors and 56% of patients with infratentorial tumors presenting with headache as their first symptom [37]. Additionally, the majority of patients with brain tumors do experience headaches at some point during their illness, with prevalence rates ranging from 60 to 90% [38]. Headaches appear to be more common in patients with a history of headache, in patients with increased ICP, and in patients with larger tumors that have more midline shift on neuroimaging [38]. Although most headaches associated with brain tumors are nonspecific, some key clinical features that are suspicious for tumors include: headache present on awakening, new-onset headache in a middle-aged or elderly patient with no prior headache history, and/or changes in character or severity of headaches in a patient with a headache history.

Vomiting with or without preceding nausea can be associated with brain tumors, particularly in the pediatric population, and is most often related to elevated ICP and resulting irritation of the vagal nuclei or the vomiting centers located in the floor of the fourth ventricle. Vomiting may or may not be accompanied by headache and this pattern can often be mistaken for migraine headache.

Table 40.3 Tumors of non-neuroepithelial origin and their WHO grade [36].

Tumors of the meninges
Meningiomas
Meningothelial meningioma I
Atypical meningioma II
Brain invasive meningioma II
Chordoid meningioma II
Clear cell meningioma II
Papillary meningioma III
Rhabdoid meningioma III
Anaplastic meningioma III
Hemangiopericytoma II
Anaplastic hemangiopericytoma III
Hemangioblastoma I
Melanocytic tumors
Melanocytoma
Melanoma
Sellar region tumors
Pituitary adenoma
Pituicytoma I
Craniopharyngioma I
Granular cell tumor I
Spindle cell oncocytoma of the adenohypophysis I
Cranial and paraspinal nerve tumors
Schwannoma
Neurofibroma
Malignant peripheral nerve sheath tumor (MPNST)
Hematolymphoid tumors
Lymphoma
Plasmacytoma
Granulocytic sarcoma
Germ cell tumors
Germinoma
Yolk sac tumor
Embryonal carcinoma
Choriocarcinoma
Mature teratoma
Immature teratoma
Metastatic tumors

Other general symptoms and signs that are reflective of increased ICP include drowsiness, changes in mental status, personality changes, cognitive impairment, papilledema, and blurred vision and/or loss of peripheral vision.

CNS tumors that involve the spinal cord can present with nonspecific back or neck pain. This pain is often at the level of the tumor; however the pain can be mistaken for radicular symptoms.

Focal Symptoms and Signs

Seizures are a common problem in patients with brain tumors, with an incidence of approximately 30% in patients with primary brain tumors [39]. Additionally, a retrospective study revealed that seizure was the presenting symptom of a brain tumor in 50 of 147 patients with intra-axial, extra-axial, and metastatic brain tumors [39]. The location and histologic grade of brain tumors correlate with seizure risk, with slow-growing, low-grade tumors and tumors located in the gray matter being most likely to produce seizures. Furthermore, lesions in the occipital lobes are the least commonly associated with seizure production, and lesions in the frontal, temporal, and parietal lobes are most commonly associated with seizure production. Seizures associated with brain tumors are most often focal in onset, but may secondarily generalize. The associated seizure semiology is directly related to location of the tumor producing the seizure.

Other focal signs can include hearing and vision problems, balance problems, weakness, sensory changes, and language disturbances. These other focal signs and symptoms are also directly related to the area affected by the brain or spinal cord tumor.

False Localizing Symptoms

False localizing symptoms generally describe neurological signs that reflect dysfunction that is distant from the expected anatomical location of the pathology. They can occur as a consequence of elevated ICP or in association with spinal cord tumors. Common examples associated with elevated ICP include cranial nerve palsies, especially diplopia secondary to effects on cranial nerve VI, and anosmia. Hemiparesis, truncal sensory levels, and muscle atrophy are examples of possible false localizing signs as a result of spinal cord tumors.

General Principles of Treatment

Surgery

Surgical resection is one of the mainstays of therapy for patients with brain or spinal cord tumors, excluding those patients with primary CNS lymphoma (PCNSL). Although surgery is rarely curative in these patients, the associated benefits are multifold and include confirmation of diagnosis, relief of mass effect, and possible improvement in seizure control. Additionally, relieving local mass effect is further beneficial to patients by often allowing a decrease in corticosteroid dose and possibly helping provide better tolerance of additional therapies such as chemotherapy and radiotherapy. Although there is some risk of focal neurologic dysfunction after surgery, improvements and refinements in surgical techniques, specifically with regards to the development of functional imaging with MRI (fMRI) and diffusion tensor imaging (DTI) tractography, have greatly reduced this potential risk. Additionally, there is increasing evidence that more extensive surgical resection is associated with longer life expectancy in patients with both low-grade and high-grade gliomas [40]. In order to evaluate the amount of residual tumor after surgical resection and to provide prognosis, radiological assessment of the postoperative tumor contrast enhancement within 3 days of resection is a more sensitive means than surgeons' intraoperative predictions of degree of resection [41, 42].

Radiotherapy

In patients with high-grade tumors, radiotherapy is the primary adjuvant treatment; it improves patient quality of life and improves survival, especially in those younger than age 65 [43]. The role of radiotherapy in patients with low-grade tumors is less clear but there is some evidence that early postoperative radiation therapy may increase progression-free survival (PFS) but not overall survival (OS) [44]. Adjuvant therapy with radiotherapy is also the general treatment for intramedullary spinal cord tumors; however dose amounts vary with the grade of the tumor and the extent of disease. Radiotherapy modalities can include brachytherapy, stereotactic fractionated radiotherapy, stereotactic radiosurgery, and three-dimensional conformal external beam radiation, which is the most common. Furthermore, proton and heavy particle therapy is being evaluated as a promising new therapeutic technique to treat brain and spinal tumors while also limiting the dose of irradiation to normal surrounding tissue [45].

Chemotherapy

The chemotherapy standard of care for treatment of patients with newly diagnosed malignant gliomas is concurrent temozolomide, a second-generation alkylating agent, with radiotherapy followed by monthly cycles of temozolomide. Several clinical trials support that temozolomide is effective against malignant gliomas and have demonstrated a statistically-significant improvement in 6-month PFS rates with temozolomide, as compared to procarbazine, another chemotherapy agent used to treat gliomas [46]. Additionally, temozolomide is also the first-line agent in treating low-grade gliomas when chemotherapy is chosen.

Anticonvulsants

There is no evidence to support the use of prophylactic antiepileptic drugs (AEDs) in patients with brain tumors who have not had a seizure. However, if patients do have focal or generalized seizures they should be treated with AEDs. Common first-line agents in these cases include levetiracetam, lamotrigine, valproic acid, and topiramate and, in general, the non-enzyme-inducing AEDs are preferred over the enzyme-inducing AEDs, such as carbamazepine and phenytoin that may alter chemotherapy metabolism unfavorably. Monotherapy is usually first-line and levetiracetam is often the chosen agent because of relatively few side effects and interactions with other medications. If this monotherapy fails to control seizures, it is generally recommended to add on a second agent rather than changing to another single agent [47]. It is important to recognize that patients with tumor-associated epilepsy can experience more side effects from AEDs and the interaction between AEDs and potential chemotherapeutic agents must be considered.

Corticosteroids

Corticosteroids are indicated in the initial treatment of all brain and spinal cord tumor patients with symptomatic vasogenic edema, except those with PCNSL, as steroid use can cause cell lysis and tumor regression and therefore should not be given until a biopsy-proven diagnosis has been made. In patients with brain and spinal cord tumors, corticosteroids can dramatically improve symptoms by relieving peritumoral edema and decreasing ICP. Patients are generally started on dexamethasone at a dose of 16 mg/day and are maintained at this dose until symptoms are improved. At this point, steroids should be tapered off or down to the lowest possible dose.

Other Modalities

Therapeutic techniques such as immunotherapy, gene therapy, and antiangiogenesis agents are currently under investigation. In particular, bevacizumab, a recombinant humanized monoclonal antibody that targets VEGF, was the first antiangiogenic agent to be approved by the US Food and Drug Administration (FDA) and, currently, its use has been extended to include recurrent cases of GBM. Further investigation into these areas will hopefully lead to other therapeutic options and, ultimately, improve survivorship.

Specific Intracranial Tumors

Astrocytic neoplasms are the most common primary brain tumor in adults. They are generally divided into focal tumors, and those that diffusely infiltrate into surrounding brain.

Focal astrocytomas include tumors such as pilocytic astrocytomas, pleomorphic xanthoastrocytomas, and subependymal giant cell astrocytomas. These tumors tend to occur in younger patients, and are found in specific regions of the neuraxis (most commonly the posterior fossa). Focal tumors are more commonly benign with a relatively indolent biological behavior, and some are amenable to surgical cure.

Diffuse astrocytomas are more varied than focal tumors in their benign or malignant nature. They include the most common primary brain tumors in adults, accounting for approximately 30–40% of all adult CNS neoplasms [48]. The diffuse astrocytic tumors carry this moniker because of their growth pattern, which involves cells diffusely infiltrating into local and distant regions of the CNS. Astrocytic neoplasms are graded based on histologic characteristics, and are divided into low-grade astrocytoma (WHO grade II), anaplastic astrocytoma (WHO III), and glioblastoma (WHO grade IV). Additional subgroups of diffuse astrocytic neoplasms include brainstem glioma. While surgery remains an important part of treatment for many diffuse tumors, additional treatment strategies are often necessary. Given diffuse astrocytomas' more common presentation in adults than focal tumors, we will consider their management first, and in more detail.

Diffuse Astrocytic Tumors

Incidence

Diffuse astrocytic neoplasms represent 30% of primary intracranial tumors, with an incidence of approximately 5–7 per 100,000 person years.

While data do not uniformly show this, there appears to be an increase in the incidence of malignant gliomas [49, 50]. Anaplastic astrocytomas and glioblastomas increased while grade II astrocytomas decreased. Thus, there is some conflict in the literature regarding an increased or stable incidence of all gliomas, with a likely increase in malignant gliomas. The reason for this apparent increase is somewhat controversial. Some of this difference may be attributed to changes in pathologic diagnosis, while the increasing longevity of the population may also be to blame [51–53]. Improved imaging with computed tomography (CT) and magnetic resonance imaging (MRI) also likely accounts for an increasing diagnosis of this entity than in the past.

Etiologic Factors

Sporadic diffuse astrocytomas typically occur *de novo* with no clear risk factor. A minority of cases are known to occur as an after effect of ionizing radiation and immunosuppression. Pettorini *et al.* found the relative risk of glioma after radiation treatment for tinea capitis was 2.6 times greater than the general population. In childhood malignancies, where higher radiation doses were given, the relative risk was 7 times greater than the general population [54]. Other risks have been implicated, but all have either been disproven or have multiple studies with conflicting results.

Familial Tumors

There are multiple familial disorders associated with astrocytomas. Optic pathway gliomas, or other astrocytomas, can occur in the setting of neurofibromatosis (NF) type 1 and 2. Tuberous sclerosis patients may rarely develop subependymal giant cell astrocytoma. Li–Fraumeni syndrome is an autosomal dominant disorder resulting from a germline *TP53* mutation (about 70% of cases), resulting in syndromic patients developing multiple primary neoplasms that may include astrocytomas (about 10% of the time) [55]. Turcot syndrome is a group of autosomal dominant disorders caused by gene alterations in a series of DNA-mismatch (MMR) genes [56]. These patients can develop multiple colorectal neoplasms, neuroblastomas, and gliomas.

Genetic Alterations

Classically, diffuse astrocytomas were often seen as a continuum from benign to malignant. Glioblastomas, in particular, were divided into primary versus secondary glioblastoma. Primary tumors arise *de novo*, typically in the sixth or seventh decade, whereas secondary glioblastomas are glioblastomas that originate as lower-grade lesions and then progress over time to glioblastoma. They tend to occur earlier, and have a better prognosis. While secondary glioblastomas often arise in patients previously diagnosed with a lower-grade lesion, they may also present after malignant transformation. In this setting, the molecular biology of these tumors helps differentiate between primary and secondary tumors.

A number of genetic mutations occur in gliomas on their path from a differentiated astrocyte or neuroepithelial precursor cell to an astrocytoma. Many of these can help to distinguish between primary and secondary tumors. The pathway to primary glioblastoma may involve a number of mutations including epidermal growth factor receptor (*EGFR*) amplification (40%), overexpression (60%), or mutation (20–30%), murine double minute 2 (*MDM2*) amplification (10%) or overexpression (>50%), loss of heterozygosity (LOH) of 10q (70%), loss of *p16Ink4a/p14ARF* (30%), mutation of phosphate and tensin homolog (*PTEN*) (40%), phosphatidylinositol 3-kinase (*PI3K*) mutation or amplification (20%), mutation of retinoblastoma (*RB*), or vascular endothelial growth factor (*VEGF*) overexpression. Low-grade astrocytomas, anaplastic astrocytomas, and secondary glioblastomas all commonly have *TP53* mutations (>65%) or overexpression of platelet-derived growth factor A (*PDGFA*) or PDGF receptor-alpha (*PDGFR-α*) (60%). Additional gene mutations associated with low-grade astrocytoma include LOH of 19q (50%), mutated *RB* (25%), amplified *CDK4* (15%), overexpressed *MDM2* (10%), loss of *P16Ink4a/P14ARF* (4%), or LOH 11p (30%). In anaplastic astrocytoma, additional gene mutations include LOH 10q (70%), loss of deleted in colorectal carcinoma (*DCC*) (50%), amplification of *PDGFR-α* (10%), mutation of *PTEN* (10%), or overexpression of *VEGF*. Secondary glioblastomas tend to carry similar markers as grade II and III astrocytomas, with additional changes that lead to progression to grade IV tumors [57].

Some genetic alterations deserve a little more attention. *TP53* mutations, as well as PDGFA and PDGFR-α abnormalities, are markers distinguishing between primary and secondary glioblastoma. The predictive relevance of PDGF and PDGFR abnormalities is unclear. However, one study of recurrent glioblastoma linked *PDGFR-α* overexpression and phosphorylation to shorter survival [58]. MGMT (O^6-methylguanine DNA methyltransferase) is a DNA repair enzyme whose methylated promoter prevents its production, impairing the cell's ability to repair DNA damage. The MGMT promoter is methylated in 40–45% of glioblastomas, and if methylated, is a strong predictor of response to temozolomide. Isocitrate dehydrogenase 1 (IDH1) is a metabolic enzyme that recently has also been implicated in a mutated form in WHO grade II astrocytoma, anaplastic astrocytoma, and secondary glioblastoma, but is rare in primary glioblastoma [59]. Additionally, *IDH1* status may be somewhat useful as a prognostic marker for glioblastoma. A randomized phase 3 trial with 318 patients with malignant gliomas found that mutated *IDH1* was prognostic for significant improvements in time to treatment failure compared to those with wild-type *IDH1*, and another study of 301 patients with newly diagnosed glioblastoma showed prolonged PFS and a trend toward longer OS in the setting of *IDH1* mutations [60, 61]. While it is unclear how mutated *IDH1* contributes to tumorigenicity, one theory states that mutated *IDH1* may convert α-ketoglutarate to 2-hydroxyglutarate, thereby blocking enzymes involved in tumor suppression and contributing to tumor growth [59].

Additional information gleaned from more recent discoveries related to genetic differences in gliomas (especially glioblastoma) has resulted in some authors proposing a new model to differentiate between glioblastoma subtypes [57, 62, 63]. The proposed subtypes include the proneural, mesenchymal, proliferative (classical), and neural subtypes. The proneural subtype is distinguished by amplification or mutation of *PDGF, IDH1/IDH2, TP53, PI3KCA*, or *PI3KR1*. The mesenchymal subtype is characterized by *NF1* deletions or mutations, along with mutations in *TP53* or *PTEN*. The proliferative subtype is characterized by *EGFR* alterations, as well as changes in *EGFRvIII, PTEN*, or $p16^{INK4A}$. These divisions may play a role in prognostication as well, as proneural subtypes have shown improved survival in comparison to proliferative or mesenchymal subtypes [64, 65]. While greater understanding of these genetic alterations has not yet led to novel treatments, they have proven useful in distinguishing between primary and secondary glioblastomas, can give useful prognostic information, and may result in successful targeted therapies in the future.

Pathology Determination

The WHO pathologic criteria for astrocytomas consist of a four-tiered system from grade I pilocytic astrocytoma (see section "Pilocytic Astrocytoma") to grade IV glioblastoma. Low-grade astrocytoma and anaplastic astrocytoma do not demonstrate endothelial proliferation or necrosis. The distinction between grade II and III lesions is based on degree of nuclear atypia and mitotic activity. The additional factors of necrosis and endothelial proliferation also aid in diagnosing glioblastoma. MIB-1 or Ki-67 is used as a cell proliferation index to help predict aggressiveness of individual tumors. A confounding factor in diffusely infiltrating astrocytomas is the "multiforme" nature of this disease, in that different regions of tumor may demonstrate significant heterogeneity in histologic appearance. This can be problematic in the setting of stereotactic needle biopsy, where a tumor may be under-graded due to sampling error. This has led to surgeons targeting biopsies, when possible, to more aggressive-appearing areas of a tumor's preoperative imaging (e.g., areas of contrast enhancement).

Astrocytomas typically are able to spread throughout the CNS, but do not readily metastasize to distant sites. Migration tends to follow white matter tracts and subependymal regions which act as highways for distant spread of tumor cells throughout the brain. This diffuse invasion limits the ability for tumors to be completely resected surgically, and allows the tumors to appear as though they present in multiple regions of the brain (multicentric gliomas, approximately 5% of tumors).

Angiogenesis is an important factor in the growth of gliomas [66, 67]. This neovasculature is fenestrated and lacks a normal blood–brain barrier, leading to contrast enhancement on MRI. This, in general, is predictive of malignant transformation, as low-grade tumors typically lack enhancement. Vascular endothelial growth factor (VEGF) is a major vasoactive factor in glial tumor angiogenesis, and has recently become a target in glioma therapy.

Diagnosis

Signs and Symptoms

Astrocytomas often present with new-onset seizures, headaches, personality changes, memory problems, altered mental status, or focal symptoms such as weakness, sensory loss, vision loss, aphasia, etc. Low-grade lesions are more likely to present with seizures without other neurological signs or symptoms, or may present incidentally, while high-grade astrocytomas are more likely to present with focal or rapidly progressive symptoms.

Anatomic Imaging

Astrocytomas are diagnosed most clearly by MRI, because a normal MRI scan essentially rules out a diffuse astrocytoma as a cause of a patient's symptoms. Low-grade astrocytoma is characterized by T2 hyperintensity with mass effect without contrast enhancement. Contrast enhancement is typically seen in the setting of anaplastic astrocytoma or glioblastoma. When following tumors over time, the development of contrast enhancement can hint at tumor progression from a low-grade lesion to a higher-grade lesion. Since low-grade astrocytomas typically do not enhance, they can sometimes be difficult to distinguish from other T2-hyperintense lesions such as vascular disease, demyelinating disease, some types of hemorrhage, etc. Typically, noting the diffuse subcortical location of a T2-hyperintense lesion causing mass effect can help secure the diagnosis. Diffusion-weighted imaging can be helpful in determining the difference between stroke and low-grade tumor, as acute strokes restrict diffusion and tumors typically do not, although increased diffusion signal can be present in the setting of malignant glioma demonstrating significant tumor cell density.

Histologic Identification

Diffuse astrocytomas require histology for definitive diagnosis. Tissue can be obtained via either open craniotomy or stereotactic needle biopsy. Tumors are graded based on their morphology (nuclear atypia), the presence or absence of necrosis, number of mitoses, and the presence of microvascular proliferation (glomerularized vessels). Astrocytic neoplasms express glial fibrillary acidic protein (GFAP). The Ki-67 or MIB-1 index helps determine the aggressive nature of the tumor by estimating proliferation.

Grading of tumors is very important, and the clinical history and imaging can be very helpful in leading to the correct pathologic diagnosis. In the setting of diffuse astrocytoma first suspected on MRI scan, the first question is whether craniotomy and tumor resection is technically feasible with an appropriate risk profile for the patient, or if a stereotactic needle biopsy would better serve the patient. In general, craniotomy and removal of as much tumor as can safely be removed makes the most sense, as extent of resection has been demonstrated to play a significant role in prognosis. It must be emphasized, however, that many outcomes, including extent of resection, often depend as much on patient factors such as age, Karnofsky performance score (KPS), comorbidities, and location of tumor, as they do on the skill of the surgeon [68–72].

When patient factors result in the necessity of a stereotactic needle biopsy, target selection is important, as sampling error may result in nondiagnostic biopsy or under-grading of tumor. Any area of the brain can potentially be targeted for needle biopsy, including the brainstem, although targeting these areas comes at higher risk to the patient for neurologic worsening after biopsy. Typically the target should include what appears to be the highest-grade area (contrast enhancement on MRI or hypermetabolism on positron emission tomography (PET)). Sufficient sample should be obtained to insure accurate tumor diagnosis and grading. One study compared open to stereotactic biopsies, and showed that obtaining six stereotactic biopsies per patient led to accurate grading in 98% of cases. In settings where a mean number of biopsies of only four was obtained, the tumor grade was underestimated in 25% of cases [73]. This demonstrates that accurate targeting of lesions and adequate tissue sampling results in appropriate diagnosis of diffuse astrocytomas even in the setting of stereotactic biopsy.

Metabolic Imaging: Positron Emission Tomography

Morphological MRI alone can sometimes have difficulty distinguishing low-grade gliomas from other diagnoses. A biopsy-controlled study showed that MRI has a high sensitivity (96%) but a low specificity (53%) [74, 75]. PET is performed using various tracers to measure metabolism in an attempt to improve diagnostic accuracy. This can be helpful in following patients for possible recurrence, or in assisting the decision for biopsy in the setting of putative low-grade diffuse astrocytoma [76]. If the PET scan is hypometabolic in comparison to normal white matter, in a patient with no neurologic signs and symptoms and a nonenhancing lesion, one might consider following the patient without biopsy. If there is an area of hypermetabolism, however, this can help target needle biopsy or signal a need for initial resection or resection in recurrence.

A recent meta-analysis assessed the accuracy of PET at the diagnosis of recurrent glioma [77]. This evaluated 26 studies where one of four tracers was used (18-fluorodeoxyglucose (^{18}F-FDG), 11-carbon methionine (^{11}C-MET), 18-fluorine fluoroethyltyrosine (^{18}F-FET), or 18-fluorine fluorothymidine (^{18}F-FLT)) in the evaluation of glioma recurrence. Data were limited on some tracers, but the authors did calculate a summary sensitivity for ^{18}F-FDG of 0.77 and a specificity of 0.78 for any glioma histology [77]. ^{11}C-MET had a summary sensitivity of 0.70 and a specificity of 0.93 for high-grade glioma [77]. The limited available studies demonstrate a lower sensitivity but higher specificity of PET in comparison to morphological MRI [78]. Both L-3,4-dihydroxy-6-^{18}F-fluorophenylalanine (^{18}F-FDopa) PET and ^{18}F-FET PET have been shown to have reasonable sensitivity and specificity in distinguishing high- from low-grade gliomas or in distinguishing recurrent disease [79, 80].

PET has also been used in an attempt to distinguish between tumor and radiation necrosis for many years. There is a wide range of sensitivities and specificities reported in the literature, with sensitivities reported typically between 0.81 and 0.86 and specificities between 0.22 and 0.92 [81]. Sensitivity and specificity may be compromised by high metabolic activity in adjacent cortex or in areas of post-treatment inflammatory change, or by partial volume effects because of small lesions [81].

Metabolic Imaging: Magnetic Resonance Spectroscopy and Magnetic Resonance Perfusion

Magnetic resonance spectroscopy (MRS) is good at distinguishing tumor from abscess, and low-grade from high-grade tumor, but is not good at distinguishing between recurrence versus radiation necrosis [82, 83]. It is, therefore, highly sensitive, but not very specific, and serves as an imaging adjunct to help improve noninvasive diagnostic accuracy [84].

MR perfusion measurement is a more recent adjunct in studying gliomas noninvasively. While three methods of MR perfusion-weighted imaging (PWI) exist (dynamic susceptibility contrast (DSC)-enhanced PWI, arterial spin labeling PWI, and dynamic contrast-enhanced PWI), DSC PWI is the most widely accepted method for glioma grading, differentiation of radiation necrosis, and distinguishing between gliomas and metastases or lymphoma [85]. The basic idea behind MR perfusion is to calculate relative changes in cerebral blood volume (rCBV). In general, high-grade gliomas have larger rCBV than low-grade gliomas, and lymphomas typically have smaller rCBV than

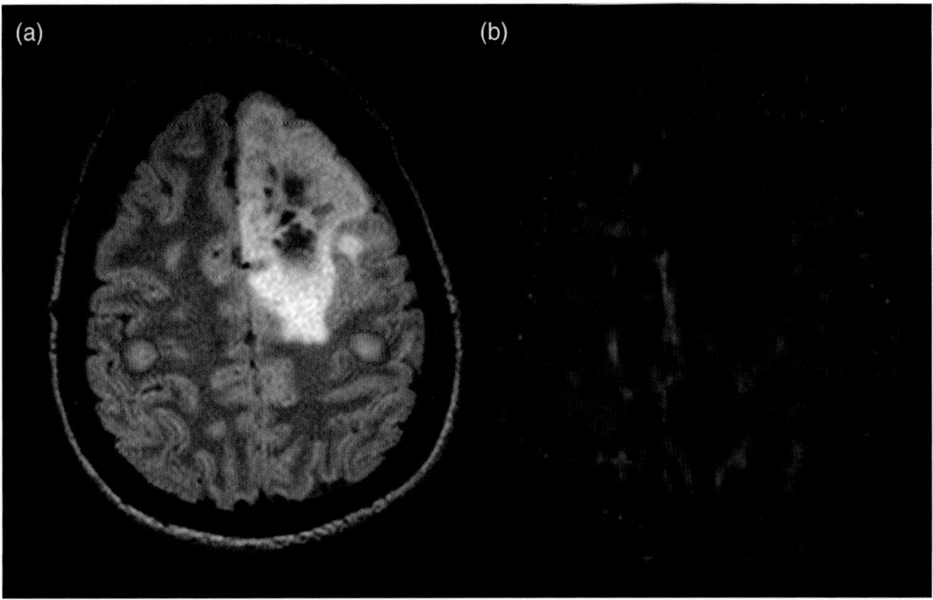

Figure 40.1 (a) T2 FLAIR image of a WHO grade II diffuse astrocytoma in the left frontal lobe with fMRI during finger tapping. (b) DTI of the same lesion demonstrating the diffusely infiltrative nature of the lesion, with it not significantly displacing surrounding fiber tracts.

gliomas or metastasis. It also helps distinguish radiation necrosis from tumor recurrence, as rCBV typically increases between scans with recurrence, but not with necrosis [86].

Functional Imaging: Functional Magnetic Resonance Imaging and Diffusion Tensor Imaging

Functional MRI and diffusion tensor imaging (DTI) both function as useful adjuncts in operative planning (Figure 40.1). Functional MRI can identify sensory, motor, or language areas to be avoided at the time of surgery. This can prove helpful to improve the safety of surgery, especially when the patient cannot tolerate awake craniotomy when the tumor affects language cortex. Functional MRI information can also be added to stereotactic image guidance to aid in surgical planning and execution. DTI can help map white matter tracts that may be displaced by tumor, helping in planning surgical approaches prior to going to the operating room [87]. This helps lower the risks associated with surgery in or near eloquent brain.

Differential Diagnosis

Many different lesions should be considered in the differential diagnosis of diffuse astrocytomas. These can include other tumors such as metastases or lymphoma, oligodendroglioma, or focal astrocytic tumors. Non-neoplastic lesions also may be confused for diffuse astrocytomas, including entities such as ischemic infarct, demyelinating lesions, old infections, or other diseases involving the white matter. This differentiation can be especially difficult in the case of low-grade gliomas that may not have significant mass effect and do not enhance with contrast.

In patients who present with focal seizures, especially if symptoms persist postictally for some time, diffuse astrocytoma may be confused with an ischemic infarct or transient ischemic attack. CT scan of the head may even confuse matters by showing an area of hypodensity incorrectly diagnosed as stroke. A contrast-enhanced MRI scan typically establishes the diagnosis. Seizures are not the only way these tumors present, and patients may also develop symptoms from mass effect or sudden hemorrhage in a high-grade lesion.

One of the important roles of noninvasive imaging is the differentiation between glioma and demyelinating disease. Like gliomas, demyelinating diseases may include large areas of T2 hyperintensity that enhance with gadolinium contrast. While they often appear with features distinct from gliomas, they can sometimes be confused, leading to biopsy in order to differentiate the two processes. Of course, histology can be confusing as well, especially on frozen section, where inflammatory cells and macrophages in a demyelinating lesion may be misinterpreted as tumor cells, resulting in misdiagnosis and inappropriate treatment plans.

Treatment

Low-Grade Astrocytoma

If observation is not chosen, treatment of low-grade astrocytoma begins with either biopsy or surgical resection. Extent of resection is often contingent on the lesion being in a surgically resectable location. Multiple retrospective studies have shown an OS benefit to greater extent of resection in low-grade astrocytoma, although no prospective trials controlling for functional and anatomic factors have been performed [88–90]. Thus, when surgery is undertaken, as extensive a resection as can safely be performed should be done.

There has been some controversy in the literature regarding the use of radiation and/or chemotherapy in these tumors. Multiple studies have investigated early versus late radiotherapy (RT) following surgical resection, two of which were phase 3 trials by the North Cancer Central Treatment Group (NCCTG)/Radiation Therapy Oncology Group (RTOG)/ Eastern Cooperative Oncology Group (ECOG) and European Organisation for Research and Treatment of Cancer (EORTC) [91–93]. The EORTC 22845 randomized 157 patients with low-grade glioma to either early RT of 54 Gy in 1.8 Gy fractions or deferred it until time of progression (control). While median PFS was better in the early RT group (5.3 vs 3.4 years), there was no difference in OS (7.4 vs 7.2 years), although patients under 40 did better than patients over 40 [88]. The NCCTG/RTOG/ECOG trial compared low- versus high-dose radiation (50.4 Gy/28 fractions vs 64.8 Gy/36 fractions) in 203 randomized patients [91]. The study found a lower survival rate and slightly higher radiation neurotoxicity incidence in the high-dose cohort. For these reasons, it is commonly recommended for patients under 40 or with radical resections and good functional status to defer RT until time of progression.

Chemotherapy was historically reserved for salvage therapy. Choices have included temozolomide (TMZ), an alkylating agent used in glioblastoma, or PCV (procarbazine, lomustine, and vincristine in combination, described prior to the advent of the common use of temozolomide). Two recent studies have started changing the role of chemotherapy for diffuse low-grade glioma (LGG). Fisher *et al.* reported preliminary results of RTOG 0424 that treated 129 high-risk LGG patients (three or more risk factors including age ≥40 years, astrocytoma histology, bihemispherical tumor, preoperative tumor diameter ≥6 cm, or a preoperative functional status of >1) with RT (54 Gy in 30 fractions) and concurrent and adjuvant temozolomide. The 3-year OS of 73.1% was higher than historical controls receiving RT alone. Buckner *et al.* have reported long-term follow-up data on RTOG 9802, a study of 251 high-risk patients with grade II astrocytoma, oligoastrocytoma, and oligodendroglioma (under 40 years old with subtotal resection or biopsy or over 40 with any biopsy or tumor resection). In this study, patients were randomized to RT alone or to RT followed by 6 cycles of combination therapy with PCV. With a median follow-up of 11.9 years, patients with combined therapy had longer median OS than those who received RT alone (13.3 vs 7.8 years, $P = 0.003$). PFS was also better – 51% at 10 years with RT plus chemotherapy versus 21% for the RT group alone. Toxicities were higher in patients with combined modality therapy. Ultimately, combined modality therapy (radiation and chemotherapy), at least in high-risk patients, is becoming more established for the treatment of LGG rather than either treatment alone. It remains unclear which chemotherapy regimen is better, PCV or temozolomide, but future randomized trials will hopefully help determine this in the next few years [94, 95].

Glioblastoma

Similar to low-grade astrocytoma, treatment of glioblastoma begins with the most extensive surgical resection that is safely possible (avoiding permanent neurologic deficit in the planned approach). This means that in some cases, only biopsy is appropriate because of multifocal brain involvement (Figure 40.2). Following surgical resection/biopsy, treatment typically consists of a combination of radiation and chemotherapy.

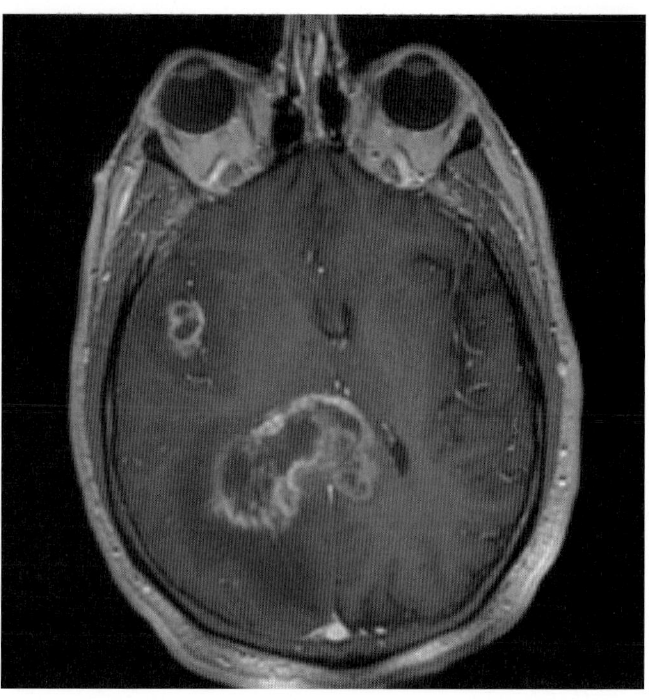

Figure 40.2 Multifocal glioblastoma. This lesion enhances with contrast, has a necrotic center, and crosses the splenium of the corpus callosum, in addition to demonstrating right temporal lobe involvement.

CNS tumors pose a unique problem: they are protected by the blood–brain barrier, so drugs must be able to penetrate the CNS and get to the tumor to be effective. This typically means drugs must be nonionized and highly lipid soluble, and have a large volume of distribution. Historically they are represented by alkylating agents such as nitrogen mustards, nitrosoureas, procarbazine, and temozolomide [96, 97]. Very little progress had been made in chemotherapy use in high-grade glioma until Stupp *et al.*, in the last decade [98]. After promising results in preclinical trials demonstrating temozolomide could function as a radiation sensitizer, Stupp *et al.* organized first a phase 2, and then a large multicenter phase 3, trial comparing concurrent and adjuvant temozolomide and radiation versus radiation alone in newly diagnosed glioblastoma in 573 patients [8, 98–100]. At median follow-up of 28 months, the median survival in the temozolomide treatment group was 14.6 months versus 12.1 months in the radiation alone group. There was no grade 3 or 4 hematologic toxicity in the control group, with grade 3/4 thrombocytopenia (3%) and neutropenia (4%) during concurrent treatment and 11% and 4%, respectively, during adjuvant chemotherapy. This has become the standard medical treatment for newly diagnosed glioblastoma. The patient undergoes 6 weeks of fractionated external beam radiation therapy to a dose of 60 Gy to the gross tumor volume plus a 2–3 cm margin as the clinical target volume (e.g., 2 Gy fractions 5 days/week) given concurrently with 42 days of daily temozolomide at 75 mg/m^2. This is followed by 6–12 cycles of 150–200 mg/m^2 temozolomide given every 5 days of a 28-day cycle after a one month off period after radiation completion. This is sometimes referred to as the "Stupp protocol." Patients are monitored for hematologic toxicity weekly. MRI is performed after concurrent therapy and then every 2 cycles of chemotherapy to evaluate treatment efficacy. Higher doses of radiation or treatment in fewer fractions have not demonstrated any benefit over the standard treatment regimen.

In recurrence, there are conflicting data as to which chemotherapy regimen should be used. Most commonly used is bevacizumab, either alone or in combination with cytotoxic agents, although multiple studies demonstrate bevacizumab alone has similar efficacy as bevacizumab in combination. Ideal timing and dosing to minimize toxicity and maximize efficacy remain to be established. Also, toxicities of antiangiogenic therapy can be significant and often require discontinuation of the drug. When bevacizumab does have to be withdrawn, rapid and substantial tumor progression seems to result [101–104].

When patients progress despite standard therapy, other regimens are sometimes used as alternative therapies. Additional therapies, such as carmustine wafers placed in the resection cavity during surgery for recurrence, may also be considered as part of therapy [105–107]. Standard therapies, along with older regimens as alternatives after failure of temozolomide and bevacizumab, that utilize agents or devices approved by the FDA, are listed in Table 40.4. Many additional targeted therapies based on the molecular biology of glioblastoma and anaplastic astrocytoma are being actively researched, although no specific therapy beyond bevacizumab has demonstrated efficacy over standard therapy.

Table 40.4 Treatment protocol for malignant glioma.

Standard treatment
Fractionated external beam radiation therapy to the gross tumor volume +2 cm clinical target volume (RT: 2 Gy fractions 5 days/week for 6 weeks for total 60 Gy)
Concurrent temozolomide 75 mg/m^2/day for 42 days during radiation. One month off, then 6–12 cycles of 150–200 mg/m^2/day every 5 days of a 28-day cycle
Chemotherapy in recurrence/progression
Bevacizumab 10 mg/kg IV infusion over 90 minutes on days 1, 15, and 29 of a 6-week cycle. May be given with a cytotoxic agent based on physician judgment
Alternative treatment options in recurrence/progression after failure of other treatments
BCNU (carmustine) 200–240 mg/m^2 IV every 6–8 weeks
PCV: Procarbazine 60 mg/m^2 PO on days 8–21, repeated every 6 weeks CCNU 110 mg/m^2 PO day 1, repeated every 6 weeks Vincristine 1.4 mg/m^2 (maximum, 2 mg) IV on days 8 and 29, repeated every 6 weeks
PCV, intensive: Procarbazine 75 mg/m^2 CCNU 130 mg/m^2 Vincristine 1.4 mg/m^2 (no cap)
Adjuncts to surgery/radiation/chemotherapy
Gliadel® wafers (polifeprosan 20 with carmustine implant) may be used in patients with newly diagnosed high-grade malignant glioma or recurrent glioblastoma as an adjunct to surgery and radiation
The NovoTTF™-100A System is a device delivering electric fields that are inferred to disrupt cell division, and may be used as monotherapy in glioblastoma recurrence after surgical and radiation options have been exhausted following chemotherapy

CCNU, 1-(2-chloroethyl)-3-cyclohexyl-1-nitrosourea (lomustine); IV, intravenous; PO, per os.

Anaplastic Astrocytoma

Anaplastic astrocytomas are much less common than glioblastomas, and are often considered together with glioblastomas in clinical trials. This has often resulted in inadequate numbers of anaplastic astrocytomas in the studies to provide meaningful statistical power for recommendations. Many advocate treating these tumors similarly to glioblastomas. Others, especially in the setting of gross total resection, or in young patients with a good KPS, recommend following surgery with RT alone with follow-up temozolomide either right away or at time of progression. There are theoretical advantages to each. Delaying temozolomide until after RT may decrease the risks of cytotoxic therapy, and has not clearly been shown to impair OS in this group of patients. Future studies need to be performed for anaplastic astrocytoma in sufficient numbers to address this issue clearly.

Brainstem Glioma

Brainstem gliomas are typically centered in the pons and present in childhood. They are usually low-grade lesions by histology and, due to their typical appearance on noninvasive imaging (e.g., MRI) and the risk associated with resection, usually are initially treated without biopsy. Patients often present with headaches, cranial nerve palsies, obstructive hydrocephalus, etc., and later may develop long-tract signs. Treatment typically involves fractionated RT. Chemotherapy usually does not improve prognosis. Survival is heavily influenced by histologic grade and infiltrative nature of the lesion. If there are features consistent with high-grade lesion, or a focal tumor such as pilocytic astrocytoma, biopsy or resection, respectively, may be indicated, but is feasible only in a small percentage of cases. In many cases, lesions are found to be diffusely infiltrating. High-grade tumors may warrant concurrent or adjuvant chemotherapy. Hydrocephalus can be treated with shunting if necessary. In children, median time to progression of diffuse lesions is 5–6 months, with a median survival of 9–12 months [108]. In adults, patients have a better prognosis, with low-grade lesions (most of which were diffusely infiltrating) having a median survival of 59–85 months [109–112].

Prognosis

Prognosis has gradually improved over the years for low-grade astrocytoma, anaplastic astrocytoma, and glioblastoma, but more research is necessary to truly make a significant difference in the lives of most individuals with these tumors. As proteomics and genetic research advance, targeted therapies, novel cytotoxic agents, immunotherapy, and other advances may all prove beneficial in the quest to improve the quality and quantity of life for diffuse astrocytoma patients.

Focal Astrocytic Tumors

Focal astrocytic tumors differ from diffuse astrocytomas in that they tend to be well circumscribed, and may be surgically curable if they are in a surgically accessible location. They predominantly affect children and young adults, and tend to be low grade despite contrast enhancement on MRI. These tumors may rarely recur aggressively in some cases.

Pilocytic Astrocytoma

Pilocytic astrocytoma is the most common primary brain tumor in children aged 5–14 and is considered a WHO grade I astrocytoma [113]. It most commonly occurs in the cerebellum, but may also occur along the optic nerve or chiasm, hypothalamus, or supratentorially. It tends to have a rather indolent course. Patients tend to present with symptoms related to the location of the tumor, which may include cranial neuropathies, ataxia, or hydrocephalus when tumors are in the posterior fossa, or seizures when occurring supratentorially. Tumors most commonly enhance vigorously with contrast, and may have a cystic component. Surgery is the mainstay of treatment, if the tumor is in a surgically accessible area, and cure may be possible from surgery alone. Radiation treatment is reserved for recurrence or progression when additional surgery is not possible [113]. Histology is characterized by pilocytes in a fibrillar background, and Rosenthal fibers (eosinophilic intracytoplasmic masses). Rare mitoses may be present without increasing the tumor grade. SEER data show inferior survival in adults versus children (5-year OS of 52.9% vs 96.5%, respectively) [114].

Pleomorphic Xanthoastrocytoma

About 90% of pleomorphic xanthoastrocytomas occur in individuals less than age 30 and generally in the temporal lobe, presenting with seizures due to cortical involvement [115]. The preferred therapy of these generally cystic lesions with a mural nodule is surgical resection, with the maneuver also helping some individuals with seizure control.

Subependymal Giant Cell Astrocytoma

Tuberous sclerosis (TS) is a genetic disorder which causes benign tumors of the brain, heart, kidney, liver, and lung. Subependymal giant cell astrocytomas (SEGA) develop in about 10–15% of individuals with tuberous sclerosis, frequently present with increasing seizures or hydrocephalus, and are best treated with surgical resection [16, 116]. Recent advances in the molecular understanding of this tumor have revealed the role of mechanistic target of rapamycin (mTOR, also known as mammalian target of rapamycin), with the mTORC inhibitor everolimus being used in patients who are not surgical candidates, with tumor stability or size reduction sometimes possible [16].

Nonastrocytic Tumors

Oligodendrogliomas

Oligodendrogliomas are slow-growing diffusely infiltrating tumors derived from the white matter of the cerebral hemispheres. Over the last 20 years, these tumors have shown a more robust response to treatment and thus a better prognosis when compared to other glial-based tumors. Oligodendrogliomas constitute nearly 20% of all glial-based tumors. The peak incidence is between the fourth and sixth decade. The presenting symptoms are nonspecific and are dependent on the location and the rate of tumor growth. The most common presenting symptoms are partial or complex seizures.

Histologically, grade II oligodendroglioma features a low to moderate cell density, with delicate branching blood vessels in a "chicken-wire" pattern. Anaplastic oligodendrogliomas (AOD) have focal or diffuse high cell density, mitosis, nuclear atypia, microvascular proliferation, and necrosis, substantiating their classification as grade III [117]. The most frequent chromosomal abnormality in oligodendroglioma is allelic loss of the 1p and 19q loci (60–70%). 1p/19q loss tumors have a more favorable clinical course and a greater response to cytotoxic regimens. AOD usually have additional deletions: LOH for 9p, deletion of CDKN2A, and deletions on chromosome 10 which correlate with poorer prognosis [118].

MRI findings are similar to astrocytic tumors. Oligodendrogliomas more often contain calcium, additionally cysts in 20%, and hemorrhage in 10%, giving the tumors a heterogeneous appearance on T1 and T2 images. Usually, oligodendrogliomas do not enhance with contrast. Enhancement is indicative of microvascular proliferation, more consistent with either AOD or a component of glioblastoma. Oligodendrogliomas rarely have extra-CNS metastases or CNS leptomeningeal spread. Routine spinal imaging or CSF sampling is not performed on newly diagnosed patients unless indicated.

The initial treatment of oligodendroglioma is surgery. If resection is not feasible, a stereotactic biopsy may be performed for diagnosis. Gross total resection (GTR) may lead to a prolonged remission. In low-grade lesions, many physicians recommend no further treatment following GTR, delaying RT until recurrence. Postsurgically, if substantial residual tumor remains, the conventional treatment is RT. Chemotherapy shows good response in patients found to have 1p19q deletion. All AOD should be treated in the postoperative period, despite the degree of resection, with RT followed by chemotherapy.

The prognosis of oligodendroglioma is relatively good with outcomes dependent on tumor location, grade, and patient age. Younger patients, with low-grade lesions centered in the frontal lobe, have the best prognosis. Patients with grade II oligodendroglioma have a median survival of 10–17 years and a 5-year survival rate of approximately 75%. AOD patients have a worse prognosis with a median survival of 4–5 years and a 5-year survival rate of approximately 40% [119].

Ependymomas

Ependymomas arise from the ependymal cells that line the ventricular system and the central canal of the spinal cord. They have a predilection for the posterior fossa, where they grow within the fourth ventricle and typically cause hydrocephalus. Supratentorial ependymomas also arise from ependymal structures but grow into the parenchyma of the hemisphere and may have no obvious intraventricular component. The most recent WHO classification divides ependymal tumors into four subtypes: subependymoma, myxopapillary ependymoma, ependymoma, and anaplastic ependymoma. They fall into three histological grades (WHO grade I–III) [120].

The incidence is bimodal, with the major peak at 5 years and a smaller peak at 35 years. Ependymomas account for 10% of childhood intracranial tumors, 60% of which occur in the posterior fossa. In adults they account for 4% of CNS tumors, and 50–60% of spinal neuroepithelial tumors. Symptoms from ependymomas are location dependent and can include headaches, nausea, emesis, changes in vision, rapid increase in head circumference in very young children, and myelopathy.

The histologic features of ependymomas are perivascular and ependymal rosettes. Generally, the tumors are low grade but they may be aggressive and spread via the CSF, seeding the meninges. They rarely metastasize to extraneural structures (primarily the lungs) [120]. A number of different mutations have been described, however, none are characteristic. Spinal cord tumors have a high incidence of LOH 22q associated with NF2. An 11q LOH, associated with the MEN1 gene, has been found with tumor recurrence and with malignant transformation to a grade III neoplasm. In pediatric ependymomas, allelic loss on the short arm of chromosome 17 has been shown.

MRI scan demonstrates a mass lesion that is heterogeneously hypointense and isointense on a T1-weighted image and hyperintense on a T2-weighted image, which may or may not have contrast enhancement. Edema may be prominent and hemorrhage may be present. Calcification, best seen on CT scan, is present in approximately 15% of ependymomas.

The initial treatment for ependymomas is maximal safe surgical resection, with adjuvant RT. The use of chemotherapy for residual tumor or as means to delay RT in children has been shown to worsen outcomes and increase recurrence [121].The prognosis of cranial ependymomas is better than most glial tumors. Five- and 10-year survival rates are approximately 80% and 50%, respectively. Anaplastic ependymomas are more invasive and more likely to spread by CSF pathways. Thus, the prognosis is worse. Eventually, most patients succumb to local recurrence rather than metastatic disease [122].

Choroid Plexus Tumors

The four segments of the CSF- producing choroid plexus are of neuroectodermal origin, each occupying either the lateral, third, or fourth ventricles. Of the choroid plexus tumors, 83% are benign choroid plexus papillomas – WHO grade I lesions. The remainder are malignant choroid plexus carcinomas (WHO grade III lesions) and atypical choroid plexus papilloma, which may represent a tumor precursor [123].

Most choroid plexus tumors cause symptoms secondary to hydrocephalus resulting from obstruction of CSF pathways, or as the result of excess production of CSF overwhelming the CSF absorptive pathways. Initial symptoms include a rapid increase in head circumference in infants, and papilledema, nausea, vomiting, seizures, ataxic gait, dysphagia, and palsy of cranial nerve VII at any age [123].

Histopathologically, the distinguishing feature between the three grades is increased mitotic activity. Choroid plexus papillomas, atypical choroid plexus papilloma, and choroid plexus carcinomas are defined by the presence of less than 2, 2–4, and 5 or more mitoses per 10 high-power fields, respectively. The diagnosis of atypical choroid plexus papilloma is important because it carries a 5-fold increase in recurrence at 5 years compared to choroid plexus papilloma [123].

Choroid plexus tumors typically exhibit a contrast-enhancing lobulated intraventricular mass. On CT, an iso- or hyperdense contrast-enhancing lesion is seen with calcification in 25–50%. MRI demonstrates a T1 and T2 isointense, homogeneously enhancing lesion with a "cauliflower appearance."

Surgical resection remains the standard of care for these tumors. Resection of choroid plexus tumors is serious, though technically possible surgery, as it almost always requires passing through normal neural structures. Chemotherapy and RT may be considered for recurrent, progressive, or metastatic lesions. Despite gross total resection, some patients will require permanent CSF diversion. Depending on the histologic group, postsurgical follow-up includes MRI from months to years. The main predictors of long-term survival in choroid plexus tumors are the degree of resection and the diagnosis of less malignant histology [124].

Neuronal and Mixed Neuronal–Glial Tumors

Central Neurocytomas

Central neurocytomas (CN) are primary neuronal tumors originating from the ventricular system.

They are composed of neuronal cells of the septum pellucidum and the subependymal cells of the lateral ventricles. The most common location is the lateral ventricle. They account for only 0.1–0.5% of all brain neoplasms, with peak incidence in the third decade of life (25%). The symptoms are location dependent [125].

Typical CT findings show large, lobulated, contrast-enhancing intraventricular tumors. Stereotypically these lesions have a base originating from the septum and extend into the ventricle. Calcium deposition can be seen in up to 50% of cases with varying distributions of deposition. Microcystic or macrocystic components cause a heterogeneous appearance. MRI demonstrates a T1 iso- to hypointense lesion that is hyperintense in T2-weighted images with a typically well-defined border.

Gross total resection and re-establishment of the CSF pathways are the primary treatment goals. Studies have shown significant improvements in local control without improvement in OS following RT and stereotactic radiosurgery (SRS) [126]. In young patients, cases with inoperable lesions, or cases where RT has been ineffective, there may be a role for chemotherapy [125].

Dysembryoplastic Neuroepithelial Tumors

Dysembryoplastic neuroepithelial tumors (DNET) are typically benign lesions of mixed neuroepithelial origin. DNETs represent 1.2% of all tumors in those under age 20. They most commonly present in infants and young children with a long history of medically refractory partial seizure that can progress to secondary generalized seizures.

Typically lesions are located within the cortex, most often as a single focus in the mesial or lateral temporal lobe. Forty percent of lesions have microscopic cystic components, and 30% are associated with subtle cortical dysplastic changes in the adjacent cortex [127].

On CT, they are hypodense, intracortical lesions with little mass effect or edema. Deformity in the overlying skull is often seen. On MRI, lesions will be hypointense on T1- and hyperintense on T2-weighted images.

DNETs rarely show malignant progression. Studies with no intervention have shown progression- free lesions up to 5 years. If DNET is suspected, stereotactic biopsy must be done with caution as the internal heterogeneity may generate an unrepresentative tissue sample and lead to an incorrect diagnosis.

In patients with medically refractory epilepsy, intolerance of AEDs, and surgically resectable lesions, gross total resection with removal of surrounding cortical dysplasia is the preferred treatment. Otherwise, close clinical and radiological surveillance is reasonable [128].

Gangliogliomas and Gangliocytomas

Gangliogliomas have both neuronal and glial cell elements and gangliocytomas are composed of ganglion cells alone. These tumors are the most common neoplastic reason for chronic, intractable, focal epilepsy in young patients [129]. They may be WHO grade I or II, are usually temporal in location, and are well circumscribed on MRI with 30–40% of cases having enhancement. Optimal treatment is gross total resection with a cure rate for seizures of 50–75%. A systematic neurophysiological workup must precede the tailored resection in order to achieve seizure control and to avoid postsurgical deficits including amnesia and/or emotional malfunctions [130].

Pineal Region Tumors

Tumors within the pineal region account for only 1–3% of primary brain tumors but include over 20 subtypes, reflecting the cell diversity found within the gland and the adjacent structures. They are 10 times more common in children, accounting for approximately 8% of childhood primary CNS tumors.

Symptoms arise from obstruction of the cerebral aqueduct and the resultant hydrocephalus, compression of the dorsal midbrain causing ocular and vision disturbances (e.g., Parinaud syndrome), and brainstem or cerebellar compression, including gait ataxia. MRI scans of pineal lesions are rarely diagnostic by themselves. Additional diagnostic evaluation of the serum and CSF for tumor markers, such as the beta subunit of human chorionic gonadotropin (β-hCG), alpha-fetoprotein, or placental alkaline phosphatase is of value.

Germ cell tumors (mainly germinomas) account for 30–85% of pineal tumors. They generally present in childhood and have a strong association with Klinefelter syndrome. They can produce drop metastases and therefore complete neural axis MRI and CSF studies are necessary at diagnosis (diagnostic in 15–75% of cases), throughout treatment, and during follow-up. Germinomas are radiosensitive and have a favorable prognosis. Five-year survival of 65–100% is reported. Teratomas arise in a similar location but are much rarer with survival dependent on degree of malignancy [131].

Pineal parenchymal tumors include primarily pineocytoma and pineoblastoma and account for 30% of tumors within the pineal region. The lower-grade pineocytoma tends to present in adults, and higher-grade pineoblastoma is more commonly seen in children. Pineocytomas are slow-growing and noninvasive, and RT to the site of the tumor is the treatment of choice after diagnosis by biopsy or surgical removal. Pineoblastoma is a WHO grade IV lesion with a 5-year survival rate with treatment of 10–50%. Case series have shown 14–43% of pineoblastomas to have concurrent spinal cord and leptomeningeal spread, requiring adjuvant cranial spinal RT and chemotherapy. Complete neuraxis MRI and CSF analysis are required at the time of diagnosis and for surveillance.

Gliomas of the pineal region are a distinct form of brainstem glioma commonly arising from the cells located within the quadrigeminal plate (i.e., a tectal glioma). Variable degrees of contrast enhancement are seen in tectal lesions and correlate with the grade of the lesion. Studies have shown PFS over 6 years in patients followed by MRI without treatment. In these cases surgical intervention is focused on CSF diversion alone [131].

Embryonal Tumors

Embryonal tumors are characterized by the WHO as undifferentiated round cell tumors with divergent patterns of differentiation. Several tumors of uncertain cell origin fit into this category. When located supratentorially, they comprise a group of tumors called CNS primitive neuroectodermal tumors (PNETs) which include medulloepithelioma, central neuroblastoma, ependymoblastoma, and CNS ganglioneuroblastoma. When primitive neuroectodermal tumors are located in the posterior fossa they are termed medulloblastoma, of which there are four variants [132, 133].

Medulloblastomas are the most common malignant solid tumor and the most common malignant brain tumor in children, accounting for 20% of childhood brain tumors. Although the peak incidence is between 5 and 8 years, a smaller peak occurs between 20 and 30 years. They have an association with Gorlin syndrome, NF, Li–Fraumeni syndrome, and tuberous sclerosis. PNETs are less common and account for 2.5% of primary CNS tumors in children and 1% of adults. Medulloblastomas and PNETs have a strong tendency to spread by subarachnoid pathways and to seed the leptomeninges producing "drop mets." CSF spread means that preoperative ventriculoperitoneal shunting is contraindicated as it may facilitate tumor deposits in the peritoneal cavity. Extraneural metastases occur in some 5% of patients, usually to bone and sometimes to lymph nodes or liver.

Symptoms are related to hydrocephalus. In addition to exhibiting signs of generalized increased intracranial pressure, patients develop gait ataxia. Dizziness, vertigo, and nystagmus also may be present. Nausea and vomiting are common in children but less so in adults.

Medulloblastomas are histologically indistinguishable from PNETs. Histologically similar tumors are also found in the pineal gland where they are categorized as pinealoblastoma and in the eyes where they are called retinoblastomas. Medulloblastomas typically arise in the vermis. Histologically classic findings are Homer Wright rosettes and palisading tumor cells [132].

The diagnosis is suggested by location and prominent enhancement of the tumor on MRI. Mutations that up-regulate the sonic hedgehog homologue pathway are common; these include *PTCH* mutations seen in Gorlin syndrome, and *SMO* and *GLI1* mutations seen in as many as 30% of sporadic cases.

The initial treatment for medulloblastoma is maximum feasible surgical resection; postsurgical adjuvant therapy is mandatory. The combination of craniospinal RT coupled with vincristine during radiotherapy and followed by 8 cycles of cisplatin, CCNU, and vincristine has shown almost 90% 5-year PFS [133].

Glomus Tumors

Glomus tumors (GT), also known as paraganglioma, chemodectoma, and glomangioma, are tumors of the neuroendocrine system most commonly found in the jugular bulb or jugular foramen, or along the tympanic branch of cranial nerve IX or the auricular branch of cranial nerve X. Symptoms are location specific and include pulsating tinnitus, otorrhea, facial nerve dysfunction, and difficulty swallowing. Therapy can include surgery; however this can be associated with high rates of morbidity and mortality. Fractionated RT and SRS are now acceptable alternative treatments. Studies of stereotactic radiosurgery have shown local tumor control in up to 100% of patients, with stable tumor volume in 60% and tumor shrinkage achieved in 40% of cases. Local tumor control can be achieved in 92% of cases treated with fractionated RT or SRS at 10 years [134].

Tumors of Cranial Nerves

Schwannomas and neurofibromas arise from the white matter producing components of peripheral and cranial nerves (CN). Schwannomas arise from Schwann cells. Neurofibromas contain cells with features of Schwann cells, fibroblasts, and perineural cells. Tumors of both types are benign and can be cured surgically if they are a component of a noncritical nerve or relatively separate from fibers of a high-function nerve projection. A significant number of patients with schwannomas and neurofibromas suffer from NF. By far the most common intracranial schwannomas encountered are those arising from the auditory nerve, vestibular schwannomas (VS). These lesions are located in the cerebellopontine angle or in the internal acoustic canal. Usually, they are tumors of middle age. Bilateral VS, present in approximately 5% of patients, is pathognomonic of NF type 2. This autosomal dominant syndrome occurs in about 1/25,000–50,000 individuals and is due to a mutation of a gene on chromosome 22q12 and loss of the NF2 protein (Merlin or schwannomin) [135].

VS are benign and grow slowly, compressing the eighth cranial nerve and causing hearing loss and tinnitus. Because vestibular function is lost slowly and is compensated for, vertigo is an uncommon symptom of VS. If the tumors grow to be large, they may compress the cerebellum and brainstem, causing gait ataxia and hydrocephalus. Numbness in the face from involvement of the trigeminal nerve and facial paralysis from involvement of the facial nerve also can be features.

On MRI, VS are well-delineated, solidly (or sometimes cystically) contrast-enhancing masses in the internal auditory canal, cerebellopontine angle, or both. Often, they are located in and expand the internal auditory meatus, a deformity not usually caused by meningiomas [136].

When these tumors are small (<1 cm) treatment with SRS alone is typical. For tumors between 1 cm and 2.5 cm, gross total resection with hearing preservation is obtainable in 75% of patients. For lesions beyond 2.5 cm, gross total resection is possible and curative; however, neurologic deficits may occur as a result of surgery [136].

Tumors of Peripheral Nerves

Benign Peripheral Nerve Lesions

In view of the ubiquitous nature of peripheral nerves, the most common representatives of this family of lesions can develop in nearly any location. Symptomatic lesions present with cosmetic deformity, pain or sensory alteration, and less often motor changes. Schwannomas and neurofibromas, making up the largest proportion of these lesions, are histologically distinct from each other but their presentation and nodular nature are generally similar in presentation. Most often they are solitary and when that is the case they are generally not associated with neurofibromatosis type 1 (NF1) [137]. Management is usually with simple observation for isolated, incidental, and minimally symptomatic lesions. However, symptomatic lesions are most often addressed with surgical resection offering the advantages of decompression and relief of deformity but at the risk of new and permanent neurologic deficits even with preoperative and intraoperative electrophysiologic monitoring. Plexiform neurofibromas are often larger, appear in younger individuals, have a distinct "bag of worms" appearance on MRI, and are more often associated with eventual diagnosis of NF1. Of serious concern is that 8–12% will develop malignant transformation [138]. Less common intraneural lesions include lipofibromatous hamartomas, granular cell tumors, and the perineurioma, that though benign, is so intimately intertwined with the parental nerve that resection is precluded without sacrifice of normal nervous structures [137, 138].

Hereditary Syndromes

Those with a genetic predisposition to these lesions, such as patients with NF1, may require multiple surgical interventions over their lifetime. NF1 has an estimated incidence of about 1 in 3,500. It is considered to be the most common cancer predisposition syndrome and to have a greater risk of mortality from malignant peripheral nerve sheath tumors (MPNST), glioma, rhabdomyosarcoma, and nonlymphocytic leukemia [135]. Neurofibromas in these patients have abnormal cells with mutations of chromosome 17q11.2 and are missing one or both alleles of *NF1* that encode for neurofibromin [135, 139]. Less common syndromes include schwannomatosis with germline mutations of the tumor suppressor gene *SMARCB1/INI1*, the Carney complex due to inactivating *PRKAR1A* mutations, and MEN2b due to activating mutations in *RET* [139].

Malignant Peripheral Nerve Sheath Tumor

Fortunately uncommon, malignant lesions of peripheral nerves are most commonly represented by malignant peripheral nerve sheath tumors. This tumor was referred to by a number of names in the older literature (e.g., malignant schwannoma, neurogenic schwannoma, and neurofibrosarcoma) but these names are now considered obsolete [135]. These tumors may have poorly defined margins with an infiltrative nature making surgical resection for cure impossible. Malignant degeneration of originally benign lesions, especially in NF1 cases with plexiform neurofibromas involving the lumbar or pelvic plexus, can attain monstrous size making therapy difficult. The risk of MPNST is

100 times that of the general population in NF1 patients. These tumors represent the fifth most common type of soft tissue sarcoma and, based on this, often become targets for fractionated RT and sometimes systemic cytotoxic regimens [136]. No reliably curative regimen is available.

Perineural Tumor Invasion

Tumors of the skin, pancreas, colon and rectum, prostate, head and neck, biliary tract, and stomach, though not primarily neural in nature, are quite capable of invading the peripheral nervous system adjacent to them and utilizing the nerves as a route for distant spread [140]. Symptoms include pain or loss of sensation or motor function in the distribution of the involved nerve. Recognition by staging and preoperative imaging is important as it may substantially limit the surgeon's ability to obtain tumor resection with clean margins and alter a surgical plan to simple biopsy in preparation for systemic therapy. In surgical specimens it is important for pathologists to pay attention to involved and adjacent nerve tissue for this process as it may provide a clue to nascent distant tumor spread [140]. Cranially, this process can be important with cutaneous squamous cell carcinoma finding its way to the cavernous sinus along branches of the trigeminal nerve. By this and other neural routes to the central nervous system leptomeningeal carcinomatosis can develop with all of its devastating effects [141]. RT can be useful and adjuvant therapy with cisplatin, doxorubicin, bleomycin, peplomycin, methotrexate, or 5-fluorouracil (depending on the primary tumor and patient characteristics) may be effective but without guaranteed tumor control [141, 142].

Chordomas

Chordomas of the skull base account for approximately 1–4% of primary bone tumors. They are considered nonmalignant tumors but are locally destructive in the skull base and tend to recur despite treatment. Due to their slow growth, the onset of signs and symptoms is insidious. Chordomas cause compression and destruction of surrounding anatomic structures in the skull base. Patients can present with headache, neck pain, diplopia, hydrocephalus, sensorimotor deficits, and endocrine abnormalities due to pituitary dysfunction.

On CT imaging, chordomas appear as a well-circumscribed soft tissue mass, slightly hyperdense with variable intratumoral calcification and surrounding lytic bone destruction. Chordomas show variable contrast enhancement both on CT and MRI. On T1-weighted MR images, chordomas appear isointense or slightly hypointense. On T2-weighted images, they have a hyperintense appearance due to high fluid content, calcifications, and their bony involvement.

The mainstay of treatment of chordomas is aggressive surgical excision. However, gross total removal cannot be achieved in many cases due to neurovascular involvement. Management of chordomas includes surgical resection followed by adjuvant radiation therapy, as chemotherapy is limited and generally ineffective [143]. Adjuvant proton beam radiotherapy is used for residual chordomas since high doses of radiation can be prescribed to the tumor site with minimal exposure to critical surrounding structures such as the brainstem [144]. Recurrent tumors are often treated surgically or with the use of SRS [145, 146].

Craniopharyngioma

Craniopharyngiomas are WHO grade I lesions that constitute 1–4% of all intracranial tumors and arise from remnants of Rathke's pouch and the craniopharyngeal duct [147]. There are two subtypes. Adamantinomatous tumors typically occur in children and have cystic and solid components containing cholesterol-rich fluid and calcifications. Papillary craniopharyngiomas occur mainly in adults and are solid masses without calcifications or cholesterol deposits. Genetic alterations in chromosomes 2 and 12 have been identified and malignant transformation has rarely been reported [147–149].

Most are suprasellar but they can also occur in intrasellar or ectopic cranial sites [150–154]. Symptoms include visual disturbances, hypothalamic–pituitary dysfunction, behavioral problems, and hydrocephalus [155–157]. Rarely, intratumoral hemorrhage or cyst rupture can result in aseptic meningitis or spontaneous nasopharyngeal drainage [158–160]. By imaging, craniopharyngiomas demonstrate mixed solid and cystic areas with calcific regions visible on CT [161].

Complete surgical resection is the desirable option for craniopharyngioma patients. However, in many cases complete surgical resection cannot be achieved safely [162]. In these cases, subtotal surgical removal followed by postoperative RT is recommended [163–168]. Various radiation options are available. SRS has been utilized for small craniopharyngiomas [169–172]. Use of proton radiotherapy has been reported in an effort to maximize treatment effect [173, 174]. Intracavitary radiotherapy with colloidal chromic phosphate or yttrium 90 has also been performed [175, 176]. RT is avoided in children younger than 3 years due to potential long-term cognitive and growth complications, and intracystic bleomycin chemotherapy has been performed in children to delay RT [177–179]. Craniopharyngiomas are known to recur and therapies include a second surgery, RT if not initially administered, or intracystic radiation or chemotherapies, depending on the anatomic details of the recurrence [171].

Epidermoid and Dermoid Cysts

Epidermoid and dermoid cysts are slow-growing benign lesions accounting for approximately 0.5–2% of all intracranial tumors. Epidermoids contain desquamated epithelial cells, keratin, and cholesterol. Dermoid cysts contain elements of the dermis such as hair follicles and apocrine, sebaceous, and sweat glands whose symptoms are related to tumor location. Symptomatic epidermoid or dermoid cysts should be approached surgically though this may not be curative [180–185].

Colloid Cysts

Colloid cysts are benign tumors that constitute 0.5–1% of all intracranial tumors. Most of them contain gelatinous viscous material and are located in the anterior third ventricle. These may cause obstructive hydrocephalus, positional headache, nausea and vomiting, dizziness, memory difficulties, and syncopal events [186, 187]. Management of colloid cysts depends on whether the patient is symptomatic. Small asymptomatic cysts can be observed. Symptomatic lesions should undergo surgical removal by endoscopic or microsurgery techniques [188–190].

Meningioma

Meningiomas originate from the CNS meninges that cover the brain and spinal cord and specifically arise from the arachnoidal cap cells. They account for approximately 20% of all primary brain tumors. The most consistent risk factor for meningioma is exposure to ionizing radiation. The relationship between hormones and meningioma risk has been demonstrated [191, 192]. The majority of benign meningiomas consistently express progesterone receptors and may also express androgen and estrogen receptors [193]. Pregnancy may alter the growth of meningiomas. Meningiomas also express a high density of somatostatin receptors, as well as dopamine (D1) and glucocorticoid receptors. The primary chromosomal abnormality in meningiomas appears to be monosomy or deletion of chromosome 22 [194–196].

Meningiomas are classified into three categories according to the WHO classification: grade I, atypical grade II, and anaplastic or malignant, based on the degree of anaplasia, number of mitoses, and presence of necrosis. WHO grade I meningiomas constitute approximately 90% of meningiomas and are associated with a low level of recurrence. Atypical and malignant meningiomas are much less common and are associated with a higher rate of recurrence and aggressive growth. Meningiomas are encapsulated tumors attached to the dura. A meningioma can take the shape of the underlying bone and in this case is called "meningioma en plaque." Meningiomas can also involve the overlying cranial bone and cause hyperostosis. Immunohistological markers positive in meningiomas are epithelial membrane antigen, vimentin, laminin, fibronectin, keratin, and S-100.

Many meningiomas grow very slowly, thus remaining asymptomatic during life, and are found incidentally. Symptomatic meningiomas commonly present as an enlarging mass that eventually leads to compression of surrounding brain structures. Most meningiomas are located intracranially and of these about 90% are supratentorial. The signs and symptoms of patients with meningiomas at presentation are slow in onset, as well as variable depending on tumor location [197]. The most common presenting symptoms are new-onset headache, personality changes, and hemiparesis, followed by seizures, visual impairment, ataxia, and aphasia [198]. Symptoms due to increased intracranial pressure may also occur with larger tumors.

CT imaging can reveal characteristic findings of meningiomas: bone hyperostosis, intratumoral calcification, osteolytic lesions, and erosion of the skull. Meningiomas are isointense on MRI T1 and T2 in most cases. They generally enhance intensely but with variable patterns dependent on location and relationship to the surrounding tissue and bone.

A dural tail adjacent to the meningioma can enhance on both CT and MRI. Meningiomas express somatostatin receptors, permitting the use of somatostatin receptor scintigraphy using octreotide [199].

Surgically accessible tumors in patients who are considered good candidates should undergo tumor resection. The goal of surgery is total removal including the dural attachment, as the completeness of surgical resection is an important prognostic factor [200]. Gross total removal alone is considered definitive treatment for grade I meningiomas [201]. Subtotal surgical removal along with aggressive pathologic features, such as dural sinus invasion or brain infiltration, is associated with higher recurrence rates. Predictors of tumor recurrence are also high levels of VEGF expression and high MIB-1 labeling index [202].

RT should be primarily considered following partial surgical resection of a meningioma or following resection of an atypical or malignant meningioma [203, 204]. RT should be also considered as monotherapy in inoperable cases of progressively symptomatic patients who are not surgical candidates. The adjuvant role of either SRS or fractionated stereotactic RT is gaining popularity in the management of small size meningiomas [205–209]. Hormonal therapy has also been investigated as a potential therapeutic modality for recurrent grade I meningiomas that cannot be managed with surgery or RT. The antiestrogen agent mepitiostane and the progesterone antagonist mifepristone (RU-486) have been studied in meningioma patients with no clear therapeutic benefit being derived [210, 211]. Finally, hydroxyurea, calcium channel blockers, somatostatin analogs, cycloxygenase-2 (COX-2) inhibitors, and recombinant interferon-alpha have all been investigated [212–216].

Hemangiopericytoma/Solitary Fibrous Tumor

Meningeal hemangiopericytoma is a malignant neoplasm that originates from meningeal capillary pericytes. Its molecular and genetic profile, and its biologic behavior, are similar to a dural-based sarcoma [217]. Hemangiopericytomas constitute approximately 3% of meningeal tumors and unlike meningiomas are more common in males. Hemangiopericytomas can be misdiagnosed as meningiomas but are more rapidly growing. Headaches and focal neurological signs related to the tumor location are the most common initial symptoms with rare spontaneous hemorrhages being described [218, 219].

On MRI, hemangiopericytomas appear isointense with gray matter on both T1- and T2-weighted MRI and nearly always enhance with gadolinium [220].

Surgical resection is considered the primary modality treatment for hemangiopericytoma [221]. If complete tumor resection cannot be achieved, adjuvant RT is recommended [222]. SRS should be considered as a therapeutic option for residual or recurrent hemangiopericytomas. Extraneural metastasis should be treated aggressively with a multimodal approach [223, 224].

Hemangioblastoma

Hemangioblastomas are benign tumors that originate almost exclusively from CNS tissue, although their exact cytologic origin remains unclear. They can occur sporadically, or in the context of von Hippel–Lindau (VHL) disease, which is characterized by hemangioblastomas in the cerebellum and retina, renal cell carcinoma, and various visceral cysts. Symptomatic disease appears earlier in VHL patients, compared with sporadic cases [225]. Hemangioblastomas are more common in males than females [226]. They are more frequently located in the pituitary stalk region, brainstem, cerebellum, and spinal cord [227]. Clinical symptoms of hemangioblastomas are due to mass effect and depend on their anatomic location [228–230].

MRI is the preferred imaging modality for CNS hemangioblastomas. Hemangioblastomas show intense enhancement on T1-weighted images after gadolinium administration, due to the fact that they are highly vascular tumors. Peritumoral edema and cysts, which are frequently associated with hemangioblastomas, can be detected on T2-weighted images. Peritumoral cyst formation is a common finding in the majority of hemangioblastomas [231].

Treatment of hemangioblastomas in the context of VHL disease is better postponed and reserved until the tumors become symptomatic. In contrast, patients with sporadic tumors often initially present with symptoms. In these patients, surgery is required both to relieve the symptoms and provide a definitive diagnosis. Because of the frequent association of hemangioblastomas with VHL disease, all patients with an isolated CNS hemangioblastoma should be screened for VHL disease. The treatment modality of choice for hemangioblastoma is complete resection, which is curative and possible for most hemangioblastomas [228–230]. In cases of incomplete surgical removal, SRS and conventional external beam RT have been investigated as potential adjuvant therapeutic modalities. SRS has better results when applied to small tumors not associated with peritumoral cysts [232, 233]. Large tumors with associated peritumoral cysts are more likely to respond better to external beam RT, although fewer data are available [234].

Primary Intraspinal Tumors

General Considerations

Spinal metastases make up the vast majority of neoplasms involving the spine. In fact, up to two-thirds of patients with systemic cancer will have spine metastasis on post mortem examination [235]. Primary intraspinal tumors make up only 10–20% of all spine tumors. In the US there are an estimated 850–1,700 new adult cases of primary spinal tumors diagnosed each year [236]. This collection of tumors is very heterogeneous and can be divided into three categories based on location relative to the dura and spinal cord: extradural (55%), intradural extramedullary (40%), and intramedullary (5%) (Table 40.5) [237].

Table 40.5 Differential diagnosis of spinal tumors relative to location.

Extradural (55%)
Metastasis (majority)
Chordoma
Osteoid osteoma
Osteoblastoma
Aneurysmal bone cyst
Chondrosarcoma
Osteochondroma
Hemangioma
Giant cell tumors
Plasmacytoma/multiple myeloma
Eosinophilic granuloma
Ewing sarcoma
Intradural extramedullary (40%)
Meningioma and schwannoma (45%)
Neurofibroma
Lipoma
Schwannoma
Hemangiopericytoma
Paraganglioma
Metastasis
Intramedullary (5%)
Astrocytoma and ependymoma (90%)
Epidermoid
Dermoid
Hemangioblastoma
Lipoma
Ganglioglioma
Metastasis (rare, less than 2%)

Clinical Findings

Back pain, although not specific to neoplasms, is the cardinal symptom of spinal tumors and is the presenting symptom in over 80% of all primary spinal tumors [235]. A detailed history and physical examination will help filter out those patients who require further workup. Pain associated with a spinal tumor is typically dull, aching, progressive, and localized over the involved vertebral level. If there is nerve root compression, these patients usually experience pain radiating into the arm, around the chest or abdomen, or down the leg. Unlike pain associated with degenerative disease, tumor pain is frequently exacerbated by bed rest and partly relieved by standing or activity. Nocturnal pain is a classic presentation of spinal tumors [237]. Coughing, sneezing, and other Valsalva maneuvers, which increase intraspinal pressure, exacerbate the tumor pain. Also, these patients frequently require increased analgesia over time. The clinician's index of suspicion should also be heightened by systemic factors such as unintended weight loss, excessive tobacco history, change in bowel or urinary function, focal weakness, prior radiation, and previously diagnosed syndromes associated with spinal tumors (i.e., neurofibromatosis) [235].

A complete physical and neurologic examination is essential for any patient suspected of having a spinal tumor. The general physical examination should focus on assessing for signs of systemic malignancy. A thorough neurological examination is critical. Testing should focus on the patient's speech, mental status, cranial nerves, strength, sensation, coordination, and reflexes. Upper motor neuron signs include spasticity, weakness, hyperreflexia, and extensor plantar responses and are present below the level of cord compression from disruption of the cortical spinal tract. Lower motor signs include atrophy, fasciculations, and hyporeflexia and are evident at the involved spinal level only from anterior horn or nerve root compression. Patients presenting with acute or rapidly progressing neurologic deficits require emergent workup. Cauda equina syndrome is caused by compression of the lumbar cauda equina and typically presents with urinary retention, diminished anal sphincter tone, "saddle anesthesia," significant asymmetric motor weakness, lower back pain, and sciatica. In addition, spinal masses may be palpable if they extend into the posterior elements, and they can cause significant deformity from vertebral fractures. It is essential to palpate the region(s) of concern and assess for scoliosis or kyphosis. Frequently, the physical examination will provide enough clues to localize potential lesions and direct imaging [235].

Diagnosis

MRI with and without contrast is now the mainstay of diagnosis. The regions scanned along the neuroaxis are dependent upon the initial history and physical examination. If lesions are discovered, imaging of the entire neuroaxis is often warranted to rule out metastasis. Individuals who cannot undergo an MRI secondary to ferromagnetic implants or pacemakers present a unique challenge. For these patients, less sensitive modalities such as technetium (^{99m}Tc) bone scans, single photon emission CT (SPECT), and standard CT myelography must be interpreted with care. Myelography is contraindicated in patients who are coagulopathic, allergic to contrast agents, or have hydrocephalus. Unfortunately, as many as 14% of patients with spinal cord compression deteriorate neurologically after lumbar myelography [235].

When an abnormality is discovered on imaging, a histologic diagnosis is essential. The location of the tumor relative to the dura and spinal cord can help guide the differential diagnosis. For extradural lesions, one should first search for signs of systemic disease since metastases are most prevalent. If no systemic disease is discovered for sampling, spinal tissue diagnosis is ultimately required and can be made through either a percutaneous image-guided needle biopsy or open surgical biopsy. Lesions extending away from the spinal canal are optimal candidates for needle biopsy; however, an open biopsy allows for concomitant decompression and stabilization if warranted.

Treatment

Given the heterogeneity of primary spinal cord tumors, there is no single treatment algorithm. Treatment strategies include surgery, RT, chemotherapy, and/or embolization depending on the anatomic and histologic characteristics [238]. Surgery is the first line of therapy for the majority of symptomatic primary spine tumors. A multidisciplinary setting is essential for optimal treatment and includes close consultation with medical oncologists, radiation oncologists, and neurosurgery or orthopedic surgery.

Specific Spinal Tumors

Primary tumors of the spinal cord, spinal nerves, and spinal meninges are identical to their intracranial counterparts. As the details of those tumors have been discussed in previous sections, only factors relevant to the spinal location are discussed here.

Chordoma

Chordomas are rare primary bone tumors developing from notochordal remnants and arise in midline structures from the skull base to the coccyx. They are most commonly located in the sacrococcygeal region (45–50%), followed by the spheno-occipital location (35–40%), and then the mobile spine (10–15%) [239]. The median age at diagnosis is 58.5 years, and they occur nearly twice as frequently in men [240]. Although slow-growing, they are locally aggressive, and roughly 30% of sacrococcygeal chordomas eventually metastasize. En bloc resection, with a margin of uninvolved tissue, is the goal of surgical intervention since extent of resection plays a major role in determining length of disease-free survival. Unfortunately, because of the large size at initial diagnosis and locally invasive nature, incomplete tumor resection is common. Some reports have shown that subtotal excision plus RT was superior to subtotal excision alone in lengthening disease-free survival [240]. Despite the use of RT as an adjuvant therapy, local recurrence is common after subtotal resection. Chemotherapy has not been shown to improve survival; however, imatinib just completed phase 2 testing with promising results [241]. Despite these efforts, the current 5-year survival is 50–68% and 10-year survival is 28–40% [240].

Schwannoma

Schwannomas are benign, slow-growing, intradural extramedullary lesions making up approximately one-third of intradural spinal tumors [242]. Most occur sporadically and are solitary, but they may also be associated with NF type 1 or 2. They are composed principally of neoplastic Schwann cells and histologically characterized by Antoni A (compact, interwoven bundles) and Antoni B (loose matrix) tissue. MRI usually demonstrates a well-encapsulated, round lesion, though they become dumbbell shaped with neuroforaminal extension (Figure 40.3). Surgical excision is the treatment of choice. While

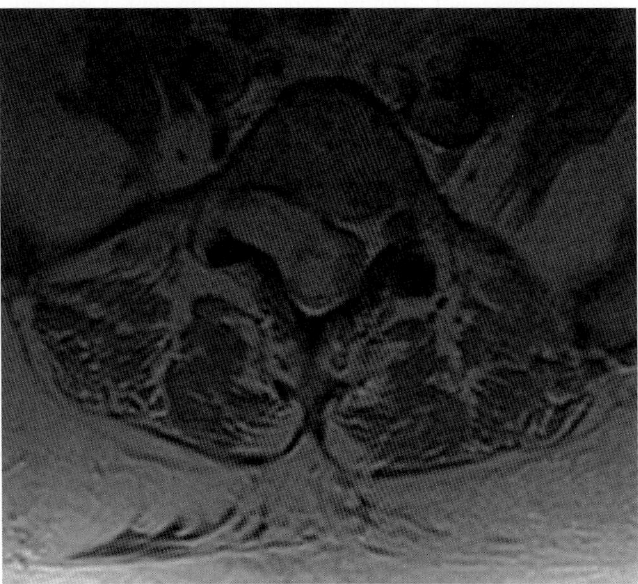

Figure 40.3 Axial contrast-enhanced MRI of the lumbar spine showing a schwannoma within the central spinal canal and extending through the neural foramen along with the right L5 nerve root.

care is taken to preserve the associated nerve root during surgery, occasionally it must be sacrificed for complete resection. This usually does not affect motor function since 75% of schwannomas arise from sensory nerve roots. Recurrence is exceedingly rare after total excision.

Meningiomas

Spinal meningiomas represent 12% of all meningiomas and one-third of intradural spine tumors [243]. There is a 4:1 female predominance and peak age at presentation is between 40 and 70 years [237]. Most tumors are sporadic; however, multiple meningiomas are often found in patients with NF2. Meningiomas are dural-based neoplastic proliferations of meningothelial cells and are usually benign, though there are rare malignant histologic subtypes. The thoracic spine is most commonly involved (greater than 80%); thus patients frequently present with upper motor neuron signs such as hyperreflexia and spasticity. On MRI a dural tail sign may be seen with homogeneous tumor enhancement. As with schwannomas, complete resection is the treatment of choice. The Simpson grading system is a useful predictor of tumor recurrence following resection (Table 40.6). Though this was written to apply primarily to cranial tumors, it generally applies well to meningiomas of the spine also [244]. In a series of 68 patients with an average follow-up of 12.5 years, there was no recurrence with grade I resection, 9.7% recurrence with grade II, and 100% recurrence with grade III or IV [243]. Therefore, any residual tumor following surgery must be watched closely with serial imaging.

Ependymomas

Ependymomas are the most common intramedullary spinal cord tumor in adults. In the spine there are two distinct histological types of ependymomas which usually present: cellular (WHO grade II and III) and myxopapillary (WHO grade I) [236]. Cellular ependymomas arise from the central canal of the cervical and thoracic cord while myxopapillary ependymomas arise from the filum terminale and usually present at, and caudal to, the conus medullaris. Most of these tumors are low grade though malignant histologic subtypes do rarely occur. On MRI these tumors show low T1-weighted signal intensity and high T2-weighted signal intensity with variable enhancement patterns. In most cases, there is a clearly defined demarcation between the tumor and spinal cord. Also, over 50% of intramedullary ependymomas have an associated syrinx. In fact, the presence of a syrinx is a good prognostic factor because it usually enables excellent operative margins between the tumor and normal cord tissue. Surgery is the treatment of choice as the local control rates are greater than 90% with gross total resection. However, the majority of patients with intramedullary tumors have some residual tumor after surgery. External beam RT at a dose of 45–54 Gy is indicated for partially resected WHO grade 2 and 3 ependymomas [236]. There are multiple trials utilizing chemotherapeutics at this time; however, none have become standard of care for patients who fail surgery and radiation.

Table 40.6 Simpson grading scale for degree of meningioma resection.

Grade I	Complete removal including resection of underlying bone and associated dura
Grade II	Complete removal and coagulation of dural attachment
Grade III	Complete removal without resection of dura or coagulation
Grade IV	Subtotal resection

Astrocytomas

Astrocytomas of the spinal cord are the second most common intramedullary glial tumors. The fibrillary subtype (WHO grade 2) presents most frequently while WHO grade 3 or 4 lesions represent 25% of cases [236]. Aside from pilocytic astrocytomas, which are WHO grade 1, spinal cord astrocytomas are infiltrative and associated with poorly characterized borders. MRI of fibrillary astrocytomas shows enlargement of the cord without enhancement, T1-weighted hypointensity, and T2-weighted hyperintensity (Figure 40.4). Pilocytic astrocytomas are typically cystic with a mural nodule while high-grade lesions have variable enhancement. It is not possible to consistently distinguish astrocytomas from ependymomas on MRI. The primary determinants of outcome are tumor histology, extent of resection, and functional status at time of presentation [236]. Treatment consists of biopsy with maximal safe surgical resection. Aside from pilocytic astrocytomas, gross total resection is extremely rare given the infiltrative nature of these tumors. RT is indicated for patients with high-grade histology, biopsied-only tumors, and progressive disease. Chemotherapy is reserved for only those patients with progression of disease following

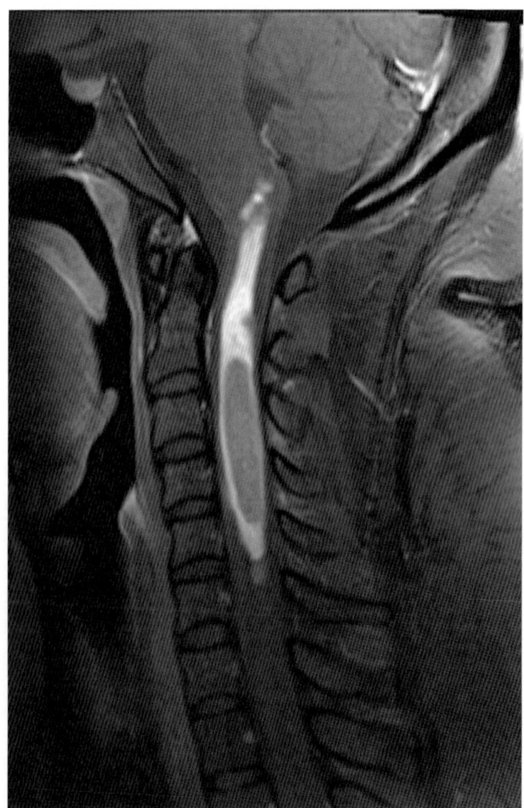

Figure 40.4 Sagittal contrast-enhanced T1-weighted MRI of the cervical spine showing a heterogeneously enhancing glioblastoma with syringomyelia in a 29-year-old female presenting with progressive right hemiparesis and pain.

surgery and RT who are no longer candidates for retreatment with these modalities. Unfortunately, there are only limited chemotherapeutic options available and studies with these agents to date have only shown a marginal benefit.

Paragangliomas

Paragangliomas of the spine are extraordinarily rare with approximately 80 cases reported since 1972 [236]. They typically present as intradural tumors within the cauda equina though there are a few cases of thoracic involvement. There is a slight male predominance with a peak incidence in the fourth to sixth decades of life. Unlike paragangliomas in the carotid and jugular bodies which are parasympathetic in type, spinal paragangliomas are predominantly of the sympathetic type. However, these tumors only rarely produce catecholamine excess. The most common clinical presentation is lumbar pain and sciatica accompanied by sensory or motor deficit in the lower extremities [245]. T2-weighted MRI produces a characteristic "salt-and-pepper" appearance secondary to the hypervascular flow voids interspersed in a matrix of increased signal intensity caused by tumor cells. Complete surgical resection is considered curative and subtotal resection often leads to recurrence. Postoperative RT for patients with incomplete resection has not been shown to decrease recurrence [245].

Other Spinal Cord Tumors

Reviewing the specific nuances of all primary spine tumors listed in Table 40.5 is beyond the scope of this text. Fortunately, the clinical presentations previously discussed are fairly consistent across all tumor subtypes. A thorough history and neurological examination will help distinguish these patients from those presenting with non-neoplastic conditions. Hemangioblastoma and gangliomas are less prevalent intramedullary tumors. They are treated with surgical resection and generally have a good prognosis following surgery. Neurofibromas are a common intradural extramedullary lesion with a presentation and treatment paradigm similar to spinal schwannomas. Resection is usually curative; however, they do rarely have malignant transformation. Finally, the primary vertebral tumors, such as Ewing sarcoma and chondrosarcoma, are treated similar to their systemic counterparts.

Spinal Metastatic Disease

Spinal metastases are a common manifestation of systemic neoplasia. More than half of all cancer patients develop spinal metastases during their disease course. Spinal metastases most frequently occur at the vertebral column, particularly the vertebral bodies. Intramedullary spinal cord tumors are more likely to be primary and are rarely metastatic. Spinal metastases are classified according to their anatomic location. Spinal metastases occur predominantly in the extradural space, whereas the remaining tumors are intradural extramedullary lesions and intramedullary metastases which are extremely rare. Breast, lung, prostate, and hematologic (e.g., lymphoma, multiple myeloma) cancers are responsible for most of the extradural spinal metastases. Intradural extramedullary spinal metastases usually arise from melanoma and lymphoma. Small cell lung carcinoma is the primary tumor responsible for the majority of intramedullary metastases. Systemic neoplasms metastasize to the spine mainly hematogenously, although direct extension of tumor is possible as well. It has also been observed that many patients with intradural extramedullary or intramedullary spinal metastases also harbor concomitant brain metastatic foci. This relationship suggests drop metastases as the responsible spread mechanism.

Clinical Findings

Once vertebral body metastasis occurs, spinal cord compression can occur leading to the patient being symptomatic. Pain is usually the initial symptom of vertebral column (bony) metastasis. Tumor-related bony pain is commonly insidious, local, and progressive. It is often described by the patients as dull and constant with characteristic worsening at night (nocturnal pain) or early in the morning. The pain is associated with tenderness on palpation over the spinous processes at the involved level. Occasionally, except for localized back pain, radicular pain can occur due to radiculopathy of the nerve root at the involved level. The radicular pain radiates to the distribution of the corresponding nerve root involved in the lesion. Vertebral destruction and resultant pathologic fracture or dislocation can lead to mechanical pain, which is characteristically aggravated by standing, movement, and coughing and alleviated when assuming a supine position or by immobility. In most patients with spinal metastases, the diagnosis is made only after signs and symptoms of spinal cord compression occur. It is an axiom in oncology that back or neck pain in a cancer patient is due to spinal metastasis until proven otherwise.

Neurological symptoms due to spinal cord compression can present either gradually within weeks, months after the onset of pain, or acutely as a neurological emergency. Neurological symptoms can be either radiculopathy or myelopathy. The latter presents initially as gait disturbance, followed by spasticity, sensory loss, weakness, and autonomic dysfunction. Autonomic dysfunction usually manifests with sphincter disturbances and results in bowel and/or bladder dysfunction, which can be present at the time of diagnosis. About half of the patients are nonambulatory at the time of diagnosis due to pain, neurological deficits, or lesions at multiple levels [246]. The presence of Brown-Séquard syndrome points to intramedullary spinal metastasis [247]. The natural history of metastatic spinal disease is gradual progression to complete and irreversible paraplegia unless adequate and timely treatment is undertaken.

Diagnosis

When spinal metastatic disease is suspected in known cancer patients, patients should undergo CT of the chest, abdomen, and pelvis, which provides information about the primary neoplasm. MRI provides optimal visualization of the spinal cord and therefore is the imaging modality of choice in patients with suspected spinal tumors, leading to early diagnosis. Spinal metastases invariably enhance after gadolinium administration. MRI, in addition to its diagnostic value, is also essential in pre-treatment planning. MRI enables the visualization of the entire vertebral axis, which is of high significance in spinal metastatic disease, given the high propensity of multiple vertebral levels of tumor infiltration [248]. MRI cannot provide optimal bone imaging, thus CT scanning is a valuable complement of MRI in the evaluation of spinal metastatic disease. Finally, radioisotope bone scan and radionucleotide CT-PET are sensitive screening or follow-up tools for assessment of the extent of disease in the body.

Treatment

The management of patients with spinal metastases is a complex process requiring a multidisciplinary approach involving the surgeon, oncologists, patient, and family members [249]. A fundamental rule in cases of symptomatic metastatic spinal disease is that treatment should be initiated as soon as possible, because neurological outcome after treatment is strongly correlated to the neurological status prior to treatment [250, 251]. The goal of treatment administration in patients with symptomatic spinal metastases is to relieve pain, preserve or restore neurological function, and maintain spinal stability. Except for cases when the spine is the sole site of metastatic disease, cure is not a realistic goal. Palliation is the reasonable expectation. The histology of the primary tumor and the post-treatment ambulatory status are the factors most consistently reported as determinants of patients' survival [252–254]. Treatment modalities involved in the management of patients with symptomatic metastatic spinal disease are medications, RT, surgery, or a combination [255].

Corticosteroids

There is strong clinical evidence supporting administration of corticosteroids intravenously or orally in patients with spinal metastases that cause spinal cord compression. The beneficial action of corticosteroids in cases of spinal cord compression can be partially attributed to the reduction of vasogenic edema and enhancement of blood flow, preventing further spinal cord ischemia and improving neurological function. Dexamethasone has been widely used in patients with metastatic spinal cord compression. Corticosteroids can also serve as an adjuvant bridging therapy during the interval between the patient's presentation and final treatment decisions. Corticosteroids administration during this crucial time interval preserves neurological function, preventing further decline of the patient's neurological status.

Radiotherapy

RT plays a vital role in the treatment of spinal metastases and it has been considered the principal therapeutic modality in many cases. Spinal irradiation is effective in cases of radiosensitive spinal metastatic tumors, such as lymphoma, multiple myeloma, small cell lung carcinoma, seminoma of the testes, and prostate carcinoma. Other RT indications are inability of the patient to tolerate surgery and multiple levels of spinal metastatic involvement. RT is effective in patients with signs and symptoms of spinal cord compression, even if the tumor is radioresistant, such as breast carcinoma and metastatic melanoma. Pretreatment neurological status and ambulatory status are the most important prognostic indicators, correlating with survival after treatment [253]. Many variations exist regarding the dose and fractionation of RT, depending on the patient's medical status and extent of metastatic spinal disease. A serious, but rare, late-onset complication of spinal irradiation is myelopathy [256]. Nonconventional RT, such as SRS, decreases the amount of radiation delivered to the normal spinal cord, leading to less significant side effects, and has been used in cases of spinal metastases [257, 258]. Intraoperative RT has also been reported, but is not widely accepted as part of standard treatment [259]. In cases of complete paraplegia, palliative pain relief should be the goal of RT.

Surgery

Surgical management of symptomatic spinal metastatic disease remains one of the main therapeutic options. The goal of surgery is preservation or restoration of neurological function and pain relief, along with aggressive spinal cord decompression and spinal stabilization/reconstruction. Any surgical approach must ensure both spinal cord decompression and stabilization of the spinal column. Decompressive laminectomy had been the preferred procedure for years, but may not provide optimal decompression. This has led to newer surgical approaches such as anterior, anteriolateral, and posterolateral exposures.

Successful surgical treatment of spinal metastatic tumors mainly depends on careful initial evaluation of patients in order to identify and select surgical candidates. Indications for surgical management of symptomatic metastatic spinal lesions include radioresistant tumors, such as sarcoma, renal cell carcinoma, and colon cancer, as well as clinically significant spinal cord compression, intractable pain not alleviated by any nonoperative intervention, and radiation failure which is defined as progression of symptoms during a course of RT. Surgery should also be selected in patients harboring a pathological vertebral fracture or dislocation leading to spinal instability. When the diagnosis of spinal metastases has not been established, surgery should be chosen. In these cases surgery serves as both a diagnostic and therapeutic procedure. Urgent surgery should be performed in the setting of paraplegia, in order to avoid complete and irreversible spinal cord compression. However, surgical intervention in these cases may not reverse paralysis established for more than 24 hours. In cases of spinal metastases that are highly vascular, such as from thyroid and renal cell carcinoma, preoperative embolization should be considered [260]. With surgical treatment (decompressive surgery with spinal reconstruction and stabilization), the benefits of spinal cord decompression and spinal stability can come at the expense of a high rate of postoperative complications, the most common of which is wound breakdown [261]. It has been shown that wound dehiscence and postoperative infections occur with even higher frequency when surgery is performed after radiotherapy [262]. As a consequence, if surgery is considered as the treatment of choice, it should be performed as soon as possible after diagnosis establishment and before radiation application.

Intracranial Metastases

Clinical Features

Brain metastases are the most common adult intracranial tumor, occurring in approximately 10–30% of adult cancer patients and causing significant morbidity and mortality in this population [263]. Risk of brain metastases differs with different primary tumor histologies, with lung cancer accounting for approximately one-half of all brain metastases [264, 265]. Metastatic disease can affect any portion of the cranial space, including the skull, dura, leptomeninges, and brain parenchyma. Hematogenous arterial spread is the typical route of dissemination, hence brain metastases tend to occur at the gray–white junction where the arterial caliber becomes smaller. The pattern of involvement reflects the distribution of blood supply and tissue volume with approximately 85% of blood supply and metastatic involvement being supratentorial and 15% of the distribution being infratentorial.

Symptoms are due to displacement of brain tissue and vasogenic edema from disruption of the blood–brain barrier (BBB). Metastases usually grow as spherical masses that push against rather than infiltrate into surrounding brain parenchyma [265]. The neurologic signs and symptoms depend on the location, size, and amount of edema associated with the lesion. Potential symptoms include headache (increased with posterior fossa or multiple brain metastases), nausea, cognitive dysfunction, gait/balance dysfunction, focal sensory or motor deficits, and visual deficits.

There have been several advances in prognostic stratification for patients with brain metastases. The recursive partitioning analysis (RPA) [266], graded prognostic assessment (GPA) [267], and most recently diagnosis-specific GPA [268] have been used to stratify patients by expected median overall survival prognosis. The diagnosis-specific GPA indicates that patients with brain metastases are a heterogeneous group and that primary site has a large influence on outcome and which patient and tumor factors should be used to accurately estimate survival.

Diagnosis

Metastatic brain disease must be distinguished from other benign and malignant processes. Though CT with contrast can be used, MRI of the brain with and without contrast is the diagnostic imaging modality of choice for brain metastases. Secondary brain neoplasms tend to be contrast enhancing, located at the gray–white junction, multiple in number, well circumscribed, and with considerable edema relative to the size of the tumor.

Biopsy should be performed whenever the diagnosis of brain metastases is in doubt, especially in cases of single brain lesions. In a study of patients with known cancer and single brain lesions on imaging, 6 of 54 patients (11%) did not have metastatic brain disease after resection or biopsy [269]. MRI can be diagnostic in certain clinical settings (i.e., in a patient with known cancer and multiple typical brain lesions).

In patients who have received previous RT, the distinction between progressive brain disease and radiation necrosis is sometimes difficult. New advanced imaging modalities, such as diffusion-weighted MRI, MRI perfusion, MR spectroscopy, and brain PET are helpful in differentiating these processes.

Treatment

Corticosteroids

Corticosteroids reduce tumor-related vasogenic edema and mass effect and are used in patients with brain metastases to relieve symptoms caused by these processes [270]. The most commonly used glucocorticoid is dexamethasone due to its relatively long half-life, low affinity for mineralocorticoid receptors, and potency (about 20 times as potent as hydrocortisone). Asymptomatic patients with small tumors and no mass effect do not need corticosteroid therapy. Since corticosteroids have a wide variety of potential short-term and long-term toxicities, dose and duration should be based on the individual patient presentation. Patients with mild symptoms are recommended a starting dose of 4–8 mg/day of dexamethasone. Patients with moderate to severe symptoms should be started on 16 mg/day or more of dexamethasone. If given, corticosteroids should be tapered over a 2-week period or longer in symptomatic patients after definitive therapy is administered.

Anticonvulsants

If a patient experiences seizures, appropriate anticonvulsant therapy should be given. There is no clear evidence for the routine use of prophylactic anticonvulsants [271]. Anticonvulsants are not uncommonly used temporarily in the perioperative period.

Radiotherapy

The standard of care for patients with poor performance status (KPS <70%) or multiple brain metastases (>4) is whole brain radiation therapy (WBRT). The most commonly used regimen is 30 Gy over 10 fractions. Due to concern for late WBRT-related leukoencephalopathy in patients with prolonged expected survival (>1 year), regimens with a lower dose per fraction (e.g., 37.5 Gy over 15 fractions or 40 Gy over 20 fractions) can be considered to reduce the risk of late toxicity. Expected control rates with WBRT alone are approximately 70% local control and 70–80% distant brain control at 1 year [272].

WBRT is also used in combination with local brain therapies, such as surgery or SRS. WBRT after surgical resection of single brain metastases significantly reduced local, distant, and total intracranial recurrence, although OS was not prolonged compared to surgery alone [273]. All randomized trials of local therapy (surgery or SRS) with or without WBRT have found improvement in intracranial control (and neurologic death in some studies) with the addition of WBRT, but none has found an improvement in OS in patients with a limited number of brain metastases [273–276]. Table 40.7 provides a summary of trials of local therapy with or without WBRT for patients with a limited number of brain metastases.

Radiosurgery

Radiosurgery, primarily SRS, as well as more recently frameless radiosurgery (FRS), has become a standard of care for patients with a limited number of brain metastases [273–273]. There have not been any randomized trials comparing SRS alone with WBRT or surgery. SRS and the combination of surgery and adjuvant WBRT are generally considered equally effective for local control of brain metastases based on retrospective data. Local control rates with SRS alone are approximately 70–90% at 1 year, depending on lesion size and histology. SRS is also effective for patients with classically radioresistant histologies, such as renal cell, melanoma, and sarcoma, with a 6-month local control rate of approximately 70% [277].

Table 40.7 Outcomes for local therapy alone versus local therapy and whole brain radiation therapy.

Study	Intervention	LC	DC	TIC	Neurologic death	Median OS
Patchell #2 [273]	Surgery	54%	63%	30%	44%	43 weeks
(crude)[1]	Surgery + WBRT	90%[2]	86%[2]	82%[2]	14%[2]	48 weeks
Chang MDACC [274]	SRS	67%	45%	27%	8 patients	15.2 months[2]
(1-year)	SRS + WBRT	100%[2]	73%[2]	73%[2]	7 patients	5.7 months
JROSG 99-1 [275]	SRS	73%	36%	24%	19%	8 months
(1-year)	WBRT + SRS	89%[2]	58%[2]	53%[2]	23%	7.5 months
EORTC [276]	SRS or surgery	41% (S)	58% (S)	22%	44%	10.9 months
(2-year)		69% (SRS)	52% (SRS)			
	Same + WBRT	73% (S)[2]	77% (S)[2]	52%[2]	28%[2]	10.7 months
		81% (SRS)[2]	67% (SRS)[2]			

[1] Crude, nonactuarial rates of recurrence.
[2] Statistically significant improvement.
DC, distant brain control; LC, local control; OS, overall survival; S, surgery; SRS, stereotactic radiosurgery; TIC, total intracranial control; WBRT, whole brain radiation therapy.

SRS is typically used for patients with a limited number of brain metastases, good performance status (KPS ≥70%), and tumor size <4 cm maximum dimension. There has been evidence that SRS therapy alone in patients with 1–4 metastases, though associated with worse intracranial control than the combination of SRS and WBRT (Table 40.7), has significantly reduced risk of neurocognitive decline. A recent study randomized patients with 1–3 brain metastases to SRS versus SRS and WBRT. Patients who received SRS and WBRT were twice as likely to develop deficits in total recall at 4-month evaluation compared to patients who underwent SRS alone (52% vs 24%, $P<0.05$) [274]. The recommended follow-up regimen for patients treated with SRS alone is close surveillance with 3-monthly MRI scans with salvage SRS as necessary for a limited number of distant brain failure sites. These data are also being extrapolated for the use of radiosurgery alone to the resection cavity for patients after surgical resection of a limited number of brain metastases [278].

The primary dose-limiting toxicity of SRS is the development of radiation necrosis. Rates of radiation necrosis can be as high as 24%, with approximately half of cases being symptomatic [279]. Reported rates of radiation necrosis after standard-dose SRS have been increasing, most likely due to increased detection of asymptomatic radiation necrosis with advancing and more frequent brain imaging.

Surgery

Surgical resection is primarily used for patients who are highly symptomatic due to mass effect or large tumors, and/or cases where the diagnosis of brain metastases is in doubt and pathologic confirmation is required. The local recurrence rate after gross total resection can be as high as 60% at 2 years [276], and multiple studies have demonstrated substantially reduced risk of local recurrence with adjuvant radiation (either WBRT or SRS). Patients with a single metastasis treated with surgery and WBRT have improved OS, improved local control, longer functionally independent period, and less dependence on corticosteroids than those treated with WBRT alone [279].

Chemotherapy

Standard chemotherapies used for metastatic solid cancers have traditionally been thought not to have significant penetrance through the blood–brain barrier and consequently to have little efficacy for brain metastases. However, this is not the rule; for example, patients with asymptomatic brain metastases with small cell lung cancer can be treated with upfront chemotherapy. Newer methods of systemic therapy, such as small molecule inhibitors and immunotherapy, have been increasingly shown to have efficacy for solid brain metastases. For melanoma brain metastases, dabrafenib (a BRAF inhibitor) has efficacy for otherwise untreated BRAF mutated melanoma brain metastases [280]. Efficacy in this setting has also been shown for ipilimumab immunotherapy for metastatic melanoma [281]. Other targeted agents with activity in brain metastases include the combination of lapatinib and capecitabine for HER-2 amplified breast cancer and erlotinib in conjunction with WBRT for EGFR-mutated adenocarcinoma of the lung [282, 283]. The integration of new systemic agents and local therapy for brain metastases is an area of ongoing research.

Primary Central Nervous System Lymphoma

Primary central nervous system lymphoma (PCNSL) is a rare form of extranodal non-Hodgkin lymphoma [284] and represents 2–3% of all primary brain tumors [285]. CNS Hodgkin lymphoma is exceedingly rare [286]. PCNSL occurs in both immunocompetent and immunocompromised hosts such as organ transplant recipients and patients with HIV-acquired immunodeficiency syndrome (HIV-AIDS). Risk of PCNSL in HIV patients is increased nearly 3,600-fold and is associated with Epstein–Barr virus infection [287, 288]. The incidence of PCNSL increased in the 1980s with the rise in HIV-AIDS [289] and has since plateaued due to effective antiretroviral strategies [290].

Clinical Presentation

In immunocompetent individuals, the median age at diagnosis is 53–57 years with a male predominance (1.2–1.7:1) [291]. Patients with PCNSL present with focal neurologic deficits (70%), signs of raised intracranial pressure (33%), seizures (14%), or ocular symptoms (4%) [292]. About 20% of patients have ocular findings at diagnosis [293]. Diffuse large B-cell lymphoma (DLBCL) accounts for 90% of PCNSL; the remaining 10% include Burkitt lymphoma, T-cell lymphomas, and other low-grade lymphomas [286]. PCNSL tumor cells, or immunoblasts, have large nuclei with coarse chromatin and tend to cluster around blood vessels [294]. Other less common presentations include neurolymphomatosis and intravascular lymphoma.

Diagnostic Evaluation

Corticosteroids induce rapid tumor lysis and should be avoided, if possible, prior to confirmation of the diagnosis. Diagnosis of PCNSL is usually made with stereotactic biopsy. Based on the International PCNSL Collaborative Group guidelines, diagnostic evaluation and staging for PCNSL should include: contrast-enhanced MRI of the brain, and spine if clinically necessary; CSF analysis, if safe to obtain, for cell count, glucose, protein, cytology, and flow cytometry; ophthalmologic evaluation with slit lamp, as up to 20% of cases may include ocular lymphoma; CT imaging of the chest, abdomen, and pelvis, or whole body PET; blood tests including basic chemistry, hepatic and renal functions, lactate dehydrogenase, and HIV serology; bone marrow biopsy and aspiration [295]. On MRI (Figure 40.5), PCNSL appears isointense/hypointense on T1-weighted imaging with homogenous contrast enhancement in 95% of cases. Lesions can be solitary (65%) or multifocal [296]. CSF findings include pleocytosis and elevated protein. CSF cytology, though negative in two-thirds of patients on first analysis, may show clumped pleomorphic cells with coarse chromatin [297]. Flow cytometry may show a monoclonal population of B cells.

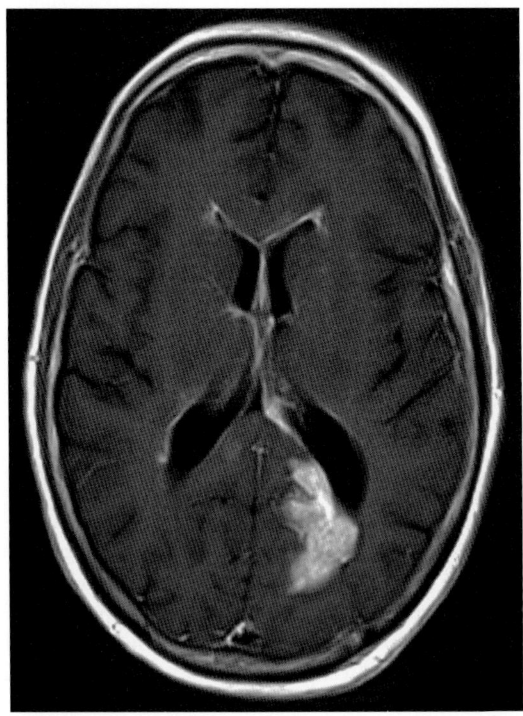

Figure 40.5 Axial T1-weighted MRI with gadolinium-based contrast demonstrating the homogeneous enhancement of a primary central nervous system lymphoma adjacent to the occipital horn of the left lateral ventricle.

Treatment

There is currently no consensus regarding the optimal treatment for PCNSL. Age, performance status, and risks of neurotoxicity should be considered while formulating treatment strategies [298]. Resection alone provides no benefit other than in emergent cases with brain herniation. WBRT alone, despite a favorable initial response, provides inadequate sustained remission and is associated with high risk for neurotoxicity, mainly in patients older than 60 years of age. High-dose ($\geq$3.5 g/m^2) methotrexate-based combination regimens are the cornerstone in the treatment of PCNSL and can achieve response rates as high as 90% with PFS between 16 and 24 months and median OS of 55 months [299, 300]. A minimum methotrexate dose of 3.5 g/m^2 is necessary to attain adequate CNS penetration. Other chemotherapy agents studied include procarbazine, vincristine, rituximab, and cytarabine and have comparable response rates [301, 302]. Despite initial favorable responses, most patients relapse and require salvage chemotherapy, including reinduction with high-dose methotrexate, or high-dose cytarabine, as well as temozolomide, rituximab, or high-dose chemotherapy with autologous stem cell rescue [302]. Favorable response to initial therapy and BCL-6 expression are associated with improved survival in PCNSL [303] while older age, poor performance status, and failure to respond to initial therapy are poor prognostic factors [304, 305]. The relative rarity of PCNSL makes it difficult to design prospective clinical trials, which are necessary to define the best treatment strategy.

Leptomeningeal Disease

Involvement of the pia and arachnoid by cancer is termed leptomeningeal disease (LMD). It is typically seen in widely metastatic or recurrent malignancies, but can also be the initial presentation of cancer in 5–10% of patients. LMD is most frequently seen in leukemia, lymphoma, breast cancer, lung cancer, and melanoma, and less commonly primitive neuroectodermal tumors (PNET) and gliomas [306]. Malignant cells can spread to the subarachnoid space by direct or hematogenous dissemination, or by extension along cranial or peripheral nerves. Approximately 8% of patients with cancer have LMD at autopsy [306, 307].

Clinical Features

Neurologic deficits develop based on the involved sites of the neuraxis. Cerebral involvement results in headache, nausea, vomiting, encephalopathy, meningismus, seizures, or weakness. Brainstem involvement may lead to cranial nerve deficits, while spinal cord or plexus involvement may result in weakness, sensory level, sphincter dysfunction, or pain [308].

Diagnosis

Definitive diagnosis is made by CSF examination that typically reveals elevated opening pressure (>25 cm water) in 50% of cases, pleocytosis, elevated protein, hypoglycorrhachia, and positive cytology (in 45–55% of cases). Additional lumbar punctures may be necessary. Flow cytometry is indicated in hematologic tumors [309]. Tumor markers in CSF, such as carcinoembryonic antigen, alpha-fetoprotein, or β-hCG, may suggest a primary source if unknown. Other nonspecific markers that are elevated in LMD include β-glucuronidase, β-microglobulin, and isoenzyme V of lactate dehydrogenase. Contrast-enhanced MRI of the entire neuraxis is the preferred imaging diagnostic modality in suspected cases of LMD, and may show dural, ependymal, or leptomeningeal enhancement, including the cord, or thickening of nerve roots (Figure 40.6) [310]. Communicating hydrocephalus may also develop. Patency of the CSF pathways can be assessed by radioisotope CSF flow studies, especially if intrathecal chemotherapy is considered [311].

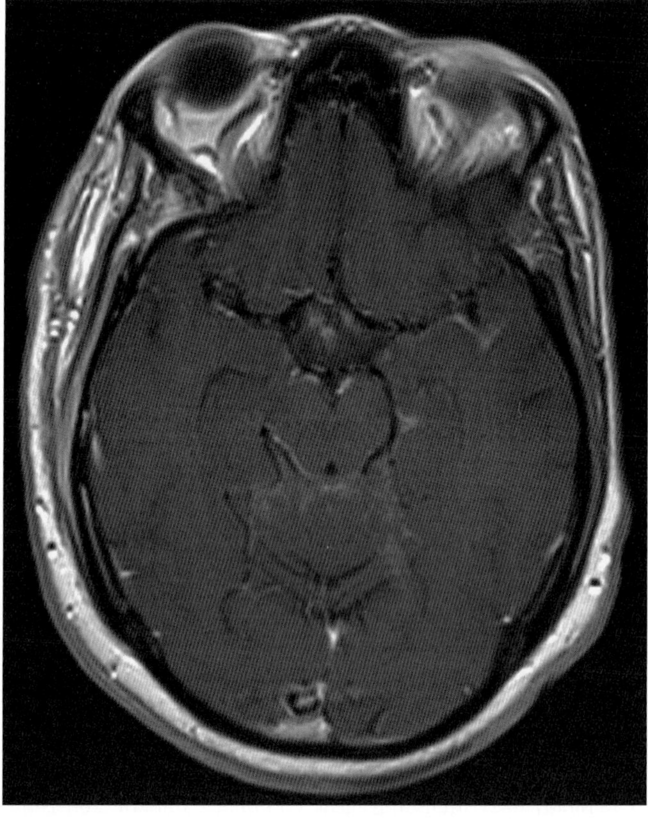

Figure 40.6 Axial T1-weighted MRI with gadolinium-based contrast in a woman with known metastatic breast carcinoma demonstrating faint leptomeningeal enhancement along the superior cerebellar folia and dorasal aspect of the midbrain in a pattern consistent with carcinomatous meningitis.

Treatment

Treatment of LMD is palliative and aimed at delaying neurologic decline and improving quality of life. In patients with high performance status and low tumor burden, a multimodal approach with focused radiotherapy to areas of bulky disease, systemic and/or intrathecal chemotherapy, or isolated intrathecal chemotherapy may be considered [312]. High-dose intravenous methotrexate, cytarabine, and thiotepa have good CSF penetration and can be used in LMD for chemosensitive tumors such as breast cancer, hematologic tumors, and small cell lung cancer [306, 313]. There is no consensus currently on the multimodal management of LMD. Intrathecal chemotherapy (by lumbar puncture or intraventricular reservoir) with methotrexate, thiotepa, cytarabine (Ara-C), or liposomal Ara-C can be used in non-bulky tumors with the advantage of decreased systemic toxicity, though significant neurotoxicity has been reported. Intra-CSF administration of monoclonal antibodies and other agents has also been attempted in LMD [314]. Palliative and hospice care must be provided to patients with poor performance status. Corticosteroids may be used for acute symptomatic relief from raised intracranial pressure or spinal cord compression. Prognosis depends on the tumor type but LMD remains a rapidly progressive and fatal condition with a median survival of 12–18 weeks based on data from clinical trials [307].

References

1 De Witt Hamer PC, Robles SG, Zwinderman AH, Duffau H, Berger MS. Impact of intraoperative stimulation brain mapping on glioma surgery outcome: a meta-analysis. *J Clin Oncol* 2012;30:2559–65.

2 Roberts DW, Valdes PA, Harris BT, *et al.* Glioblastoma multiforme treatment with clinical trials for surgical resection (aminolevulinic acid). *Neurosurg Clin N Am* 2012;23:371–7.

3 Kuhnt D, Ganslandt O, Schlaffer SM, *et al.* Quantification of glioma removal by intraoperative high-field magnetic resonance imaging: an update. *Neurosurgery* 2011;69:852–62.

4 Horska A, Barker PB. Imaging of brain tumors: MR spectroscopy and metabolic imaging. *Neuroimaging Clin N Am* 2010;20:293–310.

5 Weaver KD, Grossman SA, Herman JG. Methylated tumor-specific DNA as a plasma biomarker in patients with glioma. *Cancer Invest* 2006;24:35–40.

6 Vlassov VV, Laktionov PP, Rykova EY. Circulating nucleic acids as a potential source for cancer biomarkers. *Curr Mol Med* 2010;10:142–65.

7 Batchelor T, Carson K, O'Neill A, *et al.* Treatment of primary CNS lymphoma with methotrexate and deferred radiotherapy: A report of NABTT 96–07. *J Clin Oncol* 2003;21:1044–9.

8 Stupp R, Hegi ME, Mason WP, *et al.* European Organisation for Research and Treatment of Cancer Brain Tumour and Radiation Oncology Groups. National Cancer Institute of Canada Clinical Trials Group: Effects of radiotherapy with concomitant and adjuvant temozolomide versus radiotherapy alone on survival in glioblastoma in a randomised phase III study: 5-year analysis of the EORTC-NCIC trial. *Lancet Oncol* 2009;10:459–66.

9 Mehta MP, Paleologos NA, Mikkelson T, *et al.* The role of chemotherapy in the management of newly diagnosed brain

metastases: A systematic review and evidence-based clinical practice guideline. *J Neurooncol* 2010;96:71–83.

10 Van Meir EG, Hadjipanayis CG, Norden AD, *et al.* Exciting new advances in neuro-oncology: the avenue to a cure for malignant glioma. *CA Cancer J Clin* 2010;60:166–93.

11 Cancer Genome Atlas Research Network. Comprehensive genomic characterization defines human glioblastoma genes and core pathways. *Nature* 2008;455:1061–8.

12 Verhaak RGW, Hoadley KA, Purdom E, *et al.* Integrated genomic analysis identifies clinically relevant subtypes of glioblastoma characterized by abnormalities in PDGFRA, IDH1, EGFR, and NF1. *Cancer Cell* 2010;17:98–110.

13 Friedman HS, Prados MD, Wen PY, *et al.* Bevacizumab alone and in combination with irinotecan in recurrent glioblastoma. *J Clin Oncol* 2009;27:4733–40.

14 Kreisl TN, Kim L, Moore K, *et al.* Phase II trial of single-agent bevacizumab followed by bevacizumab plus irinotecan at tumor progression in recurrent glioblastoma. *J Clin Oncol* 2009;27:740–5.

15 Franz DN, Leonard J, Tudor C, *et al.* Rapamycin causes regression of astrocytomas in tuberous sclerosis complex. *Ann Neurol* 2006;59:490–8.

16 Jóźwiak S, Nabbout R, Curatolo P; participants of the TSC Consensus Meeting for SEGA and Epilepsy Management. Management of subependymal giant cell astrocytoma (SEGA) associated with tuberous sclerosis complex (TSC): Clinical recommendations. *Eur J Paediatr Neurol* 2013;17:348–52.

17 Jin JY, Wen N, Ren L, *et al.* Advances in treatment techniques: arc-based and other intensity modulated therapies. *Cancer J* 2011;17:166–76.

18 Amelio D, Lorentini S, Schwarz M, Amichetti M. Intensity-modulated radiation therapy in newly diagnosed glioblastoma: a systematic review on clinical and technical issues. *Radiother Oncol* 2010;97:361–9.

19 Kohler BA, Ward E, McCarthy BJ, *et al.* Annual report to the nation on the status of cancer, 1975–2007, featuring tumors of the brain and other nervous system. *J Natl Cancer Inst* 2011;103:714–36.

20 Siegel RL, Miller KD, Jemal A. Cancer statistics, 2017. *CA Cancer J Clin* 2017;67:7–30.

21 Langley RR, Fidler IJ. The biology of brain metastasis. *Clin Chem* 2013;59:180–9.

22 Posner JB. Neurologic Complications of Cancer. *Philadelphia: Davis*, 1995:482.

23 Braganza MZ, Kitahara CM, Berrington de Gonzalez A, *et al.* Ionizing radiation and the risk of brain and central nervous system tumors: a systematic review. *Neuro Oncol* 2012;14:1316–24.

24 Gerstner ER, Batchelor TT. Primary central nervous system lymphoma. *Arch Neurol* 2010;67:291–7.

25 Farrell CJ, Plotkin SR. Genetic causes of brain tumors: neurofibromatosis, tuberous sclerosis, von Hippel-Lindau, and other syndromes. *Neurol Clin* 2007;25:925–46.

26 Asa SL, Somers K, Ezzat S. The MEN-1 gene is rarely down-regulated in pituitary adenomas. *J Clin Endocrinol Metab* 1998;83:3210–2.

27 Mulligan G, Jacks T. The retinoblastoma gene family: cousins with overlapping interests. *Trends Genet* 1998;14:223–9.

28 Chow EY, Haley LP, Vickars LM. Essential thrombocythemia in pregnancy: platelet count and pregnancy outcome. *Am J Hematol* 1992;41:249–51.

29 Scheurer ME, Etzel CJ, Liu M, *et al.* Familial aggregation of glioma: a pooled analysis. *Am J Epidemiol* 2010;172:1099–107.

30 Perry A, Brat DJ. *Practical Surgical Neuropathology: A Diagnostic Approach.* Philadelphia: Churchill Livingstone, 2010.

31 Louis DN, Ohgaki H, Weistler OD, Cavenee WK. *WHO Classification of Tumours of the Central Nervous System*, 4th edn. Lyon: International Agency for Research, 2007.

32 Jiao Y, Killela PJ, Reitman ZJ, *et al.* Frequent ATRX, CIC, FUBP1, and IDH1 mutations refine the classification of malignant gliomas. *Oncotarget* 2012;3:709–22.

33 Killela PJ, Pirozzi CJ, Healy P, *et al.* Mutations in IDH1, IDH2, and in the TERT promoter define clinically distinct subgroups of adult malignant gliomas. *Oncotarget* 2014;5:1515–25.

34 Yan H, Parsons DW, Jin G, *et al.* IDH1 and IDH2 mutations in gliomas. *N Engl J Med* 2009;360:765–73.

35 Cancer Genome Atlas Research Network. Comprehensive, integrative genomic analysis of diffuse lower-grade gliomas. *N Engl J Med* 2015;372:2481–98.

36 Louis DN, Ohgaki H, Weistler OD, Cavenee WK, *et al. WHO Classification of Tumours of the Central Nervous System, revised 4th edn.* Lyon: International Agency for Research on Cancer, 2016.

37 Kunkle EC, Ray BS, Wolff HG. Studies on headache: the mechanisms and significance of the headache associated with brain tumor. *Bull N Y Acad Med* 1942;18:400–22.

38 Purdy R, Kirby S. Headaches and brain tumors. *Neurol Clin* 2004;22:39–53.

39 Lynam LM, Lyons MK, Drazkowski JF, *et al.* Frequency of seizures in patients with newly diagnosed brain tumors: a retrospective review. *Clin Neurol Neurosurg* 2007;109:634–8.

40 Sanai N, Berger MS. Recent surgical management of gliomas. *Adv Exp Med Biol* 2012;746:12–25.

41 Ekinci G, Akpinar IN, Baltacioglu F, *et al.* Early-postoperative magnetic resonance imaging in glial tumors: prediction of tumor regrowth and recurrence. *Eur J Radiol* 2003;45:99–107.

42 Albert FK, Forsting M, Sartor K, *et al.* Early postoperative magnetic resonance imaging after resection of malignant glioma: objective evaluation of residual tumor and its influence on regrowth and prognosis. *Neurosurgery* 1994;34:45–60.

43 Leibel SA, Sheline GE. Radiation therapy for neoplasms of the brain. *J Neurosurg* 1987;66:1–22.

44 Karim AB, Afra D, Cornu P, *et al.* Randomized trial on the efficacy of radiotherapy for cerebral low-grade glioma in the adult: European Organization for Research and Treatment of Cancer Study 22845 with the Medical Research Council study BRO4: an interim analysis. *Int J Radiat Oncol Biol Phys* 2002;52:316–24.

45 Patel TR, Yu JB, Piepmeier JM. Role of neurosurgery and radiation therapy in the management of brain tumors. *Hematol Oncol Clin North Am* 2012;26:757–77.

46 Yung WK, Albright RE, Olson J, *et al.* A phase II study of temozolomide vs. procarbazine in patients with glioblastoma multiforme at first relapse. *Br J Cancer* 2000;83:588–93.

47 Vecht CJ, Wilms EB. Seizures in low- and high-grade gliomas: current management and future outlook. *Expert Rev Anticancer Ther* 2010;10:663–9.

48 Schneider T, Mawrin C, Scherlach C, *et al.* Gliomas in adults. *Dtsch Arztebl Int* 2010;107:799–808.

49 Radhakrishnan K, Mokri B, Parisi JE, *et al.* The trends in incidence of primary brain tumors in the population of Rochester, Minnesota. *Ann Neurol* 1995;37:67–73.

50 Olney JW, Farber NB, Spitznagel E, *et al.* Increasing brain tumor rates: is there a link to aspartame? *J Neuropathol Exp Neurol* 1996;55:1115–23.

51 Dubrow R, Darefsky AS. Demographic variation in incidence of adult glioma by subtype, United States, 1992–2007. *BMC Cancer* 2011;11:325.

52 Werner MH, Phuphanich S, Lyman GH. The increasing incidence of malignant gliomas and primary central nervous system lymphoma in the elderly. *Cancer* 1995;76:1634–42.

53 Riggs JE. Rising primary malignant brain tumor mortality in the elderly. A manifestation of differential survival. *Arch Neurol* 1995;52: 571–5.

54 Pettorini BL, Park YS, Caldarelli M, *et al.* Radiation-induced brain tumours after central nervous system irradiation in childhood: a review. *Childs Nerv Syst* 2008;24:793–805.

55 Varley JM,McGown G, Thorncroft M, *et al.* Germ-line mutations of TP53 in Li-Fraumeni families: an extended study of 39 families. *Cancer Res* 1997;57:3245–52.

56 Hamilton SR, Liu B, Parsons RE, *et al.* The molecular basis of Turcot's syndrome. *N Engl J Med* 1995;332:839–47.

57 Parsons DW, Jones S, Zhang X, *et al.* An integrated genomic analysis of human glioblastoma multiforme. *Science* 2008;321:1807–12.

58 Paulsson J, Lindh MB, Jarvius M, *et al.* Prognostic but not predictive role of platelet-derived growth factor receptors in patients with recurrent glioblastoma. *Int J Cancer* 2011;128:1981–8.

59 von Deimling A, Korshunov A, Hartmann C. The next generation of glioma biomarkers: MGMT methylation, BRAF fusions and IDH1 mutations. *Brain Pathol* 2011;21:74–87.

60 Wick W, Hartmann C, Engel C, *et al.* NOA-04 randomized phase III trial of sequential radiochemotherapy of anaplastic glioma with procarbazine, lomustine, and vincristine or temozolomide. *J Clin Oncol* 2009;27:5874–80.

61 Weller M, Felsberg J, Hartmann C, *et al.* Molecular predictors of progression-free and overall survival in patients with newly diagnosed glioblastoma: a prospective translational study of the German Glioma Network. *J Clin Oncol* 2009;27:5743–50.

62 Huse JT, Holland EC. Targeting brain cancer: advances in the molecular pathology of malignant glioma and medulloblastoma. *Nat Rev Cancer* 2010;10:319–31.

63 Kong J, Cooper LA, Wang F, *et al.* Integrative, multimodal analysis of glioblastoma using TCGA molecular data, pathology images, and clinical outcomes. *IEEE Trans Biomed Eng* 2011;58:3469–74.

64 Gravendeel LAM, Kouwenhoven MCM, Gevaert O, *et al.* Intrinsic gene expression profiles of gliomas are a better predictor of survival than histology. *Cancer Res* 2009;69:9065–72.

65 Phillips HS, Kharbanda S, Chen R, *et al.* Molecular subclasses of high-grade glioma predict prognosis, delineate a pattern of disease progression, and resemble stages in neurogenesis. *Cancer Cell* 2006;9:157–73.

66 Wesseling P, Ruiter DJ, Burger PC. Angiogenesis in brain tumors; pathobiological and clinical aspects. *J Neurooncol* 1997;32:253–65.

67 Roberts WG, Palade GE. Neovasculature induced by vascular endothelial growth factor is fenestrated. *Cancer Res* 1997;57:765–72.

68 Burger PC, Vogel FS, Green SB, *et al.* Glioblastoma multiforme and anaplastic astrocytoma, pathologic criteria and prognostic implications. *Cancer* 1985;56:1106–11.

69 Grant R, Liang BC, Page MA, *et al.* Age influences chemotherapy response in astrocytomas. *Neurology* 1995;45:929–33.

70 Nelson JS, Tsukada Y, Schoenfeld D, *et al.* Necrosis as a prognostic criterion in malignant supratentorial, astrocytic gliomas. *Cancer* 1983;52:550–4.

71 Schold SC Jr, Burger PC, Mendelsohn DB, *et al. Primary Tumors of the Brain and Spinal Cord.* Boston: Butterworth-Heinemann, 1997:51–4.

72 Wood JR, Green SB, Shapiro WR, *et al.* The prognostic importance of tumor size in malignant gliomas: A computed tomographic scan study by the Brain Tumor Cooperative Group. *J Clin Oncol* 1988;6:338–43.

73 Daumas-Duport C. Histological grading of gliomas. *Curr Opin Neurol Neurosurg* 1992;5:923–31.

74 Pauleit D, Floeth F, Hamacher K, *et al.* O-(2-[18 F] fluoroethyl)-L-tyrosine PET combined with MRI improves the diagnostic assessment of cerebral gliomas. *Brain* 2005;128:678–87.

75 Möller-Hartmann W, Herminghaus S, Krings T, *et al.* Clinical application of proton magnetic resonance spectroscopy in the diagnosis of intracranial mass lesions. *Neuroradiology* 2002;44:371–81.

76 Roelcke U. PET: brain tumor biochemistry. *J Neurooncol* 1994;22:275–9.

77 Nihashi T, Dahabreh IJ, Terasawa T. Diagnostic accuracy of PET for recurrent glioma diagnosis: a meta-analysis. *AJNR Am J Neuroradiol* 2013;34:944–50.

78 Rapp M, Floeth FW, Felsberg J, *et al.* Clinical value of O-(2-[18 F]-fluoroethyl)-L-tyrosine positron emission tomography in patients with low-grade glioma. *Neurosurgery Focus* 2013;34:E3.

79 Nioche C, Soret M, Gontier E, *et al.* Evaluation of quantitative criteria for glioma grading with static and dynamic ^{18}F-FDopa PET/CT. *Clin Nucl Med* 2013;38:81–7.

80 Rapp M, Heinzel A, Galldiks N, *et al.* Diagnostic performance of 18 F-FET PET in newly diagnosed cerebral lesions suggestive of glioma. *J Nucl Med* 2013;54:229–35.

81 Enslow MS, Zollinger LV, Morton KA, *et al.* Comparison of 18 F-fluorodeoxyglucose and 18 F-fluorothymidine PET in differentiating radiation necrosis from recurrent glioma. *Clin Nucl Med* 2012;37:854–61.

82 Rao PJ, Jyoti R, Mews PJ, *et al.* Preoperative magnetic resonance spectroscopy improves diagnostic accuracy in a series of neurosurgical dilemmas. *Br J Neurosurg* 2013;27:646–53.

83 Porto L, Kieslich M, Franz K, *et al.* MR spectroscopy differentiation between high and low grade astrocytomas:

A comparison between paediatric and adult tumours. *Eur J Paediatr Neurol* 2011;15:214–21.
84 Bulik M, Jancalek R, Vaniceka J, *et al.* Potential of MR spectroscopy for assessment of glioma grading. *Clin Neurol Neurosurg* 2013;115:146–53.
85 Lee S. Diffusion tensor and perfusion imaging of brain tumors in high-field MR imaging. *Neuroimaging Clin N Am* 2012;22:123–34.
86 Hakyemez B, Erdogan C, Bolca N, *et al.* Evaluation of different cerebral mass lesions by perfusion-weighted MR imaging. *J Magn Reson Imaging* 2006;24:817–24.
87 Bagadia A, Purandare H, Misra BK, *et al.* Application of magnetic resonance tractography in the perioperative planning of patients with eloquent region intra-axial brain lesions. *J Clin Neurosci* 2011;18:633–9.
88 McGirt MJ, Chaichana KL, Attenello FJ, *et al.* Extent of surgical resection is independently associated with survival in patients with hemispheric infiltrating low-grade gliomas. *Neurosurgery* 2008;63:700–7.
89 Ahmadi R, Dictus C, Hartmann C, *et al.* Long-term outcome and survival of surgically treated supratentorial low-grade glioma in adult patients. *Acta Neurochir* 2009;151:1359–65.
90 Smith JS, Chang EF, Lamborn KR, *et al.* Role of extent of resection in the long-term outcome of low-grade hemispheric gliomas. *J Clin Oncol* 2008;26:1338–45.
91 Shaw E, Arusell R, Scheithauer B, *et al.* Prospective randomized trial of low- versus high-dose radiation therapy in adults with supratentorial low-grade glioma: Initial report of a North Cancer Central Treatment Group/Radiation Therapy Oncology Group/Eastern Cooperative Oncology Group study. *J Clin Oncol* 2002;20:2267–76.
92 Hanzely Z, Polgar C, Fodor J, *et al.* Role of early radiotherapy in the treatment of supratentorial WHO Grade II astrocytomas: long-term results of 97 patients. *J Neurooncol* 2003;63:305–12.
93 van den Bent MJ, Afra D, de Witte O, *et al.* Long-term efficacy of early versus delayed radiotherapy for low-grade astrocytoma and oligodendroglioma in adults: the EORTC 22845 randomised trial. *Lancet* 2005;366:985–90.
94 Fisher BJ, Hu C, Macdonald DR, *et al.* Phase 2 study of temozolomide-based chemoradiation therapy for high-risk low-grade gliomas: Preliminary results of Radiation Therapy Oncology Group 0424. *Int J Radiat Oncol Biol Phys* 2015;91:497–504.
95 Buckner JC, Shaw EG, Pugh SL, *et al.* Radiation plus procarbazine, CCNU, and vincristine in low-grade glioma. *N Engl J Med* 2016;374:1344–55.
96 French JD, West PM, Von Amerongen FK, *et al.* Effects of intracarotid administration of nitrogen mustard on normal brain and brain tumors. *J Neurosurg* 1952;9:378–89.
97 Becker KP, Yu J. Status quo-standard-of-care medical and radiation therapy for glioblastoma. *Cancer J* 2012;18:12–19.
98 Stupp R, Dietrich PY, Ostermann-Kraljevic S, *et al.* Promising survival for patients with newly diagnosed glioblastoma multiforme treated with concomitant radiation plus temozolomide followed by adjuvant temozolomide. *J Clin Oncol* 2002;20:1375–82.
99 Stupp R, Mason WP, van den Bent MJ, *et al.* Radiotherapy plus concomitant and adjuvant temozolomide for glioblastoma. *N Engl J Med* 2005;352:987–96.
100 Uyl-de Groot CA, Stupp R, van der Bent M. Cost-effectiveness of temozolomide for the treatment of newly diagnosed glioblastoma multiforme. *Expert Rev Pharmacoecon Outcomes Res* 2009;9:235–41.
101 Norden AD, Drappatz J, Wen PY. Antiangiogenic therapies for high-grade glioma. *Nat Rev Neurology* 2009;5:610–20.
102 Chamberlain MC, Raizer J. Antiangiogenic therapy for high-grade gliomas. *CNS Neurol Disord Drug Targets* 2009;8:184–94.
103 Chamberlain MC. Emerging clinical principles on the use of bevacizumab for the treatment of malignant gliomas. *Cancer* 2010;116:3988–99.
104 Vredenburgh JJ, Desjardins A, Herndon JE 2, *et al.* Phase II trial of bevacizumab and irinotecan in recurrent malignant glioma. *Clin Cancer Res* 2007;13:1253–9.
105 Brem H, Piantadosi S, Burger PC, *et al.* Placebo-controlled trial of safety and efficacy of intraoperative controlled delivery by biodegradable polymers of chemotherapy for recurrent gliomas. *The Polymer-brain Tumor Treatment Group. Lancet* 1995;345:1008–12.
106 McGirt MJ, Than KD, Weingart JD, *et al.* Gliadel (BCNU) wafer plus concomitant temozolomide therapy after primary resection of glioblastoma multiform. *J Neurosurg* 2009;110:583–8.
107 Westphal M, Hilt DC, Bortey E, *et al.* A phase 3 trial of local chemotherapy with biodegradable carmustine (BCNU) wafers (Gliadel wafers) in patients with primary malignant glioma. *Neuro Oncol* 2003;5:79–88.
108 Roujeau T, Di Rocco F, Dufour C, *et al.* Shall we treat hydrocephalus associated to brain stem glioma in children? *Childs Nerv Syst* 2011;27:1735–9.
109 Landolfi JC, Thaler HT, DeAngelis LM. Adult brainstem gliomas. *Neurology* 1998;51:1136–9.
110 Kesari S, Kim RS, Markos V, *et al.* Prognostic factors in adult brainstem gliomas: a multicenter, retrospective analysis of 101 cases. *J Neurooncol* 2008;88:175–83.
111 Salmaggi A, Fariselli L, Milanesi I, *et al.* Natural history and management of brainstem gliomas in adults. A retrospective Italian study. *J Neurol* 2008;255:171–7.
112 Guillamo JS, Monjour A, Taillandier L, *et al.* Association des Neuro-Oncologues d'Expression Francaise (ANOCEF). Brainstem gliomas in adults: prognostic factors and classification. *Brain* 2001;124:2528–39.
113 Dirven CM, Mooij JJ, Molenaar WM. Cerebellar pilocytic astrocytoma: a treatment protocol based upon analysis of 73 cases and a review of the literature. *Childs Nerv Syst* 1997;13:17–23.
114 Johnson DR, Brown PD, Galanis E, *et al.* Pilocytic astrocytoma survival in adults: analysis of the Surveillance, Epidemiology, and End Results Program of the National Cancer Institute. *J Neurooncol* 2012;108:187–93.
115 Tonn JC, Paulus W, Warmuth-Metz M, *et al.* Pleomorphic xanthoastrocytoma: report of six cases with special consideration of diagnostic and therapeutic pitfalls. *Surg Neurol* 1997;47:162–9.
116 Nabbout R, Santos M, Rolland Y, *et al.* Early diagnosis of subependymal giant cell astrocytoma in children with tuberous sclerosis. *J Neurol Neurosurg Psychiatry* 1999;66:370–5.

117 Van den Bent MJ. Diagnosis and management of oligodendroglioma. *Semin Oncol* 2004;31:645–52.
118 Zalatimo O, Zoccoli CM, Patel A, *et al.* Impact of genetic targets on primary brain tumor therapy: what's ready for prime time? *Adv Exp Med Biol* 2013;779:267–89.
119 Van den Bent MJ, Reni M, Gatta G, *et al.* Oligodendroglioma. *Crit Rev Oncol Hematol* 2008;66:262–72.
120 Amirian ES, Armstrong TS, Aldape KD, *et al.* Predictors of survival among pediatric and adult ependymoma cases: a study using Surveillance, Epidemiology, and End Results Data from 1973 to 2007. *Neuroepidemiology* 2012;39:116–24.
121 Shonka NA. Targets for therapy in ependymoma. *Targeted Oncology* 2011;6:163–9.
122 Pollack IF. Multidisciplinary management of childhood brain tumors: a review of outcomes, recent advances, and challenges. *J Neurosurg Pediatr* 2011;8: 135–48.
123 Safaee M, Oh MC, Bloch O, *et al.* Choroid plexus papillomas: advances in molecular biology and understanding of tumorigenesis. *Neuro Oncol* 2013;15:255–67.
124 Ogiwara H, Dipatri AJ, Alden TD, *et al.* Choroid plexus tumors in pediatric patients. *Br J Neurosurg* 2012;26:32–7.
125 Choudhari KA, Kaliaperumal C, Jain A, *et al.* Central neurocytoma: A multi-disciplinary review. *Br J Neurosurg* 2009;23:585–95.
126 Rades D, Schild SE. Value of postoperative stereotactic radiosurgery and conventional radiotherapy for incompletely resected typical neurocytomas. *Cancer* 2006;106:1140–3.
127 O'Brien DF, Farrell M, Delanty M, *et al.* The Children's Cancer and Leukaemia Group Guidelines for the Diagnosis and Management of Dysembryoplastic Neuroepithelial Tumours. *Br J Neurosurg* 2007;21:539–49.
128 Ray WZ, Blackburn SL, Casavilca-Zambrano S, *et al.* Clinicopathologic features of recurrent dysembryoplastic neuroepithelial tumor and rare malignant transformation: a report of 5 cases and review of the literature. *J Neurooncol* 2009;94:283–92.
129 Blumcke I, Wiestler OD. Gangliogliomas: an intriguing tumor entity associated with focal epilepsies. *J Neuropathol Exp Neurol* 2002;61:575 – 84.
130 DeMarchi R, Abu-Abed S, Munoz D, *et al.* Malignant ganglioglioma: case report and review of literature. *J Neurooncol* 2011;101:311–8.
131 Blakeley JO, Grossman SA. Management of pineal region tumors. *Curr Treat Options Oncol* 2006;7:505–16.
132 Pomeroy SL, Tamayo P, Gaasenbeek M. Prediction of central nervous system embryonal tumor outcome based on gene expression. *Nature* 2002;415:436–42.
133 Packer RJ. Embryonal Tumors: Neuro-oncology, 1st edn. *Wiley*, 2007:643–7.
134 Winn HR. Glomus tumors. In: RH Winn (ed.) *Youmans Neurological Surgery, 6th edn.* Elsevier, 2011.
135 Cates JMM, Coffin CM. Neurogenic tumors of soft tissue. Pediatr Dev Pathol 2012;15 Supplement:62–107.
136 Pollock BE, Lunsford LD, Noren G. Vestibular schwannoma management in the next century: a radiosurgical perspective. *Neurosurgery* 1998;43:475–81.
137 Woertler K. Tumors and tumor-like lesions of peripheral nerves. *Semin Musculoskelet Radiol* 2010;14:547–58.
138 Clarke SE, Kaufmann RA. Nerve tumors. *J Hand Surg* 2010;35A:1520–2.
139 Rodriguez FJ, Stratakis CA, Evans DG. Genetic predisposition to peripheral nerve neoplasia: diagnostic criteria and pathogenesis of neurofibromatoses, Carney complex, and related syndromes. *Acta Neuropathol* 2012;123:349–67.
140 Leibig C, Ayala G, Wilks JA, *et al.* Perineural invasion in cancer. *Cancer* 2009;115:3379–91.
141 Dunn M, Morgan MB, Beer TW. Perineural invasion: identification, significance and a standardized definition. *Dermatol Surg* 2009;35:214–21.
142 Limawararut V, Leibovitch I, Sullivan T, Selva D. Periocular squamous cell carcinoma. *Clin Exp Ophthalmol* 2007;35:174–85.
143 Muro K, Das S, Raizer JJ. Chordomas of the craniospinal axis: multimodality surgical, radiation and medical management strategies. *Expert Rev Neurother* 2007;7:1295–312.
144 Igaki H, Tokuuye K, Okumura T, *et al.* Clinical results of proton beam therapy for skull base chordoma. *Int J Radiat Oncol Biol Phys* 2004;60:1120–6.
145 Martin JJ, Niranjan A, Kondziolka D, *et al.* Radiosurgery for chordomas and chondrosarcomas of the skull base. *J Neurosurg* 2007;107:758–64.
146 Chang SD, Martin DP, Lee E, *et al.* Stereotactic radiosurgery and hypofractionated stereotactic radiotherapy for residual or recurrent cranial base and cervical chordomas. *Neurosurg Focus* 2001;10:E5.
147 Prabhu VC, Brown HG. The pathogenesis of craniopharyngiomas. *Childs Nerv Syst* 2005;21:622–7.
148 Gorski GK, McMorrow LE, Donaldson MH, *et al.* Multiple chromosomal abnormalities in a case of craniopharyngioma. *Cancer Genet Cytogenet* 1992;60:212–3.
149 Virik K, Turner J, Garrick R, Sheehy JP. Malignant transformation of craniopharyngioma. *J Clin Neurosci* 1999;6(6):527–530.
150 Karavitaki N, Brufani C, Warner JT, *et al.* Craniopharyngiomas in children and adults: systematic analysis of 121 cases with long-term follow-up. *Clin Endocrinol* 2005;62:397–409.
151 Koral K, Weprin B, Rollins NK. Sphenoid sinus craniopharyngioma simulating mucocele. *Acta Radiol* 2006;47:494–6.
152 Shuman AG, Heth JA, Marentette LJ, *et al.* Extracranial nasopharyngeal craniopharyngioma: case report. *Neurosurgery* 2007;60:E780–1.
153 Kawamata T, Kubo O, Kamikawa S, *et al.* Ectopic clival craniopharyngioma. *Acta Neurochir* 2002;144:1221–4.
154 Banczerowski P, Balint K, Sipos L: Temporal extradural ectopic craniopharyngioma. *Case report. J Neurosurg* 2007;107:178–80.
155 Karavitaki N, Cudlip S, Adams CB, *et al.* Craniopharyngiomas. *Endocr Rev* 2006;27:371–97.
156 de Vries L, Lazar L, Phillip M. Craniopharyngioma: presentation and endocrine sequelae in 36 children. *J Pediatr Endocrinol Metab* 2003;16:703–10.
157 Van Effenterre R, Boch AL. Craniopharyngioma in adults and children: a study of 122 surgical cases. *J Neurosurg* 2002;97:3–11.

158 Yamamoto T, Yoneda S, Funatsu N. Spontaneous haemorrhage in craniopharyngioma. *J Neurol Neurosurg Psychiatry* 1989;52:803–4.
159 Yasumoto Y, Ito M. Asymptomatic spontaneous rupture of craniopharyngioma cyst. *J Clin Neurosci* 2008;15:603–6.
160 Maier HC. Craniopharyngioma with erosion and drainage into the nasopharynx. An autobiographical case report. *J Neurosurg* 1985;62:132–4.
161 Choi SH, Kwon BJ, Na DG, *et al.* Pituitary adenoma, craniopharyngioma, and Rathke cleft cyst involving both intrasellar and suprasellar regions: differentiation using MRI. *Clin Radiol* 2007;62:453–62.
162 Hofmann BM, Hollig A, Strauss C, *et al.* Results after treatment of craniopharyngiomas: further experiences with 73 patients since 1997. *J Neurosurg* 2012;116:373–384.
163 Merchant TE, Kiehna EN, Sanford RA, *et al.* Craniopharyngioma: the St. Jude Children's Research Hospital experience 1984–2001. *Int J Radiat Oncol Biol Phys* 2002;53:533–42.
164 Merchant TE, Kiehna EN, Kun LE, *et al.* Phase II trial of conformal radiation therapy for pediatric patients with craniopharyngioma and correlation of surgical factors and radiation dosimetry with change in cognitive function. *J Neurosurg* 2006;104(2 Suppl):94–102.
165 Kiehna EN, Merchant TE. Radiation therapy for pediatric craniopharyngioma. *Neurosurg Focus* 2010;28:E10.
166 Moon SH, Kim IH, Park SW, *et al.* Early adjuvant radiotherapy toward long-term survival and better quality of life for craniopharyngiomas – a study in single institute. *Childs Nerv Syst* 2005;21:799–807.
167 Jose CC, Rajan B, Ashley S, *et al.* Radiotherapy for the treatment of recurrent craniopharyngioma. *Clin Oncol* 1992;4:287–9.
168 Habrand JL, Ganry O, Couanet D, *et al.* The role of radiation therapy in the management of craniopharyngioma: a 25-year experience and review of the literature. *Int J Radiat Oncol Biol Phys* 1999;44:255–63.
169 Lee M, Kalani MY, Cheshier S, *et al.* Radiation therapy and CyberKnife radiosurgery in the management of craniopharyngiomas. *Neurosurg Focus* 2008;24:E4.
170 Schulz-Ertner D, Frank C, Herfarth KK, *et al.* Fractionated stereotactic radiotherapy for craniopharyngiomas. *Int J Radiat Oncol Biol Phys* 2002;54:1114–20.
171 Chiou SM, Lunsford LD, Niranjan A, *et al.* Stereotactic radiosurgery of residual or recurrent craniopharyngioma, after surgery, with or without radiation therapy. *Neuro Oncol* 2001;3:159–66.
172 Kobayashi T, Kida Y, Mori Y, *et al.* Long-term results of gamma knife surgery for the treatment of craniopharyngioma in 98 consecutive cases. *J Neurosurg* 2005;103(6 Suppl):482–8.
173 Fitzek MM, Linggood RM, Adams J, *et al.* Combined proton and photon irradiation for craniopharyngioma: long-term results of the early cohort of patients treated at Harvard Cyclotron Laboratory and Massachusetts General Hospital. *Int J Radiat Oncol Biol Phys* 2006;64: 1348–1354.
174 Winkfield KM, Linsenmeier C, Yock TI, *et al.* Surveillance of craniopharyngioma cyst growth in children treated with proton radiotherapy. *Int J Radiat Oncol Biol Phys* 2009;73:716–21.
175 Shahzadi S, Sharifi G, Andalibi R, *et al.* Management of cystic craniopharyngiomas with intracavitary irradiation with 32P. *Arch Iran Med* 2008;11:30–4.
176 Julow J, Lanyi F, Hajda M, *et al.* Stereotactic intracavitary irradiation of cystic craniopharyngiomas with yttrium-90 isotope. *Prog Neurol Surg* 2007;20:289–96.
177 Scott RM. Craniopharyngioma: a personal (Boston) experience. *Childs Nerv Syst* 2005;21: 773–7.
178 Hukin J, Steinbok P, Lafay-Cousin L, *et al.* Intracystic bleomycin therapy for craniopharyngioma in children: the Canadian experience. *Cancer* 2007;109:2124–31.
179 Hader WJ, Steinbok P, Hukin J, *et al.* Intratumoral therapy with bleomycin for cystic craniopharyngiomas in children. *Pediatr Neurosurg* 2000;33:211–8.
180 Agarwal S, Rishi A, Suri V, *et al.* Primary intracranial squamous cell carcinoma arising in an epidermoid cyst – a case report and review of literature. *Clin Neurol Neurosurg* 2007;109:888–91.
181 Osborn AG, Preece MT. Intracranial cysts: radiologic-pathologic correlation and imaging approach. *Radiology* 2006;239:650–64.
182 Li F, Zhu S, Liu Y, *et al.* Hyperdense intracranial epidermoid cysts: a study of 15 cases. *Acta Neurochir* 2007;149:31–9.
183 Kumari R, Guglani B, Gupta N, *et al.* Intracranial epidermoid cyst: magnetic resonance imaging features. *Neurol India* 2009;57:359–60.
184 Brown JY, Morokoff AP, Mitchell PJ, *et al.* Unusual imaging appearance of an intracranial dermoid cyst. *Am J Neuroradiol* 2001;22:1970–2.
185 Akar Z, Tanriover N, Tuzgen S, *et al.* Surgical treatment of intracranial epidermoid tumors. *Neurol Med Chir* 2003;43:275–80.
186 Demirci S, Dogan KH, Erkol Z, *et al.* Sudden death due to a colloid cyst of the third ventricle: report of three cases with a special sign at autopsy. *Forensic Sci Int* 2009;189:e33–6.
187 Humphries RL, Stone CK, Bowers RC. Colloid cyst: a case report and literature review of a rare but deadly condition. *J Emerg Med* 2011;40: e5–9.
188 Choudhari KA. Treatment options for third ventricular colloid cysts: comparison of open microsurgical versus endoscopic resection. *Neurosurgery* 2008;62:e1384.
189 Horn EM, Feiz-Erfan I, Bristol RE, *et al.* Treatment options for third ventricular colloid cysts: comparison of open microsurgical versus endoscopic resection. *Neurosurgery* 2007;60:613–8.
190 Grondin RT, Hader W, MacRae ME, *et al.* Endoscopic versus microsurgical resection of third ventricle colloid cysts. *Can J Neurol Sci* 2007;34:197–207.
191 Lee E, Grutsch J, Persky V, *et al.* Association of meningioma with reproductive factors. *Int J Cancer* 2006;119:1152–7.
192 Custer B, Longstreth WT, Jr., Phillips LE, *et al.* Hormonal exposures and the risk of intracranial meningioma in women: a population-based case-control study. *BMC Cancer* 2006;6:152.
193 Roser F, Nakamura M, Bellinzona M, *et al.* The prognostic value of progesterone receptor status in meningiomas. *J Clin Pathol* 2004;57:1033–7.
194 Sanson M, Cornu P. Biology of meningiomas. *Acta Neurochir* 2000;142:493–505.

195 Lamszus K. Meningioma pathology, genetics, and biology. *J Neuropathol Exp Neurol* 2004;63:275–86.

196 Perry A, Gutmann DH, Reifenberger G: Molecular pathogenesis of meningiomas. *Journal of Neurooncology* 2004;70: 183–202.

197 Chamberlain MC, Blumenthal DT. Intracranial meningiomas: diagnosis and treatment. *Expert Rev Neurother* 2004;4:641–8.

198 Rockhill J, Mrugala M, Chamberlain MC. Intracranial meningiomas: an overview of diagnosis and treatment. *Neurosurg Focus* 2007;23:E1.

199 Klutmann S, Bohuslavizki KH, Brenner W, *et al.* Somatostatin receptor scintography in postsurgical follow-up examinations of meningioma. *J Nucl Med* 1998;39:1913–7.

200 Stafford SL, Perry A, Suman VJ, *et al.* Primarily resected meningiomas: outcome and prognostic factors in 581 Mayo Clinic patients, 1978 through 1988. *Mayo Clin Proc* 1998;73:936–42.

201 Condra KS, Buatti JM, Mendenhall WM, *et al.* Benign meningiomas: primary treatment selection affects survival. *Int J Radiat Oncol Biol Phys* 1997;39: 427–436.

202 Yamasaki F, Yoshioka H, Hama S, *et al.* Recurrence of meningiomas. *Cancer* 2000;89:1102–10.

203 Goldsmith BJ, Wara WM, Wilson CB, *et al.* Postoperative irradiation for subtotally resected meningiomas. A retrospective analysis of 140 patients treated from 1967 to 1990. *J Neurosurg* 1994;80:195–201.

204 Milosevic MF, Frost PJ, Laperriere NJ, *et al.* Radiotherapy for atypical or malignant intracranial meningioma. *Int J Radiat Oncol Biol Phys* 1996;34:817–22.

205 Flickinger JC, Kondziolka D, Maitz AH, *et al.* Gamma knife radiosurgery of imaging-diagnosed intracranial meningioma. *Int J Radiat Oncol Biol Phys* 2003;56:801–6.

206 Lee JY, Niranjan A, McInerney J, *et al.* Stereotactic radiosurgery providing long-term tumor control of cavernous sinus meningiomas. *J Neurosurg* 2002;97:65–72.

207 Dufour H, Muracciole X, Metellus P, *et al.* Long-term tumor control and functional outcome in patients with cavernous sinus meningiomas treated by radiotherapy with or without previous surgery: is there an alternative to aggressive tumor removal? *Neurosurgery* 2001;48:285–94.

208 Aichholzer M, Bertalanffy A, Dietrich W, *et al.* Gamma knife radiosurgery of skull base meningiomas. *Acta Neurochir* 2000;142:647–52.

209 Starke RM, Williams BJ, Hiles C, *et al.* Gamma knife surgery for skull base meningiomas. *J Neurosurg* 2012;116:588–97.

210 Oura S, Sakurai T, Yoshimura G, *et al.* Regression of a presumed meningioma with the antiestrogen agent mepitiostane. *Case report. J Neurosurg* 2000;93:132–5.

211 Grunberg SM, Weiss MH, Spitz IM, *et al.* Treatment of unresectable meningiomas with the antiprogesterone agent mifepristone. *J Neurosurg* 1991;74:861–6.

212 Newton HB. Hydroxyurea chemotherapy in the treatment of meningiomas. *Neurosurg Focus* 2007;23:E11.

213 Ragel BT, Couldwell WT, Wurster RD, *et al.* Chronic suppressive therapy with calcium channel antagonists for refractory meningiomas. *Neurosurg Focus* 2007;23:E10.

214 Chamberlain MC, Glantz MJ, Fadul CE. Recurrent meningioma: salvage therapy with long-acting somatostatin analogue. *Neurology* 2007;69:969–73.

215 Ragel BT, Jensen RL, Couldwell WT. Inflammatory response and meningioma tumorigenesis and the effect of cyclooxygenase-2 inhibitors. *Neurosurg Focus* 2007;23:E7.

216 Kaba SE, DeMonte F, Bruner JM, *et al.* The treatment of recurrent unresectable and malignant meningiomas with interferon alpha-2B. *Neurosurgery* 1997;40:271–5.

217 Rajaram V, Brat DJ, Perry A. Anaplastic meningioma versus meningeal hemangiopericytoma: immunohistochemical and genetic markers. *Hum Pathol* 2004;35:1413–8.

218 Schroder R, Firsching R, Kochanek S. Hemangiopericytoma of meninges. II. General and clinical data. *Zentralbl Neurochir* 1986;47:191–199.

219 Maruya J, Seki Y, Morita K, *et al.* Meningeal hemangiopericytoma manifesting as massive intracranial hemorrhage – two case reports. *Neurol Med Chir* 2006;46:92–7.

220 Chiechi MV, Smirniotopoulos JG, Mena H. Intracranial hemangiopericytomas: MR and CT features. *Am J Neuroradiol* 1996;17:1365–71.

221 Guthrie BL, Ebersold MJ, Scheithauer BW, *et al.* Meningeal hemangiopericytoma: histopathological features, treatment, and long-term follow-up of 44 cases. *Neurosurgery* 1989;25:514–22.

222 Fountas KN, Kapsalaki E, Kassam M, *et al.* Management of intracranial meningeal hemangiopericytomas: outcome and experience. *Neurosurg Rev* 2006;29:145–53.

223 Chang SD, Sakamoto GT. The role of radiosurgery for hemangiopericytomas. *Neurosurg Focus* 2003;14:e14.

224 Soyuer S, Chang EL, Selek U, *et al.* Intracranial meningeal hemangiopericytoma: the role of radiotherapy: report of 29 cases and review of the literature. *Cancer* 2004;100:1491–7.

225 Lonser RR, Glenn GM, Walther M, *et al.* von Hippel-Lindau disease. *Lancet* 2003;361:2059–67.

226 Conway JE, Chou D, Clatterbuck RE, *et al.* Hemangioblastomas of the central nervous system in von Hippel-Lindau syndrome and sporadic disease. *Neurosurgery* 2001;48:55–62.

227 Wanebo JE, Lonser RR, Glenn GM, *et al.* The natural history of hemangioblastomas of the central nervous system in patients with von Hippel-Lindau disease. *J Neurosurg* 2003;98:82–94.

228 Jagannathan J, Lonser RR, Smith R, *et al.* Surgical management of cerebellar hemangioblastomas in patients with von Hippel-Lindau disease. *J Neurosurg* 2008;108:210–22.

229 Weil RJ, Lonser RR, DeVroom HL, *et al.* Surgical management of brainstem hemangioblastomas in patients with von Hippel-Lindau disease. *J Neurosurg* 2003;98:95–105.

230 Lonser RR, Weil RJ, Wanebo JE, *et al.* Surgical management of spinal cord hemangioblastomas in patients with von Hippel-Lindau disease. *J Neurosurg* 2003;98:106–16.

231 Ammerman JM, Lonser RR, Dambrosia J, *et al.* Long-term natural history of hemangioblastomas in patients with von Hippel-Lindau disease: implications for treatment. *J Neurosurg* 2006;105:248–55.

232 Tago M, Terahara A, Shin M, *et al.* Gamma knife surgery for hemangioblastomas. *J Neurosurg* 2005;102 Suppl:171–4.

233 Wang EM, Pan L, Wang BJ, *et al.* The long-term results of gamma knife radiosurgery for hemangioblastomas of the brain. *J Neurosurg* 2005;102 Suppl:225–9.

234 Koh ES, Nichol A, Millar BA, *et al.* Role of fractionated external beam radiotherapy in hemangioblastoma of the central nervous system. *Int J Radiat Oncol Biol Phys* 2007;69:1521–6.
235 Sundaresan N. *Tumors of the spine: diagnosis and clinical management.* Philadelphia: Saunders, 1990.
236 Chamberlain MC, Tredway TL. Adult primary intradural spinal cord tumors: a review. *Curr Neurol Neurosci Rep* 2011;11:320–8.
237 Greenberg MS, Greenberg MS. *Handbook of Neurosurgery.* Tampa: Thieme Medical Publishers, 2010.
238 Ropper AE, Cahill KS, Hanna JW, *et al.* Primary vertebral tumors: a review of epidemiologic, histological and imaging findings, part II: locally aggressive and malignant tumors. *Neurosurgery* 2012;70:211–9.
239 Wald JT. Imaging of spine neoplasm. *Radiol Clin North Am* 2012;50:749–76.
240 Sciubba DM, Chi JH, Rhines LD. Chordoma of the spinal column. *Neurosurg Clin North Am* 2008;19:5–15.
241 Stacchiotti S, Longhi A, Ferraresi V, *et al.* Phase II study of imatinib in advanced chordoma. *J Clin Oncol* 2012;30:914–20.
242 Conti P, Pansini G, Mouchaty H, *et al.* Spinal neurinomas: retrospective analysis and long-term outcome of 179 consecutively operated cases and review of the literature. *Surg Neurol* 2004;61:34–43.
243 Nakamura M, Tsuji O, Fujiyoshi K, *et al.* Long-term surgical outcomes of spinal meningiomas. *Spine* 2012;37:E617–23.
244 Simpson D. The recurrence of intracranial meningiomas after surgical treatment. *J Neurol Neurosurg Psychiatry* 1957;20:22–39.
245 Yang S-Y, Jin YJ, Park SH, *et al.* Paragangliomas in the cauda equina region: clinicopathoradiologic findings in four cases. *J Neurooncol* 2005;72:49–55.
246 Zaidat OO, Ruff RL. Treatment of spinal epidural metastasis improves patient survival and functional state. *Neurology* 2002;58:1360–6.
247 Schiff D, O'Neill BP. Intramedullary spinal cord metastases: clinical features and treatment outcome. *Neurology* 1996;47:906–12.
248 Heldmann U, Myschetzky PS, Thomsen HS. Frequency of unexpected multifocal metastasis in patients with acute spinal cord compression. Evaluation by low-field MR imaging in cancer patients. *Acta Radiol* 1997;38:372–5.
249 Abrahm JL, Banffy MB, Harris MB. Spinal cord compression in patients with advanced metastatic cancer: "all I care about is walking and living my life". *JAMA* 2008;299:937–46.
250 Poortmans P, Vulto A, Raaijmakers E. Always on a Friday? Time pattern of referral for spinal cord compression. *Acta Oncol* 2001;40:88–91.
251 Levack P, Graham J, Collie D, *et al.* Don't wait for a sensory level – listen to the symptoms: a prospective audit of the delays in diagnosis of malignant cord compression. *Clin Oncol* 2002;14:472–80.
252 Rades D, Veninga T, Stalpers LJ, *et al.* Improved posttreatment functional outcome is associated with better survival in patients irradiated for metastatic spinal cord compression. *Int J Radiat Oncol Biol Phys* 2007;67:1506–9.
253 Helweg-Larsen S, Sorensen PS, Kreiner S. Prognostic factors in metastatic spinal cord compression: a prospective study using multivariate analysis of variables influencing survival and gait function in 153 patients. *Int J Radiat Oncol Biol Phys* 2000;46:1163–9.
254 North RB, LaRocca VR, Schwartz J, *et al.* Surgical management of spinal metastases: analysis of prognostic factors during a 10-year experience. *J Neurosurg Spine* 2005;2:564–73.
255 Cole JS, Patchell RA. Metastatic epidural spinal cord compression. *Lancet Neurol* 2008;7:459–66.
256 Koehler PJ, Verbiest H, Jager J, *et al.* Delayed radiation myelopathy: serial MR-imaging and pathology. *Clin Neurol Neurosurg* 1996;98:197–201.
257 Finn MA, Vrionis FD, Schmidt MH. Spinal radiosurgery for metastatic disease of the spine. *Cancer Control* 2007;14:405–411.
258 Gerszten PC, Burton SA, Belani CP, *et al.* Radiosurgery for the treatment of spinal lung metastases. *Cancer* 2006;107:2653–61.
259 Seichi A, Kondoh T, Hozumi T, *et al.* Intraoperative radiation therapy for metastatic spinal tumors. *Spine* 1999;24:470–3.
260 Manke C, Bretschneider T, Lenhart M, *et al.* Spinal metastases from renal cell carcinoma: effect of preoperative particle embolization on intraoperative blood loss. *Am J Neuroradiol* 2001;22:997–1003.
261 Jansson KA, Bauer HC. Survival, complications and outcome in 282 patients operated for neurological deficit due to thoracic or lumbar spinal metastases. *Eur Spine J* 2006;15:196–202.
262 Ghogawala Z, Mansfield FL, Borges LF. Spinal radiation before surgical decompression adversely affects outcomes of surgery for symptomatic metastatic spinal cord compression. *Spine* 2001;26:818–24.
263 DeVita VT, Lawrence TS, Rosenberg SA, *et al.* (eds). Cancer: Principles & Practice of Oncology, 9th edn. Philadelphia: Wolters Kluwer Health/Lippincott Williams & Wilkins, 2011:xlvii, 2638.
264 Zimm S, Wampler GL, Stablein D, *et al.* Intracerebral metastases in solid-tumor patients: natural history and results of treatment. *Cancer* 1981;48:384–94.
265 Raore B, Schniederjan M, Prabhu R, *et al.* Metastasis infiltration: an investigation of the postoperative brain-tumor interface. *Int J Radiat Oncol Biol Phys* 2011;81:1075–80.
266 Gaspar L, Scott C, Rotman M, *et al.* Recursive partitioning analysis (RPA) of prognostic factors in three Radiation Therapy Oncology Group (RTOG) brain metastases trials. *Int J Radiat Oncol Biol Phys* 1997;37:745–51.
267 Sperduto PW, Berkey B, Gaspar LE, *et al.* A new prognostic index and comparison to three other indices for patients with brain metastases: an analysis of 1,960 patients in the RTOG database. *Int J Radiat Oncol Biol Phys* 2008;70:510–4.
268 Sperduto PW, Kased N, Roberge D, *et al.* Summary report on the graded prognostic assessment: an accurate and facile diagnosis-specific tool to estimate survival for patients with brain metastases. *J Clin Oncol* 2012;30:419–25.
269 Patchell RA, Tibbs PA, Walsh JW, *et al.* A randomized trial of surgery in the treatment of single metastases to the brain. *N Engl J Med* 1990;322:494–500.
270 Ryken TC, McDermott M, Robinson PD, *et al.* The role of steroids in the management of brain metastases: a systematic

review and evidence-based clinical practice guideline. *J Neurooncol* 2010;96:103–14.

271 Mikkelsen T, Paleologos NA, Robinson PD, *et al.* The role of prophylactic anticonvulsants in the management of brain metastases: a systematic review and evidence-based clinical practice guideline. *J Neurooncol* 2010;96:97–102.

272 Andrews DW, Scott CB, Sperduto PW, *et al.* Whole brain radiation therapy with or without stereotactic radiosurgery boost for patients with one to three brain metastases: phase III results of the RTOG 9508 randomised trial. *Lancet* 2004;363:1665–72.

273 Patchell RA, Tibbs PA, Regine WF, *et al.* Postoperative radiotherapy in the treatment of single metastases to the brain: a randomized trial. *JAMA* 1998;280:1485–9.

274 Chang EL, Wefel JS, Hess KR, *et al.* Neurocognition in patients with brain metastases treated with radiosurgery or radiosurgery plus whole-brain irradiation: a randomised controlled trial. *Lancet Oncol* 2009;10:1037–44.

275 Aoyama H, Shirato H, Tago M, *et al.* Stereotactic radiosurgery plus whole-brain radiation therapy vs stereotactic radiosurgery alone for treatment of brain metastases: a randomized controlled trial. *JAMA* 2006;295:2483–91.

276 Kocher M, Soffietti R, Abacioglu U, *et al.* Adjuvant whole-brain radiotherapy versus observation after radiosurgery or surgical resection of one to three cerebral metastases: results of the EORTC 22952-26001 study. *J Clin Oncol* 2011;29:134–41.

277 Manon R, O'Neill A, Knisely J, *et al.* Phase II trial of radiosurgery for one to three newly diagnosed brain metastases from renal cell carcinoma, melanoma, and sarcoma: an Eastern Cooperative Oncology Group study (E 6397). *J Clin Oncol* 2005;23:8870–6.

278 Prabhu R, Shu H-K, Hadjipanayis C, *et al.* Current dosing paradigm for stereotactic radiosurgery alone after surgical resection of brain metastases needs to be optimized for improved local control. *Int J Radiat Oncol Biol Phys* 2012;83:e61–e6.

279 Minniti G, Clarke E, Lanzetta G, *et al.* Stereotactic radiosurgery for brain metastases: analysis of outcome and risk of brain radionecrosis. *Radiat Oncol* 2011;6:48.

280 Long GV, Trefzer U, Davies MA, *et al.* Dabrafenib in patients with Val600Glu or Val600Lys BRAF-mutant melanoma metastatic to the brain (BREAK-MB): a multicentre, open-label, phase 2 trial. *Lancet Oncol* 2012;13:1087–95.

281 Margolin K, Ernstoff MS, Hamid O, *et al.* Ipilimumab in patients with melanoma and brain metastases: an open-label, phase 2 trial. *Lancet Oncol* 2012;13:459–65.

282 Batchelor T, Romieu G, Campone M, *et al.* Lapatinib plus capecitabine in patients with previously untreated brain metastases from HER2-positive metastatic breast cancer (LANDSCAPE): a single-group phase 2 study. *Lancet Oncol* 2013;14:64–71.

283 Welsh JW, Komaki R, Amini A, *et al.* Phase II trial of erlotinib plus concurrent whole-brain radiation therapy for patients with brain metastases from non-small-cell lung cancer. *J Clin Oncol* 2013;31:895–902.

284 Batchelor T, Loeffler JS. Primary CNS lymphoma. *J Clin Oncol* 2006;24:1281–8.

285 Abrey LE, Yahalom J, DeAngelis LM. Treatment for primary CNS lymphoma: The next step. *J Clin Oncol* 2000;18:3144–50.

286 Gerstner ER, Abrey LE, Schiff D, *et al.* CNS Hodgkin Lymphoma. *Blood* 2008;112:1658–61.

287 Cote TR, Manns A, Hardy CR, *et al.* Epidemiology of brain lymphoma among people with or without acquired immunodeficiency syndrome. AIDS/cancer study group. *J Natl Cancer Inst* 1996;88:675–9.

288 Bayraktar S, Bayraktar UD, Ramos JC, *et al.* Primary CNS lymphoma in HIV positive and negative patients: Comparison of clinical characteristics, outcome and prognostic factors. *J Neurooncol* 2011;101:257–65.

289 Eby NL, Grufferman S, Flannelly CM, *et al.* Increasing incidence of primary brain lymphoma in the US. *Cancer* 1988;62:2461–5.

290 Kadan-Lottick NS, Skluzacek MC, Gurney JG. Decreasing incidence rates of primary central nervous system lymphoma. *Cancer* 2002;95:193–202.

291 Schabet M. Epidemiology of primary CNS lymphoma. *J Neurooncol* 1999;43:199–201.

292 Bataille B, Delwail V, Menet E, *et al.* Primary intracerebral malignant lymphoma: Report of 248 cases. *J Neurosurg* 2000;92:261–6.

293 Algazi AP, Kadoch C, Rubenstein JL. Biology and treatment of primary central nervous system lymphoma. *Neurotherapeutics* 2009;6:587–97.

294 Miller DC, Hochberg FH, Harris NL, *et al.* Pathology with clinical correlations of primary central nervous system non-hodgkin's lymphoma. The Massachusetts General Hospital Experience 1958-1989. *Cancer* 1994;74:1383–97.

295 Abrey LE, Batchelor TT, Ferreri AJ, *et al.* Report of an international workshop to standardize baseline evaluation and response criteria for primary CNS lymphoma. *J Clin Oncol* 2005;23:5034–43.

296 Kuker W, Nagele T, Korfel A, *et al.* Primary central nervous system lymphomas (PCNSL): MRI features at presentation in 100 patients. *J Neurooncol* 2005;72:169–77.

297 Baraniskin A, Deckert M, Schulte-Altedorneburg G, *et al.* Current strategies in the diagnosis of diffuse large B-cell lymphoma of the central nervous system. *Br J Haematol* 2012;156:421–32.

398 Ekenel M, Iwamoto FM, Ben-Porat LS, *et al.* Primary central nervous system lymphoma: The role of consolidation treatment after a complete response to high-dose methotrexate-based chemotherapy. *Cancer* 2008;113:1025–31.

399 Poortmans PM, Kluin-Nelemans HC, Haaxma-Reiche H, *et al.* High-dose methotrexate-based chemotherapy followed by consolidating radiotherapy in non-AIDS-related primary central nervous system lymphoma: European Organization for Research and Treatment of Cancer Lymphoma Group Phase II Trial 20962. *J Clin Oncol* 2003;21:4483–8.

300 DeAngelis LM, Seiferheld W, Schold SC, *et al.* Combination chemotherapy and radiotherapy for primary central nervous system lymphoma: Radiation Therapy Oncology Group study 93-10. *J Clin Oncol* 2002;20:4643–8.

301 Birnbaum T, Stadler EA, von Baumgarten L, *et al.* Rituximab significantly improves complete response rate in patients with primary CNS lymphoma. *J Neurooncol* 2012;109:285–91.

302 Gerstner ER, Batchelor TT. Primary central nervous system lymphoma. *Arch Neurol* 2010;67:291–7.

303 Braaten KM, Betensky RA, de Leval L, *et al.* Bcl-6 expression predicts improved survival in patients with primary central nervous system lymphoma. *Clin Cancer Res* 2003;9:1063–9.

304 Abrey LE, Ben-Porat L, Panageas KS, *et al.* Primary central nervous system lymphoma: The Memorial Sloan-Kettering cancer center prognostic model. *J Clin Oncol* 2006;24:5711–5.

305 Hodson DJ, Bowles KM, Cooke LJ, *et al.* Primary central nervous system lymphoma: A single-centre experience of 55 unselected cases. *Clin Oncol* 2005;17:185–91.

306 Leal T, Chang JE, Mehta M, *et al.* Leptomeningeal metastasis: Challenges in diagnosis and treatment. *Curr Cancer Ther Rev* 2011;7:319–27.

307 Drappatz J BT. Leptomeningeal metastasis. *American Society of Clinical Oncology Educational Book* 2009:100–5.

308 Wasserstrom WR, Glass JP, Posner JB. Diagnosis and treatment of leptomeningeal metastases from solid tumors: Experience with 90 patients. *Cancer* 1982;49:759–72.

309 Hegde U, Filie A, Little RF, *et al.* High incidence of occult leptomeningeal disease detected by flow cytometry in newly diagnosed aggressive B-cell lymphomas at risk for central nervous system involvement: The role of flow cytometry versus cytology. *Blood* 2005;105:496–502.

310 Chamberlain MC, Sandy AD, Press GA. Leptomeningeal metastasis: A comparison of gadolinium-enhanced mr and contrast-enhanced ct of the brain. *Neurology* 1990;40:435–8.

311 Chamberlain MC. Radioisotope CSF flow studies in leptomeningeal metastases. *J Neurooncol* 1998;38:135–140.

312 Berg SL, Chamberlain MC. Systemic chemotherapy, intrathecal chemotherapy, and symptom management in the treatment of leptomeningeal metastasis. *Curr Oncol Rep* 2003;5:29–40.

313 Aiello-Laws L, Rutledge DN. Management of adult patients receiving intraventricular chemotherapy for the treatment of leptomeningeal metastasis. *Clin J Oncol Nurs* 2008;12:429–35.

314 Shapiro WR, Young DF, Mehta BM. Methotrexate: Distribution in cerebrospinal fluid after intravenous, ventricular and lumbar injections. *N Engl J Med* 1975;293:161–6.

315 Tomlinson GE. Familial cancer syndromes and genetic counselling. *Cancer Treat Res* 1997;92:63–97.

316 Young J, Povey S. The genetic basis of tuberous sclerosis. *Mol Med Today* 1998;4:313–19.

317 Gutmann DH1, Aylsworth A, Carey JC, *et al.* The diagnostic evaluation and multidisciplinary management of neurofibromatosis 1 and neurofibromatosis 2. *JAMA* 1997;278:51–57.

318 Feldkamp MM, Gutmann DH, Guha A. Neurofibromatosis type 1: piecing the puzzle together. *Can J Neurol Sci* 1998;25:181–91.

319 Pollack IF, Mulvihill JJ. Neurofibromatosis 1 and 2. *Brain Pathol* 1997;7:823–36.

320 Wicking C, Bale AE. Molecular basis of the nevoid basal cell carcinoma syndrome. *Curr Opin Pediatr* 1997;9: 630–5.

321 Foulkes WD. A tale of four syndromes: familial adenomatous polyposis, Gardner syndrome, attenuated APC and Turcot syndrome. *QJM* 1998;88:853–63.

322 Decker HJ, Weidt EJ, Brieger J. The von Hippel-Lindau tumor suppressor gene. A rare and intriguing disease opening new insight into basic mechanisms of carcinogenesis. *Cancer Genet Cytogenet* 1997;93(1):74–83.

323 Eng C. Genetics of Cowden syndrome: through the looking glass of oncology. *Int J Oncol* 1998;12:701–10.

41

Malignant Tumors of the Eye

Devron H. Char[1,2] and Tia B. Cole[1]

[1] The Tumori Foundation, San Francisco, California, USA
[2] University of California San Francisco, San Francisco, California, USA

Introduction

Ophthalmic oncology encompasses malignant neoplasms, or lesions that simulate them that involve the eyelids, conjunctiva, intraocular contents, and orbit [1]. We have truncated this review; eyelid lesions are not covered and tumors that affect them are discussed under cutaneous neoplasms. Similarly, retinoblastoma, which occurs predominately in children under 5 years of age, is covered in Chapter 47.

Statistical data are compiled by the National Cancer Institute's Surveillance, Epidemiology, and End Results (SEER) Program for the category of "cancer of the eye and orbit" [1]. Approximately 3,130 new cancers of the eye and orbit are diagnosed and approximately 330 deaths from these cancers occur annually in the United States (US) [2]. The age-adjusted incidence rate of cancers of eye and orbit, overall, based on cases diagnosed in 2009–2013, was approximately 0.8 per 100,000 persons per year. During the same time period, the age-adjusted death rate was 0.1 per 100,000 per year [1]. These overall statistics largely reflect those of melanoma, which is the most common cancer of the eye and orbit. However, because of the great diversity of other eye and orbit cancers, this chapter presents their risk factors, diagnosis, and treatment separately for the most common of these cancers.

Conjunctival Lesions

Conjunctival malignancies are most common in older men who have been exposed to excess ultraviolet (UV) radiation [3]. The most frequent are squamous cell carcinomas, followed by melanomas, lymphomas, and Kaposi sarcoma. A myriad of benign-simulating lesions can occur in this anatomic location. In addition, cutaneous malignancy such as sebaceous carcinoma or, rarely, basal cell carcinoma, can involve the conjunctiva. The two most common conjunctival malignancies (squamous cell carcinoma and melanoma) arise from the epithelium. Therefore, if one places a drop of tetracaine in the conjunctiva and with a cotton tip applicator can move the conjunctival epithelium, and the lesion does not move (i.e., is subepithelial), it is not one of these processes.

Conjunctival squamous cell neoplasms initially arise as an intraepithelial process, usually occurring at the junction of the cornea and the conjunctiva (the limbus). Typically, these occur in older people who are exposed to excess UV radiation (hence the predilection of men over women). Other risk factors are excess exposure to petroleum products, light skin pigmentation, and human papillomavirus (HPV) and human immunodeficiency virus (HIV) exposure. Several studies have documented that patients with HIV disease have a much higher risk of developing this tumor. In fact, in a patient <50 years old who presents with a squamous cell carcinoma, HIV disease must be ruled out [4]. Carcinoma *in situ* (CIN) usually occurs demographically in a 5 years younger age cohort than the invasive tumor.

In the management of conjunctival carcinomas, the hallmark is an incisional or, if easily obtainable, an excisional biopsy. There are no data that an incisional biopsy adversely affects prognosis in any conjunctival malignancy. Most of these tumors remain superficial and rarely (<5%), in the invasive form, invade into the globe itself.

The management of these intraepithelial lesions has changed markedly over the last decade [5, 6]. Most squamous cell carcinomas that are *in situ* can be managed with topical agents. There is a paucity of randomized prospective control data comparing different topical agents. Historically, most patients were treated with mitomycin (0.04%) topically, but we and others have seen significant problems both in terms of punctal stenosis (stenosis of the drainage duct of the conjunctiva to the nose) resulting in tearing, as well as a limbal stem cell deficiency (the source of cells populating the normal cornea) in long-term follow-up of these patients. If one topical agent is not effective often another with a different mechanism of action will control the tumor. Most centers favor topical interferon with possibly a better control rate with less morbidity [7].

The American Cancer Society's Oncology in Practice: Clinical Management, First Edition. Edited by The American Cancer Society.

Unfortunately, topical agents have first-order pharmacokinetics of diffusion thus, in a thick lesion that is invasive, this is not a good option for treatment. Invasive carcinomas are treated by surgical resection, usually with frozen section control of the margins, followed with either adjunctive cryotherapy or topical agents to the resection bed of the tumor. In both settings the local control rate should be >95%. Radiation is usually limited to patients with multiple recurrences or deep invasion; although in some of those cases we and others have reported surgical ocular salvage with good vision [3].

Conjunctival Pigmented Lesions

Conjunctival melanomas most frequently arise from primary acquired melanosis (PAM) or *de novo*. In approximately 10% of cases they arise from a pre-existing nevus [8]. PAM is a unilateral condition (which must be distinguished from simple racial pigmentation in heavily pigmented patients) that generally develops in patients between 20 and 50 years of age. Incisional biopsy to assess the cellular atypia of melanocytes at the basal layer is highly predictive of whether or not these lesions will undergo malignant degeneration. In patients with PAM with significant atypia, many ophthalmic oncologists are treating such flat *in situ* lesions with topical agents (see prior comments regarding conjunctival squamous cell neoplasms).

Conjunctival melanomas have approximately one-twentieth the frequency of melanomas arising in the uveal tract [3]. They appear to be increasing in incidence, although the reasons for that have not been well delineated. Several features of a conjunctival melanoma are associated with systemic prognosis [3]. Important prognostic parameters include: tumor location (worse prognosis in lesions that involve the palpebral (eyelid) conjunctiva, the fornix, or the caruncle); tumors that are recurrent; histologically aggressive lesions; thicker tumors; and those associated with a positive sentinel node biopsy. Sentinel node biopsy is not indicated in low-risk lesions such as relatively thin tumors on the bulbar conjunctiva.

The treatment of conjunctival melanoma is surgical resection with adjunctive cryotherapy or adjunctive topical therapy. Since as many as 50% of conjunctival melanomas can recur after therapy, and up to 25% develop metastatic disease, molecular studies at the time of biopsy are useful. Unlike uveal melanomas, *BRAF* mutations are not uncommon in conjunctival melanomas and this should be tested, especially in high-risk lesions [9]. We limit the use of radiation to diffuse lesions that have recurred after the above techniques. Radiation has included conventional external beam, brachytherapy, and charged particle treatments, usually with retention of the eye.

Conjunctival Lymphoid Lesions

Conjunctival lymphoid lesions are divided into those which are benign and are a polymorphous collection of lymphoid tissue (often requiring either flow cytometry or Southern blot analysis to differentiate them from a low-grade lymphoma) versus malignant lymphomas which most often arise locally and have a relatively low propensity for systemic spread. Typically, these conjunctival lymphoid lesions are salmon pink subepithelial lesions (Figure 41.1). Unfortunately, many ophthalmologists have demonstrated that the clinical appearance is not diagnostic, nor can it be used to differentiate a benign from a malignant lymphoid lesion. We routinely biopsy these lesions with preparation for standard histopathology as well as flow cytometry and molecular analysis of antigen receptor gene rearrangement, although the latter are often not necessary. If it is a benign lymphoid lesion, it is important to realize that some of these will recur and/or undergo malignant change. If it is a lymphoma on the basis of the above studies, we will routinely obtain a full body positron emission tomography-computed tomography (PET-CT) scan.

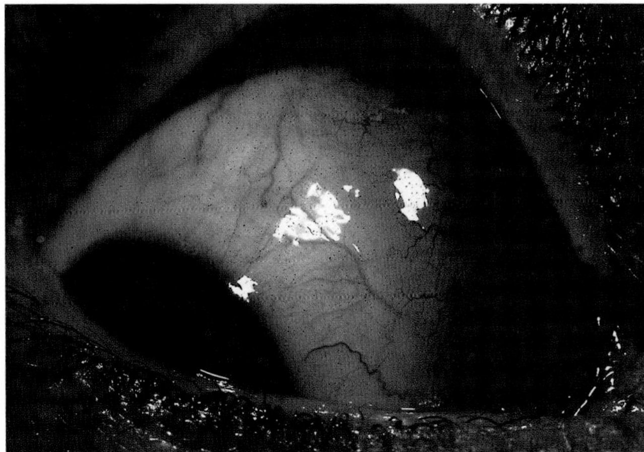

Figure 41.1 Conjunctival lymphoid lesion. Conjunctival lymphomas are typically salmon pink and subepithelial.

The management of both benign and malignant conjunctival lymphoid lesions is in flux. There were a few papers suggesting that some were due to Chlamydia, but most studies have now shown that to be a localized phenomenon in a few European geographic areas. Most studies from the US have not been able to replicate those results. In terms of management, if the lesion is focal one can treat with excision, and if it is more diffuse (the usual scenario) one can treat with either radiation, systemic medication (such as a monoclonal antibody towards B cell markers), or intralesional interferon [10]. All are effective. Obviously in cases with simultaneous systemic involvement (which fortunately is very rare), systemic chemotherapy would be required.

Conjunctival Kaposi Sarcoma and Miscellaneous Tumors

Kaposi sarcoma was very prevalent in the full-blown AIDS syndrome before the modern antiretroviral drug era. Fortunately, since the development of those agents it has become a very uncommon entity. There are a number of other rare malignancies that can involve the conjunctiva; the key point mentioned earlier is, when in doubt, a biopsy makes sense. If it is a superficial lesion one can obtain a cytological sample (typically, a scraping analogous to a cervical Pap smear) and send to a laboratory with experience in the cytopathology of eye lesions.

Orbital Tumors

Pediatric orbital tumors are covered in Chapter 47. In adults, the most common cause of either bilateral or unilateral proptosis is thyroid-related eye disease [11]. This diagnosis can be challenging, as only approximately 60% of patients will have systemic hyperthyroidism manifest at the time they present with eye findings. The evaluation of those patients is well described in several textbooks [11].

The most straightforward manner to characterize and delineate different processes that involve the orbit is based on the orbital anatomic structures involved by the process. As an example, a tumor in the intraconal (inside the muscle cone involving or not involving the optic nerve) space will often produce axial (straightforward) proptosis. An extraconal superior tumor will produce downward and forward displacement of the eye. A tumor involving the ethmoid sinuses or medial orbit will produce lateral and outward displacement of the eye, and so on. We usually characterize orbital processes as those that involve the orbital bones, the extraocular muscles, the extraconal space (the space outside of the extraocular muscles between those structures and the orbital wall), and the intraconal space including the optic nerve. Tumors in these different areas have relatively characteristic clinical and imaging patterns [3].

Signs suggestive of malignancy are rapid growth of a lesion (without a history suggestive of an infection with orbital cellulitis), a patient with marked systemic illness and weight loss, severe pain associated with the orbital process, or extensive orbital bony erosion. As a general rule, orbital MRI with a 3 Tesla magnet gives more information than a CT scan, unless there is orbital bony involvement as a primary site of pathology, in which case CT may be useful [3].

Orbital bone involvement can be due to either benign or malignant conditions although the imaging patterns are quite disparate. In adults, if there is bony erosion it almost always is a neoplastic process – either primary, such as a lacrimal gland adenoid cystic carcinoma, or a metastasis. Other intrinsic malignancies such as lymphomas or dermoid cysts involving the orbit usually only expand or smoothly erode the orbital walls. Obviously, sinus carcinomas or a CNS tumor can also secondarily erode through an orbital wall.

Benign conditions can involve the orbital bones in several ways. Some metabolic conditions will involve the orbital bone. A dermoid or hematic cyst of the orbit will often produce a "scalloped" change in the orbital bony wall, especially superiortemporally. Intraosseous hemangiomas can also arise in the orbital bone and rarely we see fibrous dysplasia or osteomas arise from the orbital bones. The most useful diagnostic test in this setting is either CT or MRI. Ultrasonography is not usually helpful in evaluating such bone lesions.

In a patient with orbital bony involvement a biopsy can be done, sometimes with a fine-needle aspiration biopsy (FNAB) under CT control, or occasionally with an open biopsy, and management depends on the nature of the process. As a general rule, benign lesions are just excised, whereas with metastatic tumors treatment usually is palliative.

Extraocular Muscle Tumors

Extraocular muscle involvement has three common etiologies. The largest group of these is thyroid-related orbitopathy. Usually the muscles involved predominantly are inferior rectus followed by medial rectus, lateral rectus, and, less commonly, either the superior recti or the obliques. Idiopathic myositis (orbital pseudotumor) has a different clinical pattern than thyroid-related myopathy. On imaging there is a tendency for thyroid-related myopathy to "spare" the tendinous portion of the muscle, while in the inflammatory or lymphomatous infiltration there is involvement of the entire muscle and tendon. Finally, small "lumpy bumpy" involvement of the muscle is more likely due to a metastatic lesion to the extraocular muscle, especially from cutaneous melanomas. We have seen a myriad of other lesions involve the extraocular muscles, but the above represent the vast majority of all cases of enlarged extraocular muscle involvement in the orbit.

Extraconal Nonosseous Tumors

Extraocular muscle tumors, especially in older people, are usually metastases, a benign lymphoid proliferation, or an orbital lymphoma. These patients usually present without systemic symptomatology and the diagnosis can often be confirmed with CT-directed FNAB. With FNAB, one can perform any of the ancillary studies which were traditionally performed on open biopsy material, although in some cases a limited yield of cells may restrict the number of such tests that can be performed.

Intraconal Tumors

Intraconal tumors can be divided into those which involve the optic nerve, those which are focal and do not involve the optic nerve, and those which are diffuse. Intrinsic optic nerve tumors in adults are most commonly optic nerve sheath meningiomas, which produce marked vision loss and relatively subtle proptosis (<3 mm of asymmetry) in middle-aged women. The MR or CT pattern of these is almost pathognomonic. Often optociliary shunt vessels are visible in the fundus.

Leukemia can involve the optic nerve, and any inflammatory process can produce swelling of the optic nerve sheath. Occasionally, uveal melanoma tracks back into the optic nerve, but in such cases a large intraocular tumor should be readily apparent either clinically or on the basis of conventional imaging studies. Rarely, in adults there are intrinsic optic nerve gliomas, especially in people who have neurofibromatosis. Metastases to the optic nerve occur, although the vast majority of ophthalmic metastases go to the posterior portion of the uveal tract.

Focal Discrete Intraconal Tumors

Most focal discrete intraconal orbital tumors are benign and present because of pressure on the optic nerve producing visual loss, or growth producing proptosis. The majority are cavernous hemangiomas, which have a typical imaging appearance (Figure 41.2). Other benign mesenchymal tumors, including solitary fibrous tumors, neurofibromas, and neurilemmomas, occur in <10% of such cases.

Diffuse involvement of the intraconal space is usually a sign of either a lymphoid process (benign or malignant) or metastases. Both of these types of processes can be adequately diagnosed with FNAB under CT control.

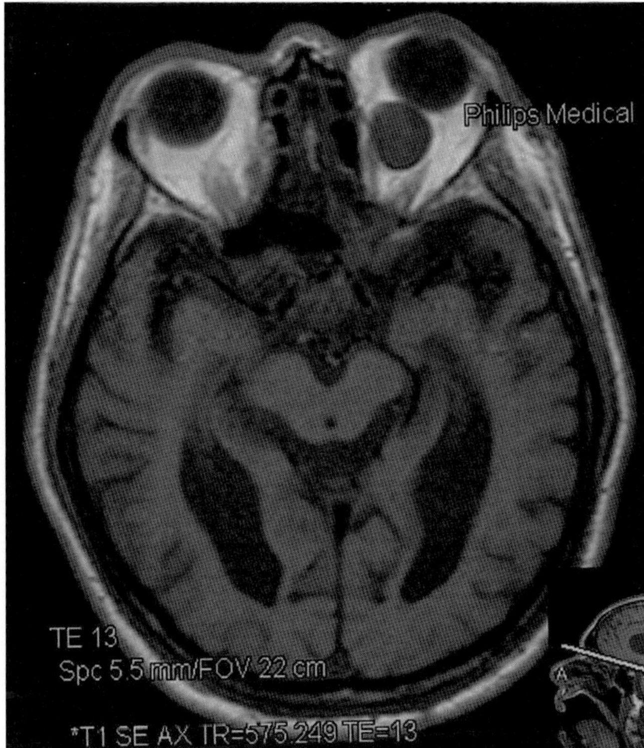

Figure 41.2 Cavernous hemangioma involving the intraconal space. Cavernous hemangiomas are the most common benign mesenchymal tumor in the orbit and typically spare the apex. They are isointense on T1-weighted MRI.

Orbital Tumor Therapy

The management of orbital neoplasms depends on their nature as well as the effect they are having on visual function. As a general rule, large benign tumors that are producing significant proptosis or vision loss are removed, usually without damage to the visually vital structures. There are several different options in terms of surgical approaches [3]. Malignant tumors involving the orbit, if they are either chemotherapy or radiation sensitive, are treated in this manner. In some cases, such as an adenoid cystic carcinoma that has not spread outside the orbit, an orbitectomy is performed to avoid tumor spread. Similarly, patients with large neglected intraocular tumors diffusely involving the orbit are often treated with surgical exenteration of the orbital tissue.

Intraocular Tumors

The most common noncutaneous ophthalmic oncologic tumor involves the intraocular structures. In adults, usually these are either pigmented benign or malignant choroidal neoplasms. The average age of patients with uveal melanomas in the US is about 60 years. Approximately 80% of these intraocular pigmented lesions involve the choroid, with approximately 10–15% involving the ciliary body and 5–10% involving the iris. Although, on a statistical basis, metastases to the choroid are more common than primary uveal melanomas, most of the former patients have widespread disease when they develop ocular findings and it is usually not a significant management issue. In contrast, choroidal melanoma is the most common primary intraocular tumor, having an incidence rate of approximately 5 per million per year in the US [12].

Choroidal melanoma is more common in light-skinned patients. There is not a strong association with environmental exposures, systemic syndromes, or family history. Most choroidal melanomas develop *de novo,* although some investigators have estimated that there is a 1 in 5,000 chance of a choroidal nevus undergoing malignant degeneration. The one variant that has a higher incidence of malignant degeneration is a nevus of Ota; individuals with this lesion have a significantly increased incidence of uveal melanomas. Families with multiple generations of uveal melanoma are rare. Associations with BAP1 gene and different environmental exposures are also uncommon [13].

A number of patients are seen each year with an indeterminate pigmented choroidal lesion, which we have labeled with the neologism "choroidal nevomas" [3]. These are lesions that are larger in both diameter and thickness than the typical nevus, and yet approximately two-thirds of them will never enlarge and do not require therapy. In this group of patients, no tumor-related mortality has been observed. One-third of these patients have manifest growth of the lesion; however, if they are rapidly identified at that point and treated, they do well. In our experience, there has been <5% 5-year mortality in that latter group of patients [3].

Over two-thirds of uveal melanomas arise within 3 mm of the optic nerve and the fovea [3]. This observation has two implications for non-ophthalmologists. One, most patients with choroidal melanomas, because of the location of the tumor, will present with visual symptoms (it is rare for a patient to present with pain unless the eye develops a quite uncommon associated scleritis or neovascular glaucoma). Two, any form of radiation therapy, even highly-focused charged particle therapies, for tumors that close to the visually vital structures usually results in poor visual outcome in those eyes.

In eyes with clear media (neither cataract or vitreous hemorrhage obscuring the view of the lesion), noninvasive diagnostic techniques have >95% accuracy in delineating a benign from a malignant pigmented lesion. We routinely perform FNAB in uveal melanoma patients for three reasons. One, in some smaller, atypical lesions there is a significant error rate (approximately 9%) in patients attempted to be managed with noninvasive diagnostic techniques. Two, we have shown in over 1,500 cases no negative effects of FNAB. Three, we can now, more accurately than with any other technique, delineate the systemic prognosis on the basis of molecular profiling of FNAB samples [14].

The molecular alterations in uveal melanoma are quite different than cutaneous melanoma [14]. Several different chromosomal abnormalities are involved; as an example, *BRAF* mutations are quite rare in uveal melanoma. In contrast, alterations on chromosomes 3, 6, 8, and 1 are relatively common in uveal melanoma. Of these, the most prognostically useful is monosomy of chromosome 3, which is associated with a worse prognosis. While *GNAQ* and *GNA11* are commonly altered early in the development of uveal melanomas, they do not have a significant association with prognosis. The most accurate means of delineating systemic prognosis is with molecular testing based on multiple gene array studies.

Based on molecular studies, a class 1A lesion has <2% 5-year tumor-related mortality, a class 1B lesion has approximately

20% 5-year mortality, and a class 2 lesion has approximately 72% 5-year tumor-related mortality [14]. The optimum management of a patient with a class 2 uveal melanoma and no evidence of systemic disease is uncertain. At the time of intraocular therapy almost none of these patients have evidence (clinical, laboratory, or imaging) of metastatic disease, yet over 5 years >70% will develop widespread melanoma. A number of centers around the country are starting trials of adjuvant therapy. In addition, the systemic post-treatment evaluation of such patients is more aggressive in terms of quarterly abdominal ultrasounds or MR scans and yearly PET-CT scans. In contrast, a class 1A or 1B lesion probably can be followed with just serum liver function tests or abdominal ultrasound.

As we demonstrated in the 1970s, the most common initial site of detection for metastatic uveal melanoma is the liver in 65% of cases. Subcutaneous nodules develop in 25%; in 7%, lung pleura or parenchyma is involved [3]. Less commonly, bone or CNS can be an initial site of metastatic disease. This pattern is very different from what is observed with metastatic cutaneous melanoma.

The management of approximately 80% of choroidal melanomas is to treat with eye-retaining radiation. The goal is to destroy the reproductive integrity of the tumor while retaining the eye and, if the tumor is away from the optic nerve and the fovea and not >6 mm thick, retaining good vision (Figure 41.3(a, b)). We have previously published a randomized dynamically balanced prospective study comparing charged particle radiation with brachytherapy and showed better control rates with charged particle therapy [15]. In our experience with particles, there is >98% local control rate, although obviously some of these patients will have already developed metastases before they are initially examined for uveal melanoma and develop clinical metastases between 6 months and 48 years later. In some centers brachytherapy, most commonly with iodine-125 radioactive plaques, is used although this does have a lower tumor control rate than charged particles. In rare cases laser is utilized, but it is usually not as effective, especially in tumors that are >3.5 mm in thickness. The results with radioactive plaques that have a similar length of follow-up with similar sizes of tumors show a higher local failure rate than is observed with proton radiation in many centers around the world. With various forms of laser or photocoagulation, failure rates of up to 50% have been reported. Some of that failure is due to a "marginal miss" where the area of eye treated has been deliberately minimized given proxmity to vital structures to avoid visual loss. The caveat to the last statement is obvious: one of the main indications for considering laser is where the clinician is trying to avoid the complications of widefield radiation; hence laser was applied to a very limited treatment area.

In approximately 20% of cases (mainly large melanomas without visual potential), primary enucleation (removal of the eye) is performed. Previous studies in a phase 3 trial comparing enucleation alone versus 20 Gy fractionated pre-enucleation radiation have demonstrated that there was no survival advantage [16].

Some more anterior tumors that involve the ciliary body and iris are treated with radiation (including some more posterior ciliary body melanomas that also involve the choroid) and some are treated with eyewall resection, iridocyclectomy, cyclectomy, or choroidectomy depending on tumor location (Figure 41.4(a, b)). The problems with eyewall resection are threefold. One, it is a technically difficult procedure and only a few of us in the world have had a large experience with these techniques. Two, it is not as reproducible in terms of being able to predict the visual or ocular outcome. Having performed over 600 such

(a)

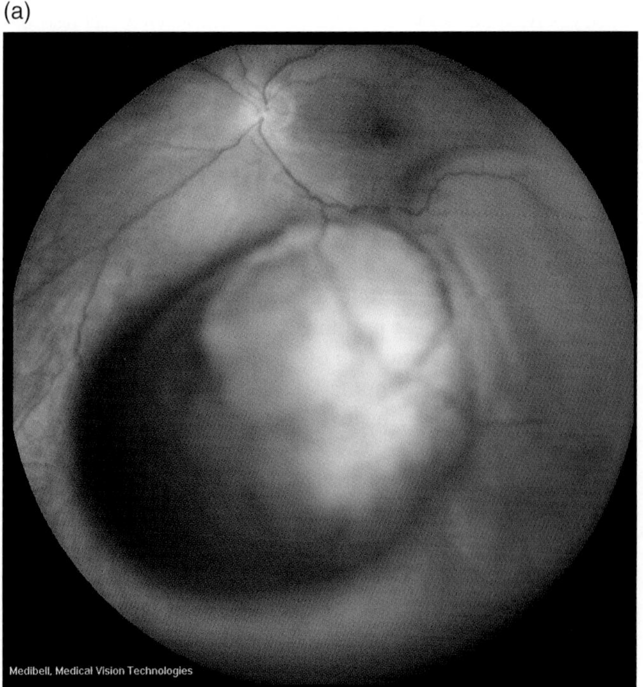

(b)

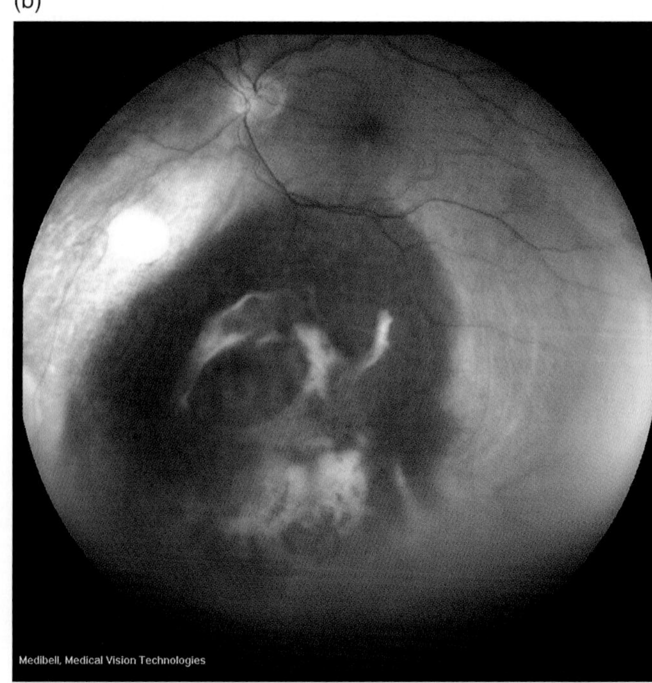

Figure 41.3 (a) Uveal melanoma prior to charged particle radiation. (b) Uveal melanoma after charged particle radiation. Onset of shrinkage is delayed until a sufficient number of cells enter the mitotic phase so that radiation-induced DNA errors result in tumor cell death.

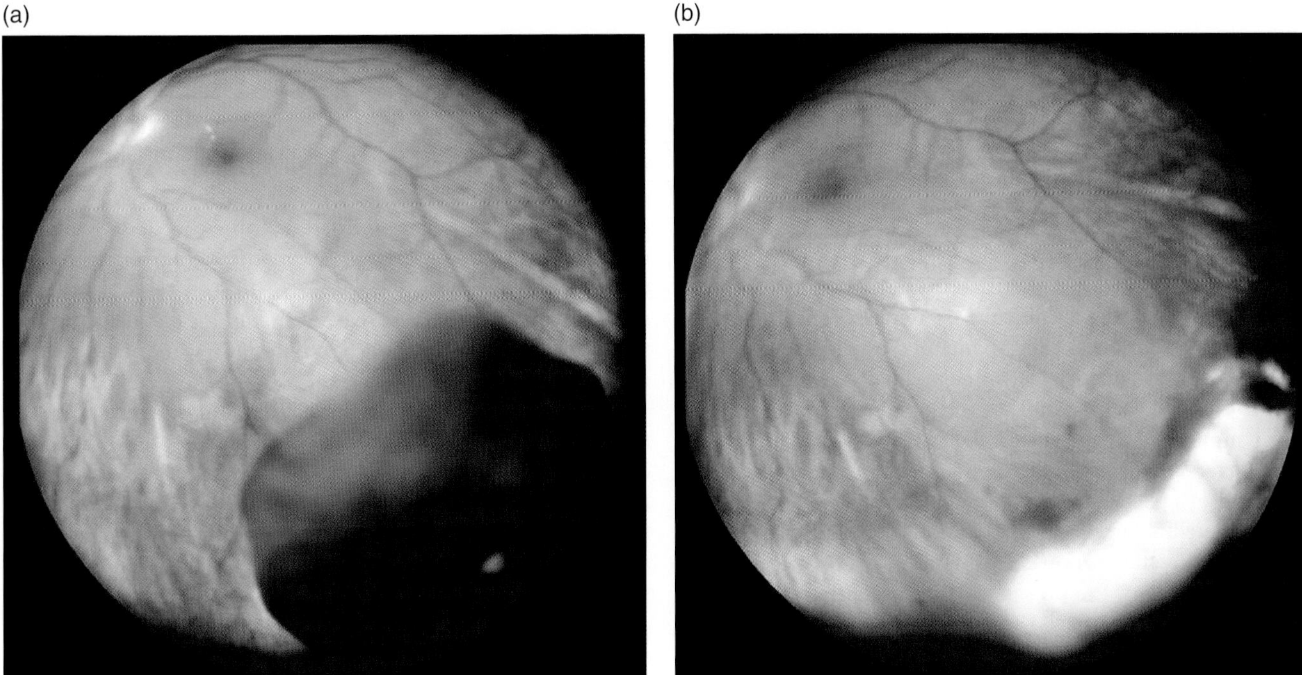

Figure 41.4 (a) Uveal melanoma prior to eyewall resection (cyclo-choroidectomy). (b) Status post cyclo-choroidectomy of a large ciliochoroidal melanoma with good visual outcome.

cases, I cannot be certain when I leave an operating room after removing a large tumor whether the eye will eventually see 20/20 or will be at "count fingers vision." Three, in three separate centers we have observed that the surgical margins are often not adequate and therefore most clinicians, even with "clear surgical margins," will use adjunctive radiation. Having said that, in very thick tumors (>8 mm in thickness) the visual results are probably better with eyewall resection than with radiation [3].

Pure iris or iris–ciliary body tumors are much less common and occur with about one-twentieth the frequency of posterior uveal melanomas (Figure 41.5). Iris tumors, for reasons that are not entirely clear, also have significantly less tumor-related mortality. Some centers have noted 12–20% tumor-related mortality in this group as compared to posterior uveal tumors.

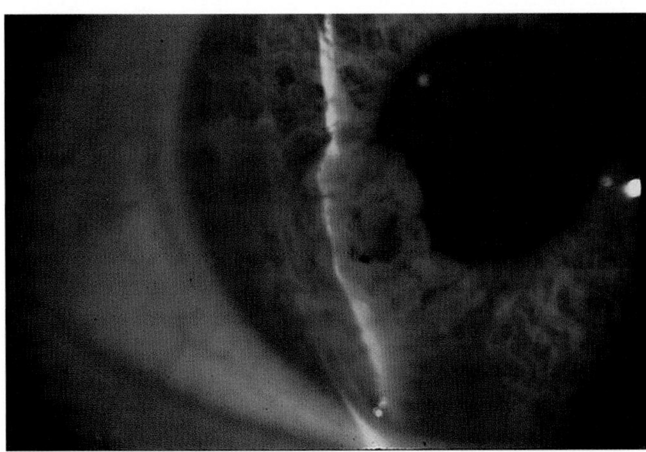

Figure 41.5 Iris melanoma.

In my personal experience, if we exclude ring melanomas (iris melanomas involving 360° of the circumference of the eye), those that also involve the ciliary body, or those in which someone has mistakenly performed a filtering operation assuming there was a benign glaucoma, we have had a <3% tumor-related mortality [17]. Generally, in iris pigmented tumors, unless they have documented growth or are actively bleeding, we recommend clinical observation without treatment. Those that have shown growth or are quite vascular we will usually resect with excellent results. Over 90% of those patients will retain 20/20 vision.

A number of other benign and malignant tumors can involve the uveal tract [3]. The three most common are choroidal nevi, choroidal hemangiomas (which are benign), and choroidal metastases. An unknown percentage of choroidal hemangiomas present because they produce exudative detachment (a retinal detachment not caused by a rhegmatogenous mechanism, i.e., one that has occurred usually because of increased vessel leakage from abnormal tumor vessels) which must be eradicated to return good vision. Usually these tumors are straightforward to diagnose with noninvasive techniques and are well treated with hematoporphyrin dye laser.

Choroidal metastases most commonly involve the posterior choroid and can be correctly diagnosed with noninvasive techniques; however adjuvant FNAB is helpful to delineate several features of these tumors that can be useful in planning therapy. The most important caveat in managing a patient with metastases to the choroid is realizing that as many as 40% [3] of such patients will have simultaneous, often "silent" metastases to the frontal lobe. It is important to re-stage any patient with a newly detected choroidal metastasis, especially including brain MRI with contrast to assess possible metastatic foci in contiguous structures. The management of choroidal metastases is similar to the management of any other metastatic lesion. There is no "blood–brain" or "blood–retinal" barrier in the choroid that would alter accessibility to drugs. While retinal metastases and metastases to the optic nerve occur, they are much less frequent than those involving the choroid.

Intraocular Lymphoma

There has been a marked increase in the occurrence of lymphomas involving the intraocular structures. Depending on the specialty one is in, approximately two-thirds of these patients are initially seen with ocular involvement and later develop CNS disease. Alternatively, patients with primary CNS lymphomas will have intraocular involvement in up to one-quarter of cases. The clinical presentation of these patients is of a pseudouveitis with decreased vision. On examination the clinician visualizes lymphoid cells, usually in the vitreous with often yellowish-white chorioretinal infiltrates. In an older patient, the presence of diffuse vitreous cells and chorioretinal infiltrates is an intraocular lymphoma until proven otherwise [18] (Figure 41.6(a, b)).

(a)

(b)

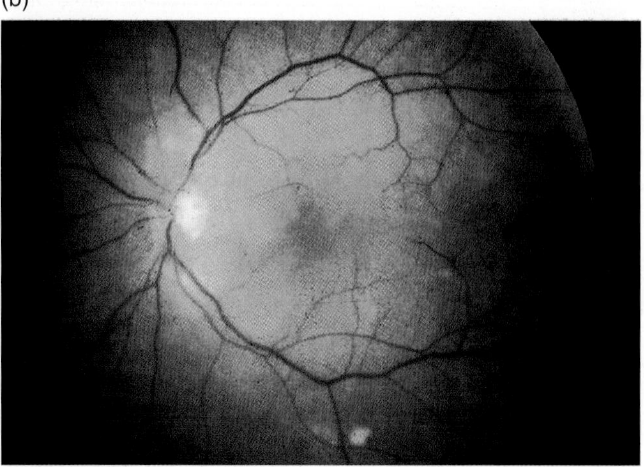

Figure 41.6 (a) Intraocular lymphoma typically has cells in the vitreous and in the retina. (b) Status post treatment of intraocular lymphoma with the return of good visual acuity.

Patients with these findings are diagnosed by a combination of vitreous biopsy and, in cases highly suggestive of a lymphoma, both cerebrospinal fluid (CSF) cytologic analysis and MRI with contrast to detect CNS involvement. The management of these patients is in flux, but is covered under treatment of CNS lymphoma. However, patients who have only eye disease with negative CSF cytology and no evidence of CNS disease on imaging can be treated with either local radiation or intravitreal chemotherapy with intraocular rituximab or intraocular methotrexate with reasonably good results. In some of these patients disease remains localized to the eye, while some will develop CNS lymphoma. All require lifelong/regular systemic evaluation [18].

Much less commonly, systemic lymphomas can recur in the eye, usually as a pseudoiritis or cyclitis with anterior chamber cells and sometimes a collection of white cells layered out in the anterior chamber angle (pseudohypopyon). The diagnosis is readily established with FNAB. These almost always harbinger a poor systemic prognosis and can be managed, depending on the systemic status of the patient, with chemotherapeutic agents or radiation. Much less commonly, systemic lymphomas can involve an isolated choroidal area, but this is rare compared to the frequency of either a primary intraocular lymphoma associated with CNS lymphoma or a systemic recurrence involving the anterior chamber angle.

Conclusion

Ophthalmic oncologic processes can usually be correctly diagnosed by an ophthalmologist with noninvasive techniques. Some of them can be serially evaluated without intervention. The systemic prognosis of a primary choroidal melanoma, the most common primary intraocular tumor, can be elegantly delineated with molecular testing. Approximately 80% of uveal melanomas can be treated with eye retention. In very large tumors, or tumors that have produced neovascular glaucoma, the eyes are removed. Intraocular lymphomas are relatively straightforward to manage but usually the patients die in 3–5 years from progressive CNS lymphoma.

Conjunctival tumors occur much less frequently but are usually amenable to treatment, although in thick, large, conjunctival melanomas there is significant tumor-related mortality.

It is easiest to establish a differential diagnosis for orbital tumors based on the orbital anatomic structure which they mainly involve. Benign lesions can often be resected if they are producing either proptosis or decreased vision. In malignant or metastatic orbital tumors usually the treatment is not surgical, although some primary aggressive carcinomas can be treated with widefield resection.

Acknowledgements

The project was supported in part by a grant from The Tumori Foundation. Dr. Char is the director of The Tumori Foundation (a nonprofit organization) and Tia Cole is a research associate.

References

1 Howlader N, Noone AM, Krapcho M, *et al.* (eds). SEER Cancer Statistics Review, 1975–2013, National Cancer Institute. Bethesda, MD, http://seer.cancer.gov/csr/1975_2013/, based on November 2015 SEER data submission, posted to the SEER web site, April 2016.
2 Siegel RL, Miler KD, Jemal A. Cancer Statistics, 2017. *CA Cancer J Clin* 2017;67:7–30.
3 Char DH. *Tumors of the Eye and Ocular Adnexa*. Hamilton: BC Decker Inc., 2001.
4 Makupa II, Swai B, Makupa WU, *et al.* Clinical factors associated with malignancy and HIV status in patients with ocular surface squamous neoplasia at Kilimanjaro Christian Medical Centre, Tanzania. *Br J Ophthalmol* 2012;96:482–4.
5 Char DH, Crawford JB. Orbital invasion despite topical anti-metabolite therapy for conjunctival carcinoma. *Graefes Arch Clin Exp Ophthalmol* 2008;246:459–61.
6 Tunc M, Char DH, Crawford B, *et al.* Intraepithelial and invasive squamous cell carcinoma of the conjunctiva: analysis of 60 cases. *Br J Ophthalmol* 1999;83:98–103.
7 Shah S, Kaliki S, Kim HJ, *et al.* Topical interferon alfa-2b for management of ocular surface squamous neoplasia in 23 cases: outcomes based on American Joint Committee on Cancer classification. *Arch Ophthalmol* 2012;130:159–64.
8 Char D. Ocular melanoma. *Surg Clin North Am* 2003;83: 253–274, vii.
9 Gear H, Williams H, Kemp EG, *et al.* BRAF mutations in conjunctival melanoma. *Invest Ophthalmol Vis Sci* 2004;45:2484–8.
10 Blasi MA, Tiberti AC, Valente P, *et al.* Intralesional interferon-alpha for conjunctival mucosa-associated lymphoid tissue lymphoma: long-term results. *Ophthalmology* 2012;119:494–500.
11 Char DH. *Thyroid Eye Disease*. Boston: Butterworth-Heinemann, 1997.
12 Gill HS, Char DH. Uveal melanoma prognostication: from lesion size and cell type to molecular class. *Can J Ophthalmol* 2012;47:246–253.
13 Höiom V, Edsgärd D, Helgadottir H, *et al.* Hereditary uveal melanoma: A report of a germline mutation in BAP1. *Genes Chromosomes Cancer* 2013;52:378–84.
14 Harbour JW. The genetics of uveal melanoma: an emerging framework for targeted therapy. *Pigment Cell Melanoma Res* 2012;25:171–81.
15 Char DH, Quivey JM, Castro JR, *et al.* Helium ions versus iodine 125 brachytherapy in the management of uveal melanoma. A prospective, randomized, dynamically balanced trial. *Ophthalmology* 1993;100:1547–54.
16 Hawkins B, Group COMS. The Collaborative Ocular Melanoma Study (COMS) randomized trial of pre-enucleation radiation of large choroidal melanoma: IV. Ten-year mortality findings and prognostic factors. COMS report number 24. *Am J Ophthalmol* 2004;138:936–51.
17 Char DH, Kemlitz AE, Miller T, *et al.* Iris ring melanoma: fine needle biopsy. *Br J Ophthalmol* 2006;90:420–2.
18 Char DH. Intraocular masquerade syndromes. In: W Tasman, EA Jaeger (eds) *Clinical Ophthalmology*. Philadelphia: JB Lippincott, 2003.

Section 12

Bone and Soft Tissue Tumors

42

Sarcomas of Bone in Adults

Mrinal Gounder, Yoshiya Yamada, and Nicola Fabbri

Memorial Sloan Kettering Cancer Center and Weill Cornell Medical College, New York, New York, USA

Incidence and Mortality

Statistical data regarding bone sarcomas are compiled by the National Cancer Institute's Surveillance, Epidemiology, and End Results (SEER) Program in the category of "bone and joint cancer." While metastatic spread to bone from carcinomas is a relatively common oncologic event, primary malignant tumors of the bones and joints are extremely rare and represent less than 0.2% of all new cancer diagnoses. In 2017, approximately 3,260 new cases will be diagnosed in the United States (US) and approximately 1,550 will die from bone and joint cancers [1]. Sarcomas comprise the vast majority of primary bone and joint cancer cases in the SEER database. Among children and adolescents younger than 20 years, the most common malignancy of bone is osteosarcoma (60%), followed by Ewing sarcoma family of tumors (ESFT) (32%), and chondrosarcoma (4%) [2]. The most common histologic types among adults aged 20 and older are chondrosarcoma (40%), osteosarcoma (28%), ESFT (8%), chordoma (10%), malignant fibrous histiocytoma (MFH) (3%), and giant cell tumor of bone (GCTB) (2%) [3].

Etiology

Bone sarcomas are classified based on the similarity of the neoplastic tissue to normal bone components. However, the pathogenesis of bone cancers remains elusive and controversial [4]. It is not clear whether the cell of origin is a true multipotential mesenchymal stem cell which differentiates or whether mature bone cells acquire stem cell-like characteristics. Chondrosarcoma has a predominant composition of cartilaginous elements, osteosarcoma has osteoid elements and when there is a predominant composition of fibrogenic elements it is termed MFH of bone, chordoma has remnants of notochord, and GCTB has both neoplastic stromal cells of osteoblastic lineage and reactive osteoclastic elements. The cell of origin remains unknown in ESFT.

Most often trauma brings attention to the new diagnosis of malignancy; however, there is no convincing evidence that trauma is a risk factor in the pathogenesis of bone and joint neoplasms. Osteosarcoma seems to have both an environmental and genetic underpinning. Genomic analysis of osteosarcoma shows complex genetic aberrations frequently involving *TP53, CDKN2A/B, MDM2, RB*, and other related genes [5,6]. External radiotherapy appears to be responsible for a very small attributable fraction of bone sarcomas with osteosarcoma representing the most common histology. Examples of historical interest documenting the association of radionuclide exposure and osteosarcoma incidence include survivors of the atomic bombs at Hiroshima and Nagasaki, radium watch dial painters, use of intravenous radium for the treatment of ankylosing spondylitis and bone tuberculosis, and use of Thorotrast for angiography. The excess incidence associated with radiotherapy is greater among survivors of childhood cancers, especially those with genetic syndromes such as hereditary retinoblastoma. Germline aberrations in *TP53* or *CHEK2* (Li–Fraumeni syndrome) or *RB1* gene (retinoblastoma) are characterized by high risk of osteosarcoma. Other genetic syndromes that predispose to sarcomas include osteogenesis imperfecta, fibrous dysplasia, multiple hereditary exostosis, and enchondromatosis. These syndromes, along with other entities such as Paget disease, can result in benign bone deformities or lesions that may give rise to osteosarcoma and chondrosarcomas. Extremely rare cases of aberrations in DNA helicases (Rothmund–Thomson syndrome and Werner syndrome) also predispose to bone sarcomas [7].

Histopathologic Classification

Classification of bone sarcomas is based largely on histological and histochemical similarity of the neoplastic tissue with normal bone components. These similarities reflect differentiation (osteogenic, chondrogenic, fibrogenic, etc.) of neoplasms that may originate from primitive multipotential mesenchymal cells, and do not imply malignant transformation of mature osteocytes, chondrocytes, fibroblasts, etc. (Table 42.1). The differential diagnosis of Ewing sarcoma, which is characterized by small round blue cells, is wide and should include desmoplastic small

The American Cancer Society's Oncology in Practice: Clinical Management, First Edition. Edited by The American Cancer Society.

Table 42.1 Common malignant bone tumors and select histologic subtypes.

Osteosarcoma:
Osteogenic
Conventional
Telangiectatic
Periosteal
Parosteal
Small cell
Paget disease- and radiation-associated
Chondrosarcoma:
Chondrogenic
Primary central (low-, intermediate-, high-grade)
Mesenchymal
Dedifferentiated
Ewing sarcoma
Chordoma:
Conventional
Dedifferentiated
Chondroid
Giant cell tumor of bone

round blue cell tumors, lymphoma, small cell osteosarcoma, medulloblastoma, and rhabdomyosarcoma. Classical techniques such as light microscopy, electron microscopy, immunohistochemistry, and fluorescent *in situ* hybridization are used to make the diagnosis, and increasingly reverse transcriptase polymerase chain reaction (RT-PCR) is used to confirm pathognomonic genetic aberrations. Ewing sarcoma has the classical chromosomal translocation of *EWS* (Chr 11) with fusion partner *FLI1* (Chr 22). Other fusion partners include *ERG, ETV1, E1A*, and *CIC-DUX*. Conventional chondrosarcomas have mutations in *IDH1* or *IDH2* in a majority of tumors. Paraosteal osteosarcoma and low-grade central osteosarcoma carry amplifications of the *MDM2* gene [8]. Nuclear expression of T brachyury, a transcription factor, occurs in nearly all chordomas and very rarely in other bone neoplasms; it also occurs in some carcinomas and germ cell tumors but these are not likely to be confused with chordoma on clinical or morphologic grounds [9]. Given the rarity of primary bone tumors it is essential to confirm their diagnosis with an expert bone sarcoma pathologist. As tumors become more undifferentiated, the diagnosis becomes additionally challenging, resulting in disagreements even among expert pathologists [6]. Molecular characteristics have not been shown to be prognostic and are thus not incorporated in staging systems. However, grade of tumor is an important prognostic criterion and part of the American Joint Committee on Cancer (AJCC) staging system.

Clinical Presentation and Diagnosis

Localized pain, fracture, or enlarging mass are the most common signs and symptoms that patients present at the time of diagnosis. Pain is often localized and described as dull, deep-seated, unremitting, and present at rest and worsened by motion or weight bearing. On examination, a localized soft tissue swelling is deep, fixed, and firm to palpation. Range of motion and gait may be affected by pain, edema, or joint effusion. Lymph node involvement is not generally seen in bone cancers. Blood studies are generally unremarkable although occasionally anemia, leukocytosis, and elevation of alkaline phosphatase and lactate dehydrogenase can be seen in osteosarcoma and Ewing sarcoma [10,11].

Sites of Presentation and Radiologic Considerations

Optimal imaging of bone sarcomas depends on the anatomic site of involvement as they can arise in any bone and within any region of the given bone [12–14]. For example, osteosarcoma typically arises as an intramedullary metaphyseal lesion and less commonly on the surface of long bones. Anatomic sites frequently involved include the lower extremities (65%), humerus (11%), pelvis (8%), and jaw (6%). ESFT often presents in extremities (49%) followed by the pelvis (23%), ribs (18%), and craniofacial (3%) areas [15]. Chondrosarcoma has a predilection for extremities, pelvis, scapula, and ribs [16]. It is important to remember that extraskeletal (or soft tissue) bone sarcomas without obvious bone involvement are not infrequently seen. Chordomas have historically been managed by orthopedic or neurosurgeons and classified as bone tumors, however they lack osteoid and arise from remnants of the embryonic notochord. Chordomas are restricted to the sacral spine (~35%), cervical or mobile spine (~30%), and clivus (~35%). Initial evaluation of a suspected bone lesion should include conventional X-ray films with biplanar views. The pattern of bone destruction, soft tissue extension, and periosteal reaction helps narrow the differential diagnosis. Involving a musculoskeletal radiologist is critical to accurate diagnosis of suspected bone neoplasms. Additional imaging of the lesion may include computed tomography (CT) which can provide excellent detail of mineralization of cortical and cancellous bones and provide detail of the interface between bone and soft tissue. Magnetic resonance imaging (MRI) is valuable in delineating anatomic relationships between tumor and normal vasculature, nerves, and joint structures and defining the extent of intramedullary involvement. A differential diagnosis based on clinical presentation and imaging of the lesion can then guide next steps in aspects of obtaining a biopsy and staging. In patients who are less than 40 years old and who present with a primary bone lesion, further workup including biopsy should be performed at the treating institution, which should include clinicians with sarcoma expertise. For patients who are older than 40 years, additional workup to exclude metastatic spread from non-bone primaries is recommended. High-grade bone sarcomas require complete staging, which includes chest X-ray and chest CT. For skeletal survey, technetium bone scans and whole-body MRI can provide excellent imaging. Similarly, high-grade sarcomas may be well visualized with PET-CT scans whereas many of the low-grade sarcomas may not exhibit ^{18}F-fluorodeoxyglucose (FDG) avidity. Metastases to brain are rare in sarcomas and therefore imaging is recommended only when there is a high clinical suspicion. Bone marrow biopsies are performed in ESFT to evaluate for marrow involvement, however there is increasing evidence that this may not be informative.

Biopsy Considerations

Biopsy is crucial for the diagnosis and management of bone sarcomas and requires experience in musculoskeletal oncology. Successful biopsy is based on accurate pre-biopsy planning and meticulous execution. Since potentially catastrophic complications may derive from a poorly performed biopsy, a treating physician lacking substantial expertise in this field should always consider referral to a musculoskeletal oncologist before the biopsy. Although technically simple, biopsy is conceptually demanding and represents an essential part of the treatment strategy, requiring expertise at a sarcoma center. Biopsy should ideally follow adequate imaging and should be the last step to complete staging of the lesion [17]. Tissue may be obtained by an open surgical biopsy or a percutaneous technique using either a core needle or a fine needle. The use of image-guided percutaneous biopsy has greatly increased during the past two decades and represents the technique of choice for the majority of lesions in most centers with sarcoma expertise. Regardless of the technique, the fundamental principle of bone tumor biopsy is that it invariably also causes contamination of surrounding tissues, and the biopsy tract needs then to be removed *en bloc* with the tumor at the time of definitive surgery [18]. Pre-biopsy planning therefore includes careful differential diagnosis, knowledge of surgical technique, and thorough discussion with the radiologist and the pathologist, in order to determine the most appropriate biopsy method and proper placement of the biopsy track to minimize contamination of uninvolved structures and ensure its removal at the time of resection (Figure 42.1).

Inappropriate placement of the biopsy tract, post-biopsy hematoma with contamination of the neurovascular bundle, and use of transverse incisions remain unfortunately common errors in the management of musculoskeletal sarcomas, complicating definitive surgery by an increased risk of wound problems and local recurrence, often requiring more extensive resections, need for plastic surgery, and sometimes amputation rather than a limb salvage procedure [19]. Hematomas may in particular infiltrate uninvolved surrounding tissues, causing extracompartmental tumor dissemination and seeding [17,18] (Figure 42.2).

Selection of the biopsy method is primarily based on the differential diagnosis, location and extent of the lesion, expertise of the involved personnel, and anticipated amount of tissue needed for conventional cytologic and/or histologic preparations, immunohistochemistry, electron microscopy, flow cytometry, molecular characterization, and possibly use in research. The importance of tumor molecular profiling is rapidly growing, particularly for soft tissue sarcomas, and progressively translating from diagnosis to selection of targeted treatment. Image-guided percutaneous biopsy techniques are today effective in establishing a diagnosis in more than 90% of cases in large high-volume referral centers for musculoskeletal sarcomas. Image-based guidance allows for proper access, avoidance of neurovascular structures, and targeting of the most viable, solid tissue for diagnosis, avoiding central areas of necrosis and cystic changes [20,21]. CT-guided core needle biopsy represents the gold standard for sampling tissue from bone lesions [21]. Even though core biopsy has shown superior diagnostic accuracy, refinement in performance and interpretation of fine-needle aspiration has allowed successful clinical application, particularly when performed during an office visit to obtain timely confirmation or exclusion of malignancy and/or recurrence [22].

Staging

The Eighth Edition AJCC TNM staging system for bone (Table 42.2) is based on primary tumor size and local extension, nodal involvement, distant metastases (lung versus other sites), and tumor grade [23]. Nodal involvement is rare in bone sarcoma and only notated when lymph nodes have disease involvement. There are four grades of differentiation: not assessable (Gx), well- (G1), moderately- (G2), and poorly- (G3) differentiated. Some histological types of bone sarcomas are graded according to cellularity, atypia, mitotic activity, necrosis, and degree of differentiation, whereas others are assigned a grade based entirely on the histological type. For example, EFST is always classified as a grade 3 tumor. The surgical staging system for bone sarcomas adopted by the Musculoskeletal Tumor Society is based on the observation

(a)

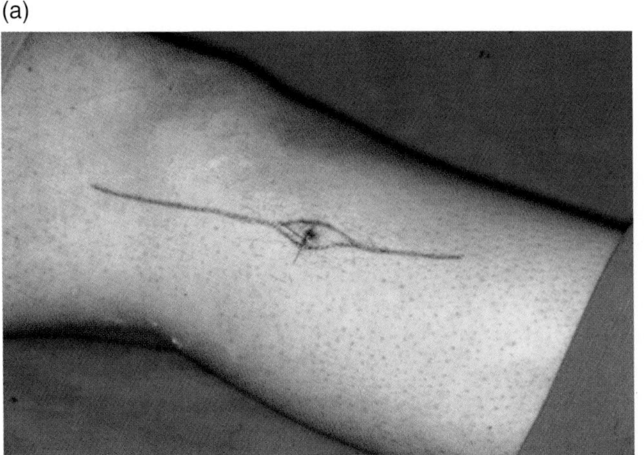

(b)

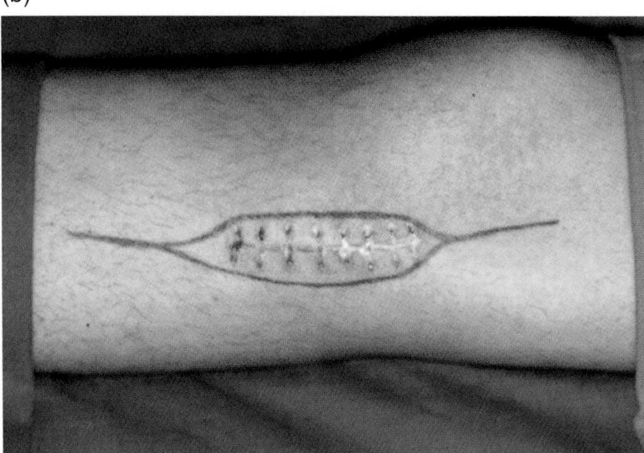

Figure 42.1 Examples of well-performed biopsy using percutaneous core needle (a) and open surgical technique (b). The biopsy tract may be easily incorporated in the ideal incision for surgical resection.

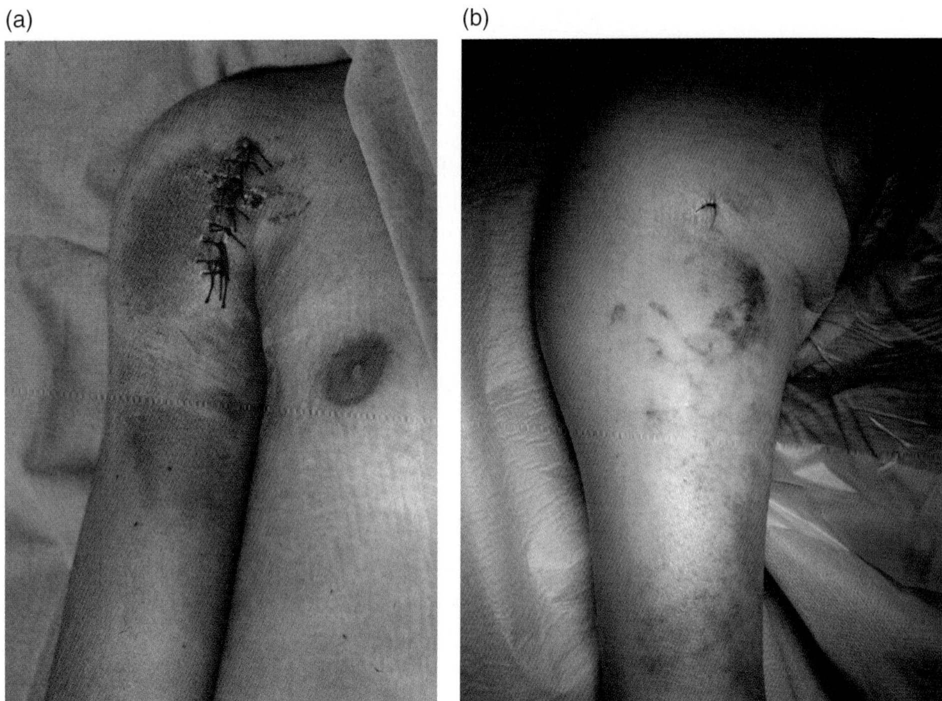

Figure 42.2 Post-biopsy hematoma and extensive contamination associated with poorly performed open biopsy of the proximal humerus (a). Even percutaneous needle biopsy may cause significant bleeding and hematoma (b). Note that the hemorrhagic subcutaneous infiltration extends distally involving the entire arm.

that bone sarcomas behave similarly regardless of histologic type [24]. The staging system is based on tumor grade (I, low-grade; II, high-grade), tumor extent (A, intraosseous involvement only; B, extraosseous extension), and presence of metastasis regardless of the extent of local tumor (III).

Primary Multimodality Treatment

Surgery

Current treatment for low-grade sarcomas is primarily surgical. However, high-grade lesions require multimodal management, including radiotherapy and/or chemotherapy. Even in high-grade tumors, however, the role of surgery remains pivotal in the overall management. In fact, curative intent in sarcomas requires an effective surgical strategy for local control of the primary tumor, with the only notable exception represented by small round blue cells tumors (EFST), for which radiotherapy is generally a reasonable alternative or complement to surgery. In order to minimize the risk of local recurrence, general surgical principles for bone and soft tissue sarcomas are *en bloc* removal of the tumor completely surrounded by normal healthy tissue [24], often referred as "wide margin" or "negative margin" (Figure 42.3).

The amount of normal tissue required as a margin to avoid local recurrence may vary according to the grade of malignancy, histologic type, and pattern of tumor growth. More importantly, it is inversely proportional to the use of a locally effective adjuvant modality of treatment in association with surgery. These principles, associated with contemporary imaging modalities and surgical reconstructive techniques, have translated in routine performance of limb salvage surgery rather than amputation in approximately 85–90% of cases in large referral centers. The goal of limb salvage is to obtain at the same time satisfactory local control of the primary tumor (the higher priority) and preservation/restoration of a functional limb. Nevertheless, amputation maintains a role in patients presenting with extensive neurovascular involvement, local recurrence, and clinical situations in which the expected function of a limb-saving procedure is no better or definitely inferior than that following amputation (Figure 42.4).

Surgery is the only treatment modality for low-grade bone sarcomas such as most chondrosarcomas and, less commonly, central or juxtacortical osteosarcomas. They are managed by wide *en bloc* excision and reconstruction as needed to restore weight-bearing bone, joints, adequate soft tissue coverage, and ultimately function. Metal implants, allografts, vascularized autografts, rotational and free flaps are variously associated to encompass a variety of different clinical settings.

Multiagent systemic chemotherapy has profoundly changed the management of high-grade classic osteosarcoma and ESFT. When compared to the pre-chemotherapy era, 5-year survival has dramatically improved from 5–15% to current 65–75% [25,26]. In addition, tumor response to preoperative chemotherapy facilitates limb-salvage surgery, and chemotherapy-induced tumor necrosis is a highly significant prognostic factor correlating with both local and distant relapse in high-grade osteosarcoma and Ewing sarcoma (Figure 42.5) [27,28].

Preoperative (or neoadjuvant) systemic chemotherapy is regarded today as the most effective means of decreasing local extent of high-grade bone sarcomas in order to facilitate limb-salvage surgery. While systemic chemotherapy improves overall

Table 42.2 AJCC TNM Eighth Edition staging of bone tumors. Used with permission of the American College of Surgeons, Chicago, Illinois. The original source for this information is the AJCC Cancer Staging Manual, Eighth Edition (2016), which is published by Springer Science + Business Media.

Definition of primary tumor (T)

Appendicular skeleton, trunk, skull, and facial bones

T category	T criteria
TX	Primary tumor cannot be assessed
T0	No evidence of primary tumor
T1	Tumor ≤8 cm in greatest dimension
T2	Tumor >8 cm in greatest dimension
T3	Discontinuous tumors in the primary bone site

Spine

T category	T criteria
TX	Primary tumor cannot be assessed
T0	No evidence of primary tumor
T1	Tumor confined to one vertebral segment or two adjacent vertebral segments
T2	Tumor confined to three adjacent vertebral segments
T3	Tumor confined to four or more adjacent vertebral segments, or any nonadjacent vertebral segments
T4	Extension into the spinal canal or great vessels
T4a	Extension into the spinal canal
T4b	Evidence of gross vascular invasion or tumor thrombus in the great vessels

Pelvis

T category	T criteria
TX	Primary tumor cannot be assessed
T0	No evidence of primary tumor
T1	Tumor confined to one pelvic segment with no extraosseous extension
T1a	Tumor ≤8 cm in greatest dimension
T1b	Tumor >8 cm in greatest dimension
T2	Tumor confined to one pelvic segment with extraosseous extension or two segments without extraosseous extension
T2a	Tumor ≤8 cm in greatest dimension
T2b	Tumor >8 cm in greatest dimension
T3	Tumor spanning two pelvic segments with extraosseous extension
T3a	Tumor ≤8 cm in greatest dimension
T3b	Tumor >8 cm in greatest dimension
T4	Tumor spanning three pelvic segments or crossing the sacroiliac joint
T4a	Tumor involves sacroiliac joint and extends medial to the sacral neuroforamen
T4b	Tumor encasement of external iliac vessels or presence of gross tumor thrombus in major pelvic vessels

Table 42.2 (Continued)

Definition of regional lymph node (N)

N category	N criteria
NX	Regional lymph nodes cannot be assessed. Because of the rarity of lymph node involvement in bone sarcomas, the designation NX may not be appropriate, and cases should be considered N0 unless clinical node involvement clearly is evident
N0	No regional lymph node metastasis
N1	Regional lymph node metastasis

Definition of distant metastasis (M)

M category	M criteria
M0	No distant metastasis
M1	Distant metastasis
M1a	Lung
M1b	Bone or other distant sites

Histologic grade (G)

G	G definition
GX	Grade cannot be assessed
G1	Well differentiated, low grade
G2	Moderately differentiated, high grade
G3	Poorly differentiated, high grade

AJCC prognostic stage groups

Appendicular skeleton, trunk, skull, and facial bones

When T is...	And N is...	And M is...	And grade is...	Then the stage group is...
T1	N0	M0	G1 or GX	IA
T2	N0	M0	G1 or GX	IB
T3	N0	M0	G1 or GX	IB
T1	N0	M0	G2 or G3	IIA
T2	N0	M0	G2 or G3	IIB
T3	N0	M0	G2 or G3	III
Any T	N0	M1a	Any G	IVA
Any T	N1	Any M	Any G	IVB
Any T	Any N	M1b	Any G	IVB

Spine and pelvis

There are no AJCC prognostic stage groupings for spine and pelvis.

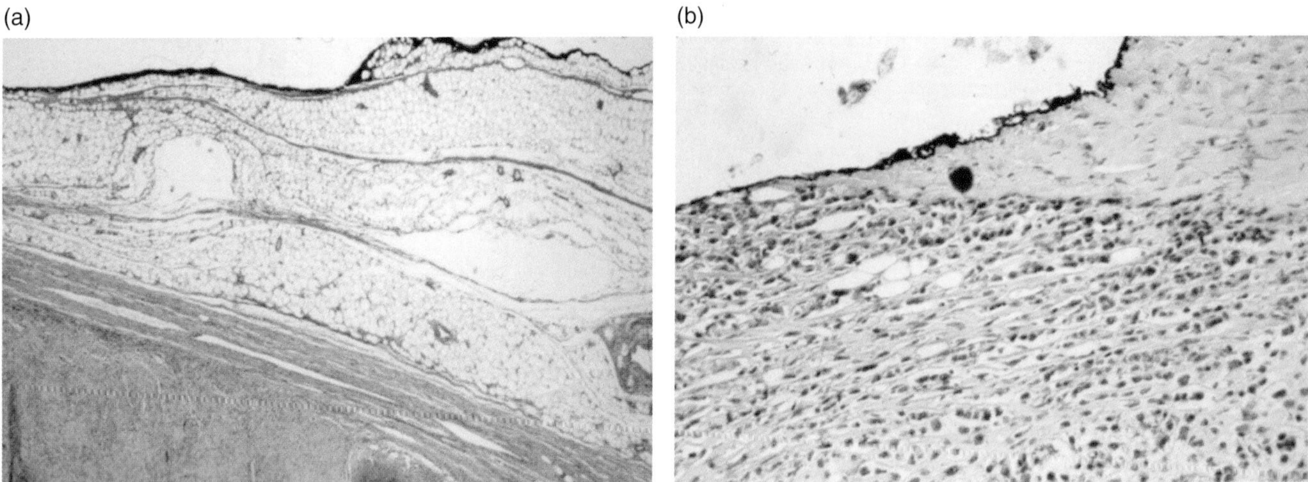

Figure 42.3 Careful histologic evaluation of the surgical margins using permanent ink is crucial for management of bone sarcomas. This requires clear communication between the surgeon and pathologist regarding orientation of the specimen. In (a), the ink is resting on normal fibro-adipose tissue, determining a "wide" or "negative" margin. In (b), the ink lies on tumor tissue, determining an "intralesional" or "positive" margin, unsatisfactory for local control because associated with increased risk of local recurrence.

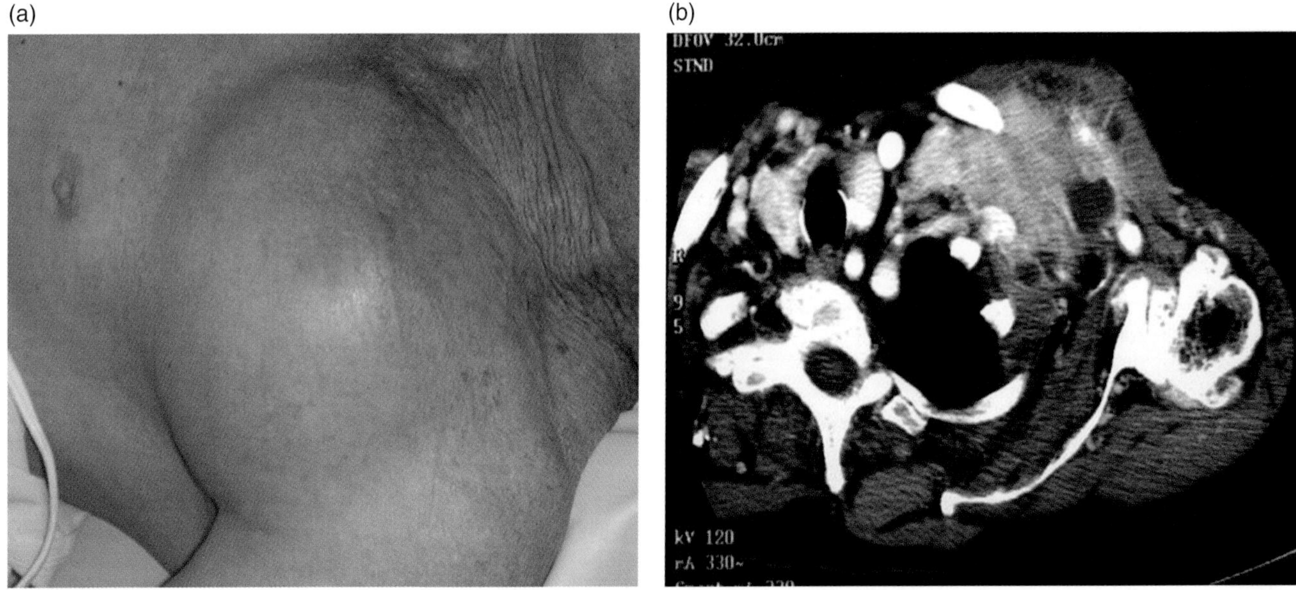

Figure 42.4 A 78 year-old man with high-grade sarcoma of the left supra- and infra-clavicular region (a), extensively involving the subclavian and axillary vessels, the brachial plexus, and the chest wall (b). This patient could not be managed by limb-salvage surgery and underwent forequarter amputation with anterosuperior chest wall resection and reconstruction.

survival, the sequence of administration (neoadjuvant or adjuvant) does not impact the gain in survival. Limb-salvage surgery after preoperative chemotherapy has become also the preferred local strategy for ESFT in most centers across the world, as an alternative to radiation therapy (Figure 42.6). Nevertheless, ESFT is exquisitely sensitive to radiotherapy and its role remains important in association with surgery to address contaminated margins, in large pelvic and axial lesions, and for local palliation of bone metastases. The surgical and reconstructive principles applied in high-grade bone sarcomas are essentially the same as for low-grade tumors. It is important to consider the advantages of surgery after induction chemotherapy (decreased tumor vascularity and down-staging) and disadvantages (higher risk of wound problems and deep infection due to the immunocompromised status of the patient). Optimization of the timing for surgery and perioperative chemotherapy administration to minimize surgical complications is therefore an important consideration in the overall patient management.

Radiotherapy

Radiotherapy is frequently considered as either an adjuvant to surgery in the management of bone sarcomas or as an upfront primary therapy in unresectable cases, although its role in the latter situation is limited in low-grade tumors and in osteosarcoma, where chemotherapy plays a much more important role.

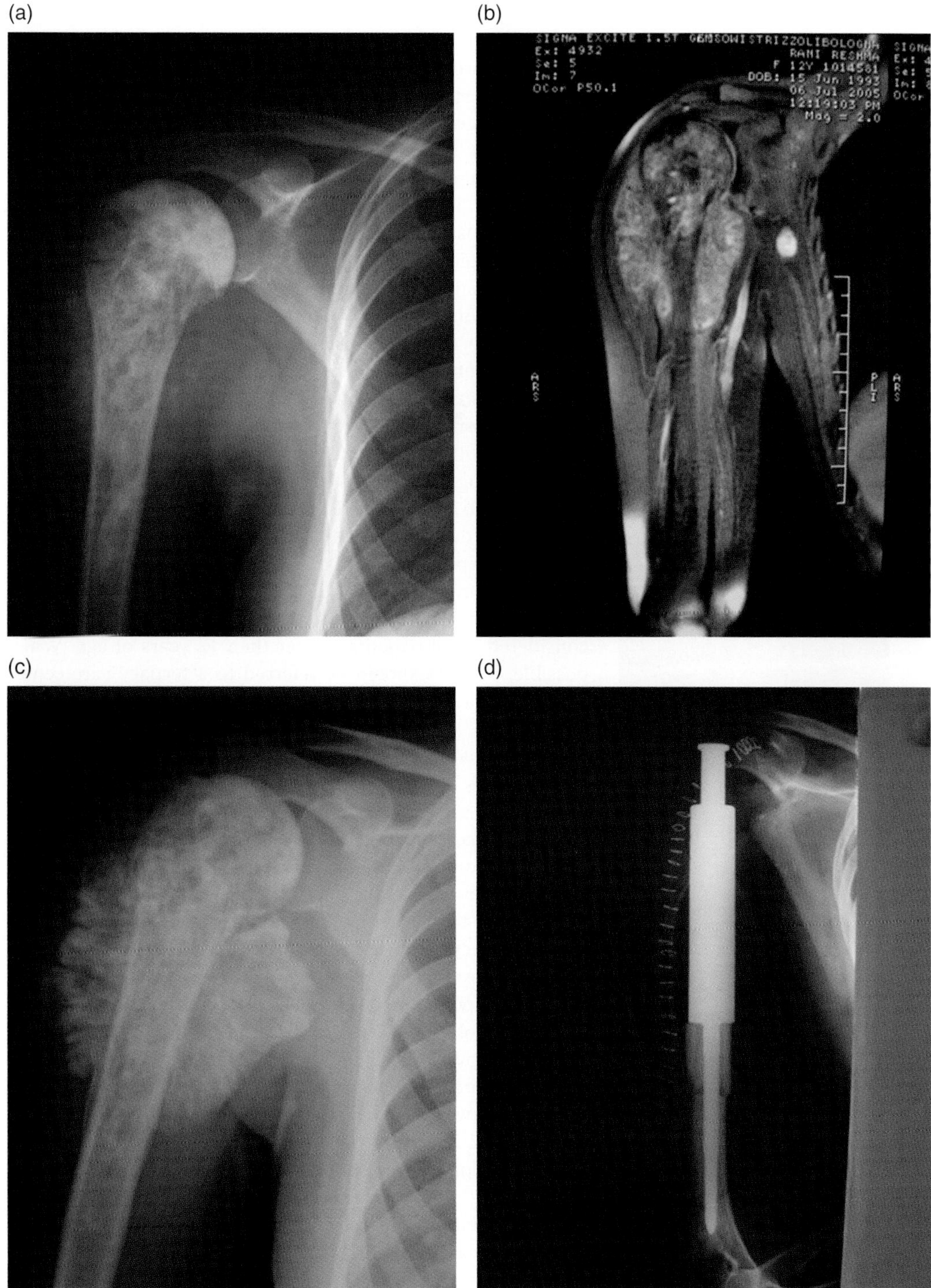

Figure 42.5 A 13-year-old boy with right proximal humerus high-grade osteosarcoma, with fuzzy limits and large soft tissue component at presentation (a). Following preoperative chemotherapy, extensive ossification (b) and delimitation of the lesion towards soft tissues has occurred (c), facilitating a difficult but possible *en bloc* excision of the proximal humerus and glenoid. This was reconstructed by a modular endoprosthesis (d).

Charged particle beams such as proton beam radiotherapy have long been utilized for the treatment of tumors of the axial skeleton such as chondrosarcomas, chordomas, and spine sarcomas [29,30]. Radiotherapy is considered definitive in the management of ESFT [10]. These small cell tumors are radiosensitive, and doses of irradiation of 45–55 Gy have been effective as primary local therapy. Radiotherapy is often recommended in lieu of surgery as local therapy for these tumors in cases where wide surgical resection would result in unacceptable loss of function or deformity [31]. Radiotherapy should especially be considered in resected tumors with positive margins. Long-term complications of radiotherapy may include soft tissue atrophy, bone necrosis, pathologic fracture, growth plate arrest with limb shortening in skeletally immature patients, soft tissue

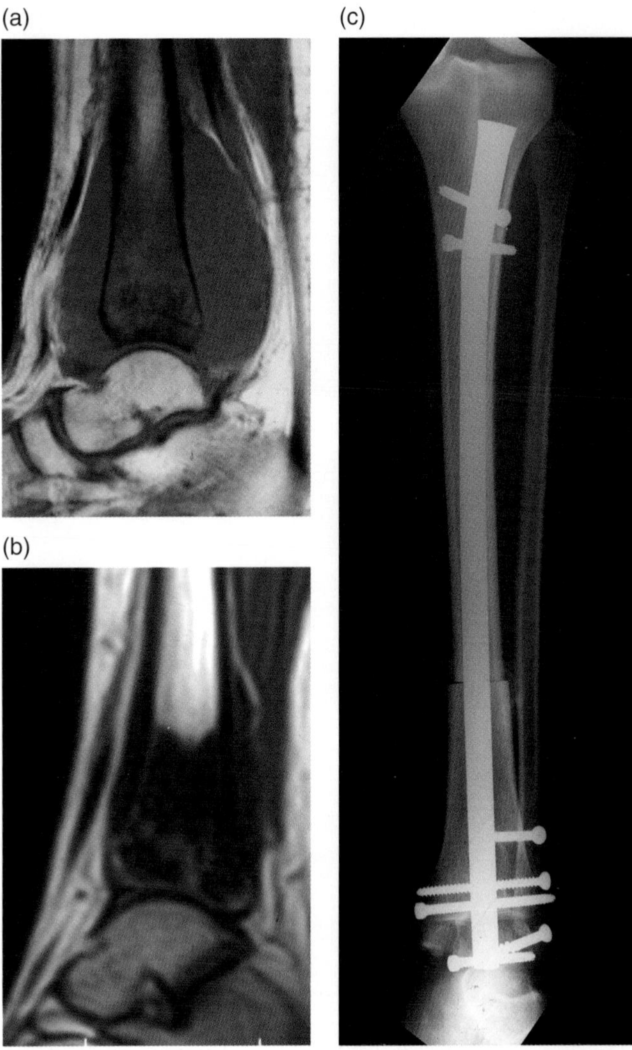

Figure 42.6 A 15-year-old girl with Ewing sarcoma of the left distal tibia. At presentation (a), there is significant soft tissue expansion visible on MRI. Dramatic response to preoperative chemotherapy (b), with substantial tumor shrinkage, particularly of the soft tissue component. Local management consisted of *en bloc* resection of the distal tibia and tibiotalar joint, followed by reconstruction with bone allograft and multiple fixation (c).

fibrosis, joint contracture, and secondary malignancies. Radiotherapy is frequently used to palliate metastases in many body sites. Both conventional and image-guided focal radiation can benefit patients who suffer from complications of metastases. High-dose focal radiotherapy in particular is emerging as an effective palliative modality for radioresistant tumors in the spine and offers benefit for patients with metastatic disease who have limited options for systemic treatment [32].

Chemotherapy

Bone sarcomas for which systemic chemotherapy is discussed here include ESFT, osteosarcoma, chondrosarcoma, chordoma, and giant cell tumors of bone. The treatment of ESFT and osteosarcoma in adults is extrapolated from the pediatric population where robust data from randomized studies are available in the management of these diseases and discussed in Chapter 47. There are few studies in adults to support this extrapolation and minimal retrospective data on the outcomes of adult patients with bone sarcomas treated with systemic chemotherapies [33]. In pediatric studies that include a wide age range of patients, increasing age is an adverse prognostic factor. In these studies, the benefits of systemic chemotherapies or dose intensity are seen in children younger than 15–18 years and less pronounced in older cohorts [34,35]. Similarly, in studies exploring dose-dense (2- vs 3-week) cycles with multiagent chemotherapies (e.g., vincristine, Adriamycin or doxorubicin, cyclophosphamide, ifosfamide and etoposide – VAC/IE:) the benefit was only seen in patients younger than 17 years of age, however the final conclusions do not reflect this subgroup analysis. Chondrosarcoma, chordoma, and giant cell tumor of bone are primarily seen in adults rather than children. Rare and more aggressive osteosarcoma subtypes such as osteosarcoma associated with Paget disease, small cell, dedifferentiated paraosteal, and high-grade surface variants are much more common in adults than in children. Since there are limited prospective or randomized data, treatment of adults with these tumors is often based on expert consensus guidelines such as those of the National Comprehensive Cancer Network [13,14]. Discussions about fertility preservation and timely referral should be considered in all patients greater than 12 years of age. When possible, patients should be referred to a tertiary care center with sarcoma expertise.

Osteosarcoma

As previously noted, in most cases low-grade osteosarcomas do not require systemic chemotherapy. In localized, high-grade osteosarcoma, the cure rate with surgery alone is less than 15–20%. Addition of multiagent chemotherapy in the neoadjuvant or adjuvant setting improves this cure rate to 50–75%, recognizing that outcomes are inferior in older patients as either a reflection of variant biology, comorbidities, or inability to receive dose-dense chemotherapy [14]. Factors that are associated with poor outcomes include older age, male sex, axial skeleton involvement, large tumor size, and poor response to chemotherapy [36]. Chemotherapy should be offered to all patients after careful consideration of comorbidities and risks of chemotherapy. The backbone of chemotherapy is a doublet of Adriamycin (doxorubicin at 60–75 mg/m^2) and cisplatin (90–120 mg/m^2) administered intravenously over several days, recognizing that there are several protocols with variable routes of administration and schedules. In pediatric protocols, the standard of care is a three-drug regimen with addition of high-dose methotrexate to Adriamycin and cisplatin. The role of high-dose methotrexate in adults is controversial. In adults, high-dose methotrexate can frequently result in delay in administering doublet due to slow clearance of methotrexate and resultant renal dysfunction, myelosuppression, and/or mucositis. In localized osteosarcoma, there is no survival difference on the sequence (neoadjuvant or adjuvant) of administering chemotherapy [37]. The advantages of chemotherapy in the neoadjuvant setting are the opportunity to gauge the effect of chemotherapy (degree of necrosis) in the resected tumor and increasing likelihood that the patient will be a candidate for limb-sparing surgery. Tumors with >90% necrosis ("good responders") have improved overall survival than those with <90% necrosis ("poor" responders) [14,36]. In an effort to improve survival outcomes in "poor" responders, various chemotherapies, notably ifosfamide and etoposide, have been used in the postoperative setting. In a large prospective, randomized EURAMOS-1 study in mostly pediatric patients, there was no improvement in survival with the addition of ifosfamide and etoposide to regimens for "poor" responders and, as expected, higher toxicities in the ifosfamide arm [38]. However, retrospective data from single institutions in adult patients suggested that addition of ifosfamide in "poor" responders improved outcomes [26,27,39]. In the metastatic setting, either at the time of initial presentation or at recurrence, active agents include doxorubicin, cisplatin, high-dose methotrexate, ifosfamide, gemcitabine, docetaxel, and the combination of oral sorafenib (a multi-tyrosine kinase inhibitor) and everolimus [14,40]. Surgery may be appropriate in select patients with a low burden of metastatic disease and who demonstrate durable disease stability [14].

Ewing Sarcoma Family of Tumors (ESFT)

There are very few studies that report on the outcomes of adult ESFT patients treated with chemotherapy. The treatment paradigm is 3–4 cycles of chemotherapy, followed by surgery for localized disease and additional chemotherapy for up to 17 cycles. ESFT are exquisitely sensitive to multiagent chemotherapy in both the localized and metastatic setting. Similar to high-grade osteosarcoma, ESFT are considered high grade and require multiregimen chemotherapy regardless of size. In localized disease, cure rates with surgery or radiation alone are less than 15% and increase to 70% with the addition of multiagent chemotherapy. Even in the metastatic setting this is a potentially curable disease, albeit spread limited to lung (stage IVA) has significantly better prognosis (30–50%) than involvement of other sites (stage IVB) where it is less than 10%. Similar to osteosarcoma, advancing age (>15 years), larger size, and axial/pelvic location are associated with worse outcomes. Chemotherapy for localized ESFT consists of vincristine, Adriamycin, cyclophosphamide (VAC) alternating with ifosfamide and etoposide (I/E) for up to 10–17 cycles [34]. Dactinomycin is substituted when the maximum dose of doxorubicin is reached. Adults rarely tolerate 17 cycles or a dose-intense regimen (2 vs 3 weeks) and treating oncologists arbitrarily consider 10–14 cycles as adequate. In contrast, in the metastatic setting, there was no advantage to alternating I/E with the three-drug regimen (VAC), using higher dose of alkylating agents, or dose intensification. The outcome of metastatic ESFT is poor. Other regimens besides VAC that have shown similar benefits are VAI (vincristine, Adriamycin, and ifosfamide) and VIDE (vincristine, ifosfamide, doxorubicin, and etoposide) [41,42]. Cyclophosphamide can have higher hematological toxicities while ifosfamide can have higher renal tubular dysfunction and therefore the choice of agents can be altered based on comorbidities. In select patients with a single site of relapse, surgery and/or radiation may be appropriate. When conventional agents fail, alternate regimens include combinations of temozolomide and irinotecan, cyclophosphamide and topotecan, and gemcitabine and docetaxel [43–45]. Early enrollment in clinical trials is critical. Agents currently being investigated include poly ADP ribose polymerase (PARP) inhibitors, insulin-like growth factor receptor-1 (IGF1R) inhibitors, and immune checkpoint inhibitors. Every effort should be made to enroll patients in appropriate clinical trials.

Chondrosarcoma

Chemotherapy is not effective in chondrosarcoma, particularly with conventional subtypes. The role of adjuvant chemotherapy is controversial in dedifferentiated and mesenchymal subtypes. Dedifferentiated chondrosarcoma is treated similarly to osteosarcoma with doxorubicin and cisplatin whereas mesenchymal chondrosarcoma is treated by EFST protocols with VAC/IE [46–49]. Chondrosarcoma is the subject of many clinical trials. Up-regulation of the Hedgehog signaling pathway led to studies with GDC-0449, a Hedgehog inhibitor, which were negative [50]. Clinical trials are ongoing with IDH1 and IDH2 inhibitors and VEGF inhibitors such as pazopanib. Clinical trials are strongly encouraged for patients who are considering systemic therapies.

Chordoma

Similar to chondrosarcoma, conventional chordomas are not sensitive to systemic chemotherapies and there may be marginal benefit in dedifferentiated chordoma [51,52]. In a phase 2 study with 9-nitro camptothecin, a topoisomerase inhibitor, only one out of 15 patients had a durable partial response and the drug was not determined to be active [53]. Up-regulation of platelet-derived growth factor receptors (PDGFR) led to a large phase 2 clinical trial with imatinib. Ten out of 51 chordoma patients with advanced disease treated with imatinib had some degree of tumor shrinkage and many had disease stability and decrease in PET avidity [54]. Small case series have shown benefit with the combination of imatinib and low-dose cisplatin, sirolimus, or everolimus. A prospective study of 27 patients treated with sorafenib showed one partial response and a median 12-month progression-free survival rate of 57% [55]. A handful of case reports showed activity with epidermal growth factor receptor (EGFR) inhibitors such as cetuximab, erlotinib, and gefitinib. A prospective trial with lapatinib showed no activity [56]. Several clinical trials targeting T brachyury and other molecular targets are currently ongoing. Clinical trials are strongly encouraged for patients who are considering systemic therapies.

Giant Cell Tumor of Bone

Localized disease can be effectively managed with serial arterial embolizations. Historically, both interferon and pegylated interferon have been used with some success. GCTB harbors cells that release receptor activator of nuclear factor κ-B ligand (RANKL) which then recruits other cells, and denosumab, a fully humanized monoclonal antibody against RANKL, showed promising activity in a small study where 86% of patients had benefit [57]. This led to a pivotal study involving 282 patients who had unresectable or resectable disease with severe surgical morbidity [58]. Denosumab induced tumor responses in 96% of patients and a significant number of patients did not undergo mutilating surgery. This led to approval of denosumab in GCTB by the US Food and Drug Administration. Denosumab has a long half-life and is a monthly injection that requires three weekly loading doses before reaching steady state levels. The optimal duration of treatment for GCTB remains to be defined.

Surveillance and Survivorship

Surveillance includes follow-up physical examination and imaging of the primary site and. if necessary. distant sites [14]. Lungs are the most common organ for distant metastases. Radiographic surveillance of bone tumors in the postoperative setting should be based on biological behavior, risk of recurrence (grade, size, site, margins), and duration of time after treatment. For example, conventional chordoma, paraosteal osteosarcoma, GCTB, and low-grade chondrosarcoma typically have local recurrence and thus extensive imaging of distant sites may not be useful. Meanwhile, ESFT and high-grade osteosarcoma have a higher propensity for distant metastases and will require more extensive surveillance. Imaging is performed every 2–4 months during the first 2 years and less frequently after that. ESFT and high-grade osteosarcoma require more frequent and longer follow-up given late recurrence. There are no surveillance tumor markers in bone sarcomas.

With advances in surgical, radiation, and chemotherapy the survival in patients with bone sarcoma has dramatically increased over the last four decades. With this gain, physicians need to pay attention to long-term consequences of treatment in survivors [59]. In the acute setting, patients suffer from both physical and psychological stress and report decreased health-related quality of life when compared to their peers. Compared to age-matched peers, survivors of bone tumors report acute psychological stress similar to post-traumatic stress disorder; however, these symptoms normalize with the passage of time (2–8 years). Attention to psychological care in the acute setting is essential. On the other hand, decrease in physical quality of life in the acute setting improves with time but never normalizes with that of peers. Patients report a variety of health issues such as loss of range of motion, weakness of extremity, diminished mineral density, chronic pain, and chemotherapy-induced infertility, neurotoxicity, and cardiac and renal impairment. Early referral to experts in physiatry and rehabilitation medicine, psychiatry, and subspecialty internal medicine is critical for the overall wellbeing of the patient in the short and long term [59].

Acknowledgement

We thank Bhavani Murugesan BA, JD, and Anita Krishnan PhD for editorial help and preparation of this manuscript.

References

1 SEER Cancer Statistics Factsheets. Bone and Joint Cancer. Bethesda, MD, National Cancer Institute.

2 American Academy of Orthopedic Surgeons. United States Bone and Joint Initiative: The Burden of Musculoskeletal Diseases in the United States. Rosemont, IL.

3 Ries LAG, Young J, Keel GE, *et al.* (eds). SEER Survival Monograph: Cancer Survival Among Adults: U.S. SEER Program, 1988-2001, Patient and Tumor Characteristics. Bethesda, MD: National Cancer Institute, SEER Program, NIH Pub. No. 07-6215, 2007.

4 Zhu L, McManus MM, Hughes DP. Understanding the biology of bone sarcoma from early initiating events through late events in metastasis and disease progression. *Front Oncol* 2013;3:230.

5 Kansara M, Teng MW, Smyth MJ, Thomas DM. Translational biology of osteosarcoma. *Nat Rev Cancer* 2014;14(11):722–35.

6 Flanagan AM, Delaney D, O'Donnell P. Benefits of molecular pathology in the diagnosis of musculoskeletal disease : Part II of a two-part review: bone tumors and metabolic disorders. *Skeletal Radiol* 2010;39(3):213–24.

7 Miller RW, Boice J, Curtis RE. Bone cancer. In: D Schottenfeld (ed.) *Cancer Epidemiology and Prevention*. New York: Oxford University Press, 2006.

8 Hameed M. Clinical applications of molecular markers in bone tumors. *Adv Anat Pathol* 2015;22(6):337–44.

9 Miettinen M, Wang Z, Lasota J, *et al.* Nuclear brachyury expression is consistent in chordoma, common in germ cell tumors and small cell carcinomas, and rare in other carcinomas and sarcomas: an immunohistochemical study of 5229 cases. *Am J Surg Pathol* 2015;39(10):1305–12.

10 Gaspar N, Hawkins DS, Dirksen U, *et al.* Ewing sarcoma: current management and future approaches through collaboration. *J Clin Oncol* 2015;33(27):3036–46.

11 Isakoff MS, Bielack SS, Meltzer P, Gorlick R. Osteosarcoma: current treatment and a collaborative pathway to success. *J Clin Oncol* 2015;3(27):3029–35.

12 Morley N, Omar I. Imaging evaluation of musculoskeletal tumors. *Cancer Treat Res* 2014;162:9–29.

13 Biermann JS. Updates in the treatment of bone cancer. *J Natl Compr Canc Netw* 2013;11(5 Suppl): 681–3.

14 Biermann JS, Adkins DR, Aquinik M, *et al.* Bone cancer. *J Natl Compr Canc Netw* 2013;11(6):688–723.

15 Bernstein M, Kovar H, Paulussen M, *et al.* Ewing's sarcoma family of tumors: current management. *Oncologist* 2006;11(5):503–19.

16 Gelderblom H, Hogendoorn PC, Dijsktra SD, *et al.* The clinical approach towards chondrosarcoma. *Oncologist* 2008; 13(3):320–9.

17 Simon MA, Biermann JS. Biopsy of bone and soft-tissue lesions. *J Bone Joint Surg Am* 1993;75(4):616–21.

18 Campanacci M, Mercuri M, Gamberini G. Biopsy. *Chir Organi Mov* 1995;80(2):113–23.

19 Mankin HJ, Mankin CJ, Simon MA. The hazards of the biopsy, revisited. Members of the Musculoskeletal Tumor Society. *J Bone Joint Surg Am* 1996;78(5):656–63.

20 Gogna A, Peh WC, Munk PL. Image-guided musculoskeletal biopsy. *Radiol Clin North Am* 2008;46(3):455–73, v.

21 Hau A, Kim I, Kattapuram S, et al. Accuracy of CT-guided biopsies in 359 patients with musculoskeletal lesions. *Skeletal Radiol* 2002;31(6):349–53.

22 Yang YJ, Damron TA. Comparison of needle core biopsy and fine-needle aspiration for diagnostic accuracy in musculoskeletal lesions. *Arch Pathol Lab Med* 2004;128(7):759–64.

23 Edge SB, American Joint Committee on Cancer. *AJCC Cancer Staging Manual*, 7th edn. New York: Springer, 2010: xiv, 648 p.

24 Enneking WF, Spanier SS, Goodman MA. A system for the surgical staging of musculoskeletal sarcoma. 1980. *Clin Orthop Relat Res* 2003;(415):4–18.

25 Meyers PA, Heller G, Healey J, *et al.* Chemotherapy for nonmetastatic osteogenic sarcoma: the Memorial Sloan-Kettering experience. *J Clin Oncol* 1992;10(1):5–15.

26 Bacci G, Ferrari S, Bertoni F, *et al.* Long-term outcome for patients with nonmetastatic osteosarcoma of the extrmity treated at the istituto ortopedico rizzoli according to the istituto ortopedico rizzoli/osteosarcoma-2 protocol: an updated report. *J Clin Oncol* 2000;18(24):4016–27.

27 Bacci G, Forni C, Longhi A, *et al.* Local recurrence and local control of non-metastatic osteosarcoma of the extremities: a 27-year experience in a single institution. *J Surg Oncol* 2007;96(2):118–23.

28 Wunder JS, Paulian G, Huvos AG, *et al.* The histological response to chemotherapy as a predictor of the oncological outcome of operative treatment of Ewing sarcoma. *J Bone Joint Surg Am* 1998;80(7):1020–33.

29 DeLaney TF, Liebsch NJ, Pedlow FX, *et al.* Phase II study of high-dose photon/proton radiotherapy in the management of spine sarcomas. *Int J Radiat Oncol Biol Phys* 2009;74(3):732–9.

30 DeLaney TF, Liebsch NJ, Pedlow FX, *et al.* Long-term results of Phase II study of high dose photon/proton radiotherapy in the management of spine chordomas, chondrosarcomas, and other sarcomas. *J Surg Oncol* 2014;110(2):115–22.

31 Schuck A, Ahrens S, von Schorlemer I, *et al.* Radiotherapy in Ewing tumors of the vertebrae: treatment results and local relapse analysis of the CESS 81/86 and EICESS 92 trials. *Int J Radiat Oncol Biol Phys* 2005;63(5):1562–7.

32 Levine AM, Coleman C, Horasek S. Stereotactic radiosurgery for the treatment of primary sarcomas and sarcoma metastases of the spine. *Neurosurgery* 2009;64(2 Suppl):A54–9.

33 Longhi A, Errani C, Gonzales-Arabio D, Ferrari C, Mercuri M. Osteosarcoma in patients older than 65 years. *J Clin Oncol* 2008;26(33):5368–73.

34 Grier HE, Krailo MD, Tarbell NJ, *et al.* Addition of ifosfamide and etoposide to standard chemotherapy for Ewing's sarcoma and primitive neuroectodermal tumor of bone. *N Engl J Med* 2003;348(8):694–701.

35 Womer RB, West DC, Krailo MD, *et al.* Randomized controlled trial of interval-compressed chemotherapy for the treatment of localized Ewing sarcoma: a report from the Children's Oncology Group. *J Clin Oncol* 2012;30(33):4148–54.

36 Bielack SS, Kempf-Bielack B, Delling G, *et al.* Prognostic factors in high-grade osteosarcoma of the extremities or trunk: an analysis of 1,702 patients treated on neoadjuvant cooperative osteosarcoma study group protocols. *J Clin Oncol* 2002;20(3):776–90.

37 Goorin AM, Schwartzentruber DJ, Devidas M, *et al.* Presurgical chemotherapy compared with immediate surgery and adjuvant chemotherapy for nonmetastatic osteosarcoma: Pediatric Oncology Group Study POG-8651. *J Clin Oncol* 2003;21(8):1574–80.

38 Marina NS, Smeland S, Bielack SS, *et al.* *MAPIE vs MAP as postoperative chemotherapy in patients with a poor response to preoperative chemotherapy for newly-diagnosed osteosarcoma: results from EURAMOS-1 (Paper 032).* Berlin: Connective Tissue Oncology Society (CTOS), 2014.

39 Benjamin RS, Patel SR. Pediatric and adult osteosarcoma: comparisons and contrasts in presentation and therapy. *Cancer Treat Res* 2009;152:355–63.

40 Grignani G, Palmerini E, Ferraresi V, *et al.* Sorafenib and everolimus for patients with unresectable high-grade osteosarcoma progressing after standard treatment: a non-randomised phase 2 clinical trial. *Lancet Oncol* 2015;16(1):98–107.

41 Paulussen M, Craft AW, Lewis I, *et al.* Results of the EICESS-92 Study: two randomized trials of Ewing's sarcoma treatment—cyclophosphamide compared with ifosfamide in standard-risk patients and assessment of benefit of etoposide added to standard treatment in high-risk patients. *J Clin Oncol* 2008;26:4385–93.

42 Le Deley MC, Paulussen M, Lewis I, *et al.* Cyclophosphamide compared with ifosfamide in consolidation treatment of standard-risk Ewing sarcoma: results of the randomized noninferiority Euro-EWING99-R1 trial. *J Clin Oncol* 2014;32(23):2440–8.

43 Casey DA, Wexler LH, Merchant MS, *et al.* Irinotecan and temozolomide for Ewing sarcoma: the Memorial Sloan-Kettering experience. *Pediatr Blood Cancer* 2009;53(6):1029–34.

44 Fox E, Patel S, Wathen JK, *et al.* Phase II study of sequential gemcitabine followed by docetaxel for recurrent Ewing sarcoma, osteosarcoma, or unresectable or locally recurrent chondrosarcoma: results of Sarcoma Alliance for Research Through Collaboration Study 003. *Oncologist* 2012;17(3):321.

45 Hunold A, Weddeling N, Paulussen M, *et al.* Topotecan and cyclophosphamide in patients with refractory or relapsed Ewing tumors. *Pediatr Blood Cancer* 2006;47(6):795–800.

46 Dickey ID, Rose PS, Fuchs B, *et al.* Dedifferentiated chondrosarcoma: the role of chemotherapy with updated outcomes. *J Bone Joint Surg Am* 2004;86-A(11):2412–8.

47 Grimer RJ, Gosheger G, Taminiau A, *et al.* Dedifferentiated chondrosarcoma: prognostic factors and outcome from a European group. *Eur J Cancer* 2007;43(14):2060–5.

48 Mitchell AD, Ayoub K, Mangham DC, *et al.* Experience in the treatment of dedifferentiated chondrosarcoma. *J Bone Joint Surg Br* 2000;82(1):55–61.

49 Cesari M, Bertoni F, Bacchini P, *et al.* Mesenchymal chondrosarcoma. An analysis of patients treated at a single institution. *Tumori* 2007;93(5):423–7.

50 Italiano A, Le Cesne A, Bellera C, *et al.* GDC-0449 in patients with advanced chondrosarcomas: a French Sarcoma Group/US and French National Cancer Institute Single-Arm Phase II Collaborative Study. *Ann Oncol* 2013;24(11):2922–6.

51 Yamada Y, Gounder M, Laufer I. Multidisciplinary management of recurrent chordomas. *Curr Treat Options Oncol* 2013;14(3):442–53.

52 Stacchiotti S, Sommer J, Chordoma Global Consensus Group. Building a global consensus approach to chordoma: a position paper from the medical and patient community. *Lancet Oncol* 2015;16(2):e71–83.

53 Chugh R, Dunn R, Zalupski MM, *et al.* Phase II study of 9-nitro-camptothecin in patients with advanced chordoma or soft tissue sarcoma. *J Clin Oncol* 2005;23(15):3597–604.

54 Stacchiotti S, Longhi A, Ferraresi V, *et al.* Phase II study of imatinib in advanced chordoma. *J Clin Oncol* 2012;30(9):914–20.

55 Amela E, Bompas E, Le Cesne A, *et al.* A phase II trial of sorafenib (SO) in advanced chordoma patients (pt). ASCO Annual Meeting 2015, Chicago.

56 Stacchiotti S, Tamborini E, Lo Vullo S, *et al.* Phase II study on lapatinib in advanced EGFR-positive chordoma. *Ann Oncol* 2013;24(7):1931–6.

57 Thomas D, Henshaw R, Skubitz K, *et al.* Denosumab in patients with giant-cell tumour of bone: an open-label, phase 2 study. *Lancet Oncol* 2010;11(3):275–80.

58 Chawla S, Henshaw R, Seeger L, *et al.* Safety and efficacy of denosumab for adults and skeletally mature adolescents with giant cell tumour of bone: interim analysis of an open-label, parallel-group, phase 2 study. *Lancet Oncol* 2013;14(9):901–8.

59 Greene M, Kobierska M, Kent PM, Piasecki P. Survivorship in young patients with bone cancer. *Curr Probl Cancer* 2013;37(4):236–43.

43

Sarcoma of Soft Tissue

Mrinal Gounder[1], Vinod Ravi[2], Yoshiya Yamada[1], Richard Carvajal[3], and Aimee Crago[1]

[1] *Memorial Sloan Kettering Cancer Center and Weill Cornell Medical College, New York, New York, USA*
[2] *The University of Texas MD Anderson Cancer Center, Houston, Texas, USA*
[3] *Columbia University Medical Center, Herbert Irving Comprehensive Cancer Center, New York, New York, USA*

Incidence and Mortality

Statistical data regarding soft tissue sarcomas are compiled by the National Cancer Institute's Surveillance, Epidemiology, and End Results (SEER) Program in the category of "soft tissue (including heart)" cancer, which includes several types of cancer originating in soft tissue, retroperitoneum and peritoneum, pleura, heart and mediastinum, and spleen [1,2]. Most, but not all, of the cancers in this category are sarcomas. The most common histologies of soft tissue sarcomas are "sarcoma, not otherwise specified" (20.6%), liposarcoma (16.8%), leiomyosarcoma (13.3%), fibrosarcoma (7.6%), and malignant fibrous histiocytoma (7.4%) [2]. Soft tissue cancer represents only 0.7% of all new cancer diagnoses; approximately 12,390 new cases occur in the United States (US) annually. There are approximately 4,990 deaths from STS annually, representing 0.8% of all deaths from cancer in the US [1]. The incidence rate of STS, overall based on cases diagnosed in 2009–2013, was approximately 3.4 per 100,000 per year. During the same time period, the age-adjusted death rate was 1.3 per 100,000 per year. The median ages at diagnosis and at death for this category were 59 years and 65 years, respectively [2].

Etiology

While sarcomas are classified according to their connective tissue of origin, it is not known whether the normal cells or mesenchymal stem cells give rise to the neoplastic component; the latter are strongly favored, however. To illustrate this, most rhabdomyosarcomas arise in locations that do not have skeletal muscle. Similarly, well-differentiated and dedifferentiated liposarcoma reside in the same tissue and have similar molecular signatures, however it is unclear whether dedifferentiated liposarcoma is a clonal evolution of well-differentiated liposarcoma or represents a unique entity. In about 20% of STS, the cell of origin cannot be determined despite extensive immunohistochemical or molecular analysis [3]. Most sarcomas are sporadic, and genetic or environmental causes have been identified in only a minority of histologies [3].

Ionizing Radiation

External radiotherapy has been associated with an increased incidence of soft tissue sarcomas in several sites, although the absolute risk appears to be relatively low. The excess incidence associated with radiotherapy is greater among survivors of childhood cancers, especially those with genetic syndromes (such as hereditary retinoblastoma which is associated with the *RB1* gene) that may increase susceptibility to radiation-associated sarcomagenesis (RAS) [4]. Although there is no well-established definition of a RAS, several factors are necessary to make the diagnosis. The sarcoma should arise in an area of previous radiation, the histology of the new lesion should be different than the originally treated tumor, and there should typically be an interval of about 3 years between the initial course of radiation and the development of a new tumor [5,6]. Malignant fibrous histiocytoma or undifferentiated pleomorphic sarcoma (MFH/UPS), angiosarcoma, and leiomyosarcoma (LMS) are the most common RAS, typically seen with radiation for breast cancers, head and neck cancers, and in hereditary retinoblastoma survivors [6].

Chemical Exposures

A recent review interpreted current evidence as suggestive of associations between STS risk and exposure to chlorophenols and certain herbicides (especially in an occupational setting) and emissions from industrial waste incinerators [7,8]. Other case control studies have not found a strong association.

Chronic Lymphedema

Chronic lymphedema is a predisposing factor to angiosarcoma which is classically seen in women who have undergone radical mastectomy for breast carcinoma and termed Stewart–Treves syndrome. In areas where filarial infections are endemic,

The American Cancer Society's Oncology in Practice: Clinical Management, First Edition. Edited by The American Cancer Society.

lymphangiosarcoma is a rare complication of filarial lymphedema. The mechanisms of vascular and lymphatic stasis and subsequent development of lymphangiosarcoma are not understood, however amplification of c-Myc has been noted.

Trauma

There are anecdotal reports that blunt trauma or surgical incision can incite STS. Many patients with newly diagnosed STS report a recent history of trauma but there is no evidence supporting trauma as the inciting factor [3,9]. Most likely, traumatic episodes bring attention to a specific body part and subsequent imaging and examination brings attention to an asymptomatic lesion. For example, trauma or surgery is often cited as an inciting factor for aggressive fibromatosis or desmoid tumors. However, discovery of recurrent somatic *CTNNB1* (encoding β-catenin) mutations and *APC* mutations in sporadic and FAP-associated desmoids weakens the link between desmoid tumors and trauma. A Scandinavian study of 100,000 patients undergoing total hip or knee replacements did not report higher incidence of sarcoma at the surgical or nonsurgical site [9].

Genetic Syndromes

Several genetic syndromes predispose affected individuals to various types of STS. STS associated with genetic syndromes account for <3% of all cases. These include type 1 neurofibromatosis (NF1) with malignant peripheral nerve sheath tumors and gastrointestinal stromal tumors (GIST), Li–Fraumeni syndrome (*TP53* or *CHEK2*) with rhabdomyosarcoma and other soft tissue sarcomas [10], familial GIST with germline mutation in *KIT or PDGFR* [11], Carney–Stratakis syndrome and GIST with mutations in succinate dehydrogenase (*SDHB*) [12], familial adenomatous polyposis/Gardner syndrome (*APC*) with desmoid tumors [13], hereditary retinoblastoma (*RB1*) with fibrosarcoma, Werner syndrome/adult progeria (*WRN*) with various soft tissue sarcomas, Gorlin syndrome/nevoid basal cell carcinoma syndrome (*PTCH1*) and rhabdomyosarcoma, tuberous sclerosis complex (*TSC1* and *TSC2*) with malignant perivascular epithelioid cell tumors and chordoma [14]. Next-generation sequencing (NGS) of sarcoma patients identified novel germline mutations in genes involved in homologous repair pathways such as *ERCC2, ATM, ATR,* and *BRCA2.* Interestingly, not all patients who were identified as having germline mutations by NGS were identified by traditional methods such as careful family history obtained by genetic counselors, underscoring the evolving importance of NGS platforms for patient management [15].

Clinical Presentation

Anatomic, Age, and Gender Distribution

Soft tissue sarcomas may develop from any site in the body. The most common locations are extremities (40%), intra-abdominal (35%), trunk (10%), head and neck (5%), and other (10%) [3,16]. The incidence of STS increases with age, with a median age at diagnosis of 65 years. Certain histologies such as Ewing, rhabdomyosarcoma, and osteosarcoma predominate in children and adolescents while synovial sarcoma, desmoid tumors, and desmoplastic small round cell tumor (DSRCT) primarily occur at a median age of 30 years. STS which have recurrent, nonrandom chromosomal translocations present earlier, in the third and fourth decades of life, while tumors with complex genomic aberrations present later in life. STS occurs equally between both genders; however a few exceptions include DSRCT which predominate in young men (9:1), Kaposi sarcoma in men, desmoid tumors in women (2:1), and angiosarcoma in women secondary to radiation and/or lymphedema for the treatment of breast carcinoma.

Natural History and Patterns of Failure

The natural history of STS is widely variable and dependent on the histology, grade, tumor size, and anatomic location. A comprehensive discussion is beyond the scope of this chapter. STS grow centrifugally along the longitudinal axis, causing compression of surrounding normal structures [3,16]. Certain STS develop a pseudocapsule from a nonspecific, inflammatory reaction. However, at microscopic evaluation finger-like projections are often found breaching the pseudocapsule and invading normal tissue. When possible, a wide surgical resection with negative margins is attempted with consideration for additional neoadjuvant or adjuvant radiation to decrease risk of local recurrence. Tumors are categorized as benign (nonrecurrent), intermediate (locally aggressive, rarely metastasizing), and malignant. High-grade malignant tumors metastasize at an overall rate of 20%, increasing to 50% when the tumor size is greater than 5 cm. Curiously, even within a particular histology there may be subtypes with wide clinical behaviors. For instance, liposarcoma has four different subtypes (well-differentiated, dedifferentiated, myxoid/round cell, and pleomorphic) with widely different natural history, treatment, and prognostic outcomes. Benign lesions such as lipoma or leiomyoma do not invade local structures, recur after surgical resection, or metastasize. Examples of intermediate STS that can occasionally metastasize include solitary fibrous tumors, myxofibrosarcoma, and well-differentiated liposarcoma. For intermediate-grade tumors, the overall rate of metastases is 3%, increasing to greater than 20% when the size exceeds 5 cm. For example, desmoid tumors are intermediate, locally aggressive tumors that often recur after surgical resection but have no metastatic potential. Hematogenous spread accounts for distant metastases with lung being the most common site of metastases (50%) followed by liver, bone/spine, skin, and peritoneum. Metastases to brain are extremely uncommon with the exception of advanced alveolar soft part sarcoma and angiosarcoma [3]. Myxoid liposarcoma has a unique propensity to metastasize to the spine. Lymphatic spread accounts for 2% of overall metastases, however certain histologies prefer this route including clear cell sarcoma (28%), epithelioid sarcoma (23%), angiosarcoma (12%), synovial sarcoma (12%), and rhabdomyosarcoma (12%) [17].

Workup and Staging

Diagnosis

Most STS arise in the extremities and patients often describe a slow-growing painless mass and less frequently a localized painful swelling [16]. Retroperitoneal (15%) and visceral (15%)

sarcomas can present with vague abdominal pain or increase in abdominal girth. Laboratory studies including tumor markers are not helpful. For extremity, head and neck, and pelvic lesions, magnetic resonance imaging (MRI) provides excellent visualization of neurovascular structures, muscle, bone, and fascial planes. For truncal, visceral, and retroperitoneal structures, computed tomography (CT) of chest, abdomen, and pelvis with contrast (when possible) provides high-quality images of the primary tumor and also serves for staging studies. CT of the lung (preferred over X-ray) should be part of initial staging as this is the most common site for metastatic spread. MRI of the thorax and abdomen may be limited by movement artifacts. Imaging of the brain should be performed if clinically indicated. A total spine MRI is indicated in myxoid/round cell liposarcoma. Positron emission tomography (PET) scans are useful when the above modalities do not provide adequate staging information. PET may also be useful in the neoadjuvant setting where a difference in maximum standardized uptake value (SUV max) of greater than 35% is correlated with chemotherapy response and improved recurrence-free survival (RFS).

Biopsy Considerations

The histology of extremity lesions varies widely and, in patients with a subset of sarcoma histologies, multimodality treatment is necessary to optimize outcomes; patients with certain types of STS may benefit from neoadjuvant chemotherapy or radiation. For this reason, most extremity tumors are biopsied prior to surgery. Exceptions to this rule include tumors consistent with well-differentiated liposarcoma on imaging or small (<2 to 3 cm in diameter), superficial lesions. The former have a pathognomonic appearance on CT and MRI (atypical lipomatous tissue with enhancing septa), obviating the need for biopsy, and the latter can be managed with excision alone [18].

In cases where biopsy of a soft tissue lesion is performed, it is essential that this procedure is carefully planned to minimize complications and to facilitate definitive treatment of a sarcoma. At the time of surgical resection, the biopsy site should ideally be resected *en bloc* with the specimen, and placement of the biopsy tract can significantly affect the ease with which this can be accomplished. Soft tissue tumors of the extremity were historically sampled with incisional biopsy. When performing a biopsy in this manner, care is taken to orient the incision along the axis of the limb to facilitate subsequent resection. Excision of an improperly, transversely-oriented scar *en bloc* with the specimen often requires removal of large islands of skin, preventing primary closure and necessitating reconstruction with a skin graft or soft tissue flap.

Because core biopsy is a less invasive procedure, most sarcoma specialists have transitioned from routine use of incisional biopsy for preoperative diagnosis of a soft tissue lesion. Analysis of core biopsies that are evaluated by an experienced pathologist demonstrated that samples obtained in this manner can be used to accurately determine both tumor histology and grade (75 and 88%, respectively) [19]. When this method of biopsy is chosen, multiple cores should be obtained from each quadrant of the tumor and the biopsy needle, as in the case of incisional biopsy, should be inserted through the skin at the site of the planned incision. When image guidance is necessary to safely perform the biopsy, direct communication between the surgeon and interventional radiologist regarding planned surgical incision can greatly facilitate proper placement of the biopsy site.

Biopsy is not always required prior to resection of retroperitoneal sarcomas; the lesions are almost universally either well- or dedifferentiated liposarcomas or leiomyosarcomas. When primary management of these tumors would be surgery, biopsy can be deferred in the context of characteristic imaging findings interpreted by an experienced radiologist. As in the extremity, well-differentiated and dedifferentiated liposarcomas are associated with regions of abnormal-appearing fat, often with enhancing septa and, in the case of dedifferentiated lesions, a solid component. If abnormal fat is not visualized on imaging, a heterogeneous, solid mass in the retroperitoneum most likely represents leiomyosarcoma, particularly when associated with the inferior vena cava or if localized to the region of the gonadal vein (generally just below the kidney). Rarely, large retroperitoneal tumors may represent lymphoma, carcinoma (renal cell, adrenal), metastatic disease, or neurogenic tumor (schwannoma or malignant peripheral nerve sheath tumor), and if the differential diagnosis includes these entities, image-guided biopsy should be performed.

Pathology

There are over 50 different histological subtypes of STS. Due to the considerable histopathological heterogeneity and rarity of STS, consultation by an expert pathologist familiar with these rare tumors is a critical first step in treatment planning. Prognosis, clinical course, and sensitivity to systemic therapy may be dependent on identifying the specific histological subtype of STS. The process of classification of sarcomas into various subtypes is based on identification of specific architectural, cytoplasmic, and nuclear characteristics that give clues to the type of connective tissue that the tumor most closely resembles. The resemblance to a normal connective tissue counterpart does not imply that the cell of origin is a mature connective tissue cell; in fact, current research suggests that sarcomas develop from primitive multipotential mesenchymal stem cells and may or may not differentiate towards a particular lineage that enables classification. Tumors that lack specific features of any particular connective tissue are often classified as unclassified sarcoma. Tumors that bear features of a particular connective tissue are classified as such: for example, tumors with features of smooth muscle are classified as leiomyosarcoma, those with features of adipose tissue are classified as liposarcoma, while those with features of cartilage are classified as chondrosarcoma, and so on. Light microscopy, immunohistochemistry, and cytogenetics are widely used to establish the pathological diagnosis. Identification of the lineage of differentiation is often a difficult task and results in differences in opinion regarding the pathological diagnosis in as high as 40% of patients, even among expert pathologists. The presence of specific clonal abnormalities of chromosome number or arrangement for certain sarcoma subtypes is often immensely useful for arriving at a specific pathological diagnosis. Characteristic translocations such as t(11;22)(q24;q12) in Ewing sarcomas, t(12;16)(q13–14;p11) in myxoid liposarcomas, t(X;18)(p11.2;q11.2) in synovial sarcoma, and so on are exceptionally useful in establishing a diagnosis of translocation-related sarcomas which account for about-one third of all sarcomas. Molecular pathology is therefore expected to play an increasing role in establishing the pathological diagnosis, predicting response to therapy, and aiding prognostication [20,21].

In addition to histologic typing, grading is extremely helpful in evaluating the degree of malignancy and is derived from multiple histologic parameters. When the diagnosis is being established from a core needle biopsy, bias introduced by preferential sampling of a heterogeneous tumor should always be considered. Grade has considerable value in predicting metastases and overall survival. Grading should not be used separate from histologic type as different histologic subtypes with the same grade can have very different risks of metastasis.

Staging

Staging of a sarcoma provides information regarding the extent of disease and has an impact on treatment planning and determining prognosis. The most commonly used model is the American Joint Committee on Cancer (AJCC) staging system that incorporates tumor size (T), grade (G), nodal status (N), and presence of metastatic disease (M). The Eighth Edition of this system has been published and can be used by clinicians to support patient care decisions starting in January 2017. The Eighth Edition definitions for the various T, N, and M categories for trunk and extremity STSare outlined in Table 43.1 and stage grouping by combination of the above-mentioned factors is outlined in Table 43.2 [22]. The Eighth Edition also includes different T categories for STS of the head and neck and for those of the abdomen and visceral organs, but prognostic stage groupings have not been developed for these sites.

Nodal metastases are unusual among STS and occur in 3–5% of cases. However, these patients have better survival compared to patients with hematogenous metastases and are thus classified as stage III. Notable exceptions for nodal involvement are rhabdomyosarcoma, synovial, clear cell, vascular, and epithelioid sarcomas. Grade (based on mitotic count, necrosis, and differentiation) is a strong predictor of metastatic potential. Patients with low- (G1), intermediate- (G2), and high- (G3) grade sarcoma have 5-year metastasis-free survival of 91–98%, 71–85%, and 44–64%, respectively. Size is an independent predictor of metastasis.

The heterogeneity of sarcomas makes it challenging to develop a system that accurately prognosticates survival. While stage is correlated with survival, several additional variables are incorporated in a nomogram derived from a prospectively maintained database at Memorial Sloan Kettering Cancer Center (MSKCC) that predicts the 12-year risk of sarcoma-specific death in the postoperative setting. This nomogram captures the different variables that predict local and distant recurrence risks and disease-specific mortality. For example, local recurrence is predicted by margin status, age (>50), local recurrence at presentation, and histology (fibrosarcoma or malignant peripheral nerve sheath) while the distant recurrence is predicted by high grade, size >5 cm, depth, local recurrence at presentation, and histology (leiomyosarcoma and non-liposarcoma) [23].

Table 43.1 Primary tumor (T), regional lymph node (N), and distant metastasis (M) category definitions for trunk and extremity soft tissue sarcomas [22]. Used with permission of the American College of Surgeons, Chicago, Illinois. The original source for this information is the AJCC Cancer Staging Manual, Eighth Edition (2016), which is published by Springer Science + Business Media.

Definition of primary tumor (T)	
T category	**T criteria**
TX	Primary tumor cannot be assessed
T0	No evidence of primary tumor
T1	Tumor 5 cm or less in greatest dimension
T2	Tumor more than 5 cm and less than or equal to 10 cm in greatest dimension
T3	Tumor more than 10 cm and less than or equal to 15 cm in greatest dimension
T4	Tumor more than 15 cm in greatest dimension
Definition of regional lymph node (N)	
N category	**N criteria**
N0	No regional lymph node metastasis or unknown lymph node status
N1	Regional lymph node metastasis
Definition of distant metastasis (M)	
M category	**M criteria**
M0	No distant metastasis
M1	Distant metastasis

Table 43.2 AJCC Prognostic Stage Groups for trunk and extremity soft tissue sarcomas [22]. Used with permission of the American College of Surgeons, Chicago, Illinois. The original source for this information is the AJCC Cancer Staging Manual, Eighth Edition (2016), which is published by Springer Science + Business Media.

When T is...	And N is...	And M is...	And grade is...	Then the stage group is...
T1	N0	M0	G1, GX	IA
T2, T3, T4	N0	M0	G1, GX	IB
T1	N0	M0	G2, G3	II
T2	N0	M0	G2, G3	IIIA
T3, T4	N0	M0	G2, G3	IIIB
Any T	N1	M0	Any G	IV
Any T	Any N	M1	Any G	IV

Primary Multimodality Treatment for Nonmetastatic Disease

Surgery

Historically, surgical resection of an STS in the extremity meant amputation of the affected limb. Randomized controlled trials have demonstrated that while this approach may minimize local recurrences, overall survival is not compromised if these tumors are managed by wide excision and selective use of radiation therapy [24]. For this reason, limb-salvage procedures are routinely employed in the management of extremity sarcomas. Fewer than 10% of patients will ultimately require amputation and in most cases this is associated with local recurrence.

Wide local excision forms the basis of the limb-sparing procedure. Unlike melanoma, STS rarely metastasizes to the lymph nodes, and surgery to evaluate the nodal basin is not required [17]. Surgery is performed with the intention of removing the sarcoma *en bloc* with the biopsy site and at least 1 cm margin of normal tissue (or fascial plane) circumferentially. The margin of normal tissue is necessary because despite the fact that many lesions appear to be well-encapsulated, microscopic disease can extend beyond this visible "pseudocapsule." It is essential to know the histologic subtype of the STS prior to planning surgical resection as in cases of dermatofibrosarcoma protuberans and myxofibrosarcoma microscopic disease can actually extend farther than 1 cm from the center of gross disease. These tumors have infiltrative borders and should be removed, when possible, with 2 cm of normal tissue circumferentially to minimize the need for re-excision [25–27]. In planning surgery for myxofibrosarcoma, it is also important to remember that this lesion can infiltrate across fascial boundaries, and in superficial lesions, unlike in surgery for other histologic subtypes, underlying muscle not just fascia should be taken with the specimen.

The surgeon may be limited in his or her ability to obtain wide margins if an STS is located directly adjacent to bone or neurovascular bundles. In this instance, the morbidity of resecting the nerve, artery, vein, or bone is not justified. Instead, the tumor should be resected by carefully skeletonizing these structures off the lesion, and radiation used as an adjunct to minimize local recurrence. Skeletonization should include removal of the neurovascular sheath, perineurium, or periosteum to optimize the margin. Encasement of neurovascular structures by a soft tissue tumor may make skeletonization difficult or impossible. When major nerves, arteries, and veins pass through a low-grade lesion, the sarcoma should be bivalved to preserve these structures (e.g., femoral or sciatic nerve, superficial femoral artery or vein). This is not feasible when the nerve, artery, and/or vein are encased by a high-grade sarcoma, however, and in these instances involved components of the neurovascular bundle should be resected with the tumor. In these situations, postoperative physical therapy can assist patients in learning to compensate for loss of femoral or ulnar nerves. Bracing can be used to assist with foot drop or radial nerve palsy [28]. Arterial bypass is performed if a major artery is resected (e.g., superficial femoral artery) while compression is used to minimize edema associated with venous resection.

Resection of these structures is more common in the context of locally recurrent tumors than in primary STS. Similar principles of management apply to locally recurrent disease as to primary lesions. The entire surgical bed should be resected in continuity with the recurrent lesion, and a margin of normal tissue should be removed with the tumor when possible. When possible, neurovascular structures should be skeletonized but encasement by a high-grade recurrence necessitates resection of major arteries, veins, or nerves. In addition, adjuvant radiation delivered during management of the patient's primary disease often increases the risk of wound healing complications; local advancement and free flaps may be used to repair the soft tissue defect created by resection, particularly if primary repair would be under significant tension or if the incision overlies major vascular structures. Rarely, limb-salvage surgery is not possible (e.g., in the context of multiple recurrences, poor reconstructive options, or certain instances of bony involvement) and amputation is required. It is important to note that local recurrence of a high-grade STS is associated with significant risk of metastasis; complete extent of disease workup should be performed prior to any morbid surgical resection or amputation and systemic therapy considered as an alternative if distal disease is detected.

As in the extremity, surgical resection is the mainstay of treatment for primary retroperitoneal tumors; however, anatomic constraints often preclude removal of retroperitoneal tumors with wide margins. In treating retroperitoneal tumors, complete R0 (no residual microscopic disease) or R1 (only microscopic residual disease) resection is the goal of operative intervention. To accomplish complete resection, adjacent organs are removed in the context of tumor invasion. Segments of colon, the spleen, and distal pancreas may be resected in continuity with the tumor if necessary. In instances where the tumor is directly adjacent to the kidney, the renal capsule can be removed to provide a margin while preserving renal function. Encasement of the renal vessels or ureter may preclude such a maneuver, however, and nephrectomy may be required to perform complete gross resection.

Controversy exists regarding whether adjacent organs should be removed in the absence of tumor invasion. Theoretically, their removal would provide an additional margin of normal tissue that might prevent local recurrence [29]. However, the limiting margin of retroperitoneal resection is often the central vessels where recurrence is often observed, and removal of adjacent organs significantly increases surgical morbidity. For these reasons, it is not clear that removal of adjacent but uninvolved organs is of clinical benefit. Generally, removal of the tumor will be performed with posterior psoas muscle, involved organs, and renal capsule as noted previously [30,31].

Recurrence is common after resection of retroperitoneal tumors. Surgery plays a limited role in the context of this clinical scenario as it is rarely curative and can carry a high rate of morbidity. In many cases, recurrence at the level of the central or mesenteric vessels makes gross resection impossible. Good clinical outcomes are observed when recurrence is detected after prolonged disease-free interval and a limited number of tumors are identified. Rapid recurrence is a contraindication to surgical resection. If tumors recur at a rate of greater than 1 cm per month after a patient's last surgery, resection is not associated with improved survival as compared to management of recurrent disease with systemic therapies [32]. As in primary disease, the goal of surgery should be complete gross resection; residual disease is associated with poor outcomes and patients undergoing R2 resection (with macroscopic residual disease) fare no better than those treated with nonoperative interventions [33].

Radiotherapy

The standard practice for the treatment of STS is radiotherapy in combination with limb-sparing surgical resection, although radiation therapy is often administered alone in cases where surgery is not feasible for technical or medical reasons [34]. Several randomized studies support the use of radiotherapy in contemporary management of STS of the extremities and trunk. These studies demonstrated a significant improvement in local disease-free survival (DFS) when radiotherapy is combined with limb-sparing surgical excision of the tumor. Improved local control is most significant for patients with high-grade sarcomas. Radiotherapy may be administered preoperatively, postoperatively, or in both periods. Most often, radiotherapy is given via external beam; however, interstitial implants (brachytherapy) also may be used to deliver irradiation locally. Considerable debate has sought to determine which method results in the best local control rate, but no randomized trials have offered a definitive conclusion. Overall, local control rates are similar for these approaches and are approximately 80–90%. Advocates of preoperative radiotherapy argue that smaller fields and lower doses are necessary (typically, 50 Gy in 25 fractions over 5 weeks), reducing acute morbidity and cost. However, preoperative external-beam radiotherapy is associated also with a four- to fivefold increase in delayed wound healing and in complications requiring intervention (e.g., infection, debridement, grafting) as compared to surgery in a nonirradiated field [35]. Preoperative radiotherapy is contraindicated when vascular reconstruction within the irradiated field is anticipated. Typically, postoperative external-beam radiotherapy is administered at doses of 60–70 Gy, with the higher doses used for positive or uncertain margins. Postoperatively, the radiotherapy field is larger because the entire surgical field with a margin of undisturbed tissue must be irradiated. Long-term complications of radiotherapy may include bone necrosis, pathologic fracture (30%), growth plate arrest with limb shortening in skeletally immature patients, soft tissue fibrosis, joint contracture, and secondary malignancies. Hence, the late complication risk, particularly fibrosis, which is associated with larger radiation fields, may be higher in the patients who receive radiation postoperatively [36].

Modern high conformal radiotherapy, such as intensity modulated radiotherapy (IMRT), may help to further reduce the risk of radiation-related complications [37]. Although a nonrandomized comparison, a recent update from MSKCC reported a significant benefit for local control in favor of IMRT over brachytherapy (95% vs 81% at 5 years, $P = 0.04$), suggesting that IMRT may be preferable to brachytherapy in the postoperative setting [38]. Radiotherapy is frequently used to palliate metastases in many body sites. Both conventional and image-guided focal radiation can benefit patients who suffer from complications of metastases. High-dose focal radiotherapy in particular is emerging as an effective palliative modality for radioresistant tumors in the spine and offers benefit for patients with metastatic disease who have limited options for systemic treatment [39].

Adjuvant Chemotherapy

The decision to initiate systemic cytotoxic chemotherapy in either the adjuvant or metastatic setting is a complex one that requires a nuanced understanding of the different sarcoma histology. Adjuvant chemotherapy for sarcoma is controversial and the decision to recommend adjuvant therapy is highly variable even between sarcoma experts [40,41]. When possible, patients should be referred to a tertiary care sarcoma center for a multidisciplinary evaluation and consideration of clinical trials. The decision to initiate adjuvant chemotherapy should be based on histology, tumor size, grade, location, age, and patient expectations. Table 43.3 provides a rough guide to chemotherapy sensitivity in the metastatic setting. Abdominal and visceral disease do not benefit from adjuvant chemotherapy. To further aid in this decision-making process, an online (https://www.mskcc.org/nomograms/sarcoma) nomogram from MSKCC is available to estimate risk of death from disease for select histology. It is important to note that small cell sarcoma, osteosarcoma, and rhabdomyosarcoma are excluded from this discussion where adjuvant therapy is standard of care.

Histology and Chemotherapy

It is clear that adjuvant chemotherapy delays local recurrence, however its benefit on overall survival (OS) is not clear. A meta-analysis of 14 randomized trials involving 1,568 patients treated with adjuvant doxorubicin-containing regimens showed a significant benefit in local and distant recurrence-free rates in extremity sarcoma with only a nonsignificant trend towards improved OS [42] (Table 43.4). At 10 years, the OS improved from 50% to 54% in the treatment arm, which represents a 4% absolute benefit; however, in extremity tumors, a 7% benefit

Table 43.3 Variable response to chemotherapy by sarcoma histology.

Response to cytotoxic chemotherapy [3]	
Resistant	Well-differentiated liposarcoma, clear cell sarcoma, alveolar soft part sarcoma, conventional chordoma, myxofibrosarcoma, GIST, dermatofibrosarcoma protuberans, solitary fibrous tumor and/or hemangiopericytoma, extraskeletal myxoid chondrosarcoma, epithelioid sarcoma
Sensitive (low–intermediate)	MFH/UPS, dedifferentiated and pleomorphic liposarcoma, radiation-associated sarcoma, MPNST, fibrosarcoma, uterine sarcoma (high grade), dedifferentiated chordoma, desmoid tumors
Sensitive (high)	Ewing sarcoma, myxoid/round cell liposarcoma, leiomyosarcoma, angiosarcoma, synovial sarcoma, rhabdomyosarcoma

GIST, gastrointestinal stromal tumor; MFH/UPS, malignant fibrous histiocytoma or undifferentiated pleomorphic sarcoma; MPNST, malignant peripheral nerve sheath tumor.

Table 43.4 Studies of adjuvant chemotherapy in sarcoma.

Clinical trial	Therapy	Special consideration	Statistical	Notes
SMAC 1997 – Sarcoma Meta-Analysis Collaboration [42]	1,568 patients randomized to doxorubicin-based regimens	Extremity lesions		Meta-analysis, FAVOR
SMAC 2008 – Sarcoma Meta-Analysis Collaboration [51]	2,170 patients randomized to different regimens	Adriamycin and ifosfamide-based regimens	RFS at 10 years (HR 0.71, $P = 0.0001$), OS (HR 0.87, $P = 0.12$)	Meta-analysis. NOT in favor
SMAC 2008 – Sarcoma Meta-Analysis Collaboration [43]	1,953 patients randomized to different regimens		10% absolute risk reduction in OS, OR 0.56	Meta-analysis, FAVOR. Did not include a large negative study
Italian study [46]	Epirubicin/ifosfamide × 5 cycles versus observation.	Large (>10 cm) extremity or pelvic lesions	5-year OS: 66% vs 44% ($P = 0.04$)	Prospective, FAVOR adjuvant Not significant in ITT analysis
French study [44]	Variable regimens		Grade 2: no benefit Grade 3: 5-year OS: 58% vs 45%, 5-year metastasis-free survival (58% vs 49%, $P = 0.01$)	Retrospective, non-standardized older regimens FAVOR in high risk
MSKCC and UCLA [45]		Large, high-grade, extremity liposarcoma	OS benefit with ifosfamide-based regimen. No benefit with doxorubicin-based regimen	Retrospective, non-randomized FAVOR for ifosfamide but not doxorubicin
EORTC [48]	IFADIC vs observation	Grade 2 or 3	RFS (39% vs 44%, $P = 0.87$), OS ($P = 0.99$)	
EORTC [47]	CYVADIC vs observation		Higher RFS (56% vs 43%, $P = 0.007$), LLR (17 vs 31%, $P = 0.004$). No difference in OS	No benefit for OS
EORTC 62931 [49]	Adriamycin and ifosfamide vs observation	351 patients, grade II–III	RFS (55% vs 53%) $P = 0.51$, OS (67% vs 68%), $P = 0.72$	No benefit for OS
Italian and Spanish sarcoma group [52]	3 vs 5 cycles of epirubicin plus ifosfamide	324 patients randomized	HR = 1	No benefit of adding two additional cycles of EI after surgery

CYVADIC, cyclophosphamide, vincristine, Adriamycin, dacarbazine; EI, epirubicin, ifosfamide; EORTC, European Organisation for Research and Treatment of Cancer; HR, hazard ratio; IFADIC, ifosfamide, Adriamycin, dacarbazine; ITT, intention-to-treat; LLR, late local recurrence; MSKCC, Memorial Sloan Kettering Cancer Center; OR, odds ratio; OS, overall survival; RFS, recurrence-free survival.

was seen in the treatment arm. In 2008, two updates to the meta-analysis were published. The first showed a statistically significant survival benefit with an odds ratio of 0.56 and an absolute OS risk reduction of 10% for anthracycline/ifosfamide combination therapy; however this did not include a large negative trial from the European Organisation for Research and Treatment of Cancer (EORTC) [43]. The second meta-analysis involving 2,170 patients showed significant improvement in relapse-free survival at 5 years (hazard ratio (HR) 0.71, $P=0.0001$) but no improvement in OS at 10 years (HR 0.87). A retrospective analysis of a prospectively maintained database by the French Sarcoma Group showed a significantly improved 5-year metastasis-free survival (58% vs 49%, $P=0.1$) and 5-year OS (58% vs-. 45% $P=0.0002$) in patients with high-grade sarcoma but no benefit in patients with low-grade sarcoma [44]. This analysis is limited due to non-randomized and non-standardized treatments during 1980–1999. A retrospective analysis from MSKCC and UCLA showed an improved OS in patients with large (>5 cm), high-grade extremity lesions with an adjuvant ifosfamide-based regimen but no survival benefit with doxorubicin [45]. In a randomized trial by the Italian Sarcoma Group, patients with high-grade or recurrent extremity sarcoma received adjuvant epirubicin and ifosfamide versus observation [46]. At a median follow-up of 59 months, there was a significant improvement in DFS (48 vs 16 months) and OS (75 vs 46 months). The absolute benefit with chemotherapy at 2 and 4 years was 13% and 19%, respectively. At longer follow-up, the estimated 5-year OS was higher in the treatment arm (66% vs 46%, $P=0.04$) but the difference was not statistically significant in the intent-to-treat analysis.

In a trial by the EORTC, patients were randomized to cyclophosphamide, vincristine, Adriamycin, and dacarbazine (CYVADIC) versus observation [47]. The treatment arm had lower local recurrence (56% vs 43%) and improved RFS rates (17% vs 31%), however there was no benefit in distant metastases or OS. A similar trial of grade 2 and 3 STS with ifosfamide, Adriamycin, dacarbazine (IFADIC) versus observation also failed to show any benefit in RFS or OS [48]. A large phase 3 study by the EORTC randomized 351 patients to observation or adjuvant doxorubicin, ifosfamide, and lenograstim [49]. No difference was seen in the 5-year RFS or OS (64% vs 69%) between the two groups. These studies were criticized for using lower doses of ifosfamide. A phase 2 study comparing doxorubicin with either 6 mg/m^2 or 12 mg/m^2 of ifosfamide showed higher toxicities in the 12 mg/m^2 cohort with no difference in DFS or OS [50]. In conclusion, there is no benefit for adjuvant chemotherapy in small, low-grade tumors while it is controversial in stage IIB and III tumors. Certain histologies and locations do not have any benefit. Any potential benefit should be discussed in the context of acute and long-term toxicities of chemotherapy. The response rates of chemotherapy in the metastatic setting are 30–40% and therefore a neoadjuvant approach would provide an opportunity to determine response while enabling limb-sparing surgery.

In summary, adjuvant chemotherapy to improve OS can only be recommended in carefully selected patients with high-risk disease that is chemotherapy sensitive after a transparent discussion with the patient regarding toxicity and small absolute benefit.

Local Recurrence or Advanced Disease

In contrast to extremity lesions (50%), retroperitoneal (40%) and head and neck sarcomas (5%) have a much higher risk of local recurrence due to anatomic constraints that limit wide surgical resections and high doses of radiation. Local recurrence has a higher risk of tumor-related mortality as recurrence is associated with distant metastases. Management of local recurrence takes into consideration numerous aspects such as anatomy, prior radiation or chemotherapy, and time from initial diagnosis to recurrence, and thus requires a multidisciplinary approach. In select cases, oligo-metastatic lesions to the lung or other organs can be surgically cured (5-year OS 10–35%) depending on number of lesions, histology, and disease-free interval [53,54]. In extremity lesions that are unresectable, isolated limb perfusion or limb infusion with melphalan or doxorubicin (or dactinomycin) with the option of adding TNF-α may be an effective modality in high-grade sarcomas [55,56]. This procedure is only approved in Europe and Canada.

Metastatic Disease

In the metastatic setting, systemic chemotherapy is not curative and is thus used for palliation. Exceptions to this rule include small round blue cell tumors (Ewing), osteosarcoma, rhabdomyosarcoma, etc. The decision to initiate chemotherapy in the metastatic setting should involve a frank discussion regarding goals of care where the benefit of palliative therapy should be balanced against potential toxicities of treatment [16]. Doxorubicin as a single agent or in combination with ifosfamide is a well-established first-line therapy [57]. The single-agent response rate is approximately 15–20% for each drug and combinations of cytotoxic therapies have an improved response rate without any benefit in PFS or OS. Cardiac toxicity can be potentially minimized by split-dose or continuous administration of doxorubicin. Pegylated doxorubicin is increasingly used when the cumulative dose of doxorubicin is exceeded or when cardiac comorbidities preclude doxorubicin. There is no standard of care for duration of treatment and thus some centers administer a fixed number of cycles followed by observation while other centers treat until the response plateaus and switch to observation [16]. The randomized phase 1/2 study of doxorubicin plus or minus olaratumab, a PDGFRA monoclonal antibody, was the first study to demonstrate a doubling of OS (26.5 vs 14.7 months, stratified HR 0.46, $P=0.0003$) [58]. This led to the US Food and Drug Administration (FDA) and European Medicines Agency (EMA) approval of doxorubicin and olaratumab in combination followed by olaratumab maintenance therapy in the first-line setting in STS. A confirmatory phase 3 study is currently underway. Other combinations include the addition of dacarbazine and cyclophosphamide with similar response rates. Gemcitabine and docetaxel are increasingly used in the first-line setting, especially in leiomyosarcoma, and the combination has improved PFS and OS when compared to single-agent gemcitabine [59]. Splitting the dose of gemcitabine and docetaxel has significantly lower toxicities and obviates the need for growth factor support. Paclitaxel has little to no activity in most STS except in angiosarcoma and Kaposi sarcoma [16]. Trabectedin, a natural compound from a marine squirt and an inhibitor of the minor groove of DNA, has potent activity in translocation-associated sarcoma and leiomyosarcoma. In a pivotal phase 3 randomized study of advanced metastatic liposarcoma and leiomyosarcoma, trabectedin resulted in a 45% risk reduction in PFS compared to dacarbazine (4.2 vs 1.5 months, HR 0.55, P <0.001), however there was no improvement in OS [60]. The benefit was notable in leiomyosarcoma and myxoid liposarcoma, but disappointing in well- and dedifferentiated liposarcoma. This led to the approval of trabectedin in the US in the second-line setting for leiomyosarcoma and liposarcoma. Eribulin, a microtubule inhibitor, was evaluated against dacarbazine in a phase 3 pivotal study in patients with advanced liposarcoma and leiomyosarcoma. The study showed no improvement in PFS but an improvement in OS in favor of eribulin (13.5 vs 11.5 months, HR 0.77, P=0.0169) [61]. This led to the FDA and EMA approval of eribulin in leiomyosarcoma and liposarcoma. The benefit of eribulin is particularly striking in pleomorphic liposarcoma.

Several other chemotherapeutic agents, including dacarbazine (DTIC), cisplatin, irinotecan, and methotrexate, have minimal activity in the majority of STS. Dactinomycin, vincristine, and etoposide are active only in small cell sarcomas, including extraskeletal Ewing sarcoma/primitive neuroectodermal tumor and rhabdomyosarcoma.

Pazopanib, an oral tyrosine kinase inhibitor (TKI) against VEGF and PDGF, was recently approved as a second-line agent in all STS except liposarcomas, embryonal rhabdomyosarcoma, chondrosarcoma, osteosarcoma, small cell sarcomas, GIST, and a few other rare histologies. A large randomized phase 3 trial showed a 4.6 versus 1.6 months and 12.5 versus 10.7 months for PFS and OS in the pazopanib and placebo arms, respectively [62]. The discovery of near universal gene amplification of *CDK4* and *MDM2* in well- and dedifferentiated liposarcoma led to evaluation of palbociclib (a CDK4 inhibitor) in dedifferentiated liposarcoma. In a single-arm phase 2 study, palbociclib demonstrated a median PFS of 18 weeks and exceeded the primary endpoint of the study [63]. An identical study design evaluating a different dosing schedule showed a median PFS of 17.9 weeks with one complete response [64]. These studies led to National Comprehensive Cancer Network (NCCN) expert panel designation of palbociclib as a therapeutic option for dedifferentiated liposarcoma.

Special Histology

Gastrointestinal Stromal Tumors (GIST)

GIST arise from the interstitial cells of Cajal and are the most common type of sarcoma with an annual incidence of about 3,000 cases in the US [3]. The most common location is stomach (65%) followed by small intestine (25%), rectum, esophagus, and abdomen. Greater than 95% of GIST express c-KIT along with DOG1 [65]. However, activating mutations in tyrosine kinase receptors occur less frequently – *KIT* (80%), *PDGFR* (8%), and *BRAF* (2%) – and most of the remaining "wild-type" GIST have recently been shown to carry mutations in *SDHB* [12,66]. Histology, immunohistochemical stains (KIT/CD117, DOG1), and mutational status are diagnostic and can guide therapy. When GIST are resectable, open or laparoscopic surgery is the primary treatment of choice so long as the pseudocapsule can be carefully preserved and tumor spillage is avoided. Prognosis of GIST is dependent on size (<2, 2–5 and >5 cm), location (gastric vs small intestine), and mitotic index (>5 per 50 high-power fields (HPF)). Small gastric lesions with low mitotic index are benign [16,65]. In large gastric GIST or those located in rectum or esophagus, a neoadjuvant approach may help achieve less morbid surgeries and negative margins and prevent rupture of the pseudocapsule and seeding. Cytotoxic chemotherapy and radiation are ineffective in GIST. In phase 3 studies, patients with metastatic GIST were randomized to a low (400 mg) or high dose (800 mg) of imatinib, an oral TKI of KIT and PDGFR, and demonstrated equivalent response, PFS, and OS rates in both arms [67–70]. The current recommendation is 400 mg daily but data suggest that GIST with *KIT* exon 9 mutations may respond to higher doses of the drug, nevertheless mutational analysis is not routinely done as it is not sufficiently discriminatory for clinical decision-making [16,71,72]. Patients typically develop resistance after 9–18 months depending on the type of *KIT* or *PDGF* mutation, and increasing the dose of imatinib to 600 or 800 mg daily may be beneficial in a subset of patients. Patients with primary or acquired resistance to imatinib may go to second-line therapy with sunitinib, also a TKI, which demonstrated improved PFS when compared to a placebo in a randomized phase 3 study with crossover at progression [73]. Regorafenib is a third-line agent which was recently approved based on significant PFS improvement over placebo (4.8 vs 0.9 months) [74]. However, when available, enrollment to clinical trials is always recommended. Other TKIs include dasatinib and sorafenib. In the adjuvant setting, intermediate- and high-risk GIST is treated with up to 3 years of imatinib [75]. High-risk patients have gastric GIST, >5 cm, and mitoses of >5/50 HPF, while those with non-gastric locations have either >5 cm or >5/50 HPF of mitoses. For more information on GIST, please refer to Chapter 11.

Desmoid Tumors

Desmoid tumors or aggressive fibromatosis (DT) are rare fibroblastic sarcomas that are locally aggressive but lack metastatic potential [76,77]. They occur at a median age of 30 with a slightly female preponderance and most often arise in the extremities, abdominal wall and cavity, thorax, and head and neck. The majority of DT are sporadic and harbor mutations in *CTNNB1*, and a minority with familial adenomatous polyposis (FAP) syndrome demonstrate *APC* mutations, both converging in the Wnt signaling pathway [78]. Evaluating estrogen receptors has no therapeutic or diagnostic benefit. In patients with FAP the risk of DT is 1000-fold higher than the general population. There are anecdotal reports of DT associated with antecedent surgery/trauma and pregnancy. The natural history of desmoids is highly variable. If asymptomatic, DT can be observed and may spontaneously regress in <2% of cases. Mortality from DT is low and is due to compromise of vital structures resulting in hydronephrosis or bowel and bladder obstruction. Adjuvant chemotherapy has no benefit in this disease. In symptomatic patients, surgery is the mainstay of therapy though recurrence rates are as high as 40% even with negative margins. Observation may be appropriate in a subgroup of patients [79]. Therefore the risks and benefits of surgery must be carefully evaluated, especially in patients with high risk of recurrence – young patients with large, extremity lesions. A nomogram is available to determine risk of recurrence [80]. Prior to any surgery, patients should be evaluated by a multidisciplinary team for radiation and/or systemic therapies in an attempt to avert mutilating surgeries where large intestinal resections are likely or limb function will be affected. Long-term consequences of radiation-induced sarcomas must be considered in young patients. Systemic therapies include tamoxifen, sorafenib, imatinib, doxorubicin, pegylated doxorubicin, dacarbazine, methotrexate, vinblastine, and cyclophosphamide [16].

Small Cell Sarcoma (Ewing, PNET, Rhabdomyosarcoma)

A clearly defined role for systemic therapy in patients with STS is limited to the subset of patients with small cell sarcomas (e.g., Ewing sarcoma, primitive neuroectodermal tumor, rhabdomyosarcoma) and to patients with recurrence or overt metastatic disease. When possible, patients should be enrolled in a clinical trial. Ewing sarcoma and PNET are described in Chapter 47. Rhabdomyosarcoma is a tumor with skeletal muscle differentiation and is primarily a pediatric cancer, described in Chapter 47. The three histologies include embryonal, alveolar, and pleomorphic. All three are represented in adults but the pleomorphic variant is over-represented in adults. Multimodal therapy with surgery, chemotherapy, and radiation is required to eradicate primary and micrometastatic disease. The outcome of adults with rhabdomyosarcoma is worse and likely due to an over-representation of the pleomorphic histology [81]. Patients who are enrolled in clinical trials appeared to benefit more than non-trial patients [82]. Chemotherapy typically used includes cyclophosphamide, dactinomycin or doxorubicin, and vincristine, with or without ifosfamide and etoposide. *ALK* translocations have been described and a phase 2 study is currently ongoing with crizotinib, an ALK inhibitor.

Surveillance

Surveillance includes follow-up physical examination and imaging of the primary site and, if necessary, distant sites. Lungs are the most common organ for distant metastases. Radiographic surveillance of STS in the postoperative setting should be based on biological behavior, risk of recurrence (grade, size, site, margins), and duration of time after treatment [16]. For example, desmoid tumors and well-differentiated liposarcoma typically have local recurrence and thus extensive imaging of distant sites may not be useful. Meanwhile, STS such as undifferentiated pleomorphic sarcoma and pleomorphic liposarcoma have a higher propensity for distant metastases and will require more extensive evaluation. There are no studies to prove that CT scans are superior to chest X-ray, however clinical judgment should be personalized. Imaging is performed every 2–4 months during the first 2 years and less frequently after that. While the risk of recurrence decreases beyond 3 years, continued surveillance is recommended for an additional 5 years. Late recurrence beyond 10 years has also been reported. There are no surveillance tumor markers in STS.

Acknowledgement

We thank Bhavani Murugesan BA, JD, for editorial suggestions and manuscript preparation.

References

1 Siegel RL, Miller KD, Jemal A. Cancer statistics, 2017. *CA Cancer J Clin* 2017;67(1):7–30.

2 Howlader N, Noone AM, Krapcho M, *et al.* (eds). SEER Cancer Statistics Review, 1975-2013, National Cancer Institute. Bethesda, MD, http://seer.cancer.gov/csr/1975_2013/, based on November 2015 SEER data submission, posted to the SEER web site, April 2016.

3 Brennan MF, Antonescu CR, Maki RG (eds). *Management of Soft Tissue Sarcoma*. New York: Springer, 2013.

4 Moppett J, Oakhill A, Duncan AW. Second malignancies in children: the usual suspects? *Eur J Radiol* 2001;37(2):95–108.

5 Arlen M, Higinbotham NL, Huvos AG, *et al.* Radiation-induced sarcoma of bone. *Cancer* 1971;28(5):1087–99.

6 Gladdy RA, Qin LX, Moraco N, *et al.* Do radiation-associated soft tissue sarcomas have the same prognosis as sporadic soft tissue sarcomas? *J Clin Oncol* 2010;28(12):2064–9.

7 Hoppin JA, Tolbert PE, Herrick RF, *et al.* Occupational chlorophenol exposure and soft tissue sarcoma risk among men aged 30–60 years. *Am J Epidemiol* 1998;148(7):693–703.

8 Kogevinas M, Becher H, Benn T, *et al.* Cancer mortality in workers exposed to phenoxy herbicides, chlorophenols, and dioxins. An expanded and updated international cohort study. *Am J Epidemiol* 1997;145(12):1061–75.

9 Visuri T, Pukkala E, Pulkkinen P, Paavolainen P. Decreased cancer risk in patients who have been operated on with total hip and knee arthroplasty for primary osteoarthrosis: a meta-analysis of 6 Nordic cohorts with 73,000 patients. *Acta Orthop Scand* 2003;74(3):351–60.

10 Malkin D. Li-fraumeni syndrome. *Genes Cancer* 2011;2(4):475–84.

11 Agarwal R, Robson M. Inherited predisposition to gastrointestinal stromal tumor. *Hematol Oncol Clin North Am* 2009;23(1):1–13, vii.

12 Janeway KA, Kim SY, Lodish M, *et al.* Defects in succinate dehydrogenase in gastrointestinal stromal tumors lacking KIT and PDGFRA mutations. *Proc Natl Acad Sci U S A* 2011;108(1):314–8.

13 Gomez Garcia EB, Knoers NV. Gardner's syndrome (familial adenomatous polyposis): a cilia-related disorder. *Lancet Oncol* 2009;10(7):727–35.

14 Wagner AJ, Malinowska-Kolodziej I, Morgan JA, *et al.* Clinical activity of mTOR inhibition with sirolimus in malignant

perivascular epithelioid cell tumors: targeting the pathogenic activation of mTORC1 in tumors. *J Clin Oncol* 2010;28(5):835–40.

15 Ballinger ML, Goode DL, Ray-Coquard I, *et al.* Monogenic and polygenic determinants of sarcoma risk: an international genetic study. *Lancet Oncol* 2016;17(9):1261–71.

16 NCCN Clinical Practice Guidelines in Oncology: Soft Tissue Sarcoma. nccn.org. (accessed 13 December 2016).

17 Fong Y, Coit DG, Woodruff JM, Brennan MF. Lymph node metastasis from soft tissue sarcoma in adults. Analysis of data from a prospective database of 1772 sarcoma patients. *Ann Surg* 1993;217(1):72–7.

18 Jelinek JS, Kransdorf MJ, Shmookler BM, Aboulafia AJ, Malawer MM. Liposarcoma of the extremities: MR and CT findings in the histologic subtypes. *Radiology* 1993;186(2):455–9.

19 Heslin MJ, Lewis JJ, Woodruff JM, Brennan MF. Core needle biopsy for diagnosis of extremity soft tissue sarcoma. *Ann Surg Oncol* 1997;4(5):425–31.

20 Randall L, Cable MG. The role of molecular testing in soft tissue sarcoma diagnosis. *Lancet Oncol* 2016;4(17):415–6.

21 Italiano A, Di Mauro I, Rapp J, *et al.* Clinical effect of molecular methods in sarcoma diagnosis (GENSARC): a prospective, multicentre, observational study. *Lancet Oncol* 2016;17(4):532–8.

22 Yoon SS, Maki RG, Asare EA, *et al.* Soft tissue sarcoma of the trunk and extremities. In: M Amin, S Edge, R Greene, D Byrd, R Brookland (eds) *AJCC Cancer Staging Manual*, 8th edn. New York: Springer, 2017.

23 Kattan MW, Leung DH, Brennan MF. Postoperative nomogram for 12-year sarcoma-specific death. *J Clin Oncol* 2002;20(3):791–6.

24 Rosenberg SA, Tepper J, Glatstein E, *et al.* The treatment of soft-tissue sarcomas of the extremities: prospective randomized evaluations of (1) limb-sparing surgery plus radiation therapy compared with amputation and (2) the role of adjuvant chemotherapy. *Ann Surg* 1982;196(3):305–15.

25 Farma JM, Ammori JB, Zager JS, *et al.* Dermatofibrosarcoma protuberans: how wide should we resect? *Ann Surg Oncol* 2010;17(8):2112–8.

26 Mentzel T, Calonje E, Wadden C, *et al.* Myxofibrosarcoma. Clinicopathologic analysis of 75 cases with emphasis on the low-grade variant. *Am J Surg Pathol* 1996;20(4):391–405.

27 Huang HY, Lal P, Qin J, Brennan MF, Antonescu CR. Low-grade myxofibrosarcoma: a clinicopathologic analysis of 49 cases treated at a single institution with simultaneous assessment of the efficacy of 3-tier and 4-tier grading systems. *Hum Pathol* 2004;35(5):612–21.

28 Brooks AD, Gold JS, Graham D, *et al.* Resection of the sciatic, peroneal, or tibial nerves: assessment of functional status. *Ann Surg Oncol* 2002;9(1):41–7.

29 Gronchi A, Miceli R, Colombo C, *et al.* Frontline extended surgery is associated with improved survival in retroperitoneal low- to intermediate-grade soft tissue sarcomas. *Ann Oncol* 2012;23(4):1067–73.

30 Singer S, Antonescu CR, Riedel E, Brennan MF. Histologic subtype and margin of resection predict pattern of recurrence and survival for retroperitoneal liposarcoma. *Ann Surg* 2003;238(3):358–70; discussion 70–1.

31 Lewis JJ, Leung D, Woodruff JM, Brennan MF. Retroperitoneal soft-tissue sarcoma: analysis of 500 patients treated and followed at a single institution. *Ann Surg* 1998;228(3):355–65.

32 Park JO, Qin LX, Prete FP, *et al.* Predicting outcome by growth rate of locally recurrent retroperitoneal liposarcoma: the one centimeter per month rule. *Ann Surg* 2009;250(6):977–82.

33 Crago AM, Singer S. Soft tissue sarcoma. In: SW Ashley SW (ed.) *ACS Surgery: Principles & Practice*. Hamilton, ON: BC Decker, 2011.

34 Kepka L, DeLaney TF, Suit HD, Goldberg SI. Results of radiation therapy for unresected soft-tissue sarcomas. *Int J Radiat Oncol Biol Phys* 2005;63(3):852–9.

35 O'Sullivan B, Davis AM, Turcotte R, *et al.* Preoperative versus postoperative radiotherapy in soft-tissue sarcoma of the limbs: a randomised trial. *Lancet* 2002;359(9325):2235–41.

36 Davis AM, O'Sullivan B, Turcotte R, *et al.* Late radiation morbidity following randomization to preoperative versus postoperative radiotherapy in extremity soft tissue sarcoma. *Radiother Oncol* 2005;75(1):48–53.

37 Alektiar KM, Brennan MF, Healey JH, Singer S. Impact of intensity-modulated radiation therapy on local control in primary soft-tissue sarcoma of the extremity. *J Clin Oncol* 2008;26(20):3440–4.

38 Alektiar KM, Brennan MF, Singer S. Local control comparison of adjuvant brachytherapy to intensity-modulated radiotherapy in primary high-grade sarcoma of the extremity. *Cancer* 2011;117(14):3229–34.

39 Levine AM, Coleman C, Horasek S. Stereotactic radiosurgery for the treatment of primary sarcomas and sarcoma metastases of the spine. *Neurosurgery* 2009;64(2 Suppl):A54–9.

40 Le Cesne A, van Glabbeke, Woll PJ, *et al.* The end of adjuvant chemotherapy (adCT) era with doxorubicin-based regimen in resected high-grade soft tissue sarcoma (STS): Pooled analysis of the two STBSG-EORTC phase III clinical trials. *J Clin Oncol* 2008;26(15 Suppl):10525.

41 Maki RG. Role of chemotherapy in patients with soft tissue sarcomas. *Expert Rev Anticancer Ther* 2004;4(2):229–36.

42 Adjuvant chemotherapy for localised resectable soft-tissue sarcoma of adults: meta-analysis of individual data. Sarcoma Meta-analysis Collaboration. *Lancet* 1997;350(9092):1647–54.

43 Pervaiz N, Colterjohn N, Farrokhyar F, *et al.* A systematic meta-analysis of randomized controlled trials of adjuvant chemotherapy for localized resectable soft-tissue sarcoma. *Cancer* 2008;113(3):573–81.

44 Italiano A, Delva F, Mathoulin-Pelissier S, *et al.* Effect of adjuvant chemotherapy on survival in FNCLCC grade 3 soft tissue sarcomas: a multivariate analysis of the French Sarcoma Group Database. *Ann Oncol* 2010;21(12):2436–41.

45 Eilber FC, Eilber FR, Eckardt J, *et al.* The impact of chemotherapy on the survival of patients with high-grade primary extremity liposarcoma. *Ann Surg* 2004;240(4):686–95; discussion 95–7.

46 Frustaci S, Gherlinzoni F, De Paoli A, *et al.* Adjuvant chemotherapy for adult soft tissue sarcomas of the extremities and girdles: results of the Italian randomized cooperative trial. *J Clin Oncol* 2001;19(5):1238–47.

47 Bramwell V, Rouesse J, Steward W, *et al.* Adjuvant CYVADIC chemotherapy for adult soft tissue sarcoma – reduced local recurrence but no improvement in survival: a study of the

European Organization for Research and Treatment of Cancer Soft Tissue and Bone Sarcoma Group. *J Clin Oncol* 1994;12(6):1137–49.

48 Brodowicz T, Schwameis E, Widder J, *et al.* Intensified Adjuvant IFADIC Chemotherapy for Adult Soft Tissue Sarcoma: A Prospective Randomized Feasibility Trial. *Sarcoma* 2000;4(4):151–60.

49 Woll PJ, Reichardt P, Le Cesne A, *et al.* Adjuvant chemotherapy with doxorubicin, ifosfamide, and lenograstim for resected soft-tissue sarcoma (EORTC 62931): a multicentre randomised controlled trial. *Lancet Oncol* 2012;13(10):1045–54.

50 Worden FP, Taylor JM, Biermann JS, *et al.* Randomized phase II evaluation of 6 g/m2 of ifosfamide plus doxorubicin and granulocyte colony-stimulating factor (G-CSF) compared with 12 g/m2 of ifosfamide plus doxorubicin and G-CSF in the treatment of poor-prognosis soft tissue sarcoma. *J Clin Oncol* 2005;23(1):105–12.

51 O'Connor JM, Chacón M, Petracci FE, Chacón RD. Adjuvant chemotherapy in soft tissue sarcoma (STS): A meta-analysis of published data. *J Clin Oncol* 2008;26(15S):10526.

52 Gronchi A, Frustaci S, Mercuri M, *et al.* Short, full-dose adjuvant chemotherapy in high-risk adult soft tissue sarcomas: a randomized clinical trial from the Italian Sarcoma Group and the Spanish Sarcoma Group. *J Clin Oncol* 2012;30(8):850–6.

53 Carballo M, Maish MS, Jaroszewski DE, Holmes CE. Video-assisted thoracic surgery (VATS) as a safe alternative for the resection of pulmonary metastases: a retrospective cohort study. *J Cardiothorac Surg* 2009;4:13.

54 Gossot D, Radu C, Girard P, *et al.* Resection of pulmonary metastases from sarcoma: can some patients benefit from a less invasive approach? *Ann Thorac Surg* 2009;87(1):238–43.

55 Moncrieff MD, Kroon HM, Kam PC, *et al.* Isolated limb infusion for advanced soft tissue sarcoma of the extremity. *Ann Surg Oncol* 2008;15(10):2749–56.

56 Deroose JP, Eggermont AM, van Geel AN, *et al.* Long-term results of tumor necrosis factor alpha- and melphalan-based isolated limb perfusion in locally advanced extremity soft tissue sarcomas. *J Clin Oncol* 2011;29(30):4036–44.

57 Lorigan P, Verweij J, Papai Z, *et al.* Phase III trial of two investigational schedules of ifosfamide compared with standard-dose doxorubicin in advanced or metastatic soft tissue sarcoma: a European Organisation for Research and Treatment of Cancer Soft Tissue and Bone Sarcoma Group Study. *J Clin Oncol* 2007;25(21):3144–50.

58 Tap WD, Jones RL, Van Tine BA, *et al.* Olaratumab and doxorubicin versus doxorubicin alone for treatment of soft-tissue sarcoma: an open-label phase 1b and randomised phase 2 trial. *Lancet* 2016;388(10043):488–97.

59 Maki RG, Wathen JK, Patel SR, *et al.* Randomized phase II study of gemcitabine and docetaxel compared with gemcitabine alone in patients with metastatic soft tissue sarcomas: results of sarcoma alliance for research through collaboration study 002 [corrected]. *J Clin Oncol* 2007;25(19):2755–63.

60 Demetri GD, von Mehren M, Jones RL, *et al.* Efficacy and safety of trabectedin or dacarbazine for metastatic liposarcoma or leiomyosarcoma after failure of conventional chemotherapy: results of a phase III randomized multicenter clinical trial. *J Clin Oncol* 2016;34(8):786–93.

61 Schöffski P, Chawla S, Maki RG, *et al.* Eribulin versus dacarbazine in previously treated patients with advanced liposarcoma or leiomyosarcoma: a randomised, open-label, multicentre, phase 3 trial. *Lancet* 2016;387(10028):1629–37.

62 van der Graaf WT, Blay JY, Chawla SP, *et al.* Pazopanib for metastatic soft-tissue sarcoma (PALETTE): a randomised, double-blind, placebo-controlled phase 3 trial. *Lancet* 2012;379(9829):1879–86.

63 Dickson MA, Tap WD, Keohan ML, *et al.* Phase II trial of the CDK4 inhibitor PD0332991 in patients with advanced CDK4-amplified well-differentiated or dedifferentiated liposarcoma. *J Clin Oncol* 2013;31(16):2024–8.

64 Dickson MA, Schwartz GK, Keohan ML, *et al.* Progression-free survival among patients with well-differentiated or dedifferentiated liposarcoma treated with CDK4 inhibitor palbociclib: a phase 2 clinical trial. *JAMA Oncol* 2016;2(7):937–40.

65 Miettinen M, Lasota J. Gastrointestinal stromal tumors: review on morphology, molecular pathology, prognosis, and differential diagnosis. *Arch Pathol Lab Med* 2006;130(10):1466–78.

66 Hirota S, Isozaki K, Moriyama Y, *et al.* Gain-of-function mutations of c-kit in human gastrointestinal stromal tumors. *Science* 1998;279(5350):577–80.

67 Demetri GD, von Mehren M, Blanke CD, *et al.* Efficacy and safety of imatinib mesylate in advanced gastrointestinal stromal tumors. *N Engl J Med* 2002;347(7):472–80.

68 Verweij J, Casali PG, Zalcberg J, *et al.* Progression-free survival in gastrointestinal stromal tumours with high-dose imatinib: randomised trial. *Lancet* 2004;364(9440):1127–34.

69 Blanke CD, Demetri GD, von Mehren M, *et al.* Long-term results from a randomized phase II trial of standard- versus higher-dose imatinib mesylate for patients with unresectable or metastatic gastrointestinal stromal tumors expressing KIT. *J Clin Oncol* 2008;26(4):620–5.

70 Blanke CD, Rankin C, Demetri GD, *et al.* Phase III randomized, intergroup trial assessing imatinib mesylate at two dose levels in patients with unresectable or metastatic gastrointestinal stromal tumors expressing the kit receptor tyrosine kinase: S0033. *J Clin Oncol* 2008;26(4):626–32.

71 Heinrich MC, Owzar K, Corless CL, *et al.* Correlation of kinase genotype and clinical outcome in the North American Intergroup Phase III Trial of imatinib mesylate for treatment of advanced gastrointestinal stromal tumor: CALGB 150105 Study by Cancer and Leukemia Group B and Southwest Oncology Group. *J Clin Oncol* 2008;26(33):5360–7.

72 Gounder MM, Maki RG. Molecular basis for primary and secondary tyrosine kinase inhibitor resistance in gastrointestinal stromal tumor. *Cancer Chemother Pharmacol* 2011;67 Suppl 1:S25–43.

73 Demetri GD, van Oosterom AT, Garrett CR, *et al.* Efficacy and safety of sunitinib in patients with advanced gastrointestinal stromal tumour after failure of imatinib: a randomised controlled trial. *Lancet* 2006;368(9544):1329–38.

74 Demetri GD, Reichardt P, Kang YK, *et al.* Efficacy and safety of regorafenib for advanced gastrointestinal stromal tumours after failure of imatinib and sunitinib (GRID): an international, multicentre, randomised, placebo-controlled, phase 3 trial. *Lancet* 2013;381(9863):295–302.

75 Joensuu H, Eriksson M, Sundby Hall K, *et al.* One vs three years of adjuvant imatinib for operable gastrointestinal stromal tumor: a randomized trial. *JAMA* 2012;307(12):1265–72.

76 Posner MC, Shiu MH, Newsome JL, *et al.* The desmoid tumor. Not a benign disease. *Arch Surg* 1989;124(2):191–6.

77 Lewis JJ, Boland PJ, Leung DH, Woodruff JM, Brennan MF. The enigma of desmoid tumors. *Ann Surg* 1999;229(6):866–72; discussion 72–3.

78 Lazar AJ, Tuvin D, Hajibashi S, *et al.* Specific mutations in the beta-catenin gene (CTNNB1) correlate with local recurrence in sporadic desmoid tumors. *Am J Pathol* 2008;173(5):1518–27.

79 Bonvalot S, Eldweny H, Haddad V, *et al.* Extra-abdominal primary fibromatosis: Aggressive management could be avoided in a subgroup of patients. *Eur J Surg Oncol* 2008;34(4):462–8.

80 Crago AM, Denton B, Salas S, *et al.* A prognostic nomogram for prediction of recurrence in desmoid fibromatosis. *Ann Surg* 2013;258(2):347–53.

81 Ogilvie CM, Crawford EA, Slotcavage RL, *et al.* Treatment of adult rhabdomyosarcoma. *Am J Clin Oncol* 2010;33(2):128–31.

82 Gerber NK, Wexler LH, Singer S, *et al.* Adult rhabdomyosarcoma survival improved with treatment on multimodality protocols. *Int J Radiat Oncol Biol Phys* 2013;86(1):58–63.

Section 13

Cancer of Unknown Primary, Paraneoplastic Syndromes, and Peritoneal Carcinomatosis

44

Cancer of Unknown Primary Site

John D. Hainsworth[1] *and F. Anthony Greco*[2]

[1] *Sarah Cannon Research Institute, Nashville, Tennessee, USA*
[2] *Sarah Cannon Cancer Center, Nashville, Tennessee, USA*

Introduction

Cancer of unknown primary site (CUP) is a heterogeneous clinical syndrome, accounting for approximately 2% of all cancer diagnoses [1]. The actual incidence is probably higher, since many of these patients are assigned other diagnoses based on suggestive clinical or pathological findings, and therefore are not recorded as CUP in tumor registries. Patients with a wide variety of cancer types are represented, so the clinical and pathologic findings vary widely.

The typical patient with CUP develops symptoms at a metastatic site, but routine clinical and pathologic evaluation fails to identify an anatomic primary site. Over the years, diagnostic techniques have improved. Therefore the spectrum of patients with CUP has evolved, and the approach to the CUP patient is in the process of changing. Foremost among these changes is the ability to predict the tissue of origin in most patients with CUP using gene expression tumor profiling.

In this chapter, management of patients with CUP is divided into three sections: (i) pathologic evaluation, including immunohistochemical (IHC) staining and gene expression tumor profiling, specialized pathological techniques that have substantially increased diagnostic capabilities; (ii) clinical evaluation of patients with CUP, with emphasis on recognizing patients with clinical syndromes requiring specific therapy; and (iii) treatment of patients with CUP.

Pathologic Evaluation

Most patients with CUP have a diagnostic biopsy of a metastatic lesion early in their evaluation. The biopsy results are frequently useful in directing further evaluation. Histologic examination remains the gold standard for initial evaluation, providing a practical classification system on which to base further testing. Four broad categories of cancer are recognized in patients with CUP: (i) adenocarcinoma, (ii) squamous cell carcinoma, (iii) neuroendocrine carcinoma, and (iv) poorly differentiated neoplasm (or carcinoma). Occasionally, metastatic melanoma or sarcoma can be diagnosed without an obvious primary tumor site; patients with these tumors should be managed following guidelines for the specific tumor type.

Further pathologic evaluation is indicated in most cancers of unknown primary site, and should be directed by the initial histologic diagnosis.

Histologic Subtypes

Poorly Differentiated Cancer

In a small percentage of patients with CUP (approximately 5%), the undifferentiated histologic features do not allow the pathologist to diagnose the tumor lineage (i.e., carcinoma vs lymphoma vs melanoma vs sarcoma); in these tumors, the histologic diagnosis is "poorly differentiated neoplasm." In a larger group (20–25%), histologic features allow the diagnosis of "carcinoma," but subcategorization is not possible; these tumors are labeled "poorly differentiated carcinoma." All patients with these histologic diagnoses require further pathologic evaluation.

It is important for the clinician to remember that optimum pathologic evaluation requires an adequate biopsy specimen in which histology can be assessed and additional studies (IHC, gene expression profiling) performed if necessary. Therefore, surgical or core needle biopsies are recommended and use of fine-needle aspiration biopsy for diagnosis should be avoided.

In patients with the initial diagnosis of "poorly differentiated neoplasm," establishment of tumor lineage is essential. Several highly treatable tumor types are contained within this group, the most common being non-Hodgkin lymphoma, present in 35–65% of cases [2, 3]. Most of the remaining patients have poorly differentiated carcinoma, including neuroendocrine carcinoma. Immunohistochemical staining is almost always successful in identifying the tumor lineage (Table 44.1); in occasional instances electron microscopy or cytogenetic analysis is also helpful.

The American Cancer Society's Oncology in Practice: Clinical Management, First Edition. Edited by The American Cancer Society.

Table 44.1 Immunohistochemical staining in the pathologic evaluation of unknown primary cancers.

	IHC Stains	
	Positive	Negative
Identifying tumor lineage		
Carcinoma	AE 1/3 (pancytokeratin) EMA	Vimentin, S-100, CLA
Lymphoma	CLA	AE 1/3, EMA, S-100
Melanoma	S-100, HMB-45, melan-A	AE 1/3, CLA
Sarcoma	Vimentin, desmin, myogen, factor VIII, CD117	AE 1/3, CLA, S-100
Neuroendocrine	Chromogranin, synaptophysin, AE 1/3	CLA, S-100, vimentin
Germ cell	OCT4, hCG, AFP, PLAP	CLA, S-100
Specific adenocarcinomas		
Colorectal	CK20, CDX2	CK7
Breast	ER, PR, HER2, GCDFP-15, mammaglobin, CK7	CK20
Lung	TTF1, CK7	CK20
Prostate	PSA	CK7, CK20
Pancreas	CK7, CA19-9, mesothelin	
Ovary	WT1, ER, CK7, mesothelin	
Renal	RCC, CD10	CK7, CK20
Liver	Hepar 1, CD10	CK7, CK20

AFP, α-fetoprotein; CK, cytokeratin; CLA, common leukocyte antigen; EMA, epithelial membrane antigen; ER, estrogen receptor; GCDFP-15, gross cystic disease fluid protein 15; hCG, human chorionic gonadotropin; PLAP, placental alkaline phosphatase; PR, progesterone receptor; PSA, prostate specific antigen; RCC, renal cell carcinoma antigen; TTF1, thyroid transcription factor; WT1, Wilms tumor 1.

Poorly differentiated carcinomas can be recognized histologically, but no further subtyping (i.e., adenocarcinoma, squamous carcinoma) is possible. All poorly differentiated carcinomas should have additional pathologic studies with IHC staining and gene expression tumor profiling (see section "Gene Expression Tumor Profiling"). Although fewer tumors of other lineages are found in this group, additional evaluation occasionally reveals an unsuspected lymphoma or a germ cell tumor.

Adenocarcinoma

Adenocarcinoma that can be easily recognized histologically (well differentiated or moderately well differentiated) is the most common diagnosis in patients with CUP (approximately 60%). Typically, patients with adenocarcinoma of unknown primary site are elderly and have widespread cancer at the time of diagnosis. Common sites of tumor involvement include lymph nodes, liver, lung, and bone.

Since adenocarcinomas share histologic features, routine histology is usually unable to predict the primary site. Although certain histologic features have been associated with particular tumor types (e.g., signet ring cells with gastric cancer, papillary features with ovarian or thyroid cancer), these features are not specific enough to identify the primary site.

As the treatment of adenocarcinomas from various primary sites improves and becomes more specific, accurate prediction of the primary site becomes increasingly important. Panels of IHC stains are often useful in suggesting a primary site (Table 44.1), although few stains are highly specific [4, 5]. Gene expression profiling also allows prediction of a site of origin in most cases, and often provides additional diagnostic information. Both modalities should now be considered in the pathologic evaluation of adenocarcinoma of unknown primary site.

Squamous Cell Carcinoma

Approximately 5% of patients with CUP have squamous cell carcinoma. Appropriate clinical evaluation is important in these patients, since many have highly effective treatment available. The diagnosis is usually made by routine histology, and additional pathologic studies are rarely necessary. In patients with atypical clinical presentations, or poorly differentiated squamous carcinoma, IHC staining or molecular studies are recommended.

Neuroendocrine Carcinoma

Neuroendocrine carcinomas account for approximately 4–5% of CUP diagnoses. A spectrum of these neoplasms is recognized in the CUP population, with varying clinical and histologic features. Improved pathologic diagnosis has resulted in increased recognition of these tumors.

Well-differentiated or low-grade neuroendocrine tumors have histologic features similar to gastrointestinal carcinoids or pancreatic neuroendocrine tumors (islet cell tumors). These tumors usually have an indolent biology, and frequently secrete bioactive substances.

Other neuroendocrine carcinomas presenting as CUP are more aggressive. One of these groups has histologic features typical of small cell carcinoma or atypical carcinoid. Other neuroendocrine carcinomas appear histologically as poorly differentiated neoplasm or poorly differentiated carcinoma, and their identification requires IHC staining.

Immunohistochemistry

Immunohistochemical staining is a widely available specialized technique for classifying neoplasms. IHC uses antibodies directed at specific cell components or products including enzymes, normal tissue components, hormones, and tumor markers. Such staining can utilize formalin-fixed paraffin-embedded tissue. Expertise is required to perform and interpret these stains reliably.

In patients with CUP who have poorly differentiated tumors, IHC staining can almost always identify tumor lineage (i.e., carcinoma, lymphoma, melanoma, sarcoma) (Table 44.1) [4–8].

In addition, germ cell tumors can be strongly suggested by IHC studies, given the appropriate clinical situation.

In patients who have CUP and a histologic diagnosis of adenocarcinoma, IHC staining can sometimes suggest the tissue of origin. The stain for prostate specific antigen (PSA) is quite specific; men with positive PSA tumor staining should be treated as if they had metastatic prostate cancer. In most patients with adenocarcinoma of unknown primary site, panels of IHC stains are used to suggest a primary site (Table 44.1). These panels often include cytokeratins (CK) 20 and 7, CDX2, thyroid transcription factor 1 (TTF1), gross cystic disease fluid protein 15 (GCDFP-15), vimentin, and neuroendocrine stains (chromogranin, synaptophysin) [9–12]. Results of IHC staining must always be interpreted in conjunction with clinical features, since none of the individual stains or staining panels is entirely specific.

Electron Microscopy

Because electron microscopy requires special tissue fixation and sectioning, and is relatively expensive, it is usually reserved for neoplasms whose lineage remains unclear after routine histology, IHC, and gene expression profiling. Electron microscopy is usually successful in identifying the lineage of poorly differentiated neoplasms, particularly in the distinction among carcinoma, lymphoma, and poorly differentiated sarcoma. However, electron microscopy cannot predict the site of origin of various adenocarcinomas.

Karyotypic/Cytogenetic Analysis

Several tumor-specific chromosomal abnormalities have been identified, including tumor-specific immunoglobulin gene rearrangements in lymphoma, chromosomal translocation (t(11:22)) in Ewing tumor and peripheral primitive neuroectodermal tumors, *BRD4-NUT* fusion oncogene (t(15:19)) in carcinoma of midline structures occurring in children and young adults, and isochrome of the short arm of chromosome 12 (i(12p)) in germ cell tumors [13–19]. In patients with poorly differentiated neoplasms who have features suggestive of one of these diagnoses, and are undiagnosed after complete pathologic evaluation, testing for a tumor-specific chromosomal abnormality should be considered. Demonstration of one of these specific abnormalities can also provide confirmation if one of these tumor types is unexpectedly identified by gene expression profiling.

Gene Expression Tumor Profiling

Specific gene expression profiles are now recognized in cancers based on their site of origin, reflecting the different gene expression profiles present in the normal tissues of origin [20]. The potential application of these findings to cancer diagnosis was first demonstrated when differences in gene expression allowed distinction of acute myeloid leukemia from acute lymphoblastic leukemia [21]. By measuring the differential expression of specific gene sets, this method of diagnosis can potentially be applied to many cancer types, and has recently been studied in the diagnosis of patients with CUP.

Several molecular cancer classifier assays are currently available, using either reverse transcription polymerase chain reaction (RT-PCR) or gene microarray techniques to measure specific gene expression patterns [22–24]. These assays measure gene expression dynamics in relation to cell lineage, rather than tumor-specific markers; this method is effective since most cancer cells retain at least part of the gene expression profile of their tissue of origin [25]. When tested in a blinded fashion, these assays were able to accurately identify the tissue of origin in 85–90% of patients with advanced cancers of known primary site.

Confirmation of similar accuracy in the prediction of tissue of origin in CUP has been difficult to obtain, since the anatomic primary site rarely becomes manifest in these patients. To date, the most direct indication of accuracy comes from a small group of CUP patients in whom primary sites became manifest later during their clinical course. In a group of 24 such patients, identified retrospectively, the prediction of tissue of origin by gene expression profiling matched the clinically identified primary site in 18 (75%) [26]. Three of the remaining 6 patients had an unsuccessful assay due to poor tissue preservation, and 3 patients had an incorrect prediction by the assay.

Several retrospective studies have also been reported, in which biopsy material from patients with CUP was tested by one of several molecular cancer classifier assays [27–31]. Although confirmation of "accuracy" was impossible in these retrospective series, since anatomic primary sites were never identified, similar findings emerged from all studies: (i) a tissue of origin was predicted in a large percentage of cases, (ii) the tissue of origin prediction was usually consistent with clinical and pathologic features, and (iii) response to empiric chemotherapy and survival were usually generally consistent with the tumor type predicted.

The clinical value of gene expression tumor profiling in the management of patients with CUP has also been addressed in a prospective study. Previously untreated patients had the CancerTYPE ID® assay (bioTheranostics, Inc.) performed on their tumor specimens, and then received site-specific therapy directed by the assay results [32]. This prospective study confirmed the ability of gene expression profiling to make a prediction of the site of tumor origin in the majority of CUP patients. Of the 289 patients enrolled in the trial, 252 (87%) had successful assays performed (unsuccessful assays were due to insufficient amounts of tumor in the biopsy specimen). When the assay was successfully performed, a site of origin was predicted in 247 of 252 patients (98%). Twenty-six different primary sites were predicted; however, the four most commonly predicted sites (biliary tract, urothelial, colorectal, and non-small cell lung cancer) accounted for 55% of all patients. The results of assay-directed, site-specific treatment are detailed in the "Treatment" section of this chapter.

The diagnostic capabilities of gene expression profiling and IHC in patients with CUP have recently been reviewed and compared [33]. In the largest trial, the results of IHC and gene expression profiling in 149 CUP patients were compared retrospectively [34]. When IHC staining suggested a single site of origin (in 35%), the molecular cancer classifier assay results were concordant in 40 of 52 (77%). However, when IHC was nonspecific or led to a prediction of two or more primary sites, concordance with the molecular cancer classifier assay prediction was poor (<50%). A group of 35 patients had additional clinical or pathologic evaluation in an attempt to confirm the molecular cancer classifier assay prediction; in 26 of these patients (74%), additional test results suggested or confirmed the profiling prediction.

Four smaller studies also showed good correlation (78%) between IHC and gene expression profiling when IHC results suggested a single primary site [35–38]. However, IHC suggested a single diagnosis in <55% of patients in all studies.

In CUP patients with poorly differentiated neoplasms, gene expression profiling has also shown substantial advantages. Thirty patients were identified retrospectively who had poorly differentiated neoplasms without a definite lineage diagnosis after complete histologic and IHC (median 18 stains) evaluation [39]. Gene expression profiling established the tumor lineage in 25 of 30 patients (83%), and suggested the tissue of origin in all 10 carcinomas. All 7 patients who received site-directed therapy based on the gene expression profiling diagnoses (germ cell 2, neuroendocrine 2, mesothelioma 2, lymphoma 1) responded, and 5 remained alive and disease-free after 25+ to 72+ months.

The current body of evidence supports several conclusions regarding gene expression profiling for diagnosis. (i) The tissue of origin can be predicted in >90% of patients with CUP, including patients with poorly differentiated neoplasms. The accuracy of these predictions (80–85%) is similar to the blinded validation studies, where the molecular cancer classifier assays were tested using metastatic lesions from cancers of known primary site. (ii) When IHC predicts a single diagnosis, the correlation with gene expression profiling results is high (>75%). In such patients, site-specific treatment based on the IHC prediction should be considered, and gene expression profiling may be unnecessary. (iii) Gene expression profiling predicts a tissue of origin in a substantial percentage of tumors in which IHC staining and other pathologic studies are nonspecific, and should be performed as part of the diagnostic evaluation. Selection of treatment based on molecular profiling assay results has now been tested, and these results are detailed in the "Treatment" section.

Clinical Evaluation

Most patients with CUP seek medical attention because of signs or symptoms of metastatic cancer. If the primary site cannot be identified by the initial clinical evaluation, it is unlikely to become apparent during the subsequent clinical course (only 5–10%). However, a primary site can be identified in approximately 75% of patients at autopsy [40, 41]. Primary sites in the gastrointestinal tract (pancreas, colorectum, liver) and lung account for approximately 60% of the primary sites identified in autopsy series, whereas primary sites in the ovary, breast, or prostate have been uncommon. Recently, primary sites predicted by molecular profiling have been generally similar, although the numbers of breast, ovarian, and urothelial cancers have been higher [32].

For patients with adenocarcinoma or poorly differentiated carcinoma, an abbreviated clinical evaluation is required before a patient can be categorized as having CUP. This initial evaluation should include a thorough history and physical examination, complete blood counts, urinalysis, basic serum chemistries, serum lactate dehydrogenase (LDH) level, and computed tomography (CT) or magnetic resonance imaging (MRI) of the chest, abdomen, and pelvis. In men, assessment should also include a prostate examination and a measurement of serum PSA. In women, the evaluation should include a pelvic examination and mammography.

Positron emission tomography (PET) is a standard diagnostic and/or staging procedure in a large number of cancer types. In retrospective series, PET identified a primary site in 30–40% of patients with CUP [42]. However, when PET was performed only after a complete diagnostic evaluation in a prospective study, results were not improved when compared to CT scanning alone [43]. Therefore, except for specific patient subgroups (see sections "Squamous Cell Carcinoma" and "Patients with a Single Site of Metastatic Carcinoma"), PET is not required in the standard clinical evaluation of CUP.

Additional clinical evaluation should be triggered in specific patients by clinical or pathologic results during the initial evaluation (Table 44.2). In these patients, additional focused evaluation may: (i) identify a primary site, (ii) narrow the spectrum of possible primary sites, or (iii) identify specific treatable subsets of patients (see section "Treatable Subsets").

Squamous Cell Carcinoma

Squamous cell carcinoma accounts for approximately 5% of all CUP diagnoses. Unlike other cancers presenting with an unknown primary site, squamous cell carcinoma almost always presents with isolated metastases in either the cervical or the inguinal lymph nodes. Patients with either of these presentations

Table 44.2 Additional diagnostic evaluation for specific patient subsets identified by initial evaluation.

Initial evaluation	Additional evaluation
Features of colon cancer (liver/peritoneal metastases; CK20+/CK7− or CDX2+)	Colonoscopy
Women with breast cancer features (axillary adenopathy; bone, lung, pleura, liver metastases)	Breast MRI, PET scan ER, GCDFP-15, HER2 stains
Women with ovarian cancer features (pelvic/peritoneal metastases; CK7+)	Pelvic ultrasound WT1 stain
Features of lung cancer (hilar/mediastinal adenopathy; TTF1+)	Bronchoscopy
Men with mediastinal/retroperitoneal mass	Testicular ultrasound Serum hCG, AFP, PLAP, OCT4 stains; FISH for i(12p)
Neuroendocrine carcinoma, low grade	OctreoScan® Upper/lower gastrointestinal endoscopy Urine 5HIAA

AFP, α-fetoprotein; CK, cytokeratin; ER, estrogen receptor; FISH, fluorescent *in situ* hybridization; GCDFP, gross cystic disease fluid protein; hCG, human chorionic gonadotropin; 5HIAA, 5-hydroxyindoleacetic acid; MRI, magnetic resonance imaging; PET, positron emission tomography; PLAP, placental alkaline phosphatase; TTF1, thyroid transcription factor; WT1, Wilms tumor 1.

frequently do well with appropriate therapy; therefore, the initial diagnostic evaluation is of particular importance.

Unilateral cervical adenopathy is the most common presentation of squamous cell carcinoma of unknown primary site. Patients often have a history of tobacco and/or alcohol use, although some of these lesions are associated with human papillomavirus infection. Upper and mid-cervical lymph nodes are most frequently involved, and in these situations a primary tumor in the head and neck region is likely. Appropriate clinical evaluation includes direct endoscopy with visual examination of the oropharynx, hypopharynx, nasopharynx, larynx, and upper esophagus, and biopsy of any suspicious areas. Computed tomography (CT) of the neck is useful in defining the extent of disease, and occasionally identifies the primary site. PET is also useful in identifying primary sites in these patients [44]. With this evaluation, primary sites in the head and neck are detected in the large majority of patients; in one study, primary sites were found in 231 of 267 patients (87%) presenting with metastatic squamous carcinoma in cervical nodes [45].

Ipsilateral tonsillectomy is recommended as a diagnostic modality in patients with metastatic involvement of a single subdigastric, mid-jugulocarotid, or submandibular lymph node. Bilateral tonsillectomy has been recommended in patients with bilateral subdigastric adenopathy [46]. In one series, 26% of patients presenting in this manner had a tonsillar primary identified at the time of tonsillectomy [47].

When lower cervical or supraclavicular nodes are involved, a primary lung cancer should be suspected. In addition to the head and neck examinations previously described, CT of the chest and fiberoptic bronchoscopy should be performed.

When squamous cell carcinoma involves inguinal lymph nodes, a primary site can usually be found in the genital or anorectal areas. Examination of the anal canal, vulva, vagina, uterine cervix, penis, and scrotum is important. Suspicious areas should be biopsied. Identification of a primary site is important in this group of patients, because curative therapy is available for carcinomas of the vulva, vagina, cervix, and anus even after spread to regional lymph nodes.

Metastatic squamous cell carcinoma involving an area other than cervical or inguinal lymph nodes is an uncommon presentation for CUP patients, and usually represents metastasis from an occult lung primary. In such cases, an evaluation as described for adenocarcinoma of unknown primary site is recommended, and fiberoptic bronchoscopy should be considered.

Neuroendocrine Carcinoma

Approximately 4–5% of CUPs are neuroendocrine carcinomas, and this diagnosis is usually made after appropriate pathologic examination. Although a variety of neuroendocrine carcinomas occur, clinical management requires their separation into low-grade and aggressive categories. This distinction can usually be made by the pathologist; low-grade tumors typically have a classical carcinoid or islet cell appearance, whereas aggressive neuroendocrine carcinomas are either small cell carcinoma or poorly differentiated carcinoma with positive neuroendocrine IHC stains. While the initial clinical evaluation should be the same as described for adenocarcinoma of unknown primary site, several additional diagnostic tests should be considered in these patients.

Low-grade neuroendocrine carcinomas presenting with an unknown primary site most frequently involve the liver. Although a large percentage of these tumors secrete bioactive substances, clinical syndromes from tumor production of bioactive substances are apparent in only a minority, and can include carcinoid syndrome, glucagonoma syndrome, Zollinger–Ellison syndrome, and VIPoma syndrome. Because the gastrointestinal tract is the most common site of origin for low-grade neuroendocrine carcinomas, evaluation should include upper and lower gastrointestinal endoscopy. If these are unrevealing, imaging of the pancreas with endoscopic ultrasonography should be considered. Since approximately 80% of low-grade neuroendocrine carcinomas have high concentrations of somatostatin receptors, somatostatin receptor scintigraphy (OctreoScan®) is frequently of value in locating a primary site [48]. Elevated urinary levels of 5-hydroxyindoleacetic acid (5-HIAA) are highly suggestive of a carcinoid tumor arising in the small bowel, and are useful for following response to therapy.

Aggressive neuroendocrine carcinomas of unknown primary site are usually widely metastatic when diagnosed and are rarely associated with clinical syndromes produced by secretion of bioactive substances. Some aggressive neuroendocrine carcinomas have a typical "small cell" histologic appearance, whereas others lack morphologic features of neuroendocrine differentiation, which is recognized only by IHC staining [49]. Clinical evaluation should be similar to that described for adenocarcinomas of unknown primary site. Brain MRI should also be considered, due to the high risk of central nervous system metastases [50]. Somatostatin receptor scintigraphy (OctreoScan®) is relatively insensitive and is not recommended in this setting. Patients with a history of cigarette smoking should be suspected of having a lung primary, particularly if the tumor has a small cell histology, and fiberoptic bronchoscopy should be performed.

The origin of these aggressive neuroendocrine carcinomas may remain unknown. Some of these patients probably have small cell lung cancer with an occult primary tumor. However, more than half of these patients have no smoking history and therefore the diagnosis of small cell lung cancer is unlikely [49]. Some of these tumors are probably anaplastic variants of well-recognized neuroendocrine carcinomas, particularly gastrointestinal carcinoid tumors. Such tumors arising in the gastrointestinal tract are well described, and have a biology and response to treatment that is distinct from their low-grade counterparts [51]. Rarely, aggressive neuroendocrine carcinomas arise from a wide variety of primary sites (so-called "extrapulmonary small cell carcinoma"). These tumors may also account for some aggressive neuroendocrine carcinomas of unknown primary site.

Treatment

After completion of the clinical and pathologic evaluations, patients with the initial diagnosis of CUP fall into three broad categories. First, patients who have an anatomic primary site defined during their initial evaluation should be treated appropriately for their defined tumor type, and should no longer be considered to have CUP. A second group of patients (approximately 15–20%) have specific treatable clinical syndromes, even though an anatomic primary site is not identified. Appropriate identification and management of these patients is important, since some have highly treatable cancers. Unfortunately, a large group of patients (approximately 80–85%) have no primary site identified and do not fit into any of the specific treatable subsets. Empiric chemotherapy has been the standard therapy for these patients for many years. Site-specific therapy, directed by the results of gene expression tumor profiling, offers a new treatment approach in many CUP patients and will likely become the new standard in the near future.

Treatable Subsets

Several subsets of patients, identifiable during the initial clinical or pathologic evaluation, require specific treatment and are summarized in Table 44.3 and discussed in the following sections. In most of these specific presentations, treatment recommendations follow guidelines for a specific cancer type, based on the presumption that a CUP presentation represents an unusual variant presentation. Clinical experience in most of these subsets has justified this presumption, and survival is similar to that achieved with standard treatment for the corresponding metastatic cancers of known primary site. In the future, the actual primary sites in these patients may be confirmed by the use of gene expression tumor profiling. However, until the utility of molecular tumor profiling is confirmed in these subsets, treatment should follow the guidelines outlined here.

Women with Axillary Lymph Node Metastases

Breast cancer should be suspected in women who have an adenocarcinoma of unknown primary site and axillary adenopathy [52]. Additional imaging and IHC studies of biopsy tissue should be performed, as outlined in Table 44.2. MRI and PET scanning can identify occult breast cancers even with normal mammography [53–55].

If detectable metastases are limited to axillary lymph nodes, these women may have stage II breast cancer, which is potentially curable with appropriate therapy. Modified radical mastectomy shows an invasive occult primary breast cancer in 44–80% of patients, even when physical examination and mammography are normal. In patients who also have normal MRI and/or PET scans, the incidence of identifying an occult breast cancer at mastectomy is probably lower, although not well studied. When detected, primary tumors are usually less than 2 cm in diameter and may measure only a few millimeters; occasionally, only noninvasive cancer is identified in the breast [56]. Radiation therapy to the breast is an alternative to mastectomy, and has provided roughly equivalent results, although no prospective comparisons have been performed [57]. Neoadjuvant or adjuvant therapy is indicated in this setting using guidelines established for the treatment of stage II breast cancer.

Women with axillary node involvement and additional sites of metastases should be managed as if they have metastatic

Table 44.3 Treatment and prognosis of specific patient subsets.

Subset	Typical histology	Therapy	Prognosis
Women, isolated axillary LN	Adeno, PDA	Treat as stage II breast cancer	Similar to stage II breast cancer
Women, axillary LN + other metastases	Adeno, PDA	Treat as metastatic breast cancer	Similar to metastatic breast cancer
Women, peritoneal carcinomatosis	Adeno (often serous) PDC	Treat as stage III ovarian cancer	Similar to stage III ovarian cancer
Men, blastic bone metastases or high serum PSA or PSA tumor staining	Adeno	Treat as metastatic prostate cancer	Similar to metastatic prostate cancer
Colon cancer profile	Adeno	Treat as metastatic colon cancer	18–20-month median survival
Single metastatic site	Adeno, PDC	Definitive local therapy	Variable; occasional long survival
Isolated cervical LN	Squamous	Combined chemoradiation (as for locally advanced H/N cancer)	30–60% 5-year survival
Isolated inguinal LN	Squamous	Inguinal node dissection, radiation therapy, ± chemotherapy	15–20% 5-year survival
Extragonadal germ cell syndrome (2 or more features; see text)	PDC	Treat for poor prognosis germ cell tumor	35–50% cure rate
Neuroendocrine carcinoma, low grade	Carcinoid/ islet cell features	Treat as advanced carcinoid	Similar to metastatic carcinoid
Neuroendocrine carcinoma, aggressive	Small cell, or PDC	Treat as small cell lung cancer	Median survival 14 months, occasional long-term survival

Adeno, adenocarcinoma; H/N, head and neck; LN, lymph node; PDA, poorly differentiated adenocarcinoma; PDC, poorly differentiated carcinoma; PSA, prostate specific antigen.

breast cancer, particularly if the sites of involvement are typical of metastatic breast cancer (e.g., multiple bone metastases, pleural involvement, lymphangitic lung involvement). Hormone receptor and *HER2* status should be determined from the initial biopsy specimen, since these patients may derive major benefit from hormonal or *HER2*-targeted therapy. In patients whose clinical features are questionable, gene expression tumor profiling may help to confirm the diagnosis of metastatic breast cancer.

Women with Peritoneal Carcinomatosis

In women, adenocarcinoma involving the peritoneum without an obvious primary site usually originates in the ovary or in extraovarian tissues with similar histogenesis. These tumors frequently have histologic features typical of ovarian cancer, including papillary or serous configuration, or psammoma bodies. Clinical features are also similar to ovarian cancer, with metastases often limited to the peritoneal surface and elevated serum levels of CA-125. These tumors are more common in women with *BRCA1* mutations or strongly positive family histories, and occasionally occur even after prophylactic oophorectomy [58, 59].

It is now clear that some of these carcinomas arise from the peritoneal surface (primary peritoneal carcinoma) or from the fimbriated ends of the fallopian tubes [60, 61]. Carcinomas arising from these sites share a similar lineage with the epithelium giving rise to ovarian carcinoma, and have gene expression profiles nearly identical to ovarian carcinoma [22].

The management of women with peritoneal carcinomatosis should follow guidelines for advanced ovarian carcinoma. Surgical cytoreduction should be considered in all patients with bulky intra-abdominal disease, either at the time of diagnosis or after initial chemotherapy [62]. Chemotherapy using a taxane/platinum combination should be administered, and produces results similar to those achieved in advanced ovarian cancer [63–67]. In fact, the similar prognosis is well enough documented that women with primary peritoneal carcinoma are now included in clinical trials evaluating new treatments for advanced ovarian cancer.

Papillary serous peritoneal carcinomatosis has occasionally been reported in men [68]; however, the rarity of these cases has precluded any study of the biology of these tumors, and some may be metastatic from other primaries. Gene expression profiles of these tumors, as compared to similar clinical syndromes in women, have not been investigated. A trial of chemotherapy, similar to that used in advanced ovarian cancer, is a reasonable approach for patients with good performance status.

Men with Elevated Serum PSA and/or PSA Tumor Staining

Serum PSA concentrations should be measured and tumor biopsies should be stained for PSA in men with adenocarcinoma of unknown primary site. The likelihood of metastatic prostate cancer is increased in men with blastic bone metastases as the predominant site of tumor involvement. However, patients with other clinical features (e.g., metastases to the lung, mediastinum, or upper abdominal lymph nodes), in the absence of concomitant bone involvement, occasionally have elevated serum PSA levels and respond to hormonal therapy for advanced prostate cancer [69, 70]. In such patients, a needle biopsy of the prostate usually confirms the primary site, but may not be necessary for optimum management. Treatment for patients with advanced prostate cancer has recently improved, and all men with CUP and elevated serum or tumor PSA should receive treatment following guidelines for advanced prostate cancer.

Patients with a Colon Cancer Profile

In autopsy series, the colon is one of the most common sites for occult primaries [40, 41]. Treatment for metastatic colon cancer has improved substantially during the last two decades, with the median expected survival increasing from 9 to 24 months [71, 72]. Since optimal treatment for metastatic colorectal cancer differs substantially from the empiric chemotherapy regimens used for patients with CUP, accurate identification of this subset of patients is particularly important.

Recently, a "colon cancer profile" has been identified, so that CUP patients likely to have metastatic colon cancer with an occult primary site can be identified and treated appropriately [73, 74]. Components of this "profile" include: (i) predominant metastatic sites in the liver and/or peritoneum, (ii) histology typical of gastrointestinal adenocarcinoma, and (iii) typical immunohistochemical staining pattern, including either positive staining with CDX2 or the combination of CK20 positive/CK7 negative staining. Seventy-four CUP patients with this profile were identified retrospectively; 53 patients had received first-line therapy with colorectal cancer regimens, and the median overall survival was 37 months [74]. Although prospective documentation of this favorable prognosis is not yet available, patients with CUP and a "colon cancer profile" should currently be considered for treatment following guidelines for metastatic colon cancer.

The prediction of a colorectal site of origin by gene expression profiling may also effectively identify patients who respond to colon cancer therapy. Two such groups of patients, retrospectively identified, have been reported [75, 76]. The large majority of patients in both series had normal colonoscopies. In both series, approximately 45% of patients had IHC staining results that were atypical for colon cancer, and therefore did not fit the "colon cancer profile" described previously. Patients who received site-specific therapy for metastatic colon cancer (first-line, second-line, or both) had median survivals of 21 months and 27 months, respectively. These results are similar to those achieved in patients with metastatic colon cancer, supporting the accuracy of the gene expression profiling predictions.

Patients with a Single Site of Metastatic Carcinoma

In occasional patients, only a single metastatic lesion is identified after a complete staging evaluation. In this situation, the possibility of an unusual primary tumor mimicking metastatic cancer should be considered. Examples of cancers that can present in this fashion include skin adnexal tumors (e.g., apocrine, sebaceous, and eccrine carcinomas), Merkel cell carcinomas, and occasional sarcomas, melanomas, or lymphomas mistakenly interpreted as poorly differentiated carcinoma. Single metastases can occur in a variety of sites including lymph nodes, lung, brain, adrenal gland, liver, and bone. Before initiating local treatment, a PET scan is helpful to exclude other unsuspected metastatic sites [77].

If no additional metastatic disease is found, resection of the solitary lesion should be considered. If resection is not feasible due to the location of the metastatic lesion, definitive local radiation therapy should be administered. In most patients with good performance status, the authors have also used either adjuvant or neoadjuvant chemotherapy with a platinum-based regimen, although data confirming the value of this approach are not available in this uncommon patient group.

In most patients, additional occult metastatic sites become manifest after disease-free intervals of varying duration. However, these patients frequently survive one year or longer, and a minority has substantially longer survival. In one group of patients presenting with isolated brain metastasis, 15% remained progression-free 5 years after definitive therapy [78]. We have treated and followed 36 patients with metastases at a single site (unpublished observation). All patients had primary treatment with either resection or radiotherapy, and many received empiric neoadjuvant or adjuvant chemotherapy. The median survival in this group is 17 months; the 3-year survival is 28%.

Extragonadal Germ Cell Cancer Syndrome

A few patients with poorly differentiated carcinoma of unknown primary site have extragonadal germ cell tumors that are not recognizable using standard histologic criteria [79, 80]. These patients typically have two or more of the following characteristics: (i) male <50 years of age; (ii) predominant tumor location in midline sites (mediastinum, retroperitoneum); (iii) elevated serum levels of human chorionic gonadotropin, α-fetoprotein, or both; (iv) short duration of symptoms, with evidence of rapid tumor growth. The diagnosis of germ cell tumor can be confirmed in some of these patients if an i(12p) chromosomal abnormality is detected by cytogenetic evaluation. Many of these patients have excellent responses to chemotherapy, and approximately 35–50% are cured with the cisplatin-based regimens used for poor-prognosis testicular cancer. All patients with this syndrome should have a trial of such therapy.

In previous years, an empiric trial of cisplatin-based chemotherapy as used for testicular cancer was recommended for a broad spectrum of patients with poorly differentiated carcinoma, even in the absence of multiple features of the extragonadal germ cell cancer syndrome. These recommendations were based on some early anecdotal reports of excellent responses with this approach [79–82], and on a large prospective study reported in 1992 [83]. In this group of 220 patients with poorly differentiated carcinoma of unknown primary site, major tumor responses were seen in 62%, 26% had complete response, and 10% had long-term, disease-free survival. In retrospect, we are now certain that this clinical trial was heavily weighted with good-prognosis patients now included in several favorable subsets. These subsets included: (i) patients with two or more features of the extragonadal germ cell syndrome, (ii) patients with poorly differentiated neoplasms otherwise not specified, (iii) patients with anaplastic lymphoma diagnosed as carcinoma in years past but now routinely recognized by specialized pathology, (iv) patients with primary peritoneal carcinoma, and (v) patients with poorly differentiated neuroendocrine carcinoma. Patients in these subsets are now recognized at the time of their initial evaluation, and should receive specific therapy (Table 44.3). After these favorable subsets are removed, the remaining patients with poorly differentiated carcinoma have a prognosis that is similar to patients with adenocarcinoma of unknown primary site, and treatment should follow similar guidelines.

Squamous Cell Carcinoma Involving Cervical or Supraclavicular Lymph Nodes

When metastatic squamous cell carcinoma is detected in cervical or supraclavicular nodes, appropriate clinical evaluation identifies a primary site in the head and neck region, or in the lung, in 85% of patients. Most of the remaining patients are presumed to have occult primary sites in the head and neck; when such patients are treated with ipsilateral radical neck dissection as the only treatment modality, primary sites in the head and neck subsequently became manifest in up to 40%.

When no primary site is identified in patients with high or mid-cervical node involvement, treatment should follow guidelines for patients with locally advanced squamous cell cancer of the head and neck. Randomized trials in patients with head and neck cancer have shown advantages for concurrent chemoradiation versus either sequential chemotherapy and radiation therapy, or treatment with local modalities alone [84]. Although similar randomized phase 3 trials have not been completed in patients without an identified primary site, a non-randomized comparison of patients treated with combined modality therapy versus local therapy alone showed a higher complete response rate (81 vs 60%, respectively) and longer median survival (>37 vs 24 months) in patients receiving combined modality treatment [85]. As in locally advanced head and neck cancer, patients with advanced cervical adenopathy (N3) or poorly differentiated carcinoma have inferior survival [86]. Five-year disease-free survival rates with combined modality therapy have usually been reported in the 50–60% range, but have been as high as 71% [87], presumably varying due to clinical characteristics in these small series.

Patients with low cervical or supraclavicular adenopathy have inferior survival using treatment guidelines for advanced head and neck cancer, presumably because more of the occult primary sites are in the lung. Although the outcome is inferior, combined modality treatment should be considered in these patients; approximately 10–15% can be expected to have a long-term, disease-free survival.

Squamous Cell Carcinoma Involving Inguinal Lymph Nodes

The vast majority (99% in one series) of patients with metastatic squamous cell carcinoma involving inguinal lymph nodes have a detectable primary site in the genital or anorectal area (including the surrounding skin) [88]. For the occasional patient in whom no primary site is identified, inguinal lymph node dissection with or without radiation therapy to the inguinal area sometimes results in long-term survival [89]. Since combined modality therapy has improved results in other regional squamous cell carcinomas (anus, cervix), neoadjuvant or adjuvant chemotherapy should also be considered.

Low-Grade Neuroendocrine Carcinoma

Patients with well-differentiated neuroendocrine tumor of unknown primary site usually have liver metastases, and clinical syndromes from tumor production of bioactive substances may be apparent. If a primary site is not revealed after a complete evaluation (Table 44.2), the treatment approach should be similar to that recommended for well-differentiated neuroendocrine tumors (carcinoids) of the gastrointestinal tract. Depending upon the clinical situation, management may include local therapy (resection of isolated metastases, cryotherapy, radiofrequency ablation, hepatic artery ligation/embolization) or systemic therapy. Initial systemic treatment should include a somatostatin analog (either long-acting octreotide or lanreotide), since this therapy increases the time to tumor progression, effectively controls symptoms from tumor-related bioactive substances, and has low toxicity [90, 91]. Everolimus and sunitinib are additional treatment options for low-grade neuroendocrine tumors [92–94]. Several cytotoxic agents also have some activity (streptozocin, doxorubicin, 5-fluorouracil, temozolomide), and sometimes provide useful palliation. Since these neoplasms are often indolent, watchful waiting is also sometimes appropriate for asymptomatic patients.

Aggressive Neuroendocrine Carcinomas

Aggressive neuroendocrine carcinomas of unknown primary site with histologic features of small cell carcinoma, and those with features of poorly differentiated carcinoma (often large cell) with neuroendocrine staining by IHC are usually responsive to combination chemotherapy. Most of these patients have clinical evidence of rapid tumor growth, and have multiple sites of metastases. Platinum/etoposide regimens, as used in extensive-stage small cell lung cancer, are currently recommended [49, 95]. These regimens have produced high overall response rates, complete response rates of 13–22%, and occasional long-term survivors.

Empiric Therapy for Carcinoma of Unknown Primary Site

Approximately 80% of patients with carcinoma of unknown primary site do not fit into any of the favorable clinical subsets. Empiric, "broad spectrum" combination chemotherapy regimens were developed for these patients, and have produced modest benefits. Although randomized trials are few, two-drug platinum-based regimens (usually paired with a taxane or gemcitabine) are generally accepted as the most efficacious. With these regimens, the median survival ranges from 7.5 to 10 months, 2-year survival is in the 7–19% range, and occasional patients (<5%) have more prolonged survival [96–99]. Details of the development and results of empiric chemotherapy have been reviewed [100].

Although empiric chemotherapy has produced modest benefits, the continued routine recommendation of this treatment for patients with CUP is becoming increasingly problematic. Empiric chemotherapy regimens, designed at a time when there was substantial overlap in the systemic therapy of different tumor types, are increasingly less effective in providing adequate "coverage" as the therapies for specific cancer types become more individualized. For example, current therapy for patients with advanced colon or kidney cancer is substantially different than therapy with any of the empiric CUP chemotherapy regimens (which have previously been shown to be ineffective in these tumor types). Even in the treatment of non-small cell lung cancer, where first-line treatment with a taxane/platinum combination (as used for empiric treatment of CUP) is still considered a reasonable treatment, optimum treatment may involve multiple other drugs (bevacizumab, erlotinib, pemetrexed, crizotinib, nivolumab) not included in empiric CUP regimens. Accurate prediction of the site of origin, even when the anatomic primary site remains undetectable, is becoming increasingly important in the management of this heterogeneous patient population.

Site-Specific Therapy Directed by Molecular Tumor Profiling

The use of site-specific therapy directed by the results of gene expression tumor profiling, as an alternative to empiric chemotherapy, is increasing. Several studies have shown that molecular cancer classifier assays can predict a tissue of origin in the large majority of CUP patients, and these predictions are usually consistent with the clinical and pathologic features [27, 29, 34]. Retrospective studies have shown that CUP patients predicted to have a site of origin in the colon or rectum have median survivals of more than 20 months when treated with colon cancer regimens [75, 76].

The results of a large, prospective phase 2 study also support the role of gene expression tumor profiling in the management of patients with CUP [32]. In this study, patients with a new diagnosis of CUP had tumor biopsy material submitted for a 92-gene RT-PCR cancer classification assay (CancerTYPE ID®). When a site of origin was predicted by the assay, patients received site-specific therapy. Of the 252 patients who had sufficient tumor in the biopsy specimen to perform the assay, 247 (98%) had a tissue of origin predicted; in the remaining 5 patients, the tumor was unclassifiable by the assay. The median survival of the 194 patients who received site-specific therapy was 12.5 months. When treatment-sensitive tumor types were predicted by the assay, treatment outcome was superior when compared to less sensitive tumor types (13.4 vs 7.6 months; $P = 0.04$). In general, the median survivals of subgroups of patients with specific tumor types were as expected: patients predicted to have traditionally resistant tumor types such as pancreas and biliary tract had short median survivals (8 and 6 months, respectively), whereas median survivals exceeded 24 months in patients predicted to have breast or ovarian cancer.

This trial demonstrated that site-specific therapy directed by gene expression tumor profiling was feasible, and resulted in a median survival that compared favorably to historical results reported with empiric chemotherapy. As anticipated, patients with sensitive tumor types had longer survival (median 13.7 months), presumably because they were able to receive optimum site-specific therapy. Although a randomized trial is the only way to provide definitive proof that assay-directed, site-specific therapy is superior to empiric chemotherapy, it is our opinion that the existing data are now strong enough that gene expression tumor profiling should be incorporated into the management of patients with CUP.

Screening for "Actionable" Molecular Alterations

Many new cancer treatments exploit cancer-specific molecular alterations critical to cancer cell growth and metastasis. Appropriate patient populations for these agents are defined not only by the tumor type but also by the presence of specific molecular alterations. Screening of patients with specific cancer types is already a standard part of clinical practice, and broader screening for potentially "actionable" alterations is becoming more common.

In a recent study, comprehensive genomic profiling in a group of 200 CUP patients revealed the presence of "actionable" molecular alterations (for which targeted therapy is currently available) in 24% of tumors [101]. Alterations seen most frequently included *HER2* (8%), *BRCA2* (6%), *BRAF* (6%), and *EGFR* (6%). Although these findings suggest new possibilities for targeted treatment, confirmation of the efficacy of such therapy in CUP awaits clinical trials.

While awaiting results of such studies, it is currently appropriate to search for specific molecular alterations based on gene expression profiling results. For example, patients with CUP predicted to have non-small cell lung cancer should be evaluated for EGFR-activating mutations and *ALK* and *ROS1* rearrangements. A few such patients were found to have *ALK* rearrangements, leading to successful treatment with crizotinib [102]. The coordinated use of gene expression profiling for diagnosis and additional molecular assays to identify "actionable" molecular alterations is the likely direction of CUP treatment in the future.

Prognostic Factors

Several retrospective analyses have identified clinical and pathologic features associated with favorable response to treatment in patients with CUP [83, 103–108]. All of these analyses involved patients receiving empiric chemotherapy of various types, and may not be applicable if empiric chemotherapy is replaced by site-specific therapy directed by gene expression profiling results. Many of the prognostic features identified are related to tumor grade or extent of disease, and have therefore been identified as prognostic factors for many types of advanced cancer. Favorable prognostic features include: tumor location (lymph nodes/soft tissue vs liver/bone), fewer sites of metastatic disease, female sex, good performance status, normal LDH level, normal serum albumin, and normal lymphocyte count.

In one report, the combination of performance status and serum LDH could be used to separate patients into "good" and "poor" risk categories. In a group of 150 patients, the median survival was 11.7 months with good performance status and normal serum LDH, versus 3.9 months with poor performance status and/or elevated LDH [106].

In another analysis, based on 317 patients seen consecutively, the combination of normal serum albumin and the absence of liver metastases identified a favorable patient subset (median survival of 12 months) when compared to patients with low serum albumin and/or liver metastases (median survival 3.5 months) [107].

Future Directions

The treatment paradigm for patients with CUP is in the process of changing. In Figure 44.1, we outline a new model for the evaluation and treatment of patients with CUP. Patients who comprise the treatable subsets should receive treatment as outlined in Table 44.3 and in the "Treatable Subsets" section. For the remaining patients, gene expression tumor profiling is usually successful in predicting the site of origin. Based on gene expression profiling predictions, tumor tissue should also be tested for well-recognized molecular alterations with therapeutic implications (e.g., *HER2* in breast cancer, *ALK/ROS1/EGFR* in lung cancer), followed by site-specific therapy. Confirmation of the superiority of molecular cancer classifier assay-directed, site-specific therapy versus empiric chemotherapy is incomplete; however, current data are strong enough to recommend this approach.

Even with successful prediction of the primary site, treatment of a substantial proportion of CUP patients will remain relatively poor, due to the inherent resistance of the tumor types involved. Site-specific treatment for pancreatic or biliary tract cancers, for example, will have relatively minor impact on survival versus the results produced by empiric CUP chemotherapy. At present, CUP patients predicted to have responsive tumor types are the ones who will benefit from this approach. Particular benefit will be derived in tumor types for which relatively specific targeted therapy is now part of standard therapy (e.g., breast, non-small cell lung, renal, melanoma). Assay-directed, site-specific therapy will also allow future improvements in treatment for specific solid tumors to be rapidly incorporated into the treatment of patients with CUP.

Although the site of tumor origin can now be predicted in most patients, it is important to remember that anatomic primary sites are infrequently found in these patients. Therefore, these patients should still be considered as a distinct group, even though many will receive site-specific therapy. Since cancers presenting with an unknown primary site have a distinct biology and clinical behavior, it is possible (and even likely) that results of site-specific treatment will differ to some extent in these patients when compared to results in patients with known primary sites. Additional experience with assay-directed, site-specific therapy, as well as more complete analysis of tumors for the presence of actionable molecular abnormalities, will further improve our understanding of these tumors, and will likely lead to further advances in therapy.

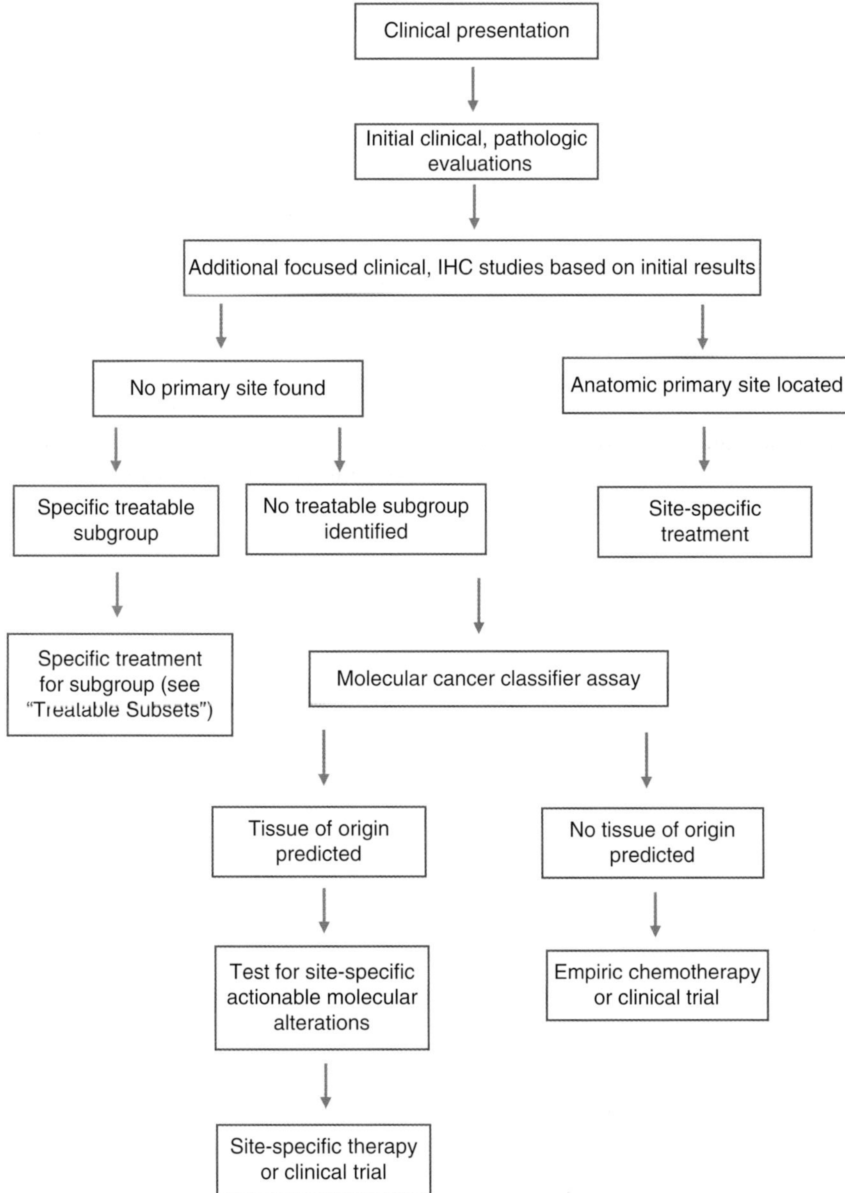

Figure 44.1 Treatment of patients with carcinoma of unknown primary site.

References

1 Urban D, Rao A, Bressel M, *et al.* Cancer of unknown primary: a population-based analysis of temporal change and socioeconomic disparities. *Br J Cancer* 2013;109:1318–24.

2 Gatter KC, Alcock C, Heryet A, Mason DY. Clinical importance of analyzing malignant tumours of uncertain origin with immunohistochemical techniques. *Lancet* 1985;1:1302–5.

3 Horning SJ, Carrier EK, Rouse RV, *et al.* Lymphomas presenting as histologically unclassified neoplasms: characteristics and response to treatment. *J Clin Oncol* 1989;7:1281–7.

4 Oien KA. Pathologic evaluation of unknown primary cancer. *Semin Oncol* 2009;36:8–37.

5 Dennis JL, Oien KA. Hunting the primary: novel strategies for defining the origin of tumours. *J Pathol* 2005;205:236–47.

6 Warnke RA, Gatter KC, Falini B, *et al.* Diagnosis of human lymphoma with monoclonal antileukocyte antibodies. *N Engl J Med* 1983;309:1275–81.

7 Battifora H, Trowbridge IS. A monoclonal antibody useful for the differential diagnosis between malignant lymphoma and nonhematopoietic neoplasms. *Cancer* 1983;51:816–21.

8 Mackey B, Ordonez NG. Pathological evaluation of neoplasms with unknown primary tumor site. *Semin Oncol* 1993;20:206–28.

9 Brown RW, Campagna LB, Dunn JK, Cagle PT. Immunohistochemical identification of tumor markers in metastatic adenocarcinoma. A diagnostic adjunct in the determination of primary site. *Am J Clin Pathol* 1997;107:12–19.

10 Kaufmann O, Deidesheimer T, Muehlenberg M, *et al.* Immunohistochemical differentiation of metastatic breast carcinomas from metastatic adenocarcinomas of other common primary sites. *Histopathology* 1996;29:233–40.

11 Lagendijk JH, Mullink H, Van Diest PJ, *et al.* Tracing the origin of adenocarcinomas with unknown primary using immunohistochemistry: differential diagnosis between colonic and ovarian carcinomas as primary sites. *Hum Pathol* 1998;29:491–7.

12 Tot T. Adenocarcinomas metastatic to the liver: the value of cytokeratins 20 and 7 in the search for unknown primary tumors. *Cancer* 1999;85:171–7.

13 Arnold A, Cossman J, Bakhshi A, *et al.* Immunoglobulin-gene rearrangements as unique clonal markers in human lymphoid neoplasms. *N Engl J Med* 1983;309:1593–9.

14 Rowley JD. Recurring chromosome abnormalities in leukemia and lymphoma. *Semin Hematol* 1990;27:122–36.

15 Turc-Carel C, Philip I, Berger MP, *et al.* Chromosomal translocation in Ewing's sarcoma. *N Engl J Med* 1983;309:497–8.

16 Whang-Peng J, Triche TJ, Knutsen T, *et al.* Chromosome translocation in peripheral neuroepithelioma. *N Engl J Med* 1984;311:584–5.

17 Gerald WL, Ladanyi M, de Alava E, *et al.* Clinical, pathologic, and molecular spectrum of tumors associated with t(11;22)(p13;q12): desmoplastic small round-cell tumor and its variants. *J Clin Oncol* 1998;16:3028–36.

18 French CA, Kutok JL, Faquin WC, *et al.* Midline carcinoma of children and young adults with NUT rearrangement. *J Clin Oncol* 2004;22:4135–49.

19 Motzer RJ, Rodriguez E, Reuter VE, *et al.* Molecular and cytogenetic studies in the diagnosis of patients with poorly differentiated carcinomas of unknown primary site. *J Clin Oncol* 1995;13:274–82.

20 Su AI, Welsh JB, Sapinoso LM, *et al.* Molecular classification of human carcinomas by use of gene expression signatures. *Cancer Res* 2001;61:7388–93.

21 Golub TR, Slonim DK, Tamayo P, *et al.* Molecular classification of cancer: class discovery and class prediction by gene expression monitoring. *Science* 1999;286:531–7.

22 Erlander MG, Ma XJ, Kesty NC, *et al.* Performance and clinical evaluation of the 92-gene real time PCR assay for tumor classification. *J Mol Diagn* 2011;13:493–503.

23 Pillai R, Deeter R, Rigl CT, *et al.* Validation and reproducibility of a microarray-based gene expression test for tumor identification in formalin-fixed, paraffin-embedded specimens. *J Mol Diagn* 2011;13:48–56.

24 Meiri E, Mueller WC, Rosenwald S, *et al.* A second-generation microRNA-based assay for diagnosing tumor tissue origin. *Oncologist* 2012;17:801–12.

25 Ma XJ, Pate R, Wang X, *et al.* Molecular classification of human cancers using a 92-gene real-time quantitative polymerase chain reaction assay. *Arch Pathol Lab Med* 2006;130:465–73.

26 Greco FA, Spigel DR, Yardley DA, *et al.* Molecular profiling in unknown primary cancer: accuracy of tissue of origin prediction. *Oncologist* 2010;15:500–6.

27 Varadhachary GR, Talantov D, Raber M, *et al.* Molecular profiling of carcinoma of unknown primary and correlation with clinical evaluation. *J Clin Oncol* 2008;26:4442–8.

28 Bridgewater J, van Laar R, Floore A, Van'T Veer L. Gene expression profiling may improve diagnosis in patients with carcinoma of unknown primary. *Br J Cancer* 2008;98:1425–30.

29 Horlings HM, van Laar RK, Kerst JM, *et al.* Gene expression profiling to identify the histogenetic origin of metastatic adenocarcinomas of unknown primary. *J Clin Oncol* 2008;26:4435–41.

30 van Laar RK, Ma XJ, de Jong D, *et al.* Implementation of a novel microarray-based diagnostic test for cancer of known primary. *Int J Cancer* 2009;125:1390–7.

31 Hainsworth JD, Pillai R, Henner WD, *et al.* Molecular tumor profiling in the diagnosis of patients with carcinoma of unknown primary site: Retrospective evaluation of a gene microarray assay. *J Mol Diagn* 2011;2:106.

32 Hainsworth JD, Rubin MS, Spigel DR, *et al.* Molecular gene expression profiling to predict the tissue of origin and direct site-specific therapy in patients with carcinoma of unknown primary site: a prospective trial of the Sarah Cannon Research Institute. *J Clin Oncol* 2013;31:217–23.

33 Hainsworth JD, Greco FA. Gene expression profiling in patients with carcinoma of unknown primary site: from translational research to standard of care. *Virchows Arch* 2014;464:393–402.

34 Greco FA, Lennington WJ, Spigel DR, Hainsworth JD. Molecular profiling diagnosis in unknown primary cancer: Accuracy and ability to complement standard pathology. *J Natl Cancer Inst* 2013;105:782–90.

35 Horlings HM, van Laar RK, Kerst JM, *et al.* Gene expression profiling to identify the histogenetic origin of metastatic adenocarcinomas of unknown primary. *J Clin Oncol* 2008;26:4435–41.

36 Monzon FA, Medeiros F, Lyons-Weiler M, Henner WD. Identification of tissue of origin in carcinoma of unknown primary with a microarray-based gene expression test. *Diagn Pathol* 2010;5:3.

37 Varadhachary GR, Spector Y, Abbruzzese JL, *et al.* Prospective gene signature study using microRNA to identify the tissue of origin in patients with carcinoma of unknown primary. *Clin Cancer Res* 2011;17:4063–70.

38 Morawietz L, Floore A, Stork-Sloots L, *et al.* Comparison of histopathological and gene expression-based typing of cancer of unknown primary. *Virchows Arch* 2010;456:23–9.

39 Greco FA, Lennington WJ, Spigel DR, Hainsworth JD. Poorly differentiated neoplasms of unknown primary site: diagnostic usefulness of a molecular cancer classifier assay. *Mol Diag Ther* 2015;19:91–7.

40 Nystrom JS, Werner JM, Heffelfinger-Juttner J, *et al.* Metastatic and histologic presentations in unknown primary cancer. *Semin Oncol* 1977;4:53–8.

41 Pentheroudakis G, Golfinopoulos V, Pavlidis N. Switching benchmarks in cancer of unknown primary: from autopsy to microarray. *Eur J Cancer* 2007;43:2026–36.

42 Sève P, Billotey C, Broussolle C, *et al.* The role of 2-deoxy-2-[F-18]fluoro-D-glucose positron emission tomography in disseminated carcinoma of unknown primary site. *Cancer* 2007;109:292–9.

43 Møller AK, Loft A, Berthelsen AK, *et al.* A prospective comparison of 18 F-FDG PET/CT and CT as diagnostic tools to identify the primary tumor site in patients with extracervical carcinoma of unknown primary site. *Oncologist* 2012;17:1146–54.

44 Rusthoven KE, Koshy M, Paulino AC. The role of fluorodeoxyglucose positron emission tomography in cervical lymph node metastases from an unknown primary tumor. *Cancer* 2004;101:2641–9.

45 Jones AS, Cook JA, Phillips DE, Roland NR. Squamous carcinoma presenting as an enlarged cervical lymph node. *Cancer* 1993;72:1756–61.

46 Varadhachary GR, Abbruzzese JL, Lenzi R. Diagnostic strategies for unknown primary cancer. *Cancer* 2004;100:1776–85.

47 Lapeyre M, Malissard L, Peiffert D, *et al.* Cervical lymph node metastasis from an unknown primary: is a tonsillectomy necessary? *Int J Radiat Oncol Biol Phys* 1997;39:291–6.

48 Catena L, Bichisao E, Milione M, *et al.* Neuroendocrine tumors of unknown primary site: Gold dust or misdiagnosed neoplasms? *Tumori* 2011;97:564–7.

49 Hainsworth JD, Johnson DH, Greco FA. Poorly differentiated neuroendocrine carcinoma of unknown primary site: A newly recognized clinicopathologic entity. *Ann Intern Med* 1988;109:364–71.

50 Hick RJ. Use of molecular targeted agents for the diagnosis, staging and therapy of neuroendocrine malignancy. *Cancer Imaging* 2010;10:S83–91.

51 Moertel CG, Kvals LK, O'Connell MJ, Rubin J. Treatment of neuroendocrine carcinomas with combined etopside and cisplatin: Evidence of major therapeutic activity in the anaplastic variants of these neoplasms. *Cancer* 1991;68:227–32.

52 Bhatia SK, Saclarides TJ, Witt TR, *et al.* Hormone receptor studies in axillary metastases from occult breast cancer. *Cancer* 1987;59:1170–2.

53 Block EF, Meyer MA. Positron emission tomography in diagnosis of occult adenocarcinoma of the breast. *Am Surg* 1998;64:906–8.

54 Schorn C, Fischer U, Luftner-Nagel S, Westerhof JP, Grabbe E. MRI of the breast in patients with metastatic disease of unknown primary. *Eur Radiol* 1999;9(3):470–3.

55 Orel SG, Weinstein SP, Schnall MD, *et al.* Breast MR imaging in patients with axillary node metastases and unknown primary malignancy. *Radiology* 1999;212:543–9.

56 Rosen PP. Axillary lymph node metastases in patients with occult noninvasive breast cancer. *Cancer* 1980;46:1298–306.

57 Ellerbroek N, Holmes F, Singletary E, *et al.* Treatment of patients with isolated axillary nodal metastases from an occult primary carcinoma consistent with breast origin. *Cancer* 1990;66:1461–7.

58 Schorge JO, Muto MG, Welch WR, *et al.* Molecular evidence for multifocal papillary serous carcinoma of the peritoneum in patients with germ-line *BRCA1* mutations. *J Natl Cancer Inst* 1998;90:841–5.

59 Tobacman JK, Greene MH, Tucker MA, *et al.* Intra-abdominal carcinomatosis after prophylactic oophorectomy in ovarian cancer-prone families. *Lancet* 1982;2:795–7.

60 Roh MH, Kindelberger D, Crum CP. Serous tubal intraepithelial carcinoma and the dominant ovarian mass: clues to a serous tumor origin? *Am J Surg Pathol* 2009;33:376–83.

61 Semmel DR, Folkins AK, Hirsch MS, *et al.* Intercepting early pelvic serous carcinoma by routine pathological examination of the fimbria. *Mod Pathol* 2009;22:985–8.

62 Dauplat J, Le Bouëdec G, Pomel C, Scherer C. Cytoreductive surgery for advanced stages of ovarian cancer. *Semin Surg Oncol* 2000;19:42–8.

63 Strnad CM, Grosh WW, Baxter J, *et al.* Peritoneal carcinomatosis of unknown primary site in women. A distinctive subset of adenocarcinoma. *Ann Intern Med* 1989;111:213–7.

64 Dalyrymple JC, Bannatyne P, Russell P, *et al.* Extraovarian peritoneal serous papillary carcinoma. A clinicopathologic study of 31 cases. *Cancer* 1989;64:110–5.

65 Ransom DT, Patel SR, Keeney GL, *et al.* Papillary serous carcinoma of the peritoneum. A review of 33 cases treated with platin-based chemotherapy. *Cancer* 1990;66:1091–4.

66 Fromm GL, Gershenson DM, Silva EG. Papillary serous carcinoma of the peritoneum. *Obstet Gynecol* 1990;75:89–95.

67 Bloss JD, Liao SY, Buller RE, *et al.* Extraovarian peritoneal serous papillary carcinoma: a case-control retrospective comparison to papillary adenocarcinoma of the ovary. *Gynecol Oncol* 1993;50:347–51.

68 Shah IA, Jayram L, Gani OS, *et al.* Papillary serous carcinoma of the peritoneum in a man: a case report. *Cancer* 1998;82:860–6.

69 Tell DT, Khoury JM, Taylor HG, Veasey SP. Atypical metastasis from prostate cancer: clinical utility of the immunoperoxidase technique for prostate-specific antigen. *JAMA* 1985;253:3574–5.

70 Gentile PS, Carloss HW, Huang TY, *et al.* Disseminated prostatic carcinoma simulating primary lung cancer. Indications for immunodiagnostic studies. *Cancer* 1988;62:711–5.

71 Saltz LB, Clarke S, Diaz-Rubio E, *et al.* Bevacizumab in combination with oxaliplatin-based chemotherapy as first-line therapy in metastatic colorectal cancer: a randomized phase III study. *J Clin Oncol* 2008;26:2013–9.

72 Grothey A, Sugrue MM, Purdie DM, *et al.* Bevacizumab beyond first progression is associated with prolonged overall survival in metastatic colorectal cancer: results from a large observational cohort study (BRiTE). *J Clin Oncol* 2008;26:5326–34.

73 Varadhachary GR, Raber MN, Matamoros A, Abbruzzese JL. Carcinoma of unknown primary with a colon-cancer profile-changing paradigm and emerging definitions. *Lancet Oncol* 2008;9(6):596–9.

74 Varadhachary GR, Karanth S, Hainsworth JD, *et al.* Patients with carcinoma of unknown primary and "colon cancer profile": clinicopathologic features and survival data. *Int J Clin Oncol* 2014;19:479–84.

75 Hainsworth JD, Schnabel CA, Erlander MG, *et al.* A retrospective study of treatment outcomes in patients with carcinoma of unknown primary site and a colorectal cancer molecular profile. *Clin Colorectal Cancer* 2012;11:112–8.

76 Greco FA, Lennington WJ, Spigel DR, *et al.* Carcinoma of unknown primary site: outcomes in patients with a colorectal molecular profile treated with site-specific chemotherapy. *J Cancer Therapy* 2012;3:37–43.

77 Rades D, Kuhnel G, Wildfang I, *et al.* Localised disease in cancer of unknown primary (CUP): The value of positron emission tomography (PET) for individual therapeutic management. *Ann Oncol* 2001;12:1605–9.

78 Nguyen LN, Maor MH, Oswald MJ. Brain metastases as the only manifestation of an undetected primary tumor. *Cancer* 1998;83:2181–4.

79 Hainsworth JD, Greco FA. Poorly differentiated carcinoma of unknown primary site. In: MF Fer, FA Greco, R Oldham (eds) *Poorly Differentiated Neoplasms and Tumors of Unknown Origin*. Orlando, FL: Grune and Stratton, Inc., 1986:189.

80 Fox RM, Woods RL, Tattersall MH, McGovern VJ. Undifferentiated carcinoma in young men: the atypical teratoma syndrome. *Lancet* 1979;1:1316–8.

81 Richardson RL, Schoumacher RA, Fer MF, *et al.* The unrecognized extragonadal germ cell cancer syndrome. *Ann Intern Med* 1981;94:181–6.

82 Greco FA, Vaughn WK, Hainsworth JD. Advanced poorly differentiated carcinoma of unknown primary site: recognition of a treatable syndrome. *Ann Intern Med* 1986;104:547–53.

83 Hainsworth JD, Johnson DH, Greco FA. Cisplatin-based combination chemotherapy in the treatment of poorly differentiated carcinoma and poorly differentiated adenocarcinoma of unknown primary site: results of a 12-year experience. *J Clin Oncol* 1992;10:912–22.

84 Wendt TG, Grabenbauer GG, Rodel CM, *et al.* Simultaneous radiochemotherapy versus radiotherapy alone in advanced head and neck cancer: a randomized multicenter study. *J Clin Oncol* 1998;16:1318–24.

85 de Braud F, Heilbrun LK, Ahmed K, *et al.* Metastatic squamous cell carcinoma of an unknown primary localized to the neck. Advantages of an aggressive treatment. *Cancer* 1989;64:510–5.

86 Fernández JA, Suárez C, Martínez JA, *et al.* Metastatic squamous cell carcinoma in cervical lymph nodes from an unknown primary tumour: prognostic factors. *Clin Otolaryngol Allied Sci* 1998;23:158–3.

87 Argiris A, Smith SM, Stenson K, *et al.* Concurrent chemoradiotherapy for N2 or N3 squamous cell carcinoma of the head and neck from an occult primary. *Ann Oncol* 2003;14:1306–11.

88 Zaren HA, Copeland EM 3rd. Inguinal node metastases. *Cancer* 1978;41:919–23.

89 Guarischi A, Keane TJ, Elkahim T. Metastatic inguinal nodes from an unknown primary neoplasm: A review of 56 cases. *Cancer* 1987;59:572–7.

90 Rinke A, Müller HH, Schade-Brittinger C, *et al.* Placebo-controlled, double-blind, prospective, randomized study on the effect of octreotide LAR in the control of tumor growth in patients with metastatic neuroendocrine midgut tumors: a report from the PROMID Study Group. *J Clin Oncol* 2009;27:4656–63.

91 Caplin ME, Pavel M, Cwikla JB, *et al.* Lanreotide in metastatic enteropancreatic neuroendocrine tumors. *N Engl J Med* 2014;371:224–33.

92 Raymond E, Dahan L, Raoul JL, *et al.* Sunitinib malate for the treatment of pancreatic neuroendocrine tumors. *N Engl J Med* 2011;364:501–3.

93 Yao JC, Shah MH, Ito T, *et al.* Everolimus for advanced pancreatic neuroendocrine tumors. *N Engl J Med* 2011;364:514–23.

94 Yao JC, Fazio N, Singh S, *et al.* Everolimus for the treatment of advanced non-functional neuroendocrine tumours of the lung or gastrointestinal tract (RADIANT-4): a randomized, placebo-controlled, phase 3 study. *Lancet* 2016;387:968–77.

95 Hainsworth JD, Spigel DR, Litchy S, Greco FA. Phase II trial of paclitaxel, carboplatin, and etoposide in advanced poorly differentiated neuroendocrine carcinoma: A Minnie Pearl Cancer Research Network Study. *J Clin Oncol* 2006;24:3548–54.

96 Briasoulis E, Kalofonos H, Bafaloukos D, *et al.* Carboplatin plus paclitaxel in unknown primary carcinoma: a phase II Hellenic Cooperative Oncology Group study. *J Clin Oncol* 2000;18:3101–7.

97 Greco FA, Erland JB Morrissey LH, *et al.* Carcinoma of unknown primary site: phase II trials with docetaxel plus cisplatin or carboplatin. *Ann Oncol* 2000;11:211–5.

98 Hainsworth JD, Spigel DR, Clark BL, *et al.* Paclitaxel/carboplatin/etoposide versus gemcitabine/irinotecan in the first-line treatment of patients with carcinoma of unknown primary site: a randomized, phase III Sarah Cannon Oncology Research Consortium Trial. *Cancer J* 2010;16:70–5.

99 Culine S, Lortholary A, Voigt JJ, *et al.* Cisplatin in combination with either gemcitabine or irinotecan in carcinomas of unknown primary site: results of a randomized phase II study – trial for the French Study Group on Carcinomas of Unknown Primary (GEFCAP101). *J Clin Oncol* 2003;21:3479–82.

100 Greco FA, Pavlidis N. Treatment for patients with unknown primary carcinoma and unfavorable prognostic factors. *Semin Oncol* 2009;36:65–74.

101 Ross JS, Wang K, Gay L, et al. Comprehensive genomic profiling of carcinoma of unknown primary site: new routes to targeted therapies. *JAMA Oncol* 2015;1:40–9.

102 Hainsworth JD, Greco FA. Lung adenocarcinoma with *ALK* rearrangement presenting as carcinoma of unknown primary site: recognition and treatment implications. *Drugs—Real World Outcomes* 2016;3:115–20.

103 Abruzzese JL, Abbruzzese MC, Hess KR, *et al.* Unknown primary carcinoma: natural history and prognostic factors in 657 consecutive patients. *J Clin Oncol* 1994;12:1272–80.

104 Saghatchian M, Fizazi K, Borel C, *et al.* Carcinoma of an unknown primary site: a chemotherapy strategy based on histological differentiation – results of a prospective study. *Ann Oncol* 2001;12:535–40.

105 van der Gaast A, Verweij J, Henzen-Logmans SC, *et al.* Carcinoma of unknown primary: identification of a treatable subset? *Ann Oncol* 1990;1:119–22.

106 Culine S, Kramar A, Saghatchian M, *et al.* Development and validation of a prognostic model to predict the length of survival in patients with carcinomas of an unknown primary site. *J Clin Oncol* 2002;20:4679–83.

107 Seve P, Ray-Coquard I, Trillet-Lenoir V, *et al.* Low serum albumin levels and liver metastasis are powerful prognostic markers for survival in patients with carcinomas of unknown primary site. *Cancer* 2006;107:2698–705.

108 Kodaira M, Takahashi S, Yamada S, *et al.* Bone metastasis and poor performance status are prognostic factors for survival of carcinoma of unknown primary site in patients treated with systemic chemotherapy. *Ann Oncol* 2010;21:1163–7.

45

Paraneoplastic Syndromes

Lorraine C. Pelosof and David E. Gerber

Harold C. Simmons Comprehensive Cancer Center, The University of Texas Southwestern Medical Center, Dallas, Texas, USA

Introduction

In 1888, Herman Oppenheim described symptoms occurring specifically in cancer patients that were not caused by direct tumor invasion or compression [1]. In the 1940s, A. Guichard and G. Vignon first called these syndromes "paraneoplastic" [2]. Paraneoplastic syndromes generally feature clinical signs and symptoms due to tumor secretion of bioactive substances or to immune cross-reactivity between normal host tissue and tumor cells. These pathophysiologic processes may affect endocrine, neurologic, dermatologic, rheumatologic, and hematologic organ systems. The prevalence of paraneoplastic syndromes among patients with cancer is estimated to be as high as 15% [3]. The most commonly associated malignancies include small cell lung cancer (SCLC), breast cancer, gynecologic tumors, and hematologic malignancies [4]. Timely recognition of paraneoplastic syndromes is essential, as these conditions may be the first manifestation of a new malignancy or may herald disease recurrence. While clinical overlap with nonparaneoplastic disorders may confound the diagnosis of these conditions, recent advances in serologic testing and radiographic imaging may aid in this process. Similarly, advances in cancer therapy, immunosuppressive regimens, and other treatments have improved clinical outcomes of paraneoplastic syndromes. This chapter will focus on the diagnosis and treatment of specific paraneoplastic syndromes, with emphasis on those most frequently encountered clinically.

Paraneoplastic Constitutional Syndromes

Tumor secretion of bioactive molecules can cause paraneoplastic constitutional symptoms such as fever, cachexia, and thrombophilia. Secretion of interleukin-6 (IL-6) has been associated with fever in renal cell carcinoma (RCC) and pheochromocytoma. Other malignancies typically associated with tumor fever include hematologic malignancies such as Hodgkin lymphoma and diffuse large B-cell lymphoma [3–7]. The diagnosis of paraneoplastic fever should only be made after other potential causes, such as infection, have been addressed. Once other causes have been ruled out, antipyretics can be employed for symptom management.

Cancer cachexia is characterized by significant decrease in body weight, largely due to adipose tissue and skeletal muscle loss [8]. Cancer cachexia is associated with poor prognosis and arises from a multifactorial process that includes the general inflammatory state and host response to insult, as also occurs in noncancer conditions such as sepsis [8]. Circulating factors implicated in the development of cancer cachexia include IL-6, tumor necrosis factor-α (TNF-α), and vascular endothelial growth factor (VEGF) [8, 9]. IL-6 and VEGF may be expressed or secreted directly by various tumors including RCC, pheochromocytoma, and pancreatic tumors [3, 6, 9, 10]. Treatment of cancer cachexia requires a multimodality approach incorporating nutrition, exercise, and tumor-directed therapy. Additionally, newer approaches use nonsteroidal anti-inflammatory drugs to decrease systemic inflammation, as well as selective androgen receptor modulators and humanized anti-IL-6 antibodies to increase lean body mass and muscle function [11, 12].

Cancer patients are estimated to be approximately five times more likely to develop venous thromboembolism (VTE) than is the general population [13, 14]. Gynecologic, pancreatic, brain, and lung cancers are considered the most thrombophilic malignancies [13, 15]. Principal mediators of this systemic hypercoagulability include tumor-associated tissue factor (TF) and cancer procoagulant [14]. TF, which is overexpressed on the surface of breast, pancreatic, and hematologic cancers, initiates the extrinsic clotting cascade [14–16]. Cancer procoagulant, a protease expressed in diverse cancer types, directly activates factor X [14]. A detailed discussion of the diagnosis and treatment of VTE is beyond the scope of this chapter and is covered in numerous reviews [17–19]. In general, low-molecular-weight heparin is preferred over warfarin for the long-term management of VTE in cancer patients, as there is a reduced incidence of VTE recurrence [20]. Newer anticoagulants, such as the anti-Xa agent rivaroxaban and the anti-IIa agent dabigatran, offer the convenience of oral administration but are not readily reversible [21].

The American Cancer Society's Oncology in Practice: Clinical Management, First Edition. Edited by The American Cancer Society.

Paraneoplastic Endocrine Syndromes

Paraneoplastic endocrine syndromes are due to ectopic secretion of peptides or glycoproteins by tumors not arising from tissues that would normally secrete these bioactive substances (eutopic secretion) [3]. In general, clinical features of ectopic secretion resemble those resulting from eutopic secretion [3]. Treating the underlying tumor often improves or resolves endocrine paraneoplastic syndromes. Additionally, various medical therapies are available to counter directly the effects of the implicated paraneoplastic substances. Typically, paraneoplastic endocrine syndromes are discovered after a cancer diagnosis and their presence does not correlate with disease stage [22]. After successful treatment of the underlying malignancy, recurrence of an endocrine paraneoplastic syndrome may herald tumor recurrence [3]. Multiple malignancies may cause paraneoplastic endocrine syndromes; the highest prevalence of these conditions is seen with neuroendocrine tumors such as SCLC. The clinical and diagnostic features, associated cancers, and treatment of the most common paraneoplastic endocrine syndromes are listed in Table 45.1.

Syndrome of Inappropriate Antidiuretic Hormone (SIADH)

One to two percent of all cancer patients develop syndrome of inappropriate antidiuretic hormone (SIADH), a hypo-osmotic, euvolemic hyponatremia caused by the ectopic secretion of either ADH or atrial natriuretic peptide (ANP). SCLC is the most commonly associated malignancy; approximately 15% of all SCLC patients develop SIADH [3, 23]. To diagnose SIADH, it is important to distinguish its euvolemic hyponatremia from the hypovolemic hyponatremia that occurs with gastrointestinal losses, cerebral salt wasting, and adrenal insufficiency [23]. Clinical manifestations of SIADH, which are primarily neurocognitive, depend on the degree of hyponatremia as well as the rate of onset. In addition to addressing the underlying tumor, treatment options include free water restriction, demeclocycline, vasopressin-receptor antagonists, and the discontinuation of any contributing drugs. The rate of correction must be proportional to the rapidity of onset of the hyponatremia to avoid overly rapid correction that can result in central pontine myelinolysis. This condition is characterized by lethargy, dysarthria, spastic quadriparesis, and pseudobulbar palsy, all of which may be permanent [24]. Symptomatic, acute-onset (within 48 hours) hyponatremia may necessitate the use of 3% saline and can normally be corrected at approximately 1–2 mmol/L/h for a maximum of 8–10 mmol/L over the first 24 hours. Chronic hyponatremia should be corrected more slowly [24]. Importantly, the administration of normal saline may *worsen* SIADH because the osmolality of normal saline (308 mOsm/L) is often less than that of the excreted urine, resulting in a further decline in the serum sodium level. Response to demeclocycline, which interferes with the renal response to ADH, is seen within days to weeks. Adverse effects are primarily gastrointestinal and renal. If used long-term, demeclocycline may result in diabetes insipidus (excretion of overly dilute urine leading to hypernatremia) and – because demeclocycline is an antibacterial agent – bacterial or yeast superinfection [23, 24].

Hypercalcemia

Approximately 10% of all patients with cancer will develop malignancy-associated hypercalcemia. Hypercalcemia in this population is associated with a high mortality rate (approximately 50% at 30 days) [24, 34]. Humoral hypercalcemia of malignancy, caused by tumor secretion of parathyroid hormone-related protein (PTHrP), causes approximately 80% of cases and is typically seen in squamous cell cancers, RCC, gynecologic malignancies, breast cancer, and certain lymphomas [26]. Other causes of hypercalcemia in cancer patients include local osteolytic hypercalcemia (approximately 20% of cases), secretion of vitamin D (less than 1% of cases, generally lymphomas), and secretion of ectopic PTH (very rare) [3, 26]. The severity of clinical features – which include gastrointestinal symptoms, neurologic changes, and renal failure – depends on the degree of hypercalcemia, the rate of onset, and the patient's baseline neurologic and renal function. Optimal therapy for malignancy-associated hypercalcemia is tumor-directed treatment. Many patients will not require other specific interventions [26]. Other common treatments include intravenous hydration with normal saline, intravenous bisphosphonates (which inhibit osteoclast bone resorption), and calcitonin (which inhibits bone resorption and increases renal calcium excretion) [26]. Loop diuretics were employed historically but should be used with caution as they may exacerbate hypercalcemia when used in patients who are not adequately hydrated [26]. After bisphosphonate infusion, serum calcium levels generally decline within 2–4 days, reach a nadir within 4–7 days, and remain suppressed for up to 3 weeks [26]. Renal dysfunction and osteonecrosis of the jaw are the main serious adverse effects associated with bisphosphonates. The risk of developing osteonecrosis is increased after prolonged use and also in the setting of recent invasive dental procedures [25]. Denosumab is a fully human monoclonal antibody against receptor activator of nuclear factor κB ligand (RANKL), the principal trigger for osteoclast function. It has been approved for the prevention of skeletal-related events in cancer patients with bone metastases and has been used to treat bisphosphonate-refractory hypercalcemia [35–37]. Calcitonin may result in a relatively rapid decline in serum calcium, but effects are short-lived and more modest than those seen with bisphosphonates [25].

Cushing Syndrome

An estimated 5–20% of Cushing syndrome (hypercortisolism) occurs as a paraneoplastic phenomenon and is caused by tumor secretion of adrenocorticotropic hormone (ACTH) or, less commonly, corticotropin-releasing hormone (CRH) [3, 29]. SCLC and bronchial carcinoid tumors account for 50–60% of these cases [3, 29, 38]. Unlike SIADH and hypercalcemia, paraneoplastic Cushing syndrome often presents symptomatically before the diagnosis of the associated malignancy [3, 28, 29]. Patients present with hypertension, hypokalemia, muscle weakness, generalized edema, and weight gain [30, 39]. Associated laboratory abnormalities include elevations in serum cortisol, urinary free cortisol, and midnight ACTH [30]. Failure to respond to high-dose dexamethasone suppression distinguishes ectopic (i.e., paraneoplastic) Cushing syndrome from a pituitary source [30].

Table 45.1 Paraneoplastic endocrine syndromes. Modified with permission from Pelosof LC, Gerber DE. Paraneoplastic syndromes: an approach to diagnosis and treatment. Mayo Clin Proc 2010; 85(9):838–54.

Syndrome	Clinical features	Laboratory values	Associated malignancies	Management[1]	References
SIADH	Gait disturbance, headache, nausea, fatigue, muscle cramps, anorexia, confusion, lethargy, seizures, respiratory depression, coma	Hyponatremia (severe symptoms seen when serum sodium falls to <125 mmol/L in less than 48 hours) Increased urine osmolality (>100 mOsm/kg in the context of euvolemic hyponatremia)	Small cell lung cancer Mesothelioma Bladder Ureteral Endometrial Prostate Oropharyngeal Thymoma Lymphoma Ewing sarcoma Brain Gastrointestinal Breast Adrenal	Free water restriction (usually <1000 mL/day) Adequate salt and protein intake Salt tablets Demeclocycline Vasopressin-receptor antagonists (conivaptan, tolvaptan) Hypertonic (3%) saline **(if acute onset)** **Goal correction rates:** *Acute onset* (*<48 hours*): increase serum sodium level 1–2 mmol/L per hour (8–10 mmol/L during first 24 hours of treatment) *Chronic*: increase serum sodium level 0.5 mmol/L per hour Discontinuation of offending drugs (e.g., opiates, antidepressants, thiazide diuretics, and certain chemotherapy drugs)	[23, 24]
Hypercalcemia	Altered mental status, weakness, ataxia, lethargy, hypertonia, renal failure, nausea/vomiting, hypertension, bradycardia	Hypercalcemia Mild (<12 mg/dL): often asymptomatic Moderate (12–14 mg/dL): symptomatic if acute; well-tolerated if chronic Severe (>14 mg/dL): progressive symptoms Low to normal PTH level Elevated PTHrP level	Breast Multiple myeloma Renal cell Squamous cell Cancers (especially lung and head and neck) Lymphoma Gynecologic	Normal saline Bisphosphonates Calcitonin Denosumab (consider if refractory to bisphosphonates) Loop diuretics (*Note*: use with caution and only if patient volume replete) Glucocorticoids (for lymphoma, myeloma) Mithramycin Gallium nitrate Hemodialysis Discontinuation of offending drugs (e.g., calcium supplements, vitamin D, thiazide diuretics, calcium-containing antacids, lithium)	[22, 25, 26]
Cushing syndrome	Muscle weakness, peripheral edema, hypertension, weight gain, centripetal fat distribution	Hypokalemia (typically less than 3.0 mmol/L) Elevated baseline serum cortisol (greater than 800 nmol/L) Normal to elevated (greater than 100 mg/L) midnight serum ACTH (not suppressed with dexamethasone) Failure to respond to high-dose dexamethasone suppression test	Small cell lung cancer Bronchial carcinoid Thymus Thyroid (medullary thyroid cancer) Adenocarcinoma (lung, colon, ovarian, esophageal)	Ketoconazole Octreotide or octreotide LAR Aminoglutethimide Metyrapone Mitotane Etomidate Mifepristone Adrenalectomy (reserved for refractory cases) Supportive measures: antihypertensives, diuretics, supplemental potassium	[27–30]
Hypoglycemia	Sweating, anxiety, tremors, palpitations, hunger, weakness, seizures, confusion, coma	For non-islet cell tumor hypoglycemia (NICTH): low serum glucose low serum insulin (often less than 10–25 pmol/L) low serum C-peptide (often less than 100 pmol/L)	Mesothelioma Sarcomas Lung Gastrointestinal	*Acute treatment* Glucose (oral and/or parenteral) *Chronic treatment* Corticosteroids Diazoxide Glucagon infusion (after assessing for adequate hepatic glycogen stores) Octreotide or octreotide LAR Human growth hormone	[22, 31–33]

[1] In addition to treating the underlying malignancy.
ACTH, adrenocorticotropic hormone; LAR, long-acting release; NICTH, non-islet cell tumor hypoglycemia; PTH, parathyroid hormone; PTHrP, PTH-related protein; SIADH, syndrome of inappropriate antidiuretic hormone secretion.

Beyond treatment of the underlying tumor, inhibiting steroidogenesis with agents such as ketoconazole is a mainstay of therapy [27]. Despite associated nausea, hepatotoxicity, and potential for drug–drug interactions, ketoconazole is generally better tolerated than other adrenal toxins such as mitotane, metyrapone, and aminoglutethimide. Other available treatments target ACTH release (octreotide) and cortisol action (mifepristone) [27]. Treatment of Cushing-associated hypertension and hypokalemia is also a critical component of management [27].

Hypoglycemia

Both pancreatic islet cell tumors (insulinomas) and certain extrapancreatic cancers may cause tumor-associated hypoglycemia [31]. Paraneoplastic non-islet cell tumor hypoglycemia (NICTH) is the more common mechanism and usually affects elderly patients with advanced-stage malignancy [31, 32]. NICTH is usually caused by tumor secretion of insulin-like growth factor 2 (IGF-2) [31]. As with other paraneoplastic endocrine syndromes, optimal therapy involves tumor resection or treatment. Medical management focuses on maintenance of adequate blood glucose levels. Acutely, this includes oral and/or parenteral dextrose. Chronic management may include diazoxide (which inhibits insulin secretion by pancreatic β cells), corticosteroids, growth hormone, octreotide, or glucagon.

Paraneoplastic Neurologic Syndromes

In contrast to paraneoplastic endocrine syndromes, patients present with paraneoplastic neurologic syndromes (PNS) prior to a cancer diagnosis in approximately 80% of cases [40]. Although PNS are rare (fewer than 1% of patients with cancer are affected) [41], certain tumors are associated with a considerably higher incidence, including thymomas (up to 15–20%), B-cell and plasma cell neoplasms (up to 10%), and SCLC (up to 5%) [42]. These and other over-represented malignancies tend to (i) produce neuroendocrine proteins (e.g., SCLC), (ii) contain neuronal components (e.g., teratomas), (iii) involve immunoregulatory organs (e.g., thymomas), or (iv) affect immunoglobulin production (e.g., lymphoma, myeloma) [42]. PNS may affect the central nervous system, the neuromuscular junction, or the peripheral nervous system. Depending on the involved nervous system compartment, clinical features of PNS may include cognitive and personality changes, ataxia, cranial nerve deficits, motor weakness, and numbness. Table 45.2 lists the clinical features, associated malignancies, diagnostic studies (which may include imaging, serologies, electromyography, nerve conduction studies, electroencephalography, and cerebrospinal fluid analysis), and treatment options (which center on immunomodulation) for PNS.

PNS most often result from immune cross-reactivity between tumor antigens and components of the nervous system. Antigenic similarity between the cancer and the neuronal proteins results in humoral (onconeural antibodies) and cellular (onconeural antigen-specific T lymphocytes) immune responses [41, 56, 57]. While onconeural antibodies may often be detected through serologic testing, in many instances they are neither sensitive nor specific for the associated PNS [58]. Interpretation of clinical and laboratory findings, particularly in patients without a prior cancer diagnosis, requires caution because many of these conditions also occur outside a cancer context. For instance, only 60% of Lambert–Eaton myasthenic syndrome (LEMS) cases are paraneoplastic [40]. Nevertheless, diagnosis of an apparent PNS should prompt a thorough search for an underlying tumor. Imaging studies including computed tomography (CT) of the chest, abdomen, and pelvis should be performed. If these are unrevealing, fluorodeoxyglucose positron emission tomography (FDG-PET) may be considered [40, 59, 60]. Patient demographics and the specific PNS identified may direct other investigations such as mammography and colonoscopy. If, despite this investigation, no cancer is identified, it is generally recommended that repeat screening be conducted in 3–6 months and then every 6 months thereafter for approximately 4 years [61]. Beyond that time, the likelihood of a subsequent cancer diagnosis decreases considerably.

Onconeural antibodies are characterized according to target antigen location. **Group 1 nuclear and cytoplasmic neuronal antigens (NCNA) antibodies** target antigens such as Yo, Ri, HuD, Ma1/2, and CRMP5/CV2 and are strongly associated with malignancy, including SCLC, ovarian cancer, and breast cancer [43]. Because these target antigens are intracellular (and therefore presumably not accessible to circulating antibodies), the pathophysiologic role of these antibodies is unclear. It is possible that antibodies may be markers of a T-lymphocyte reaction to these antigens [43]. Immunomodulatory treatment of PNS associated with group 1 antibodies has historically had limited success [43]. More recently, however, T-cell-directed treatments such as tacrolimus have demonstrated promise [41]. **Group 2 cell-surface synaptic antigens (CSSA) antibody** targets include the NMDA receptor, voltage-gated calcium channel (VGCC), $GABA_BR$, and GluR1/2 [43, 56]. These antibodies are less strongly associated with cancer than are group 1 antibodies. Many of the previously characterized "seronegative" PNS cases are now felt to be due to group 2 antibodies [56]. Clinical manifestations arise from antibody interference with synaptic transmission. The associated PNS are more likely to respond to immunotherapy than are PNS associated with group 1 antibodies [43]. **Group 3 intracellular synaptic antigens (ISA) antibodies** are directed against the intracellular synaptic antigens GAD65 (glutamic acid decarboxylase 65 kDa) and amphiphysin in presynaptic terminals. These antibodies have variable associations with malignancy. The associated PNS have an intermediate response to immunotherapies [43].

In addition to treating the underlying malignancy, immune modulation represents the mainstay of PNS therapy. Specific approaches include corticosteroids, corticosteroid-sparing agents such as azathioprine and cyclophosphamide, the anti-CD20 monoclonal antibody rituximab, intravenous immunoglobulin (IVIG), and plasma exchange (plasmapheresis). Treatment-induced reduction in onconeural antibody titers has been associated with clinical improvement [46, 62]. After successful treatment of the associated malignancy, recurrence of detectable antibody titers may indicate tumor relapse [63, 64].

Table 45.2 Paraneoplastic neurologic syndromes. Modified with permission from Pelosof LC, Gerber DE. Paraneoplastic syncromes: an approach to diagnosis and treatment. © 2010 Mayo Foundation for Medical Education and Research. Published by Elsevier Inc.

Syndrome	Clinical features	Associated antibodies	Diagnostic studies	Associated malignancies	Management[1]	References
Limbic encephalitis (LE)	Mood changes, hallucinations, memory loss, seizures, less commonly hypothalamic symptoms; onset over days to months	anti-Hu (with small cell lung cancer), anti-Ma2 (with testicular cancer), anti-CRMP5/ CV2, anti-amphiphysin	**EEG** epileptic foci in temporal lobe(s); focal or generalized slow activity **FDG-PET** increased metabolism in temporal lobe(s) **MRI** hyperintensity in medial temporal lobe(s) **CSF** pleocytosis, elevated protein, elevated IgG, oligoclonal bands	Small cell lung cancer Testicular Breast Thymoma Teratoma Hodgkin lymphoma	IVIG Corticosteroids Plasma exchange Cyclophosphamide Rituximab	[40, 42–45]
Paraneoplastic cerebellar degeneration (PCD)	Ataxia, diplopia, dysphagia/dysarthria; prodrome of dizziness, nausea, vomiting	anti-Hu, anti-Yo, anti-CRMP5/CV2, anti-Ma, anti-Tr, anti-Ri, anti-VGCC, anti-mGluR1	**FDG-PET** increased metabolism (early stage) and then decreased metabolism (late stage) in cerebellum **MRI** cerebellar atrophy (late stage)	Small cell lung cancer Gynecologic Hodgkin lymphoma Breast	IVIG Corticosteroids Plasma exchange Cyclophosphamide Rituximab	[40, 42–45]
Lambert–Eaton myasthenia syndrome (LEMS)	Proximal lower extremity muscle weakness, fatigue, diaphragmatic weakness, bulbar symptoms (usually milder than in myasthenia gravis); later in course, autonomic symptoms in most patients	anti-VGCC	**EMG** low compound muscle action potential amplitude; decremental response with low-rate stimulation but incremental response with high-rate stimulation	Small cell lung cancer Extrapulmonary small cell carcinoma (e.g., cervix, prostate) Lymphoma Adenocarcinomas	3,4- Diaminopyridine (DAP) Pyridostigmine (with or without guanidine) Corticosteroids Azathioprine IVIG Plasma exchange	[40, 42, 43, 46, 47]
Myasthenia gravis (MG)	Fatigable weakness of voluntary muscles (ocular-bulbar and limbs), diaphragmatic weakness	anti-AchR	**EMG** decremental response to repetitive nerve stimulation	Thymoma (in ~15% of MG patients)	Thymectomy (for thymic malignancy) Pyridostigmine Corticosteroids Azathioprine Cyclosporine Tacrolimus Mycophenolate mofetil Rituximab Cyclophosphamide Plasma exchange IVIG	[46, 48–50]

(Continued)

Table 45.2 (Continued)

Syndrome	Clinical features	Associated antibodies	Diagnostic studies	Associated malignancies	Management[1]	References
Autonomic neuropathy	Panautonomic neuropathy, often subacute (weeks) onset, involving sympathetic, parasympathetic, and enteric systems: orthostatic hypotension, GI dysfunction, dry eyes/mouth, bowel/bladder dysfunction, altered pupillary light reflexes, loss of sinus arrhythmia *Chronic gastrointestinal pseudo-obstruction* (*CGP*): constipation, nausea/vomiting, dysphagia, weight loss, abdominal distension	anti-Hu, anti-CRMP5/CV2, anti-nAchR, anti-amphiphysin	**Abdominal X-ray/barium studies/CT** GI dilatation but no mechanical obstruction (for CGP) **Esophageal manometry** achalasia or spasms (for CGP)	Small cell lung cancer Thymoma	*For orthostatic hypotension* Water, salt intake Fludrocortisone Midodrine Ibuprofen Caffeine Erythropoietin (if anemic) *For pseudo-obstruction* Neostigmine	[40, 46, 51–53]
Subacute (peripheral) sensory neuropathy	Multifocal and asymmetric distribution of paresthesias/pain (usually upper extremities before lower), ataxia, decreased or absent deep tendon reflexes	anti-Hu, anti-CRMP5/CV2, anti-amphiphysin	**NCS** reduced/absent sensory nerve action potentials **CSF** pleocytosis, high IgG, oligoclonal bands	Lung (~70–80%) – usually small cell lung cancer Breast Ovarian Sarcomas Hodgkin lymphoma	Corticosteroids Cyclophosphamide IVIG Plasma exchange	[40, 46, 54, 55]

[1] In addition to treating the underlying malignancy.

AchR, acetylcholine receptor; CGP, chronic gastrointestinal pseudo-obstruction; CRMP, collapsin response mediator proteins; CSF, cerebrospinal fluid; DAP, diaminopyridine; EEG, electroencephalogram; EMG, electromyelogram; FDG-PET, fluorodeoxyglucose positron emission tomography; IVIG, intravenous immunoglobulin; LEMS, Lambert–Eaton myasthenia syndrome; mGluR1, metabotropic glutamate receptor-subtype 1; MRI, magnetic resonance imaging; nAchR, nicotinic acetylcholine receptor; NCS, nerve conduction study; NMDA, N-methyl-D-aspartate; VGCC, voltage-gated calcium channel.

Table 45.3 Paraneoplastic dermatologic and rheumatologic syndromes. Modified with permission from Pelosof LC, Gerber DE. Paraneoplastic syndromes: an approach to diagnosis and treatment. © 2010 Mayo Foundation for Medical Education and Research. Published by Elsevier Inc.

Syndrome	Clinical features	Diagnostic studies	Associated malignancies	Management[1]	References
Acanthosis nigricans	Velvety, hyperpigmented skin (usually on flexural regions) Papillomatous changes involving mucous membranes and mucocutaneous junctions Rugose changes on palms and dorsal surface of large joints (e.g., tripe palms)	Skin biopsy: hyperkeratosis and papillomatosis	Adenocarcinoma of abdominal organs, especially gastric	Retinoids Topical corticosteroids and cyproheptadine	[69, 72, 75, 76]
Dermatomyositis (DM)	Heliotrope rash (violaceous, edematous rash on upper eyelids) Gottron papules (scaly papules on bony surfaces) Erythematous rash on face, neck, chest or back, shoulders ("shawl sign"); rash may be photosensitive Proximal muscle weakness Swallowing difficulty Respiratory difficulty Muscle pain	Elevated serum CK, AST, ALT, LDH, and aldolase EMG: increased spontaneous activity with fibrillations, complex repetitive discharges, and positive sharp waves Muscle biopsy: perivascular or interfascicular septal inflammation and perifascicular atrophy	(15–20% of cases paraneoplastic) Ovarian Breast Prostate Lung Colorectal Non-Hodgkin lymphoma Nasopharyngeal	Corticosteroids Azathioprine Methotrexate Cyclosporine Mycophenolate mofetil Cyclophosphamide IVIG	[69, 77]
Erythroderma	Erythematous, exfoliating, diffuse rash (often pruritic)	Skin biopsy (histology shows dense perivascular lymphocytic infiltrate)	Chronic lymphocytic leukemia Cutaneous T-cell lymphoma (including mycosis fungoides) Gastrointestinal Adult T-cell leukemia/lymphoma Myeloproliferative disorders	Topical corticosteroids Narrowband UVB phototherapy	[78–81]
Hypertrophic osteoarthropathy (HOA)	Subperiosteal new bone formation on phalangeal shafts ("clubbing") Periosteal reaction along long bones Synovial effusions (mainly large joints) Pain, swelling along affected bones, joints	Nuclear bone scan showing intense and symmetric uptake in long bones	(90% of cases paraneoplastic) Intrathoracic tumors Metastases to lung Metastases to bone Nasopharyngeal carcinoma Sarcoma	Bisphosphonates Localized radiation therapy	[69, 71, 82, 83]
Leukocytoclastic vasculitis	Usually small and medium vessel involvement Ulceration, cyanosis, pain over affected regions (especially digits) Palpable purpura often over lower extremities Renal impairment Peripheral neuropathy	Skin biopsy: fibrinoid necrosis of vessel walls, endothelial swelling, leukocytoclasis, RBC extravasation	Leukemia/lymphoma Myelodysplastic syndrome Gastrointestinal Lung Urologic Multiple myeloma Rhabdomyosarcoma	Corticosteroids Dapsone Colchicine Methotrexate Azathioprine IVIG	[69, 84–88]
Paraneoplastic pemphigus (PNP)	Severe cutaneous blisters and erosions (predominantly on trunk, soles, palms) Severe mucosal erosions including stomatitis	Skin biopsy: keratinocyte necrosis, epidermal acantholysis, IgG and complement deposition in epidermal and basement membrane zones Serum autoantibodies to epithelia (including against plakin proteins and desmogleins)	Non-Hodgkin lymphoma (PNP is largely associated with B-cell diseases) Chronic lymphocytic leukemia Thymoma Castleman disease Follicular dendritic cell sarcoma	Systemic corticosteroids Azathioprine Cyclophosphamide Cyclosporine IVIG Mycophenolate mofetil Plasma exchange Rituximab	[69, 78, 89–95,]

(Continued)

Table 45.3 (Continued)

Syndrome	Clinical features	Diagnostic studies	Associated malignancies	Management[1]	References
Polymyalgia rheumatica (PMR)	Limb girdle and neck pain and stiffness	Elevated serum ESR (but often not as high as in nonparaneoplastic PMR) Elevated CRP Anemia	Myelodysplastic syndrome Leukemia/lymphoma Colon Lung Renal Prostate Breast	Prednisone (typically less responsive to steroid therapy than nonparaneoplastic PMR) Methotrexate	[68, 96–98]
Sweet syndrome (acute febrile neutrophilic dermatosis)	Painful, erythematous nodules, papules, plaques, or pustules on extremities, face, or upper trunk (acute onset) Neutrophilia Fever Malaise	Skin biopsy: polymorphonuclear cell dermal infiltrate	Leukemia (especially AML) Non-Hodgkin lymphoma Myelodysplastic syndrome Genitourinary Breast Gastrointestinal Multiple myeloma Gynecologic Testicular Melanoma	Corticosteroids (topical, intralesional, systemic) Potassium iodide (topical) Colchicine Dapsone	[69, 70, 73, 99–101]

[1] In addition to treating the underlying malignancy.
ALT, alanine aminotransferase; AML, acute myeloid leukemia; AST, aspartate aminotransferase; CK, creatine kinase; CRP, C-reactive protein; EMG, electromyography; ESR, erythrocyte sedimentation rate; IVIG, intravenous immunoglobulin; LDH, lactate dehydrogenase; RBC, red blood cell; UV, ultraviolet.

For certain PNS, treatments directed at the resulting neuropathophysiologic properties are key components of management. These include pyridostigmine (an acetylcholinesterase inhibitor) for myasthenia gravis and 3,4-diaminopyridine (a potassium channel blocker) for Lambert–Eaton myasthenic syndrome.

The overall impact of PNS on clinical outcomes reflects numerous factors [65]. Recognition of a PNS may lead to detection and treatment of an otherwise clinically occult and highly treatable tumor. Additionally, onconeural antibodies may indicate an antitumor immunologic effect. For instance, patients with SCLC who have circulating anti-Hu antibodies have higher complete response rates (odds ratio 5.4) and longer overall survival than those patients without anti-Hu antibodies [66]. Although such observations raise the hypothetical concern than treatment of PNS with immune modulation may result in cancer progression, this phenomenon has not been observed clinically. Separately, PNS may impart substantial neurologic toxicity. Because PNS may cause irreversible damage to the nervous system, treatment often results in symptom stability rather than improvement. These outcomes stand in contrast to those of endocrine paraneoplastic syndromes, which frequently resolve entirely with successful treatment of the associated malignancy. Finally, the advent of immune checkpoint inhibitors as effective treatment for multiple cancer types has introduced concerns that these agents may cause or exacerbate immune-related paraneoplastic syndromes [67].

Paraneoplastic Dermatologic and Rheumatologic Syndromes

Paraneoplastic dermatologic and rheumatologic syndromes generally have similar presentations to their nonparaneoplastic counterparts. Because these conditions may be the first sign of an internal malignancy or the initial manifestation of tumor recurrence, expedited age- and risk factor-guided cancer screening is indicated in these patients [68, 69]. Rheumatologic syndromes refractory to standard treatments may indicate a paraneoplastic association [68]. Successful cancer treatment often results in symptom improvement or resolution, but many of these conditions also warrant and respond to specific therapies [68–70]. Among the various syndromes, the proportion of cases with paraneoplastic etiology varies widely. For instance, up to 90% of patients with acanthosis nigricans of the palms (tripe palms) and up to 90% of patients with hypertrophic osteoarthropathy have an associated malignancy [71, 72]. Conversely, only 10–25% of dermatomyositis cases and 20% of Sweet syndrome (febrile neutrophilic dermatosis) cases are paraneoplastic [69, 73, 74]. Table 45.3 details the clinical presentation, diagnostic studies, associated malignancies, and treatment of the more common paraneoplastic dermatologic and rheumatologic syndromes. Selected paraneoplastic dermatologic syndromes are depicted in Figures 45.1, 45.2, 45.3, and 45.4.

Paraneoplastic Hematologic Syndromes

With the exception of thrombophilia, paraneoplastic hematologic syndromes are generally asymptomatic and do not require specific treatment. These conditions typically present in patients with advanced or metastatic disease and subside with effective antitumor therapy [102, 103]. Paraneoplastic eosinophilia, which results from tumor production of IL-3, IL-5, and granulocyte–macrophage colony-stimulating factor (GM-CSF), is seen in less than 1% of malignancies overall but occurs in approximately 10% of all lymphoma cases and in 3% of lung cancer cases; it is often a marker of advanced disease [102, 103].

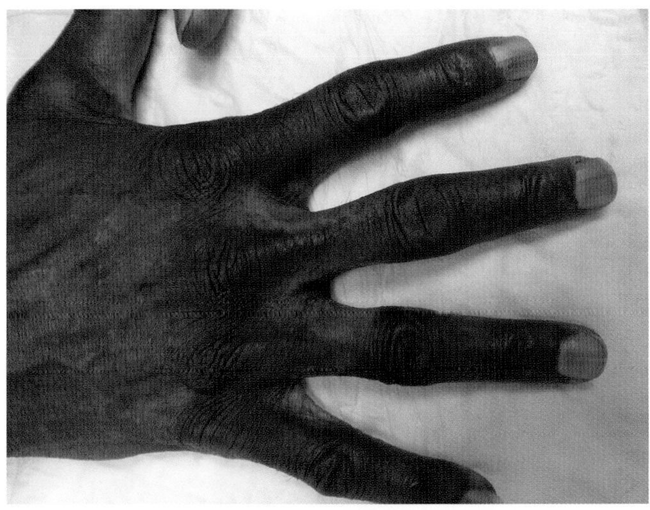

Figure 45.1 Acanthosis nigricans. *Source:* Christopher Sayed, MD, Department of Dermatology, The University of North Carolina School of Medicine. Reproduced with permission of Dr Sayed.

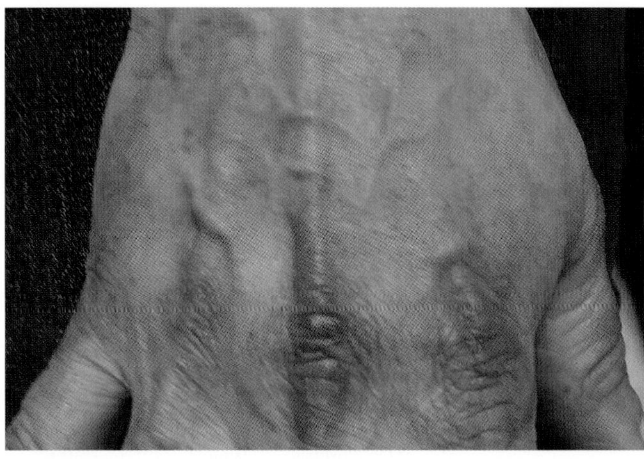

Figure 45.2 Dermatomyositis (Gottron papules). *Source:* Benjamin Chong, MD, Department of Dermatology, The University of Texas Southwestern Medical Center.

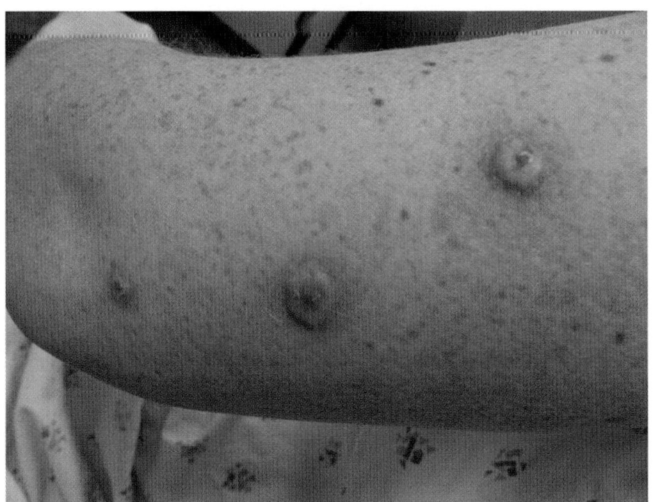

Figure 45.3 Sweet syndrome. *Source:* Christopher Sayed, MD, Department of Dermatology, The University of North Carolina School of Medicine. Reproduced with permission of Dr Sayed.

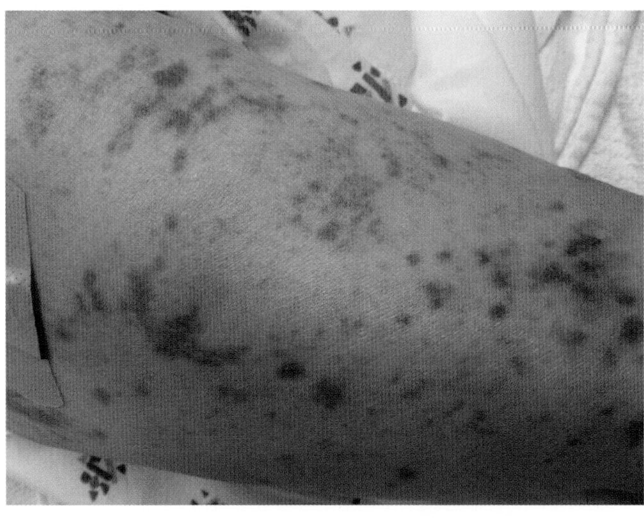

Figure 45.4 Leukocytoclastic vasculitis. *Source:* Christopher Sayed, MD, Department of Dermatology, The University of North Carolina School of Medicine. Reproduced with permission of Dr Sayed.

In contrast to primary eosinophilia (a clonal phenomenon arising from a hematologic neoplastic process), paraneoplastic and other secondary eosinophilias are not usually associated with end-organ damage such as infiltrative cardiomyopathy [102]. Both paraneoplastic granulocytosis (attributed to tumor secretion of cytokines such as granulocyte colony-stimulating factor) and paraneoplastic thrombocytosis (possibly due to thrombopoietin-like molecules or IL-6) are associated with advanced disease and poor prognosis [103, 104]. Elevated serum levels of IL-6 may distinguish secondary (including paraneoplastic) thrombocytosis from a primary myeloproliferative disorder [105]. Pure red cell aplasia (PRCA) is most often seen with thymic malignancies. Due to the severity of the associated normocytic anemia, supportive measures including transfusions are often required. Additionally, immunosuppressive agents may be employed [106, 107]. The clinical features, associated tumors, and treatments of common hematologic paraneoplastic syndromes are detailed in Table 45.4.

Conclusion

Early recognition of paraneoplastic syndromes may facilitate the timely diagnosis of cancer. Effective treatment of these syndromes may improve quality of life and facilitate the administration of cancer-directed therapy.

Table 45.4 Paraneoplastic hematologic syndromes. Modified with permission from Pelosof LC, Gerber DE. Paraneoplastic syndromes: an approach to diagnosis and treatment. © 2010 Mayo Foundation for Medical Education and Research. Published by Elsevier Inc.

Syndrome	Clinical features	Laboratory data	Associated malignancies	Management[1]	References
Eosinophilia	Dyspnea Wheezing	Hypereosinophilia Elevated serum IL-5, IL-3, IL-2, GM-CSF Absence of mutations in *FIP1L1*, *PDGFR* α and β, or *FGFR1*	Lymphomas Leukemias Lung Thyroid Gastrointestinal Renal Breast Gynecologic	Inhaled or systemic corticosteroids (if symptomatic)	[102, 108–110]
Granulocytosis	Asymptomatic (no symptoms or signs of leukostasis such as neurological deficits or dyspnea)	Granulocyte (neutrophil) count $>8 \times 10^9$/L Typically with no shift to immature neutrophil forms Elevated leukocyte alkaline phosphatase (LAP) Elevated serum G-CSF	Gastrointestinal Lung Breast Gynecologic GU Brain Hodgkin lymphoma Sarcomas	Specific treatment not indicated	[103, 110–112]
Thrombocytosis	Asymptomatic (no bleeding or clotting abnormalities)	Elevated platelet count greater than $\sim 400 \times 10^9$/L Elevated serum IL-6 Absence of mutations in *JAK2* and *MPL*	Gastrointestinal Lung Breast Gynecologic Renal cell Prostate Mesothelioma Glioblastoma Head and neck	Specific treatment not indicated	[103, 104, 113–115]
Pure red cell aplasia (PRCA)	Dyspnea, pallor, fatigue, syncope	Severe anemia Low/absent reticulocytes Bone marrow with nearly absent erythroid precursors Platelet and white blood cell counts often in normal ranges	Thymoma Leukemia (large granular lymphocyte leukemia) Lymphoma Myelodysplastic syndrome	Blood transfusions Corticosteroids Anti-thymocyte globulin Cyclosporine Cyclophosphamide Rituximab Alemtuzumab Plasma exchange Splenectomy Thymectomy (for thymoma) (*Use immunosuppressive agents with caution in patients with lymphoid malignancies/MDS.*)	[106, 107, 116–118]

[1] In addition to treating the underlying malignancy.

FGFR1, fibroblast growth factor receptor 1; FIP1L1, factor interacting with PAP1-like 1; G-CSF, granulocyte colony-stimulating factor; GM-CSF, granulocyte-macrophage colony-stimulating factor; GU, genitourinary; IL, interleukin; JAK2, Janus kinase 2; LAP, leukocyte alkaline phosphatase; MPL, myeloproliferative leukemia protein; PDGFR, platelet-derived growth factor receptor.

References

1 Oppenheim H. Über Hirnsymptome bei Carcinomatose ohne nachweisbare Veränderungen im Gehirn. *Charité-Annalen (Berlin)* 1888;(13):335–44.

2 Guichard A, Vignon G. La polyradiculonéurite cancéreuse métastatique. *J Med Lyon* 1949;30(700):197–207.

3 Kaltsas G, Androulakis II, de Herder WW, Grossman AB. Paraneoplastic syndromes secondary to neuroendocrine tumours. *Endocr Relat Cancer* 2010;17(3):R173–93.

4 Miret M, Horvath-Puho E, Deruaz-Luyet A, *et al.* Potential paraneoplastic syndromes and selected autoimmune conditions in patients with non-small cell lung cancer and small cell lung cancer: a population-based cohort study. *PLoS One* 2017;12(8):e0181564.

5 Ben-Baruch S, Canaani J, Braunstein R, *et al.* Predictive parameters for a diagnostic bone marrow biopsy specimen in the work-up of fever of unknown origin. *Mayo Clin Proc* 2012;87(2):136–42.

6 Blay JY, Rossi JF, Wijdenes J, *et al.* Role of interleukin-6 in the paraneoplastic inflammatory syndrome associated with renal-cell carcinoma. *Int J Cancer* 1997;72(3):424–30.
7 Kim HL, Belldegrun AS, Freitas DG, *et al.* Paraneoplastic signs and symptoms of renal cell carcinoma: implications for prognosis. *J Urol* 2003;170(5):1742–6.
8 Fearon KC, Glass DJ, Guttridge DC. Cancer cachexia: mediators, signaling, and metabolic pathways. *Cell Metab* 2012;16(2):153–66.
9 Ding GX, Feng CC, Song NH, *et al.* Paraneoplastic symptoms: Cachexia, polycythemia, and hypercalcemia are, respectively, related to vascular endothelial growth factor (VEGF) expression in renal clear cell carcinoma. *Urol Oncol* 2012;31(8):1820–5.
10 Martignoni ME, Kunze P, Hildebrandt W, *et al.* Role of mononuclear cells and inflammatory cytokines in pancreatic cancer-related cachexia. *Clin Cancer Res* 2005;11(16):5802–8.
11 Fearon K, Arends J, Baracos V. Understanding the mechanisms and treatment options in cancer cachexia. *Nat Rev Clin Oncol* 2013;10(2):90–9.
12 Crawford J, Prado CM, Johnson MA, *et al.* Study design and rationale for the phase 3 clinical development program of enobosarm, a selective androgen receptor modulator, for the prevention and treatment of muscle wasting in cancer patients (POWER trials). *Curr Oncol Rep* 2016;18(6):37.
13 Gerber DE, Grossman SA, Streiff MB. Management of venous thromboembolism in patients with primary and metastatic brain tumors. *J Clin Oncol* 2006;24(8):1310–8.
14 Park HJ, Ranganathan P. Neoplastic and paraneoplastic vasculitis, vasculopathy, and hypercoagulability. *Rheum Dis Clin North Am* 2011;37(4):593–606.
15 Welsh J, Smith JD, Yates KR, *et al.* Tissue factor expression determines tumour cell coagulation kinetics. *Int J Lab Hematol* 2012;34(4):396–402.
16 Nagy JA, Benjamin L, Zeng H, Dvorak AM, Dvorak HF. Vascular permeability, vascular hyperpermeability and angiogenesis. *Angiogenesis* 2008;11(2):109–19.
17 Lee AY. Treatment of venous thromboembolism in cancer patients. *Best Pract Res Clin Haematol* 2009;22(1):93–101.
18 Streiff MB. Diagnosis and initial treatment of venous thromboembolism in patients with cancer. *J Clin Oncol* 2009;27(29):4889–94.
19 Ay C, Pabinger I, Cohen AT. Cancer-associated venous thromboembolism: Burden, mechanisms, and management. *Thromb Haemost* 2017;2:219–30.
20 Lee AY, Levine MN, Baker RI, *et al.* Low-molecular-weight heparin versus a coumarin for the prevention of recurrent venous thromboembolism in patients with cancer. *N Engl J Med* 2003;349(2):146–53.
21 Soff GA. A new generation of oral direct anticoagulants. *Arterioscler Thromb Vasc Biol* 2012;32(3):569–74.
22 Spinazze S, Schrijvers D. Metabolic emergencies. *Crit Rev Oncol Hematol* 2006;58(1):79–89.
23 Raftopoulos H. Diagnosis and management of hyponatremia in cancer patients. *Support Care Cancer* 2007;15(12):1341–7.
24 Ellison DH, Berl T. Clinical practice. The syndrome of inappropriate antidiuresis. *N Engl J Med* 2007;356(20):2064–72.
25 Lumachi F, Brunello A, Roma A, Basso U. Medical treatment of malignancy-associated hypercalcemia. *Curr Med Chem* 2008;15(4):415–21.
26 Stewart AF. Clinical practice. Hypercalcemia associated with cancer. *N Engl J Med* 2005;352(4):373–9.
27 Nieman LK. Medical therapy of Cushing's disease. *Pituitary* 2002;5(2):77–82.
28 Morandi U, Casali C, Rossi G. Bronchial typical carcinoid tumors. *Semin Thorac Cardiovasc Surg* 2006;18(3):191–8.
29 Barbosa SL, Rodien P, Leboulleux S, *et al.* Ectopic adrenocorticotropic hormone-syndrome in medullary carcinoma of the thyroid: a retrospective analysis and review of the literature. *Thyroid* 2005;15(6):618–23.
30 Teves D. Clinical approach of Cushing syndrome resulting from ACTH-producing metastatic neuroendocrine tumor. *Endocrinologist* 2005;15(6):401–4.
31 Nayar M, Lombard, MG, Furlong, NJ, *et al.* Diagnosis and management of nonislet cell tumor hypoglycemia case series and review of the literature. *Endocrinologist* 2006;16(4):227–30.
32 Teale JD, Marks V. Glucocorticoid therapy suppresses abnormal secretion of big IGF-II by non-islet cell tumours inducing hypoglycaemia (NICTH). *Clin Endocrinol (Oxf)* 1998;49(4):491–8.
33 Hoff AO, Vassilopoulou-Sellin R. The role of glucagon administration in the diagnosis and treatment of patients with tumor hypoglycemia. *Cancer* 1998;82(8):1585–92.
34 Ralston SH, Gallacher SJ, Patel U, Campbell J, Boyle IT. Cancer-associated hypercalcemia: morbidity and mortality. Clinical experience in 126 treated patients. *Ann Intern Med* 1990;112(7):499–504.
35 Fizazi K, Carducci M, Smith M, *et al.* Denosumab versus zoledronic acid for treatment of bone metastases in men with castration-resistant prostate cancer: a randomised, double-blind study. *Lancet* 2011;377(9768):813–22.
36 Boikos SA, Hammers HJ. Denosumab for the treatment of bisphosphonate-refractory hypercalcemia. *J Clin Oncol* 2012;30(29):e299.
37 Rosner MH, Dalkin AC. Onco-nephrology: the pathophysiology and treatment of malignancy-associated hypercalcemia. *Clin J Am Soc Nephrol* 2012;7(10):1722–9.
38 Nagy-Mignotte H, Shestaeva O, Vignoud L, *et al.* Prognostic impact of paraneoplastic cushing's syndrome in small-cell lung cancer. *J Thorac Oncol* 2014;9(4):497–505.
39 Nimalasena S, Freeman A, Harland S. Paraneoplastic Cushing's syndrome in prostate cancer: a difficult management problem. *BJU Int* 2008;101(4):424–7.
40 Honnorat J, Antoine JC. Paraneoplastic neurological syndromes. *Orphanet J Rare Dis* 2007;2:22.
41 Orange D, Frank M, Tian S, *et al.* Cellular immune suppression in paraneoplastic neurologic syndromes targeting intracellular antigens. *Arch Neurol* 2012;69(9):1132–40.
42 Dalmau J, Rosenfeld MR. Paraneoplastic syndromes of the CNS. *Lancet Neurol* 2008;7(4):327–40.
43 Viaccoz A, Honnorat J. Paraneoplastic neurological syndromes: general treatment overview. *Curr Treat Options Neurol* 2013;15(2):150–68.

44 Shams'ili S, de Beukelaar J, Gratama JW, *et al.* An uncontrolled trial of rituximab for antibody associated paraneoplastic neurological syndromes. *J Neurol* 2006;253(1):16–20.
45 Keime-Guibert F, Graus F, Fleury A, *et al.* Treatment of paraneoplastic neurological syndromes with antineuronal antibodies (Anti-Hu, anti-Yo) with a combination of immunoglobulins, cyclophosphamide, and methylprednisolone. *J Neurol Neurosurg Psychiatry* 2000;68(4):479–82.
46 de Beukelaar JW, Sillevis Smitt PA. Managing paraneoplastic neurological disorders. *Oncologist* 2006;11(3):292–305.
47 Oh SJ, Kim DS, Head TC, Claussen GC. Low-dose guanidine and pyridostigmine: relatively safe and effective long-term symptomatic therapy in Lambert-Eaton myasthenic syndrome. *Muscle Nerve* 1997;20(9):1146–52.
48 Richman DP, Agius MA. Treatment of autoimmune myasthenia gravis. *Neurology* 2003;61(12):1652–61.
49 Zebardast N, Patwa HS, Novella SP, Goldstein JM. Rituximab in the management of refractory myasthenia gravis. *Muscle Nerve* 2010;41(3):375–8.
50 van Sonderen A, Wirtz PW, Verschuuren JJ, Titulaer MJ. Paraneoplastic syndromes of the neuromuscular junction: therapeutic options in myasthenia gravis, lambert-eaton myasthenic syndrome, and neuromyotonia. *Curr Treat Options Neurol* 2013;15(2):224–39.
51 Calvet X, Martinez JM, Martinez M. Repeated neostigmine dosage as palliative treatment for chronic colonic pseudo-obstruction in a patient with autonomic paraneoplastic neuropathy. *Am J Gastroenterol* 2003;98(3):708–9.
52 Gupta V, Lipsitz LA. Orthostatic hypotension in the elderly: diagnosis and treatment. *Am J Med* 2007;120(10):841–7.
53 Vernino S, Low PA, Lennon VA. Experimental autoimmune autonomic neuropathy. *J Neurophysiol* 2003;90(3):2053–9.
54 Oh SJ, Dropcho EJ, Claussen GC. Anti-Hu-associated paraneoplastic sensory neuropathy responding to early aggressive immunotherapy: report of two cases and review of literature. *Muscle Nerve* 1997;20(12):1576–82.
55 Vernino S, O'Neill BP, Marks RS, O'Fallon JR, Kimmel DW. Immunomodulatory treatment trial for paraneoplastic neurological disorders. *Neuro Oncol* 2004;6(1):55–62.
56 Graus F, Dalmau J. Paraneoplastic neurological syndromes. *Curr Opin Neurol* 2012;25(6):795–801.
57 Albert ML, Austin LM, Darnell RB. Detection and treatment of activated T cells in the cerebrospinal fluid of patients with paraneoplastic cerebellar degeneration. *Ann Neurol* 2000;47(1):9–17.
58 Sculier C, Bentea G, Ruelle L, *et al.* Autoimmune paraneoplastic syndromes associated to lung cancer: a systematic review of the literature: Part 5: neurological auto-antibodies, discussion, flow chart, conclusions. *Lung Cancer* 2017;111:164–75.
59 Subramaniam RM, Shields AF, Sachedina A, *et al.* Impact on Patient Management of [18 F]-Fluorodeoxyglucose-Positron Emission Tomography (PET) Used for Cancer Diagnosis: Analysis of Data From the National Oncologic PET Registry. *Oncologist* 2016;21(9):1079–84.
60 Sheikhbahaei S, Marcus C, Fragomeni RS, *et al.* Whole Body FDG-PET and FDG-PET/CT in Patients with Suspected Paraneoplastic Syndrome: A Systematic review and Meta-analysis of Diagnostic Accuracy. *J Nucl Med* 2017;58(7):1031–6.
61 Titulaer MJ, Soffietti R, Dalmau J, *et al.* Screening for tumours in paraneoplastic syndromes: report of an EFNS task force. *Eur J Neurol* 2011;18(1):19–e3.
62 Dalmau J, Gleichman AJ, Hughes EG, *et al.* Anti-NMDA-receptor encephalitis: case series and analysis of the effects of antibodies. *Lancet Neurol* 2008;7(12):1091–8.
63 Jarius S, Hoffmann LA, Stich O, *et al.* Relative frequency of VGKC and 'classical' paraneoplastic antibodies in patients with limbic encephalitis. *J Neurol* 2008;255(7):1100–1.
64 Chatterjee M, Hurley LC, Levin NK, Stack M, Tainsky MA. Utility of paraneoplastic antigens as biomarkers for surveillance and prediction of recurrence in ovarian cancer. *Cancer Biomark* 2017;3(11). doi: 10.3233/CBM-170652. [Epub ahead of print].
65 Padda SK, Yao X, Antonicelli A, *et al.* Paraneoplastic syndromes and thymic malignancies: an examination of the international thymic malignancy interest group retrospective database. *J Thorac Oncol* 2017;27(11). [Epub ahead of print]. PMID 29191778.
66 Graus F, Dalmou J, Rene R, *et al.* Anti-Hu antibodies in patients with small-cell lung cancer: association with complete response to therapy and improved survival. *J Clin Oncol* 1997;15(8):2866–72.
67 Yshii LM, Hohlfeld R, Liblau RS. Inflammatory CNS disease caused by immune checkpoint inhibitors: status and perspectives. *Nat Rev Neurol* 2017;13(12):755–63.
68 Azar L, Khasnis A. Paraneoplastic rheumatologic syndromes. *Curr Opin Rheumatol* 2013;25(1):44–9.
69 Thiers BH, Sahn RE, Callen JP. Cutaneous manifestations of internal malignancy. *CA Cancer J Clin* 2009;59(2):73–98.
70 Cohen PR. Sweet's syndrome – a comprehensive review of an acute febrile neutrophilic dermatosis. *Orphanet J Rare Dis* 2007;2:34.
71 Ali N, Abbasi AN, Karsan F, *et al.* A case of finger clubbing associated with nasopharyngeal carcinoma in a young girl, and review of pathophysiology. *J Pak Med Assoc* 2009;59(4):253–4.
72 Mekhail TM, Markman M. Acanthosis nigricans with endometrial carcinoma: case report and review of the literature. *Gynecol Oncol* 2002;84(2):332–4.
73 Franco M, Giusti C, Malieni D, *et al.* Sweet's syndrome associated with neoplasms. *An Bras Dermatol* 2006;81(5):473–82.
74 Koh ET, Seow A, Ong B, *et al.* Adult onset polymyositis/dermatomyositis: clinical and laboratory features and treatment response in 75 patients. *Ann Rheum Dis* 1993;52(12):857–61.
75 Anderson SH, Hudson-Peacock M, Muller AF. Malignant acanthosis nigricans: potential role of chemotherapy. *Br J Dermatol* 1999;141(4):714–6.
76 Katz RA. Treatment of acanthosis nigricans with oral isotretinoin. *Arch Dermatol* 1980;116(1):110–1.
77 Dalakas MC, Hohlfeld R. Polymyositis and dermatomyositis. *Lancet* 2003;362(9388):971–82.
78 Robak E, Robak T. Skin lesions in chronic lymphocytic leukemia. *Leuk Lymphoma* 2007;48(5):855–65.

79 Chong VH, Lim CC. Erythroderma as the first manifestation of colon cancer. *South Med J* 2009;102(3):334–5.

80 Pezeshkpoor F, Yazdanpanah MJ, Shirdel A. Specific cutaneous manifestations in adult T-cell leukemia/ lymphoma. *Int J Dermatol* 2008;47(4):359–62.

81 Takatsuka Y, Komine M, Fujita E, *et al.* Erythroderma associated with leukocytosis in premalignant myeloproliferative disorder. *Int J Dermatol* 2009;48(3):324–6.

82 Garganese MC, De Sio L, Serra A, *et al.* Rhabdomyosarcoma associated hypertrophic osteoarthropathy in a child: detection by bone scintigraphy. *Clin Nucl Med* 2009;34(3):155–7.

83 Mauricio O, Francis L, Athar U, *et al.* Hypertrophic osteoarthropathy masquerading as lower extremity cellulitis and response to bisphosphonates. *J Thorac Oncol* 2009;4(2):260–2.

84 Pelajo CF, de Oliveira SK, Rodrigues MC, Torres JM. Cutaneous vasculitis as a paraneoplastic syndrome in childhood. *Acta Reumatol Port* 2007;32(2):181–3.

85 Solans-Laque R, Bosch-Gil JA, Perez-Bocanegra C, *et al.* Paraneoplastic vasculitis in patients with solid tumors: report of 15 cases. *J Rheumatol* 2008;35(2):294–304.

86 Jain P, Kumar P, Parikh PM. Multiple myeloma with paraneoplastic leucocytoclastic vasculitis. *Indian J Cancer* 2009;46(2):173–4.

87 Gupta S, Handa S, Kanwar AJ, Radotra BD, Minz RW. Cutaneous vasculitides: clinico-pathological correlation. *Indian J Dermatol Venereol Leprol* 2009;75(4):356–62.

88 Chen KR, Carlson JA. Clinical approach to cutaneous vasculitis. *Am J Clin Dermatol* 2008;9(2):71–92.

89 Ahmed AR, Spigelman Z, Cavacini LA, Posner MR. Treatment of pemphigus vulgaris with rituximab and intravenous immune globulin. *N Engl J Med* 2006;355(17):1772–9.

90 Gergely L, Varoczy L, Vadasz G, Remenyik E, Illes A. Successful treatment of B cell chronic lymphocytic leukemia-associated severe paraneoplastic pemphigus with cyclosporin A. *Acta Haematol* 2003;109(4):202–5.

91 Lapidoth M, David M, Ben-Amitai D, *et al.* The efficacy of combined treatment with prednisone and cyclosporine in patients with pemphigus: preliminary study. *J Am Acad Dermatol* 1994;30(5 Pt 1):752–7.

92 Borradori L, Lombardi T, Samson J, *et al.* Anti-CD20 monoclonal antibody (rituximab) for refractory erosive stomatitis secondary to CD20(+) follicular lymphoma-associated paraneoplastic pemphigus. *Arch Dermatol* 2001;137(3):269–72.

93 Hertzberg MS, Schifter M, Sullivan J, Stapleton K. Paraneoplastic pemphigus in two patients with B-cell non-Hodgkin's lymphoma: significant responses to cyclophosphamide and prednisolone. *Am J Hematol* 2000;63(2):105–6.

94 Williams JV, Marks JG, Jr, Billingsley EM. Use of mycophenolate mofetil in the treatment of paraneoplastic pemphigus. *Br J Dermatol* 2000;142(3):506–8.

95 Kridin K, Zelber-Sagi S, Comaneshter D, *et al.* Pemphigus and hematologic malignancies: a population-based study of 11,859 patients. *J Am Acad Dermatol* 2017;30(11). [Epub ahead of print]. PMID 29198780.

96 Keith MP, Gilliland WR. Polymyalgia rheumatica and breast cancer. *J Clin Rheumatol* 2006;12(4):199–200.

97 Anton E. More on polymyalgia rheumatica (PMR) as a paraneoplastic rheumatic syndrome in the elderly (bicytopenia and PMR preceding acute myeloid leukemia). *J Clin Rheumatol* 2007;13(2):114.

98 Hernandez-Rodriguez J, Cid MC, Lopez-Soto A, Espigol-Frigole G, Bosch X. Treatment of polymyalgia rheumatica: a systematic review. *Arch Intern Med* 2009;169(20):1839–50.

99 Horio T, Imamura S, Danno K, Furukawa F, Ofuji S. Treatment of acute febrile neutrophilic dermatosis (Sweet's Syndrome) with potassium iodide. *Dermatologica* 1980;160(5):341–7.

100 Suehisa S, Tagami H. Treatment of acute febrile neutrophilic dermatosis (Sweet's syndrome) with colchicine. *Br J Dermatol* 1981;105(4):483.

101 Maillard H, Leclech C, Peria P, Avenel-Audran M, Verret JL. Colchicine for Sweet's syndrome. A study of 20 cases. *Br J Dermatol* 1999;140(3):565–6.

102 Anagnostopoulos GK, Sakorafas GH, Kostopoulos P, *et al.* Disseminated colon cancer with severe peripheral blood eosinophilia and elevated serum levels of interleukine-2, interleukine-3, interleukine-5, and GM-CSF. *J Surg Oncol* 2005;89(4):273–5.

103 Jameson JL, Longo DL. *Chapter 121. Paraneoplastic syndromes: endocrinologic/hematologic. In: DL Kasper, AS Fauci, SL Hauser, et al. (eds) Harrison's Principles of Internal Medicine, 19th edn.* New York: McGraw Hill Education, 2015.

104 Sierko E, Wojtukiewicz MZ. Platelets and angiogenesis in malignancy. *Semin Thromb Hemost* 2004;30(1):95–108.

105 Tefferi A, Ho TC, Ahmann GJ, Katzmann JA, Greipp PR. Plasma interleukin-6 and C-reactive protein levels in reactive versus clonal thrombocytosis. *Am J Med* 1994;97(4):374–8.

106 Sawada K, Hirokawa M, Fujishima N. Diagnosis and management of acquired pure red cell aplasia. *Hematol Oncol Clin North Am* 2009;23(2):249–59.

107 Thompson CA. Pure red cell aplasia and thymoma. *J Thorac Oncol* 2007;2(4):263–4.

108 Valent P. Pathogenesis, classification, and therapy of eosinophilia and eosinophil disorders. *Blood Rev* 2009;23(4):157–65.

109 Tefferi A, Patnaik MM, Pardanani A. Eosinophilia: secondary, clonal and idiopathic. *Br J Haematol* 2006;133(5):468–92.

110 Ashdhir P, Jain P, Pokharna R, Nepalia S, Sharma SS. Pancreatic cancer manifesting as liver metastases and eosinophilic leukemoid reaction: a case report and review of literature. *Am J Gastroenterol* 2008;103(4):1052–4.

111 Ahn HJ, Park YH, Chang YH, *et al.* A case of uterine cervical cancer presenting with granulocytosis. *Korean J Intern Med* 2005;20(3):247–50.

112 Araki K, Kishihara F, Takahashi K, *et al.* Hepatocellular carcinoma producing a granulocyte colony-stimulating factor: report of a resected case with a literature review. *Liver Int* 2007;27(5):716–21.

113 Blay JY, Favrot M, Rossi JF, Wijdenes J. Role of interleukin-6 in paraneoplastic thrombocytosis. *Blood* 1993;82(7):2261–2.

114 Chen MH, Chang PM, Chen PM, *et al.* Prognostic significance of a pretreatment hematologic profile in patients with head and neck cancer. *J Cancer Res Clin Oncol* 2009;135(12):1783–90.

115 Tefferi A. Essential thrombocythemia, polycythemia vera, and myelofibrosis: current management and the prospect of targeted therapy. *Am J Hematol* 2008;83(6):491–7.

116 Tanna S, Ustun C. Immunosuppressive treatment in patient with pure red cell aplasia associated with chronic myelomonocytic leukemia: harm or benefit? *Int J Hematol* 2009;90(5):597–600.

117 Robak T. Monoclonal antibodies in the treatment of autoimmune cytopenias. *Eur J Haematol* 2004;72(2):79–88.

118 Clark DA, Dessypris EN, Krantz SB. Studies on pure red cell aplasia. XI. Results of immunosuppressive treatment of 37 patients. *Blood* 1984;63(2):277–86.

46

Peritoneal Surface Malignancies

Kiran K. Turaga

University of Chicago, Chicago, Illinois, USA

Introduction

The peritoneum is remarkably resistant to the development of primary malignancies but is often the site of metastatic disease. The most common adult primary peritoneal malignancies are primary peritoneal carcinomas and malignant mesotheliomas. Malignancies secondarily involving the peritoneum are much more common with an estimated 8–15% of all colorectal carcinomas and 60–70% of all ovarian malignancies developing peritoneal disease [1, 2]. Although the etiopathogenesis of such conditions is disparate, the development of a common phenotypic expression of metastases leads to common management paradigms that have been adopted in these disease processes.

The most dramatic condition that is associated with peritoneal surface malignancy is pseudomyxoma peritonei, which is often confused with a disease while in fact it is a syndrome. This syndrome consists of mucinous ascites that leads to abdominal distension, bowel obstruction, malnutrition, inanition, and eventually death. This is usually the consequence of mucinous tumors of the stomach, ovary, pancreas, and appendix.

Primary Peritoneal Malignancies

Primary Peritoneal Cancer

Serous carcinomas that arise from the ovary, fallopian tubes, or peritoneum are often treated as a single entity. This approach is supported by the finding of intraepithelial carcinoma in the fallopian tubes in patients with *BRCA* mutations undergoing prophylactic salpingo-oophorectomy, and it has been proposed that most cases of these three malignancies might have a fallopian tube origin [3–5]. The incidence rate of primary peritoneal cancer in the United States (US) is approximately 0.46 per 100,000 women per year [6].

Malignant Mesothelioma

Malignant peritoneal mesothelioma comprises 10–15% of all mesotheliomas and although most widely known for its association with asbestos, is also associated with other chemical and physical carcinogens [7–10]. It is a relatively rare yet lethal malignancy with around 400–800 new cases annually in the US. The three main histological types of malignant mesothelioma are epithelioid, biphasic, and sarcomatoid, with the first having the most favorable prognosis and the last the least favorable [7].

Peritoneal Sarcomatosis

Desmoplastic small round cell tumors (DSRCT) are exceedingly uncommon cancers of primary peritoneal origin, unlike sarcomatosis occurring from rhabdomyosarcomas, gastrointestinal stromal tumors (GIST) tumors, or leiomyosarcomas which are usually spread by dissemination from spillage of tumor during surgical resection. DSRCT is generally associated with a poor prognosis, and multimodality therapy with intraperitoneal chemotherapy has played an important role in the management of these patients, especially in the pediatric population [11, 12]. Although secondary peritoneal sarcomatosis has been treated with cytoreductive surgical techniques and chemoperfusion, the results have not been as encouraging and clinical trial participation is generally encouraged [13].

Secondary Malignancies

The mechanism of development of peritoneal disease from a primary site cancer is poorly understood although decreased expression of E-cadherin and up-regulation of cadherin repressors have been demonstrated [14–16]. The distribution of cancer cells has been proposed to be due to the constant circulation of peritoneal fluid, diaphragmatic excursions, and intestinal peristalsis [17, 18]. Preference for these tumor subtypes to metastasize to the omentum is frequently seen and this is explained by propensity of tumor cells to attach to "milky spots," which are immune aggregates with vascular endothelial growth factor (VEGF)-A production [19].

The American Cancer Society's Oncology in Practice: Clinical Management, First Edition. Edited by The American Cancer Society.

Epithelial Appendiceal Neoplasms (EAN)

Mucinous neoplasms of the appendix occur with a frequency of about 1,500 new cases per year in the US alone [20, 21]. Genomic signatures of appendiceal neoplasms with peritoneal dissemination are remarkably different than colorectal cancer with peritoneal disease [22]. Appendiceal neoplasms form a heterogeneous spectrum of diseases from benign lesions to aggressive malignant disease.

When associated with peritoneal dissemination, these diseases have been grouped into three variants: disseminated peritoneal adenomucinosis, peritoneal mucinous carcinomatosis, and peritoneal mucinous carcinomatosis intermediate/discordant, with a significant correlation with prognosis [23]. Primary mucinous tumors of the appendix are divided into four groups: mucinous adenoma (including hyperplasia, retention cysts, and cystadenomas), low-grade mucinous neoplasms with low risk of recurrence, low-grade mucinous neoplasms with high risk of recurrence, and mucinous adenocarcinoma [24]. While patients with mucinous adenomas and those with acellular mucin (no epithelial cells) outside the appendix do remarkably well with no peritoneal failures, presence of epithelial cells outside the appendix suggests high risk of peritoneal recurrence with a 10-year survival of 46%. The group with mucinous adenocarcinoma had the worst survival (5-year survival of 28%) [24]. The World Health Organization (WHO) classification has incorporated all mucinous histologies with peritoneal dissemination into mucinous adenocarcinomas, being differentiated into their prognostic groups by the grade, which can make prognostic information difficult to ascertain from pathology alone.

The natural history of appendiceal mucinous neoplasms with peritoneal dissemination usually leads to the development of the pseudomyxoma peritonei syndrome with ascites, malnutrition, and bowel obstruction [25]. Historical series that have examined serial cytoreductions for these patients found a relatively lower survival as compared to cytoreduction combined with hyperthermic intraperitoneal chemotherapy (HIPEC) [25–28]. The application of HIPEC with or without bidirectional chemotherapy (IV + IP) or EPIC (early postoperative intraperitoneal chemotherapy) is now considered standard of care in the management of these neoplasms although level I evidence is not available [25]. The role of systemic chemotherapy in these neoplasms is rather controversial, and the groups that have been shown to have benefit include patients with high-grade histologies (such as signet ring cell tumors) and patients with non-cytoreducible disease [29–31].

A right hemicolectomy is not always necessary for patients who present with peritoneal disease since the prognosis is usually defined by the peritoneal disease burden and the extent of cytoreduction [32, 33].

Colorectal Carcinomas

In a large Swedish series of patients with colorectal carcinoma, approximately 8% developed peritoneal disease [1]. Recent autopsy studies have revealed that the incidence of peritoneal metastases (with or without concomitant other sites of metastases) could be as high as 51%, with 15% being peritoneal alone [34]. Patients with aggressive disease at diagnosis such as American Joint Committee on Cancer/Union for International Cancer Control (AJCC/UICC) T4 tumors, patients with limited peritoneal disease, and those with perforated lesions are at a high risk for developing subsequent peritoneal disease and this has been associated with BRAF mutations in these subtypes [35, 36]. Patients with peritoneal metastases may develop bowel obstructions during the course of the disease and thus often die earlier than patients with visceral metastases [37]. Patients from the Eindhoven (Netherlands) registry treated with palliative chemotherapy demonstrated a trend towards improvement in survival; in the same series, patients with other metastases (in addition to peritoneal carcinomatosis) had shorter survival [38]. A subset analysis of the North Central Cancer Treatment Group (NCCTG) and Aide et Recherche en Cancérologie Digestive (ARCAD) trials that examined the role of systemic chemotherapy for stage IV colon cancer found that patients with peritoneal disease had a shorter median survival than those with other sites of metastatic disease [32, 37, 39].

One challenge concerning peritoneal disease with colorectal cancer is the inability to accurately measure the disease burden and accurately assess response, which makes it difficult to manage patients who are often considered as having minimal disease, when in fact the true burden of disease is high. The peritoneal cancer index (PCI, or simplified PCI) has been most commonly used as staging system for peritoneal disease, but this can only be applied at laparoscopy or laparotomy (Figure 46.1). Systems for noninvasive staging, such as the peritoneal surface disease severity score (PSDSS), have been proposed to accurately stratify patients into groups that might identify peritoneal disease, and the PSDSS has been validated in multi-institutional studies [40, 41].

Cytoreductive surgery and hyperthermic intraperitoneal chemotherapy (CRS + HIPEC) has been proposed as an adjunctive therapy to improve survival in colorectal cancer patients with peritoneal disease. A randomized trial in 2003 examined 105 patients treated with CRS + HIPEC versus systemic chemotherapy (5-FU) and found the median survival improved from 12.6 months to 22.3 months [42]. The trial was criticized for not having a contemporary comparison arm although recent updates and numerous registry studies have demonstrated durability of survival benefit [43]. Recent reports have suggested that the possibility of cure might be considered in a subset of patients who achieve long-term disease-free survival (>10 years) [44].

The goal of preventing peritoneal carcinomatosis has led researchers to apply CRS + HIPEC to high-risk tumors, since almost 56% of such patients had peritoneal disease on a systematic second look [36]. Early application of CRS + HIPEC has been proposed in high-risk patients (perforated tumors, or patients with limited peritoneal/ovarian metastases) and is the subject of ongoing trials, as is the effect of the actual chemoperfusion.

Gastric Cancer

Approximately 19.5% of patients with gastric cancer will have free intraperitoneal cancer cells, as seen in the EVOCAPE study [45]. Patients with positive peritoneal cytology have a uniformly worse prognosis and although all patients with gastric cancer can develop peritoneal disease, the risk is higher in those with

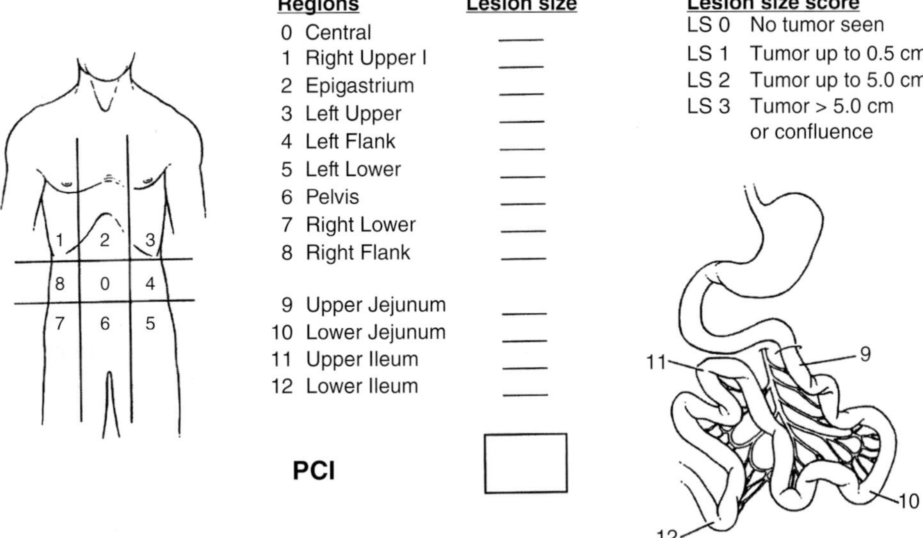

Figure 46.1 Peritoneal cancer index (PCI). The abdomen is divided into nine zones, and the intestines into four zones. A score of 0–3 is assigned to each zone based on the size of the tumor burden assessed intraoperatively. The score can vary from 0 to 39. *Source:* Jacquet 1996 [66]. Reproduced with permission of Springer.

diffuse gastric cancer (linitis plastica), signet cell morphology, and perforated gastric tumors [46].

Development of peritoneal disease portends a poor prognosis, and with limited benefit from systemic therapy, especially in the HER2/neu negative tumors, alternate regional therapies have been considered for this disease [47]. The role of intraperitoneal chemotherapy in combination with extensive intraperitoneal lavage has been evaluated in a randomized controlled trial of 88 patients with cytology positive disease, which found a 43.8% 5-year survival in the study arm as compared to other arms which either received intraperitoneal chemotherapy alone (4.6%) or neither (0%). When compared to cytoreduction alone, CRS + HIPEC added a modest survival benefit (11.0 vs 6.5 months) in patients with gastric cancer with peritoneal disease in another phase 3 randomized controlled trial [48].

Ovarian Cancer

Epithelial ovarian cancer is discussed in Chapter 19. When intraperitoneal disease is present, patients are best treated in a multidisciplinary fashion and surgical cytoreduction to less than 1 cm combined with intravenous and intraperitoneal chemotherapy has shown significant survival benefit in two randomized trials – the GOG 172 (median survival 128 months) and GOG 114 (median survival 110 months) – as compared to IV alone arms (82.4 months) [49, 50].

Other Malignancies

Aggressive upper gastrointestinal malignancies such as esophageal carcinoma, hepatopancreatobiliary carcinomas, and melanomas can also present with peritoneal dissemination which is rapidly fatal. Systemic therapy and clinical trials are the mainstay for the treatment of such conditions.

Diagnosis

The diagnosis of peritoneal carcinomatosis by imaging methods is not just difficult but rather impossible unless disease is widespread. This is because the morphology of the lining of the peritoneal surface is such that there are natural undulations and respiratory variation that make it difficult to determine presence of disease. Additionally, the morphology of early implants along with their size of a few millimeters can make it difficult for reconstruction software to discriminate these lesions. The gold standard for diagnosis of peritoneal disease is direct visual examination via a laparotomy or laparoscopy, confirmed by histology [51]. Cross-sectional imaging with the application of diffusion-weighted magnetic resonance technology has shown promise to discriminate early disease [33]. However, for patients with advanced disease, imaging has a useful role in predicting both the ability to cytoreduce and outcome. Large lesions (>5 cm), disease in the portal hepatis, malignant bowel obstruction, and ascites (nonmucinous) generally predict inability to cytoreduce completely [52, 53]. While positron emission tomography (PET) imaging usually has a limited role in mucinous disease, it does have a negative prognostic value. When PET imaging is avid, it does suggest inability to cytoreduce [54]. Although it is important to stage the chest in all patients, neoplasms of low malignant potential such as appendiceal mucinous neoplasms rarely spread to the lungs.

The importance of tumor markers in the management of epithelial appendiceal neoplasms is paramount, with CA-19-9, CA-125, and carcinoembryonic antigen (CEA) all being important for these patients. High levels of these tumor markers can predict inability to cytoreduce and high burden of disease [55–57]. For individual histological subtypes, tumor markers can be used appropriately (CA-125 for primary peritoneal, CEA for colon cancer). C-reactive protein has also been suggested as a useful prognostic marker [55–57].

Treatment of Patients with Peritoneal Disease

Certain histologies such as appendiceal mucinous neoplasms, colorectal adenocarcinomas, mesothelioma, and epithelial ovarian carcinomas lend themselves to treatment with intraperitoneal therapy. Multidisciplinary evaluation with use of systemic chemotherapy in the management of patients with high-grade disease is often necessary (Table 46.1). Intraperitoneal (IP) chemotherapy is attractive in the treatment of patients with peritoneal metastases because these metastases have a very poor blood supply and the concentration of drugs in these lesions from chemotherapy administered systemically is usually extremely low [18, 58]. Intraperitoneal chemotherapy has the advantage of delivery of high doses with minimal systemic absorption [58]. This has been postulated to overcome platinum resistance for tumors previously treated with chemotherapy. While IP chemotherapy is effective, the need for specialized expertise and the limited dissemination of current knowledge has constrained its widespread use. Consensus standardization efforts, guidelines, and future prospective randomized trials are changing the way IP chemotherapy is being applied.

With the evolution of metastasectomy leading to survival benefit in patients with hepatic metastases, the application of cytoreduction to patients with peritoneal metastases seems intuitive [59]. The peritoneum acts as a barrier to dissemination of disease and a metastasectomy with oncological principles yields similar survival benefit as seen with metastasectomies in the liver which are now more well accepted [60]. However, peritonectomy techniques require careful removal of parietal

Table 46.1 Common treatment strategies employed in the management of patients with peritoneal surface malignancies.

Histological subtype	Systemic therapy	Cytoreductive surgery	Regional therapy
Primary			
Primary peritoneal	Taxane/carboplatin (neoadjuvant/adjuvant)	Optimal cytoreduction (<1 cm residual disease)	Intraperitoneal chemotherapy (cisplatin/paclitaxel) for optimally debulked patient ± HIPEC (cisplatin/carboplatin)
Malignant mesothelioma	Cisplatin/pemetrexed	Optimal cytoreduction (<2.5 mm residual disease)	HIPEC (cisplatin /Adriamycin/ mitomycin-C)
DSRCT	Cyclophosphamide, doxorubicin, vincristine alternating with ifosfamide and etoposide Autologous stem cell rescue Whole abdominal radiation	Optimal cytoreduction (<2.5 mm residual disease)	HIPEC (cisplatin)
Secondary			
Low-grade appendiceal neoplasms	—	Optimal cytoreduction (<2.5 mm residual disease)	HIPEC (mitomycin-C)
High-grade appendiceal neoplasms (including goblet cell carcinoid, signet ring cell histology)	Fluoropyrimidine, oxaliplatin, irinotecan, anti-EGFR antibodies (cetuximab/ panitumumab), anti-VEGF antibodies (bevacizumab)	Optimal cytoreduction (<2.5 mm residual disease)	HIPEC (mitomycin-C)
Colorectal carcinomas	Fluoropyrimidine, oxaliplatin, irinotecan, anti-EGFR antibodies (cetuximab/ panitumumab), anti-VEGF antibodies (bevacizumab)	Optimal cytoreduction (<2.5 mm residual disease)	HIPEC (mitomycin-C/ oxaliplatin/ irinotecan)
Ovarian carcinoma	Taxane/carboplatin (neoadjuvant/adjuvant)	Optimal cytoreduction (<1 cm residual disease)	Intraperitoneal chemotherapy (cisplatin/paclitaxel) for optimally debulked patient ± HIPEC (cisplatin)
Gastric carcinoma	Cisplatin/fluoropyrimidine docetaxel/epirubicin trastuzumab for HER2/neu + tumors	± Optimal cytoreduction (<2.5 mm residual disease)	± HIPEC (cisplatin/mitomycin-C) ± IP docetaxel/paclitaxel
Esophageal/pancreatic/ hepatobiliary	Fluoropyrimidine/oxaliplatin/irinotecan Gemcitabine/cisplatin Nab-paclitaxel gastric regimens	—	—
Sarcomas (non-GIST)	Adriamycin/ifosfamide	Optimal cytoreduction (<2.5 mm residual disease)	± HIPEC (cisplatin/Adriamycin)
Sarcomas (GIST)	Tyrosine kinase inhibitors imatinib/sunitinib/ pazopanib/regorafenib	—	—

DSRCT, desmoplastic small round cell tumors; EGFR, epidermal growth factor receptor; GIST, gastrointestinal stromal tumors; HIPEC, hyperthermic intraperitoneal chemotherapy; IP, intraperitoneal; VEGF, vascular endothelial growth factor.

peritoneum with visceral sparing if possible, or organ resection if necessary to achieve a complete cytoreduction. Numerous studies have demonstrated the favorable impact of a complete cytoreduction on survival [25]. Intraoperative peritoneal staging with the PCI is performed to measure the burden of disease. The PCI score can be used to prognosticate patients and also select patients who would benefit maximally from cytoreductive surgery [61, 62]. For instance, a PCI score of ≤5 was associated with a 5-year survival of 72% after cytoreductive surgery and HIPEC [63]. Upon incidental detection of peritoneal disease, the surgeon is best served by carefully quantifying the disease burden and referring the patient to a specialized peritoneal surface malignancy unit where appropriate care can be performed.

After a complete cytoreduction, the patient undergoes hyperthermic intraperitoneal chemoperfusion or, in histologies best treated with IP chemotherapy, a port is placed in the peritoneal cavity. HIPEC is performed by placing cannulas in the abdomen and circulating warm (42° Celsius) fluid at high flow rates (600–1500 mL/minute) for 60–110 minutes after an optimal cytoreduction. At an advanced peritoneal surface disease unit, the mortality from CRS + HIPEC should be less than 2%, with a major morbidity similar to any major abdominal surgery [64]. The use of chemotherapy leads to hematologic and anastomotic complications with a higher frequency, yet with careful surveillance and operative techniques these can be managed with low risk to patients. Patients who are planned to receive IP chemotherapy receive this on a 2- to 3-week cycle which is given with or without systemic chemotherapy.

Malignant Bowel Obstruction

While the therapy directed against peritoneal surface disease is aimed at improving survival, the natural progression of disease often leads to malignant bowel obstructions. Management of malignant bowel obstruction is difficult in patients with peritoneal disease and requires a treatment algorithm that incorporates medical management including somatostatin and antiemetics, surgical or endoscopic management including gastrostomy tubes, stents, and bypass surgery, and palliative care. Surgical palliation such as resection or bypass has been considered for the management of patients with malignant bowel obstructions. It is the author's experience that while endoscopic stents are favorable for the management of locally advanced lesions, they are usually problematic for patients with peritoneal disease [65].

Summary

Numerous advances in the management of peritoneal surface malignancies including better detection with diffusion-weighted magnetic resonance imaging and laparoscopy, along with application of intraperitoneal therapies, have improved the prognosis of patients significantly. Early second look operations for high-risk tumors such as perforated colon cancer and prophylactic HIPEC show much promise in preventing and treating early disease. Multidisciplinary care with palliative therapy is critical to ensuring best outcomes for patients.

References

1 Segelman J, Granath F, Holm T, *et al.* Incidence, prevalence and risk factors for peritoneal carcinomatosis from colorectal cancer. *Br J Surg* 2012;99(5):699–705.
2 Teo MC. Update on the management and the role of intraperitoneal chemotherapy for ovarian cancer. *Curr Opin Obstet Gynecol* 2014;26(1):3–8.
3 Leeper K, Garcia R, Swisher E, *et al.* Pathologic findings in prophylactic oophorectomy specimens in high-risk women. *Gynecol Oncol* 2002;87(1):52–6.
4 Powell CB, Kenley E, Chen LM, *et al.* Risk-reducing salpingo-oophorectomy in BRCA mutation carriers: role of serial sectioning in the detection of occult malignancy. *J Clin Oncol* 2005;23(1):127–32.
5 Reitsma W, de Bock GH, Oosterwijk JC, *et al.* Support of the 'fallopian tube hypothesis' in a prospective series of risk-reducing salpingo-oophorectomy specimens. *Eur J Cancer* 2013;49(1):132–41.
6 Goodman MT, Shvetsov YB. Rapidly increasing incidence of papillary serous carcinoma of the peritoneum in the United States: fact or artifact? *Int J Cancer* 2009;124(9):2231–5.
7 Teta MJ, Mink PJ, Lau E, Sceurman BK, Foster ED. US mesothelioma patterns 1973-2002: indicators of change and insights into background rates. *Eur J Cancer Prev* 2008;17(6):525–34.
8 Boffetta P. Epidemiology of peritoneal mesothelioma: a review. *Ann Oncol* 2007;18(6):985–90.
9 Rodriguez D, Cheung MC, Housri N, Koniaris LG. Malignant abdominal mesothelioma: defining the role of surgery. *J Surg Oncol* 2009;99(1):51–7.
10 Farioli A, Ottone M, Morganti AG, *et al.* Radiation-induced mesothelioma among long-term solid cancer survivors: a longitudinal analysis of SEER database. *Cancer Med* 2016;5(5):950–9.
11 Hayes-Jordan A, Green HL, Lin H, *et al.* Complete cytoreduction and HIPEC improves survival in desmoplastic small round cell tumor. *Ann Surg Oncol* 2014;21(1):220–4.
12 Mora J, Modak S, Cheung NK, *et al.* Desmoplastic small round cell tumor 20 years after its discovery. *Future Oncol* 2015;11(7):1071–81.
13 Baratti D, Pennacchioli E, Kusamura S, *et al.* Peritoneal sarcomatosis: is there a subset of patients who may benefit from cytoreductive surgery and hyperthermic intraperitoneal chemotherapy? *Ann Surg Oncol* 2010;17(12):3220–8.
14 Bai F, Guo X, Yang L, *et al.* Establishment and characterization of a high metastatic potential in the peritoneum for human gastric cancer by orthotopic tumor cell implantation. *Dig Dis Sci* 2007;52(6):1571–8.
15 Terauchi M, Kajiyama H, Yamashita M, *et al.* Possible involvement of TWIST in enhanced peritoneal metastasis of epithelial ovarian carcinoma. *Clin Exp Metastasis* 2007;24(5):329–39.

16 Yoshida J, Horiuchi A, Kikuchi N, *et al.* Changes in the expression of E-cadherin repressors, Snail, Slug, SIP1, and Twist, in the development and progression of ovarian carcinoma: the important role of Snail in ovarian tumorigenesis and progression. *Med Mol Morphol* 2009;42(2):82–91.

17 Carmignani CP, Sugarbaker TA, Bromley CM, Sugarbaker PH. Intraperitoneal cancer dissemination: mechanisms of the patterns of spread. *Cancer Metastasis Rev* 2003;22(4):465–72.

18 Ceelen WP, Bracke ME. Peritoneal minimal residual disease in colorectal cancer: mechanisms, prevention, and treatment. *Lancet Oncol* 2009;10(1):72–9.

19 Gerber SA, Rybalko VY, Bigelow CE, *et al.* Preferential attachment of peritoneal tumor metastases to omental immune aggregates and possible role of a unique vascular microenvironment in metastatic survival and growth. *Am J Pathol* 2006;169(5):1739–52.

20 Misdraji J. Mucinous epithelial neoplasms of the appendix and pseudomyxoma peritonei. *Mod Pathol* 2015;28:S67–79.

21 Sugarbaker PH. New standard of care for appendiceal epithelial neoplasms and pseudomyxoma peritonei syndrome? *Lancet Oncol* 2006;7(1):69–76.

22 Levine EA, Blazer DG, 3rd, Kim MK, *et al.* Gene expression profiling of peritoneal metastases from appendiceal and colon cancer demonstrates unique biologic signatures and predicts patient outcomes. *J Am Coll Surg* 2012;214(4):599–606; discussion 606–7.

23 Ronnett BM, Yan H, Kurman RJ, *et al.* Patients with pseudomyxoma peritonei associated with disseminated peritoneal adenomucinosis have a significantly more favorable prognosis than patients with peritoneal mucinous carcinomatosis. *Cancer* 2001;92(1):85–91.

24 Pai RK, Beck AH, Norton JA, Longacre TA. Appendiceal mucinous neoplasms: clinicopathologic study of 116 cases with analysis of factors predicting recurrence. *Am J Surg Pathol* 2009;33(10):1425–39.

25 Sugarbaker PH. The natural history, gross pathology, and histopathology of appendiceal epithelial neoplasms. *Eur J Surg Onco* 2006;32(6):644–7.

26 Gough DB, Donohue JH, Schutt AJ, *et al.* Pseudomyxoma peritonei. Long-term patient survival with an aggressive regional approach. *Ann Surg* 1994;219(2):112–9.

27 Minor AA. Management of malignant pseudomyxoma: can anyone help? *Can J Surg* 1982;25(4):364.

28 Misdraji J, Yantiss RK, Graeme-Cook FM, Balis UJ, Young RH. Appendiceal mucinous neoplasms: a clinicopathologic analysis of 107 cases. *Am J Surg Pathol* 2003;27(8):1089–103.

29 Shapiro JF, Chase JL, Wolff RA, *et al.* Modern systemic chemotherapy in surgically unresectable neoplasms of appendiceal origin: a single-institution experience. *Cancer* 2010;116(2):316–22.

30 Farquharson AL, Pranesh N, Witham G, *et al.* A phase II study evaluating the use of concurrent mitomycin C and capecitabine in patients with advanced unresectable pseudomyxoma peritonei. *Br J Cancer* 2008;99(4):591–6.

31 Lieu CH, Lambert LA, Wolff RA, *et al.* Systemic chemotherapy and surgical cytoreduction for poorly differentiated and signet ring cell adenocarcinomas of the appendix. *Ann Oncol* 2012;23(3):652–8.

32 Franko J, Goldman CD, Turaga KK. Role of chemotherapy in peritoneal carcinomatosis in metastatic colorectal cancer. *Curr Colorectal Cancer Rep* 2013;9:242–9.

33 Foster JM, Gupta PK, Carreau JH, *et al.* Right hemicolectomy is not routinely indicated in pseudomyxoma peritonei. *Am Surg* 2012;78(2):171–7.

34 Hugen N, van de Velde CJ, de Wilt JH, Nagtegaal ID. Metastatic pattern in colorectal cancer is strongly influenced by histological subtype. *Ann Oncol* 2014;25(3):651–7.

35 Yokota T, Ura T, Shibata N, *et al.* BRAF mutation is a powerful prognostic factor in advanced and recurrent colorectal cancer. *Br J Cancer* 2011;104(5):856–62.

36 Elias D, Goere D, Di Pietrantonio D, *et al.* Results of systematic second-look surgery in patients at high risk of developing colorectal peritoneal carcinomatosis. *Ann Surg* 2008;247(3):445–50.

37 Franko J, Shi Q, Goldman CD, *et al.* Treatment of colorectal peritoneal carcinomatosis with systemic chemotherapy: a pooled analysis of north central cancer treatment group phase III trials N9741 and N9841. *J Clin Oncol* 2012;30(3):263–7.

38 Klaver YL, Lemmens VE, Creemers GJ, *et al.* Population-based survival of patients with peritoneal carcinomatosis from colorectal origin in the era of increasing use of palliative chemotherapy. *Ann Oncol* 2011;22(10):2250–6.

39 Franko J, Shi Q, Meyers JP, *et al.* Prognosis of patients with peritoneal metastatic colorectal cancer given systemic therapy: an analysis of individual patient data from prospective randomised trials from the Analysis and Research in Cancers of the Digestive System (ARCAD) database. *Lancet Oncol* 2016;17(12):1709–19.

40 Esquivel J, Lowy AM, Markman M, *et al.* The American Society of Peritoneal Surface Malignancies (ASPSM) Multiinstitution Evaluation of the Peritoneal Surface Disease Severity Score (PSDSS) in 1,013 Patients with Colorectal Cancer with Peritoneal Carcinomatosis. *Ann Surg Oncol* 2014;21(13):4195–201.

41 Pelz JO, Chua TC, Esquivel J, *et al.* Evaluation of best supportive care and systemic chemotherapy as treatment stratified according to the retrospective peritoneal surface disease severity score (PSDSS) for peritoneal carcinomatosis of colorectal origin. *BMC Cancer* 2010;10:689.

42 Verwaal VJ, van Ruth S, de Bree E, *et al.* Randomized trial of cytoreduction and hyperthermic intraperitoneal chemotherapy versus systemic chemotherapy and palliative surgery in patients with peritoneal carcinomatosis of colorectal cancer. *J Clin Oncol* 2003;21(20):3737–43.

43 Verwaal VJ, Bruin S, Boot H, van Slooten G, van Tinteren H. 8-year follow-up of randomized trial: cytoreduction and hyperthermic intraperitoneal chemotherapy versus systemic chemotherapy in patients with peritoneal carcinomatosis of colorectal cancer. *Ann Surg Oncol* 2008;15(9):2426–32.

44 Goere D, Malka D, Tzanis D, *et al.* Is there a possibility of a cure in patients with colorectal peritoneal carcinomatosis amenable to complete cytoreductive surgery and intraperitoneal chemotherapy? *Ann Surg* 2013;257(6):1065–71.

45 Cotte E, Peyrat P, Piaton E, *et al.* Lack of prognostic significance of conventional peritoneal cytology in colorectal and gastric cancers: results of EVOCAPE 2 multicentre prospective study. *Eur J Surg Oncol* 2013;39(7):707–14.

46 Mezhir JJ, Shah MA, Jacks LM, *et al.* Positive peritoneal cytology in patients with gastric cancer: natural history and outcome of 291 patients. *Ann Surg Oncol* 2010;17(12):3173–80.

47 Bang YJ, Van Cutsem E, Feyereislova A, *et al.* Trastuzumab in combination with chemotherapy versus chemotherapy alone for treatment of HER2-positive advanced gastric or gastro-oesophageal junction cancer (ToGA): a phase 3, open-label, randomised controlled trial. *Lancet* 2010;376(9742):687–97.

48 Yang XJ, Huang CQ, Suo T, *et al.* Cytoreductive surgery and hyperthermic intraperitoneal chemotherapy improves survival of patients with peritoneal carcinomatosis from gastric cancer: final results of a phase III randomized clinical trial. *Ann Surg Oncol* 2011;18(6):1575–81.

49 Armstrong DK, Bundy B, Wenzel L, *et al.* Intraperitoneal cisplatin and paclitaxel in ovarian cancer. *N Engl J Med* 2006;354(1):34–43.

50 Landrum LM, Java J, Mathews CA, *et al.* Prognostic factors for stage III epithelial ovarian cancer treated with intraperitoneal chemotherapy: a Gynecologic Oncology Group study. *Gynecol Oncol* 2013;130(1):12–8.

51 Jayakrishnan TT, Zacharias AJ, Sharma A, *et al.* Role of laparoscopy in patients with peritoneal metastases considered for cytoreductive surgery and hyperthermic intraperitoneal chemotherapy (HIPEC). *World J Surg Oncol* 2014;12:270.

52 Dowdy SC, Mullany SA, Brandt KR, Huppert BJ, Cliby WA. The utility of computed tomography scans in predicting suboptimal cytoreductive surgery in women with advanced ovarian carcinoma. *Cancer* 2004;101(2):346–52.

53 Jacquet P, Jelinek JS, Chang D, Koslowe P, Sugarbaker PH. Abdominal computed tomographic scan in the selection of patients with mucinous peritoneal carcinomatosis for cytoreductive surgery. *J Am Coll Surg* 1995;181(6):530–8.

54 Passot G, Glehen O, Pellet O, *et al.* Pseudomyxoma peritonei: role of 18 F-FDG PET in preoperative evaluation of pathological grade and potential for complete cytoreduction. *Eur J Surg Oncol* 2010;36(3):315–23.

55 Kusamura S, Hutanu I, Baratti D, Deraco M. Circulating tumor markers: predictors of incomplete cytoreduction and powerful determinants of outcome in pseudomyxoma peritonei. *J Surg Oncol* 2013;108(1):1–8.

56 Baratti D, Kusamura S, Deraco M. Circulating CA125 and diffuse malignant peritoneal mesothelioma. *Eur J Surg Oncol* 2009;35(11):1198–9.

57 Baratti D, Kusamura S, Martinetti A, *et al.* Prognostic value of circulating tumor markers in patients with pseudomyxoma peritonei treated with cytoreductive surgery and hyperthermic intraperitoneal chemotherapy. *Ann Surg Oncol* 2007;14(8):2300–8.

58 Ceelen WP, Flessner MF. Intraperitoneal therapy for peritoneal tumors: biophysics and clinical evidence. *Nat Rev Clin Oncol* 2010;7(2):108–15.

59 Pawlik TM, Schulick RD, Choti MA. Expanding criteria for resectability of colorectal liver metastases. *Oncologist* 2008;13(1):51–64.

60 Elias D, Quenet F, Goere D. Current status and future directions in the treatment of peritoneal dissemination from colorectal carcinoma. *Surg Oncol Clin North Am* 2012;21(4):611–23.

61 Glehen O, Gilly FN, Boutitie F, *et al.* Toward curative treatment of peritoneal carcinomatosis from nonovarian origin by cytoreductive surgery combined with perioperative intraperitoneal chemotherapy: a multi-institutional study of 1,290 patients. *Cancer* 2010;116(24):5608–18.

62 Maggiori L, Elias D. Curative treatment of colorectal peritoneal carcinomatosis: current status and future trends. *Eur J Surg Oncol* 2010;36(7):599–603.

63 Elias D, Faron M, Iuga BS, *et al.* Prognostic similarities and differences in optimally resected liver metastases and peritoneal metastases from colorectal cancers. *Ann Surg* 2015;261(1):157–63.

64 Chua TC, Yan TD, Saxena A, Morris DL. Should the treatment of peritoneal carcinomatosis by cytoreductive surgery and hyperthermic intraperitoneal chemotherapy still be regarded as a highly morbid procedure?: a systematic review of morbidity and mortality. *Ann Surg* 2009;249(6):900–7.

65 Shariat-Madar B, Jayakrishnan TT, Gamblin TC, Turaga KK. Surgical management of bowel obstruction in patients with peritoneal carcinomatosis. *J Surg Oncol* 2014;110(6):666–9.

66 Jacquet P, Sugarbaker PH. Clinical research methodologies in diagnosis and staging of patients with peritoneal carcinomatosis. In: PH Sugarbaker (ed.) *Peritoneal Carcinomatosis: Principles of Management.* Boston, MA: Kluwer Academic Publishers, 1996:359–374.

Section 14

Pediatric and Adolescent Oncology

47

Pediatric Cancers

Stephanie B. Dixon[1], Lisa M. Force[1], Pratiti Bandopadhayay[2], Peter Manley[2], Carlos Rodriguez-Galindo[1], Lewis B. Silverman[2], and Karen J. Marcus[2]

[1] *St. Jude Children's Research Hospital, Memphis, Tennessee, USA*
[2] *Dana-Farber/Boston Children's Cancer and Blood Disorders Center, Boston, Massachusetts, USA*

Introduction to Pediatric Oncology

Every year in the United States (US) there are approximately 10,270 new cases of cancer and 1,190 cancer deaths among children aged 0–14 years [1]. Cancer is the second leading cause of mortality for children in the US. Childhood cancers differ from adult cancers in their sites of origins and histologic subtypes, etiologic characteristics, response to treatment, and outcome. In the adult population, carcinomas comprise the largest group of cancers and most often arise in the lung, breast, prostate, colon, and rectum. The distribution of the most common pediatric malignancies is quite different: leukemias (30%), brain and other nervous system cancers (26%), soft tissue sarcomas (7%), neuroblastoma (6%), non-Hodgkin lymphomas (6%), Wilms tumor (5%), and Hodgkin lymphoma (3%) [1]. Many cancers of adults are related to carcinogenic exposures such tobacco, poor diet, obesity, physical inactivity, alcohol, and certain microorganisms (human papillomavirus, *Helicobacter pylori*, hepatitis viruses, etc.). Less is known regarding the etiology of most childhood malignancies, although some are associated with recognized genetic syndromes.

This chapter reviews the epidemiologic factors, pathologic features, clinical presentation, and treatment of the more common pediatric malignancies – acute lymphoblastic leukemia, acute myeloid leukemia, rhabdomyosarcoma, germ cell tumors, retinoblastoma, Wilms tumor, osteosarcoma, Ewing sarcoma, Hodgkin lymphoma, non-Hodgkin lymphoma, neuroblastoma, medulloblastoma, and central nervous system gliomas. Despite the rarity of childhood cancers, encouraging progress has been made in the treatment of childhood cancer. Major advances in cancer genetics and the molecular biological characteristics of cancer have been gained through research on these tumors. The improvements in the treatment of childhood cancers have come about largely through cooperative groups both in North America and internationally. It is this collaboration of expertise and effort that will continue to improve the outcome of childhood cancer. Successful treatment of childhood cancer also demands knowledge of the potential for late treatment toxicities that can have devastating consequences as surviving children mature. Among these late effects are growth abnormalities, cardiac sequelae, neurocognitive effects, sterility, and the development of second, treatment-induced cancers. Many of these toxicities are unavoidable, depending on the treatment required to eradicate disease; however, every attempt to minimize such late effects must be made in parallel with improvements in cancer treatment.

Acute Lymphoblastic Leukemia

Definition

Acute lymphoblastic leukemia (ALL) is characterized by replacement of normal marrow elements with malignant lymphoblasts (cancerous cells derived from lymphoid precursor cells).

Incidence

ALL is the most common childhood cancer, representing 26% of the cancers diagnosed in children under 15 years of age. There has been an average increase in incidence of ALL from 1975 to 2010 of 0.7% per year. The peak incidence of ALL in the US and other industrialized countries occurs in children between the ages of 2 and 4 years. There is a slight male predominance, with a male:female ratio of 1.3:1. In the US, the incidence of ALL is higher in White and Hispanic children than in Black children [2]. In marked contrast to the increasing incidence rate, there was an average annual decrease of 3.1% in the ALL mortality rate during 1988–2010 [2,3].

Etiology and Risk Factors

In the vast majority of cases of ALL, causative factors cannot be identified. However, there are a few underlying conditions which are associated with an increased risk of developing ALL.

The American Cancer Society's Oncology in Practice: Clinical Management, First Edition. Edited by The American Cancer Society.

For instance, children with Down syndrome (trisomy 21) are 10–20 times more likely to develop acute leukemia than non-Down syndrome children [4]. Although AML predominates in the first few years of life, ALL is the more common leukemia observed in Down syndrome. Other genetic conditions that have been associated with an increased risk of developing ALL include neurofibromatosis and ataxia-telangiectasia [5,6]. Some environmental exposures, including pre- and post-natal exposures to very high doses of radiation (such as those experienced by victims of the atomic bomb in Japan during World War II), have also been linked to the development of ALL; however, data are conflicting regarding the association between other environmental exposures (including lower-dose ionizing radiation and electromagnetic fields) and subsequent development of ALL [7]. Rarely, ALL may arise as a secondary leukemia in patients who have received chemotherapy (especially topoisomerase II inhibitors, such as epipodophyllotoxins) for other malignancies [8].

Classification

Based on expression of cell surface markers, ALL is typically divided into two distinct immunophenotypic subtypes: B-ALL (~85% of cases) and T-ALL (~15% of cases).

B-ALL is characterized by the expression of CD79a, CD19, HLA-DR, and other B cell-associated antigens. Approximately 90% of precursor B-cell ALL cases express the CD10 surface antigen. Absence of CD10 is associated with the presence of rearrangement of the *MLL* gene on chromosome 11, a cytogenetic abnormality that has been associated with a poor prognosis [9]. The presence of surface immunoglobulin (observed in 1–2% of cases of childhood ALL) is diagnostic of mature B-cell ALL, a subtype that is biologically indistinguishable from Burkitt lymphoma. Patients with mature B-cell ALL should be treated with regimens for advanced-stage Burkitt lymphoma rather than those designed for other types of ALL [10].

T-ALL is characterized by expression of cytoplasmic CD3, and surface expression of T-cell antigens, such as CD2, CD5, and CD7. It is more common in adolescents than in younger children, and is associated with higher presenting leukocyte counts than B-ALL [11]. Patients with T-ALL may present with a mediastinal mass, which can lead to airway compression at diagnosis. Mediastinal masses are almost never observed in B-ALL. A subset of T-ALL, known as early T-precursor (ETP) phenotype, is characterized by a distinctive immunophenotype (CD1a and CD8 negativity, with weak expression of CD5 and coexpression of stem cell or myeloid markers). It has been identified in 10–15% of pediatric T-ALL, and, in retrospective analyses, has been associated with a poorer prognosis [12].

Diagnosis

Many patients present with fatigue, pallor, bone pain, or bleeding and are found to have cytopenias and/or hepatosplenomegaly or lymphadenopathy. Evaluation of the bone marrow by aspirate and biopsy is essential to make the diagnosis of ALL. The definition of ALL includes at least 25% marrow involvement by lymphoblasts (confirmed by flow cytometry and/or immunohistochemistry); however, most children with ALL present with well over 50% of the marrow replaced by lymphoblasts (typically 80–90%). In addition to morphologic evaluation, marrow aspirate should also be examined by flow cytometry to define immunophenotype, as well as karyotype analysis and fluorescent *in situ* hybridization (FISH) studies to screen for prognostically relevant chromosomal abnormalities.

A lumbar puncture should be performed in patients with newly diagnosed ALL. However, the initial lumbar puncture should only be performed in conjunction with the administration of intrathecal chemotherapy; therefore, this procedure should be done only after the diagnosis of ALL has been confirmed by marrow and/or peripheral blood studies.

Outcome and Prognostic Factors

The 5-year survival rate for children younger than 15 years with ALL has improved dramatically in the US, from approximately 57% for those diagnosed between 1975 and 1979 to 90% for those diagnosed between 2003 and 2009 [2].

A number of clinical and biologic factors have been identified as prognostically important in ALL, including the following:

1) *Age at diagnosis*: Children aged 1–10 years have a better prognosis than older and younger patients; infants have the worst prognosis [13]. The prognostic relevance of age is related, at least in part, to age-related differences in the frequencies of various ALL subtypes. For instance, there is a much higher frequency of B-precursor ALL with "favorable" cytogenetic abnormalities, including high hyperdiploidy and the *ETV6-RUNX1* (also known as *TEL-AML1*) fusion, in children aged 1–10 years [13]. Conversely, approximately 80% of infants with ALL present with a rearrangement of the *MLL* gene on chromosome 11, which has been associated with a very high risk of relapse [14].
2) *Presenting leukocyte count*: Higher presenting leukocyte counts are associated with a higher risk of subsequent relapse. Most current treatment protocols use a leukocyte count of 50,000/μL as the cut-off point to define patients at higher and lower risk of relapse [15].
3) *CNS status*: The presence of CNS leukemia at diagnosis (defined as cerebrospinal fluid samples with 5 or more white blood cells (WBC)/μL and cytospin slides positive for blasts) has been identified as an adverse prognostic factor [16].
4) *Immunophenotype*: Historically, patients with T-cell phenotype (T-ALL) had a higher risk of relapse than those with B-precursor phenotype (B-ALL). However, with more intensive regimens, children and adolescents with T-ALL appear to fare as well as those with B-ALL [11].

   In approximately 15–30% of patients with newly diagnosed ALL, flow cytometry reveals coexpression of at least one myeloid antigen on the cell surface. Myeloid antigen coexpression in ALL does not appear to be an independent predictor of outcome [17]. However, such cases need to be distinguished from leukemia of ambiguous lineage, an uncommon subtype of acute leukemia that may have features of both myeloid and lymphoid precursor cells, but whose predominant lineage cannot be determined. In the World Health Organization (WHO) classification, the presence of myeloperoxidase in a blast cell with lymphoid-associated surface antigens is consistent with a diagnosis of leukemia of ambiguous lineage [18].

5) *Cytogenetics*: Several recurrent chromosomal abnormalities are observed in lymphoblasts of patients with ALL and are important prognostic factors, especially in B-precursor ALL.

Chromosomal abnormalities associated with more favorable outcomes include high hyperdiploidy (51–65 chromosomes), observed in ~25% cases of B-ALL [19]. For patients with high hyperdiploidy, those who have trisomies of chromosomes 4, 10, and 17 may have especially favorable outcomes [20]. The *ETV6-RUNX1* (*TEL-AML1*) fusion has also been associated with a favorable outcome [19,21]. This translocation, involving chromosomes 12 and 21, is observed in ~20% of cases of B-ALL and is, in general, only detectable by FISH or polymerase chain reaction (PCR) screening studies [21]. Neither of these chromosomal abnormalities commonly occurs in T-ALL.

Rearrangements of the *MLL* gene (chromosome 11q23) are seen in ~5% of childhood ALL cases and in approximately 80% of infant cases. This abnormality has been associated with a poor prognosis, and patients with *MLL* gene rearrangements are usually treated with intensified therapy. Low hypodiploidy (<44 chromosomes), observed in 1–2% of pediatric ALL patients, has also been associated with a poor prognosis [22]. In some studies, patients with another uncommon genetic abnormality, intrachromosomal amplification of the *RUNX1* gene on chromosome 21 (iAMP21), have been reported to have an increased risk of relapse [23].

The Philadelphia chromosome (t9(;22)(q34;q11.2)) occurs in 3–5% of pediatric ALL and is more common in older children and adolescents [13]. Historically, it was associated with an extremely poor prognosis, and was considered an indication for allogeneic hematopoietic stem cell transplant (SCT) in first complete remission [24]. However, results from more recent clinical trials have suggested that the combination of a tyrosine kinase inhibitor and cytotoxic chemotherapy (without SCT) may be associated with a relatively favorable outcome in patients with Philadelphia chromosome-positive ALL [25].

6) *Early response to therapy*: The level of residual disease in the peripheral blood and marrow after the first few days to weeks of therapy strongly correlates with long-term outcome. For instance, inferior event-free survival (EFS) rates have been observed in patients with a poor prednisone response, defined as a peripheral blood absolute blast count above 1,000/μL after a steroid prophase consisting of 7 days of prednisone and a single dose of intrathecal methotrexate [26].

Minimal residual disease (MRD) testing is now used as standard to detect submicroscopic levels of leukemia in patients after the initiation of therapy. MRD may be assessed by multiparameter flow cytometry or PCR [27,28]. Several studies have shown that the level of MRD at the end of the first 4 weeks of therapy is the strongest independent predictor of outcome [29,30]. Patients who are in a complete morphologic remission but have a high level of MRD at the end of the initial induction phase have a high risk of subsequent relapse. MRD levels at earlier (e.g., day 8 of induction) and later time points (e.g., week 12) have also been shown to have prognostic significance [29–31].

7) *Novel prognostic factors:* Recent research utilizing genomic profiling and other genetic/epigenetic techniques has identified a biologically distinctive subset of patients with a high risk of relapse. These patients have a gene expression signature similar to patients with BCR-ABL-positive ALL, but lack that translocation [32,33]. This B-ALL subset is characterized by a high frequency of deletions in the *IKZF1* (a gene that encodes a transcription factor), overexpression of *CRLF2* (a cytokine receptor gene), and mutations of *JAK* (a tyrosine kinase involved in the activation of transcription factors) [33–35]. These factors are not yet screened as standard in patients with ALL, and further studies are necessary to determine whether they should be incorporated into risk classification schema.

Treatment

Risk-Stratified Therapy

Most regimens for childhood ALL stratify therapy utilizing a risk-adapted strategy. Patients are assigned to a risk group based on the prognostic factors outlined in the previous section. Those with "higher risk" features are treated with more intensive, potentially more toxic, treatments in order to improve their cure rates, while patients with more favorable clinical and biologic features are treated with less intensive regimens in order to spare them some of the more morbid components of therapy.

Pediatric ALL patients are typically assigned an initial risk group at the time of diagnosis based on their age and initial leukocyte count. Most regimens use the National Cancer Institute (NCI) criteria to stratify patients [15]. A patient who is age 1 to younger than 10 years old and has an initial leukocyte count less than 50,000/μL is considered standard risk by the NCI criteria. All other patients are considered high risk. On some regimens, leukemia immunophenotype (B-cell vs T-cell) and central nervous system (CNS) status are also used to determine therapy at the time of diagnosis. After therapy has been started, the initial risk group status may be modified based on leukemia cytogenetics and early response to therapy (e.g., MRD). A final risk group status is then assigned and used to determine the intensity of postinduction therapy.

Treatment Phases

Nearly all children and adolescents with newly diagnosed ALL are treated with chemotherapy for 2–3 years. In general, treatment is divided into several phases, including remission induction, consolidation/intensification, and continuation (maintenance).

Remission Induction

This generally lasts 4–6 weeks and includes treatment with vincristine, a corticosteroid, L-asparaginase, and often an anthracycline (daunorubicin or doxorubicin), as well as intrathecal chemotherapy. The goal of this phase is to induce a complete remission (absence of microscopically detectable leukemia in the presence of normal or near-normal peripheral blood counts). More than 95% of newly diagnosed children and adolescents with ALL will achieve a complete remission at the end of this phase [36,37]. Most patients with persistent, morphologically detectable leukemia at the end of the remission induction phase will ultimately achieve complete remission with alternative agents; however, such patients have a poor prognosis and may benefit from an allogeneic hematopoietic SCT once complete remission is achieved [38].

Consolidation/Intensification

This phase begins as soon as complete remission is achieved, and, in general, lasts for several months. The specific agents and schedules during this phase vary amongst different ALL treatment regimens. Drugs typically include high-dose methotrexate with leucovorin rescue, cyclophosphamide, cytarabine, and thiopurines, as well as the agents used during the remission induction phase, such as vincristine, corticosteroids, anthracyclines, and L-asparaginase [36,37,39]. It is during this phase that treatment differs the most between standard- (or low-) risk and high-risk patients, with higher-risk patients typically receiving a more intensive consolidation regimen.

Continuation (Maintenance)

Continuation, which commences after completion of consolidation, is the least intensive of the treatment phases. It consists of low-dose, weekly methotrexate, nightly oral 6-mercaptopurine, and often vincristine and corticosteroid pulses given on a regular basis [40].

CNS-Directed Treatment

Not all the chemotherapy agents administered by mouth or intravenously to treat ALL are able to effectively penetrate into the CNS. Because of this, the CNS is considered a "sanctuary site"; unless specific therapy is directed toward the CNS, the majority of children (even those without detectable lymphoblasts in their spinal fluid at diagnosis) will develop a relapse in their CNS. Thus, all current ALL regimens incorporate CNS-directed treatments during some or all of the treatment phases. Options for CNS-directed treatments include intrathecal chemotherapy, systemically administered chemotherapy that is known to be CNS-penetrant (such as high-dose methotrexate), or cranial radiation [41]. Intrathecal chemotherapy is a universal component of ALL treatment regardless of risk group; cranial radiation is typically reserved for those patients considered at highest risk of CNS relapse (e.g., patients with CNS leukemia at diagnosis) [42].

Relapsed ALL

Approximately 15–20% of children and adolescents with ALL experience a relapse. Most relapses occur within the first 5 years after initial diagnosis, but rarely relapses may occur at later time points; relapses almost never occur after a patient has been in complete remission for 10 years [37]. The majority of relapses involve the bone marrow, but up to 5% of patients experience an isolated extramedullary relapse, primarily involving the CNS but sometimes involving other sites, such as the testes.

The most important prognostic factors after leukemia recurrence are site and timing of relapse [43]. Isolated extramedullary relapses have a better prognosis than those that involve the marrow. Also, the longer the duration of complete remission before a relapse occurs, the higher the chance of cure.

When a patient relapses, reinduction chemotherapy is administered with the goal of achieving a second complete remission. For patients who are able to achieve a second remission, postinduction treatment options include intensive chemotherapy regimens (usually including agents that are not typically given at the time of initial diagnosis) and allogeneic SCT. The decision to proceed to SCT or not depends upon site and timing of relapse. For instance, patients with a late isolated CNS relapse are effectively treated with intensive chemotherapy combined with cranial radiation, and typically do not receive allogeneic SCT [44]. Conversely, those with an early marrow relapse have a better chance of cure if they proceed to SCT in second complete remission rather than receiving treatment with chemotherapy alone [45]. Emerging data suggest that end-reinduction MRD levels may have strong prognostic significance in relapsed ALL, especially in patients with a late marrow relapse [46]. Investigators are studying whether end-reinduction MRD may be used to identify late-relapsing patients who might benefit from an allogeneic SCT and those who might fare as well with chemotherapy alone [47].

Follow-up and Late Effects

With the successful improvement in survival of children diagnosed with ALL, the late effects of treatment have become more apparent. Early mortality from cardiac disease, second malignant neoplasms (SMNs), and pulmonary disease have been described in survivors of childhood ALL [48]. Anthracycline exposure during ALL treatment has decreased over time with newer treatment protocols, but even at lower cumulative doses there is an increased risk of congestive heart failure (CHF) compared to the general population [49,50]. The cumulative incidence of SMNs varies widely from 1 to 10% depending on the antileukemic regimen used and follow-up duration, and include hematologic malignancies such as acute myeloid leukemia, myelodysplastic syndrome, non-Hodgkin lymphoma and Hodgkin lymphoma, CNS tumors, especially if the patient received prior CNS radiation, and various other carcinomas or other malignancies [51]. Obesity, insulin resistance, and bony morbidity in the forms of osteopenia, fractures, and/or avascular necrosis have been consistently described, with a likely role of corticosteroids in the dysregulation of weight and a clear causal role of corticosteroid exposure in bony complications [52].

Cranial radiation is being used very rarely in current practice due to the efficacy of intrathecal chemotherapy, but was the standard of care for a period of time. The sequelae, in addition to cranial SMNs and head and neck cancers, include long-term neuropsychological effects, particularly in younger children, and decreased adult height due to direct impairment of bone and muscle growth in addition occasionally to growth hormone deficiency [53]. Even without cranial radiation, ALL systemic chemotherapy includes treatment with dexamethasone and high-dose methotrexate, which may have late neuropsychological effects [54]. As late effects of therapy have become more apparent, ALL treatment has adapted and continues to attempt to minimize therapies that have particularly toxic late effects.

Acute Myeloid Leukemia

Definition

Acute myeloid leukemia (AML, also known as acute myelogenous leukemia) is a clonal disorder in which a hematopoietic stem cell or progenitor cell undergoes malignant transformation, gaining the ability to be self-renewing with decreased capacity for differentiation. In order to be defined as "acute," the bone marrow typically must have >20% myeloid blasts. Additional myeloid malignancies include:

- Chronic myelogenous leukemia (CML), a clonal malignancy involving all hematopoietic cell lineages that is nearly always associated with the 9;22 translocation and has three distinct clinical stages including a chronic phase, accelerated phase, and blast crisis [55,56].
- Juvenile myelomonocytic leukemia (JMML), which typically presents with hepatosplenomegaly, lymphadenopathy, and a skin rash in addition to elevated peripheral monocytes, and is often associated with an elevated fetal hemoglobin level, monosomy 7, and leukemic cell mutations in the RAS pathway [57,58].
- Transient myeloproliferative disorder (TMD), a clonal expansion of myeloblasts that occurs in infants with trisomy 21 and is associated with *GATA1* gene mutations, which spontaneously regresses in most cases although 20% of patients ultimately develop AML [59,60].
- Myelodysplastic syndrome (MDS), a heterogeneous group of disorders characterized by ineffective hematopoiesis, dysplastic hematopoietic cells, progressive cytopenias, cytogenetic abnormalities such as deletions of the long arm of chromosome 5 or 7 (particularly in therapy-related MDS), and which have an increased propensity to transform into AML [61–63].

Incidence

AML is less common than ALL during childhood, with approximately 24% of of leukemias diagnosed in patients <15 years of age classified as myeloid [1]. The annual AML incidence rates among children and adolescents <20 years of age are 7.9 cases per million boys and 8.0 cases per million girls, with the highest incidence in the first 2 years of life, decreasing until age 6, and then increasing during the remainder of childhood and adolescence [2,64]. The incidence is similar for boys and girls as well as for Caucasians and African Americans, but there is a possible increased overall incidence in Hawaiians and a possible higher incidence of acute promyelocytic leukemia (M3), a subtype of AML, in Hispanic children [65].

Etiology and Risk Factors

Various genetic and environmental factors have been associated with increased risk for development of pediatric AML. However, the majority of pediatric AML diagnoses do not have clear causative factors. Hereditary conditions with an observed increase in AML incidence in childhood include inherited disorders with dysfunctional DNA repair mechanisms and increased chromosome fragility such as Bloom syndrome and Fanconi anemia, in addition to disorders of myelopoiesis such as congenital neutropenia and Shwachman–Diamond syndrome [66–69]. Germline mutations in *RUNX1, CEBPA,* and *GATA2* are associated with increased risk of developing MDS or AML [70–73]. The most common genetic condition predisposing to the development of AML, however, is trisomy 21 (Down syndrome), where there is an increased risk of both AML and ALL and a notable 500 times increased risk of acute megakaryocytic leukemia (M7), a specific subtype of AML, as compared to the general pediatric population [74].

Many environmental risk factors have been associated with an increased risk of AML in childhood, although the data in support of these associations continue to evolve. Prenatally, older maternal age, maternal consumption of alcohol during pregnancy, and ionizing radiation exposure have been associated with an increased risk of AML, as well as potentially pesticide and dietary DNA topoisomerase II inhibitor exposure (soy, beans, coffee, black or green tea, cocoa, wine) *in utero* [65,75–79]. Postnatal treatment with alkylating agents is associated with an increased risk of MDS and secondary AML, particularly with therapy-related AML that demonstrates deletions of chromosomes 5 or 7 [80,81]. Treatment with topoisomerase II inhibitors is associated with increased risk of developing therapy-related AML that carries 11q23 alterations in the mixed-lineage leukemia (MLL) gene [82]. These therapy-related acute myeloid leukemias generally have a worse prognosis than AML that develops without prior therapy.

Presentation

Children with AML present similarly to those with ALL, with the majority of their signs and symptoms secondary to bone marrow infiltration by myeloid blast cells. These symptoms include pallor, fatigue, bone pain, fever, and bleeding. Approximately 10–20% of patients present with hyperleukocytosis (defined in AML as a leukocyte count >100,000/uL), a finding that increases potential for leukostasis, a congestion of leukocytes in small vessels of the brain and lungs [83]. This is an emergency in pediatric oncology due to the associated morbidity and mortality, and may be treated with leukapheresis or cytoreductive agents such as low-dose cytarabine or hydroxyurea. Children with AML may present with increased, normal, or decreased leukocyte counts, but regardless of the number these blast cells do not function appropriately and patients are at increased risk of serious and fatal bacterial infections.

AML has several presenting features that differ from classic ALL presentations. All subtypes of AML can cause disseminated intravascular coagulation (DIC), but this complication is most commonly described in acute promyelocytic leukemia (APL, M3) and improves with the use of all-trans retinoic acid (ATRA) in induction treatment. Extramedullary leukemic infiltration is fairly common in AML, occurring in approximately 20% of children, and may involve the skin (leukemia cutis), gingiva (often with bleeding), liver or spleen (particularly in infants), testes, or chloromas (solid tumors made of myeloblasts that may occur throughout the body but have a predilection for the orbit and epidural regions) [84]. CNS involvement (defined as $>5 \times 10^6$ white blood cells in the CSF with a nontraumatic spinal tap and cytology positive for blasts) may occur in up to 20% of patients at diagnosis, although the range reported in the literature is quite broad [85,86]. Up to 3.5% of patients die during the first two weeks of treatment from leukostasis or bleeding complications, emphasizing the importance of excellent supportive care [87].

Diagnosis, Classification, and Evaluation

Diagnosis of AML should begin with a good history and physical examination with attention to any syndromic features, then an assessment of peripheral blood counts and examination of a peripheral blood smear for cell morphology. If the presenting leukocyte count is low, peripheral myeloid blasts may not always be present; regardless, a definitive diagnosis of AML requires bone marrow assessment for morphology with cytochemistry, immunophenotyping (flow cytometry), and cytogenetics (karyotype, FISH, and molecular genetic testing). This testing is typically obtained via bone marrow aspirate and trephine biopsy; a myeloid blast percentage >20% in the bone marrow confirms a diagnosis of AML [18]. However, in children MDS can present with between 20 and 30% blasts in the bone marrow, an important differential diagnosis, as MDS is an indication for SCT [88]. The genetic testing performed on the bone marrow sample plays an important role in confirming a diagnosis of AML in equivocal cases, in addition to being important for initial risk stratification. If the bone marrow sample is inadequate (a "dry tap") or there is high suspicion for MDS, analysis of the bone marrow trephine specimen may be useful; thus, it is recommended to perform both a bone marrow aspirate and trephine biopsy during the initial diagnostic procedure. CNS status is also important to assess at diagnosis, although the lumbar puncture may be delayed if a patient is in active DIC or has a significant bleeding risk that is not correctable with a platelet transfusion.

The morphologic classification of AML is still based on the French–American–British (FAB) system[89], which divides AML subtypes by phenotype along a spectrum from the least differentiated (FAB M0) to the most differentiated/mature (FAB M7) (Table 47.1). Auer rods are cytoplasmic deposits that form needle shapes, are azurophilic with a classic Wright–Giemsa stain, and are myeloperoxidase (MPO) positive. They are specific to AML but variably present among the FAB subtypes.

Immunophenotyping is important for accurate lineage classification, both in distinguishing AML from ALL as well as determining AML M0 and M7, which can be difficult to delineate by morphology alone, and identifying mixed phenotype or ambiguous lineage leukemias [90]. Cytogenetics have become essential for risk stratification and appropriate treatment for hematopoietic malignancies; conventional cytogenetics may detect abnormalities in approximately 75% of pediatric AML [88]. The most recent WHO classification of myeloid neoplasms and acute leukemia acknowledges the relevance of genetic features by including a category for AML with recurrent genetic abnormalities. This category includes AML with t(8;21), inv(16), *PML-RARA* (usually t(15;17)), mutated *NPM1*, and *CEBPA* mutations (all known to be associated with a more favorable prognosis), as well as t(6;9) (known to be associated with adverse prognosis). Additional cytogenetic alterations that are associated with adverse prognosis include monosomy 5 or 7, FLT3-ITD with high allelic ratio, and AML with a complex karyotype (generally indicating three or more unrelated cytogenetic changes). If a patient does not carry a prognostic cytogenetic or molecular abnormality they are typically classified as intermediate risk.

While risk stratification traditionally relied on pathologic and genetic features, the role of response to induction therapy in further refining risk is under investigation; MRD assessed by flow cytometry of the bone marrow following the first induction course of chemotherapy may identify intermediate-risk patients at risk of relapse [91]. Various trials have chosen different MRD cut-offs and it is yet to be determined whether MRD will be prognostic in children with known favorable or unfavorable genetic features [92,93].

Table 47.1 FAB Classification of acute myeloid leukemia.

FAB subtype	Description
M0	Acute myeloblastic leukemia with minimal differentiation
M1	Acute myeloblastic leukemia without maturation
M2	Acute myeloblastic leukemia with maturation
M3	Acute promyelocytic leukemia (APL)
M4	Acute myelomonocytic leukemia
M5	Acute monocytic leukemia
M6	Acute erythrocytic leukemia
M7	Acute megakaryoblastic leukemia (AMKL)

Source: Bennett 1985 [89].

Treatment

Therapy for children with AML is risk-adapted based on biologic factors in order to cure patients with the least toxicity and late effects possible, but overall is one of the most intensive chemotherapy regimens used for children with cancer. Remission induction therapy generally includes a backbone of cytarabine and an anthracycline such as daunorubicin, idarubicin, or mitoxantrone. A third drug, either etoposide or 6-thioguanine, is commonly added to this backbone, and with two courses of a three-drug regimen approximately 90% of patients will enter remission [90,94,95]. Various strategies to increase rates of remission have included decreased time between cycles or increased dosing of cytarabine or anthracyclines. In general, this intensification results in more durable disease-free survival, although with potential increased treatment-related toxicity, highlighting the importance of quality supportive care [88,90].

Following induction, postremission therapy is necessary for remission to be durable, and typically consists of 2–3 courses of chemotherapy comprised of drugs with different mechanisms such as L-asparaginase, etoposide, and mitoxantrone, in addition to cytarabine [96,97]. CNS treatment is administered to all children with AML, even if they are CNS negative at diagnosis, given concern that systemic chemotherapy does not adequately treat any AML blasts that enter the CSF. CNS treatment consists of intrathecal cytarabine or methotrexate (or triple intrathecal therapy at St. Jude Children's Research Hospital) in combination with a steroid, between 4 and 12 times during therapy; the optimal number of intrathecal treatments is not known [88]. Generally CNS radiation is now avoided as prophylaxis given the significant side effects associated with radiation to the developing brain. In regard to SCT, allogeneic SCT is only recommended in first complete remission (CR) if the child does not have favorable risk factors or if the benefit is felt to outweigh the potential toxicity. In many studies the availability of a HLA-matched sibling donor played a role in whether allogeneic SCT was considered as postremission therapy [90]. In second CR or therapy-related AML in first CR, allogeneic SCT is typically recommended [88]. The 5-year overall survival (OS) for pediatric AML is approximately 64% [2].

Treatment for APL differs from generic AML treatment, and ATRA is initiated immediately on diagnosis given the risk of significant and fatal bleeding [88]. Children who present with elevated leukocyte counts (typically defined as $>10 \times 10^9$/L) qualify as high risk and are initiated on chemotherapy as well as ATRA in order to decrease the risk of APL differentiation syndrome [98]. ATRA induces blast maturation and in combination with anthracycline ± cytarabine chemotherapy has a 5-year OS of >80% [99,100]. ATRA is continued in maintenance in combination with 6-thioguanine and methotrexate; APL is currently the only subtype of AML where maintenance therapy is used. Arsenic trioxide (ATO) has also shown much promise to act as an anthracycline-sparing agent, and is actively being studied in children with APL [101].

Follow-Up and Late Effects

Late effects reported in survivors of pediatric AML who did not undergo SCT include significant cardiac toxicities as well as second malignancies and renal, hepatic, and gastrointestinal adverse effects [102–104]. Higher doses of anthracyclines are currently being used than in the past, raising concern that cardiac toxicities will be a larger issue in the future for childhood AML survivors [105]. In survivors at one institution who underwent allogeneic SCT as part of their treatment, growth abnormalities, neurocognitive deficits, transfusion-acquired hepatitis, infertility, endocrinopathies, and cataracts were observed in addition to cardiac abnormalities and second malignancies [103]. The significant late effects of HSCT underscore the importance of optimizing therapeutic approaches that do not require HSCT.

Hodgkin Lymphoma

Definition

Hodgkin lymphoma is characterized by the presence of multinucleated giant cells known as Reed–Sternberg cells or large mononuclear cell variants known as lymphocytic and histiocytic cells, in a background of inflammatory cells.

Incidence

Hodgkin lymphoma (HL) represents approximately 4% of childhood (ages 1–14 years) cancers, and 8% of cancers in adolescents (ages 15–19 years). Incidence rates are highest among young adults aged 20–34. The incidence rates for HL in children and adolescents in the US are approximately 9% higher for males than females, and are highest among non-Hispanic whites and lowest among Asian Americans and Pacific Islanders. Observed 15-year survival is approximately 91% [2,106].

Etiology and Risk Factors

Risk of HL is increased among individuals with a history of Epstein–Barr virus (EBV) and/or human immunodeficiency virus (HIV) infection. Additionally, the risk that a close relative of a patient with HL will develop the disease is increased slightly; most such cases involve two siblings or a parent and child [2,107].

Classification of Hodgkin Lymphoma

Reed–Sternberg cells or large mononuclear Reed–Sternberg cell variants (known as lymphocytic and histiocytic cells) are the clonal, neoplastic cells of HL, and are found in varying numbers among a polymorphous background of inflammatory cells. Hodgkin lymphoma is divided into two broad pathological classes: classical HL and nodular lymphocyte-predominant HL [108]. Classical HL is divided into four subtypes:

1) Lymphocyte-rich classical Hodgkin lymphoma.
2) Nodular sclerosis Hodgkin lymphoma.
3) Mixed-cellularity Hodgkin lymphoma.
4) Lymphocyte-depleted Hodgkin lymphoma.

This subclassification is histologic and based on the number of Reed–Sternberg cells, the characteristics of the inflammatory background, and the presence or absence of fibrosis.

Presentation and Evaluation

Most cases of HL arise in lymph nodes or extranodal lymphoid tissue such as Waldeyer ring. Patients usually present with enlarged lymph nodes, which in children is also a frequent physical finding secondary to benign causes. Usually, the lymph nodes involved with HL are non-tender and are described as firm and rubbery. Nodes may be enlarged for several weeks or months. Suspicious lymph nodes must be subjected to biopsy. A thorough history is important, with special attention to the presence of "B" symptoms: unexplained weight loss of 10% over 6 months, drenching night sweats, and unexplained fevers of 101 °F or higher on three occasions.

A careful physical examination should be performed, and a biopsy of the suspicious node or mass is required to establish the diagnosis. All patients undergo laboratory studies, including complete blood counts, renal function tests, liver function tests, and erythrocyte sedimentation rate (ESR) analysis. Patients with HL have altered cellular immunity but relatively normal humoral immunity. Radiographic imaging with plain-film chest radiography and computed tomography (CT) of the chest, abdomen, and pelvis are recommended. CT of the neck is performed for patients with any neck adenopathy. Positron emission tomography (PET) scanning now is being used by most institutions. PET-CT integrates functional and anatomic imaging and is used to stage and monitor response to treatment in HL. Bone scanning is performed for patients with bony pain or elevated alkaline phosphatase levels. The staging system used for HL is the Ann Arbor Staging System [109]. This system does not include an assessment of bulk of disease.

Treatment

The treatment of pediatric HL is risk stratified and response based. Following the diagnostic staging evaluation, children are classified into risk groups to determine the appropriate treatment. Patients are classified into low-, intermediate-, and high-risk groups. This classification varies among the many different pediatric cooperative groups and consortia. The stratifications generally consider stage, presence of B symptoms, extranodal disease, and, in some stratification systems, bulk of disease. Treatment consists of initial multiagent chemotherapy with a response evaluation done after 2–3 cycles. Many of the agents in the MOPP and ABVD regimens originally developed to treat HL are still used. The concept of non-cross-resistant chemotherapy incorporates several factors: each agent is individually active; the agents differ in their mechanisms of action; and toxicities do not overlap. The agents in MOPP consist of nitrogen mustard, vincristine (Oncovin), procarbazine, and prednisone; ABVD includes doxorubicin, bleomycin, vinblastine, and dacarbazine. Etoposide has been used as an effective alternative to procarbazine to decrease gonadal toxicity.

The rapidity of the early response to chemotherapy has been used to determine extent of chemotherapy and the need for involved-field radiotherapy. Survival rates of more than 90% are expected for such children. Children with more advanced disease are also treated with combined-modality therapy. Trials are ongoing to limit the use of radiotherapy, especially in pediatric patients. Patients who relapse can often be salvaged with high-dose chemotherapy and stem cell rescue.

Follow-Up and Late Effects

The recommended follow-up of children treated for HL includes recording a history and performing a physical examination, chest radiography, and complete blood counts every 3 months for the first year, quarterly for the second 2 years, and semiannually thereafter. Continued use of chest, neck, and abdominal-pelvic CT scans for follow-up is controversial as a retrospective report from the Children's Oncology Group reported that 86% of relapses were detected by clinical symptoms, physical examination, and laboratory studies [110].

Any female patient who received thoracic irradiation should undergo screening for breast cancer starting 8–10 years after treatment and annually thereafter; screening with MRI may be beneficial for younger women [111]. The current goals of treating HL are to improve the outcome for poor-risk patients and to minimize late toxicities in patients whose outcome is favorable. The acute toxicities of HL treatment in children include nausea and vomiting, myelosuppression, mucositis, and hair loss and are similar to those in adults. The late effects of therapy include thyroid dysfunction, musculoskeletal abnormalities, reproductive difficulties, cardiac toxicity, pulmonary toxicity, and second tumors. Second cancers after pediatric HL include solid tumors and secondary leukemias and lymphomas. The median time to the development of leukemias is shorter than that to the development of solid tumors. The incidence of leukemia is related to the administration of chemotherapy, and that of solid tumors is associated with irradiation. Most commonly, the solid tumors are breast tumors (in females), sarcomas, melanomas, and thyroid cancers. The actuarial risk at 20 years (reported from Stanford) is 9.7% for males, 16.8% for females, and 9.2% for breast cancer. Relapse of HL increased the risk of a second cancer, further emphasizing the important goal of initial cure of disease [112].

Non-Hodgkin Lymphoma

Definition

Non-Hodgkin lymphomas (NHL) are a heterogeneous group of cancers showing varying degrees of B-cell, T-cell, and NK-cell differentiation.

Incidence

NHLs comprise approximately 6% of cancers among children younger than 15 years and 8% of cancers among adolescents aged 15–19 years. NHL incidence rates in the US for male children and adolescents are more than double those of females. Incidence rates for NHL overall increase steadily during the first two decades of life. However, age at diagnosis varies substantially among various types of NHL. The average annual percentage increase for NHL incidence rates for children and adolescents was 1.1 from 1975 to 2010 [2].

Etiology and Risk Factors

Numerous factors have been linked to an increased risk of NHL. Immunodeficiency syndromes, such as severe combined immunodeficiency syndrome, Wiskott–Aldrich syndrome, common variable immunodeficiency, ataxia-telangiectasia, and the X-linked lymphoproliferative syndrome, are associated with an increased risk of developing a lymphoma [6,113]. Children with an acquired immunodeficiency, such as that secondary to human immunodeficiency virus (HIV) infection or immunosuppressive therapy after solid-organ or bone marrow transplantation, are at increased risk of developing a malignant lymphoma or a lymphoproliferative disorder [114–116]. Most of the lymphomas that occur in patients with abnormalities of the immune system (either constitutional or acquired) are large B-cell or Burkitt tumors in subtype. Monoclonal Epstein–Barr virus (EBV) DNA has been identified in tumor tissue from many such patients, implicating an early role for the virus in tumor development [117]. One potential explanation of this is the activation of activation-induced deaminase (AID) and polymerase-n by EBV infection as well as HIV and malaria infections. These enzymes assist in immunoglobulin gene class switching leading to antibody diversity; however, given their role in DNA mutagenesis this can also lead to oncogene mutation promotion and translocation. This, in addition to the ability of EBNA-1 to induce breaks in DNA, may assist in the explanation of the development of EBV-positive Burkitt lymphoma as well as their higher mutation rates in antigen receptor gene (VDJ) sequences [118].

Pathologic Classification

The NHLs that occur in children are almost always high grade. Using the WHO 2016 classification, NHL is divided by cell type (B-lineage, T-lineage, or natural killer (NK) cell lineage) and differentiation (precursor vs mature). Pediatric NHLs generally fall into the following categories: lymphoblastic lymphoma including precursor T-cell and precursor B-cell lymphoma; mature B-cell lymphoma including Burkitt, Burkitt-like, and diffuse large B-cell lymphoma (DLBCL); or anaplastic large cell lymphoma (T- and null-cell types) [119]. The frequency, immunophenotype, and associated chromosomal translocations are shown in Table 47.2.

Table 47.2 Major histopathological categories of non-Hodgkin lymphoma in children and adolescents.

WHO classification	Immunophenotype	Clinical presentation	Chromosome abnormalities	Genes affected
Burkitt and Burkitt-like lymphoma/leukemia	Mature B cell	Intra-abdominal (sporadic), head and neck (non-jaw, sporadic), jaw (endemic), bone marrow, CNS	t(8;14)(q24;q32), t(2;8)(p11;q24), t(8;22)(q24;q11)	*C-MYC, IGH, IGK, IGL*
Diffuse large B-cell lymphoma	Mature B cell	Nodal, abdominal, bone, primary CNS (when associated with immunodeficiency), mediastinal	No consistent cytogenetic abnormality identified	–
Primary mediastinal B-cell lymphoma	Mature B cell, often CD30+	Mediastinal, but may also have other nodal or extranodal disease (i.e., abdominal, often kidney)	9p and 2p gains	*JAK2, C-rel, SOCS1*
Lymphoblastic lymphoma, precursor T-cell leukemia, or precursor B-cell lymphoma	Pre-T cell Pre-B cell	Mediastinal, bone marrow Skin, bone, head and neck	*MTS1*/p16ink4a; deletion *TAL1* t(1;14)(p34;q11), t(11;14)(p13;q11)	*TAL1, TCRAO, RHOMB1, HOX11, NOTCH1*
Anaplastic large cell lymphoma, systemic	CD30+ (Ki-1+) T cell/null cell	Variable, but systemic symptoms often prominent	t(2;5)(p23;q35); less common variant translocations involving *ALK*	*ALK, NPM*
Anaplastic large cell lymphoma, cutaneous	CD30+ (Ki-usually)	Skin only; single or multiple lesions	Lacks t(2;5)	–

Presentation and Diagnosis

The clinical presentation of NHL in children depends on the histologic background, the extent of disease, and the primary site of disease. NHLs in children are more often extranodal than in adults. They involve abdominal structures in approximately one-third of cases, the mediastinum in one-third of cases, and the head and neck in one-third of cases. The majority of patients, almost two-thirds, will have advanced disease at diagnosis due to rapid growth and spread by hematogenous dissemination. Cranial nerve palsies or cerebrospinal fluid pleocytosis are indicative of CNS involvement while cytopenias suggest bone marrow infiltration. Patients who have lymphoblastic lymphoma or Burkitt lymphoma with greater than 25% marrow involvement are generally considered to have acute lymphoblastic leukemia and can be treated on leukemia clinical trials [120].

The most common sites are related to the histologic subtypes. Sporadic Burkitt lymphoma typically involves the abdomen or the head and neck. Endemic Burkitt lymphoma presents as a jaw mass in over 50% of cases, although primary abdominal tumors are also common. These tumors grow rapidly, and patients are at risk of developing tumor lysis syndrome, particularly when therapy is begun. Alkalinization, vigorous hydration, and the administration of allopurinol are indicated to decrease the risk of development of this syndrome [121]. Additionally, patients can present with abdominal pain and vomiting due to bowel obstruction from tumor compression of bowels, intussusception, or with symptoms of compression at other primary sites, such as spinal cord compression with an epidural mass [120].

Often, lymphoblastic lymphoma presents with a mediastinal mass, frequently with an associated pleural effusion. The mediastinal mass can grow rapidly, causing airway compromise or compression of the superior vena cava. Prompt initiation of chemotherapy is indicated after diagnostic material has been obtained. Although the occurrence of a primary abdominal tumor in patients with lymphoblastic lymphoma is rare, involvement of such abdominal organs as the liver and spleen can occur. These lymphomas, representing 30% of childhood NHL, most often are of the T-cell immunophenotype. Some patients with a non-T-cell immunophenotype present with peripheral adenopathy or isolated bone involvement [120].

Large cell lymphomas in children can present with an anterior mediastinal mass, an abdominal mass, skin involvement, or bone involvement. Less frequently, large cell lymphomas occur in other extranodal or nodal sites. Spread to the bone marrow or to the CNS is less frequent than in Burkitt lymphomas or lymphoblastic lymphomas. Large cell lymphomas in children can be of T-cell, B-cell, or indeterminate phenotype. Pediatric DLBCL differ from those in adults as they are not typically associated with *BCL-2* gene translocations; additionally, a small subset contains t(8;14) which suggests biologic similarities to Burkitt lymphoma [122]. Thirty percent of childhood large cell lymphomas have anaplastic features, including abundant cytoplasm, atypical lobulated nuclei, and prominent nucleoli [123]. Generally, systemic anaplastic large cell lymphomas in children are of T-/null cell lineage, strongly CD30-positive, and have a chromosomal translocation involving the anaplastic lymphoma kinase (*ALK*) gene in 90% of cases, most often t(2;5). Often, these lymphomas present in advanced stage with extranodal sites of involvement including bone, bone marrow, lung, and skin. However, it is rare to see CNS disease [123,124].

Evaluation and Staging

The evaluation of patients with NHL includes complete blood counts with differential counts; analysis of serum electrolyte levels, calcium, phosphorus, uric acid, and lactate dehydrogenase; a test for HIV; cerebrospinal fluid analysis; bilateral bone marrow biopsies and aspirates; and renal and liver function tests. Radiographic imaging should include CT of the chest,

Table 47.3 St. Jude (Murphy) staging system for non-Hodgkin lymphoma.

Stage	Definition
I	Single tumor of nodal area, excluding abdomen and mediastinum
II	Disease extent is limited to a single tumor with regional node involvement, two or more tumors or nodal areas involved on one side of the diaphragm, or a primary gastrointestinal tract tumor (completely resected) with or without regional node involvement
III	Tumors or involved lymph node areas occur on both sides of the diaphragm. Stage III NHL also includes any primary intrathoracic (mediastinal, pleural, or thymic) disease, extensive primary intra-abdominal disease, or any paraspinal or epidural tumors
IV	Tumors involve bone marrow and/or CNS, regardless of other sites of involvement

Source: Murphy 1980 [125].

abdomen, and pelvis. PET scans or bone scans are performed as part of the initial staging evaluations.

While the Ann Arbor staging system is used in pediatric HL and for all adult lymphomas, it is less accurate for pediatric NHL, and the Murphy staging system is typically used (Table 47.3) [125]. This system differs from that used in staging adult NHL and reflects such patterns of presentation and involvement as frequent extranodal disease, CNS disease, bone marrow disease, and noncontiguous spread of disease. Accurate staging and pathologic classification are critical in determining the appropriate therapy, including the duration, intensity, and expected outcome.

Treatment and Outcome

Owing to the systemic nature of NHL, chemotherapy is the mainstay of treatment for all patients. Surgery plays a limited role except for obtaining diagnostic material and for biopsy of areas suspicious for residual disease. CNS prophylaxis is given with intrathecal chemotherapy for the majority of patients. Radiotherapy is used for such emergent situations such as intracranial involvement, spinal cord compression, airway compromise, or compression of the superior vena cava. In addition, patients who have CNS disease at diagnosis receive intensified intrathecal therapy and often cranial irradiation, except in the case of Burkitt lymphoma. The treatment regimens differ on the basis of histology and the stage of disease.

Burkitt and Diffuse Large B-Cell Lymphoma

Burkitt lymphoma (BL) and diffuse large B-cell lymphoma (DLBCL) represent 19% and 22% of NHL among children and adolescents, respectively [2]. Patients with stage I or stage II Burkitt lymphoma or large cell lymphoma receive cyclophosphamide, vincristine, prednisone, doxorubicin (Adriamycin), and methotrexate. Protocols may vary, with some differences in which agents are used and in the length of therapy. The 5-year EFS for patients with early-stage, large cell NHL or with early-stage Burkitt lymphoma is 85–95% [126]. Randomized trials in children with early-stage NHL have shown the absence of benefit of involved-field irradiation [126]. Patients with stage III and stage IV Burkitt lymphoma receive similar agents with the addition of high-dose methotrexate, high-dose cytarabine, etoposide, and intensive triple intrathecal therapy, which has been effective in eliminating the need for cranial irradiation. In some patients, the use of the anti-CD20 antibody rituximab has been shown to add benefit. The expected EFS at 5 years is 84–92% [127]. Typically children with DLBCL are treated on the same protocols as those with Burkitt lymphoma with similar outcomes though the duration of chemotherapy is often longer and relapse may occur at longer intervals after therapy. Relapse of B-cell NHL is rare, but chance of cure after relapse remains <30%. In this population, high-dose chemotherapy with high-dose cytarabine and etoposide (CYVE) or rituximab, ifosfamide, carboplatin, and etoposide are used, with autologous SCT if complete remission is achieved [128].

Lymphoblastic Lymphoma

Lymphoblastic lymphoma accounts for approximately 20% of NHL among children and adolescents [2]. The vast majority of lymphoblastic lymphomas are of T-cell origin. Children with early-stage lymphoblastic lymphoma receive Adriamycin, vincristine, prednisone, and cyclophosphamide, as well as oral mercaptopurine and oral methotrexate for maintenance therapy. CNS prophylaxis is given with intrathecal therapy for children with low-stage NHL and head and neck primary lesions. Patients with advanced-stage lymphoblastic lymphoma are treated with regimens similar to therapy for ALL including multiple chemotherapeutic agents followed by maintenance therapy for up to 2 years. Despite advances in therapies for ALL and improved outcomes with the use of agents such as high-dose methotrexate and asparaginase, outcomes for lymphoblastic lymphoma have remained stagnant since the 1980s with most studies reporting EFS of 75–80%. Similar to other NHL subtypes, relapse occurs infrequently but when it does the chance of cure is less than 30%. Unfortunately, there has been limited effectiveness of new agents such as nelarabine or clofarabine for T-cell disease. Ongoing studies of blinatumomab, a bi-specific CD19/CD3 antibody, may show promise for B-cell disease [128].

Anaplastic Large Cell Lymphoma

Anaplastic large cell lymphoma (ALCL) accounts for approximately 10–15% of NHL among children and adolescents. Up to 50% of pediatric patients present with mediastinal disease, and almost all have lymph node involvement. It is much less common in the pediatric population to have isolated, cutaneous ALCL. In North America, treatment typically consists of the APO regimen (doxorubicin, prednisone, vincristine, 6-mercaptopurine and methotrexate), which is a 12-month outpatient regimen. It has demonstrated efficacy and safety in a series of North American cooperative group studies, but does have a 300 mg/m^2 cumulative anthracycline dose. European regimens contain a lower cumulative dose of anthracycline and include high-dose methotrexate and alkylating agents. Across regimens it has been observed that approximately 30% of patients will have recurrence or progression of disease; however, unlike other NHLs, it typically remains sensitive to chemotherapy after recurrence. In fact, the majority of patients obtain a second complete remission with weekly vinblastine therapy. Recently, the Children's Oncology Group (COG) evaluated whether substitution of weekly vinblastine for every 3-week vincristine improved EFS using ANHL0131; unfortunately, outcomes in the traditional APO and vinblastine substitution arm were similar with increased toxicity in the vinblastine arm. EFS remained at near 75% with OS of approximately 85% at 3 years. Current COG studies are evaluating the safety and efficacy of brentuximab vedotin (a CD-30 antibody–drug conjugate) and crizotinib (an ALK-inhibitor used in *ALK*+ non-small cell lung cancer) in patients with newly diagnosed ALCL [124].

Follow-Up and Late Effects

The recommended follow-up of children treated for NHL includes a history, physical examination, and complete blood counts, with a decrease in frequency of evaluations over time. In many patients screening for recurrence will also include imaging such as contrast-enhanced CT or PET scans. Recent studies have questioned this practice in subtypes such as Burkitt lymphoma and DLBCL where relapse is rare and often not initially detected by imaging; surveillance imaging can lead to significant exposure to ionizing radiation and may not provide additional benefit [129]. The 5-year OS for pediatric NHL has increased from 45% in 1975 to >85% in 2016 [130]. From 1975 through 2010, there was an average annual percentage decrease of 4.1% in NHL mortality rates. Observed 15-year survival is approximately 76% [2]. With this improved survival, long-term effects of therapy have become more apparent and mitigation of late effects by risk adaptation of therapies, such as omission of radiation from most regimens, has become a focus of treatment.

The most common late effects noted in this diverse population include increased cardiovascular risk factors such as obesity and hypertension, decreased physical function, and impaired neurocognitive function; however, given the heterogeneity of disease and treatment, follow-up must be individualized. High-dose anthracycline is not uncommon as part of treatment and these patients remain at risk of acute and long-term cardiac toxicity requiring close monitoring with EKG and echocardiogram. Although cranial radiation has been eliminated from many regimens, the effects of CNS-directed chemotherapy such as high-dose methotrexate and cytarabine used in many regimens likely contribute to the high rates of neurocognitive impairment reported. Additionally, many survivors experience infertility and although pelvic irradiation is less common, the continued use of high-dose alkylating agents in current regimens remains a significant risk factor for gonadal failure and azoospermia. Finally, the rate of secondary neoplasms in this group was found to be six times that of the general population, though this appears to be a risk primarily in patients treated with radiation therapy. Follow-up of patients by a provider who is aware of the potential late effects of treatment and focused on early identification of chronic health conditions in this population is necessary [130].

Osteosarcoma

Definition

Osteosarcoma is the most common malignant tumor of bone in children. The tumor is of mesenchymal origin, most commonly occurring in the metaphysis of long bones.

Incidence

Primary malignant tumors of bone represent approximately 4% of cancers among children younger than 15 years and 7% of cancers among adolescents aged 15–19. More than half (56%) of these primary bone cancers among children and adolescents are osteosarcomas [2]. They are uncommon among children younger than 5 years. The incidence rate peaks at 15 years, as appearance of the tumor is associated with the adolescent growth spurt [106].

Etiology and Risk Factors

Osteosarcoma arises from primitive bone or osteoid-producing mesenchymal cells, typically found in long bones near the metaphysis [131].

Children with heritable retinoblastoma, due to *RB1* gene mutation, have a markedly increased risk of developing osteosarcoma, up to 500 times the general population. However, this may be slightly overestimated; historically treatment for retinoblastoma more frequently included radiation therapy, which greatly increases these patients' risk for development of osteosarcoma [132–134]. Patients with germline *TP53* mutations (Li–Fraumeni syndrome) are at increased risk for many cancers; the second most common malignancy in this patient population is osteosarcoma, with up to 12% of patients affected. Other populations at increased risk include patients with disorders due to germline mutations in the RecQ helicases, involved in maintenance of genomic stability by separation of complementary DNA strands for replication and repair. These disorders include Bloom syndrome, Rothmund–Thompson syndrome, and Werner syndrome [134].

As indicated by the high incidence of osteosarcoma in these familial syndromes, somatic mutations of the tumor suppressor genes *RB1* and *TP53* are the most common alterations documented. Multiple other genes have been implicated in the development or spread of osteosarcoma, such as the association of amplification of the proto-oncogene MYC in many osteosarcomas, particularly in metastatic disease [134,135].

Pathology

Most osteosarcomas arise in the medullary canal, spread centrifugally, break through the cortex and the periosteum, and develop a soft tissue mass. The notable exceptions, parosteal and periosteal osteosarcomas, both arise in the cortex. The majority of osteosarcomas are classic, further categorized as osteoblastic, fibroblastic, or chondroblastic. The other less frequently occurring types of osteosarcoma include telangiectatic, periosteal, and parosteal tumors. The last form is more common in adults, often presenting in the femur and associated with a more indolent biology. The periosteal type may occur at any age and progresses at a rate intermediate between that of the parosteal and that of the remaining types of osteosarcoma [131,136].

Presentation

Most children and adolescents with osteosarcoma present with pain, a swelling secondary to a soft tissue mass, or, occasionally, a pathologic fracture. The pain or swelling may be attributed erroneously to sports-related trauma, which in some studies occurred in nearly half of patients later diagnosed with osteosarcoma. Diagnostic delays are less frequent than in Ewing sarcoma and are typically less than 2 months from symptoms onset. More than 60% of osteosarcomas occur around the knee, including the distal femur, proximal tibia, or fibula; 10% occur in the proximal humerus; 10% occur in the proximal femur or pelvis; and the remainder occur in other bones such as the skull and mandible [137].

Diagnosis and Evaluation

The initial evaluation includes plain-film radiographs of the primary site, often revealing the sunburst sign, characteristic of horizontal bony spicules of new bone surrounding the tumor as it has broken through the cortex. Also typical on plain radiograph is the Codman triangle resulting from the periosteal new bone formation at the margin of the tumor. CT scans demonstrate cortical destruction, and MRI scans can best delineate the soft tissue component, the presence of skip metastases, and intramedullary spread [131,138,139].

The initial biopsy should be planned by a surgeon experienced in bone tumors and limb-sparing techniques. Depending on location and imaging features, an open biopsy or a core needle biopsy may be performed by the surgeon or an experienced interventional radiologist [140]. If a soft tissue mass is present, that tissue is subjected to biopsy, as it most likely contains viable tumor. Most tumors are of high histologic grade at diagnosis.

The most common site of osteosarcoma metastases is the lung, with other bones being the second most common site. One to two percent of patients present with skip metastases, synchronous regional bone metastases in the primary bone or transarticularly, which are important to identify prior to surgical management. Metastatic disease, most commonly in the lungs, followed by bones, will be found in up to 20% of patients at the time of initial diagnosis. Hence, a CT scan to seek pulmonary metastases and nuclear imaging for other bony lesions are indicated in the initial evaluations. Previously nuclear bone scan was used to evaluate for bony metastatic disease; however, PET-CT scan has been found to be more sensitive and accurate and is increasingly used [138,139,141]. Negative prognostic indicators include metastatic disease at diagnosis, axial skeletal location of primary disease, and poor histologic response to therapy [142].

Treatment

The current management of osteosarcoma includes neoadjuvant chemotherapy prior to complete surgical resection of the primary tumor and metastatic sites followed by adjuvant chemotherapy. Radiation therapy may be used when complete tumor resection is not possible [143].

Two prospective, randomized controlled trials in the 1980s demonstrated the improvement in survival with the use of adjuvant systemic chemotherapy in osteosarcoma over surgery alone [144,145]. While cisplatin and doxorubicin can result in cure rates in excess of 50% for patients with localized disease, studies have shown superior results with three-drug regimens, most notably with the addition of high doses of methotrexate; the current standard regimen is MAP (high-dose methotrexate, Adriamycin (doxorubicin) and cisplatin) [146]. Due to toxicity as well as cost and complexity of treatment associated with methotrexate and cisplatin, a study demonstrated similar outcome results with a three-drug regimen of carboplatin, doxorubicin, and ifosfamide [147]. A trial evaluating if interval-compressed chemotherapy improved outcomes similarly to that seen in Ewing sarcoma demonstrated no survival advantage [143].

The recently reported EURAMOS trial for patients with localized osteosarcoma used a MAP backbone and randomized patients with good response (<10% viable tumor after two MAP cycles) to the addition of interferon alpha 2b, and patients with poor response (≥10% viable tumor) to the addition of ifosfamide and etoposide. Neither intervention resulted in improved outcomes over the standard MAP; the 3-year EFS estimates for good responders were 75% and 77% for MAP and MAP plus interferon alpha 2b, respectively, and the 3-year EFS estimates for poor responders were 55% and 53% for MAP and MAP plus ifosfamide and etoposide, respectively [143,148,149].

While historically amputations were used for primary tumors in the extremities, today the use of limb-sparing procedures has become widespread. The use of endoprosthetics has not been shown to negatively impact survival when adequate surgical margins are achieved (≥1.5 cm). While surgery is key in the management of osteosarcoma, 80% of patients ultimately would succumb to metastatic disease if no systemic chemotherapy were administered [145,150,151].

Radiotherapy in the management of the primary tumor in osteosarcoma is reserved for unresectable lesions or, in some selected cases, for perioperative treatment or palliation of symptoms. The vast majority of osteosarcoma patients will undergo surgical resection; however, for those patients who have unresectable disease or in whom wide surgical margins cannot be achieved, high-dose ionizing radiation therapy adds to local control. Proton irradiation is also becoming more widely used for unresectable cases. This is especially useful in younger patients as it allows lower doses of radiation to nontarget tissue, minimizing side effects and risk of secondary malignancy [152].

Patients with close surgical margins (<1.5 cm) and a poor response to presurgical chemotherapy may be at higher risk for local recurrence. Multiple studies have demonstrated that patients with a good histologic response have better outcomes, with 5-year EFS above 75% in patients with ≥90% necrosis noted by histopathology following surgical tumor removal, compared to only 50–60% 5-year survival in patients with <90% necrosis [142,143,153]. There continue to be ongoing investigations of novel therapeutic targets that have demonstrated biologic activity though currently none has been shown to improve outcomes.

Follow-Up and Late Effects

The OS for nonmetastatic osteosarcoma in the modern chemotherapeutic era is 60–70%, while that for patients with metastatic disease remains poor with a 5-year OS of less than 40%. Patients with pulmonary metastases can have long-term survival if all overt metastatic occurrences can be resected surgically [142,154].

After completion of therapy, patients who remain disease free are followed closely for evidence of recurrence, typically with continued clinic visits and imaging. Imaging includes a minimum of radiographs of the primary site and interval chest CT due to the risk of metastatic lung disease [139]. The interval between visits increases over time and children should eventually be transitioned to a long-term follow-up clinic. This typically occurs after 5 years, as recurrence after this time is very rare. Additional clinical monitoring is needed for secondary neoplasms as a proportion of patients have an inherited cancer predisposition syndrome, such as Li–Fraumeni syndrome or heritable retinoblastoma [134,155].

Survivors of osteosarcoma treated with multiagent chemotherapy and surgery are at risk for late complications of therapy [144]. These sequelae include cardiotoxicity related to doxorubicin, which can occur either acutely or decades after completion of therapy. Recent studies suggest that dexrazoxane can be used to attempt to decrease cardiotoxicity of anthracyclines without negatively impacting tumor response or survival [156]. Other therapy-related toxicities include hearing loss due to ototoxicity from cisplatin, and renal tubular and glomerular damage from ifosfamide and cisplatin. Fertility also may be affected after the use of alkylating agents such as cyclophosphamide and ifosfamide [157]. Musculoskeletal complications of limb-sparing surgery, such as fracture of a prosthesis or leg-length discrepancy, also can occur.

Though much progress has been made in the treatment of osteosarcoma and in the understanding of this tumor's cancer biology, still more work lies ahead to improve the outcome and to diminish the late sequelae of this tumor.

Ewing Sarcoma

Definition

Ewing sarcoma, also referred to as the "Ewing sarcoma family of tumors," is the second most common bone cancer in children and adolescents. It is an aggressive neoplasm of the bone or soft tissues that arises from primitive neuroectodermal cells. The Ewing sarcoma family of tumors includes classic Ewing sarcoma of the bone and extraosseous Ewing sarcoma as well as older terms such as peripheral primitive neuroectodermal tumor or Askin tumor (Ewing sarcoma of the chest wall) [158–160].

Incidence

Ewing sarcoma is the second most common malignancy of bone. Primary malignant bone tumors represent approximately 4% of cancers among children younger than 15 years and 7% of cancers among adolescents aged 15–19 years. One-third of primary bone cancers among children and adolescents are Ewing sarcoma [2]. The majority of patients diagnosed with Ewing sarcoma are adolescents, with less than 25% diagnosed under the age of 10 years. Ewing sarcoma is much more common in White children than Black with incidence rates nearly 7.5 times higher in Whites. There is also lower incidence in Asian/Pacific Islanders and Hispanic children. In addition, there is a difference in incidence between genders with approximately 60% of cases occurring in males [2,160].

Etiology and Risk Factors

Ewing sarcoma is believed to arise from mesodermal and neural crest progenitor cells that have undergone malignant transformation. Ewing sarcoma is characterized by the presence of fusion oncogenes involving the *EWS* gene and commonly a member of the ETS family of transcription factor genes (such as *FLI1* or *ERG*) [161]. There are no known genetic predispositions to Ewing sarcoma, and unlike osteosarcoma, it is not seen as part of the Li–Fraumeni syndrome. There are no clear associations with environmental risk factors such as radiation exposure [162].

Classification

Ewing sarcoma is a member of the group of small round blue cell tumors. The tumor cells are uniform and undifferentiated. Despite their rapid clinical growth, these cells have a low mitotic index. By molecular analysis, Ewing sarcoma is characterized by chimeric fusion transcripts of the *EWS* gene, such as a translocation involving the EWSR1 gene, located on chromosome 22 band q12. A t(11;22)(q24;q12) translocation, forming the *EWS-FLI1* gene fusion, occurs in over 85% of cases [162,163].

Presentation

Patients with Ewing sarcoma typically present with tumor-related symptoms. These often include pain or a palpable mass. Less often patients will have associated symptoms of fever or weight loss. The time from symptom onset to diagnosis can be prolonged, typically between 2 and 5 months; however, duration of symptoms prior to diagnosis has not been shown to be associated with metastatic disease at diagnosis or with survival [164]. Most tumors occur in the lower extremities or pelvis. About 25% of Ewing sarcomas arise in soft tissue (extraosseous). In a recent study, patients who presented with extraosseous Ewing sarcoma were more likely to be female, older age, and have nonpelvic primary sites [165]. About one-quarter of patients have detectable metastatic disease at diagnosis with the lungs being the most common site, followed by bone and bone marrow [158].

Diagnosis and Evaluation

Initial workup includes imaging, preferably with MRI of the primary site, which is most helpful when performed prior to any biopsy to avoid changes in imaging from bleeding and edema. If Ewing sarcoma is suspected based on history, examination, and imaging, biopsy should be performed. These are often core biopsies with image guidance but can also be an open biopsy. Because these tumors can have significant necrosis, it is important to ensure adequate tissue is obtained, which may necessitate several core samples.

Pathologic confirmation demonstrates the small round tumor cells with the classic *EWS-FLI1* gene fusion characteristic of the t(11;22) translocation or an alternate EWS fusion product [163]. Staging workup includes PET-CT or bone scintigraphy for metastatic disease as well as a chest CT due to a high incidence of pulmonary metastatic disease relative to other sites. Additionally, bone marrow aspirates and biopsies are performed. In some trials, patients with metastatic disease are classified in risk groups as localized, pulmonary metastatic disease only versus multisite metastatic disease [158].

Treatment

Treatment of Ewing sarcoma involves a multidisciplinary approach that includes a combination of chemotherapy, radiation therapy, and surgery.

Local control of the primary site is typically performed after the first few cycles of chemotherapy. Surgical resection is the preferred modality for local control when it is felt a complete resection is possible. Surgical bone prosthetics such as endoprosthetics and allografts have helped increase the number of patients receiving surgical control while working to minimize late effects. Radiation is used as definitive local control only when a lesion is inoperable. Radiation is used postoperatively for incomplete resections; other indications for postoperative radiation therapy, such as poor tumor response to chemotherapy histologically, are controversial [166].

The addition of chemotherapy in the 1960s greatly improved the survival for patients with localized Ewing sarcoma. The current standard of care for patients with localized Ewing sarcoma in North America is interval-compressed VDC-IE (vincristine, doxorubicin, cyclophosphamide, alternated with ifosfamide and etoposide) and filgrastim (G-CSF) support for count recovery, with cycles given every 2 weeks instead of every 3 weeks. The most recent COG trial for localized Ewing sarcoma, AEWS0031, demonstrated improved EFS without increased toxicity for patients with localized Ewing sarcoma receiving interval-compressed therapy [167]. Multiple studies have looked at the addition of megadose chemotherapy and/or total body irradiation (TBI) with autologous stem cell rescue for metastatic or relapsed Ewing sarcoma without consistently demonstrating a survival benefit over standard-dose chemotherapy; however, some European studies suggest subsets of patients with primary multifocal disease who may benefit from these regimens [166,168].

Follow-Up and Late Effects

Patients with a complete response who have finished therapy are closely followed for evidence of recurrence, typically with careful history, examination, and imaging. The interval between visits will increase and children should be transitioned to long-term follow-up clinics after 2–5 years. Overall survival for patients with localized Ewing sarcoma is 65–75%; children with metastatic disease at diagnosis have poorer outcomes with overall survival of 20–35% [2,160,161].

There are many therapy-related toxicities and long-term effects. Close follow-up for survivors of Ewing sarcoma involves monitoring for secondary malignancies as well as other therapy-related toxicities. Secondary malignancies include treatment-related AML, typically associated with etoposide use, as well as radiation-associated osteosarcoma, soft tissue sarcomas, or breast cancer. Additionally, appropriate monitoring for late cardiac toxicity with periodic EKG and echocardiogram is important given many patients receive moderate- to high-dose anthracycline therapy. Infertility associated with high-dose alkylating therapy or radiation fields is also a common issue, making fertility preservation when possible an important part of the initial evaluation of these patients [169].

Neuroblastoma

Definition

Neuroblastoma (NBL) is an embryonal malignancy derived from primitive neural crest cells of the sympathetic nervous system and may arise at any point along the sympathetic ganglia chain or adrenal medulla. It is the most common extracranial solid tumor of childhood.

Incidence

Neuroblastoma accounts for approximately 7% of cancers among children younger than 15 years. Incidence rates are slightly higher for boys than for girls, and are substantially higher among non-Hispanic Whites in comparison with other racial and ethnic groups in the US [2]. However, due at least in part to differences in tumor biology, African American children are more likely to have high-risk neuroblastoma and more likely to have poor outcomes [170,171]. Neuroblastoma is the most common cancer diagnosed in the first year of life, representing half of all malignancies diagnosed in the first month of life and one-third of all malignancies diagnosed in the first year [172]. The incidence rates among boys and girls <20 years old are 8.5 and 7.6 cases per million individuals each year, with highest rates among infants <1 year of age [2,106].

Presentation

Neuroblastoma is unique among human cancers in its ability to undergo spontaneous differentiation and regression. Disseminated neuroblastoma can regress spontaneously in a subset of infants with metastatic disease involving the liver, skin, and limited infiltration of the bone marrow (known as stage 4S disease) [173]. Furthermore, residual microscopic disease after a resected localized neuroblastoma rarely results in disease recurrence. This interesting natural history is one reason that screening for neuroblastoma is not recommended, in addition to a lack of reduction in overall mortality demonstrated in prior screening studies [174,175]. A family history is present in approximately 1–2% of new neuroblastoma cases, and a genetic predisposition to neuroblastoma has been associated with germline mutations of *ALK* as well as germline deletions at the 1p36 or 11q14-23 locus [176–178]. No environmental risk factors have consistently been associated with increased risk of developing neuroblastoma.

Neuroblastoma can occur in the abdomen or thorax and patients may present with an abdominal or flank mass (the most common presentation), with respiratory symptoms from a thoracic primary tumor, with Horner syndrome from a cervicothoracic primary lesion, or with bladder symptoms resulting from a pelvic primary tumor. Children with advanced disease involving the bone marrow may present with pallor or easy bruising or can experience bone pain, fever, and failure to thrive. When neuroblastoma originates in the stellate ganglion Horner syndrome (ptosis, miosis, and anhidrosis) can occur, and neuroblastoma originating in paraspinal ganglia can invade neural foramina and compress the spinal cord, requiring immediate treatment in order to avoid paralysis [179]. Metastases to the orbit may result in proptosis or periorbital ecchymosis ("raccoon eyes"), and metastases to subcutaneous tissue may result in a "blueberry rash." A syndrome combining opsoclonus (rapid multidirectional eye movements) and myoclonus (truncal ataxia) occurs in approximately 5% of patients, generally with early-stage neuroblastoma [180]. The opsoclonus/myoclonus syndrome is thought to be caused by an as yet incompletely understood immunologic mechanism; corticosteroid treatment, plasmapheresis, and intravenous immunoglobulin (IVIG) have shown to be effective in managing this syndrome, although improvement may only be partial [181–183].

Diagnosis and Evaluation

The diagnostic evaluation of patients in whom neuroblastoma is suspected often begins with an investigation of the primary tumor. An abdominal ultrasound may demonstrate a mass if the primary tumor is abdominal, and plain-film radiography may show calcifications. The diagnosis of neuroblastoma is established if an unequivocal pathologic diagnosis is made from tumor tissue or if the bone marrow contains unequivocal tumor cells and the urine contains increased catecholamine metabolites (vanillylmandelic acid (VMA) or homovanillic acid (HVA) levels greater than 3 standard deviations above the mean per milligram of creatinine for age) [184]. Neuroblastoma is one of several small round blue cell tumors of childhood; thus, if neuronal differentiation is not clearly present on conventional hematoxylin–eosin staining, additional immunohistochemical staining may be performed and typically will be positive for chromogranin A, neuron-specific enolase (NSE), and synaptophysin. Monoclonal antibodies against neural-specific antigens such as GD2 increase detection sensitivity, and reverse transcriptase polymerase chain reaction (RT-PCR) of neuroblastoma-specific markers such as GD2 synthase further increase sensitivity, although the clinical utility and prognostic significance of this information is still being investigated.

More extensive imaging of the primary tumor either by CT scan or MRI is performed, with preference for MRI if the primary lesion is paraspinal with potential for extension into the spinal canal. Neuroblastoma is capable of metastasizing hematogenously or via the lymphatic system, and the majority of patients present with regional or distant spread at diagnosis. Either CT or MRI may also be utilized to evaluate for metastatic disease to solid organs such as the liver, and bilateral bone marrow aspirates and biopsies are performed as part of the assessment for metastatic disease. An MIBG (meta-iodobenzylguanidine) scan is performed, usually with the ^{123}I isotope; MIBG avidity is present in >90% of neuroblastomas but when a neuroblastoma is not MIBG avid, a bone scan (with ^{99}Tc) or FDG-PET should be performed [185,186].

Tumor Biology

Evaluation of the neuroblastoma tumor tissue by pediatric pathologists is critical for assigning risk group and treatment category. The Shimada International Neuroblastoma Pathology Classification (INPC) defines tumors as "favorable" or "unfavorable" histology on the basis of the stroma (stroma-rich vs stroma-poor, according to the presence or absence of schwannian spindle cell stroma), the extent of tumor differentiation, and the mitotic–karyorrhectic index (MKI) [187,188]. In addition to histological classification, the assessment of biological markers has become an important component of the workup and a critical determinant in guiding therapy, particularly *MYCN* amplification and DNA ploidy.

Amplification of the *MYCN* oncogene, defined as >10 copies per diploid genome, is found in approximately 25% of primary tumors and is strongly correlated with advanced disease [189–191]. *MYCN* amplification has been associated in several studies with rapid tumor progression and poor clinical outcome independent of patient age or stage [189,190,192–196]. In regard to DNA ploidy, neuroblastomas are classified as either diploid (DNA index of 1) or hyperdiploid (DNA index >1), with hyperdiploidy generally known to be associated with more favorable biology. The majority of tumors have karyotypes in the diploid range, but many are hyperdiploid or near-triploid. Often, the hyperdiploid and near-triploid tumors in infants have increased chromosomal numbers without any identifiable structural rearrangements and these patients have a relatively favorable prognosis. Frequently, patients with near-diploid tumors and older patients with hyperdiploid tumors do have structural rearrangements that predict a more aggressive course [197–201].

Many biological characteristics of neuroblastoma tumors are not currently used in determining therapy; however, as clinical research matures, these characteristics may be found useful as therapeutic targets or as clinically important prognostic factors. Segmental chromosomal abnormalities such as the deletion of chromosome 1p or 11q, and the gain of 17q, have been associated with a poor prognosis [202]. However, the utility of assessing these abnormalities is as yet unclear given that more conventional prognostic indicators such as age and stage appear to be more significant [203]. The *ALK* gene, thought to be important in the development of the nervous system, has been noted to be mutated in approximately 10% of patients with neuroblastoma, and correlates with poorer outcomes in intermediate- and high-risk neuroblastoma [204]. Finally, the *ATRX* gene is more commonly mutated in adolescents and young adults with neuroblastoma, who typically have a more indolent presentation than infants and younger children [205].

Staging

Prior to the development of the classic International Neuroblastoma Staging System (INSS) in 1987, three major staging systems had been used worldwide. Although these various systems provided similar results in distinguishing low-stage patients from high-stage patients, they embodied substantial differences that precluded comparisons. In addition to a new, mutually accepted staging system, the INSS established criteria for the diagnosis of neuroblastoma and strict definitions of response [184]. The staging system recommended for neuroblastoma is now in the process of likely transitioning from the INSS (Table 47.4), a primarily surgical-based classification [184,206], to the International Neuroblastoma Risk Group (INRG) staging system, a primarily imaging-based classification [207]. Image-defined risk factors in the INRG staging system vary by the anatomic site of the primary tumor but generally include tumor encasement of major vessels or nerves and extension into bone or adjacent organs.

Table 47.4 International Neuroblastoma Staging System. Adapted from Brodeur 1988 [184].

Stage	Definition
1	Localized tumor with complete gross excision, with or without microscopic residual disease; representative ipsilateral lymph nodes negative for tumor microscopically (lymph nodes adherent to and removed with primary possibly positive)
2A	Localized tumor with incomplete gross excision; representative ipsilateral nonadherent lymph nodes negative for tumor microscopically
2B	Localized tumor with or without complete gross excision, with ipsilateral nonadherent lymph nodes positive for tumor; enlarged contralateral lymph nodes negative microscopically
3	Unresectable unilateral tumor infiltrating across the midline, with or without regional lymph node involvement; or localized unilateral tumor with contralateral regional lymph node involvement; or midline tumor with bilateral extension by infiltration (unresectable) or by lymph node involvement
4	Any primary tumor with dissemination to distant lymph nodes, bone, bone marrow, liver, skin, other organs (except as defined for stage 4S)
4S	Limited to infants younger than 1 year and localized primary tumor (as defined for stage 1, 2A, or 2B) with dissemination limited to skin, liver, or bone marrow (or all). Bone marrow involvement must be 10% of total nucleated cells identified as malignant on bone marrow biopsy or aspirate; more extensive bone marrow involvement stage 4

In addition to tumor stage, prognostic factors for neuroblastoma include patient age, as well as primary tumor site, tumor histopathologic features, tumor biologic features such as amplification of the *MYCN* oncogene and DNA index (ploidy), and tumor response to treatment [2]. Primary adrenal tumors are more likely to be associated with unfavorable prognostic features, and older age is known to be a particularly poor prognostic indicator in high-risk neuroblastoma especially in adolescents and young adults, regardless of stage [208,209]. The INRG classification system uses the most clinically relevant and statistically significant factors, including INRG stage, patient age, tumor histology and grade of differentiation, tumor ploidy, *MYCN* and 11q status [196].

Treatment

Neuroblastoma can be divided into genetically distinct groups on the basis of biological properties. When these biological characteristics are combined with clinical properties, patients can be stratified into risk groups, and therapy can be tailored for patients on the basis of these clinical and biological groupings. The treatment modalities employed in the management of neuroblastoma include surgery, chemotherapy, radiotherapy, antibody therapy, biological differentiating agents, and at times observation alone. Surgery may be needed to establish the diagnosis, obtain sufficient tissue for biological studies, and classify pathologic and molecular characteristics of a tumor, as well as to excise a primary tumor when feasible.

Treatment is determined by risk group; age, stage, *MYCN* status, DNA ploidy, and Shimada pathologic classification are used to classify patients into low-, intermediate-, and high-risk strata, but the potential treatment categories and specific risk factors used for treatment determination are actively evolving.

Low-risk patients generally include patients with lowstage tumors (INSS stage 1 or 2) without *MYCN* amplification as well as specific patients with stage 4S disease (without *MYCN* amplification, <1 year of age, favorable histology, and DNA ploidy >1). Treatment is most commonly surgical resection alone, with excellent outcomes (OS 97% in a recent COG study) [210]. A complete or even good partial resection of a primary tumor is sufficient therapy and is the treatment of choice in favorable patients. Second-look surgery or postinduction chemotherapy is used in situations in which an initial tumor is deemed unresectable but can be rendered resectable with chemotherapy. Neuroblastoma is also sensitive to ionizing irradiation, and very low-dose radiotherapy (3–6 Gy in 3–4 fractions) has been given to neonates with stage IVS disease and respiratory compromise secondary to massive hepatomegaly [211]. In infants <6 months with small adrenal tumors (<5 cm in diameter) thought most likely to be neuroblastoma, close observation without biopsy or surgery is currently being recommended. In a prospective study, this expectant approach resulted in 3-year EFS and OS of 97.7% and 100%, respectively, and avoidance of surgery in 81% of the infants [212].

Intermediate-risk patients are those under 1 year of age with non-*MYCN* amplified stage III tumors or patients over 1 year with favorable Shimada, non-*MYCN* amplified stage III tumors. Infants with non-*MYCN* amplified disease who are under 1 year of age with stage IVS disease or under 18 months with stage IV disease are also considered intermediate risk [213]. Intermediate-risk patients have been successfully treated with surgery and chemotherapy. Chemotherapy may be given before surgical resection, and patients whose tumors have unfavorable biology receive twice as many cycles of chemotherapy as those with favorable biology (8 compared to 4 cycles). Neuroblastomas respond to several chemotherapeutic agents, including doxorubicin, cisplatin, melphalan, cyclophosphamide, etoposide (VP-16), and teniposide (VM-26). Combination chemotherapy has been used to exploit differences in mechanism of action and toxicities in order to avoid development of drug resistance. However, the OS for intermediate-risk patients was approximately 96% in a COG trial published in 2010 that reduced chemotherapy dose and duration compared to earlier trials; thus future protocols aim to reduce chemotherapy even more while maintaining the excellent outcomes [214].

Children with *MYCN* amplified tumors (other than the very unusual case of a patient with a stage 1 amplified tumor or an infant with stage II favorable Shimada) are considered high risk, in addition to patients >1 year of age with stage III non-*MYCN* amplified disease and patients >18 months of age with stage IV disease. Children with high-risk neuroblastoma require more intensive treatment, typically in the form of cisplatin-based induction chemotherapy, surgical resection, and consolidation therapy with myeloablation and autologous stem cell rescue followed by focal radiotherapy delivered to the primary tumor bed as well as to residual metastatic sites. Post-consolidation therapy is given to treat potential minimal residual disease and includes immunotherapy with monoclonal antibodies against GD2, and differentiating therapy with cis-retinoic acid [215,216]. Using this approach, the 2-year EFS and OS for high-risk patients that respond to induction therapy and can successfully complete treatment have shown to be 66% and 86%, respectively [216].

Follow-Up and Late Effects

In general, improved outcomes for neuroblastoma have required high-dose chemotherapy, increasing the risk of late effects. The use of platinum-based chemotherapy increases the risk of severe sensorineural hearing loss, which is particularly notable among children treated for high-risk neuroblastoma [217,218]. This hearing loss is typically permanent and may ultimately contribute to learning difficulties or impaired social interactions in the future. The use of alkylating agents such as cyclophosphamide, particularly at high cumulative doses, is associated with ovarian failure as well as second malignant neoplasms (SMNs) [219]. Current high-risk neuroblastoma protocols also use topoisomerase II inhibitors which are associated with an increased risk of treatment-related myelodysplasia and leukemia [220].

A review of outcomes from nearly 1,000 neuroblastoma survivors diagnosed between 1970 and 1986 in the US and Canada was published in 2009 and found that the most common cause of late mortality (>5 years after diagnosis) was disease recurrence, followed by SMNs and pulmonary and cardiac complications [221]. This study also described that neuroblastoma survivors were eight times more likely to have chronic health conditions as compared to a sibling cohort, with nearly a third developing neurologic issues such as extremity weakness, abnormal sensation, or difficulties with balance [222]. While the current standard of care in the US does not include TBI in preparatory regimens for children requiring autologous stem cell transplantation, TBI was utilized in the past and was associated with increased risk of cataracts, thyroid insufficiency, and growth delays in addition to SMNs [222]. Additional late effects experienced by children with high-risk neuroblastoma who underwent autologous SCT include renal impairment and musculoskeletal complications such as osteochondromas, kyphoscoliosis, and fractures [223]. Thus, as advances continue to be made for the effective treatment of high-risk neuroblastoma, it will be important to closely follow patients after treatment completion so that these late effects are appropriately addressed, in addition to working towards treatment regimens that may be able to minimize the potential for late effects.

Wilms Tumor

Definition

Wilms tumor (WT), also known as nephroblastoma, is the most common primary malignant renal tumor of children. Wilms tumor can arise from either the renal medulla or cortex, and is typically well delineated from the renal parenchyma, often compressing the parenchyma surrounding it [224]. Other primary renal tumors that can affect children include clear cell sarcoma of the kidney, congenital mesoblastic nephroma (the most common renal tumor between 0 and 1 month of age), malignant rhabdoid tumor of the kidney, primary neuroectodermal tumor (PNET) of the kidney, and renal carcinomas such as renal cell carcinoma (the most common renal tumor among individuals ≥15 years) and renal medullary carcinoma [225].

Incidence

Wilms tumor accounts for almost 5% of cancers in children younger than 15 years. Among children and adolescents younger than 20 years in the US, annual incidence rates are 5.3 per million boys and 6.3 per million girls [1,2,226]. Relative to Whites, incidence rates are highest among Blacks and lower among other racial and ethnic groups in the US [2]. Most cases of Wilms tumor are diagnosed in children less than 5 years old; median age at diagnosis for unilateral cases is 41.5 months (~3.5 years) in boys and 46.9 months (~3.9 years) in girls [227]. Approximately 5% of Wilms tumor cases are bilateral and these cases typically present earlier in life, at a median age of 29.5 months (~2.5 years) and 32.6 months (~2.7 years) for boys and girls, respectively [227].

Etiology and Risk Factors

The study of Wilms tumor has played an important role in revealing mechanisms of tumor development, with the discovery of the *WT1* tumor suppressor gene at 11p13 contributing to Knudson's two-hit hypothesis for tumor formation [228]. In contrast to effects of other tumor suppressor genes such as *RB1*, the consequences of *WT1* gene deletion are restricted to those tissues that normally express the gene. *WT1* expression may be required for appropriate renal tissue differentiation and morphogenesis, as these cells in the kidney normally express the *WT1* gene [229,230].

There are multiple additional genes that have been implicated in the etiology of Wilms tumor including *WT2* (IGF2 locus of 11p15), β-catenin (*CTNNB1*), *WTX*, and *TP53*, although many cases of Wilms tumor have unclear genetic origins [231]. WT2 functions in the insulin-like growth factor pathway, β-catenin and WTX function in the Wnt signaling pathway, and TP53 functions as a tumor suppressor gene. There are two key somatic defects at 11p15: *IGF2* loss of imprinting (also known as the H19 epimutation) and paternal uniparental disomy [231]. These 11p15 defects are the most common abnormalities identified thus far in Wilms tumor, occurring in 50–75% of tumors [231,232]. However, the precise interactions and relative contributions of these various genetic abnormalities to the development of Wilms tumor are being actively studied.

There are several recognized syndromes associated with an increased risk of Wilms tumor, most of which are associated with genetic alterations of the aforementioned genes [233,234]. Table 47.5 describes the genetic etiology and clinical manifestations of these syndromes in further detail.

In addition to the syndromes listed in Table 47.5, Li–Fraumeni syndrome, a hereditary cancer predisposition syndrome associated with *TP53* mutations, Perlman syndrome, Sotos syndrome, and Bloom syndrome also increase the risk for development of Wilms tumor [233]. Several chromosomal abnormalities have also been reported with Wilms tumor, including the interstitial deletion of chromosome 11 at band p13, trisomy 13, and trisomy 18 [233]. Finally, some Wilms tumor cases have been found within families and a portion are attributable to Wilms tumor predisposition genes with variable penetrance, *FWT1* and *FWT2* [233,235].

Table 47.5 Syndromes associated with an increased risk of Wilms tumor.

Syndrome	Genetic origin	Clinical manifestations
Beckwith–Wiedemann syndrome	Loss of heterozygosity (LOH) at 11p15, associated with genetic or epigenetic alterations in the IGF2 locus	Wilms tumor susceptibility, macrosomia, macroglossia, neonatal hypoglycemia, organomegaly, anterior abdominal wall defects (umbilical hernias, omphaloceles, etc.), and hemihypertrophy
Denys–Drash syndrome	Congenital point mutations in *WT1*	Wilms tumor susceptibility, genitourinary abnormalities in males (highly variable in severity but can exhibit pseudohermaphroditism), renal disease (classically a nephropathy from mesangial sclerosis, may present with hypertension or nephrotic syndrome, typically progressing to renal failure)
WAGR syndrome	Heterozygous constitutional deletions at 11p13 that encompass *WT1* and the contiguous *PAX6* gene (which when absent leads to aniridia)	*W*ilms tumor, *a*niridia, *g*enitourinary anomalies (ambiguous external genitalia and cryptorchidism in males), and mental *r*etardation
Frasier syndrome	Congenital splice-site mutation in *WT1*	Wilms tumor susceptibility, progressive glomerulopathy (typically focal segmental glomerulosclerosis which progresses to renal failure), genitourinary abnormalities (typically severe/male pseudohermaphroditism), increased risk of gonadoblastomas
Simpson–Golabi–Behmel syndrome	Mutations or deletions of the *GPC3* gene at Xq26. *GPC3* is a cell surface proteoglycan that interacts with growth factors and the Wnt pathway	Wilms tumor susceptibility, coarse facial features, cardiac and skeletal abnormalities, intellectual impairment, accessory nipples

While many syndromes are associated with Wilms tumor susceptibility, surveillance is generally recommended for children who are at >5% risk of developing a Wilms tumor and following review by a geneticist. Typically screening is via abdominal ultrasound every 3 months beginning at diagnosis of the syndrome and continuing until the child is 5–8 years old [236,237].

Classification

Wilms tumor is thought to be derived from primitive metanephric blastemic cells. Although most Wilms tumors are single tumors, 7% are multifocal in one kidney and 5% are bilateral [238]. Bilateral involvement is associated with an increased risk of an underlying genetic abnormality and should raise suspicion for an underlying syndrome. Precursor lesions to Wilms tumor, nephrogenic rests, are found in the normal kidney of patients with Wilms tumor, and when there is diffuse or multifocal involvement of the kidneys with nephrogenic rests this is known as "nephroblastomatosis" [239].

Classic Wilms tumor is triphasic, composed of the three cell types that comprise embryonic renal tissue: blastemic, stromal (mesenchymal), and epithelial. The histology is classified as favorable, indicating well-differentiated components, and unfavorable. Unfavorable histology Wilms tumors are defined by the presence of anaplasia, containing cells with giant polypoid nuclei, hyperchromasia, irregular mitotic figures, and poor differentiation, and have an adverse prognosis in comparison to those with favorable histology [240,241]. Anaplastic Wilms tumor is associated with a high rate of *TP53* mutations; focal anaplasia is defined by the confinement of the anaplasia strictly to a single focus within the tumor while tumors with more extensive anaplasia are considered to be diffusely anaplastic [242]. In general, patients with focal anaplasia have a better prognosis than those with diffuse anaplasia [240]. Within classic favorable histology Wilms tumor, evidence has emerged demonstrating that loss of heterozygosity for chromosome 1p or 16q in tumor tissue is associated with a poorer prognosis [243].

Two separate renal tumors were previously grouped with Wilms tumor in initial studies but are now considered distinct histopathologic entities, associated with higher rates of relapse and death with different patterns of metastasis than classic Wilms tumor. These renal tumors are clear cell sarcoma of the kidney and malignant rhabdoid tumor of the kidney. Clear cell sarcoma tends to invade the surrounding kidney tissue and is associated with a higher rate of bone metastases. The cell of origin of rhabdoid tumors remains elusive but this tumor is known to be aggressive and associated with separate rhabdoid tumors of the brain [244,245]. Finally, congenital mesoblastic nephroma is a tumor of infancy separate from Wilms tumor, related to infantile fibrosarcoma, and curable by nephrectomy [246].

Presentation, Diagnosis, and Evaluation

Wilms tumor most often presents as an abdominal mass in a relatively well-appearing child. Abdominal pain, microscopic or gross hematuria, fever, and hypertension may occur, and more rarely bleeding within the tumor can result in a child presenting with a quickly enlarging abdominal mass associated with pallor, anemia, fatigue, and pain. The presence of genitourinary anomalies or other associated characteristics, such as aniridia, macroglossia, or hemihypertrophy, should be noted as they can suggest certain genetic syndromes. Often, obtaining abdominal ultrasonography is the first and easiest step, and this radiographic study will differentiate a solid from a cystic mass and frequently can identify the origin of any mass present. Abdominal ultrasonography also can demonstrate the patency of the inferior vena cava (IVC), an important finding given that Wilms tumor is associated with venous thrombosis that may extend into the IVC and in limited cases to the heart [247]. A complete blood count, test of liver and renal functions, determination of serum calcium levels, and urinalysis should be performed. An MRI or CT scan of the abdomen is obtained to evaluate the mass further and to assess the presence of lymph nodes and extension of the tumor into other structures, including the liver or spleen. CT of the chest is required to identify pulmonary metastases (the most common site of metastasis); for equivocal lesions, a biopsy may be indicated.

Diagnosis of the primary tumor is based on histology, and in the US surgical removal of the involved kidney with tumor intact is preferred at diagnosis when feasible. However, the International Society of Paediatric Oncology (SIOP) treatment protocols typically recommend chemotherapy without initial biopsy or nephrectomy unless there is evidence of tumor rupture, and histology is evaluated at the future nephrectomy. Staging for Wilms tumor also varies by whether National Wilms Tumor Study Group (NWTS, now the Renal Tumor Committee of the Children's Oncology Group (COG)) protocols or SIOP protocols are used; the COG staging for Wilms tumor is described in Table 47.6 [248].

A bone scan should be obtained for patients with clear cell sarcoma and for all patients who have Wilms tumor with pulmonary or hepatic metastases or bony symptoms. MRI of the brain is indicated for children with clear cell sarcoma or malignant rhabdoid tumors, as both have a propensity to develop metastases to the brain.

Table 47.6 Children's Oncology Group Wilms Tumor Staging System. Adapted from Perlman 2005 [248].

Stage	Definition
I	Tumor limited to the kidney, completely excised; renal capsule with an intact outer surface; tumor not ruptured or sampled for biopsy prior to removal (fine-needle aspiration excluded); vessels of renal sinus not involved; no evidence of tumor at or beyond the margins of resection
II	Tumor extended beyond kidney but completely excised; regional extension (e.g., penetration of renal capsule or extensive invasion of renal sinus); blood vessels outside renal parenchyma, including vessels of renal sinus, with possible tumor; no evidence of tumor at or beyond the margins of resection
III	Residual nonhematogenous tumor present, confined to the abdomen; any of the following: biopsy performed prior to resection, including fine-needle aspiration; spillage before or during surgery confined to the flank and not involving the peritoneal surface; lymph nodes within the abdomen or pelvis involved by tumor; intrathoracic or other extra-abdominal lymph nodes considered stage IV; tumor penetrating peritoneal surface tumor; implants found on peritoneal surface; gross or microscopic tumor remaining postoperatively; tumor not completely resectable because of local infiltration into vital structures; or tumor spillage not confined to the flank before or during surgery
IV	Hematogenous metastases (lung, liver, bone, brain, etc.) or lymph node metastases outside the abdominopelvic region
V	Bilateral renal involvement present at diagnosis; each side staged individually

Treatment and Outcomes

The NWTS Group, now the Renal Tumor Committee of COG, performed a series of prospective randomized trials with multifactorial design [249]. These trials have included thousands of children with Wilms tumor and have progressively attempted to maintain excellent cure rates while reducing therapy intensity or duration based on surgical stage and histopathologic evaluation. In general, in North America surgery is performed immediately following diagnosis unless the tumor is invading surrounding organs, has a tumor thrombus associated that extends beyond the hepatic veins, or presents as bilateral disease or with pulmonary metastases associated with significant respiratory compromise. During surgery lymph nodes are sampled in order to accurately stage, and every effort is made to remove the tumor without breaking the capsule, as intraoperative spillage of tumor increases the risk of tumor recurrence [250].

Postoperative therapy for children with favorable histology is outlined below:

- Stage I and II favorable histology: vincristine and dactinomycin; no abdominal irradiation.
- Stage III and IV favorable histology: vincristine, dactinomycin, and doxorubicin; abdominal irradiation for an abdominal tumor at stage III; bilateral whole lung irradiation for patients with pulmonary metastases unless lung metastases only are present and metastases have completely responded to induction chemotherapy; irradiation to other sites of metastases such as liver or bone.

If necessary, radiation therapy to the flank or abdomen is administered within 14 days of surgery in COG protocols, and classically patients with metastatic disease to the lungs received whole lung radiation at this time as well, although guidelines for the management of pulmonary metastatic disease are evolving [251]. Children with unfavorable histology Wilms tumor require more intensive treatment as well as abdominal radiotherapy. Agents such as doxorubicin, cyclophosphamide, and etoposide are used for those with higher than stage I disease with unfavorable histology. Clear cell sarcoma of the kidney and rhabdoid tumor of the kidney are also treated with more aggressive chemotherapy as well as radiotherapy.

The outcome for children with favorable histology Wilms tumor is excellent; children with Wilms tumor have a 5-year OS of 92% in the US [2]. However, children with high-risk renal tumors (non-favorable Wilms tumor and most other types of renal tumors in children) have a worse outcome, which has been the impetus for intensification of treatment for these children [252].

Follow-Up and Late Effects

Given the excellent overall prognosis for Wilms tumor, limiting the late effects of treatment is an important consideration for the development of new protocols in addition to the monitoring of previously treated patients.

Cardiotoxicity is a known complication of anthracycline chemotherapy, particularly doxorubicin. Congestive heart failure has been found to occur in approximately 4.4% of patients initially treated with doxorubicin for Wilms tumor at 20 years post diagnosis, with increased risk in females and patients who received lung or left abdominal radiation [253]. SMNs were noted in 1.6% of Wilms tumor survivors treated in NWTS Group protocols over a 15-year period, and included sarcomas, carcinomas, leukemias, lymphomas, and brain tumors [254]. In this study abdominal radiation increased risk of SMNs and was potentiated by receiving doxorubicin. Radiation treatment in growing children also results in the potential for musculoskeletal effects such as kyphosis, scoliosis, and an overall decrease in adult height. The relative risk of these effects depends on the total dose, fractionation, and field of radiation therapy delivered [255]. Finally, radiation therapy to the abdomen has been associated with infertility, particularly if the radiation field includes the lower abdomen, as well as premature birth and fetal growth restriction [255,256].

Renal dysfunction following Wilms tumor treatment is a concern, but the cumulative incidence of end-stage renal disease (ESRD) 20 years following diagnosis of unilateral nonsyndromic Wilms tumor is very low at 0.6% [257]. In the setting of bilateral Wilms tumor, WAGR syndrome, Denys–Drash syndrome, or other genitourinary anomalies (hypospadias or cryptorchidism) the risk is much higher, highlighting the importance of nephron-sparing surgery in bilateral disease, as well as minimizing nephrotoxic chemotherapy and radiation to the remaining kidney if possible [255,257].

Rhabdomyosarcoma

Definition

The rhabdomyosarcoma (RMS) cell of origin is a mesenchymal cell, which normally matures into skeletal muscle, smooth muscle, fat, fibrous tissue, bone, or cartilage. Rhabdomyosarcomas are believed to develop from those mesenchymal cells that were committed to the skeletal muscle lineage, although these tumors can display evidence of multilineage phenotype.

Incidence

The most common malignant tumor of soft tissues in children is rhabdomyosarcoma, which comprises approximately 3% of all cancers among children in the US younger than 15 years [1]. The incidence rate is highest among children less than 5 years old. Among children and adolescents in the US younger than 20 years, incidence rates for boys and girls are 5.4 and 4.2 cases per million individuals per year, respectively. Among racial and ethnic groups in the US, rhabdomyosarcoma incidence rates are highest in African Americans and lowest in Asian Americans and Pacific Islanders [2].

Etiology and Risk Factors

Rhabdomyosarcoma has been associated with familial cancer syndromes and other predisposing conditions, such as Li–Fraumeni, Beckwith–Wiedemann, neurofibromatosis type I, *DICER-1*, Costello, and Noonan syndromes [258–263].

Pathology

Rhabdomyosarcomas are identified on the basis of characteristic light-microscopical, immunohistochemical, electron-microscopical, and molecular genetic features. These tumors are composed of small, round, blue cells that often exhibit cross-striations under the light microscope. The immunohistochemical features include positive staining for the muscle proteins actin and myosin and for desmin, myoglobin, MyoD, and Z-band protein. The two major variants of rhabdomyosarcoma are the embryonal and alveolar subtypes, which have characteristic appearances under the light microscope and distinguishing molecular markers. The chromosomal translocations characteristic of the alveolar subtype are t(2;13)(q35;q14) and t(1;13)(p36;q14), which result in the fusion of genes *PAX3* and *PAX7*, respectively, with *FOXO1* and that can be identified using RT-PCR [264]. This tool provides confirmatory evidence of the alveolar subtype. The loss of heterozygosity of chromosome 11p15 can be used to identify the embryonal subtype [265]. Approximately 20% of alveolar rhabdomyosarcomas lack the defining *PAX-FOX01* translocation; the clinical behavior and prognosis for these patients is similar to cases presenting with the embryonal subtype [266].

Diagnosis and Evaluation

Rhabdomyosarcoma can originate from many sites. The most frequent region of origin is the head and neck (35%); the most common site within the head and neck is the orbit [267]. Other head and neck sites are the parameninges, which include the nasopharynx, paranasal sinuses, middle ear, mastoid, and pterygoid-infratemporal fossa; the scalp; the buccal mucosa; the oropharynx; the larynx; and the neck [268]. Tumors in the orbit present with proptosis and, occasionally, with ophthalmoplegia or periorbital edema. Tumors in nonorbital parameningeal sites produce nasal or sinus obstruction, sinusitis, epistaxis, and aural obstruction. Cranial nerve palsies can occur with invasion of the base of the skull and meningeal extension. The histology of rhabdomyosarcoma of the head and neck is usually embryonal. Regional nodal involvement from rhabdomyosarcoma arising in the head and neck is infrequent, although proper clinical and radiological exploration of the cervical nodal chains is always recommended.

The second most frequent site for rhabdomyosarcoma is the genitourinary tract, accounting for more than 20% of all cases [267]. Tumors can arise in the bladder and prostate, the paratesticular area, the vagina, and the uterus. Bladder tumors grow intraluminally and can produce urinary obstruction and hematuria. Often, children with genitourinary rhabdomyosarcoma present with a pelvic mass, a mass in the scrotum in patients with paratesticular tumors, or grapelike masses in the vagina (botryoid tumors), which can break off and appear in the diaper. Abdominal masses may be present in patients with retroperitoneal primary lesions or owing to the involvement of para-aortic nodes. Nodal involvement is present in 26% of cases arising in the paratesticular area and in 20–40% of cases in such other genitourinary sites as the bladder and prostate. The majority of rhabdomyosarcomas in the genitourinary tract are of the embryonal subtype [267].

Most often, rhabdomyosarcoma of the extremity leads to a mass or swelling of the affected limb. The mass may be painful, but the presence of pain varies. Tumors arising in the extremity represent 20% of rhabdomyosarcomas. Regional nodal involvement is common (approximately 12%), particularly if the histology of the tumor is alveolar, which is the more likely subtype in extremity tumors. Rhabdomyosarcoma can occur in the trunk, perineal–perianal region, biliary tract, heart, breast, and ovary. In some cases, a primary site cannot be determined [267].

The most common metastatic sites of rhabdomyosarcoma are the lung, bone marrow, bones, liver, and brain. In addition, the regional nodes can be targets of tumor spread, the frequency of which varies by site and histology.

Evaluation and Staging

Evaluation of children with rhabdomyosarcoma requires participation by pathologists, radiologists, surgeons, pediatric oncologists, and irradiation oncologists. The diagnostic studies include: complete blood count; liver function tests; CT scanning and MRI of the primary tumor; CT scanning of the lungs and of the abdomen and pelvis for primaries arising in these sites; bone scan; and bone marrow aspirates and biopsies. Biopsy is required for all patients for whom future resection is planned. Immediate surgical excision is recommended only if it will not cause significant functional morbidity. Lymph node biopsy is performed for clinically enlarged or suspicious nodes. The site of the primary tumor influences the likelihood of nodal disease and will be a determining factor also in surgical management. Even in the absence of enlarged lymph nodes, a sentinel node biopsy is usually recommended for primaries of the extremities, particularly those of alveolar histology.

The staging of rhabdomyosarcoma is critical in determining appropriate treatment and the prognosis. Patients with localized tumors that can be resected completely have a better prognosis than do those with regional or distant disease. The clinical grouping system (Table 47.7) was developed by the Intergroup Rhabdomyosarcoma Study (IRS) group in 1972 and is based on the results of initial surgical resection [269]. A revised staging system has been developed on the basis of the TNM (tumor–node–metastasis) system (Table 47.8) [269]. This system is less dependent on such factors as surgical excision at diagnosis, which can be affected by the aggressiveness of a local surgeon. It also takes into consideration the site of the primary tumor and its size, and nodal involvement. The clinical grouping system is used in conjunction with the TNM system to determine the role of radiotherapy.

Table 47.7 Soft tissue sarcoma clinical grouping classification.

Group	Definition
I	Localized disease, completely resected a) Confined to muscle/organ or origin b) Contiguous involvement–infiltration outside the muscle or organ of origin, as through fascial planes
II	Total gross resection with evidence of regional spread a) Grossly resected tumor with microscopic residual disease b) Regional disease with involved nodes, completely resected with no microscopic residual c) Regional disease with involved nodes, grossly resected, but with evidence of microscopic residual and/or histologic involvement of the most distal regional node (from the primary site) in the dissection
III	Incomplete resection with gross residual disease a) After biopsy only b) After gross major resection of the primary (>50%)
IV	Distant metastatic disease present at onset • Lung, liver, bones, bone marrow, brain, distant muscle/nodes • The presence of positive cytology in CSF, pleural or abdominal fluid, as well as implants on pleural or peritoneal surfaces place patients in clinical group IV

Source: Lawrence 1997 [269]. Reproduced with permission of John Wiley & Sons.
CSF, cerebrospinal fluid.

Table 47.8 TNM pre-treatment staging classification for rhabdomyosarcoma.

Stage	Sites	T	Size	N	M
I	Orbit, head and neck (excluding parameningeal)	T1 or T2	a or b	N0 or N1 or Nx	M0
II	Parameningeal	T1 or T2	a	N0 or Nx	M0
III	Parameningeal	T1 or T2	a	N1	M0
			b	N0 or N1 or Nx	M0
IV	All	T1 or T2	a or b	N0 or N1	M1

Source: Lawrence 1997 [269]. Reproduced with permission of John Wiley & Sons.
Tumor:
T1 – confined to anatomic site of origin
T2 – extension and/or fixative to surrounding tissues
a) ≤5 cm in diameter in size
b) >5 cm in diameter in size
Regional nodes:
N0 – regional nodes not clinically involved
N1 – regional nodes clinically involved by neoplasm
Nx – clinical status of regional nodes unknown

Treatment

The treatment of RMS involves resection of the primary tumor, chemotherapy for cytoreduction of the primary tumor and treatment of microscopic and gross metastases, and radiotherapy for control of local or regional residual disease. The randomized clinical trials carried out by the IRS and the Children's Oncology Group have helped to determine the current therapeutic recommendations. Combination chemotherapy is a component of treatment for all patients [36,270]. These trials have found vincristine, dactinomycin, and cyclophosphamide to be among the most active agents against rhabdomyosarcoma, and they would be considered standard therapy outside of a protocol [267,270–272]. The IRS-IV compared the standard VAC (vincristine, actinomycin D, and cyclophosphamide) with VIE (vincristine, ifosfamide, and etoposide) and VAI (vincristine, actinomycin D, and ifosfamide) and showed that there were no statistically significant differences in outcome, establishing VAC as the gold standard [273]. The subsequent IRS studies (now COG studies) have explored risk-adapted therapies (Table 47.9). For patients with low-risk disease, outcomes are excellent with standard VAC therapy, with survival rates in excess of 90%. A subset of these patients (subset 1) can be treated without alkylators [272]. For patients in the intermediate-risk category, treatment usually includes intensive alkylator

Table 47.9 Children's Oncology Group rhabdomyosarcoma risk group classification. Adapted from Raney 2011 [272].

Risk group	Histology	Stage	Group
Low (35%)[1]	Embryonal	I	I, II, III
	Embryonal	II, III	II, III
Intermediate (50%)	Embryonal	II, III	III, IV[2]
	Alveolar	I, II, III	I, II, III
High (15%)	Embryonal or alveolar	IV	IV[3]

[1] Two subsets of low risk:
Subset 1 (lowest risk): stage I or II, group I, II, *or* stage I, group III (orbit only).
Subset 2: stage I, group III, *or* stage 3, group I, II.
[2] Intermediate risk includes: metastatic embryonal rhabdomyosarcoma <10 years of age.
[3] High risk includes: metastatic embryonal rhabdomyosarcoma >10 years of age.

therapy with standard VAC; in conjunction with radiation therapy, survival rates for this group of patients are 60–70% [274]. Patients with metastatic disease have a very poor prognosis, with survival rates below 30%; however, children younger than 10 years with embryonal histology have a more favorable outcome [275].

Radiotherapy is indicated for all patients with microscopic or macroscopic residual disease. Failure to comply with radiation guidelines is associated with a high risk of local or regional disease recurrence [276]. Radiation therapy is an essential part of all treatment protocols, except for low-risk tumors that are completely resected. Patients with completely resected alveolar tumors should still receive radiation therapy (3,600 cGy), as the risk of local relapse after surgery only is high [277]. Patients with microscopic residual disease receive 4,140 cGy in standard fractions (180 cGy per fraction), whereas patients with gross residual or unresectable disease receive 5,040 cGy with standard fractionation. The IRS-IV trial failed to show any advantage to the use of hyperfractionated radiotherapy, and thus standard fractionation is recommended [278].

With this approach, therapy can be tailored to maximize tumor control and to minimize late effects in patients with favorable characteristics, while identifying patients with unfavorable characteristics for whom more intensive therapy is indicated.

Follow-Up and Late Effects

Monitoring for recurrence usually follows similar guidelines to other solid malignancies, with imaging of the primary site and potential metastatic sites, usually lungs, at regular intervals. While most schedules are imaging intensive, the impact of such an approach on survival has not been clearly documented [279]. Long-term survivors of rhabdomyosarcoma require close follow-up for proper monitoring of late effects [280]. In addition to the well-known long-term effects of chemotherapy, particularly those associated with intensive alkylator and anthracycline use, survivors of rhabdomyosarcoma are at risk of developing severe sequelae related to the local treatments used. This is particularly important for young children with genitourinary and head and neck primaries [281–283]. Finally, children with rhabdomyosarcoma are at high risk of developing SMNs; this risk is higher for young children with embryonal primaries, particularly if anaplastic features are present [259].

Germ Cell Tumors

Definition

Germ cell tumors (GCT) are neoplasms that derive from the totipotential primordial germ cells. These tumors can be germinomatous or embryonal.

Incidence

Germ cell, trophoblastic, and other gonadal tumors comprise approximately 3% of cancers among children younger than 15 years. Incidence is higher among adolescents aged between 15 and 19 years, representing 15% of cancers in that group [284]. Incidence rates during adolescence are approximately 20% higher for girls than for boys. The median ages at diagnosis for boys and girls in Germany are approximately 3 years and 9 years, respectively [285]. Additionally, intracranial germ cell tumors comprise approximately 3–5% of all central nervous system tumors and are most commonly germinomatous [284].

Etiology and Risk Factors

The only two well-established predisposing factors are cryptorchidism in males and disorders of sexual development (especially those with gonadal dysgenesis and hypovirilization). This includes patients with chromosomal imbalances such as Turner syndrome and forms of mosaicism. Frequently, children with presacral or sacrococcygeal teratomas have congenital anomalies of the vertebrae, the genitourinary system, or the anorectum [286]. Although there is no known cause identified, the incidence of intracranial germ cell tumors is increased in the Japanese population compared to the US and Europe by up to five times; however, there is no increase in testicular germ cell tumors in this population [287].

Pathology

Pure germ cell tumors are called germinomatous and are either seminomas (if presenting in testes) or dysgerminomas (if presenting in ovarian tissue). Nonseminomatous germ cell tumors can be made up of different elements, which include embryonal carcinoma (stem cell component), teratoma (somatically differentiated component), endodermal sinus (yolk sac) tumor, and choriocarcinoma (extraembryonic differentiation). Tumors with embryonal differentiation can be embryonal carcinomas, teratomas, endodermal sinus (yolk sac) tumors, or choriocarcinomas [286]. Germ cell tumors containing a mixture of neoplastic germ cells and embryonal cells are termed mixed germ cell tumors. Additionally, the histology can be suggested by the tumor markers they secrete. Tumors with a component of choriocarcinoma secrete the β-subunit of human chorionic gonadotropin (β-hCG) while elevated alpha-fetoprotein (AFP) is associated with yolk sac tumors; however, embryonal carcinomas and teratomas can secrete small amounts of AFP, and some elevation of β-hCG can be seen in embryonal carcinomas and germinomas containing syncytiotrophoblasts [284,287].

Presentation

The location of these tumors along the midline is a manifestation of the migration of the germ cells during embryonic development. Extragonadal tumors can present in the sacrococcygeal area, the retroperitoneum, the mediastinum, the neck, and the pineal gland. The presacral and sacrococcygeal teratomas that occur in newborns and young infants almost always are benign, whereas 65% of those occurring after age 6 months are malignant.

Gonadal Germ Cell Tumors

In children and adolescents, ovarian tumors account for approximately 25% of all GCT, and usually develop in pubertal and postpubertal girls, who typically present with acute or chronic pain and an enlarged abdomen. Testicular tumors account for 18–20% of all GCT. In infants, they usually present as a painless mass in the scrotum, and distant metastases are rare. In contrast, in older boys and adolescents, testicular tumors tend to disseminate early into the retroperitoneal lymph nodes and lung [288].

Extragonadal Germ Cell Tumors

Over half of germ cell tumors are extragonadal, and these tumors have worse prognosis than gonadal germ cell tumors [289]. The most common site is the sacrococcygeal area (25% of germ cell tumors), where tumors may be present at birth. Many sacrococcygeal tumors have an external component, and obstruction of the rectum or urinary tract is a common presenting problem. The second most common site of extragonadal germ cell tumors is the brain (18–20%), where tumors develop in the pineal area. Patients present with nonspecific signs of increased intracranial pressure or with Parinaud syndrome. Germinomas account for 60% of these pineal tumors, followed by mature and immature teratomas (30%). The more malignant embryonal carcinoma, endodermal sinus tumor, and choriocarcinoma account for the remaining 10% of brain germ cell tumors Intracranial germinomas have a high tendency for craniospinal dissemination [290]. Less frequently encountered extragonadal germ cell tumors are located in mediastinal and retroperitoneal sites.

Germ cell tumors have an infiltrative growth pattern and may disseminate by both lymphogenous and hematogenous routes. The most common sites of metastases are the lungs but metastatic disease can occur in the bone, liver, and brain. Approximately 20% of patients present with distant metastatic disease [287].

Diagnosis and Evaluation

Radiographic evaluation after thorough history and physical examination includes imaging of the primary tumor site, which can include ultrasound in testicular disease or MRI or CT for other primary sites. All patients should have a CT of the chest, and a bone scan is usually recommended to complete staging.

Serum markers such as β-hCG and AFP are very useful for diagnosis, monitoring of response, and prediction of recurrence. Not all germ cell tumors secrete these markers; AFP elevation reflects a yolk sac tumor component, whereas β-hCG is secreted by the syncytiotrophoblastic component of choriocarcinomas, although it can also be elevated in up to 20% of germinomas [288]. Additionally, normal newborns have elevated levels of AFP, which remain elevated above adult levels during most of the first year of life. Also, hepatoblastoma, pancreatoblastoma, and other conditions, such as liver damage, may result in elevation of the serum AFP levels.

Histology provides definitive diagnosis. Surgical approach for diagnosis is important as it can affect staging, for example a trans-scrotal approach should never be used and up-stages the patient due to disruption of lymphatic channels. For testicular tumors in prepubertal boys, if AFP is elevated radical orchiectomy should be performed; testis-sparing surgery is acceptable with normal AFP if a benign teratoma is suspected. In postpubertal males, radical orchiectomy is indicated for all testicular tumors. For ovarian masses suspected to be germ cell tumor due to elevated AFP or β-hCG levels or to radiologic features, the ovary should be resected intact, inspection of surrounding tissue and the other ovary performed, and peritoneal washings obtained for cytology. For extragonadal tumors, complete surgical resection at diagnosis reduces the risk of recurrence. Additionally, as there is no clear difference in patients achieving cure with upfront resection, neoadjuvant chemotherapy can be used to reduce morbidity if aggressive resection would be needed at presentation [287].

Treatment

The successful treatment of germ cell tumors includes a multimodal strategy, where surgery, chemotherapy, and radiotherapy play a role. The histological subentities differ in their response to chemotherapy and radiotherapy.

Mature and Immature Teratomas

A complete surgical resection is curative for mature teratomas. For immature gonadal and extragonadal teratomas, the outcome is also excellent with surgery alone, and chemotherapy should only be used for the rare patient whose disease recurs [291].

Malignant Germ Cell Tumors

Different chemotherapeutic agents and combinations are effective in the treatment of malignant germ cell tumors. However, platinum-based regimens are considered to be the standard of therapy. In the US, the intergroup POG-CCG studies have prospectively explored the PEB (cisplatin, etoposide, and bleomycin) regimen [292,293]. For patients with stage II testicular or stages I/II ovarian tumors, 4 courses of PEB result in excellent outcome, with survival rates >90% [293]. For patients with gonadal stages III–IV and extragonadal stages I–IV malignant germ cell tumors, the North American cooperative groups explored the role of cisplatin intensification, and patients were randomized to receive standard (20 mg/m^2/day for 5 days) or high-dose (40 mg/m^2/day for 5 days) cisplatin [292]. Overall, there was a trend towards improved outcome for patients receiving high-dose PEB; however, the OS was not significantly different (>80% in both arms) and the high-dose arm was significantly more toxic. An alternative to the PEB regimen is the JEB regimen where carboplatin is used instead of cisplatin; this regimen appears to have comparable efficacy and less toxicity [294]. An international randomized study comparing the efficacy of the PEB and JEB regimens is currently underway.

Based on these results, a more refined risk-adapted therapy, based on stage and site, is possible. The classification proposed by the COG stratifies patients into three groups:

1) *Low risk*: Patients with stage I immature teratomas (with or without malignant elements) and gonadal malignant germ cell tumors, which can be cured with surgery alone. Boys with stage I testicular tumors and girls with stage I ovarian tumors originally treated with surgical resection and observation can usually be salvaged (>95%) if relapse occurs by using further surgical excision and standard PEB chemotherapy [293,295,296]. Therefore, surgery alone is an option for stage I gonadal tumors; however, close follow-up observation to document a normalization of the tumor markers after surgery is mandatory.
2) *Intermediate risk*: Patients with stage II–IV gonadal, and stage I–II extragonadal tumors have an excellent outcome (survival >90%) with the standard PEB or JEB regimens. Studies exploring reduced therapy have shown decreased survival with 3 versus 4 cycles of PEB; therefore, 4 cycles remains the standard of therapy [287].
3) *High risk*: Patients with stage III/IV extragonadal tumors. For these patients, survival with the standard PEB or JEB regimens is not better than 80%. Although high-dose PEB may provide some advantage, the incidence and severity of long-term toxicities are very significant and cannot be decreased with the use of amifostine. Therefore, new strategies are needed. The most recent completed COG study (AGCT1P1) explored the addition of cyclophosphamide to standard PEB; however, numbers were insufficient to demonstrate an improved EFS or OS [297].

With the more widespread use of cisplatin-based regimens, the previously used prognostic factors like histology, site, and tumor stage have in part lost their prognostic relevance. Although the majority of patients can be cured, patients who are older (>11 years), have ovarian stage IV disease, or extragonadal stage II–IV disease have a significantly worse prognosis with <70% long-term disease-free (LTDF) survival. Within this group, patients >11 years with stage IV extragonadal disease had <40% LTDF survival [298].

Follow-Up and Late Effects

For teratomas, surveillance with determination of serum levels of AFP for 3–5 years after surgery is recommended. For low-risk patients treated with surgery alone, close follow-up to observe normalization of tumor markers is necessary. After completion of therapy, tumor markers should be frequently monitored initially and intermittent imaging of at least the primary site performed. Most recurrences happen within the first 2 years; however, later recurrences at 5 or more years post therapy have been reported [288].

Follow-up is also needed for monitoring late effects of therapy. As most patients are cured, many recent and upcoming trials are focused on therapy modifications or reductions to mitigate these late effects. Therapy-related toxicities related to cisplatin most commonly include hearing loss, nephrotoxicity with decreased glomerular function, and potential for neurotoxicity in adulthood related to heavy metal exposure. Pulmonary toxicity occurs in up to 50% of patients with bleomycin exposure, and although it is often reversible some survivors develop restrictive lung disease or other permanent complications. Finally, there is an increased risk of secondary malignancy in patients treated for germ cell tumors, and close monitoring in adulthood is needed as some studies have suggested the rate occurs at 1% per year with no plateau [287].

Retinoblastoma

Definition

Retinoblastoma is a childhood malignancy that develops from immature neuroectodermal cells in the eye.

Incidence

Retinoblastoma is the most common malignant ocular tumor afflicting children. It generally occurs in children younger than 5 years, and comprises approximately 5% of malignant neoplasms of that age group. Incidence rates in the US do not vary substantially by sex, race, or ethnicity, and have remained stable over time [2].

Etiology and Risk Factors

Two-thirds of retinoblastoma cases are unilateral, and the remainder are bilateral. The median age at diagnosis of unilateral retinoblastoma is approximately 2 years while the median age at diagnosis of bilateral disease is less than 1 year. Patients with bilateral disease carry a germline mutation of the *RB1* gene. This mutation is inherited from an affected parent in only 25% of the cases; in the remainder of cases, the mutation occurs *in utero*, usually in early embryogenesis. Approximately 10% of patients with unilateral disease also have the heritable form with a germline mutation and are capable of transmitting the disease to their offspring [299]. The genetic defect is the loss of heterozygosity at the retinoblastoma gene (RB) locus that predisposes the child to the development of retinoblastoma. Alteration of both copies of the retinoblastoma gene leads to malignant tumor development. Patients with the inherited form of the disease possess a germline mutation at the *RB1* locus. The second mutation ("hit") at the RB1 site leads to malignant tumor growth [300]. These patients are also at high risk of developing second malignancies [133]. Patients with sporadic (nonheritable) disease have two somatic mutations. In 1971, based on the mathematical analysis of the age at presentation of bilateral (hereditary) and unilateral (mostly nonhereditary) cases of retinoblastoma, Knudson proposed the "two-hit hypothesis," in which two mutational events in a developing retinal cell lead to the development of retinoblastoma [300]. This hypothesis was subsequently extended to suggest that the two events could be mutations of both alleles of the *RB1* gene. *RB1*, located in chromosome 13q14, was identified and cloned in 1986 [301]. Its product, pRb, is a key substrate for G1 cyclin-cdk complexes, which phosphorylate target gene products required for the transition of the cell through the G1 phase of the cell cycle. The active pRb functions as a tumor suppressor and stands as the major gatekeeper to control this critical point in growth regulation. The lack of pRb or its inactivation will remove the pRb constraint on cell cycle control, with the consequence of deregulated cell proliferation. Biallelic loss of *RB1* function is required for tumor development; this loss is germline and somatic for patients with bilateral disease, and somatic in a single cell in patients with unilateral disease. However, additional events may be required for tumor progression. Approximately two-thirds of tumors have MDM4/MDM2 amplification leading to inactivation of the p53 pathway [302]. Other genes and pathways are probably also involved; studies using comparative genomic hybridization have consistently shown chromosomal gains and amplifications at 6p and 1q, and losses at 16 q1. Finally, a very small proportion of tumors appear to develop in the context of normal *RB1*; amplification of *N-MYC* has been described in those cases [303].

Pathology

A retinoblastoma is composed of small round cells with scant cytoplasm and a deeply staining nucleus, resembling embryonal retinal cells. It appears grossly as a white, friable tumor with dense calcifications. Tumors that arise from the internal nuclear layer, the nerve fiber layer, the ganglion cell layer, or the external nuclear layer grow toward the subretinal space, pushing the retina inward and leading to retinal detachment [304]. This type of retinoblastoma is known as the exophytic type. Tumors that arise from the inner layers of the retina and grow toward the vitreous are known as the endophytic type.

Presentation, Diagnosis, and Evaluation

Frequently, children present with leukocoria (white-eye reflex), strabismus, conjunctival erythema, and decreased visual acuity; conversely, the disorder may be detected on routine eye examination. Leukocoria can result also from non-neoplastic conditions, such as *Toxocara canis* infection, retrolental fibroplasia secondary to prolonged oxygen administration at birth, congenital cataracts, and Coats disease [305].

The physical examination of children with retinoblastoma can reveal a white pupillary reflex, esotropia, exotropia, decreased acuity, or pain due to glaucoma or uveitis after tumor necrosis. Tumors near the macula can be seen with direct ophthalmoscopy; tumors at the periphery of the retina may not be apparent with direct visualization. All children with suspected retinoblastoma must undergo examination of both eyes under general anesthesia. In addition to the examination under anesthesia, a complete blood count, urinalysis, and renal and liver function tests should be performed. Ultrasound of the eye is usually also performed, and it is particularly useful in cases of massive retinal detachment where visualization of the entire retina is impaired. MRI of the brain is useful in defining the extent of the intraocular tumor and in assessing extraocular spread.

Retinoblastoma can metastasize to the CNS and bone marrow in patients with advanced intraocular disease. A lumbar puncture and bone marrow aspiration and biopsy can be performed under anesthesia at the time of the examination. Radionuclide bone scanning is indicated for patients with extensive ocular disease, positive bone marrow, or bony symptoms that could suggest bone metastases.

"Trilateral retinoblastoma" refers to the association of bilateral retinoblastoma with an asynchronous intracranial tumor, which occurs in less than 10% of bilateral cases [306]. Tumors comprising trilateral retinoblastoma are primitive neuroectodermal tumors (PNETs) exhibiting varying degrees of neuronal or photoreceptor differentiation, suggesting an origin from the germinal layer of primitive cells. The majority of these tumors are pineal region PNETs (pineoblastomas), but in 20–25% of the cases the tumors are suprasellar or parasellar. The median age at diagnosis of trilateral retinoblastoma is 23–48 months and the interval between the diagnosis of bilateral retinoblastoma and the diagnosis of the brain tumor is usually more than 20 months [307].

Staging

All patients undergo examination of both eyes under anesthesia; each eye is staged separately. The staging system traditionally used is that of Reese and Ellsworth [308]. However, developments in the conservative management of intraocular retinoblastoma have made the Reese–Ellsworth grouping system less predictable of eye salvage, and less helpful in guiding treatment. A new staging system (international classification of retinoblastoma) has been developed, with the goal of providing a simpler, user-friendly classification more applicable to current therapies. This new system is based on extent of tumor seeding within the vitreous cavity and subretinal space, rather than on tumor size and location, and seems to be a better predictor of treatment success (Table 47.10) [309].

Treatment

Treatment of retinoblastoma aims to save life and preserve vision, and thus needs to be individualized. Factors that need to be considered include unilaterality or bilaterality of the disease, potential for preserving vision, and intraocular and extraocular staging [310].

Surgery

Enucleation is indicated for large tumors filling the vitreous, for which there is little or no likelihood of restoring vision, and in cases of tumor present in the anterior chamber or in the presence of neovascular glaucoma. Enucleation should be performed by an experienced ophthalmologist; the eye must be removed intact, without seeding the malignancy into the orbit, and avoiding globe perforation [311]. For optimal staging, a long section (10–15 mm) of the optic nerve needs to be removed with the globe. An orbital implant is usually fitted during the same procedure, and the extraocular muscles are attached to it.

Focal Therapies

Focal treatments are used for small tumors (less than 3–6 mm), usually in patients with bilateral disease, and in combination with chemotherapy. **Photocoagulation** with argon laser is used for the treatment of tumors situated at or posterior to the equator of the eye, and for the treatment of retinal neovascularization

Table 47.10 International classification for intraocular retinoblastoma.

Group A
Small tumors away from foveola and disc
• Tumors ≤3 mm in greatest dimension confined to the retina, *and* • Located at least 3 mm from the foveola and 1.5 mm from the optic disc
Group B
All remaining tumors confined to the retina
• All other tumors confined to the retina not in group A • Subretinal fluid (without subretinal seeding) ≤3 mm from the base of the tumor
Group C
Local subretinal fluid or seeding
• Local subretinal fluid alone >3 to ≤6 mm from the tumor • Vitreous seeding or subretinal seeding ≤3 mm from the tumor
Group D
Diffuse subretinal fluid or seeding
• Subretinal fluid alone >6 mm from the tumor • Vitreous seeding or subretinal seeding >3 mm from the tumor
Group E
Presence of any or more of these poor prognosis features
• More than two-thirds of globe filled with tumor • Tumor in anterior segment • Tumor in or on the ciliary body • Iris neovascularization • Neovascular glaucoma • Opaque media from hemorrhage • Tumor necrosis with aseptic orbital cellulitis • Phthisis bulbi

Source: Shields 2006 [309]. Reproduced with permission of Elsevier.

due to radiation therapy [312]. This technique is limited to tumors measuring no greater than 4.5 mm in base, and no greater than 2.5 mm in thickness. The treatment is directed to coagulate all blood supply to the tumor. **Cryotherapy** is used for the treatment of small equatorial and peripheral lesions, measuring no more than 3.5 mm in base and no more than 2 mm in thickness [313]. One or two monthly sessions of triple freeze and thaw are performed, and tumor control rates are usually excellent. Finally, an important focal method is **transpupillary thermotherapy**, which applies focused heat at sub-photocoagulation levels, usually with a diode laser [314]. In thermotherapy, the goal is to deliver a temperature of 42–60 °C for 5–20 minutes to the tumor, sparing retinal vessels from photocoagulation. The use of focal treatments is especially important in conjunction with chemotherapy; the two treatment modalities appear to have a synergistic effect. In general, local control rates of 70–80% can be achieved. Complications of focal treatments include transient serous retinal detachment, retinal traction and tears, and localized fibrosis.

Chemotherapy

Chemotherapy is indicated in patients with extraocular disease, in the subgroup of patients with intraocular disease with high-risk histological features, and in patients with bilateral disease, in conjunction with aggressive focal therapies. Agents effective in the treatment of retinoblastoma include platinum compounds, etoposide, cyclophosphamide, doxorubicin, vincristine, and ifosfamide [310].

Radiotherapy

The goal of radiation therapy is to minimize integral dose to the patient to avoid the risk of complications: late normal tissue damage and SMNs. The incidence of second cancer in this patient population is very high even if radiation is not used. Radiation therapy can be delivered in the form of brachytherapy or external-beam radiation. Brachytherapy is used for the control of small tumors, usually in conjunction with other therapies; implants of radioactive material are placed in the form of episcleral plaques for a period of time to deliver high doses of radiation well focused to the tumor, sparing the normal structures. The majority of implants today use iodine-125 (^{125}I). Many other agents can be used, such as gold, cobalt, palladium, ruthenium, and others [315–318]. External-beam technique is used for treatment of the entire eye globe for ocular salvage, or for the management of extraocular disease to the orbit, CNS, or metastatic sites. Photons are commonly used; however, the use of proton therapy has significant advantages for patients with bilateral disease in terms of potentially lower risk of second malignancies [319,320].

Treatment of Intraocular Retinoblastoma

Unilateral Retinoblastoma

In the absence of extraocular disease, enucleation alone is curative for 85–90% of children with unilateral retinoblastoma. The outcome for patients with unilateral disease that has been enucleated is excellent, with good functional results and minimal long-term effects [321]. In view of the apparent success in treating bilateral intraocular disease with chemoreduction, a conservative approach with chemotherapy and focal measures is being increasingly used. With the use of intra-arterial chemotherapy, ocular salvage rates above 70–80% can be achieved [322]. For patients undergoing enucleation, adjuvant chemotherapy is indicated in those patients with massive choroidal involvement, scleral invasion, and invasion of the optic nerve past the lamina cribrosa. Different chemotherapy regimens have been proposed. Six-month treatment with VDC (vincristine, cyclophosphamide, and doxorubicin), VCE (vincristine, carboplatin, and etoposide), or a hybrid, with alternating courses of both regimens, appears to be effective. Radiation therapy is only indicated when there is transscleral disease or involvement of the cut end of the optic nerve.

Bilateral Retinoblastoma

In the past, the treatment for patients with bilateral retinoblastoma has been enucleation of those eyes with advanced intraocular disease and no visual potential, and the use of external-beam radiation therapy for the remaining eyes. However, there are several complications associated with radiation therapy. Irradiation of the orbit during a period of rapid growth results in a major decrease in orbital volume, resulting in mid-facial deformities. More important, however, is the greatly increased risk for the development of a sarcoma within the radiation therapy field, compared to the underlying increased risk of secondary neoplasms in these predisposed individuals. This risk may be age related, and decreases as irradiation is delayed [323]. These concerns have resulted in the development of more conservative approaches. The treatment of patients with bilateral retinoblastoma now incorporates upfront chemotherapy, which is intended to achieve maximum chemoreduction of the intraocular tumor burden early in the treatment, followed by aggressive focal therapies. This approach has resulted in an increase in the eye salvage rates and in a decrease (and delay) in the use of radiation therapy. Different chemotherapy combinations are used, although the best results are achieved with a combination of vincristine, carboplatin, and etoposide. Salvage rates for group A and B eyes approach 100% using these techniques. For patients with advanced intraocular tumors (groups C and D), ocular salvage rates above 70%, with minimal use of radiation therapy, can be achieved with intensive chemotherapy and aggressive local control [324].

Intravitreal and Intra-Arterial Chemotherapy for Intraocular Retinoblastoma

Japanese investigators have pioneered the administration of intravitreal and intra-arterial melphalan for patients with advanced or recurrent intraocular retinoblastoma [325]. Good clinical responses in patients with progressive retinoblastoma were obtained using intravitreal melphalan followed by hyperthermia [325]. Kaneko *et al.* initially reported the feasibility of injecting melphalan into the ipsilateral carotid artery, with documented efficacy [325]. The technique was later perfected by Mohri using a balloon catheter inflated in the distal internal carotid artery that allowed for selective flow into the ophthalmic artery [326]. More recently, Abramson *et al.* reported a variation of this technique that includes a direct cannulation of the ophthalmic artery using a microcatheter [327]. Using this approach, high ocular salvage rates can now be achieved after the administration of 3–5 mg of intra-arterial melphalan, although other agents such as topotecan and carboplatin are also used [2,327,328]. Ocular salvage rates using intra-arterial chemotherapy are now in excess of 80% [329]; the use of this new treatment modality is being progressively incorporated into the front line of ocular salvage for intraocular retinoblastoma. Direct administration of melphalan into the vitreous is also a promising approach for cases with vitreous disease [330].

Treatment of Extraocular Retinoblastoma

Extraocular dissemination of retinoblastoma is a product of the socio-economic conditions that result in delayed diagnosis and treatment. In Europe and the US, fewer than 5% of patients present with extraocular disease, in contrast to up to 40–80% in less developed countries [331,332].

Orbital and Loco-Regional Retinoblastoma

Orbital retinoblastoma occurs as a result of progression of the tumor through the emissary vessels and sclera. For this reason, scleral disease is considered to be extraocular, and should be treated as such. Orbital retinoblastoma is isolated in 60–70% of cases; lymphatic, hematogenous, and CNS metastases occur in the remaining patients [333]. Treatment should include systemic chemotherapy and radiation therapy; with this approach, 60–85% of patients can be cured. Since most recurrences occur in the CNS, regimens using drugs with well-documented CNS penetration are recommended. Different chemotherapy regimens have proven to be effective, including vincristine, cyclophosphamide, and doxorubicin, platinum- and epipodophyllotoxin-based regimens, or a combination of both [310]. For patients with macroscopic orbital disease, it is recommended that surgery be delayed until response to chemotherapy has been obtained (usually 2 or 3 courses of treatment). Enucleation should then be performed, and an additional 4–6 courses of chemotherapy administered. Local control should then be consolidated with orbital irradiation (40–45 Gy). Using this approach, orbital exenteration can be avoided [334]. Patients with isolated involvement of the optic nerve at the transection level should also receive similar systemic treatment, and irradiation should include the entire orbit (36 Gy) with 9–10 Gy boost to the chiasm (total 45–46 Gy). The pre-auricular and cervical lymph nodes should be explored carefully, since 20% of patients with orbital retinoblastoma have lymphatic metastases [333]. Lymphatic dissemination does not carry a worse prognosis, provided that the involved lymph nodes are also irradiated.

Central Nervous System Disease

Intracranial dissemination occurs by direct extension through the optic nerve, and its prognosis is dismal [331,334]. Treatment for these patients should include platinum-based intensive systemic chemotherapy and CNS-directed therapy. Although intrathecal chemotherapy has been traditionally used, there is no preclinical or clinical evidence to support its use. Although the use of irradiation in these patients is controversial, responses have been observed with craniospinal irradiation, using 23.4–36 Gy to the entire craniospinal axis, with a boost to achieve up to 45 Gy to sites of measurable disease. Therapeutic intensification with high-dose, marrow-ablative chemotherapy and autologous hematopoietic progenitor cell rescue has been explored, but its role is not yet clear [335,336].

(Extra-Cranial) Metastatic Retinoblastoma

Hematogenous metastases may develop in the bones, bone marrow, and, less frequently, the liver. Although long-term survivors have been reported with conventional chemotherapy, these reported cures should be considered anecdotal. In recent years, however, it has been shown in small series of patients that metastatic retinoblastoma can be cured using high-dose, marrow-ablative chemotherapy and autologous hematopoietic progenitor cell rescue. The approach is similar to metastatic neuroblastoma; patients receive short and intensive induction regimens usually containing alkylating agents, anthracyclines, etoposide, and platinum compounds, and are then consolidated with marrow-ablative chemotherapy and autologous hematopoietic cell rescue. Using this approach, the outcome appears to be excellent [336].

Follow-Up and Late Effects

Follow-up after treatment of retinoblastoma varies from patient to patient. In general, evaluation for recurrence, typically at the primary site, includes ophthalmologic examination, often performed under anesthesia, and examination of the surrounding tissue or orbit in patients who have undergone enucleation or radiation therapy.

The cumulative incidence of second cancers in patients with germline mutations of the *RB1* gene is greatly elevated with the use and increasing dose of radiation therapy, and this incidence is reported to increase steadily with age, reaching up to 40–60% at 40–50 years of age (though a more recent study estimates a considerably lower risk) [337,338]. Conversely, patients with nonhereditary retinoblastoma are not inherently at an increased risk. Almost every neoplasm type has been reported in survivors of retinoblastoma, and 60–70% of the tumors occur in the head and neck areas [337,338]. The most common second tumor is osteogenic sarcoma, arising both inside and outside the irradiation field, which accounts for approximately one-third of all cases of second cancers. Soft tissue sarcomas and melanomas are second in frequency, accounting for 20–25% of cases. In recent years, it has become apparent that patients with hereditary retinoblastoma are also at risk of developing epithelial cancers late in adulthood [133]. Of those, lung cancer appears to be the most common.

Because their orbital growth is still in progress, children treated for retinoblastoma are at risk of functionally and cosmetically significant bony orbital abnormalities. These sequelae become evident by early adolescence, when orbital growth is largely complete, and result in the "hour-glass facial deformity." Both enucleation, which causes orbital contraction, and radiotherapy, which induces arrest of bone growth, adversely affect orbital growth. In children treated for bilateral retinoblastoma, the impact of enucleation in orbital development is not different from that of irradiation. However, final orbital volumes after enucleation correlate with the size of the prosthetic implant.

Gliomas

Definition

Gliomas are a diverse group of CNS tumors that are commonly defined as arising from glial or glial precursor cells. Ependymomas arise from the ependymal cells, which line the ventricular system, and can arise throughout the CNS [339].

Incidence

Primary brain tumors represent approximately 21% of cancers among children younger than 15 years and 10% of cancers among adolescents aged 15–19 years [2]. Gliomas are the most common type of primary CNS tumors in all age groups and account for approximately 52.9% of all brain and CNS tumors (malignant and benign) of children younger than 15 years. Of these, approximately 60% are pilocytic astrocytomas and other low-grade gliomas (33.2% and 27.1%, respectively). High-grade gliomas account for 21% of all gliomas and approximately 11.1% of all brain and CNS tumors but account for the greatest proportion of deaths (43.8%). Ependymal tumors represent 10.4% of gliomas [339,340]. Incidence rates of gliomas are higher in White and Asian-Pacific Islander children compared to Black and American Indian-Alaskan Native children [339,340].

Etiology and Risk Factors

The etiology of most childhood brain tumors remains unknown. Ionizing radiation and cancer predisposition syndromes are the only known risk factors; however, factors such as parental age, birth defects, and environmental factors are being investigated [341]. Neurofibromatosis type 1 carries an increased risk primarily for pilocytic astrocytoma, most often involving the optic nerve (also known as an "optic glioma") while neurofibromatosis type 2 has an increased risk of spinal intramedullary and cauda equina gliomas, primarily ependymomas. Patients with tuberous sclerosis carry an increased risk of developing subependymal giant cell astrocytomas (SEGA), which are low-grade gliomas, often arising from the wall of the lateral ventricles. Patients with Turcot syndrome due to mismatch repair mutations in hereditary nonpolyposis colon cancer or *APC* mutations in familial adenomatous polyposis are at increased risk of anaplastic astrocytoma and glioblastoma as well as medulloblastoma. Patients with Li–Fraumeni syndrome and *TP53* germline mutations are at increased risk for bone and soft tissue sarcomas, breast cancer, adrenocortical carcinoma, and brain tumors. Most brain tumors in this population are astrocytic, including low-grade and anaplastic astrocytomas as well as glioblastomas [342,343]. Little is known regarding risk factors for childhood ependymoma [344].

Classification

While there is no standard definition for gliomas, the Central Brain Tumor Registry of the United States (CBTRUS) includes astrocytoma, glioblastoma, oligodendroglioma, ependymoma, mixed, and not otherwise specified glioma as well as a few rare histologic subtypes in their reports [339]. Gliomas are often categorized as low-grade (WHO grade I–II) which includes pilocytic astrocytoma, and high-grade (WHO grade III–IV) which includes anaplastic astrocytoma and glioblastoma or most ependymomas. An alternate categorization is by site; this is particularly relevant when discussing brainstem gliomas such as diffuse intrinsic pontine gliomas.

Low-grade gliomas include a number of different subtypes and lack high-grade histologic features such as vascular proliferation and palisading necrosis. It has been recently recognized that the majority of pediatric low-grade gliomas harbor genomic alterations that affect the MAPK pathway. Most commonly these include alterations of *BRAF*, with tandem duplication in grade I pilocytic astrocytomas or the presence of the *BRAF* V600E mutation in grade II pediatric low-grade gliomas [345].

High-grade gliomas are those showing high-grade features such as anaplasia, increased mitotic activity, and microvascular proliferation or necrosis [346]. The most common high-grade gliomas are anaplastic astrocytoma and glioblastoma [339,340]. Additionally, the most recent 2016 WHO Classification of Tumors of the Central Nervous System uses molecular features in addition to histology in the hope of improving classification and diagnosis in order to tailor patient therapy [346,347].

Brainstem gliomas are glial tumors arising in the midbrain, pons, or medulla. They can be either diffusely infiltrative or focally discrete lesions. Pontine lesions are more commonly diffusely infiltrative with expansion into the midbrain, medulla, and cerebellopontine peduncles. These infiltrative pontine tumors are called diffuse intrinsic pontine gliomas (DIPG). Histologically the tumors comprise WHO grade II–IV gliomas. Dorsally exophytic brainstem tumors tend to be low-grade, juvenile pilocytic astrocytomas (JPAs) [348].

Ependymomas arise from the ependymal cells of the ventricular system and can arise throughout the CNS. The majority of ependymomas occur intracranially, with two-thirds located in the posterior fossa. Approximately 10% arise along the spinal cord. Ependymomas are classified as myxopapillary ependymoma (WHO grade I), nonanaplastic ependymoma (WHO grade II), or anaplastic ependymoma (WHO grade III) [344].

Presentation

Clinical findings in patients with brain tumors are most often nonspecific such as headache, fatigue, vomiting, or lethargy [349]. Children with pediatric gliomas can present with signs and symptoms related to the location of the tumor. With low-grade gliomas, there can be a long period of gradual onset of symptoms. Children may present with signs of increased intracranial pressure due to infiltration or compression of normal structures or obstruction of CSF flow. These symptoms include headaches, vomiting, and papilledema but often begin as more vague complaints such as mood changes or fatigue [344,349,350]. Symptoms may also be localizing though these are less frequent, and vision loss or endocrinopathies can be the presenting signs of optic pathway or hypothalamic tumors [349,351]. Children may present with seizures, even long-standing epilepsy if the tumor is low grade [352]. Children with a brainstem glioma commonly present with symptoms of cranial nerve dysfunction, cerebellar signs such as ataxia, and long tract signs such as hyperreflexia or clonus [353].

Diagnosis and Evaluation

A brain tumor can be diagnosed with CT or MRI. MRI provides more information and can be helpful to identify typical features of certain brain tumors. Low-grade gliomas are typically iso- or hypointense on T1-weighted imaging and may appear cystic, while ependymomas can have variable signal characteristics but often have heterogeneous enhancement with contrast [354,355]. DIPG are T1 hypointense and T2 hyperintense on MRI with minimal contrast enhancement [348,356]. Spinal MRI and CSF cytologic examination are necessary in the workup of posterior fossa ependymomas because they are more likely to spread; however, a spinal MRI concurrent with brain imaging is often performed to rule out metastatic deposits in low-grade gliomas [344,354,357].

Surgical resection is important for tissue diagnosis and to reduce tumor burden and potentially relieve symptoms. Diagnostic classification is primarily based on histology; however, the 2016 WHO classification system does incorporate some molecular genetic features [347]. Traditionally DIPG have not been routinely biopsied at diagnosis, due to their difficult location. With recent advances in neurosurgical techniques allowing for stereotactic biopsy, the tumors are being increasingly biopsied, especially when they have atypical features and in the setting of research for better understanding of biological characteristics and targeting treatment [353,358].

Treatment

Treatment of gliomas includes surgical resection, chemotherapy, and radiation, and differs based on grade, histologic and at times molecular subtype, and tumor location. For pediatric low-grade gliomas that can be safely resected, a complete resection is most commonly curative [355]. For those that cannot be fully resected, treatment is reserved for progressive or symptomatic tumors. Because OS is high, the aim is thus to achieve disease control while minimizing tumor- and therapy-related morbidity.

Chemotherapy is used for progressive tumors that cannot be safely resected. The two most commonly used regimens include the combination of vincristine and carboplatin, or a combination of four drugs (6-thioguanine, CCNU (lomustine), procarbazine, and vincristine, also known by the acronym TPCV). Recently these were examined in a randomized clinical trial by COG, which found that both regimens had activity in pediatric low-grade gliomas [354,359]. While there was a trend to increased responses to the TPCV regimen, this was not statistically significant. Many oncologists use vincristine and carboplatin as the first-line chemotherapy regimen for progressive pediatric low-grade gliomas, due to its low side effect profile. Dorsally exophytic brainstem tumors can be associated with a 5-year survival rate of 75% after subtotal resection. Pathologically, such tumors tend to be juvenile pilocytic astrocytomas (JPAs) [348]. Chemotherapy regimens for pediatric low-grade gliomas can be used to treat these tumors.

Chemotherapy is used to achieve disease stability, although it is not expected to be curative. Many children require treatment with more than one course of chemotherapy. The tumors are expected to stabilize after children transition to adulthood. The aim is thus to achieve disease control with minimal morbidity. Radiation therapy does not confer survival advantage for children with pediatric low-grade gliomas, and is associated with significant morbidity. For this reason, radiation therapy, which was once standard treatment, is now typically avoided. With the discovery of BRAF alterations and activation of the MAPK pathway, novel agents targeting these alterations and pathway are currently being investigated in clinical trials and may represent targeted therapeutic options for pediatric low-grade gliomas [360].

Children with low-grade gliomas and neurofibromatosis 1 have a superior prognosis to children with sporadic low-grade gliomas. Pediatric low-grade gliomas have even been reported to spontaneously regress in children with NF1 [361]. In these children, particularly those with optic pathway gliomas, therapy is reserved for lesions causing symptoms such as visual compromise.

Similarly, the initial treatment of pediatric high-grade gliomas involves maximal surgical resection that can be safely achieved without causing neurological sequelae. The amount of resection is a prognostic variable [362,363]. Unlike low-grade gliomas, adjuvant therapy is necessary due to the poor prognosis of these tumors. For most patients, radiation therapy is administered to the tumor with doses of 54–60 Gy in conventional fractionation [363,364].

The combination of chemotherapy concurrently with radiation therapy and as maintenance therapy following completion of radiation therapy has been investigated with variable results. Although some studies previously reported improvement in progression-free survival with adjuvant chemotherapy, recent protocols have not demonstrated a significant survival advantage [365]. Currently, maximal surgical resection followed by radiation therapy with temozolomide and/or bevacizumab (a monoclonal antibody that inhibits VEGF-A and thus angiogenesis) is the accepted treatment. This is despite no evidence for a survival benefit; however, temozolomide is well tolerated and easy to administer. Children less than 3 years have a better outcome with high-grade gliomas and should be considered for treatment with surgery followed by chemotherapy alone due to the long-term side effects of radiation therapy. Many children are treated on clinical trials and current focuses include molecular classification and development of novel, targeted therapeutics [363,364].

The role of surgical resection of DIPG is extremely limited given the tumor location. The current standard of care is local radiation therapy; however, as this has been shown only to prolong survival by 3–6 months it is considered aggressive palliative therapy. To date, no chemotherapy has been shown to improve survival of these aggressive tumors. Additionally, there has been no significant survival benefit in hyper- or hypo-fractionated radiation therapy over conventional radiation. It is hoped that, with increasing numbers of diagnostic biopsies and molecular profiling, the biology of these tumors will be greater understood, leading to the development of novel therapeutic strategies that will ultimately improve patient survival [353,366].

Follow-Up and Late Effects

Prognosis varies greatly depending on location of tumor, degree of resection, histologic grade, and metastatic spread. While pilocytic astrocytomas and other low-grade gliomas have 10-year survival rates of >95% and >84% respectively, over 90% of patients diagnosed with DIPG die within 2 years of diagnosis and patients with other high-grade gliomas have a 28% 5-year OS [340,341]. Following completion of therapy, surveillance with imaging is important to monitor for recurrence or progression of incompletely resected disease.

Long-term survivors of pediatric gliomas are at risk for many therapy-related late effects. This is most well studied in patients with low-grade glioma given the high survival rates for these tumors. Over two-thirds of patients treated with radiation therapy will develop some long-term complication. While patients may have motor dysfunction or functional impairments related to their resection or tumor itself, most long-term effects are related to craniospinal radiation therapy. Patients treated for CNS tumors are at risk for neurocognitive deficits, which are more profound in patients treated with cranial radiation at younger ages (often defined as <5 years old). Additionally, patients treated with cranial radiation often develop endocrinopathies including thyroid hormone, growth hormone, or ACTH deficiency, and obesity. These patients are also at risk of vasculopathy and have higher rates of first time stroke as well as recurrent stroke than the general population. Hearing loss is also reported in approximately one-third of patients treated for CNS tumors. Finally, patients are at risk of secondary neoplasm related to radiation or chemotherapy, most commonly a secondary glioma or AML. Due to the significant morbidity of treatment-related late effects, patients with a history of childhood CNS tumors benefit from long-term follow-up that specifically monitors for and addresses these concerns [367–371].

Medulloblastoma

Definition

Medulloblastoma is an embryonal tumor that arises in the cerebellum, and is the most common malignant CNS tumor of childhood [372].

Incidence

Primary brain tumors represent approximately 21% of cancers among children younger than 15 years and 10% of cancers among adolescents aged 15–19 years [2]. Medulloblastomas account for approximately 20% of malignant brain and other CNS tumors among children younger than 15 years. The age distribution is bimodal, with peaks at 3–4 years and 8–10 years. Medulloblastoma is more common among boys than girls (incidence rates 0.60 and 0.38 cases per 100,000 children per year, respectively). Among racial and ethnic groups in the US, incidence is highest among non-Hispanic Whites and lowest among African Americans [340,373].

Etiology and Risk Factors

Medulloblastoma is associated with genetic predisposition syndromes. Gorlin syndrome (nevoid basal cell carcinoma syndrome), which is caused by *PTCH* gene mutations, is associated with medulloblastoma in addition to basal cell carcinoma and macrocephaly. Medulloblastoma is typically desmoplastic, with a more favorable prognosis than sporadic tumors, and occurs in approximately 5% of patients with Gorlin syndrome. Patients with Turcot syndrome due to mismatch repair mutations in hereditary nonpolyposis colon cancer or *APC* mutations in familial adenomatous polyposis are at increased risk of anaplastic astrocytoma and glioblastoma as well as medulloblastoma. Patients with Li–Fraumeni syndrome and *TP53* germline mutations are at increased risk for bone and soft tissue sarcomas, breast cancer, adrenocortical carcinoma, and brain tumors. Although most brain tumors in this population are astrocytic, other pediatric brain tumors including medulloblastoma can occur [343,373].

Classification

Histologically, medulloblastomas are small round blue cell tumors. A number of histological subtypes have been described, including nodular desmoplastic medulloblastoma (which carries an excellent prognosis), classical histology medulloblastoma, and large cell variant or anaplastic medulloblastoma (which are associated with a poor prognosis).

Recently, through profiling of genomic alterations and gene expression, it has been recognized that medulloblastoma encompasses a heterogeneous group of tumors. Four distinct subtypes have been characterized [374]. These include the Wnt positive group, the Sonic Hedgehog group, group 3, and group 4. Each subgroup has distinct genomic profiles and is characterized by differences in clinical features and prognosis.

Wnt positive medulloblastomas are characterized by mutations of β-catenin, which result in up-regulation of the Wnt pathway. These tumors usually occur in older children, are of the classical histological subtype, and are associated with an excellent prognosis, with OS rates of greater than 90%.

The Sonic Hedgehog group of medulloblastomas is characterized by mutations in the sonic hedgehog pathway. This subgroup can include any histological subtype; however nodular desmoplastic medulloblastomas are most likely to belong to the Sonic Hedgehog group. These tumors can have amplification of the *MYC* or *MYCN* oncogenes. Children with Sonic Hedgehog medulloblastomas have an intermediate prognosis, with an inferior prognosis compared to those with tumors in the Wnt subgroup but a superior prognosis compared to those tumors from group 3 or 4.

Group 3 and group 4 tumors are characterized by a poorer prognosis. Group 3 tumors have a high incidence of amplification of the *MYC* oncogene, and these tumors have often metastasized at diagnosis. Group 4 tumors are commonly characterized by the presence of *MYCN* amplification [347,374,375].

Presentation

The most common presenting symptoms of medulloblastoma result from obstructive hydrocephalus, which presents with headache, vomiting, and nausea. In particular, elevated intracranial pressure often causes early morning headaches and vomiting. Most frequently, the observed signs result from increased intracranial pressure or cerebellar dysfunction. These signs include papilledema, ataxia and other gait disturbance, and cranial nerve deficits. Patients with suspected brain tumors should undergo MRI with and without contrast [375].

Diagnosis and Evaluation

Diagnostic workup begins with imaging. Medulloblastomas are seeding tumors with a propensity to disseminate throughout the neuraxis. Spinal MRI with and without contrast should be performed at diagnosis (preferably before surgery) and cerebrospinal fluid evaluation should be performed on all patients (usually at least 2 weeks after surgery but prior to commencement of therapy) [357].

The staging of medulloblastoma is based on the surgical assessment of the tumor's extent and on radiographic imaging (Table 47.11) [376]. In the Langston modification of the Chang staging system, children with total or near-total resection (<1.5 cm^2 residual tumor post resection) are considered to be standard risk. Patients with more advanced disease are classified as high risk.

Table 47.11 Langston modification of Chang staging for medulloblastoma. Source: Halperin 1996 [376].

Stage	Definition
T1	Tumor <3 cm in diameter
T2	Tumor >3 cm in diameter
T3a	Tumor >3 cm with extension into aqueduct of Sylvius or foramen of Luschka (or both)
T3b	Tumor >3 cm with extension into brainstem
T4	Tumor >3 cm with extension past aqueduct of Sylvius or foramen magnum
M0	No gross subarachnoid or hematogenous metastasis
M1	Microscopic tumor cells in cerebrospinal fluid
M2	Gross nodular seeding beyond primary site in the cerebellar or cerebral subarachnoid space
M3	Gross nodular spinal seeding
M4	Extracranial metastasis

Treatment

Maximal surgical resection of the tumor is the initial component of the care of a child with a medulloblastoma, and where safely possible a complete resection should be achieved. A complete resection improves the prognosis and reduces the subsequent therapy required [377]. Surgical morbidity can include the posterior fossa syndrome, which consists of mutism, pharyngeal dysfunction, respiratory dysfunction, and ataxia [378]. Generally, these operative sequelae are reversible over the months after surgery.

Children are staged and risk stratified postoperatively. Children with no evidence of metastatic disease who have undergone a complete resection (<1.5 cm^2 residual tumor post resection), with no evidence of high-risk pathological features such as large cell/anaplastic medulloblastoma, are designated "standard risk." Those who have metastatic disease, postsurgical residual disease >1.5 cm^2, or high-risk histopathological features are designated "high risk" and are treated with higher doses of radiation therapy and chemotherapy. Future clinical trials will endeavor to incorporate the molecular and genetic characteristics into the risk stratification for children with newly diagnosed medulloblastoma.

Following maximal surgical resection, children above the age of 3 years are treated initially with craniospinal irradiation (CSI), with a local boost to the posterior fossa/tumor bed. Medulloblastomas are relatively radiosensitive and with the increasing recognition of dose-dependent and severe neurocognitive deficits associated with radiation therapy, efforts have been made to reduce the dose of CSI. The current dose of CSI for children with standard-risk medulloblastoma is 23.4 Gy, with a large cooperative clinical trial underway to examine the safety of reducing this further to 18 Gy. Children with high-risk disease still receive 36 Gy.

Medulloblastomas are chemosensitive, with high response rates to alkylating agents such as cyclophosphamide and platinum-based agents [379,380]. Children receive maintenance chemotherapy following the completion of radiation therapy.

Prognosis varies by molecular subtype, location, resectability, and presence of metastatic disease. Overall 10-year survival rates for children with medulloblastoma are 64%. Children with standard-risk medulloblastoma treated with maximal surgical resection, CSI, and maintenance chemotherapy generally respond well to treatment, with 10-year OS rates near 80% [2,339,374].

The treatment of infants with medulloblastoma presents specific and significant challenges due to devastating long-term neurocognitive sequelae after treatment with CSI. Strategies that incorporate surgery and chemotherapy only or focal radiation therapy to the tumor bed have been utilized [381–383]. These protocols have reduced OS compared to strategies that incorporate CSI; however, there appears to be a subset of patients who remain disease free after chemotherapy alone. Due to the devastating morbidity associated with such therapy, priority is given to delaying or avoiding radiation therapy in trials for children under 3 years of age [378].

Follow-Up and Late Effects

Surveillance imaging after resection and/or treatment should be performed using MRI. Patients who have recurrent disease detected by surveillance prior to the onset of symptoms have been shown to have increased rates of successful salvage therapy. Imaging is typically spaced out after 1 year of relapse-free survival but should continue at least 5 years as most recurrences occur within 5 years [384]. These children remain at risk of long-term side effects of therapy including the development of secondary cancers, neurocognitive deficits, endocrinopathies, growth deficits, and vasculopathy, similar to children with gliomas or other CNS tumors [368–370].

References

1 Siegel RL, Miller KD, Jemal A. Cancer statistics, 2017. *CA Cancer J Clin* 2017;67(1):7–30.

2 Ward E, DeSantis C, Robbins A, Kohler B, Jemal A. Childhood and adolescent cancer statistics, 2014. *CA Cancer J Clin* 2014;64(2):83–103.

3 Shah A, Coleman MP. Increasing incidence of childhood leukaemia: a controversy re-examined. *Br J Cancer* 2007;97(7):1009–12.

4 Hasle H. Pattern of malignant disorders in individuals with Down's syndrome. *Lancet Oncol* 2001;2(7):429–36.

5 Stiller CA, Chessells JM, Fitchett M. Neurofibromatosis and childhood leukaemia/lymphoma: a population-based UKCCSG study. *Br J Cancer* 1994;70(5):969–72.

6 Taylor AM, Metcalfe JA, Thick J, Mak YF. Leukemia and lymphoma in ataxia telangiectasia. *Blood* 1996;87(2):423–38.

7 Inaba H, Greaves M, Mullighan CG. Acute lymphoblastic leukaemia. *Lancet* 2013;381(9881):1943–55.

8 Andersen MK, Christiansen DH, Jensen BA, *et al.* Therapy-related acute lymphoblastic leukaemia with MLL rearrangements following DNA topoisomerase II inhibitors, an increasing problem: report on two new cases and review of the literature since 1992. *Br J Haematol* 2001;114(3):539–43.

9 Behm FG, Raimondi SC, Frestedt JL *et al.* Rearrangement of the MLL gene confers a poor prognosis in childhood acute lymphoblastic leukemia, regardless of presenting age. *Blood* 1996;87(7):2870–7.

10 Patte C, Auperin A, Michon J, *et al.* The Societe Francaise d'Oncologie Pediatrique LMB89 protocol: highly effective multiagent chemotherapy tailored to the tumor burden and initial response in 561 unselected children with B-cell lymphomas and L3 leukemia. *Blood* 2001;97(11):3370–9.

11 Goldberg JM, Silverman LB, Levy DE, *et al.* Childhood T-cell acute lymphoblastic leukemia: the Dana-Farber Cancer Institute acute lymphoblastic leukemia consortium experience. *J Clin Oncol* 2003;21(19):3616–22.

12 Coustan-Smith E, Mullighan CG, Onciu M, *et al.* Early T-cell precursor leukaemia: a subtype of very high-risk acute lymphoblastic leukaemia. *Lancet Oncol* 2009;10(2):147–56.

13 Moricke A, Zimmermann M, Reiter A, *et al.* Prognostic impact of age in children and adolescents with acute lymphoblastic leukemia: data from the trials ALL-BFM 86, 90, and 95. *Klin Padiatr* 2005;217(6):310–20.

14 Pieters R, Schrappe M, De Lorenzo P, *et al.* A treatment protocol for infants younger than 1 year with acute lymphoblastic leukaemia (Interfant-99): an observational study and a multicentre randomised trial. *Lancet* 2007;370(9583):240–50.

15 Smith M, Arthur D, Camitta B, *et al.* Uniform approach to risk classification and treatment assignment for children with acute lymphoblastic leukemia. *J Clin Oncol* 1996;14(1):18–24.

16 Burger B, Zimmermann M, Mann G, *et al.* Diagnostic cerebrospinal fluid examination in children with acute lymphoblastic leukemia: significance of low leukocyte counts with blasts or traumatic lumbar puncture. *J Clin Oncol* 2003;21(2):184–8.

17 Pui CH, Rubnitz JE, Hancock ML, et al. Reappraisal of the clinical and biologic significance of myeloid-associated antigen expression in childhood acute lymphoblastic leukemia. *J Clin Oncol* 1998;16(12):3768–73.

18 Vardiman JW, Thiele J, Arber DA, *et al.* The 2008 revision of the World Health Organization (WHO) classification of myeloid neoplasms and acute leukemia: rationale and important changes. *Blood* 2009;114(5):937–51.

19 Moorman AV, Ensor HM, Richards SM, *et al.* Prognostic effect of chromosomal abnormalities in childhood B-cell precursor acute lymphoblastic leukaemia: results from the UK Medical Research Council ALL97/99 randomised trial. *Lancet Oncol* 2010;11(5):429–38.

20 Sutcliffe MJ, Shuster JJ, Sather HN, *et al.* High concordance from independent studies by the Children's Cancer Group (CCG) and Pediatric Oncology Group (POG) associating favorable prognosis with combined trisomies 4, 10, and 17 in children with NCI Standard-Risk B-precursor Acute Lymphoblastic Leukemia: a Children's Oncology Group (COG) initiative. *Leukemia* 2005;19(5):734–40.

21 Rubnitz JE, Wichlan D, Devidas M, *et al.* Prospective analysis of TEL gene rearrangements in childhood acute lymphoblastic leukemia: a Children's Oncology Group study. *J Clin Oncol* 2008;26(13):2186–91.

22 Nachman JB, Heerema NA, Sather H, *et al.* Outcome of treatment in children with hypodiploid acute lymphoblastic leukemia. *Blood* 2007;110(4):1112–5.

23 Moorman AV, Richards SM, Robinson HM, *et al.* Prognosis of children with acute lymphoblastic leukemia (ALL) and intrachromosomal amplification of chromosome 21 (iAMP21). *Blood* 2007;109(6):2327–30.

24 Arico M, Schrappe M, Hunger SP, *et al.* Clinical outcome of children with newly diagnosed Philadelphia chromosome-positive acute lymphoblastic leukemia treated between 1995 and 2005. *J Clin Oncol* 2010;28(31):4755–61.

25 Schultz KR, Bowman WP, Aledo A, *et al.* Improved early event-free survival with imatinib in Philadelphia chromosome-positive acute lymphoblastic leukemia: a children's oncology group study. *J Clin Oncol* 2009;27(31):5175–81.

26 Schrappe M, Reiter A, Ludwig WD, *et al.* Improved outcome in childhood acute lymphoblastic leukemia despite reduced use of anthracyclines and cranial radiotherapy: results of trial ALL-BFM 90. *German-Austrian-Swiss ALL-BFM Study Group. Blood* 2000;95(11):3310–22.

27 Coustan-Smith E, Sancho J, Behm FG, *et al.* Prognostic importance of measuring early clearance of leukemic cells by flow cytometry in childhood acute lymphoblastic leukemia. *Blood* 2002;100(1):52–8.

28 Zhou J, Goldwasser MA, Li A, *et al.* Quantitative analysis of minimal residual disease predicts relapse in children with B-lineage acute lymphoblastic leukemia in DFCI ALL Consortium Protocol 95-01. *Blood* 2007;110(5):1607–11.

29 Conter V, Bartram CR, Valsecchi MG, *et al.* Molecular response to treatment redefines all prognostic factors in children and adolescents with B-cell precursor acute lymphoblastic leukemia: results in 3184 patients of the AIEOP-BFM ALL 2000 study. *Blood* 2010;115(16):3206–14.

30 Borowitz MJ, Devidas M, Hunger SP, *et al.* Clinical significance of minimal residual disease in childhood acute lymphoblastic leukemia and its relationship to other prognostic factors: a Children's Oncology Group study. *Blood* 2008;111(12):5477–85.

31 Schrappe M, Valsecchi MG, Bartram CR, *et al.* Late MRD response determines relapse risk overall and in subsets of childhood T-cell ALL: results of the AIEOP-BFM-ALL 2000 study. *Blood* 2011;118(8):2077–84.

32 Mullighan CG, Su X, Zhang J, *et al.* Deletion of IKZF1 and prognosis in acute lymphoblastic leukemia. *N Engl J Med* 2009;360(5):470–80.

33 Den Boer ML, van Slegtenhorst M, De Menezes RX, *et al.* A subtype of childhood acute lymphoblastic leukaemia with poor treatment outcome: a genome-wide classification study. *Lancet Oncol* 2009;10(2):125–34.

34 Mullighan CG, Collins-Underwood JR, Phillips LA, *et al.* Rearrangement of CRLF2 in B-progenitor- and Down syndrome-associated acute lymphoblastic leukemia. *Nat Genet* 2009;41(11):1243–6.

35 Harvey RC, Mullighan CG, Chen I-M, *et al.* Rearrangement of CRLF2 is associated with mutation of JAK kinases, alteration of IKZF1, Hispanic/Latino ethnicity, and a poor outcome in pediatric B-progenitor acute lymphoblastic leukemia. *Blood* 2010;115(26):5312–21.

36 Moricke A, Zimmermann M, Reiter A, *et al.* Long-term results of five consecutive trials in childhood acute lymphoblastic leukemia performed by the ALL-BFM study group from 1981 to 2000. *Leukemia* 2010;24(2):265–84.

37 Silverman LB, Stevenson KE, O'Brien JE, *et al.* Long-term results of Dana-Farber Cancer Institute ALL Consortium protocols for children with newly diagnosed acute lymphoblastic leukemia (1985-2000). *Leukemia* 2010;24(2):320–34.

38 Schrappe M, Hunger SP, Pui C-H, *et al.* Outcomes after induction failure in childhood acute lymphoblastic leukemia. *N Engl J Med* 2012;366(15):1371–81.

39 Gaynon PS, Angiolillo AL, Carroll WL, *et al.* Long-term results of the children's cancer group studies for childhood acute lymphoblastic leukemia 1983-2002: a Children's Oncology Group Report. *Leukemia* 2010. ;24(2):285–97.

40 Eden T, Pieters R, Richards S. Systematic review of the addition of vincristine plus steroid pulses in maintenance treatment for childhood acute lymphoblastic leukaemia – an individual patient data meta-analysis involving 5,659 children. *Br J Haematol* 2010;149(5):722–33.

41 Richards S, Pui CH, Gayon P. Systematic review and meta-analysis of randomized trials of central nervous system directed therapy for childhood acute lymphoblastic leukemia. *Pediatr Blood Cancer* 2013;60(2):185–95.

42 Pui CH, Howard SC. Current management and challenges of malignant disease in the CNS in paediatric leukaemia. *Lancet Oncol* 2008;9(3):257–68.

43 Nguyen K, Devidas M, Cheng SC, *et al.* Factors influencing survival after relapse from acute lymphoblastic leukemia: a Children's Oncology Group study. *Leukemia* 2008;22(12):2142–50.

44 Barredo JC, Devidas M, Lauer SJ, *et al.* Isolated CNS relapse of acute lymphoblastic leukemia treated with intensive systemic chemotherapy and delayed CNS radiation: a pediatric oncology group study. *J Clin Oncol* 2006;24(19):3142–9.

45 Eapen M, Raetz E, Zhang MJ, *et al.* Outcomes after HLA-matched sibling transplantation or chemotherapy in children with B-precursor acute lymphoblastic leukemia in a second remission: a collaborative study of the Children's Oncology Group and the Center for International Blood and Marrow Transplant Research. *Blood* 2006;107(12):4961–7.

46 Eckert C, von Stackelberg A, Seeger K, *et al.* Minimal residual disease after induction is the strongest predictor of prognosis in intermediate risk relapsed acute lymphoblastic leukaemia – long-term results of trial ALL-REZ BFM P95/96. *Eur J Cancer* 2013;49(6):1346–55.

47 Eckert C, Henze G, Seeger K, *et al.* Use of allogeneic hematopoietic stem-cell transplantation based on minimal residual disease response improves outcomes for children with relapsed acute lymphoblastic leukemia in the intermediate-risk group. *J Clin Oncol* 2013. ;31(21):2736–42.

48 Armstrong GT, Liu Q, Yasui Y, *et al.* Late mortality among 5-year survivors of childhood cancer: a summary from the Childhood Cancer Survivor Study. *J Clin Oncol* 2009;27(14):2328–38.

49 Kremer LCM, van Dalen EC, Offringa M, *et al.* Anthracycline-induced clinical heart failure in a cohort of 607 children: long-term follow-up study. *J Clin Oncol* 2001;19(1):191–6.

50 Ness KK, Armenian SH, Kadan-Lottick N, *et al.* Adverse effects of treatment in childhood acute lymphoblastic leukemia: general overview and implications for long-term cardiac health. *Exp Rev Hematol* 2011;4(2):185–197.

51 Schmiegelow K, Levinsen MF, Attarbaschi A, *et al.* Second malignant neoplasms after treatment of childhood acute lymphoblastic leukemia. *J Clin Oncol* 2013;31(19):2469–76.

52 Van Dongen-Melman JEWM, Hokken-Koelega AC, Hählen K, *et al.* Obesity after successful treatment of acute lymphoblastic leukemia in childhood. *Pediatr Res* 1995;38(1):86–90.

53 Chow CW, Tabrizi SN, Tiedemann K, Waters KD. Squamous cell carcinomas in children and young adults: a new wave of a very rare tumor? *J Pediatr Surg* 2007;42(12):2035–9.
54 Krull KR, Brinkman TM, Li C, *et al.* Neurocognitive outcomes decades after treatment for childhood acute lymphoblastic leukemia: a report from the St Jude Lifetime Cohort Study. *J Clin Oncol* 2013;31(35):4407–15.
55 Rowley JD. Letter: A new consistent chromosomal abnormality in chronic myelogenous leukaemia identified by quinacrine fluorescence and Giemsa staining. *Nature* 1973;243(5405):290–3.
56 Hijiya N, Schultz KR, Metzler M, Millot F, Suttorp M.Pediatric chronic myeloid leukemia is a unique disease that requires a different approach. *Blood* 2016;127(4):392–9.
57 Loh ML. Recent advances in the pathogenesis and treatment of juvenile myelomonocytic leukaemia. *Br J Haematol* 2011;152(6):677–87.
58 Chan RJ, Cooper T, Kratz CP, Weiss B, Loh ML. Juvenile myelomonocytic leukemia: a report from the 2nd International JMML Symposium. *Leuk Res* 2009;33(3):355–62.
59 Hitzler JK, Cheung J, Li Y, Scherer SW, Zipursky A. GATA1 mutations in transient leukemia and acute megakaryoblastic leukemia of Down syndrome. *Blood* 2003;101(11):4301–4.
60 Massey GV, Zipursky A, Chang MN, *et al.* A prospective study of the natural history of transient leukemia (TL) in neonates with Down syndrome (DS): Children's Oncology Group (COG) study POG-9481. *Blood* 2006;107(12):4606–13.
61 Pedersen-Bjergaard J, Andersen MT, Andersen MK. Genetic pathways in the pathogenesis of therapy-related myelodysplasia and acute myeloid leukemia. Hematology Am Soc Hematol Educ Program 2007:392–7.
62 Vardiman J. The classification of MDS: from FAB to WHO and beyond. *Leuk Res* 2012;36(12):1453–8.
63 Heaney ML, Golde DW. Myelodysplasia. *N Engl J Med* 1999;340(21):1649–60.
64 Howlader N, *et al.* SEER Cancer Statistics Review, 1975-2010, National Cancer Institute. Bethesda, MD, http://seer.cancer.gov/csr/1975_2010/ based on November 2012 SEER data submission.
65 Puumala SE, Ross JA, Aplenc R, Spector LG. Epidemiology of childhood acute myeloid leukemia. *Pediatr Blood Cancer* 2013;60(5):728–33.
66 Poppe B, Van Limbergen H, Van Roy N, *et al.* Chromosomal aberrations in Bloom syndrome patients with myeloid malignancies. *Cancer Genet Cytogenet* 2001;128(1):39–42.
67 Peffault de Latour R, Soulier J. How I treat MDS and AML in Fanconi anemia. *Blood* 2016;127(24):2971–9.
68 Freedman MH, Alter BP. Risk of myelodysplastic syndrome and acute myeloid leukemia in congenital neutropenias. *Semin Hematol* 2002;39(2):128–33.
69 Dror Y, Freedman MH. Shwachman-Diamond syndrome: An inherited preleukemic bone marrow failure disorder with aberrant hematopoietic progenitors and faulty marrow microenvironment. *Blood* 1999;94(9):3048–54.
70 Owen CJ, Toze CL, Koochin A, *et al.* Five new pedigrees with inherited RUNX1 mutations causing familial platelet disorder with propensity to myeloid malignancy. *Blood* 2008;112(12):4639–45.
71 Wang X, Muramatsu H, Okuno Y, *et al.* GATA2 and secondary mutations in familial myelodysplastic syndromes and pediatric myeloid malignancies. *Haematologica* 2015;100(10):e398–401.
72 Tawana K, Fitzgibbon J. CEBPA-Associated Familial Acute Myeloid Leukemia (AML) 2010 Oct 21 [Updated 2016 Apr 28]. In: Adam MP, Ardinger HH, Pagon RA, *et al.* (eds) *GeneReviews® [Internet].* Seattle (WA): University of Washington, Seattle; 1993-2017. Available from: https://www.ncbi.nlm.nih.gov/books/NBK47457/ (accessed 2 November 2017).
73 Godley LA. Inherited predisposition to acute myeloid leukemia. *Semin Hematol* 2014;51(4):306–21.
74 Xavier AC, Ge Y, Taub JW. Down syndrome and malignancies: a unique clinical relationship: a paper from the 2008 william beaumont hospital symposium on molecular pathology. *J Mol Diagn* 2009;11(5):371–80.
75 Shu XO, Ross JA, Pendergrass TW, *et al.* Parental alcohol consumption, cigarette smoking, and risk of infant leukemia: a Childrens Cancer Group study. *J Natl Cancer Inst* 1996;88(1):24–31.
76 Latino-Martel P, Chan DS, Druesne-Pecollo N, *et al.* Maternal alcohol consumption during pregnancy and risk of childhood leukemia: systematic review and meta-analysis. *Cancer Epidemiol Biomarkers Prev* 2010;19(5):1238–60.
77 Johnson KJ, Carozza SE, Chow EJ, *et al.* Parental age and risk of childhood cancer: a pooled analysis. *Epidemiology* 2009;20(4):475–83.
78 Belson M, Kingsley B, Holmes A. Risk factors for acute leukemia in children: a review. *Environ Health Perspect* 2007;115(1):138–45.
79 Spector LG, Xie Y, Robison LL, *et al.* Maternal diet and infant leukemia: the DNA topoisomerase II inhibitor hypothesis: a report from the children's oncology group. *Cancer Epidemiol Biomarkers Prev* 2005;14(3):651–5.
80 Tucker MA, Meadows AT, Boice JD Jr, *et al.* Leukemia after therapy with alkylating agents for childhood cancer. *J Natl Cancer Inst* 1987;78(3):459–64.
81 Andersen MK, Pedersen-Bjergaard J. Increased frequency of dicentric chromosomes in therapy-related MDS and AML compared to de novo disease is significantly related to previous treatment with alkylating agents and suggests a specific susceptibility to chromosome breakage at the centromere. *Leukemia* 2000;14(1):105–11.
82 Andersen MK, Christiansen DH, Kirchhoff M, Pedersen-Bjergaard J.Duplication or amplification of chromosome band 11q23, including the unrearranged MLL gene, is a recurrent abnormality in therapy-related MDS and AML, and is closely related to mutation of the TP53 gene and to previous therapy with alkylating agents. *Genes Chromosomes Cancer* 2001;31(1):33–41.
83 Abla O, Angelini P, Di Giuseppe G, *et al.* Early complications of hyperleukocytosis and leukapheresis in childhood acute leukemias. *J Pediatr Hematol Oncol* 2016;38(2):111–7.
84 Kobayashi R, Tawa A, Hanada R, *et al.* Extramedullary infiltration at diagnosis and prognosis in children with acute myelogenous leukemia. *Pediatr Blood Cancer* 2007;48(4):393–8.

85 Pui CH, Dahl GV, Kalwinsky DK, *et al.*, Central nervous system leukemia in children with acute nonlymphoblastic leukemia. *Blood* 1985;66(5):1062–7.

86 Johnston DL, Alonzo TA, Gerbing RB, Lange BJ, Woods WG. The presence of central nervous system disease at diagnosis in pediatric acute myeloid leukemia does not affect survival: a Children's Oncology Group study. *Pediatr Blood Cancer* 2010;55(3):414–20.

87 Creutzig U, Zimmermann M, Reinhardt D, *et al.* Early deaths and treatment-related mortality in children undergoing therapy for acute myeloid leukemia: analysis of the multicenter clinical trials AML-BFM 93 and AML-BFM 98. *J Clin Oncol* 2004;22(21):4384–93.

88 Creutzig U, van den Heuvel-Eibrink MM, Gibson B, *et al.* Diagnosis and management of acute myeloid leukemia in children and adolescents: recommendations from an international expert panel. *Blood* 2012;120(16):3187–205.

89 Bennett JM, Catovsky D, Daniel MT, *et al.* Proposed revised criteria for the classification of acute myeloid leukemia: a report of the French-American-British Cooperative Group. *Ann Intern Med* 1985;103(4):620–5.

90 Pui CH, Schrappe M, Ribeiro RC, Niemeyer CM. Childhood and adolescent lymphoid and myeloid leukemia. Hematology Am Soc Hematol Educ Program 2004:118–45.

91 Loken MR, Alonzo TA, Pardo L, *et al.* Residual disease detected by multidimensional flow cytometry signifies high relapse risk in patients with de novo acute myeloid leukemia: a report from Children's Oncology Group. *Blood* 2012;120(8):1581–8.

92 Paietta E. When it comes to MRD, AML not equal ALL. *Blood* 2012;120(8):1536–7.

93 MRD-AML-BFM Study Group, Langebrake C, Creutzig U, *et al.* Residual disease monitoring in childhood acute myeloid leukemia by multiparameter flow cytometry: the MRD-AML-BFM Study Group. *J Clin Oncol* 2006;24(22):3686–92.

94 Stevens RF, Hann IM, Wheatley K, Gray RG. Marked improvements in outcome with chemotherapy alone in paediatric acute myeloid leukemia: results of the United Kingdom Medical Research Council's 10th AML trial. MRC Childhood Leukaemia Working Party. *Br J Haematol* 1998;101(1):130–40.

95 Abrahamsson J, Forestier E, Heldrup J, *et al.* Response-guided induction therapy in pediatric acute myeloid leukemia with excellent remission rate. *J Clin Oncol* 2011;29(3):310–5.

96 Gibson BE, Webb DK, Howman AJ, *et al.* Results of a randomized trial in children with Acute Myeloid Leukaemia: medical research council AML12 trial. *Br J Haematol* 2011;155(3):366–76.

97 Hann IM, Webb DK, Gibson BE, Harrison CJ. MRC trials in childhood acute myeloid leukaemia. *Ann Hematol* 2004;83 Suppl 1:S108–12.

98 Sanz MA, Grimwade D, Tallman MS, *et al.* Management of acute promyelocytic leukemia: recommendations from an expert panel on behalf of the European LeukemiaNet. *Blood* 2009;113(9):1875–91.

99 Bally C, Fadlallah J, Leverger G, *et al.* Outcome of acute promyelocytic leukemia (APL) in children and adolescents: an analysis in two consecutive trials of the European APL Group. *J Clin Oncol* 2012;30(14):1641–6.

100 Testi AM, D'Angiò M, Locatelli F, Pession A, Lo Coco F. Acute promyelocytic leukemia (APL): comparison between children and adults. *Mediterr J Hematol Infect Dis* 2014;6(1):e2014032.

101 Abla O, Ribeiro RC. How I treat children and adolescents with acute promyelocytic leukaemia. *Br J Haematol* 2014;164(1):24–38.

102 Mulrooney DA, Dover DC, Li S, *et al.* Twenty years of follow-up among survivors of childhood and young adult acute myeloid leukemia: a report from the Childhood Cancer Survivor Study. *Cancer* 2008;112(9):2071–9.

103 Leung W, Hudson MM, Strickland DK, *et al.* Late effects of treatment in survivors of childhood acute myeloid leukemia. *J Clin Oncol* 2000;18(18):3273–9.

104 Skou AS, Glosli H, Jahnukainen K, *et al.* Renal, gastrointestinal, and hepatic late effects in survivors of childhood acute myeloid leukemia treated with chemotherapy only – a NOPHO-AML study. *Pediatr Blood Cancer* 2014;1(9):1638–43.

105 Orgel E, Zung L, Ji L, *et al.* Early cardiac outcomes following contemporary treatment for childhood acute myeloid leukemia: a North American perspective. *Pediatr Blood Cancer* 2013;60(9):1528–33.

106 Ries LAG, Smith MA, Gurney JG, *et al.* (eds). Cancer Incidence and Survival among Children and Adolescents: United States SEER Program 1975-1995, National Cancer Institute, SEER Program. Bethesda, MD: NIH, 1999:99–4649.

107 Fraumeni JF, Jr. Family studies in Hodgkin's disease. *Cancer Res* 1974;34(5):1164–5.

108 Harris NL. Hodgkin's lymphomas: classification, diagnosis, and grading. *Semin Hematol* 1999;36(3):220–32.

109 Carbone PP, Kaplan HS, Musshoff K, Smithers DW, Tubiana M. Report of the Committee on Hodgkin's Disease Staging Classification. *Cancer Res* 1971;31(11):1860–1.

110 Voss SD, Chen L, Constine LS, *et al.* Surveillance computed tomography imaging and detection of relapse in intermediate- and advanced-stage pediatric Hodgkin's lymphoma: a report from the Children's Oncology Group. *J Clin Oncol* 2012;30(21):2635–40.

111 Saslow D, Boetes C, Burke W, *et al.* American Cancer Society guidelines for breast screening with MRI as an adjunct to mammography. *CA Cancer J Clin* 2007;57(2):75–89.

112 O'Brien MM, Donaldson SS, Balise RR, Whittemore AS, Link MP. Second malignant neoplasms in survivors of pediatric Hodgkin's lymphoma treated with low-dose radiation and chemotherapy. *J Clin Oncol* 2010;28(7):1232–9.

113 Filipovich AH, Mathur A, Kamat D, Shapiro RS. Primary immunodeficiencies: genetic risk factors for lymphoma. *Cancer Res* 1992;52(19 Suppl):5465 s–5467 s.

114 Fischer A, Blanche S, Le Bidois J, *et al.* Anti-B-cell monoclonal antibodies in the treatment of severe B-cell lymphoproliferative syndrome following bone marrow and organ transplantation. *N Engl J Med* 1991;324(21):1451–6.

115 Reynolds P, Saunders LD, Layefsky ME, Lemp GF.The spectrum of acquired immunodeficiency syndrome (AIDS)-associated malignancies in San Francisco, 1980-1987. *Am J Epidemiol* 1993;137(1):19–30.

116 Stefan DC, Wessels G, Poole J, *et al.* Infection with human immunodeficiency virus-1 (HIV) among children with cancer in South Africa. *Pediatr Blood Cancer* 2011;56(1):77–9.
117 Anagnostopoulos I, Herbst H, Niedobitek G, Stein H. Demonstration of monoclonal EBV genomes in Hodgkin's disease and Ki-1-positive anaplastic large cell lymphoma by combined Southern blot and in situ hybridization. *Blood* 1989;74(2):810–6.
118 Gruhne B, Kamranvar SA, Masucci MG, Sompallae R. EBV and genomic instability – a new look at the role of the virus in the pathogenesis of Burkitt's lymphoma. *Semin Cancer Biol* 2009;19(6):394–400.
119 Swerdlow SH, Campo E, Pileri SA, *et al.* The 2016 revision of the World Health Organization classification of lymphoid neoplasms. *Blood* 2016;127(20):2375–90.
120 Sandlund JT, Downing JR, Crist WM. Non-Hodgkin's lymphoma in childhood. *N Engl J Med* 1996;334 (19):1238–48.
121 Sandlund JT, Hutchison RE, Crist WM. Non-Hodgkin's lymphoma. In: DJ Fernbach, TJ Vietti (eds) *Clinical Pediatric Oncology*. St. Louis: CRC Press, 1991:337–53.
122 Goldsby RE, Carroll WL. The molecular biology of pediatric lymphomas. *J Pediatr Hematol Oncol* 1998;20(4):282–96.
123 Sandlund JT, Pui CH, Santana VM, *et al.* Clinical features and treatment outcome for children with CD30+ large-cell non-Hodgkin's lymphoma. *J Clin Oncol* 1994;12(5):895–8.
124 Alexander S, Kraveka JM, Weitzman S, *et al.* Advanced stage anaplastic large cell lymphoma in children and adolescents: results of ANHL0131, a randomized phase III trial of APO versus a modified regimen with vinblastine: a report from the children's oncology group. *Pediatr Blood Cancer* 2014;61(12):2236–42.
125 Murphy SB. Classification, staging and end results of treatment of childhood non-Hodgkin's lymphomas: dissimilarities from lymphomas in adults. *Semin Oncol* 1980;7(3):332–9.
126 Link MP, Shuster JJ, Donaldson SS, Berard CW, Murphy SB. Treatment of children and young adults with early-stage non-Hodgkin's lymphoma. *N Engl J Med* 1997;337(18):1259–66.
127 Gore L, Trippett TM. Emerging non-transplant-based strategies in treating pediatric non-Hodgkin's lymphoma. *Curr Hematol Malig Rep* 2010;5(4):177–84.
128 Minard-Colin V, Brugières L, Reiter A, *et al.* Non-Hodgkin lymphoma in children and adolescents: progress through effective collaboration, current knowledge, and challenges ahead. *J Clin Oncol* 2015;33(27):2963–74.
129 Eissa HM, Allen CE, Kamdar K, *et al.* Pediatric Burkitt's lymphoma and diffuse B-cell lymphoma: are surveillance scans required? *Pediatr Hematol Oncol* 2014;31(3):253–7.
130 Ehrhardt MJ, Sandlund JT, Zhang N, *et al.* Late outcomes of adult survivors of childhood non-Hodgkin lymphoma: A report from the St. Jude Lifetime Cohort Study. *Pediatr Blood Cancer* 2017;64(6):e26338.
131 Klein MJ, Siegal GP. Osteosarcoma: anatomic and histologic variants. *Am J Clin Pathol* 2006;125(4):555–81.
132 Wong FL, Boice JD Jr, Abramson DH, *et al.* Cancer incidence after retinoblastoma. Radiation dose and sarcoma risk. *JAMA* 1997;278:1262–7.
133 Fletcher O, Easton D, Anderson K, *et al.* Lifetime risks of common cancers among retinoblastoma survivors. *J Natl Cancer Inst* 2004;96(5):357–63.
134 Kansara M, Thomas DM. Molecular pathogenesis of osteosarcoma. *DNA Cell Biol* 2007;26(1):1–18.
135 Lavigueur A, Maltby V, Mock D, *et al.* High incidence of lung, bone, and lymphoid tumors in transgenic mice overexpressing mutant alleles of the p53 oncogene. *Mol Cell Biol* 1989;9(9):3982–91.
136 Schajowicz F, Sissons HA, Sobin LH. The World Health Organization's histologic classification of bone tumors. A commentary on the second edition. *Cancer* 1995;75(5):1208–14.
137 Widhe B, Widhe T. Initial symptoms and clinical features in osteosarcoma and Ewing sarcoma. *J Bone Joint Surg Am* 2000;82(5):667–74.
138 Kager L, Zoubek A, Kastner U, *et al.* Skip metastases in osteosarcoma: experience of the Cooperative Osteosarcoma Study Group. *J Clin Oncol* 2006;24(10):1535–41.
139 Meyer JS, Nadel HR, Marina N, *et al.* Imaging guidelines for children with Ewing sarcoma and osteosarcoma: a report from the Children's Oncology Group Bone Tumor Committee. *Pediatr Blood Cancer* 2008;51(2):163–70.
140 Ward WG, Savage P, Boles CA, Kilpatrick SE., Fine-needle aspiration biopsy of sarcomas and related tumors. *Cancer Control* 2001;8(3):232–8.
141 Byun BH, Kong CB, Lim I, *et al.* Comparison of (18)F-FDG PET/CT and (99 m)Tc-MDP bone scintigraphy for detection of bone metastasis in osteosarcoma. *Skeletal Radiol* 2013;42(12):1673–81.
142 Janeway KA, Barkauskas DA, Krailo MD, *et al.* Outcome for adolescent and young adult patients with osteosarcoma: a report from the Children's Oncology Group. *Cancer* 2012;118(18):4597–605.
143 Isakoff MS, Bielack SS, Meltzer P, Gorlick R. Osteosarcoma: current treatment and a collaborative pathway to success. *J Clin Oncol* 2015;33(27):3029–35.
144 Link MP, Goorin AM, Miser AW, *et al.* The effect of adjuvant chemotherapy on relapse-free survival in patients with osteosarcoma of the extremity. *N Engl J Med* 1986;314:1600–6.
145 Eilber F, Giuliano A, Eckardt J, *et al.* Adjuvant chemotherapy for osteosarcoma: a randomized prospective trial. *J Clin Oncol* 1987;5(1):21–6.
146 Anninga JK, Gelderblom H, Fiocco M, *et al.* Chemotherapeutic adjuvant treatment for osteosarcoma: where do we stand? *Eur J Cancer* 2011;47(16):2431–45.
147 Daw NC, Neel MD, Rao BN, *et al.* Frontline treatment of localized osteosarcoma without methotrexate: results of the St. Jude Children's Research Hospital OS99 trial. *Cancer* 2011;117(12):2770–8.
148 Marina NM, Smeland S, Bielack SS, *et al.* Comparison of MAPIE versus MAP in patients with a poor response to preoperative chemotherapy for newly diagnosed high-grade osteosarcoma (EURAMOS-1): an open-label, international, randomised controlled trial. *Lancet Oncol* 2016;17(10):1396–408.
149 Rodriguez-Galindo C. Pharmacological management of Ewing sarcoma family of tumours. *Expert Opin Pharmacother* 2004;5(6):1257–70.

150 Dome JS, Schwartz CL. Osteosarcoma. *Cancer Treat Res* 1997.;92:215–51.

151 Loh AH, Wu H, Bahrami A, *et al.* Influence of bony resection margins and surgicopathological factors on outcomes in limb-sparing surgery for extremity osteosarcoma. *Pediatr Blood Cancer* 2015;62(2):246–51.

152 Ciernik IF, Niemierko A, Harmon DC, *et al.* Proton-based radiotherapy for unresectable or incompletely resected osteosarcoma. *Cancer* 2011;117(19):4522–30.

153 Davis AM, Bell RS, Goodwin PJ. Prognostic factors in osteosarcoma: a critical review. *J Clin Oncol* 1994;12(2):423–31.

154 Ottaviani G, Jaffe N. The epidemiology of osteosarcoma. *Cancer Treat Res* 2009;152:3–13.

155 Bernthal NM, Federman N, Eilber FR, *et al.* Long-term results (>25 years) of a randomized, prospective clinical trial evaluating chemotherapy in patients with high-grade, operable osteosarcoma. *Cancer* 2012;118(23):5888–93.

156 Schwartz CL, Wexler LH, Krailo MD, *et al.* Intensified chemotherapy with dexrazoxane cardioprotection in newly diagnosed nonmetastatic osteosarcoma: a report from the Children's Oncology Group. *Pediatr Blood Cancer* 2016;63(1):54–61.

157 Nagarajan R, Kamruzzaman A, Ness KK, *et al.* Twenty years of follow-up of survivors of childhood osteosarcoma: a report from the Childhood Cancer Survivor Study. *Cancer* 2011;117(3):625–34.

158 Balamuth NJ, Womer RB. Ewing's sarcoma. *Lancet Oncol* 2010;11(2):184–92.

159 De Ioris MA, Prete A, Cozza R, *et al.* Ewing sarcoma of the bone in children under 6 years of age. *PLoS One* 2013;8(1):e53223.

160 Esiashvili N, Goodman M, Marcus RB, Jr. Changes in incidence and survival of Ewing sarcoma patients over the past 3 decades: Surveillance Epidemiology and End Results data. *J Pediatr Hematol Oncol* 2008;30(6):425–30.

161 Lawlor ER, Sorensen PH. Twenty years on: what do we really know about Ewing sarcoma and what is the path forward? *Crit Rev Oncog* 2015;20(3-4):155–71.

162 Carvajal R, Meyers P. Ewing's sarcoma and primitive neuroectodermal family of tumors. *Hematol Oncol Clin North Am* 2005;19(3):501–25, vi–vii.

163 Delattre O, Zucman J, Melot T, *et al.* The Ewing family of tumors – a subgroup of small-round-cell tumors defined by specific chimeric transcripts. *N Engl J Med* 1994;331(5):294–9.

164 Brasme JF, Chalumeau M, Oberlin O, Valteau-Couanet D, Gaspar N. Time to diagnosis of Ewing tumors in children and adolescents is not associated with metastasis or survival: a prospective multicenter study of 436 patients. *J Clin Oncol* 2014;32(18):1935–40.

165 Applebaum MA, Worch J, Matthay KK, *et al.* Clinical features and outcomes in patients with extraskeletal Ewing sarcoma. *Cancer* 2011;117(13):3027–32.

166 Gaspar N, Hawkins DS, Dirksen U, *et al.* Ewing sarcoma: current management and future approaches through collaboration. *J Clin Oncol* 2015;33(27):3036–46.

167 Womer RB, West DC, Krailo MD, *et al.* Randomized controlled trial of interval-compressed chemotherapy for the treatment of localized Ewing sarcoma: a report from the Children's Oncology Group. *J Clin Oncol* 2012;30(33):4148–54.

168 Ladenstein R, Pötschger U, Le Deley MC, *et al.* Primary disseminated multifocal Ewing sarcoma: results of the Euro-EWING 99 trial. *J Clin Oncol* 2010;28(20):3284–91.

169 Ginsberg JP, Goodman P, Leisenring W, *et al.* Long-term survivors of childhood Ewing sarcoma: report from the childhood cancer survivor study. *J Natl Cancer Inst* 2010;102(16):1272–83.

170 Charlton J, Pritchard-Jones K. WT1 mutation in childhood cancer. *Methods Mol Biol* 2016;1467:1–14.

171 Gurney JG, Ross JA, Wall DA, *et al.* Infant cancer in the U.S.: histology-specific incidence and trends, 1973 to 1992. *J Pediatr Hematol Oncol* 1997;19(5):428–32.

172 Cohn SL, Meitar D, Kletzel M. Neuroblastoma: solving a biologic puzzle. *Cancer Treat Res* 1997;92:125–62.

173 Nickerson HJ, Matthay KK, Seeger RC, *et al.* Favorable biology and outcome of stage IV-S neuroblastoma with supportive care or minimal therapy: a Children's Cancer Group study. *J Clin Oncol* 2000;18(3):477–86.

174 Woods WG, Gao RN, Shuster JJ, *et al.* Screening of infants and mortality due to neuroblastoma. *N Engl J Med* 2002;346(14):1041–6.

175 Schilling FH, Spix C, Berthold F, *et al.* Neuroblastoma screening at one year of age. *N Engl J Med* 2002;346(14):1047–53.

176 Mosse Y, Greshock J, King A, *et al.* Identification and high-resolution mapping of a constitutional 11q deletion in an infant with multifocal neuroblastoma. *Lancet Oncol* 2003;4(12):769–71.

177 Mosse YP, Laudenslager M, Longo L, *et al.* Identification of ALK as a major familial neuroblastoma predisposition gene. *Nature* 2008;455(7215):930–5.

178 Satge D, Moore SW, Stiller CA, *et al.* Abnormal constitutional karyotypes in patients with neuroblastoma: a report of four new cases and review of 47 others in the literature. *Cancer Genet Cytogenet* 2003;147(2):89–98.

179 Mahoney NR, Liu GT, Menacker SJ, *et al.* Pediatric horner syndrome: etiologies and roles of imaging and urine studies to detect neuroblastoma and other responsible mass lesions. *Am J Ophthalmol* 2006;142(4):651–9.

180 Altman AJ, Baehner, RL. Favorable prognosis for survival in children with coincident opso-myoclonus and neuroblastoma. *Cancer* 1976;37(2):846–52.

181 Pranzatelli MR. The neurobiology of the opsoclonus-myoclonus syndrome. *Clin Neuropharmacol* 1992;15(3):186–228.

182 Connolly AM, Pestronk A, Mehta S, Pranzatelli MR 3rd, Noetzel MJ. Serum autoantibodies in childhood opsoclonus-myoclonus syndrome: an analysis of antigenic targets in neural tissues. *J Pediatr* 1997;130(6):878–84.

183 Russo C, Cohn SL, Petruzzi MJ, de Alarcon PA. Long-term neurologic outcome in children with opsoclonus-myoclonus associated with neuroblastoma: a report from the Pediatric Oncology Group. *Med Pediatr Oncol* 1997;28(4):284–8.

184 Brodeur GM, Seeger RC, Barrett A, *et al.* International criteria for diagnosis, staging, and response to treatment in patients with neuroblastoma. *J Clin Oncol* 1988. ;6(12):1874–81.

185 Hero B, Hunneman DH, Gahr M, Berthold F. Evaluation of catecholamine metabolites, mIBG scan, and bone marrow cytology as response markers in stage 4 neuroblastoma. *Med Pediatr Oncol* 2001;36(1):220–3.
186 Bleeker G, Tytgat GA, Adam JA, *et al.* 123I-MIBG scintigraphy and 18 F-FDG-PET imaging for diagnosing neuroblastoma. *Cochrane Database Syst Rev* 2015(9):Cd009263.
187 Shimada H, Chatten J, Newton WA Jr, *et al.* Histopathologic prognostic factors in neuroblastic tumors: definition of subtypes of ganglioneuroblastoma and an age-linked classification of neuroblastomas. *J Natl Cancer Inst* 1984;73(2):405–16.
188 Shimada H, Ambros IM, Dehner LP, *et al.* The International Neuroblastoma Pathology Classification (the Shimada system). *Cancer* 1999;86(2):364–72.
189 Brodeur GM, Seeger RC, Schwab M, Varmus HE, Bishop JM. Amplification of N-myc in untreated human neuroblastomas correlates with advanced disease stage. *Science* 1984;224(4653):1121–4.
190 Seeger RC, Brodeur GM, Sather H, *et al.* Association of multiple copies of the N-myc oncogene with rapid progression of neuroblastomas. *N Engl J Med* 1985;313(18):1111–6.
191 Ambros PF, Ambros IM, Brodeur GM, *et al.* International consensus for neuroblastoma molecular diagnostics: report from the International Neuroblastoma Risk Group (INRG) Biology Committee. *Br J Cancer* 2009;100(9):1471–82.
192 Brodeur GM, Seeger RC, Sather H, *et al.* Clinical implications of oncogene activation in human neuroblastomas. *Cancer* 1986;58(2 Suppl):541–5.
193 Seeger RC, Wada R, Brodeur GM, et al. Expression of N-myc by neuroblastomas with one or multiple copies of the oncogene. *Prog Clin Biol Res* 1988;271:41–9.
194 Brodeur GM. Patterns and significance of genetic changes in neuroblastomas. In: TP Pretlow, TG Pretlow (eds) *Biochemical and Molecular Aspects of Selected Tumors*, Orlando, FL: Academic Press, 1991: 251–76.
195 Brodeur GM, Hayes FA, Green AA, *et al.* Consistent N-myc copy number in simultaneous or consecutive neuroblastoma samples from sixty individual patients. *Cancer Res* 1987;47(16):4248–53.
196 Cohn SL, Pearson AD, London WB, et al. The International Neuroblastoma Risk Group (INRG) classification system: an INRG Task Force report. *J Clin Oncol* 2009;27(2):289–97.
197 Look AT, Hayes FA, Shuster JJ, *et al.* Clinical relevance of tumor cell ploidy and N-myc gene amplification in childhood neuroblastoma: a Pediatric Oncology Group study. *J Clin Oncol* 1991;9(4):581–91.
198 Christiansen H, Lampert F. Tumour karyotype discriminates between good and bad prognostic outcome in neuroblastoma. *Br J Cancer* 1988;57(1):121–6.
199 Look AT, Hayes FA, Nitschke R, McWilliams NB, Green AA. Cellular DNA content as a predictor of response to chemotherapy in infants with unresectable neuroblastoma. *N Engl J Med* 1984;311(4):231–5.
200 Gansler T, Chatten J, Varello M, Bunin GR, Atkinson B. Flow cytometric DNA analysis of neuroblastoma. Correlation with histology and clinical outcome. *Cancer* 1986;58(11):2453–8.
201 Oppedal BR, Storm-Mathisen I, Lie SO, Brandtzaeg P. Prognostic factors in neuroblastoma. Clinical, histopathologic, and immunohistochemical features and DNA ploidy in relation to prognosis. *Cancer* 1988;62(4):772–80.
202 Bown N, Cotterill S, Lastowska M, *et al.* Gain of chromosome arm 17q and adverse outcome in patients with neuroblastoma. *N Engl J Med* 1999;340(25):1954–61.
203 Schleiermacher G, Mosseri V, London WB, *et al.* Segmental chromosomal alterations have prognostic impact in neuroblastoma: a report from the INRG project. *Br J Cancer* 2012;107(8):1418–22.
204 Bresler SC, Weiser DA, Huwe PJ, *et al.* ALK mutations confer differential oncogenic activation and sensitivity to ALK inhibition therapy in neuroblastoma. *Cancer Cell* 2014;26(5):682–94.
205 Cheung NK, Zhang J, Lu C, *et al.* Association of age at diagnosis and genetic mutations in patients with neuroblastoma. *JAMA* 2012;307(10):1062–71.
206 Brodeur GM, Pritchard J, Berthold F, *et al.* Revisions of the international criteria for neuroblastoma diagnosis, staging, and response to treatment. *J Clin Oncol* 1993;11(8):1466–77.
207 Monclair T, Brodeur GM, Ambros PF, *et al.* The International Neuroblastoma Risk Group (INRG) staging system: an INRG Task Force report. *J Clin Oncol* 2009;27(2):298–303.
208 Vo KT, Matthay KK, Neuhaus J, *et al.* Clinical, biologic, and prognostic differences on the basis of primary tumor site in neuroblastoma: a report from The International Neuroblastoma Risk Group Project. *J Clin Oncol* 2014;32(28):3169–76.
209 Mosse YP, Deyell RJ, Berthold F, *et al.* Neuroblastoma in older children, adolescents and young adults: a report from the International Neuroblastoma Risk Group project. *Pediatr Blood Cancer* 2014;61(4):627–35.
210 Strother DR, London WB, Schmidt ML, *et al.* Outcome after surgery alone or with restricted use of chemotherapy for patients with low-risk neuroblastoma: results of Children's Oncology Group study P9641. *J Clin Oncol* 2012;30(15):1842–8.
211 Deacon JM, Wilson PA, Peckham MJ. The radiobiology of human neuroblastoma. *Radiother Oncol* 1985;3(3):201–9.
212 Nuchtern JG, London WB, Barnewolt CE, *et al.* A prospective study of expectant observation as primary therapy for neuroblastoma in young infants: a Children's Oncology Group study. *Ann Surg* 2012;256(4):573–80.
213 London WB, Castleberry RP, Matthay KK, *et al.* Evidence for an age cutoff greater than 365 days for neuroblastoma risk group stratification in the Children's Oncology Group. *J Clin Oncol* 2005;23(27):6459–65.
214 Baker DL, Schmidt ML, Cohn SL, *et al.* Outcome after reduced chemotherapy for intermediate-risk neuroblastoma. *N Engl J Med* 2010;363(14):1313–23.
215 Matthay KK, Villablanca JG, Seeger RC, *et al.* Treatment of high-risk neuroblastoma with intensive chemotherapy, radiotherapy, autologous bone marrow transplantation, and 13-cis-retinoic acid. *N Engl J Med* 1999;341:1165–73.
216 Yu AL, Gilman AL, Ozkaynak MF, *et al.* Anti-GD2 antibody with GM-CSF, interleukin-2, and isotretinoin for neuroblastoma. *N Engl J Med* 2010;363(14):1324–34.

217 Gurney JG. Neuroblastoma, childhood cancer survivorship, and reducing the consequences of cure. *Bone Marrow Transplant* 2007;40(8):721–2.

218 Landier W, Knight K, Wong FL, *et al.* Ototoxicity in children with high-risk neuroblastoma: prevalence, risk factors, and concordance of grading scales – a report from the Children's Oncology Group. *J Clin Oncol* 2014;32(6):527–34.

219 Laverdiere C, Cheung NK, Kushner BH, *et al.* Long-term complications in survivors of advanced stage neuroblastoma. *Pediatr Blood Cancer* 2005;45(3):324–32.

220 Kushner BH, Cheung NK, Kramer K, Heller G, Jhanwar SC. Neuroblastoma and treatment-related myelodysplasia/leukemia: the Memorial Sloan-Kettering experience and a literature review. *J Clin Oncol* 1998;16(12):3880–9.

221 Laverdiere C, Liu Q, Yasui Y, *et al.* Long-term outcomes in survivors of neuroblastoma: a report from the Childhood Cancer Survivor Study. *J Natl Cancer Inst* 2009;101(16):1131–40.

222 Flandin I, Hartmann O, Michon J, *et al.* Impact of TBI on late effects in children treated by megatherapy for Stage IV neuroblastoma. A study of the French Society of Pediatric oncology. *Int J Radiat Oncol Biol Phys* 2006;64(5):1424–31.

223 Trahair TN, Vowels MR, Johnston K, *et al.* Long-term outcomes in children with high-risk neuroblastoma treated with autologous stem cell transplantation. *Bone Marrow Transplant* 2007;40(8):741–6.

224 Cost NG, Lubahn JD, Granberg CF, *et al.* Pathological review of Wilms tumor nephrectomy specimens and potential implications for nephron sparing surgery in Wilms tumor. *J Urol* 2012;188(4 Suppl):1506–10.

225 van den Heuvel-Eibrink MM, Grundy P, Graf N, *et al.* Characteristics and survival of 750 children diagnosed with a renal tumor in the first seven months of life: A collaborative study by the SIOP/GPOH/SFOP, NWTSG, and UKCCSG Wilms tumor study groups. *Pediatr Blood Cancer* 2008;50(6):1130–4.

226 Howlader N, Noone AM, Krapcho M, *et al.* (eds). SEER Cancer Statistics Review, 1975–2013. National Cancer Institute. Bethesda, MD, https://seer.cancer.gov/csr/1975_2013/, based on November 2015 SEER data submission, posted to the SEER web site, April 2016.

227 Breslow N, Olshan A, Beckwith JB, Green DM. Epidemiology of Wilms tumor. *Med Pediatr Oncol* 1993;21(3):172–81.

228 Knudson AG. Hereditary cancer: two hits revisited. *J Cancer Res Clin Oncol* 1996;122(3):135–40.

229 Fanni D, Fanos V, Monga G, *et al.* Expression of WT1 during normal human kidney development. *J Matern Fetal Neonatal Med* 2011;24 Suppl 2:44–7.

230 Ozdemir DD, Hohenstein P. Wt1 in the kidney – a tale in mouse models. *Pediatr Nephrol* 2014;29(4):687–93.

231 Scott RH, Murray A, Baskcomb L, *et al.* Stratification of Wilms tumor by genetic and epigenetic analysis. *Oncotarget* 2012;3(3):327–35.

232 Hohenstein P, Pritchard-Jones K, Charlton J. The yin and yang of kidney development and Wilms' tumors. *Genes Dev* 2015;29(5):467–82.

233 Scott RH, Stiller CA, Walker L, Rahman N. Syndromes and constitutional chromosomal abnormalities associated with Wilms tumour. *J Med Genet* 2006;43(9):705–15.

234 Dome JS, Mullen EA, Argani P. Pediatric renal tumors. In: DG Nathan, SH Orkin, D Ginsburg, *et al.* (eds) *Nathan and Oski's Hematology and Oncology of Infancy and Childhood*, Philadelphia, PA: W.B. Saunders, 2015.

235 Rahman N, Abidi F, Ford D, *et al.* Confirmation of FWT1 as a Wilms' tumour susceptibility gene and phenotypic characteristics of Wilms' tumour attributable to FWT1. *Hum Genet* 1998;103(5):547–56.

236 Scott RH, Walker L, Olsen Ø E, *et al.* Surveillance for Wilms tumour in at-risk children: pragmatic recommendations for best practice. *Arch Dis Child* 2006;91(12):995–9

237 Gracia Bouthelier R, Lapunzina P. Follow-up and risk of tumors in overgrowth syndromes. *J Pediatr Endocrinol Metab* 2005;18 Suppl 1:1227–35.

238 Breslow N, Beckwith JB, Ciol M, Sharples K. Age distribution of Wilms' tumor: report from the National Wilms' Tumor Study. *Cancer Res* 1988;48(6):1653–7.

239 Beckwith JB, Kiviat NB, Bonadio JF. Nephrogenic rests, nephroblastomatosis, and the pathogenesis of Wilms' tumor. *Pediatr Pathol* 1990;10(1-2):1–36.

240 Dome JS, Cotton CA, Perlman EJ, et al. Treatment of anaplastic histology Wilms' tumor: results from the fifth National Wilms' Tumor Study. *J Clin Oncol* 2006;24(15):2352–8.

241 Bonadio JF, Storer B, Norkool P, *et al.* Anaplastic Wilms' tumor: clinical and pathologic studies. *J Clin Oncol* 1985;3(4):513–20.

242 Bardeesy N, Falkoff D, Petruzzi MJ, *et al.* Anaplastic Wilms' tumour, a subtype displaying poor prognosis, harbours p53 gene mutations. *Nat Genet* 1994;7(1):91–7.

243 Grundy PE, Breslow NE, Li S, et al. Loss of heterozygosity for chromosomes 1p and 16q is an adverse prognostic factor in favorable-histology Wilms tumor: a report from the National Wilms Tumor Study Group. *J Clin Oncol* 2005;23(29):7312–21.

244 Weeks DA, Beckwith JB, Mierau GW, Luckey DW. Rhabdoid tumor of the kidney. A report of 111 cases from the National Wilms' Tumor Study Pathology Center. *Am J Surg Pathol* 1989;13(6):439–58.

245 Bonnin JM, Rubinstein LJ, Palmer NF, Beckwith JB. The association of embryonal tumors originating in the kidney and in the brain. A report of seven cases. *Cancer* 1984;54(10):2137–46.

246 Howell CG, Othersen HB, Kiviat NE, *et al.* Therapy and outcome in 51 children with mesoblastic nephroma: a report of the National Wilms' Tumor Study. *J Pediatr Surg* 1982;17(6):826–31.

247 Shamberger RC, Ritchey ML, Haase GM, *et al.* Intravascular extension of Wilms tumor. *Ann Surg* 2001;234(1):116–21.

248 Perlman EJ. Pediatric renal tumors: practical updates for the pathologist. *Pediatr Dev Pathol* 2005;8(3):320–38.

249 D'Angio GJ, Breslow N, Beckwith JB, *et al.* Treatment of Wilms' tumor. Results of the Third National Wilms' Tumor Study. *Cancer* 1989;64(2):349–60.

250 Shamberger RC, Guthrie KA, Ritchey ML, *et al.* Surgery-related factors and local recurrence of Wilms tumor in National Wilms Tumor Study 4. *Ann Surg* 1999;229(2):292–7.

251 Green DM. The treatment of stages I-IV favorable histology Wilms' tumor. *J Clin Oncol* 2004;22(8):1366–72.

252 Wilms' tumor: status report, 1990. By the National Wilms' Tumor Study Committee. *J Clin Oncol* 1991;9(5):877–87.

253 Green DM, Grigoriev YA, Nan B, *et al.* Congestive heart failure after treatment for Wilms' tumor: a report from the National Wilms' Tumor Study group. *J Clin Oncol* 2001;19(7):1926–34.

254 Breslow NE, Takashima JR, Whitton JA, *et al.* Second malignant neoplasms following treatment for Wilm's tumor: a report from the National Wilms' Tumor Study Group. *J Clin Oncol* 1995;13(8):1851–9.

255 Wright KD, Green DM, Daw NC. Late effects of treatment for wilms tumor. *Pediatr Hematol Oncol* 2009;26(6):407–13.

256 Signorello LB, Cohen SS, Bosetti C, *et al.* Female survivors of childhood cancer: preterm birth and low birth weight among their children. *J Natl Cancer Inst* 2006;98(20):1453–61.

257 Breslow NE, Collins AJ, Ritchey ML, *et al.*, End stage renal disease in patients with Wilms tumor: results from the National Wilms Tumor Study Group and the United States Renal Data System. *J Urol* 2005;174(5):1972–5.

258 Doros L, Yang J, Dehner L, *et al.* DICER1 mutations in embryonal rhabdomyosarcomas from children with and without familial PPB-tumor predisposition syndrome. *Pediatr Blood Cancer* 2012;59(3):558–60.

259 Archer NM, Amorim RP, Naves R, *et al.* An increased risk of second malignant neoplasms after rhabdomyosarcoma: population-based evidence for a cancer predisposition syndrome? *Pediatr Blood Cancer* 2016;63(2):196–201.

260 Cohen MM. Beckwith-Wiedemann syndrome: historical, clinicopathological, and etiopathogenetic perspectives. *Pediatr Dev Pathol* 2005;8(3):287–304.

261 Kratz CP, Franke L, Peters H, *et al.* Cancer spectrum and frequency among children with Noonan, Costello, and cardio-facio-cutaneous syndromes. *Br J Cancer* 2015;112(8):1392–7.

262 Crucis A, Richer W, Brugières L, *et al.* Rhabdomyosarcomas in children with neurofibromatosis type I: A national historical cohort. *Pediatr Blood Cancer* 2015;62(10):1733–8.

263 Hettmer S, Archer NM, Somers GR, *et al.* Anaplastic rhabdomyosarcoma in TP53 germline mutation carriers. *Cancer* 2014;120(7):1068–75.

264 Sorensen PH, Lynch JC, Qualman SJ, *et al.* PAX3-FKHR and PAX7-FKHR gene fusions are prognostic indicators in alveolar rhabdomyosarcoma: a report from the children's oncology group. *J Clin Oncol* 2002;20(11):2672–9.

265 Mao L, Lee DJ, Tockman MS, *et al.* Microsatellite alterations as clonal markers for the detection of human cancer. *Proc Natl Acad Sci U S A* 1994;91(21):9871–5.

266 Skapek SX, Anderson J, Barr FG, *et al.* PAX-FOXO1 fusion status drives unfavorable outcome for children with rhabdomyosarcoma: A children's oncology group report. *Pediatr Blood Cancer* 2013;60(9):1411–7.

267 Crist W, Gehan EA, Ragab AH, *et al.* The Third Intergroup Rhabdomyosarcoma Study. *J Clin Oncol* 1995;13(3):610–30.

268 Rodary C, Gehan EA, Flamant F, *et al.* Prognostic factors in 951 nonmetastatic rhabdomyosarcoma in children: a report from the International Rhabdomyosarcoma Workshop. *Med Pediatr Oncol* 1991;19(2):89–95.

269 Lawrence W, Anderson JR, Gehan EA, Maurer H. Pretreatment TNM staging of childhood rhabdomyosarcoma. *Cancer* 1997;80(6):1165–70.

270 Maurer HM, Gehan EA, Beltangady M, *et al.* The Intergroup Rhabdomyosarcoma Study-II. *Cancer* 1993;71:1904–22.

271 Pappo AS, Shapiro DN, Crist WM, Maurer HM. Biology and therapy of pediatric rhabdomyosarcoma. *J Clin Oncol* 1995;13:2123–39.

272 Raney RB, Walterhouse DO, Meza JL, *et al.* Results of the Intergroup Rhabdomyosarcoma Study Group D9602 protocol, using vincristine and dactinomycin with or without cyclophosphamide and radiation therapy, for newly diagnosed patients with low-risk embryonal rhabdomyosarcoma: a report from the Soft Tissue Sarcoma Committee of the Children's Oncology Group. *J Clin Oncol* 2011;29(10):1312–8.

273 Crist WM, Anderson JR, Meza JL, et al. Intergroup rhabdomyosarcoma study-IV: results for patients with nonmetastatic disease. *J Clin Oncol* 2001;19(12):3091–102.

274 Arndt CAS, Stoner JA, Hawkins DS, *et al.* Vincristine, actinomycin, and cyclophosphamide compared with vincristine, actinomycin, and cyclophosphamide alternating with vincristine, topotecan, and cyclophosphamide for intermediate-risk rhabdomyosarcoma: children's oncology group study D9803. *J Clin Oncol* 2009;27(31):5182–8.

275 Weigel BJ, Lyden E, Anderson JR, *et al.* Intensive multiagent therapy, including dose-compressed cycles of ifosfamide/etoposide and vincristine/doxorubicin/cyclophosphamide, irinotecan, and radiation, in patients with high-risk rhabdomyosarcoma: a report from the Children's Oncology Group. *J Clin Oncol* 2016;34(2):117–22.

276 Million L, Anderson J, Breneman J, *et al.* Influence of noncompliance with radiation therapy protocol guidelines and operative bed recurrences for children with rhabdomyosarcoma and microscopic residual disease: a report from the Children's Oncology Group. *Int J Radiat Oncol Biol Phys* 2011;80(2):333–8.

277 Breneman J, Meza J, Donaldson SS, *et al.* Local control with reduced-dose radiotherapy for low-risk rhabdomyosarcoma: a report from the Children's Oncology Group D9602 study. *Int J Radiat Oncol Biol Phys* 2012;83(2):720–6.

278 Donaldson SS, Meza J, Breneman JC, *et al.* Results from the IRS-IV randomized trial of hyperfractionated radiotherapy in children with rhabdomyosarcoma – a report from the IRSG. *Int J Radiat Oncol Biol Phys* 2001;51(3):718–28.

279 Lin JL, Guillerman RP, Russell HV, *et al.* Does routine imaging of patients for progression or relapse improve survival in rhabdomyosarcoma? *Pediatr Blood Cancer* 2016;63(2):202–5.

280 Stevens MCG. Treatment for childhood rhabdomyosarcoma: the cost of cure. *Lancet Oncol* 2005;6(2):77–84.

281 Seitz G, Dantonello TM, Int-Veen C, *et al.* Treatment efficiency, outcome and surgical treatment problems in patients suffering from localized embryonal bladder/prostate rhabdomyosarcoma: A report from the cooperative soft tissue sarcoma trial CWS-96. *Pediatr Blood Cancer* 2011;56(5):718–24.

282 Walterhouse DO, Meza JL, Breneman JC, *et al.* Local control and outcome in children with localized vaginal rhabdomyosarcoma: A report from the Soft Tissue Sarcoma committee of the Children's Oncology Group. *Pediatr Blood Cancer* 2011;57(1):76–83.

283 Raney RB, Asmar L, Vassilopoulou-Sellin R, *et al.* Late complications of therapy in 213 children with localized, nonorbital soft-tissue sarcoma of the head and neck: A descriptive report from the Intergroup Rhabdomyosarcoma Studies (IRS)-II and - III. *Med Pediatr Oncol* 1999;33(4):362–71.

284 Plant AS, Chi SN, Frazier L. Pediatric malignant germ cell tumors: A comparison of the neuro-oncology and solid tumor experience. *Pediatr Blood Cancer* 2016;63(12):2086–95.

285 Kaatsch P, Häfner C, Calaminus G, Blettner M, Tulla M. Pediatric germ cell tumors from 1987 to 2011: incidence rates, time trends, and survival. *Pediatrics* 2015;135(1):e136–43.

286 Hersmus R, de Leeuw BH, Wolffenbuttel KP, *et al.* New insights into type II germ cell tumor pathogenesis based on studies of patients with various forms of disorders of sex development (DSD). *Mol Cell Endocrinol* 2008;291(1-2):1–10.

287 Shaikh F, Murray MJ, Amatruda JF, *et al.* Paediatric extracranial germ-cell tumours. *Lancet Oncol* 2016;17(4):e149–62.

288 Gobel U, Schneider DT, Calaminus G, *et al.* Germ-cell tumors in childhood and adolescence. GPOH MAKEI and the MAHO study groups. *Ann Oncol* 2000;11(3):263–71.

289 Baranzelli MC, Kramar A, Bouffet E, *et al.* Prognostic factors in children with localized malignant nonseminomatous germ cell tumors. *J Clin Oncol* 1999;17(4):1212.

290 Packer RJ, Cohen BH, Cooney K. Intracranial germ cell tumors. *Oncologist* 2000;5(4):312–20.

291 Marina NM, Cushing B, Giller R, *et al.* Complete surgical excision is effective treatment for children with immature teratomas with or without malignant elements: Pediatric Oncology Group/Children's Cancer Group intergroup study. *J Clin Oncol* 1999;17(7):2137–43.

292 Cushing B, Giller R, Cullen JW, *et al.* Randomized comparison of combination chemotherapy with etoposide, bleomycin, and either high-dose or standard-dose cisplatin in children and adolescents with high-risk malignant germ cell tumors: a pediatric intergroup study – Pediatric Oncology Group 9049 and Children's Cancer Group 8882. *J Clin Oncol* 2004;22(13):2691–700.

293 Rogers PC, Olson TA, Cullen JW, *et al.* Treatment of children and adolescents with stage II testicular and stages I and II ovarian malignant germ cell tumors: A Pediatric Intergroup Study – Pediatric Oncology Group 9048 and Children's Cancer Group 8891. *J Clin Oncol* 2004;22(17):3563–9.

294 Mann JR, Raafat F, Robinson K, *et al.* The United Kingdom Children's Cancer Study Group's second germ cell tumor study: carboplatin, etoposide, and bleomycin are effective treatment for children with malignant extracranial germ cell tumors, with acceptable toxicity. *J Clin Oncol* 2000;18(22):3809–18.

295 Schlatter M, Rescorla F, Giller R, et al. Excellent outcome in patients with stage I germ cell tumors of the testes: a study of the Children's Cancer Group/Pediatric Oncology Group. *J Pediatr Surg* 2003;38(3):319–24; discussion 319–24.

296 Billmire DF, Cullen JW, Rescorla FJ, *et al.* Surveillance after initial surgery for pediatric and adolescent girls with stage I ovarian germ cell tumors: report from the Children's Oncology Group. *J Clin Oncol* 2014;32(5):465–70.

297 Malogolowkin MH, Krailo M, Marina N, Olson T, Frazier AL. Pilot study of cisplatin, etoposide, bleomycin, and escalating dose cyclophosphamide therapy for children with high risk germ cell tumors: a report of the children's oncology group (COG). *Pediatr Blood Cancer* 2013;60(10):1602–5.

298 Frazier AL, Hale JP, Rodriguez-Galindo C, *et al.* Revised risk classification for pediatric extracranial germ cell tumors based on 25 years of clinical trial data from the United Kingdom and United States. *J Clin Oncol* 2015;33(2):195–201.

299 Vogel F. Genetics of retinoblastoma. *Hum Genet* 1979;52(1):1–54.

300 Knudson A. Mutation and Cancer: statistical study of retinoblastoma. *PNAS* 1971;68:820–3.

301 Lee WH, Bookstein R, Hong F, *et al.* Human retinoblastoma susceptibility gene: cloning, identification, and sequence. *Science* 1987;235(4794):1394–9.

302 Laurie NA, Donovan SL, Shih CS, *et al.* Inactivation of the p53 pathway in retinoblastoma. *Nature* 2006;444(7115):61–6.

303 Rushlow DE, Mol BM, Kennett JY, *et al.* Characterisation of retinoblastomas without RB1 mutations: genomic, gene expression, and clinical studies. *Lancet Oncol* 2013;14(4):327–34.

304 Zimmerman LE. Retinoblastoma and retinocytoma. In: WH Spencer (ed.) *Ophthalmic Pathology: An Atlas and Textbook*. Philadelphia, PA: Saunders, 1983:1292.

305 Nelson LB. Abnormalities of the pupil and iris. In: RE Behrman, RM Kliegman, AM Arvin (eds) *Nelson Texbook of Pediatrics*. Philadelphia, PA: Saunders, 1996:1770–2.

306 Holladay DA, Holladay A, Montebello JF, Redmond KP. Clinical presentation, treatment, and outcome of trilateral retinoblastoma. *Cancer* 1991;67(3):710–5.

307 Kivelä T. Trilateral retinoblastoma: a meta-analysis of hereditary retinoblastoma associated with primary ectopic intracranial retinoblastoma. *J Clin Oncol* 1999;17(6):1829–37.

308 Reese AB, Ellsworth RM. The evaluation and current concept of retinoblastoma therapy. *Trans Am Acad Ophthalmol Otolaryngol* 1963;67:164–72.

309 Shields C, Mashayekhi A, Au AK, *et al.* The International Classification of Retinoblastoma predicts chemoreduction success. *Ophthalmology* 2006;113(12):2276–80.

310 Rodriguez-Galindo C, Chantada GL, Haik BG, Wilson MW. Treatment of retinoblastoma: current status and future perspectives. *Curr Treat Options Neurol* 2007;9(4):294–307.

311 Shields CL, Shields JA. Recent developments in the management of retinoblastoma. *J Pediatr Ophthalmol Strabismus* 1999;36(1):8–18.

312 Shields JA, Shields CL, DePotter P. Photocoagulation of retinoblastoma. *Int Ophthalmol Clin* 1993;33(3):95–9.

313 Shields JA, Parsons H, Shields CL, Giblin ME. The role of cryotherapy in the management of retinoblastoma. *Am J Ophthalmol* 1989;108(3):260–4.

314 Shields CL, Santos MC, Diniz W, *et al.* Thermotherapy for retinoblastoma. *Arch Ophthalmol* 1999;117(7):885–93.

315 Fass D, McCormick B, Abramson D, Ellsworth R. Cobalt60 plaques in recurrent retinoblastoma. *Int J Radiat Oncol Biol Phys* 1991;21(3):625–7.

316 Freire JE, De Potter P, Brady LW, Longton WA. Brachytherapy in primary ocular tumors. *Semin Surg Oncol* 1997;13(3):167–76.

317 Al-Haj AN, Lobriguito AM, Lagarde CS. Radiation dose profile in 125I brachytherapy: an 8-year review. *Radiat Prot Dosimetry* 2004;111(1):115–9.

318 Abouzeid H, Moekli R, Gaillard M-C, *et al.* ^{106}Ruthenium brachytherapy for retinoblastoma. *Int J Radiat Oncol Biol Phys* 2008;71(3):821–8.

319 Reisner ML, Viégas CM, Grazziotin RZ, *et al.* Retinoblastoma – comparative analysis of external radiotherapy techniques, including an IMRT technique. *Int J Radiat Oncol Biol Phys* 2007; 67(3):933–41.

320 Sethi RV, Shih HA, Yeap BY, *et al.* Second nonocular tumors among survivors of retinoblastoma treated with contemporary photon and proton radiotherapy. *Cancer* 2014;120(1):126–33.

321 Ross G, Lipper EG, Abramson D, Preiser L. The development of young children with retinoblastoma. *Arch Pediatr Adolesc Med* 2001;155(1):80–3.

322 Gobin Y, Dunkel IJ, Marr BP, Brodie SE, Abramson DH. Intra-arterial chemotherapy for the management of retinoblastoma: Four-year experience. *Arch Ophthalmol* 2011;129(6):732–7.

323 Abramson DH, Frank CM. Second nonocular tumors in survivors of bilateral retinoblastoma. A possible age effect on radiation-related risk. *Ophthalmology* 1998; 105(4):573–80.

324 BrennanRC, Qaddoumi I, Mao S, *et al.* Ocular salvage and vision preservation using a topotecan-based regimen for advanced intraocular retinoblastoma. *J Clin Oncol* 2017;35(1):72–7.

325 Kaneko A, Suzuki S. Eye-preservation treatment of retinoblastoma with vitreous seeding. *Jpn J Clin Oncol* 2003;33(12):601–7.

326 Mohri M. The technique of selective ophthalmic arterial infusion for conservative treatment of recurrent intraocular retinoblastoma. *Keio Igaku* 1993;70:679–87.

327 Abramson DH, Dunkel IJ, Brodie SE, Kim JW, Gobin YP. A phase I/II study of direct intraarterial (ophthalmic artery) chemotherapy with melphalan for intraocular retinoblastoma: initial results. *Ophthalmology* 2008;115(8):1398–404.

328 Abramson DD, Dunkel IJ, Brodie SE, Marr B, Gobin YP. Bilateral superselective ophthalmic artery chemotherapy for bilateral retinoblastoma: Tandem therapy. *Arch Ophthalmol* 2010;128(3):370–2.

329 Abramson DH, Marr BP, Dunkel IJ, *et al.* Intra-arterial chemotherapy for retinoblastoma in eyes with vitreous and/or subretinal seeding: 2-year results. *Br J Ophthalmol* 2012;96(4):499–502.

330 Munier FL, Gaillard MC, Balmer A, *et al.* Intravitreal chemotherapy for vitreous disease in retinoblastoma revisited: from prohibition to conditional indications. *Br J Ophthalmol* 2012;96(8):1078–83.

331 Antonelli CBG, Steinhorst F, de Cássia Braga Ribeiro K, *et al.* Extraocular retinoblastoma: A 13-year experience. *Cancer* 2003;98(6):1292–8.

332 Menon BS, Reddy SC, Maziah WM, Ham A, Rosline H. Extraocular retinoblastoma. *Med Pediatr Oncol* 2000;35(1)75–6.

333 Doz F, Khelfaoui F, Mosseri V, *et al.* The role of chemotherapy in orbital involvement of retinoblastoma. *Cancer* 1994;74(2):722–32.

334 Chantada G, Fandiño A, Casak S, *et al.* Treatment of overt extraocular retinoblastoma. *Med Pediatr Oncol* 2003;40(3)158–61.

335 Namouni F, Doz F, Tanguy ML, *et al.* High-dose chemotherapy with carboplatin, etoposide and cyclophosphamide followed by a haematopoietic stem cell rescue in patients with high-risk retinoblastoma: a SFOP and SFGM study. *Eur J Cancer* 1997;33(14)2368–75.

336 Dunkel IJ, Khakoo Y, Kernan NA, *et al.* Intensive multimodality therapy for patients with stage 4a metastatic retinoblastoma. *Pediatr Blood Cancer* 2010;55(1):55–9.

337 Kleinerman RA, Tucker MA, Tarone RE, *et al.* Risk of new cancers after radiotherapy in long-term survivors of retinoblastoma: An extended follow-up. *J Clin Oncol* 2005;23(10)2272–9.

338 Kleinerman RA, Tucker MA, Abramson DH, *et al.* Risk of soft tissue sarcomas by individual subtype in survivors of hereditary retinoblastoma. *J Natl Cancer Inst* 2007;99(1):24–31.

339 Ostrom QT, Gittleman H, Liao P, *et al.* CBTRUS statistical report: primary brain and central nervous system tumors diagnosed in the United States in 2007-2011. *Neuro Oncol* 2014;16 Suppl 4:iv1–63.

340 Ostrom QT, de Blank PM, Kruchko C, *et al.* Alex's Lemonade Stand Foundation Infant and Childhood Primary Brain and Central Nervous System Tumors Diagnosed in the United States in 2007-2011. *Neuro Oncol* 2015;16 Suppl 10:x1–x36.

341 Johnson KJ, Cullen J, Barnholtz-Sloan JS, *et al.* Childhood brain tumor epidemiology: a brain tumor epidemiology consortium review. *Cancer Epidemiol Biomarkers Prev* 2014;23(12):2716–36.

342 Tao ML, Barnes PD, Billett AL, *et al.* Childhood optic chiasm gliomas: radiographic response following radiotherapy and long-term clinical outcome. *Int J Radiat Oncol Biol Phys* 1997;39(3):579–87.

343 Stefanaki K, Alexiou GA, Stefanaki C, Prodromou N. Tumors of central and peripheral nervous system associated with inherited genetic syndromes. *Pediatr Neurosurg* 2012;48(5):271–85.

344 Reni M, Gatta G, Mazza E, Vecht C. Ependymoma. *Crit Rev Oncol Hematol* 2007;63(1):81–9.

345 Zhang J, Wu G, Miller CP, *et al.*, Whole-genome sequencing identifies genetic alterations in pediatric low-grade gliomas. *Nat Genet* 2013;45(6):602–12.

346 Louis DN, Ohgaki H, Wiestler OD, *et al.* The 2007 WHO classification of tumours of the central nervous system. *Acta Neuropathol* 2007;114(2):97–109.

347 Louis DN, Perry A, Reifenberger G, *et al.* The 2016 World Health Organization Classification of Tumors of the Central Nervous System: a summary. *Acta Neuropathol* 2016;131(6):803–20.

348 Barkovich AJ, Krischer J, Kun LA, *et al.* Brain stem gliomas: a classification system based on magnetic resonance imaging. *Pediatr Neurosurg* 1990;16(2):73–83.

349 Chu TP, Shah A, Walker D, Coleman MP. Pattern of symptoms and signs of primary intracranial tumours in children and young adults: a record linkage study. *Arch Dis Child* 2015;100(12):1115–22.

350 Honig PJ, Charney EB. Children with brain tumor headaches. *Distinguishing features. Am J Dis Child* 1982;136(2):121–4.

351 Campagna M, Opocher E, Viscardi E, *et al.* Optic pathway glioma: long-term visual outcome in children without neurofibromatosis type-1. *Pediatr Blood Cancer* 2010;55(6):1083–8.

352 Drake J, Hoffman HJ, Kobayashi J, Hwang P, Becker LE. Surgical management of children with temporal lobe epilepsy and mass lesions. *Neurosurgery* 1987;21(6):792–7.

353 Vanan MI, Eisenstat DD. DIPG in children – what can we learn from the past? *Front Oncol* 2015;5:237.

354 Bonfield CM, Steinbok P. Pediatric cerebellar astrocytoma: a review. *Childs Nerv Syst* 2015;31(10):1677–85.

355 Pollack IF, Claassen D, al-Shboul Q, Janosky JE, Deutsch M. Low-grade gliomas of the cerebral hemispheres in children: an analysis of 71 cases. *J Neurosurg* 1995;82(4):536–47.

356 Brandao LA, Poussaint TY. Pediatric brain tumors. *Neuroimaging Clin N Am* 2013;23(3):499–525.

357 Pollack IF. Brain tumors in children. *N Engl J Med* 1994;331(22):1500–7.

358 Walker DA, Liu J, Kieran M, *et al.* A multi-disciplinary consensus statement concerning surgical approaches to low-grade, high-grade astrocytomas and diffuse intrinsic pontine gliomas in childhood (CPN Paris 2011) using the Delphi method. *Neuro Oncol* 2013;15(4):462–8.

359 Ater JL, Zhou T, Holmes E, *et al.* Randomized study of two chemotherapy regimens for treatment of low-grade glioma in young children: a report from the Children's Oncology Group. *J Clin Oncol* 2012;30(21):2641–7.

360 Nageswara Rao AA, Packer RJ. Advances in the management of low-grade gliomas. *Curr Oncol Rep* 2014;16(8):398.

361 Perilongo G, Moras P, Carollo C, *et al.* Spontaneous partial regression of low-grade glioma in children with neurofibromatosis-1: a real possibility. *J Child Neurol* 1999;14(6):352–6.

362 Campbell JW, Pollack IF, Martinez AJ, Shultz B. High-grade astrocytomas in children: radiologically complete resection is associated with an excellent long-term prognosis. *Neurosurgery* 1996;38(2):258–64.

363 Fangusaro J. Pediatric high grade glioma: a review and update on tumor clinical characteristics and biology. *Front Oncol* 2012;2:105.

364 Vanan MI, Eisenstat DD. Management of high-grade gliomas in the pediatric patient: Past, present, and future. *Neurooncol Pract* 2014;1(4):145–57.

365 Sposto R, Ertel IJ, Jenkin RD, *et al.* The effectiveness of chemotherapy for treatment of high grade astrocytoma in children: results of a randomized trial. A report from the Childrens Cancer Study Group. *J Neurooncol* 1989;7(2):165–77.

366 Hargrave D, Bartels U, Bouffet E. Diffuse brainstem glioma in children: critical review of clinical trials. *Lancet Oncol* 2006;7(3):241–8.

367 Brinkman TM, Bass JK, Li Z, *et al.* Treatment-induced hearing loss and adult social outcomes in survivors of childhood CNS and non-CNS solid tumors: Results from the St. *Jude Lifetime Cohort Study. Cancer* 2015;121(22):4053–61.

368 Brinkman TM, Krasin MJ, Liu W, *et al.* Long-Term Neurocognitive Functioning and Social Attainment in Adult Survivors of Pediatric CNS Tumors: Results From the St Jude Lifetime Cohort Study. *J Clin Oncol* 2016;34(12):1358–67.

369 Fullerton HJ, Stratton K, Mueller S, *et al.* Recurrent stroke in childhood cancer survivors. *Neurology* 2015;85(12):1056–64.

370 Tsui K, Gajjar A, Li C, *et al.* Subsequent neoplasms in survivors of childhood central nervous system tumors: risk after modern multimodal therapy. *Neuro Oncol* 2015;17(3):448–56.

371 Williams NL, Rotondo RL, Bradley JA, *et al.* Late effects after radiotherapy for childhood low-grade glioma. Am J Clin Oncol 2016 [Epub ahead of print].

372 Kun LE. Brain tumors. Challenges and directions. *Pediatr Clin North Am* 1997;44(4):907–17.

373 Chintagumpala M, Gajjar A. Brain tumors. *Pediatr Clin North Am* 2015;62(1):167–78.

374 Taylor MD, Northcott PA, Korshunov A, *et al.*, Molecular subgroups of medulloblastoma: the current consensus. *Acta Neuropathol* 2012;123(4):465–72.

375 Bartlett F, Kortmann R, Saran F. Medulloblastoma. *Clin Oncol (R Coll Radiol)* 2013;25(1):36–45.

376 Halperin EC, Friedman HS. Is there a correlation between duration of presenting symptoms and stage of medulloblastoma at the time of diagnosis? *Cancer* 1996;78(4):874–80.

377 Jenkin D, Goddard K, Armstrong D, *et al.* Posterior fossa medulloblastoma in childhood: treatment results and a proposal for a new staging system. *Int J Radiat Oncol Biol Phys* 1990;19(2):265–74.

378 Cochrane DD, Gustavsson B, Poskitt KP, Steinbok P, Kestle JR. The surgical and natural morbidity of aggressive resection for posterior fossa tumors in childhood. *Pediatr Neurosurg* 1994;20(1):19–29.

379 Friedman HS, Oakes WJ. The chemotherapy of posterior fossa tumors in childhood. *J Neurooncol* 1987;5(3):217–29.

380 Heideman RL, Kovnar EH, Kellie SJ, *et al.* Preirradiation chemotherapy with carboplatin and etoposide in newly diagnosed embryonal pediatric CNS tumors. *J Clin Oncol* 1995;13(9):2247–54.

381 Ashley DM, Merchant TE, Strother D, et al. Induction chemotherapy and conformal radiation therapy for very young children with nonmetastatic medulloblastoma: Children's Oncology Group study P9934. *J Clin Oncol* 2012;30(26):3181–6.

382 Dhall G, Grodman H, Ji L, Sands S, *et al.* Outcome of children less than three years old at diagnosis with non-metastatic medulloblastoma treated with chemotherapy on the "Head Start" I and II protocols. *Pediatr Blood Cancer* 2008;50(6):1169–75.

383 von Bueren AO, von Hoff K, Pietsch T, *et al.* Treatment of young children with localized medulloblastoma by chemotherapy alone: results of the prospective, multicenter trial HIT 2000 confirming the prognostic impact of histology. *Neuro Oncol* 2011;13(6):669–79.

384 Saunders DE, Hayward RD, Phipps KP, Chong WK, Wade AM. Surveillance neuroimaging of intracranial medulloblastoma in children: how effective, how often, and for how long? *J Neurosurg* 2003;99(2):280–6.

Index

Page numbers in *italics* refer to illustrations; those in **bold** refer to tables

The American Cancer Society's Oncology in Practice: Clinical Management, First Edition. Edited by The American Cancer Society.

c

t

u